Contents in Brief

EVOLVE STUDENT RESOURCES

Go to http://evolve.elsevier.com/Leifer for access to the following resources.

Animations

Chapter 2
Breasts
Female External Genitalia
Female Reproductive Ducts
Male External Genitalia
Menstrual Cycle
Ovarian Cycle
Ovarian Cyst
Ovarian Torsion
Ovaries
Spermatozoa

Chapter 3
Fertilization to Implantation
Fetal Circulation
Function of the Placenta
Maternal–Fetal Circulation
Oogenesis
Ovulation
Oxygenated Fetal Circulation
Pregnancy Stages, Trimesters
Sex Determination
Spermatogenesis

Chapter 4
Fetal Development, First Trimester
Fetal Development, Second Trimester
Fetal Development, Third Trimester

Chapter 5
Abruptio Placentae
Sickle Cell Anemia
Ectopic Pregnancy
Placenta Previa
Rh Compatibility
Seizure in Pregnancy

Chapter 6
Birth or Parturition
Breech Delivery, Arms
Breech Delivery, Face
Breech Presentation Examination
Breech Presentation with Sonogram
Membrane Rupture
Normal Delivery
Placental Delivery

Chapter 8
Bleeding Complications
Cesarean Section
Placental Abruption (Abruptio Placentae)
Postterm Pregnancy: Internal and External
  Changes to Fetus
Shoulder Dystocia: Suprapubic Pressure in Delivery
Umbilical Cord Prolapse
Vacuum Extraction

Chapter 9
Umbilical Vein Catheter Placement

Chapter 11
Breast Cancer
Breast Cancer Metastasis
Hemorrhagic Ovarian Cyst
Pelvic Inflammatory Disease
Ruptured Ovarian Cyst
Speculum Exam

Chapter 14
Fetal Hypoxia
Ventriculoperitoneal Shunt for Hydrocephalus VP

Chapter 17
CPR for the Child

Chapter 22
Tracheostomy

Chapter 23
Meningitis
Seizure in an Infant
Spinal Tap in a Child

Chapter 24
Osteomyelitis

Chapter 25
Anoxic Brain Injury
Asthma
Bag Ventilation, Correct
Bag Ventilation, Inefficient
Endotracheal Intubation
Intubation, Correct and Incorrect
Oxygen Desaturation
Pediatric Pneumonia (Streptococcal Pneumonia)
Tracheostomy

Chapter 26
Cardiac Tamponade

Chapter 28
Abdominal Anatomy
Bowel Resection
Esophageal Intubation
Inguinal Hernia Repair
Intussusception
Volvulus, Pediatric

Chapter 31
Type 1 Diabetes
Type 2 Diabetes

Chapter 32
Chicken Pox (Varicella Zoster)
Mumps

Patient Teaching Plans in English and Spanish

Chapter 9
Breastfeeding Your Infant

Chapter 11
Breast Self-Exam

Chapter 12
Bathing Your Infant

Chapter 30
Skin Care for Infants, Children, and Adolescents

Skills Performance Checklists

Chapter 6
Skill 6-1	Assisting with an Emergency Birth
Skill 6-2	Determining Fetal Heart Rate
Skill 6-3	External Electronic Fetal Monitoring
Skill 6-4	Testing for the Presence of Amniotic Fluid (Nitrazine Paper Test)
Skill 6-5	Determining Contractions by Palpation
Skill 6-6	Administering Eye Ointment to the Newborn
Skill 6-7	Administering Intramuscular Injections to the Newborn

Chapter 9
Skill 9-1	Observing and Massaging the Uterine Fundus
Skill 9-2	Estimating the Volume of Lochia
Skill 9-3	Assessing the Perineum
Skill 9-4	Assisting with a Sitz Bath
Skill 9-5	Performing Perineal Care
Skill 9-6	Providing Umbilical Cord Care
Skill 9-7	Bottle Feeding the Infant

Chapter 11
Skill 11-1	How to Perform Breast Self-Examination
Skill 11-2	How to Use a Diaphragm
Skill 11-3	How to Use the Male Condom

Chapter 12
Skill 12-1	Taking Head and Chest Measurements
Skill 12-2	Bulb Suctioning
Skill 12-3	Swaddling the Newborn
Skill 12-4	Assessing for Jaundice
Skill 12-5	Bathing the Newborn

Chapter 13
Skill 13-1	Applying a Pulse Oximeter
Skill 13-2	Kangaroo Care

Chapter 14
Skill 14-1	Technique for Turning the Child in a Body Cast

Chapter 15
Skill 15-1	Assessing the Length and Height of Infants and Children
Skill 15-2	Calculating Body Mass Index (BMI)

Chapter 22
Skill 22-1	The Mummy Restraint (Swaddling)
Skill 22-2	Blood Pressure Measurement in Children
Skill 22-3	Axillary Temperature Technique
Skill 22-4	Tympanic Temperature Technique
Skill 22-5	Collecting a Urine Specimen in Infants
Skill 22-6	Administering Oral Medications
Skill 22-7	Administering Nose Drops
Skill 22-8	Administering Ear Drops
Skill 22-9	Removal of a Peripheral Intravenous Catheter
Skill 22-10	Gastrostomy Tube Feeding

Chapter 23
Skill 23-1	General Modifications and Precautions in Pediatric Feeding Techniques for Children with Cerebral Palsy

Chapter 24
Skill 24-1	Neurovascular Checks

Chapter 25
Skill 25-1	Using the Peak Flow Meter
Skill 25-2	Using a Metered-Dose Inhaler

Videos

Chapter 4
Assessment of the Pregnant Patient

Chapter 6
Nursing Care during Labor and Birth

Chapter 8
Cesarean Delivery

Chapter 12
Assessment of the Newborn

Chapter 17
Assessment of the Toddler

Chapter 18
Assessment of the Preschool Child

Chapter 19
Assessment of the School-Age Child

Chapter 20
Assessment of the Adolescent

Additional Resources

Chapter 1
Leading Causes and Number of Deaths in the United
  States by Age

Chapter 15
Dietary Reference Intakes (DRIs) and Recommended
  Dietary Allowances (RDAs)
Tips for Reducing Childhood Obesity in English and
  Spanish

Resources in Every Chapter

Answer Guidelines for Critical Thinking Questions
Answers and Rationales for Review Questions for the
  NCLEX® Examination
Calculators
• Body Mass Index (BMI)
• Body Surface Area
• Fluid Deficit
• Glasgow Coma Scale
• IV Dosage
• Units Conversion
Glossary with English and Spanish Pronunciations
Fluids and Electrolytes Tutorial
Interactive Review Questions for the NCLEX®
  Examination

Camille Lindsey Killough, RN, MSN
Nursing Instructor
Pearl River Community College—Forrest County Campus
Hattiesburg, Mississippi

Hana Malik, RN, MSN, FNP
Professor and Academic Director
Illinois College of Nursing
Lombard, Illinois

Terri Peterson, RN, MSN/Ed
Associate Professor
Bauder College
Atlanta, Georgia

Janet Pinkelman, RNC, MSN
Professor of Nursing
Owens Community College
Toledo, Ohio

Susan K. Rice, PhD, RN, CPNP, CNS
Professor
College of Nursing
University of Toledo
Toledo, Ohio

Sandra Secord, RN, MSN
Nursing Instructor
Sheridan College
Oakville, Ontario, Canada

Amelia Sherinski, RN, BSN
Medical Oncology Nurse
Medical University of South Carolina
Charleston, South Carolina

Dr. Crystal R. Sherman, DNP, CNP, FNP-BC, APHN-BC
Assistant Professor of Nursing
Shawnee State University
Portsmouth, Ohio

Kristine Simoni, RN, MSN
Nursing Instructor
Anoka Technical College
Anoka, Minnesota

Russlyn A. St. John, RN, MSN
Professor and Coordinator, Practical Nursing
Practical Nursing Department
St. Charles Community College
Cottleville, Missouri

Eileen Tracy Stork, MS, RNC-OB
Instructor
Cincinnati State Technical and Community College
Cincinnati, Ohio

Elizabeth Summers, RN, MSN, CNE
Nursing Instructor
Cass Career Center
Harrisonville, Missouri

Laura Travis, MSN, RN
Health Careers Coordinator
Tennessee College of Applied Technology—Dickson
Dickson, Tennessee

Peggy Valentine, RN, BSN, MSNC, DON
Director of Nursing
Skyline College
Roanoke, Virginia

Elise Webb, RN, MSN
CE Health Programs Coordinator
Wilson Community College
Wilson, North Carolina

Karmen Culver Williams, RN, MSN
Nursing Professor
Helena College—University of Montana
Helena, Montana

LPN Threads and Advisory Board

LPN THREADS

The seventh edition of *Introduction to Maternity and Pediatric Nursing* shares some features and design elements with other Elsevier LPN/LVN textbooks. The purpose of these *LPN Threads* is to make it easier for students and instructors to use the variety of books required by the relatively brief and demanding LPN/LVN curriculum. The following features are included in the *LPN Threads*.

- The **full-color design, cover, photos,** and **illustrations** are visually appealing and pedagogically useful.
- **Objectives** (numbered) begin each chapter, provide a framework for content, and are especially important in providing the structure for the TEACH Lesson Plans for the textbook.
- **Key Terms** with phonetic pronunciations and page-number references are listed at the beginning of each chapter. Key terms appear in color in the chapter and are defined briefly, with full definitions in the **Glossary.** The goal is to help the student with limited proficiency in English to develop a greater command of the pronunciation of scientific and nonscientific English terminology.
- A wide variety of **special features** relate to critical thinking, clinical practice, health promotion, safety, patient teaching, complementary and alternative therapies, communication, home health care, and more. Refer to the To the Student section of this introduction on p. xiii for descriptions and examples of these features.
- **Critical Thinking Questions** presented at the ends of chapters and with Nursing Care Plans provide students with opportunities to practice critical thinking and clinical decision-making skills with realistic patient scenarios. Answers are provided in the Student Resources section on the Evolve website.
- **Key Points** at the end of each chapter correlate to the objectives and serve as useful chapter reviews.
- A full suite of **Instructor Resources** is available, including TEACH Lesson Plans and PowerPoint Slides, Test Bank, Image Collection, and Open-Book Quizzes.
- A **reading-level evaluation** is performed on every chapter of the manuscript during the book's development to increase the consistency among chapters and to ensure that the text is easy to understand.
- In addition to consistent content, design, and support resources, these textbooks benefit from the advice and input of the **Elsevier LPN/LVN Advisory Board**.

LPN ADVISORY BOARD

Tawne D. Blackful, RN, MSN, MEd
Instructor, Associate Degree Nursing
Blinn College
Bryan, Texas

Nancy Bohnarczyk, MA
Adjunct Instructor
College of Mount St. Vincent
New York, New York

Sharon Boyle, MSN, RN-BC
LPN Instructor
Passaic County Technical Institute
Wayne, New Jersey

Dolores Cotton, RN, MSN
Practical Nursing Coordinator
Meridian Technology Center
Stillwater, Oklahoma

Shelly R. Hovis, RN, MS
Director, Practical Nursing
Kiamichi Technology Centers
Antlers, Oklahoma

Dawn Johnson, RN, MSN/Ed
Practical Nurse Administrator and Nurse
  Educator
Erie Business Center PN Program
Erie, Pennsylvania

Patty Knecht, PhD, RN, ANEF
Director of Practical Nursing
Practical Nursing Program and West
  Grove Satellite
Chester County Intermediate Unit
Downingtown, Pennsylvania

Nancy Maebius, PhD, RN
Community Relations Liaison &
  Education Consultant
Galen College of Nursing
San Antonio, Texas

Hana Malik, RN, MSN, FNP-BC
Academic Director
Illinois College of Nursing
Lombard, Illinois

Barb Ratliff, RN, MSN
Associate Director of Health Programs
Butler Technology and Career
Development Schools
Hamilton, Ohio

Faye Silverman, RN, MSN/Ed, PHN, WOCN
Director of Nursing
Kaplan College
North Hollywood, California

Russlyn A. St. John, RN, MSN
Professor and Coordinator, Practical
  Nursing
Practical Nursing Department
St. Charles Community College
Cottleville, Missouri

Fleur de Liza S. Tobias-Cuyco, BSc, CPhT
Dean, Director of Student Affairs, and
  Instructor
Preferred College of Nursing
Los Angeles, California

To the Instructor

EDUCATION OF THE LICENSED PRACTICAL/ VOCATIONAL NURSE

Depth with simplicity continues to be the theme of this text, which is based on current health care practices and the need to adapt to advances in medicine and technology to maintain quality patient care. The role of the nurse is changing at every level, and the curriculum of educational programs for the licensed practical/ vocational nurse (LPN/LVN) also must change to prepare graduates adequately for entry-level positions. In years past, completion of the LPN/LVN program was considered a terminal certificate. Today, however, many LPN/LVN programs are considered "ladders" into the associate degree nursing (ADN) RN program. LPNs/LVNs progressing to the ADN program often do not repeat specialty content such as maternity and pediatric nursing at the ADN level. This text contains the most accurate, current, and clinically relevant information within the scope of practice for the LPN/LVN but with sufficient depth of knowledge and concepts essential to facilitate student success in the RN ladder program.

ABOUT THE TEXT

As in previous editions, this combined maternity and pediatrics text highlights the ways in which infants and children differ from adults. Because of differences in anatomy, physiology, and psychology, techniques for caring for the infant, child, or pregnant woman may vary from those used for the adult medical-surgical patient. Principles of physiology and pathophysiology are presented in this text as a review to help students understand and identify normal and abnormal health.

The changing health care delivery system, the current I.O.M. goals, and the objectives of *Healthy People 2020* focus on health promotion and risk reduction. In response, this text provides comprehensive discussions of family-centered care, wellness, health promotion, illness prevention, women's health issues, and the growth and development of the child *and the parent*. **This information forms one continuum of knowledge that flows from conception to adulthood and is organized from simple to complex and health to illness.**

The normal process of growth and development—from conception to adulthood—is the core of maternity and pediatric knowledge. Therefore, it is integrated as an essential feature of this text. The nurse must be able to provide parents with an awareness of the changing developmental needs of the growing fetus and child to promote healthy parenting.

The effects of illness and medication in the pregnant woman are influenced by the presence of a fetus; dosages are determined by the age and weight of the infant or young child, and illness or injury at a specific phase of growth and development may have an impact on the achievement of normal developmental tasks. Nothing is *standard* among these populations, and these are some of the unique challenges of maternity and pediatric nursing.

The systems approach is maintained in presenting physiological illness (with the exception of congenital anomalies present at birth and communicable diseases of children). **The organization of this text is designed to facilitate its use in a combined maternity and pediatric course, a maternity course followed by a separate pediatric course, or a medical-surgical course that integrates maternity and pediatric concepts.**

This edition encompasses the core aspects of evidence-based maternal–child nursing in health and illness, incorporating updates in clinical care and technology. LPN/LVN education includes tasks and technology used in acute-care hospitals. However, the modern trend of health care reform is moving the focus from the institution to the population. In addition, many parents use complementary or alternative therapies for themselves and their children. Chapter 34 fills the gap between traditional Western therapies and common alternative or complementary therapies for which there is standard scientific evidence, as well as some readily available over-the-counter remedies. All nurses need a working knowledge of the actions, interactions, and safety of these interventions related to the growing fetus and child. An understanding of the trend toward active participation in one's own health care requires knowledge that can help the patient choose safe self-care practices.

Managed health care gave rise to the clinical pathway, and LPNs/LVNs must understand their role in the plan of care. The reader is encouraged to approach clinical problems using critical thinking rather than predetermined habit or memorization of fact. The strong base of knowledge provided by this text focuses on abilities (skills) and beginning concepts of critical thinking. Critical thinking is the basis of clinical decision making and is an essential part of nursing education at every level. Critical thinking questions are included in most chapters with answer guidelines available to the student on the Evolve website. Also, the four different types of care plan styles presented in this text (standard patient care plan, family care plan, pictorial pathway, and clinical pathway) are designed to assist readers in adapting to the style used in the area in which they practice. The unfolding case study is introduced in this edition to challenge the student to apply concepts discussed in the text, using critical thinking that is enhanced by the open-ended questions relating to the presenting family in the chapter. Answers to the open-ended questions can be found in the student's resource materials provided online. Each chapter also offers credible online resources for students to use to enhance their evidence-based knowledge and critical thinking skills.

Positive communication skills are an essential part of caring nursing interventions. Cultural differences related to various perceptions of health and illness and traditional health practices are presented to enable the student nurse to begin developing cultural competence with the community served.

Clinical rotations, particularly in obstetrics and pediatrics, seem to be shortened each year because sites for hands-on clinical experiences are difficult to find, especially for LPN/LVN nursing students. This text is designed to bridge the gap between the classroom and the clinical arena by presenting current facts, concepts, and principles that promote learning through comprehension rather than memorization. Careful consideration of LPN/LVN nurse practice acts and the NCLEX-PN® Test Plan have guided the inclusion of 42 detailed Skills—in addition to many photos and drawings of specific procedures—unique to obstetrics and pediatrics and designed to emphasize nursing actions and responsibilities. Each Skill includes several icons that symbolize common steps for *any* skill in *any* area of general medical-surgical nursing—checking the order, introducing yourself, identifying the patient, performing hand hygiene, and so forth (see p. xiv). It is essential for the student to understand the importance of these steps and to know when to perform each. Presented as a continuum of related images, these icons become engrained in the students' minds as steps that must be considered before performing any intervention. However, these icons also are standard and require critical thinking for students to determine the specific supplies and equipment they may need and when it is necessary to don gloves or other protective equipment.

Every effort has been made to provide a readable text in a simplified format with an array of tables, figures and new photographs and illustrations that allow a comprehensive understanding of techniques essential for effective maternity and pediatric nursing care. It is hoped that the information presented in this text will help the LPN/LVN handle challenging clinical situations that require the use of a broad knowledge base and the ability to think critically, to prioritize, and to use specific clinical skills. This book, with its theme of *depth with simplicity,* is designed to prepare the LPN/LVN student for mobility in the profession as well as to enable the LPN/LVN to provide evidence-based quality maternity and pediatric nursing care to a diverse population in a rapidly changing world.

NEW AND UPDATED CONTENT

The seventh edition has been thoroughly revised with the most recent research and information, including guidelines based on the World Health Organization's Baby-Friendly Hospital Initiative (BFHI), complementary and alternative therapies used in maternal–child care, the impact of body piercings and tattoos on diagnostic imaging and surgery, nonpharmacological prevention and treatment of hypertension, updated immunization mandates, emergency preparedness, and preventing medication errors, among others.

In this edition, newborn care has been divided into three transitional phases with nursing responsibilities outlined for each:
- Phase 1: Care in the delivery room (Chapter 6)
- Phase 2: Assessment during the first few hours after birth (Chapter 9)
- Phase 3: Care of the parent(s) before discharge from the hospital (Chapter 12)

The women's health section also has been updated. The intent is that the information provided will improve the understanding of women's health problems related to maternal–child care and therefore help the nurse improve the quality of women's lives by reducing pain, stress, and illness resulting from delayed treatment, or lack of knowledge, or lack of preventive care.

Chapter 32 has been expanded to meet the cutting-edge need for discussion of the nurse's role in natural and man-made disasters. Floods, hurricanes, tornados, and tsunamis have hit cities in the United States, and terrorism has pierced the U.S. borders. Nurses at all levels need to know their role and responsibilities in such events and since the maternal–child patient has unique needs and susceptibilities, this is included in this text.

HALLMARK FEATURES

The following are hallmark features of this book:
- Content that spans the **developmental continuum** is organized from **simple to complex** and from **health to illness,** making it easy to locate information.
- Focus is on **family-centered care, health promotion and illness prevention, women's health issues, and growth and development of child and parent.**

- **Obstetric content** includes exercise during pregnancy, routine screening tests done during pregnancy, in-depth complementary and alternative therapy content, nursing interventions and responsibilities for analgesia during childbirth, latest update of Bishop score, pediatric language milestones and communication problems in pediatric growth and development, therapeutic play, and sickle cell crises.
- **Pictorial story of vaginal and cesarean births** includes photographs through delivery, followed by delivery of placenta.
- Table 4-6 explains in detail the **physiological and psychosocial changes during trimesters** of pregnancy, signs and symptoms, and nursing interventions.
- **Cultural practices** as they relate to pregnancy and delivery, maternal/infant care, and pediatric care are presented in detailed tables.
- **Cultural Assessment Data Collection Tool** (Chapter 4) checklist assists the nurse in developing an individualized plan of care.
- **MyPlate for Young Children, and the Portion Plate for Kids** (Chapter 15) can help teach children about balanced diets and portion control that will promote healthy growth and development.
- **Bioterrorism** is related to the pregnant woman and children.
- **Loss, death, and grief** and children's responses to death at various ages are presented.
- **Skills** unique to obstetrics and pediatrics (with Performance Checklists for each on Evolve) cover a wide range of maternal and pediatric nursing interventions.
- **Nursing Care Plans** provide expected outcomes, interventions, and rationales for nursing interventions.
- **Unfolding Case Study** with open-ended critical thinking questions to assess application of content to practice as students follow one family through the conception and birth process.
- **Nursing Tips** throughout highlight pertinent information applicable in the clinical setting.
- **Advances in technology** and a peek into the near future are discussed throughout the text.
- **Pediatric laboratory values** have been included in Appendix I as a reference tool because they are not always standard content in lab books.
- **A multilingual glossary of symptoms** is presented in Appendix F to enhance the nurse's data collection in 15 languages.

TEACHING AND LEARNING PACKAGE

For the Instructor

The comprehensive **Evolve Resources with TEACH Instructor Resource** include the following:

- Test Bank with approximately 1025 multiple-choice and alternate-format questions with topic, step of the nursing process, objective, cognitive level, NCLEX® category of client needs, correct answer, rationale, and text page reference
- TEACH Instructor Resource with Lesson Plans and PowerPoint slides that correlate each text and ancillary component
- Image Collection that contains all the illustrations and photographs in the textbook
- Open-Book Quizzes and Answer Keys for each chapter

For the Student

The Evolve **Student Resources** (see p. ii for a detailed list) include the following assets and more:

- Animations depicting anatomy and physiology
- Answers and Rationales for Review Questions for the NCLEX® Examination
- Answer Guidelines for Critical Thinking Questions
- Audio Glossary with pronunciations in English and Spanish
- Calculators for determining body mass index (BMI), body surface area, fluid deficit, Glasgow coma score, IV dosages, and conversion of units
- Fluids and Electrolytes Tutorial
- Interactive Review Questions for the NCLEX® Examination with immediate feedback, including answers, rationales, and page references
- Patient Teaching Plans in English and Spanish
- Skills Performance Checklists for each Skill in the textbook
- Tips for Reducing Childhood Obesity in English and Spanish
- Videos of patient assessment and vaginal and caesarean births

The **Study Guide,** once again written by Emily McKinney, is a valuable supplement to help students understand and apply the content of the text. *Learning Activities, Thinking Critically, Review Questions, Crossword Puzzles, Case Studies,* and *Applying Knowledge* sections provide students with various learning tools for reinforcement and exploration of text material. The Study Guide includes text page number references for each question, and an Answer Key is provided for students on the Evolve website.

To the Student

READING AND REVIEW TOOLS

- **Objectives** introduce the chapter topics.
- **Key Terms** are listed with page numbers. Difficult medical, nursing, or scientific terms are accompanied by simple phonetic pronunciations. Key Terms are considered essential to understanding chapter content and are in color the first time they appear. Key Terms are briefly defined in the text, with complete definitions in the Glossary.
- Each chapter ends with a *Get Ready for the NCLEX® Examination!* section that includes: (1) **Key Points** that reiterate the chapter objectives and serve as a useful review of concepts; (2) a list of **Additional Resources** including the Study Guide, Evolve Resources, and Online Resources; (3) an extensive set of **Review Questions for the NCLEX® Examination** with answers located on Evolve; and (4) **Critical Thinking Questions** for many chapters with answer guidelines located on Evolve.
- A complete **Bibliography and Reader References** in the back of the text cite evidence-based information and provide resources for enhancing knowledge.

CHAPTER FEATURES

Skills are presented in a logical format with defined *purpose,* relevant *illustrations,* and detailed and numbered nursing *steps.* Each Skill includes icons that serve as reminders to perform the basic steps applicable to *all* nursing interventions:

 Check orders.

 Gather necessary equipment and supplies.

 Introduce yourself.

 Check patient's identification.

 Provide privacy.

 Explain the procedure/intervention.

 Perform hand hygiene.

 Don gloves (if applicable).

Not listing the exact supplies or equipment needed encourages you to think critically about what you might need to do or to gather according to hospital protocol before performing the specific Skill.

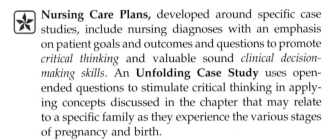 **Nursing Care Plans,** developed around specific case studies, include nursing diagnoses with an emphasis on patient goals and outcomes and questions to promote *critical thinking* and valuable sound *clinical decision-making skills.* An **Unfolding Case Study** uses open-ended questions to stimulate critical thinking in applying concepts discussed in the chapter that may relate to a specific family as they experience the various stages of pregnancy and birth.

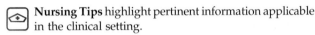 **Nursing Tips** highlight pertinent information applicable in the clinical setting.

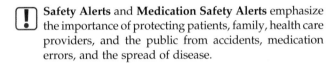 **Safety Alerts** and **Medication Safety Alerts** emphasize the importance of protecting patients, family, health care providers, and the public from accidents, medication errors, and the spread of disease.

Health Promotion boxes emphasize a healthy lifestyle, preventive behaviors, and screening tests to assist in the prevention of accidents and illness.

Medication tables provide quick access to information about commonly used medications related to maternity or pediatric nursing care.

Cultural Considerations boxes explore select cultural preferences and how to address the needs of a culturally diverse patient and family when planning care.

Nutrition Considerations provide important nutrition information for the pregnant woman, infant, and growing child.

Patient Teaching boxes appear frequently in the text to help develop awareness of the vital role of patient/family teaching in health care today.

Communication boxes focus on communication strategies with real-life examples of nurse–patient dialogue.

Legal & Ethical Considerations present pertinent information about the legal issues and ethical dilemmas that may face the practicing nurse.

Home Care Considerations boxes discuss the issues facing patients and caregivers in the home setting.

Memory Joggers provide easy-to-remember mnemonics and acronyms for remembering specific information.

Contents

UNIT VI THE CHANGING HEALTH CARE ENVIRONMENT, 760

34 Complementary and Alternative Therapies in Maternity and Pediatric Nursing, 760

APPENDIXES

The Past, Present, and Future

http://evolve.elsevier.com/Leifer

Objectives

1. Recall the contributions of persons in history to the fields of maternity and pediatric care.
2. List the organizations concerned with setting standards for the nursing care of maternity and pediatric patients.
3. Name two international organizations concerned with maternity and pediatric care.
4. State the influence of the federal government on maternity and pediatric care.
5. List three federal programs that assist mothers and infants.
6. Understand the legal responsibilities of the nurse to report certain diseases or conditions to the public health authorities.
7. Contrast present-day concepts of maternity and child care with those of the past.
8. Discuss how culture affects childbirth and child care.
9. Discuss common terms used in expressing vital statistics.
10. List four reasons why statistics are important.
11. State two types of health care delivery systems in the United States.
12. Discuss the role of the advanced practice nurse.
13. List the five steps of the nursing process.
14. Contrast a nursing care plan with a clinical pathway.
15. Define the Nursing Interventions Classification (NIC) and its relationship to the nursing process.
16. Describe the Nursing Outcomes Classification (NOC) and its influence on the nursing process.
17. Compare and contrast nursing and medical diagnosis frameworks with focus on North American Nursing Diagnosis Association International (NANDA-I) taxonomy.
18. Define critical thinking.
19. Discuss the role of critical thinking in the nursing process and in clinical judgment.
20. Discuss the role of critical thinking as it relates to test taking and lifelong learning.
21. Discuss the objectives of *Healthy People 2020* as it relates to maternity and pediatric care.
22. Examine the importance of documentation as a nursing responsibility.
23. Describe the role of the community health nurse as a health care provider.

Key Terms

advanced practice nurses (p. 10)
advocate (p. 10)
birthing centers (p. 6)
clinical nurse specialist (CNS) (p. 10)
clinical pathways (p. 12)
cost containment (p. 6)
critical thinking (p. 14)
cultural awareness (p. 7)
cultural competence (p. 7)
cultural sensitivity (p. 7)
culture (p. 6)
diagnosis-related groups (DRGs) (p. 8)
documentation (p. 15)
empowerment (p. 2)
evidence-based practice (p. 14)
family care plan (p. 17)
full inclusion (p. 10)
genomics (p. 8)
Health Information Portability and Accountability Act (HIPAA) (p. 4)

health maintenance organizations (HMOs) (p. 9)
Healthy People 2020 (p. 16)
labor, delivery, and recovery (LDR) rooms (p. 6)
mainstream (p. 10)
midwives (p. 6)
morbidity (mŏr-BĬD-ĭ-tē, p. 3)
mortality (mŏr-TĂL-ĭ-tē, p. 3)
nursing care plan (p. 11)
nursing process (p. 11)
obstetrician (ŏb-stĕ-TRĬSH-ĕn, p. 2)
obstetrics (ŏb-STĔT-rĭks, p. 2)
pediatric nurse practitioner (PNP) (p. 10)
pediatrics (pē-dē-ĂT-rĭks, p. 2)
preferred provider organizations (PPOs) (p. 9)
puerperium (pū-ĕr-PĒ-rē-ŭm, p. 2)
statistics (stă-TĬS-tĭks, p. 12)
SBAR (or S-BAR) (ĔS-băr) p. 16)

The word **obstetrics** is derived from the Latin term *obstetrix*, which means "stand by." It is the branch of medicine that pertains to the care of women during pregnancy, childbirth, and the postpartum period (**puerperium**). Maternity nursing is the care given by the nurse to the expectant family before, during, and following birth.

A physician specializing in the care of women during pregnancy, labor, birth, and the postpartum period is an **obstetrician**. These physicians perform cesarean deliveries and treat women with known or suspected obstetric problems as well as attend normal deliveries. Many family physicians and certified nurse-midwives also deliver babies.

Pediatrics is defined as the branch of medicine that deals with the child's development and care and the diseases of childhood and their treatment. The word is derived from the Greek *pais, paidos,* meaning "child," and *iatreia,* "cure."

Family-centered care recognizes the strength and integrity of the family and places it at the core of planning and implementing health care. The family members as caregivers and decision makers are an integral part of both obstetric and pediatric nursing. The philosophy, goals, culture, and ethnic practices of the family contribute to their ability to accept and maintain *control* over the health care of family members. This control is called **empowerment**. The nurse's role in maternity and pediatric family-centered care is to enter into a contract or partnership with the family to achieve the goals of health for its members.

THE PAST

OBSTETRICS

The skill and knowledge related to obstetrics have evolved over centuries. The earliest records concerning childbirth are in the Egyptian papyruses (circa 1550 BC). Soranus, a Greek physician who practiced in second-century Rome and who is known as the father of obstetrics, made later advances. He instituted the practice of podalic version, a procedure used to rotate a fetus to a breech, or feet-first, position. Podalic version is important in the vaginal delivery of the second infant in a set of twins. In this procedure the physician reaches into the uterus and grasps one or both of the infant's feet to facilitate delivery. Planned cesarean birth is safer than podalic version and today is used more often.

With the decline of the Roman Empire and the ensuing Dark Ages, scientific exploration and associated medical improvements came to a halt. During the nineteenth century, however, Karl Credé (1819-1892) and Ignaz Semmelweis (1818-1865) made contributions that improved the safety and the health of mother and child during and after childbirth. In 1884 Credé recommended instilling 2% silver nitrate into the eyes of newborns to prevent blindness caused by gonorrhea. Credé's innovation has saved the eyesight of incalculable numbers of babies.

Semmelweis's story is a classic in the history of maternity care. In the 1840s he worked as an assistant professor in the maternity ward of the Vienna general hospital. There he discovered a relationship between the incidence of puerperal fever (or "childbed fever"), which caused many deaths among women in lying-in wards, and the examination of new mothers by student doctors who had just returned from dissecting cadavers. Semmelweis deduced that puerperal fever was septic, contagious, and transmitted by the *unwashed hands* of physicians and medical students. Semmelweis's outstanding work, written in 1861, is titled *The Causes, Understanding, and Prevention of Childbed Fever.* Tragically, his teaching was not finally accepted until 1890.

Louis Pasteur (1822-1895), a French chemist, confirmed that puerperal fever was caused by bacteria and could be spread by improper hand washing and contact with contaminated objects. The simple, but highly effective, procedure of hand washing continues to be one of the most important means of preventing the spread of infection in the hospital and the home today.

Joseph Lister (1827-1912), a British surgeon influenced by Pasteur, experimented with chemical means of preventing infection. He revolutionized surgical practice by introducing antiseptic surgery.

PEDIATRICS

Methods of childcare have varied throughout history. The culture of a society has a strong influence on standards of childcare. Many primitive tribes were nomads. Strong children survived, whereas the weak were left to die. This practice of infanticide (French and Latin *infans,* "infant," and *caedere,* "to kill") helped to ensure the safety of the group. As tribes became settled, more attention was given to children, but they were still frequently valued only for their productivity. Certain peoples, such as the Egyptians and the Greeks, were advanced in their attitudes. The Greek physician Hippocrates (460-370 BC) wrote of illnesses peculiar to children.

In the Middle Ages, the concept of childhood did not exist. Infancy lasted until about age 7 years, at which time the child was assimilated into the adult world. The art of that time depicts children wearing adult clothes and wigs. Most children did not attend school.

Christianity had a considerable impact on childcare. In the early seventeenth century, Saint Vincent de Paul founded several children's asylums. Many of these eventually became hospitals, although their original concern was for the abandoned. The first children's hospital was founded in Paris in 1802. In the United States, the Children's Aid Society, founded in New York City in 1853, cared for numerous homeless children. In 1855 the first pediatric hospital in the United States, The Children's Hospital of Philadelphia, was founded.

Abraham Jacobi (1830-1919) is known as the father of pediatrics because of his many contributions to the field. The establishment of pediatric nursing as a specialty paralleled that of departments of pediatrics in medical schools, the founding of children's hospitals, and the development of separate units for children in foundling homes and general hospitals. By the 1960s, separate pediatric units were also common in hospitals. Parents were restricted by rigid visiting hours that allowed parent–infant contact for only a few hours each day; when medically indicated, nursing mothers were allowed to enter the pediatric unit for 1 hour at a time to breastfeed their infants.

OBSTETRIC AND PEDIATRIC CARE IN THE UNITED STATES

The immigrants who reached the shores of North America brought with them a wide variety of practices and beliefs about the birth process. Many practices were also contributed by the Native American nations. A midwife or relative attended to most deliveries in the early United States. One physician, Samuel Bard, who was educated outside the United States, is credited with writing the first American textbook for midwives in 1807.

As a young Harvard physician, Oliver Wendell Holmes (1809-1894) wrote a paper detailing the contagious nature of puerperal fever, but he, like Semmelweis, was widely criticized by his colleagues. Eventually, the "germ theory" became accepted, and more mothers and babies began to survive childbirth in the hospital.

Before the 1900s most babies were born at home. Only very ill patients were cared for in lying-in hospitals. Maternal and child **morbidity** and **mortality** were high in such institutions because of crowded conditions and unskilled nursing care. Hospitals began to develop training programs for nurses. As the medical profession grew, physicians developed a closer relationship with hospitals. This, along with the advent of obstetric instruments and anesthesia, caused a shift to hospital care during childbirth. By the 1950s, hospital practice in obstetrics was well established. By 1960, more than 90% of births in the United States occurred in hospitals.

However, hospital care during that time did not embrace the family-centered approach. Often the father waited in a separate room during the labor and birth of his child. The mother was often sedated with "twilight sleep" and participated little during labor and delivery. After birth, the infant was not reunited with the parents for several hours, which resulted in a delay of parent–infant bonding.

Organizations concerned with setting standards for maternity and pediatric nursing were developed. These included the American College of Nurse-Midwives (ACNM); the Association of Women's Health, Obstetric, and Neonatal Nurses (AWHONN), which was formerly the Nurses Association of the American College of Obstetricians and Gynecologists (NAACOG); and the Division of Maternal Nursing within the American Nurses Association (ANA). The American Academy of Pediatrics (AAP), made up of pediatricians from across the nation, has established a position of leadership in setting health standards for children.

Legal & Ethical Considerations

The ANA develops standards of practice that serve as a guide to meet some current challenges. These standards are used when policies and procedures are established. Also, each state has a nurse practice act that determines the scope of practice for the registered nurse, the practical nurse, and the certified nurse assistant. Because these descriptions vary from state to state, nurses must stay informed about the laws in the state where they are employed.

Government Influences in Maternity and Pediatric Care

Legislation. The high mortality of mothers and infants motivated action by the federal government to improve care. The following is a chronological list of some of the important milestones in United States history related to maternity and pediatric care and safety:

- The Sheppard-Towner Act of 1921 provided funds for state-managed programs for maternity care.
- Title V of the Social Security Act, passed in 1935, provided funds for maternity care.
- The Fair Labor Standards Act, passed in 1938, established a general minimum working age of 16 years and a minimum working age of 18 years for jobs considered hazardous. More importantly, this act paved the way for the establishment of national minimum standards for child labor and provided a means of enforcement.
- The National Institutes of Health (NIH) established support for maternity research and education (1962).
- Head Start programs were established to increase educational exposure for preschool children (1966).
- The Women, Infants, and Children (WIC) Program was established to provide supplemental food and education for families in need of assistance (1966).
- The National Center for Family Planning was established to provide contraceptive information (1970).
- In 1974, the government passed the Child Abuse Prevention and Treatment Act (CAPTA).
- In 1975, the Education for All Handicapped Children Act provided for support and public education of handicapped children.
- The Title V amendment of the Public Health Services Act established maternal–infant care centers in public clinics (1981).
- In 1982, the Community Mental Health Center was funded; and the Missing Children's Act was passed, providing a nationwide clearinghouse for missing children.
- The Family and Medical Leave Act (FMLA) of 1993 enabled employees to take 12 weeks of unpaid leave to care for newborns or ill family members without losing benefits or pay status in their jobs.

- Title XIX of the Medicaid program increased access to care by indigent women (1993).
- The **Health Information Portability and Accountability Act (HIPAA)**, enacted in 2003, set standards to protect patients' health information. Patients are allowed access to their medical records and control over how their personal information is disclosed.
- The Health Information Technology for Economic and Clinical Health Act (HITECH) was enacted in 2009 to extend HIPAA regulations by protecting electronic health records.
- The Health Care Reform Bill of 2010, known as the Health Care Affordability Act, is supposed to expand health care coverage to millions of Americans who were previously uninsured.

⚖ Legal & Ethical Considerations

HIPAA and HITECH

Health care personnel are expected to maintain strict confidentiality concerning all patient information. HIPAA regulations mandate that the names and personal information of patients be kept in a secure and private place. Nurses and other health care personnel must maintain strict confidentiality concerning all patient information. The HITECH addition to HIPAA, enacted in July 2009, includes confidentiality requirements involving the monitoring and management of access to electronic health records.

In 2010 President Obama signed the Patient Protection and Affordable Care Act into law that focuses on preventive health care. In 2012 the Supreme Court upheld the constitutionality of the Affordable Health Care Act, which is to increase accessibility to health care in America and will be in full effect by 2014.

Laws requiring the licensing of physicians and pharmacists indirectly affect the health of children and of the general public. Protection is also afforded by the Pure Food and Drug Act, which has allowed for governmental control over medicines, poisons, and the purity of foods. Programs for disaster relief, care and rehabilitation of handicapped children, foster child care, family counseling, family day care, protective services for abused or neglected children, and education of the public are maintained and supported by governmental and private agencies. State licensing bureaus control the regulation of motor vehicles. Car seats for infants and children are currently mandatory. Protection of the public by law enforcement agencies is important, because automobile accidents rank among the leading causes of injury and death in children.

The Children's Bureau. Lillian Wald, a nurse who was interested in the welfare of children, is credited with suggesting the establishment of a federal children's bureau. After the Children's Bureau was established in 1912, it focused attention on the problem of infant mortality. A program that dealt with maternal mortality then followed this program. These programs eventually led to birth registration in all states. In the 1930s, the Children's Bureau investigations led to the development of hot lunch programs in many schools. Today the Children's Bureau is administered under the auspices of the Department of Health and Human Services.

⌂ Nursing Tip

Community programs such as foster grandparents' programs, home health or parent aides, and telephone hotlines for children who are home alone after school are of particular value to dysfunctional or isolated families.

White House Conferences. President Theodore Roosevelt called for the First White House Conference on Children and Youth in 1909. This conference continues to be held every 10 years. In the White House Conference on Child Health and Protection of 1930, the Children's Charter was written (Box 1-1). The charter lists 17 statements related to the needs of children in the areas of education, health, welfare, and protection, and it is considered one of the most important documents in child care history. This declaration has been widely distributed throughout the world.

The 1980 White House Conference on Families focused on involving the states at the grassroots level. A series of statewide hearings were held to identify the most pressing problems of families in the various localities. A tremendous range of viewpoints on many subjects was shared, and specific recommendations were made.

International Year of the Child. The year 1979 was designated as the International Year of the Child (IYC). Its purpose was to focus attention on the critical needs of the world's 1.5 billion children and to inspire the nations, organizations, and individuals of the world to consider how well they provide for children (U.S. Commission of the International Year of the Child, 1980). At this time, the United Nations reaffirmed the Declaration of the Rights of the Child (Box 1-2). Two international organizations concerned with children are the United Nations International Children's Fund (UNICEF) and the World Health Organization (WHO).

Department of Public Health. The Department of Public Health bears a great deal of responsibility for the prevention of disease and death during childhood. Preventive efforts are made on national, state, and local levels. This department sees to the inspection of the water, milk, and food supplies of communities and enforces the maintenance of proper sewage and garbage disposal. Epidemics are investigated and, when necessary, persons capable of transmitting diseases are isolated. The Department of Public Health is also concerned with the inspection of housing and, also, offers services to mothers and infants through programs such as Women, Infants, and Children (WIC).

Box 1-1   The Children's Charter of 1930*

I. For every child spiritual and moral training to help him or her to stand firm under the pressure of life.

II. For every child understanding and the guarding of personality as a most precious right.

III. For every child a home and that love and security which a home provides; and for those children who must receive foster care, the nearest substitute for their own home.

IV. For every child full preparation for the birth; the mother receiving prenatal, natal, and postnatal care; and the establishment of such protective measures as will make childbearing safer.

V. For every child protection from birth through adolescence, including periodic health examinations and, where needed, care of specialists and hospital treatment; regular dental examinations and care of the teeth; protective and preventive measures against communicable diseases; the ensuring of pure food, pure milk, and pure water.

VI. For every child from birth through adolescence, promotion of health, including health instruction and health programs, wholesome physical and mental recreation, with teachers and leaders adequately trained.

VII. For every child a dwelling place safe, sanitary, and wholesome, with reasonable provisions for privacy; free from conditions which tend to thwart development; and a home environment harmonious and enriching.

VIII. For every child a school which is safe from hazards, sanitary, properly equipped, lighted, and ventilated. For younger children nursery schools and kindergartens to supplement home care.

IX. For every child a community which recognizes and plans for needs; protects against physical dangers, moral hazards, and disease; provides safe and wholesome places for play and recreation; and makes provision for cultural and social needs.

X. For every child an education, which, through the discovery and development of individual abilities, prepares the child for life and through training and vocational guidance prepares for a living, which will yield the maximum of satisfaction.

XI. For every child such teaching and training as will prepare him or her for successful parenthood, homemaking, and the rights of citizenship and, for parents, supplementary training to fit them to deal wisely with the problems of parenthood.

XII. For every child education for safety and protection against accidents to which modern conditions subject the child—those to which the child is directly exposed and those which, through loss or maiming of the parents, affect the child directly.

XIII. For every child who is blind, deaf, crippled, or otherwise physically handicapped and for the child who is mentally handicapped, such measures as will early discover and diagnose his handicap, provide care and treatment, and so train the child that the child may become an asset to society rather than a liability. Expenses of these services should be borne publicly where they cannot be privately met.

XIV. For every child who is in conflict with society the right to be dealt with intelligently as society's charge, not society's outcast; with the home, the school, the church, the court, and the institution when needed, shaped to return the child whenever possible to the normal stream of life.

XV. For every child the right to grow up in a family with an adequate standard of living and the security of a stable income as the surest safeguard against social handicaps.

XVI. For every child protection against labor that stunts growth, either physical or mental, that limits education that deprives children of the right of comradeship, of play, and of joy.

XVII. For every rural child as satisfactory schooling and health services as for the city child, and an extension to rural families of social, recreational, and cultural facilities.

*National White House Conference: *White House Conference on Child Health and Protection, 1930*, College Park, Md., 1930, U.S. Children's Bureau Files, National Archives.

Box 1-2   The United Nations Declaration of the Rights of the Child*

The General Assembly proclaims that the child is entitled to a happy childhood and that all should recognize these rights and strive for their observance by legislative and other means:

1. All children without exception shall be entitled to these rights regardless of race, color, sex, language, religion, politics, national or social origin, property, birth, or other status.

2. The child should be protected so that he or she may develop physically, mentally, morally, spiritually, and socially in freedom and dignity.

3. The child is entitled at birth to a name and nationality.

4. The child is entitled to healthy development, which includes adequate food, housing, recreation, and medical attention. He or she shall receive the benefits of Social Security.

5. The child who is handicapped physically, mentally, or emotionally shall receive treatment, education, and care according to his or her need.

6. The child is entitled to love and a harmonious atmosphere, preferably in the environment of his or her parents. Particular love, care, and concern need to be extended to children without families and to the poor.

7. The child is entitled to a free education and opportunities for play and recreation and to develop his or her talents.

8. The child shall be the first one protected in times of adversity.

9. The child shall be protected against all forms of neglect, cruelty, and exploitation. He or she should not be employed in hazardous occupations or before the minimum age.

10. The child shall not be subjected to racial or religious discrimination. The environment should be peaceful and friendly.

*Adapted from U.N. General Assembly Resolution 1386 (XIV), November 20, 1959.

Legal & Ethical Considerations

Reportable Situations

The nurse has a legal responsibility to report certain diseases or conditions to the local public health authorities. A reportable disease is an illness that poses a health hazard to the public, such as a foodborne infection, tuberculosis, sexually transmitted infection (STI), or other communicable condition (see Chapter 32). Suspected child abuse or suicidal behavior must be reported immediately to protect the child from further harm. Required reporting forms are available from the employer or the public health department. The nurse must have a basic understanding of legal and ethical responsibilities and the role of the health care team to be able to use critical thinking skills and provide meaningful support to the family.

THE PRESENT

FAMILY-CENTERED CARE

In family-centered childbearing, the family is recognized as a unique system. Every family member is affected by the birth of a child; therefore, family involvement during pregnancy and birth is seen as constructive and, indeed, necessary for bonding and support. To accommodate family needs, alternative birth centers, birthing rooms, rooming-in units, and mother–infant coupling have been developed. These arrangements are alternatives to the previous standard of separate areas for labor and delivery, which made it necessary to transport a mother from one area to another and fragmented her care.

The three separate sections of the maternity unit—labor-delivery, postpartum, and newborn nursery—have merged. The whole sequence of events may take place in one suite of **labor, delivery, and recovery (LDR) rooms**. The patient is not moved from one area to another, but receives care during labor and delivery and then remains in the same room to recover and care for her new infant. The rooms are often decorated to look homelike.

Freestanding **birthing centers** outside the traditional hospital setting are popular with low-risk maternity patients. These birthing centers provide comprehensive care, including antepartum, labor-delivery, postpartum, mothers' classes, lactation classes, and follow-up family planning. Home birth using midwives is not currently a widespread practice, because malpractice insurance is expensive, and emergency equipment for unexpected complications is not available.

FINANCIAL CONSIDERATIONS

Cost containment is the efficient and effective use of resources. It includes monitoring and regulating expenditures of funds and involves the institution's budget. At first, cost containment influenced maternity care by requiring the discharge of mother and newborn in 24 hours or less after delivery. As a result of problems that occurred, current legislation allows a 48-hour hospital stay for vaginal deliveries and a stay of 4 days for a cesarean section.

CHANGING PERCEPTIONS OF CHILDBEARING

Current maternity practice focuses on a high-quality family experience. *Childbearing is seen as a normal and healthy event.* Parents are prepared for the changes that take place during pregnancy, labor, and delivery. They are also prepared for changes in family dynamics after the birth. Treating each family according to its individual needs is considered paramount.

During the 1950s, the hospital stay for labor and delivery was 1 week. The current average stay in uncomplicated cases is 1 to 2 days. Routine follow-up of the newborn takes place within 2 weeks. A nurse visits the homes of infants and mothers who appear to be at high risk.

MIDWIVES

Throughout history, women have played an important role as birth attendants or **midwives**. The first school of nurse-midwifery opened in New York City in 1932. There are many accredited programs across the United States, all located in or affiliated with institutions of higher learning. The certified nurse-midwife (CNM) is a registered nurse who has graduated from an accredited midwife program and is nationally certified by the American College of Nurse-Midwives. The CNM provides comprehensive prenatal and postnatal care and attends uncomplicated deliveries. The CNM ensures that each patient has a backup physician who will assume her care should a problem occur.

ROLE OF THE CONSUMER

Consumerism has played an important part in family-centered childbirth. In the early 1960s, the natural childbirth movement awakened expectant parents to the need for education and involvement. Prepared childbirth, La Leche League (breastfeeding advocates), and Lamaze classes gradually became accepted. Parents began to question the routine use of anesthesia and the exclusion of fathers from the delivery experience.

Today, a father's attendance at birth is common. Visiting hours are liberal, and extended contact with the newborn is encouraged. The consumer continues to be an important instigator of change. Consumer groups, with the growing support of professionals, have helped to revise restrictive policies previously thought necessary for safety. It has been demonstrated that informed parents can make wise decisions about their own care during this period if they are adequately educated and given professional support.

CULTURAL CONSIDERATIONS

Culture is a body of socially inherited characteristics that one generation hands down to the next. Culture consists of values, beliefs, and practices shared by members of the group. Culture becomes a patterned expression of the thoughts and actions (called traditions) and affects the way patients respond to health care.

The United States is a culturally diverse nation, and nurses must develop **cultural awareness** and **cultural sensitivity** to practices and values that differ from their own. Only this way can nurses develop the **cultural competence** that will enable them to adapt health care practices to meet the needs of patients from various cultures.

The cultural background of the expectant family strongly influences its adaptation to the birth experience. Nursing Care Plan 1-1 lists nursing interventions for selected diagnoses that pertain to cultural diversity. One way in which the nurse gains important information about an individual's culture is to ask the pregnant

---

Nursing Care Plan 1-1 — Care of Childbearing Families Related to Potential or Actual Stress Caused by Cultural Diversity

PATIENT DATA A 22-year-old, para 0, gravida 1, is admitted to the labor room in active early labor. Her partner is with her, and they do not speak English.

EXAMPLES OF NIC AND NOC
NIC: presence; touch
NOC: communication ability

Selected Nursing Diagnosis: Impaired verbal communication related to language barriers

Goals	Nursing Interventions	Rationales
The woman will have an opportunity to understand communication in her own language.	Arrange for a family or staff member interpreter as needed.	Interpreter can provide support for woman and help to lessen her anxieties. Poor communication can result in time delays, errors, and misinterpretation of intent.
	Clearly define instructions in woman's language of origin.	A common language is necessary for communication to take place.
	Provide written instructions in woman's language whenever possible.	Written instructions can be reviewed at a less stressful time by patient. In some cases it is necessary to determine if person can read.
	Explain the use and purpose of all instruments and equipment, along with the effects or possible effects on the mother and fetus.	Education of family lessens anxiety and provides family with a sense of control.
	Provide opportunities for clarification and questions.	Learning takes time; repetition of important material promotes learning. Nurse can determine woman's understanding of information and clarify misconceptions.

EXAMPLES OF NIC AND NOC
NIC: spiritual support
NOC: anxiety control, coping

Selected Nursing Diagnosis: Compromised family coping related to isolation, different customs, attitudes, or beliefs

Goals	Nursing Interventions	Rationales
Family members will state that they feel welcome and safe in the environment provided.	Encourage orientation visit to the maternity unit before delivery.	Families who have clear, accurate information can better participate in labor and delivery. Viewing the delivery setting before using it decreases anxiety about the unknown.
	Inform families about routines, visiting hours, significant persons who can assist in labor and delivery, and location of newborn after delivery.	Families have different expectations of the health care system. They may hesitate to ask questions because of shyness or fear of "losing face."
	Determine and respect practices and values of family and incorporate them into nursing care plans as much as possible.	Clarification of culturally specific values and practices will prevent misunderstanding and conflict with the nurse's value system. Nursing care plans promote organization of care and communication among staff members.

Critical Thinking Questions
1. The extended family of a patient in the labor room requests permission to stay with the patient and the husband throughout labor. What should the nurse's response be?
2. A patient admitted to the labor room refuses to let a male physician perform a vaginal examination. What should the nursing role be?
   See p. 12 for an explanation of NIC, NOC, and NANDA.

woman what she considers normal practice. Data collection questions might include the following:

- How does the woman view her pregnancy (as an illness, a vulnerable time, or a healthy time)?
- Does she view the birth process as dangerous? Why?
- Is birth a public or private experience for her?
- In what position does she expect to deliver (i.e., squatting, lithotomy, or some other position)?
- What type of help does she need before and after delivery?
- What role does her immediate or extended family play in relation to the pregnancy and birth?

Such information helps to promote understanding and individualizes patient care. It also increases the satisfaction of the patient and the nurse regarding the quality of care provided. Cultural influences on nursing care are discussed in Chapter 6.

TECHNOLOGY AND SPECIALTY EXPERTISE

Technological advances have enabled many infants to survive who might otherwise have died (Figure 1-1). High-risk prenatal clinics and the neonatal intensive care unit offer the 1-lb preemie an opportunity to survive. A pediatric cardiologist now treats children with heart problems. The pediatric surgeon provides much of the complex surgery needed by the newborn with a congenital defect. Pediatric psychiatrists manage emotional problems. Many hospital laboratories are well equipped to test pediatric specimens. Chromosomal studies and biochemical screening have made identification of risks and family counseling more significant than ever. The field of perinatal biology has advanced to the forefront of pediatric medicine.

The medical profession and allied health agencies work as a team to ensure the total well-being of the

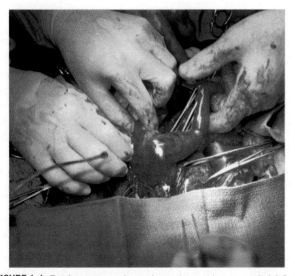

FIGURE 1-1 Fetal surgery can be performed to repair a congenital defect before birth. (From Harrison MR, Globus MS, Filly RA, eds: *The unborn patient: prenatal diagnosis and treatment*, ed 2, Philadelphia, 1991, Saunders.)

patient. Children with defects previously thought to be incompatible with life are taken to special diagnostic and treatment centers where they receive expert attention and care. After discharge, many of these children are cared for in their homes. The number of chronically disabled children is growing. Some are dependent on sophisticated hospital equipment such as ventilators and home monitors. The required nursing care at home may call for the suctioning of a tracheostomy, central line care, and other highly technical skills. Parents must be carefully educated and continually supported. Although this type of care is cost-effective and psychologically sound for the child, respite care is extremely important, because 24-hour-a-day care is extremely taxing for the family, both physically and psychologically.

GENOMICS

Genomics is the study of the functions of all of the genes in the human body, with a focus on their interactions with each other and the environment. The *Human Genome Project* has identified all genetic material present in the human body. The door is now open as medical researchers have identified genes responsible for specific congenital disorders and can develop "gene therapy" to replace missing genes or alter defective genes (Figure 1-2). This knowledge, combined with technological advances, can result in earlier diagnosis, earlier intervention, and an integration of genomic knowledge in patient education as well as therapy.

HEALTH CARE DELIVERY SYSTEMS

Cost containment is a major motivating factor in current health care, especially when health costs rise without decreases in morbidity and mortality. Many hospitals are merging to increase their buying power and reduce duplication of services.

Insurance reimbursement has become an important consideration in health care. The federal government has had to revise its Medicare and Medicaid programs. Among other changes, it instituted **diagnosis-related groups (DRGs)**. These refer to a Medicare system that determines payment for a hospital stay based on the patient's diagnosis. This mandate has had a tremendous impact on health care delivery. Patients are being discharged earlier from the hospital, and more care is being given in skilled nursing facilities and in the home. Some insurance companies are employing nurses in the role of case managers. Nurses remaining in institutions also may be required to assume the role of case managers and to become more flexible through cross-training. Nurses are expected to be concerned with keeping hospital costs down while maintaining the quality of care. Many suggest that the future of nursing may depend on how well nurses can demonstrate their value and cost-effectiveness.

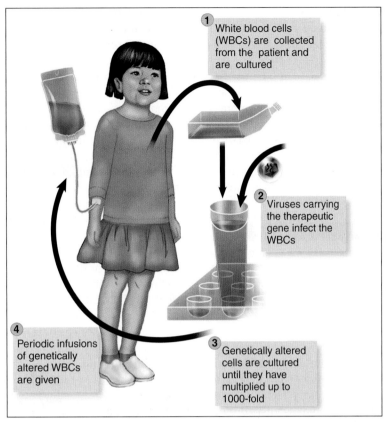

FIGURE 1-2 Gene therapy. One goal of gene replacement therapy is to alter the existing body cells to eliminate the cause of a genetic disease. The therapeutic or missing gene can be combined with a virus that can enter the infant's system. This is called gene augmentation. In gene replacement therapy, new therapeutic genes are combined with viruses that can enter the human genome. (From Patton KT, Thibodeau GA: *Anatomy & physiology*, ed 7, St Louis, 2010, Mosby.)

Inside the figure:

1. White blood cells (WBCs) are collected from the patient and are cultured

2. Viruses carrying the therapeutic gene infect the WBCs

3. Genetically altered cells are cultured until they have multiplied up to 1000-fold

4. Periodic infusions of genetically altered WBCs are given

Health maintenance organizations (HMOs) and **preferred provider organizations (PPOs)** have emerged as alternative medical care delivery systems. Insurers and providers of care have united to hold costs down yet remain competitive. Historically, a two-tiered system evolved: one tier (private insurance, HMOs, and PPOs) served people with greater financial resources, and the other tier (Medicare and Medicaid) served people with fewer resources. With recent federal legislative changes, a large percentage of persons who were uninsured will have access to health care via the Healthcare Reform Act of 2010. Box 1-3 defines managed care systems.

Box 1-3 **Health Care Delivery Systems**

managed care: Integrates financing with health care for members; for a monthly "capitation" fee, contracts with physicians and hospitals to provide health care with strict utilization review for cost containment

HMO: A health maintenance organization that offers health services for a fixed premium

PPO: A preferred provider organization contracts with providers for services on a discounted fee-for-service basis for members

utilization review: Reviews appropriateness of health care services and guidelines for physicians for treatment of illness, controlling management of care to achieve cost containment

---

NURSING CARE

Procedural modifications for the nurse have been made, including adherence to standard precautions during the labor and delivery process (see Appendix A), during umbilical cord care, and in the nursery. More emphasis on data entry and retrieval makes it necessary for nursing personnel to be computer literate. Sociologically, families have become smaller, the number of single parents is increasing, child and spouse abuse is rampant, and more mothers work outside of the home to help support the family. These developments present special challenges to maternal and child health nurses. Careful assessment and documentation to detect abuse are necessary, and nurses must be familiar with community support services for women and children in need. Nurses must also be flexible and promote policies that make health care more available for working parents. Teaching must be integrated into care plans and individually tailored to the family's needs and its cultural and ethnic background.

Cultural Considerations

Perception of Health and Illness

Cultural beliefs today, as in the past, affect how a family perceives health and illness. Holistic nursing includes being alert for cultural diversity and incorporating this information into the plan for nursing care.

Pediatric Nurses as Advocates

An **advocate** is a person who intercedes or pleads on behalf of another. Pediatric nurses are increasingly assuming the role of child advocate. Advocacy may be required for the child's physical and emotional health and may include other family members. Hospitalized children frequently cannot determine or express their needs. When nurses believe that the child's best interests are not being met, they must seek assistance. This usually involves taking the problem to the multidisciplinary team. Nurses must document their efforts to seek instruction and direction from their head nurse, supervisors, or the physician.

> **Nursing Tip**
>
> It is a nursing responsibility to collect data; it is vital for the nurse to initiate interventions for abnormal findings or refer for follow-up care and document findings and the follow-up provided.

Health Promotion

Health promotion continues to assume increased importance, and it is the basis of the 2010 Health Care Reform Act implemented by President Obama. Preventing illness or disability is cost effective; more important, it saves the family from stress, disruptions, and financial burden. Healthy children spend fewer days in the hospital. Many conditions are treated in same-day surgery, ambulatory settings, or emergency departments. Rather than being distinct, hospital and home care have become interdependent.

Many chronically ill children are living into adulthood, creating the need for more support services. Medically fragile and technology-dependent children may change the typical profile of chronically ill children. The nurse is often the initiator of support services to these patients through education and referral. Ideally these services will assist the child to become as independent as possible, lead a productive life, and be integrated into society. In the past, the term **mainstream** was used to describe the process of integrating a physically or mentally challenged child into society. The term **full inclusion**, signifying an expansion of the mainstream policy, is being used more frequently today. Early infant intervention programs for children with developmental disabilities attempt to reduce or minimize the effects of the disability. These services may be provided in a clinic or in the home. The need for in-home, family-centered pediatric care will continue to grow with the number of children with chronic illness who survive.

Quality of life is particularly relevant. Organ transplants have saved some children; however, the complications, limited availability, and expense of these transplants create moral and ethical dilemmas. Older children with life-threatening conditions must be included in planning modified advance directives with their families and the medical team.

These developments, along with the explosion of information, an emphasis on individual nurses' accountability, new technology, and the use of computers in health care, make it especially imperative for nurses to maintain their knowledge and skills at the level necessary to provide safe care. Employers often offer continuing education classes for their employees. Most states require proof of continuing education for the renewal of nursing licenses.

> **Nursing Tip**
>
> Expanded nursing roles include the clinical nurse specialist, the pediatric nurse practitioner, the school nurse practitioner, the family nurse practitioner, and the certified nurse-midwife.

Advanced Practice Nurses

In keeping with the current practice of focusing on prevention of illness and maintenance of health rather than the treatment of illness, the specialty of **pediatric nurse practitioner (PNP)** was born. The PNP provides ambulatory and primary care for patients. The school nurse or child life specialist expands the accessibility of preventive health care to the well child.

> **Health Promotion**
>
> ### *Healthy People 2020:* Specific Contributions of School Nurses
>
> The expanding role of the school nurse will include these interventions:
>
> 1. Reviewing participation in and effectiveness of physical education programs for normal and disabled students
> 2. Providing nutritional education and guidance
> 3. Supervising school nutrition programs
> 4. Participating in maintaining a drug- and tobacco-free environment for students
> 5. Providing education in the prevention of sexually transmitted infections
> 6. Providing guidance to students and staff concerning prevention of injuries
> 7. Providing oral health education
> 8. Providing age-appropriate human immunodeficiency virus (HIV) education
> 9. Reviewing immunization laws and records
> 10. Assessing the community needs in relation to the child population and reassessing or revising roles in relation to prevention, screening, monitoring, teaching, and follow-up of health needs or problems
>
> Modified from the U.S. Department of Health and Human Services: *Healthy People 2020: national health promotion and disease prevention objectives.* Washington, DC, 2010.

The **clinical nurse specialist (CNS)** provides care in the hospital or community to specific specialty patients, such as cardiac, neurological, or oncological care. CNSs conduct primary research and facilitate necessary changes in health care management of their patients. Often the PNP and the CNS are called **advanced practice nurses**, and they have a registered nurse (RN) license, as well as an advanced degree. Advanced

Box 1-4   Advanced Practice Nursing Specialties

OGNP: Obstetric-gynecology nurse practitioner
WHNP: Women's health care nurse practitioner
NNP: Neonatal nurse practitioner
FPNP: Family planning nurse practitioner
IBCLC: International board-certified lactation consultant
CDDN: Certified developmental disabilities nurse
CNM: Certified nurse-midwife
CPN: Certified pediatric nurse
CPON: Certified pediatric oncology nurse
CRNA: Certified registered nurse anesthetist

From Hamric A, Spross J, Hanson C: *Advanced practice nursing: an integrative approach,* ed 4, Philadelphia, 2008, Elsevier; "What's in a name?" *Adv Nurs* 55-56, 2005; Cherry B, Jacob S: *Contemporary nursing: issues, trends and management,* St Louis, 2011, Mosby.

practice nurses can specialize in obstetrics, pediatrics, or neonatal care. Box 1-4 lists some specialties that have developed in maternal–child care.

Nursing Tip

An important role of the nurse is that of being a patient advocate.

Nursing Tools

The Nursing Process. The **nursing process** was developed in 1963. This term referred to a series of steps describing the systematic problem-solving approach nurses used to identify, prevent, or treat actual or potential health problems. In 1973, the ANA developed standards relating to this nursing process that have been nationally accepted and include the following:

1. *Assessment:* Collection of patient data, both subjective and objective
2. *Diagnosis:* Analysis of data in terms of NANDA nursing diagnoses (see inside back cover)
3. *Planning:* Preparation of a plan of care designed to achieve stated outcomes
4. *Outcomes identification:* Identification of individualized expected patient outcomes
5. *Implementation:* Carrying out of interventions identified in the plan of care
6. *Evaluation:* Evaluation of outcome progress and redesigning of the plan if necessary

The nursing process is a framework of action designed to meet the individual needs of patients. It is problem-oriented and goal-directed and involves the use of critical thinking, problem solving, and decision making. The nursing process is expressed in an individualized nursing care plan. Diagnoses approved by NANDA-I are listed on the inside back cover. Table 1-1 differentiates between medical and nursing diagnoses.

Nursing Care Plans. The **nursing care plan** is developed as a result of the nursing process. It is a written instrument of communication among staff members that focuses on individualized patient care. See Nursing Care Plan 1-1 for an example of a care plan. Other sample

Table 1-1   Comparison of Medical and Nursing Diagnoses

MEDICAL DIAGNOSIS	NURSING DIAGNOSIS
Acquired immunodeficiency syndrome (AIDS)	Imbalanced nutrition: less than body requirements related to anorexia and evidenced by weight loss
Gestational diabetes mellitus	Deficient knowledge related to gestational diabetes mellitus (GDM) and its effects on pregnant woman and fetus; manifested by crying, anxiety
Cystic fibrosis	Ineffective airway clearance related to mucus accumulation; manifested by rales, fatigue

care plans for maternity and pediatric nursing are provided throughout this text. Certain terms used in care plans are important to understand (Box 1-5).

A nursing care plan is a "picture" of a typical clinical situation that may be encountered by the graduate nurse. Specific data concerning the patient are obtained. These data can be used as clues to solve the mystery or problem concerning the patient (this phase is called

Box 1-5   Common Terms Used in Nursing Care Plans

patient: An individual, group, family, or community that is the focus of a nursing intervention
nursing activity: An action that implements an intervention to assist the patient toward a desired outcome (a series of activities may be needed to implement an intervention)
nursing diagnosis: A clinical judgment about a patient's response to an actual or potential health problem; nursing diagnosis provides basis for selection of nursing interventions to achieve an outcome for which the nurse is accountable (North American Nursing Diagnosis Association [NANDA], 2008)
nursing intervention: Any treatment or nursing activity based on clinical judgment and knowledge that a nurse performs to achieve a specific outcome for the patient; includes direct or indirect patient care or community or public health activities
scope of practice: The range of specific activities related to health care or health promotion that a health care provider has legal authority to perform. Performance of these activities requires substantial knowledge or technical skill. Specific activities are listed by the state nurse practice act, and nurses must practice within the limitations of the nurse practice act of their state. For example, a licensed practical nurse/licensed vocational nurse (LPN/LVN) cannot perform surgery; that activity is within the scope of a medical doctor.
standards of practice: Established minimum criteria for competent nursing care approved by nursing practice organizations such as the state board of nursing, The Joint Commission (TJC), and the American Nurses Association (ANA)

collection). These clues help the nurse identify the problems of the patient. By organizing all the clues and identifying several problems, the nurse then prioritizes the problems identified. This phase of care planning is called *analysis.* When the priority problem is identified, the nurse can use knowledge, experience, and resources such as doctors' prescriptions, textbooks, journals, or the Internet to decide on a plan of action to solve the problem. This phase is called *planning.* The actual nursing activities necessary to solve the problem are called nursing interventions. The nursing interventions are planned with specific outcomes or goals in mind. An outcome or goal is the positive resolution of the patient's problem. The nursing interventions are the basis of the nursing or bedside care provided to the patient. After the nursing care is provided, the nurse re-evaluates the original problem to determine whether the goal was met or the outcome achieved. If goals have not been met, the nurse suggests revision of interventions.

Clinical Pathways. **Clinical pathways,** also known as *critical pathways, care maps,* or *multidisciplinary action plans,* are collaborative guidelines that define multidisciplinary care in terms of outcomes within a timeline. Fundamentally, the pathway identifies expected progress within a set timeline and benchmarks by which to recognize this progress. This expected progress of the patient becomes a standard of care; therefore, clinical pathways are based on research rather than on tradition. By setting specific recovery goals that the patient is expected to reach each day, deviations are readily identified. These deviations are called *variances.* If the patient's progress is slower than expected, the outcome (goal) is not achieved within the timeline and a negative variance occurs, and discharge from the hospital may be delayed. The use of clinical pathways improves the quality of care and reduces unnecessary hospitalization time. It is an essential component of managed care and promotes coordination of the entire health care team. Sample clinical pathways are presented throughout the chapters in this text.

Statistics. **Statistics** refers to the process of gathering and analyzing numerical data. Statistics concerning birth, illness (*morbidity*), and death (*mortality*) provide valuable information for determining or projecting the needs of a population or subgroup and for predicting trends. In the United States, vital statistics are compiled for the country as a whole by the National Center for Health Statistics and are published in the Centers for Disease Control and Prevention (CDC) annual report, *Vital Statistics of the United States,* and in the pamphlet *Morbidity and Mortality Weekly Report (MMWR).* Each state's bureaus of vital statistics issue statistics as well. Other independent agencies also supply statistics regarding various specialties.

A maternity nurse may use statistical data to become aware of reproductive trends, to determine populations

---

| Box 1-6 | Common Vital Statistics Terms |

birth rate: The number of live births per 1000 population in 1 year

fertility rate: The number of births per 1000 women ages 15 to 44 years in a given population

fetal mortality rate: The number of fetal deaths (fetuses weighing 500 g or more) per 1000 live births per year

infant mortality rate: The number of deaths of infants under age 1 year per 1000 live births per year

maternal mortality rate: The number of maternal deaths per 100,000 live births that occur as a direct result of pregnancy (includes the 42-day postpartum period)

neonatal mortality rate: The number of deaths of infants less than age 28 days per 1000 live births per year

perinatal mortality rate: Includes both fetal and neonatal deaths per 1000 live births per year

---

at risk, to evaluate the quality of prenatal care, or to compare relevant information from state to state and country to country. Box 1-6 lists some frequently used terms in vital statistics.

Statistics show, for example, that sudden infant death syndrome (SIDS) was the second leading cause of death under the age of 1 year in 1980, but was the third in 2010. Respiratory distress syndrome was the third leading cause of death under 1 year of age in 1980 and the eighth leading cause of death in 2007 through 2010 (NIH, 2012). *Go to the Evolve website for more detailed information on infant deaths in the United States.* Research, education, and nursing care account for many of the positive changes in these statistical reports.

Table 1-2 compares the national birth rates per 1000 women between the ages of 15 and 44 as of July 1, 2011, and the percentage that were preterm (less than 37 completed weeks of gestation) and the percentage born by cesarean section. One of the goals of *Healthy People 2020* is to reduce the number of cesarean section births and reduce the number of preterm births by the year 2020. The percent of preterm births decreased from 12.0 to 11.7 between 2010 and 2011, but the number of late preterm births (37 to 38 weeks' gestation) has remained at approximately 8.3%. See Chapter 13 for details concerning the health problems related to premature and preterm infants.

NIC, NOC, and NANDA. Nursing Interventions Classification (NIC) by Bulechek and colleagues (2012), *Nursing Outcomes Classification (NOC)* by Moorhead and colleagues (2012), and the North American Nursing Diagnosis Association International (NANDA-I, 2011) *Nursing Diagnoses: Definitions and Classification* are companions that aid in the critical-thinking aspect of patient care. They provide a standardization of language concerning patient status and nursing activities that enables nurses to work in the managed care environment, improve quality of care, reduce costs, promote research, and facilitate the development of a reimbursement system for nursing services rendered.

Table 1-2   Birth Statistics in the United States, 2011

AREA	NUMBER OF BIRTHS	BIRTH RATE (%)	CESAREAN SECTIONS (%)	PRETERM* (%)
United States	**3,953,593**	**12.7**	**32.8**	**11.7**
Alabama	59,347	12.4	35.1	14.9
Alaska	11,455	15.8	22.4	10.4
Arizona	85,543	13.2	27.6	12.1
Arkansas	38,713	13.2	34.3	13.2
California	502,118	13.3	33.2	9.8
Colorado	65,055	12.7	25.3	10.3
Connecticut	37,280	10.4	35.8	10.1
Delaware	11,257	12.4	32.5	11.2
District of Columbia	9,314	15.1	33.9	13.7
Florida	213,344	11.2	38.1	13.0
Georgia	132,488	13.5	33.6	13.2
Hawaii	18,957	13.8	26.0	12.3
Idaho	22,305	14.1	24.5	10.2
Illinois	161,312	12.5	31.7	12.1
Indiana	83,702	12.8	30.6	11.6
Iowa	38,213	12.5	30.5	11.1
Kansas	39,642	13.8	30.2	11.2
Kentucky	55,377	12.7	36.3	13.4
Louisiana	61,889	13.5	39.9	15.6
Maine	12,704	9.6	30.9	9.6
Maryland	73,086	12.5	34.8	12.5
Massachusetts	73,225	11.1	32.6	10.5
Michigan	114,004	11.5	32.8	12.0
Minnesota	68,411	12.8	26.8	9.9
Mississippi	39,856	13.4	38.0	16.9
Missouri	76,117	12.7	31.4	11.6
Montana	12,069	12.1	29.5	10.8
Nebraska	25,720	14.0	30.8	10.6
Nevada	35,295	13.0	33.8	13.2
New Hampshire	12,852	9.7	30.8	9.5
New Jersey	105,886	12.0	39.1	11.7
New Mexico	27,289	13.1	23.0	11.8
New York	241,290	12.4	34.3	10.9
North Carolina	120,385	12.5	30.4	12.6
North Dakota	9,527	13.9	28.7	9.9
Ohio	137,916	11.9	31.2	12.0
Oklahoma	52,274	13.8	34.2	13.2
Oregon	45,157	11.7	28.9	9.1
Pennsylvania	143,148	11.2	31.4	11.0
Rhode Island	10,960	10.4	32.8	10.4
South Carolina	57,368	12.3	35.2	14.1
South Dakota	11,849	14.4	25.3	11.2
Tennessee	79,588	12.4	33.5	12.8
Texas	377,449	14.7	35.3	12.8
Utah	51,223	18.2	22.7	10.9

Continued

Table 1-2 Birth Statistics in the United States, 2011—cont'd

AREA	NUMBER OF BIRTHS	BIRTH RATE (%)	CESAREAN SECTIONS (%)	PRETERM (%)
Vermont	6,078	9.7	27.8	8.8
Virginia	102,648	12.7	34.1	11.2
Washington	86,976	12.7	28.8	9.8
West Virginia	20,720	11.2	36.8	12.7
Wisconsin	67,811	11.9	25.8	10.4
Wyoming	7,398	13.0	27.0	10.2
Puerto Rico	42,153	11.3	46.7	17.6

Data from *National Vital Statistics Reports* 62(1):June 28, 2013.
*Preterm births are births less than 37 completed weeks of gestation.

NIC and NOC codes make possible the collection of electronic data for the purposes of research and reimbursement. Nursing Care Plan 1-1 includes NIC and NOC entries to demonstrate how they are incorporated into the typical care plan. The specific codes assigned to NIC and NOC are not included in this text, because the registered nurse is responsible for the coding. However, the LPN/LVN is responsible for understanding and working with NIC and NOC terminology.

NIC. NIC specifies actions that nurses perform to help patients toward a goal or outcome. The focus is on the action of the nurse. Physiological interventions such as suctioning and psychosocial interventions such as reducing fears and anxieties are useful in the prevention, as well as the treatment, of illness. There is a relationship among nursing diagnosis (NANDA-I), nursing interventions (NIC), and nursing outcomes (NOC). Nursing outcomes are different from nursing goals, because nursing goals are either met or unmet. Nursing outcomes are described on a continuum. This makes it possible to measure *outcomes* as nursing actions influence them.

NOC. NOC was developed to identify outcomes of nursing care that are directly influenced by nursing actions (Moorhead et al, 2012). *Outcomes* are defined as the behaviors and feelings of the patient in response to the nursing care given.

Critical Thinking. Nurses have job-specific knowledge and skills they incorporate into their daily nursing practice by applying thought. *General thinking* involves random or memorized thoughts. An example of general thinking would be memorizing the steps of a clinical procedure or skill. *Critical thinking,* however, is purposeful, goal-directed thinking based on scientific evidence rather than assumption or memorization.

The way a nurse solves the problems of a patient is not always found in a textbook or in class lectures. Sometimes the nurse must consider factors that are specific to the individual patient or affected by the individual situation. For example, the cultural background of the patient or the age of the patient influences how effective a given intervention will be. If the problem

Box 1-7 Steps in Preparing a Nursing Care Plan

1. Collect data from chart, medical order sheet, laboratory reports, history and physical examination, progress notes, and so on.
2. Review medical diagnosis of patient in text.
3. Assess patient; interview patient.
4. Select appropriate nursing diagnosis from the North American Nursing Diagnosis Association (NANDA) list. Note the etiology and the evidence related to each choice.
5. Select measurable Nursing Outcomes Classifications (NOC) that are realistic for the patient, stating the timeline for achieving the outcomes.
6. Identify Nursing Interventions Classification (NIC) that will facilitate outcomes.
7. Identify nursing actions within these interventions.
8. Evaluate outcome; revise care plan as needed.

is a protein deficiency and the nurse selects the intervention to teach the importance of meat in the diet, the intervention will be ineffective—that is, it will not have a positive outcome—if this patient is a vegetarian, because meat will not be eaten. Thus **critical thinking** must enter the picture for optimum nursing care to be provided. Critical thinking entails applying creativity and ingenuity to solve a problem: combining basic standard principles with data specific to the patient. The basic steps in preparing a care plan involve critical thinking and are outlined in Box 1-7.

Critical thinking organizes the approach to discovery and involves the reflection and integration of

Nursing Tip

Evidence-based practice starts when the nurse uses the best evidence obtained from current, valid, published research. When the nurse combines that information with his or her critical thinking process, experiences, and patients' needs, it is then possible to plan safe, effective nursing care for the patient. Two nursing journals focusing on maternal and child health are the *Journal of Obstetric, Gynecologic, and Neonatal Nursing* (JOGNN) and the *American Journal of Maternal Child Nursing* (MCN).

information that enables the nurse to arrive at a conclusion or make a judgment. An example of critical thinking would be modifying the steps in a clinical procedure or skill so that the individual patient's needs are met but the basic principles of the skill are not violated (e.g., sterile technique). With critical thinking, *problem solving* is effective and *problem prevention* occurs. General thinking can occur naturally, but critical thinking is a skill that must be learned.

Because critical thinking is an active process, the regular use of critical thinking can assist in moving general information into long-term memory and can increase creativity. Critical thinking skills help the nurse adapt to new situations that occur every day and aid in clinical decision making about care. Critical thinking can improve the care nurses give to patients, improve test scores (through critical thinking about a scenario in the question), and improve working conditions by enabling the nurse to analyze and find creative ways to improve existing policies and practices.

The nursing process and critical thinking. The nursing process (assessment, diagnosis, outcomes identification, planning, implementation, and evaluation) is a tool for effective critical thinking. When a nurse uses the nursing process in critical thinking, a clinical judgment can be made that is specific to the data collected and the clinical situation. In every clinical contact, a nurse must identify actual and potential problems and make decisions about a plan of action that will result in a positive patient outcome; know why the actions are appropriate; differentiate between those problems that the nurse can handle independently and those that necessitate contacting other members of the health care team; and prioritize those actions (Box 1-8).

Differentiating between actions that can be performed independently and those requiring collaboration with other health care providers is based on the *scope of practice* of the licensed practical or vocational nurse (LPN/LVN). The state board of nursing publishes the scope of practice of the LPN/LVN.

Using critical thinking to improve test scores. Attending class, reading the text, and studying are the basis of learning, and evaluation of learning is achieved by testing. Weekly tests evaluate short-term learning. Final examinations evaluate long-term learning or retention of learning. Retained learning is subject to later recall

and therefore is most useful in nursing practice after graduation from nursing school. Recalling facts that have been retained is what makes critical thinking in nursing practice possible. For a nurse to recognize or analyze abnormal findings, the normal findings must be recalled and used for comparison. An intervention can then be formulated.

Using critical thinking in studying involves the following:
- *Understanding* facts before trying to memorize them
- *Prioritizing* information to be memorized
- *Relating* facts to other facts (clusters, patterns, groups)
- *Using all five senses* to study (read, write, draw, listen to audio, see pictures of symptoms)
- *Reviewing* before tests
- *Reading critically* (identifying key concepts and using critical thinking) when working with sample questions during study

Documentation

Documentation, or charting, has always been a legal responsibility of the nurse and continues to be a National Patient Safety Goal of The Joint Commission (TJC). When a medication is given or a treatment performed, it must be accurately documented on the patient's chart. Charting responsibilities also include head-to-toe assessment of the patient and a recording both of data pertinent to the diagnosis and the response to treatment.

⚖ Legal & Ethical Considerations

Documentation

For legal purposes, if the nurse does not document an intervention, the intervention was not done. Documentation must be detailed and accurate.

There have been many forms of charting required by different hospitals in different areas of the country that have guided the nurse toward comprehensive charting. A traditional problem was when several members of the multidisciplinary health care team would access the chart at the same time. While the nurse was recording a medication administered, the medication record was "tied up" until the recording was complete. While a physician was reviewing the chart and the progress of the patient, the records were tied up until the conference was completed.

Electronic documentation was developed to decrease the number of medical errors caused by illegible handwriting and is now used by most hospitals in the country. Electronic documentation is paperless, and a bar-coding system is often used to document medication administration at the patient's bedside. Security features are usually built in, and integrated prompts

---

Box 1-8 Process of Critical Thinking

1. Identify the problem.
2. Differentiate fact from assumption.
3. Check reliability and accuracy of data.
4. Determine relevant from irrelevant.
5. Identify possible conclusions or outcomes.
6. Set priorities and goals.
7. Evaluate response of patient.

encourage accurate and comprehensive documentation by requiring certain entries be made before the user can progress further through the system. Critical ranges can be programmed into the computer so the nurse is alerted to deviations from the norm as information is recorded. Using electronic documentation, all caregivers have simultaneous access to patient records on all patients at all times from various locations. The adaptation of computer-based programs and their application in the hospital setting has motivated all nurses to become computer literate.

SBAR Communication

Another TJC National Patient Safety goal involves improving communication between members of the health care team. One technique of communication concerning the patient among the members of the health care team is the use of **SBAR** (or **S-BAR**), a formal method of providing end-of-shift reports. The SBAR process includes discussion of these elements:

- *Situation:* The status of the patient on the unit
- *Background:* The background or relevant history of the patient that may influence care
- *Assessment:* An analysis of the problem or continuing patient need based on assessments made or orders written
- *Recommendation:* What the current patient need is and the outcome goals

HEALTHY PEOPLE 2020

Healthy People 2020 updates the previous decade's statement of national health promotion and disease prevention objectives facilitated by the federal government (U.S. Department of Health and Human Services, 2010). The report identifies objectives designed to use the vast knowledge and technology of health care that was developed in the twentieth century to improve the health and quality of life for Americans in the twenty-first century. The objectives fall under broad categories of effort: health promotion, health protection, preventive services, and the development of surveillance and data systems. The specific goals include increasing the span of healthy life, reducing health disparities among Americans, and achieving access to preventive care for all Americans. Some priority areas include maternal and infant health, immunizations, prevention of sexually transmitted infections, oral health, nutrition, and physical fitness. It is a "vision for the new century" to achieve a nation of healthy people (see Health Promotion box on p. 10). The *Healthy People 2010* goal of reducing the maternal mortality rate of 3.3 per 100,000 was not achieved, as the maternal mortality rate was 12.1 per 100,000 in 2010. More coordination and effort is needed to achieve this goal by the year 2020.

THE FUTURE

HEALTH CARE REFORM

The revolution in health care involves the conflict between cost containment and quality of care. When health care became a profitable business industry, cost containment and managed care were born. Managed care openly and continuously evaluates care given and can result in increased quality. Quality assurance committees are investigating the routine management of patients, especially in the area of preventive care and tests.

The federal government enacted a health care reform plan in 2010 to reduce the cost of health care while making it more accessible to all. Access to care also depends on the availability of resources within a community. Health insurance has played an important role in health care delivery. Having health insurance does not necessarily ensure access to care, because the insurance company often must approve (or deny) the expenditure before a test or care is provided. Historically, families that could not afford health insurance often did not seek preventive health care such as prenatal care, infant immunizations, and well-baby check-ups. More than 5% of all children in the United States have no regular health care provider and therefore may not receive preventive care or follow-up care (Child and Family Statistics, 2011). The Healthcare Reform Act of 2010 proposes to facilitate access to health care that was previously unavailable for preventive care and follow-up care. Managed care and utilization review committees that evaluate the appropriateness of health care services also have an impact on physicians' management of patients. Continued study is needed to determine the effect of managed care on the quality of health care and cost containment. Nurses are involved as patient advocates in the health care reform movement to ensure quality of care.

 Safety Alert!

According to standards recommended by the American Congress of Obstetricians and Gynecologists (ACOG), pregnant women should ideally make about 13 prenatal visits during the course of a normal, full-term pregnancy.

FUTURE ROLES FOR NURSES

Community-Based Nursing

Nursing care within the community and in the home is not a new concept in maternal–child nursing. In the first part of the twentieth century, the work of Lillian Wald, founder of the Henry Street Settlement, brought home health care to poor children. Margaret Sanger's work as a public health nurse opened access to care for poor pregnant women and was the seed for the development of modern Planned Parenthood programs.

The community is now the major health care setting for patients, and the challenge is to provide safe, caring, cost-effective, high-quality care to mothers, infants, and families. This challenge involves the nurse, who can advocate on behalf of patients and influence government, business, and the community to recognize the need for supporting preventive care of maternal–infant patients to ensure a healthy population for the future. The nurse must work with the interdisciplinary health care team to identify needs within the community and create cost-effective approaches to comprehensive preventive and therapeutic care.

Involving schools, churches, health fairs, websites, and the media facilitate the role of the nurse as an educator within the community. Some registered nurses are branching out into the community as private practitioners, such as lactation consultants for new mothers. The nursing care plan is expanding to become a **family care plan,** because the nurse is providing care to the patient in the home. Growth and development of the family and family lifestyles are discussed in Chapter 15, and the family care plan is presented in Chapter 9. Creativity, problem solving, coordination of multidisciplinary caregivers, case management, assessment, and referral are just some of the essential skills required of a nurse providing community-based care to maternal–infant patients.

Preventive care is only one aspect of current and future home care and community-based nursing. Therapeutic care is also provided in the home setting, and the nurse must educate the family concerning care, monitoring, and the potential needs for professional referral. Specialized care such as fetal monitoring of high-risk pregnant women, apnea monitoring of high-risk newborns, diabetic glucose monitoring, heparin therapy, and total parenteral nutrition can be safely accomplished in the home setting, often supported by telephone/computer access to a nurse manager.

The home health care team, as advocated by the American Academy of Pediatrics Committee on Children with Disabilities, includes a pediatrician; nurses; occupational, physical, and respiratory therapists; speech therapists; home teachers; social workers; and home health aides. The American Academy of Home Health Care Physicians has expressed a medical commitment to the concept of home care for the future.

The future role of the nurse will involve providing health care in a variety of settings and working closely with the multidisciplinary health care team. The nurse will function as a caregiver, teacher, collaborator, advocate, manager, and researcher. Competence in care and accountability to patient, family, community, and profession are core responsibilities of the nurse of today and tomorrow. Nurses will take a key role in shaping the health care picture of tomorrow. For this reason the Institute of Medicine (IOM) recommended a blueprint for the nurse of the future to include a widening of the scope of practice to provide more accessibility to health care. The IOM also set a goal of having 80% of nurses be BSN prepared by the year 2020, and the number of faculty prepared with a doctorate degree needs to double by the year 2020. The IOM has suggested guidelines for the education and practice of the nurse of tomorrow.

THE BROADENING PARADIGM OF MATERNAL–CHILD CARE

Maternal–child care has traditionally been focused on reduction of morbidity and mortality of mothers and the survival of the newborn. Many newborns survive today that just a few years ago had no chance of survival. Early prenatal care, fetal surgery, use of prenatal glucocorticoids, technology, and NICU care have all played a role in increasing the positive outcome of pregnancy, and the goals of *Healthy People 2020* may well be met. There now is an added focus concerning an increased awareness of the developmental origins of adult disease. One of the best-known studies many years ago concerned the use of a drug called DES during pregnancy that resulted in vaginal adenocarcinoma of the offspring as an adult. We are beginning to realize that "gestational programming" signifies that the nutrition, hormonal, and metabolic environment in utero permanently alters metabolic physiology and gene expression in the offspring (Gabbe, 2012). The role of nutrition is known to be of increasing importance, because data evidenced the relationship of prenatal iodine supplementation to the elimination of cretinism and its associated defects, and also related the prenatal supplementation of folic acid to the reduction of the occurrence of neural tube defects such as spina bifida in the newborn. Data have also shown that many low–birth-weight infants develop cardiac disease and hypertension as adults (Kliegman, 2011). Maternal obesity during pregnancy and the large-for-gestational-age newborn have been shown as associated with the infant developing altered liver function as an adult; and the exposure of the fetus to betamethasone used during pregnancy has shown a relationship to the development of insulin resistance and cardiac pathology in adulthood. Studies even have shown that a high ingestion of licorice during pregnancy is related to verbal disabilities and personality problems such as aggression in the adult offspring (Raikkonen, 2009).

Therefore the focus of prenatal care must not only be the healthy outcome of mother and fetus, but must now also include reducing the long-term consequences of the prenatal environment that impacts the prevention or reduction of adult-onset diseases.

Get Ready for the NCLEX® Examination!

Key Points

- In 1840 Ignaz Semmelweis suggested that handwashing was an important concept in preventing infection. This simple procedure is still a cornerstone of nursing care.
- The American Nurses Association (ANA) has written standards of maternal–child health practices.
- HIPAA regulations mandate maintaining confidentiality concerning patient medical records and personal information.
- The Fair Labor Standards Act, passed in 1938, regulates the use of child labor.
- Lillian Wald, a nurse, is credited with suggesting the establishment of the Children's Bureau.
- The White House Conferences on Children and Youth investigate and report on matters pertaining to children and their families among all classes of people.
- The Children's Charter of 1930 is considered one of the most important documents in child care history.
- The United Nations Declaration of the Rights of the Child calls for freedom, equality of opportunity, social and emotional benefits, and enhancement of each child's potential.
- Labor, delivery, and recovery (LDR) rooms provide family-centered birthing and promote early parent–infant bonding.
- The culture of a society has a strong influence on family and child care.
- The cultural background of the expectant family plays an important role in its members' adaptation to the birth experience.
- The educational focus for the childbearing family is that childbirth is a normal and healthy event.
- The nurse must understand the culture and tradition of the family and its influence on health practices.
- Advanced practice nurses are registered nurses with advanced degrees who are certified and specialize, manage patient care, and conduct research.
- The nursing process consists of five steps: assessment, nursing diagnosis, planning (with outcomes identification), implementation, and evaluation. It is an organized method in nursing practice and a means of communication among staff members.
- Diagnosis-related groups (DRGs), a form of cost containment, continue to affect nursing practice.
- The nursing care plan is a written instrument of communication that uses the nursing process to formulate a plan of care for a specific patient. It uses nursing diagnoses and involves critical thinking and problem solving.
- Clinical pathways are collaborative guidelines that define multidisciplinary care in terms of outcomes within a timeline.
- *Statistics* refers to gathering and analyzing numerical data.
- *Birth rate* refers to the number of live births per 1000 population in 1 year.

- In the United States, vital statistics are compiled for the country as a whole by the National Center for Health Statistics.
- Critical thinking is an active process that involves recall of information that is stored in long-term memory so that judgments based on facts can be analyzed and prioritized for use in clinical decision making.
- The use of critical thinking skills increases the ability of the nurse to make clinical decisions that meet individual needs of patients. The use of critical thinking skills can also improve test scores. The use of critical thinking also stimulates creativity that can improve quality of care and the work environment.
- Utilization review committees, quality assurance committees, the American Academy of Pediatrics Committee on Children with Disabilities, the American Academy of Home Care Physicians, and the Association of Women's Health Obstetric and Neonatal Nurses (AWHONN) are some of the organizations that set and maintain standards of maternity and pediatric care.
- Nurses have legal and ethical responsibilities to report specific conditions to local public health agencies to protect the patient and the community.
- Charting is the legal responsibility of the nurse and includes a head-to-toe assessment and data pertinent to the diagnosis and the response of the patient to treatment.
- SBAR is a technique of communicating patient information among staff at the end of one shift and the beginning of the next.
- *Healthy People* is a statement of national health promotion that is a vision for the twenty-first century. The objectives are designed to use technology and knowledge to improve health care and quality of life.
- Home health care involves therapy, monitoring, teaching, and referral.
- The focus of prenatal care is not only the outcome of a healthy family, mother, and fetus, but also the management of the prenatal environment to achieve the reduction of adult onset diseases.

Additional Learning Resources

SG Go to your Study Guide for additional learning activities to help you master this chapter content.

evolve Go to your Evolve website (http://evolve.elsevier.com/Leifer) for the following learning resources:
- Animations
- Answer Guidelines for Critical Thinking Questions
- Answers and Rationales for Review Questions for the NCLEX® Examination
- Glossary with English and Spanish pronunciations
- Interactive Review Questions for the NCLEX® Examination
- Patient Teaching Plans in English and Spanish
- Skills Performance Checklists
- Video clips and more!

Online Resources
- American Academy of Home Care Physicians: www.aahcp.org
- American Academy of Pediatrics: www.aap.org
- National Center for Health Statistics: www.cdc.gov/nchs
- National Human Genome Research Institute: www.genome.gov
- World Health Organization: www.who.int

Review Questions for the NCLEX® Examination

1. The number of deaths of infants younger than age 28 days per 1000 live births is termed the:
   1. infant death rate.
   2. neonatal birth rate.
   3. neonatal morbidity rate.
   4. neonatal mortality rate.

2. Which nursing action is the priority when a patient arrives at the clinic?
   1. Prepare a plan of care.
   2. Select the appropriate NANDA diagnoses.
   3. Administer medications as ordered.
   4. Determine and document history and vital signs.

3. An organization that sets standards of practice for nursing is the:
   1. American Medical Association (AMA).
   2. American Nurses Association (ANA).
   3. utilization review committee.
   4. American Academy of Pediatrics (AAP).

4. The nurse is providing "evidence based care" when she:
   1. adheres to hospital procedure book guidelines.
   2. carries out protocols learned in nursing school.
   3. carries out the practice requested by the charge nurse or health care provider.
   4. knows that the practice has been published in a professional journal or text.

5. Which source would the nurse use to determine whether a specific nursing activity is within the scope of practice of an LPN/LVN?
   1. Doctor's prescription record
   2. Nursing procedure manual
   3. Head nurse or nurse manager
   4. The Nurse Practice Act

Human Reproductive Anatomy and Physiology

http://evolve.elsevier.com/Leifer

Objectives

1. Define each key term listed.
2. Describe changes of puberty in males and females.
3. Identify the anatomy of the male reproductive system.
4. Explain the functions of the external and internal male organs in human reproduction.
5. Describe the influence of hormones in male reproductive processes.
6. Identify the anatomy of the female reproductive system.
7. Explain the functions of the external, internal, and accessory female organs in human reproduction.
8. Discuss the importance of the pelvic bones to the birth process.
9. Explain the menstrual cycle and the female hormones involved in the cycle.

Key Terms

biischial diameter (bī-ĬS-kē-ŭl dī-ĂM-ĭ-tĕr, p. 26)
climacteric (klī-MĂK-tĕr-ĭk, p. 27)
diagonal conjugate (p. 26)
dyspareunia (dĭs-păh-RŪ-nē-ă, p. 23)
embryo (ĔM-brē-ō, p. 23)
external os (p. 24)
follicle-stimulating hormone (FSH) (p. 27)
internal os (p. 24)
luteinizing hormone (LH) (p. 22)
menarche (mĕ-NĂR-kē, p. 27)
menopause (MĔN-ō-păwz, p. 27)
obstetric conjugate (p. 26)

obstetrical perineum (p. 22)
oxytocin (ŏk-sē-TŌ-sĭn, p. 29)
ovulation (p. 27)
ovum (p. 25)
prostate gland (p. 22)
puberty (p. 20)
rugae (RŪ-jē, p. 23)
semen (p. 22)
smegma (SMĔG-mă, p. 21)
spermatogenesis (spuĭr-maĭ-tō-JĔN-ĕ-sĭs, p. 21)
transverse diameter (p. 26)
zygote (ZĪ-gōt, p. 25)

Understanding childbirth requires an understanding of the structures and functions of the body that make childbearing possible. This knowledge includes anatomy, physiology, sexuality, embryology of the growing fetus, and the psychosocial changes that occur in both the male and the female. This chapter addresses the anatomy and physiology of the male and female reproductive systems.

PUBERTY

Before puberty, male and female children appear very much alike except for their genitalia. Puberty involves changes in the whole body and the psyche as well as in the expectations of society toward the individual.

Puberty is a period of rapid change in the lives of boys and girls during which the reproductive systems mature and become capable of reproduction. Puberty begins when the secondary sex characteristics (e.g., pubic hair)

appear. Puberty ends when mature sperm are formed or when regular menstrual cycles occur. This transition from childhood to adulthood has been identified and often celebrated by various rites of passage. Some cultures have required demonstrations of bravery, such as hunting wild animals or displays of self-defense. Ritual circumcision is another rite of passage in some cultures and religions. In the United States today, some adolescents participate in religious ceremonies such as bar or bat mitzvah or confirmation, but for others, these ceremonies are unfamiliar. The lack of a universal "rite of passage" to identify adulthood has led to confusion for some contemporary adolescents in many industrialized nations.

MALE

Male hormonal changes normally begin between 10 and 16 years of age. Outward changes become apparent when the size of the penis and testes increases and there is a general growth spurt. Testosterone, the primary male sex hormone, causes the boy to grow taller, become more muscular, and develop secondary sex characteristics such as pubic hair, facial hair, and a deeper voice. The voice deepens but is often characterized by squeaks or cracks before reaching its final pitch. Testosterone levels are constant, not cyclical as are female hormones, although levels may decrease with age to 50% of peak levels by age 80 years. Nocturnal emissions ("wet dreams") may occur without sexual stimulation. These emissions usually do not contain sperm.

FEMALE

The first outward change of puberty in females is development of the breasts (see Figure 2-7). The first menstrual period (menarche) occurs 2 to 2½ years later (age 11 to 15 years). Female reproductive organs mature to prepare for sexual activity and childbearing. The female experiences a growth spurt, but her growth spurt ends earlier than the male's. Her hips broaden as her pelvis assumes the wide basin shape needed for birth. Pubic hair and axillary hair appear. The quantity varies, as it does in males.

REPRODUCTIVE SYSTEMS

MALE

The male reproductive system consists of external and internal organs (Figure 2-1).

External Genitalia

The penis and the scrotum, which contains the testes, are the male external genitalia.

Penis. The penis consists of the glans and the body. The glans is the rounded, distal end of the penis. It is visible on a circumcised penis but is hidden by the foreskin on an uncircumcised one. **Smegma** is a cheeselike sebaceous substance that collects under the foreskin and is easily removed with basic hygiene. At the tip of the glans is an opening called the urethral meatus. The body of the penis contains the urethra (the passageway for sperm and urine) and erectile tissue (the corpus spongiosum and two corpora cavernosa). The usually flaccid penis becomes erect during sexual stimulation when blood is trapped within the spongy erectile tissues. The erection allows the male to penetrate the female's vagina during sexual intercourse. The penis has two functions:

1. Provides a duct to expel urine from the bladder
2. Deposits sperm in the female's vagina to fertilize an ovum

Scrotum. The scrotum is a sac that contains the testes. The scrotum is suspended from the perineum, keeping the testes away from the body and thereby lowering their temperature, which is necessary for normal sperm production (**spermatogenesis**).

Internal Genitalia

The internal genitalia include the testes, vas deferens, prostate, seminal vesicles, ejaculatory ducts, urethra, and accessory glands.

Testes. The testes (testicles) are a pair of oval glands housed in the scrotum. They have two functions:

1. Manufacture male germ cells (spermatozoa or sperm)
2. Secrete male hormones *(androgens)*

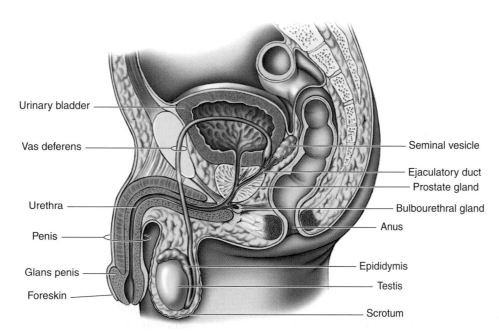

Urinary bladder
Vas deferens
Urethra
Penis
Glans penis
Foreskin

Seminal vesicle
Ejaculatory duct
Prostate gland
Bulbourethral gland
Anus
Epididymis
Testis
Scrotum

FIGURE 2-1 The male reproductive organs. (From Herlihy B, Maebius NK: *The human body in health and illness*, ed 4, Philadelphia, 2011, Saunders.)

Sperm are made in the convoluted seminiferous tubules that are contained within the testes. Sperm production begins at puberty and continues throughout the life span of the male.

The production of *testosterone,* the most abundant male sex hormone, begins with the anterior pituitary gland. Under the direction of the hypothalamus, the anterior pituitary gland secretes follicle-stimulating hormone (FSH) and **luteinizing hormone (LH)**. FSH and LH initiate the production of testosterone in the Leydig cells of the testes.

Testosterone has the following effects not directly related to sexual reproduction:

- Increases muscle mass and strength
- Promotes growth of long bones
- Increases basal metabolic rate (BMR)
- Enhances production of red blood cells
- Produces enlargement of vocal cords
- Affects the distribution of body hair

These effects result in the greater strength and stature and a higher hematocrit level in males than in females. Testosterone also increases the production of sebum, a fatty secretion of the sebaceous glands of the skin, and it may contribute to the development of acne during early adolescence. However, as the skin adapts to the higher levels of testosterone, acne generally recedes.

Ducts. Each epididymis, one from each testicle, stores and carries the sperm to the penis. The sperm may remain in the epididymis for 2 to 10 days, during which time they mature and then move on to the vas deferens. Each vas deferens passes upward into the body, goes around the symphysis pubis, circles the bladder, and passes downward to form (with the ducts from the seminal vesicles) the ejaculatory ducts. The ejaculatory ducts then enter the back of the **prostate gland** and connect to the upper part of the urethra, which is in the penis. The urethra transports both urine from the bladder and semen from the prostate gland to the outside of the body, although not at the same time.

Accessory Glands. The accessory glands are the *seminal vesicles,* the *prostate gland,* and the *bulbourethral glands,* also called *Cowper's glands.* The accessory glands produce secretions (seminal plasma). The secretions of these glands have three functions:

1. Nourish the sperm
2. Protect the sperm from the acidic environment of the woman's vagina
3. Enhance the motility (movement) of the sperm

The combined seminal plasma and sperm are called **semen**. Semen may be secreted during sexual intercourse before ejaculation. Therefore pregnancy may occur even if ejaculation occurs outside the vagina. Increased heat in the environment around the sperm (testes) increases the motility but shortens the life span of the sperm. A constant increase in temperature around the testes can prevent spermatogenesis and lead to permanent sterility. (Refer to a medical-surgical nursing textbook for the testicular self-examination procedure.)

FEMALE

The female reproductive system consists of external genitalia, internal genitalia, and accessory structures such as the mammary glands (breasts). The bony pelvis is also discussed in this chapter because of its importance in the childbearing process.

External Genitalia

The female external genitalia are collectively called the *vulva.* They include the mons pubis, labia majora, labia minora, fourchette, clitoris, vaginal vestibule, and perineum (Figure 2-2).

Mons Pubis. The mons pubis (*mons veneris*) is a pad of fatty tissue covered by coarse skin and hair. It protects the symphysis pubis and contributes to the rounded contour of the female body.

Labia Majora. The labia majora are two folds of fatty tissue on each side of the vaginal vestibule. Many small glands are located on the moist interior surface.

Labia Minora. The labia minora are two thin, soft folds of tissue that are seen when the labia majora are separated. Secretions from sebaceous glands in the labia are bactericidal to reduce infection and also lubricate and protect the skin of the vulva.

Fourchette. The fourchette is a fold of tissue just below the vagina, where the labia majora and the labia minora meet. It is also known as the **obstetrical perineum**. Lacerations in this area often occur during childbirth.

Clitoris. The clitoris is a small, erectile body in the most anterior portion of the labia minora. It is similar in structure to the penis. Functionally, it is the most erotic, sensitive part of the female genitalia, and it produces smegma. Smegma is a cheeselike secretion of the sebaceous glands.

Vaginal Vestibule. The vaginal vestibule is the area seen when the labia minora are separated and includes five structures:

1. The *urethral meatus* lies approximately 2 cm below the clitoris. It has a foldlike appearance with a slit type of opening, and it serves as the exit for urine.
2. *Skene's ducts* (paraurethral ducts) are located on each side of the urethra and provide lubrication for the urethra and the vaginal orifice.
3. The *vaginal introitus* is the division between the external and internal female genitalia.
4. The *hymen* is a thin elastic membrane that closes the vagina from the vestibule to various degrees.

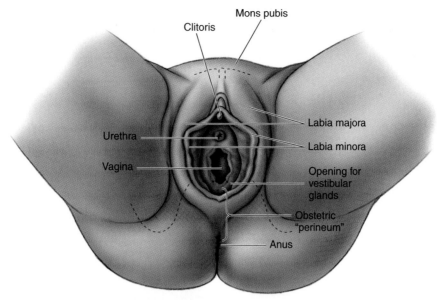

FIGURE 2-2 The external female reproductive organs. (From Herlihy B, Maebius NK: *The human body in health and illness,* ed 4, Philadelphia, 2011, Saunders.)

5. The *ducts of the Bartholin glands* (vulvovaginal glands) provide lubrication for the vaginal introitus during sexual arousal and are normally not visible.

Perineum. The perineum is a strong, muscular area between the vaginal opening and the anus. The elastic fibers and connective tissue of the perineum allow stretching to permit the birth of a full-term infant. The perineum is the site of the episiotomy (incision) if performed or potential tears during childbirth. Pelvic weakness or painful intercourse (**dyspareunia**) may result if this tissue does not heal properly.

Internal Genitalia

The internal genitalia are the vagina, uterus, fallopian tubes, and ovaries. Figure 2-3 illustrates the side view of these organs, and Figure 2-4 illustrates the frontal view.

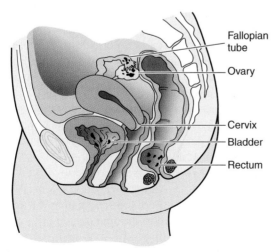

FIGURE 2-3 Side view of the internal female reproductive organs. (From Herlihy B, Maebius NK: *The human body in health and illness,* ed 4, Philadelphia, 2011, Saunders.)

Vagina. The vagina is a tubular structure made of muscle and membranous tissue that connects the external genitalia to the uterus. Because it meets with the cervix at a right angle, the anterior wall is about 2.5 cm (1 inch) shorter than the posterior wall, which varies from 7 to 10 cm (approximately 2.8 to 4 inches). The marked stretching of the vagina during delivery is made possible by the **rugae**, or transverse ridges of the mucous membrane lining. The vagina is self-cleansing and during the reproductive years maintains a normal acidic pH of 4 to 5. Antibiotic therapy, frequent douching, and excessive use of vaginal sprays, deodorant sanitary pads, or deodorant tampons may alter the self-cleansing activity.

The vagina has three functions:
1. Provides a passageway for sperm to enter the uterus
2. Allows drainage of menstrual fluids and other secretions
3. Provides a passageway for the infant's birth

Strong pelvic floor muscles stabilize and support the internal and external reproductive organs. The most important of these muscles is the levator ani, which supports the three structures that penetrate it: urethra, vagina, and rectum.

> **⬧ Nursing Tip**
>
> An excellent opportunity to reinforce knowledge about the self-cleansing function of the vagina, menstruation, and reproduction is when teaching women about feminine hygiene or while discussing family planning.

Uterus. The uterus (womb) is a hollow muscular organ in which a fertilized ovum is implanted, an **embryo** forms, and a fetus develops. It is shaped like an upside-down pear or light bulb. In a mature,

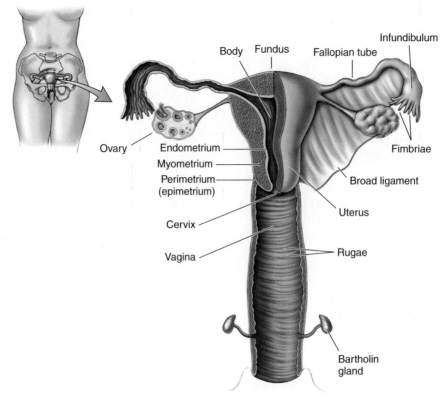

FIGURE 2-4 Frontal view of the internal female reproductive organs. (From Herlihy B, Maebius NK: *The human body in health and illness,* ed 4, Philadelphia, 2011, Saunders.)

nonpregnant female, it weighs approximately 60 g (2 oz) and is 7.5 cm (3 inches) long, 5 cm (2 inches) wide, and 1 to 2.5 cm (0.4 to 1 inch) thick. The uterus lies between the bladder and the rectum above the vagina.

Several ligaments support the uterus. The *broad ligament* provides stability to the uterus in the pelvic cavity; the *round ligament* is surrounded by muscles that enlarge during pregnancy and keep the uterus in place; the *cardinal ligaments* prevent uterine prolapse; and the *uterosacral ligaments* are surrounded by smooth muscle and contain sensory nerve fibers that may contribute to the sensation of dysmenorrhea (painful menstruation). Stretching of the uterine ligaments as the uterus enlarges during pregnancy can cause minor discomfort to the mother.

Nerve supply. Because the autonomic nervous system innervates the reproductive system, its functions are not under voluntary (conscious) control. Therefore even a paraplegic woman can have adequate contractions for labor. Sensations for uterine contractions are carried to the central nervous system (CNS) via the eleventh and twelfth thoracic nerve roots. Pain from the cervix and the vagina passes through the pudendal nerves. The motor fibers of the uterus arise from the seventh and eighth thoracic vertebrae. This separate motor and sensory nerve supply allows for the use of a local anesthetic without interfering with uterine contractions and is important in pain management during labor.

Anatomy. The uterus is separated into three parts: fundus, corpus, and cervix. The fundus (upper part) is broad and flat. The fallopian tubes enter the uterus on each side of the fundus. The corpus (body) is the middle portion, and it plays an active role in menstruation and pregnancy.

The fundus and the corpus have three distinct layers:
1. The *perimetrium* is the outermost or serosal layer that envelops the uterus.
2. The *myometrium* is the middle muscular layer that functions during pregnancy and birth. It has three involuntary muscle layers: a longitudinal outer layer, a figure-of-eight interlacing middle layer, and a circular inner layer that forms sphincters at the fallopian tube attachments and at the internal opening of the cervix.
3. The *endometrium* is the inner or mucosal layer that is functional during menstruation and implantation of the fertilized ovum. It is governed by cyclical hormonal changes.

The *cervix* (lower part) is narrow and tubular and opens into the upper vagina. The cervix consists of a cervical canal with an internal opening near the uterine corpus (the **internal os**) and an opening into the vagina (the **external os**). The mucosal lining of the cervix has four functions:
1. Lubricates the vagina
2. Acts as a bacteriostatic agent

3. Provides an alkaline environment to shelter deposited sperm from the acidic pH of the vagina
4. Produces a mucous plug in the cervical canal during pregnancy

Fallopian Tubes. The fallopian tubes, also called uterine tubes or oviducts, extend laterally from the uterus, one to each ovary (see Figure 2-4). They vary in length from 8 to 13.5 cm (3 to 5.3 inches). Each tube has four sections:

1. The *interstitial* portion extends into the uterine cavity and lies within the wall of the uterus.
2. The *isthmus* is a narrow area near the uterus.
3. The *ampulla* is the wider area of the tube and is the usual site of fertilization.
4. The *infundibulum* is the funnel-like enlarged distal end of the tube. Fingerlike projections from the infundibulum, called *fimbriae*, hover over each ovary and "capture" the **ovum** (egg) as it is released by the ovary at ovulation.

The four functions of the fallopian tubes are to provide the following:

1. A passageway in which sperm meet the ovum
2. The site of fertilization (usually the outer ⅓ of the tube)
3. A safe, nourishing environment for the ovum or **zygote** (fertilized ovum)
4. The means of transporting the ovum or zygote to the corpus of the uterus

Cells within the tubes have *cilia* (hairlike projections) that beat rhythmically to propel the ovum toward the uterus. Other cells secrete a protein-rich fluid to nourish the ovum after it leaves the ovary.

Ovaries. The ovaries are two almond-shaped glands, each about the size of a walnut. They are located in the lower abdominal cavity, one on each side of the uterus, and are held in place by ovarian and uterine ligaments. The ovaries have two functions:

1. Production of hormones, chiefly estrogen and progesterone
2. Stimulation of an ovum's maturation during each menstrual cycle

At birth, every female infant has all the ova (oocytes) that will be available during her reproductive years (approximately 2 million cells). These degenerate significantly so that by adulthood the remaining oocytes number only in the thousands. Of these, only a small percentage is actually released (about 400 during the reproductive years). Every month, one ovum matures and is released from the ovary. Any ova that remain after the climacteric (the time surrounding menopause) no longer respond to hormonal stimulation to mature.

Pelvis

The bony pelvis occupies the lower portion of the trunk of the body. Four bones attached to the lower spine form it:

- Two innominate bones
- Sacrum
- Coccyx

Each innominate bone is made up of an *ilium, pubis,* and *ischium,* which are separate during childhood but fuse by adulthood. The ilium is the lateral, flaring portion of the hip bone; the pubis is the anterior hip bone. These two bones join to form the symphysis pubis. The curved space under the symphysis pubis is called the pubic arch. The ischium is *below* the ilium and supports the seated body. An ischial spine, one from each ischium, juts inward to varying degrees. These ischial spines serve as a reference point for descent of the fetus during labor. The posterior pelvis consists of the sacrum and the coccyx. Five fused, triangular vertebrae at the base of the spine form the sacrum. The sacrum may jut into the pelvic cavity, causing a narrowing of the birth passageway. Below the sacrum is the coccyx, the lowest part of the spine.

The bony pelvis has three functions:

1. Supports and distributes body weight
2. Supports and protects pelvic organs
3. Forms the birth passageway

Types of Pelves. There are four basic types of pelves (Figure 2-5). Most women have a combination of pelvic characteristics rather than having one pure type. Each type of pelvis has implications for labor and birth:

- The *gynecoid* pelvis is the classic female pelvis, with rounded anterior and posterior segments. This type is most favorable for vaginal birth.
- The *android* pelvis has a wedge-shaped inlet with a narrow anterior segment; it is typical of the male anatomy.

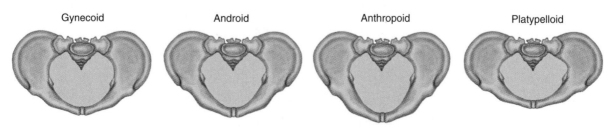

Gynecoid   Android   Anthropoid   Platypelloid

FIGURE 2-5 Four types of pelves. The gynecoid pelvis is the typical female pelvis and is optimum for passage of the fetal head. (From Murray SS, McKinney ES, Gorrie TM: *Foundations of maternal–newborn nursing,* ed 3, Philadelphia, 2002, Saunders.)

- The *anthropoid* pelvis has an anteroposterior diameter that equals or exceeds its transverse diameter. The shape is a long, narrow oval. Women with this type of pelvis can usually deliver vaginally, but their infant is more likely to be born in the occiput posterior (back of the fetal head toward the mother's sacrum) position.
- The *platypelloid* pelvis has a shortened anteroposterior diameter and a flat, transverse oval shape. This type is unfavorable for vaginal birth.

False and True Pelves. The pelvis is divided into the false and true pelves by an imaginary line (the linea terminalis) that extends from the sacroiliac joint to the anterior iliopubic prominence. The upper, or false, pelvis supports the enlarging uterus and guides the fetus into the true pelvis. The lower, or true, pelvis consists of the pelvic inlet, the pelvic cavity, and the pelvic outlet. The true pelvis is important, because it dictates the bony limits of the birth canal.

Pelvic Diameters. The diameters of the pelvis must be adequate for passage of the fetus during birth (Figure 2-6).

Pelvic inlet. The pelvic inlet, just below the linea terminalis, has obstetrically important diameters. The anteroposterior diameter is measured between the symphysis pubis and the sacrum and is the shortest inlet diameter. The transverse diameter is measured across the linea terminalis and is the largest inlet diameter. The oblique diameters are measured from the right or left sacroiliac joint to the prominence of the linea terminalis.

Measurements of the pelvic inlet (Table 2-1) include the following:

- **Diagonal conjugate:** The distance between the suprapubic angle and the sacral promontory. The health care provider assesses this measurement during a manual pelvic examination.

Table 2-1	Average Pelvic Measurements
MEASUREMENT	**DIAMETER (cm)**
Inlet	
Diagonal conjugate	11.5
Obstetric conjugate (true)	9.5-10
Transverse	13.5
Oblique	12.75
Outlet	
Anteroposterior	9.5
Biischial	10-12
Posterior sagittal	7.5

- **Obstetric conjugate** (the smallest inlet diameter): Estimated by subtracting 1.5 to 2 cm from the diagonal conjugate (the approximate thickness of the pubic bone). This measurement determines whether the fetus can pass through the birth canal.
- **Transverse diameter:** The largest diameter of the inlet. It determines the inlet's shape.

Pelvic outlet. The *transverse* diameter of the outlet is a measurement of the distance between the inner surfaces of the ischial tuberosities and is known as the **biischial diameter**. The anteroposterior measurement of the outlet is the distance between the lower border of the symphysis pubis and the tip of the sacrum. It can be measured by vaginal examination. The *sagittal* diameters are measured from the middle of the transverse diameter to the pubic bone anteriorly and to the sacrococcygeal bone posteriorly. The coccyx can move or break during the passage of the fetal head, but an immobile coccyx can decrease the size of the pelvic outlet and make vaginal birth difficult. A narrow pubic arch can also affect the passage of the fetal head through the birth canal.

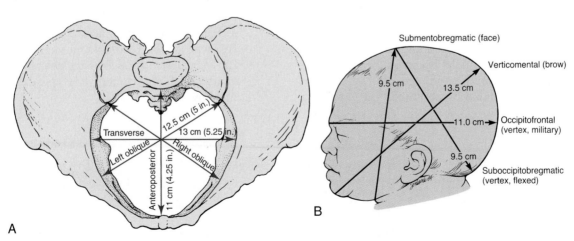

FIGURE 2-6 A, Four important pelvic inlet diameters are the anteroposterior, the transverse, and the right and left oblique diameters. **B,** The measurements of the fetal skull determine the reason the fetal head must turn and change position during birth process to enable the smallest diameter of the infant head to pass through the smallest diameter of the mother's pelvis. (**A,** Modified from *Stedman's illustrated medical dictionary,* ed 25, Baltimore, 1990, Williams & Wilkins. **B,** From Gabbe SG et al: *Obstetrics: normal and problem pregnancies,* ed 6, Philadelphia, 2012, Saunders.)

Adequate pelvic measurements are essential for a successful vaginal birth. Problems that can cause a pelvis to be small (e.g., a history of a pelvic fracture or rickets) potentially indicate that delivery by cesarean section will be necessary.

Breasts

Female breasts (mammary glands) are accessory organs of reproduction. They produce milk after birth to provide nourishment and maternal antibodies for the infant (Figure 2-7). The nipple, in the center of each breast, is surrounded by a pigmented areola. Montgomery's glands (Montgomery's tubercles) are small sebaceous glands in the areola that secrete a substance to lubricate and protect the breasts during lactation.

Each breast is made of 15 to 24 lobes arranged like the spokes of a wheel. Adipose (fatty) and fibrous tissues separate the lobes. The adipose tissue affects size and firmness and gives the breasts a smooth outline. Breast size is primarily determined by the amount of fatty tissue and is unrelated to a woman's ability to produce milk.

Alveoli (lobules) are the glands that secrete milk. They empty into approximately 20 separate lactiferous (milk-carrying) ducts. Milk is stored briefly in widened areas of the ducts, called ampullae or lactiferous sinuses.

Reproductive Cycle and Menstruation

The female reproductive cycle consists of regular changes in secretions of the anterior pituitary gland, the ovary, and the endometrial lining of the uterus (Figure 2-8). The anterior pituitary gland, in response to the hypothalamus, secretes **follicle-stimulating hormone (FSH)** and luteinizing hormone (LH). FSH stimulates maturation of a follicle in the ovary that contains a single ovum. Several follicles start maturing during each cycle, but usually only one reaches final maturity. The maturing ovum and the corpus luteum (the follicle left empty after the ovum is released) produce increasing amounts of estrogen and progesterone, which leads to enlargement of the endometrium. A surge in LH stimulates final maturation and the release of an ovum. Approximately 2 days before ovulation, the vaginal secretions increase noticeably.

Ovulation occurs when a mature ovum is released from the follicle about 14 days before the onset of the next menstrual period. The corpus luteum turns yellow (luteinizing) immediately after ovulation and secretes increasing quantities of progesterone to prepare the uterine lining for a fertilized ovum. Approximately 12 days after ovulation, the corpus luteum degenerates if fertilization has not occurred, and progesterone and estrogen levels decrease. The drop in estrogen and progesterone levels causes the endometrium to break down, resulting in menstruation. The anterior pituitary gland secretes more FSH and LH, beginning a new cycle.

The beginning of menstruation, called **menarche**, occurs at about age 11 to 15 years. Early cycles are often irregular and may be anovulatory. Regular cycles are usually established within 6 months to 2 years of the menarche. In an average cycle, the flow (menses) occurs every 28 days, plus or minus 5 to 10 days. The flow itself lasts from 2 to 5 days, with a blood loss of 30 to 40 mL and an additional loss of 30 to 50 mL of serous fluid. Fibrinolysin is contained in the necrotic endometrium being expelled, and therefore clots are not normally seen in the menstrual discharge.

The **climacteric** is a period of years during which the woman's ability to reproduce gradually declines. **Menopause** refers to the final menstrual period, although in casual use the terms *menopause* and *climacteric* are often used interchangeably.

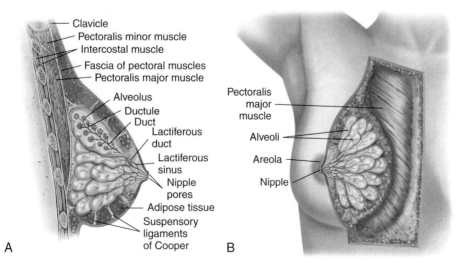

FIGURE 2-7 The female breast. **A,** Side view of a lactating breast. Each lobule of glandular tissue is drained by a lactiferous duct that eventually opens through the nipple. **B,** Anterior view of a lactating breast. Overlying skin and connective tissue have been removed from the medial side to show the internal structure of the breast and the underlying skeletal muscle. In nonlactating breasts, the glandular tissue is much less prominent, with adipose tissue comprising most of each breast. (From Seidel HM et al: *Mosby's guide to physical examination*, ed 7, St Louis, 2011, Mosby.)

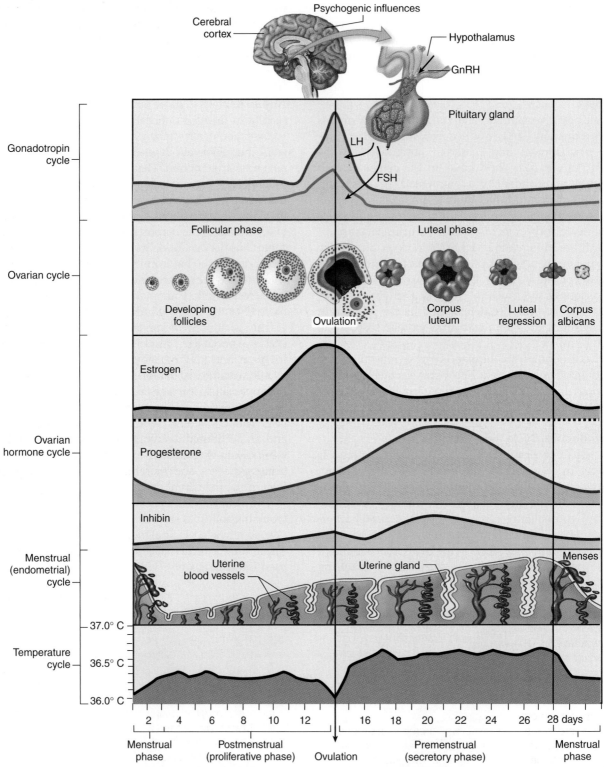

FIGURE 2-8 Female reproductive cycles. This diagram illustrates the interrelationships among the hypothalamic, pituitary, ovarian, and uterine functions throughout a standard 28-day menstrual cycle. The variations in basal body temperature are also illustrated. *FSH,* Follicle-stimulating hormone; *GnRH,* gonadotropic releasing hormone; *LH,* luteinizing hormone. (From Patton KT, Thibodeau GA: *Anatomy & physiology,* ed 8, St Louis, 2013, Mosby.)

THE HUMAN SEXUAL RESPONSE

There are four phases of the human sexual response:

1. *Excitement:* Heart rate and blood pressure increase; nipples become erect

2. *Plateau:* Skin flushes; erection occurs; semen appears on tip of penis

3. *Orgasmic:* Involuntary muscle spasms of the rectum, the vagina, and the uterus occur; ejaculation occurs

4. *Resolution:* Engorgement resolves; vital signs return to normal

PHYSIOLOGY OF THE MALE SEX ACT

The male psyche can initiate or inhibit the sexual response. The massaging action of intercourse on the glans penis stimulates sensitive nerves that send impulses to the sacral area of the spinal cord and to the brain. Stimulation of nerves supplying the prostate and scrotum enhances sensations. The parasympathetic nerve fibers cause relaxation of penile arteries, which fill the cavernous sinuses of the shaft of the penis that stretch the erectile tissue so that the penis becomes firm and elongated (erection). The same nerve impulses cause the urethral glands to secrete mucus to aid in lubrication for sperm motility. The sympathetic nervous system then stimulates the spinal nerves to contract the vas deferens and cause expulsion of the sperm into the urethra (emission). Contraction of the muscle of the prostate gland and seminal vesicles expels prostatic and seminal fluid into the urethra, contributing to the flow and motility of the sperm. This full sensation in the urethra stimulates nerves in the sacral region of the spinal cord that cause rhythmical contraction of the penile erectile tissues and urethra and skeletal muscles in the shaft of the penis, which expel the semen from the urethra (ejaculation). The period of emission and ejaculation is called male orgasm.

Within minutes, erection ceases (*resolution*), the cavernous sinuses empty, penile arteries contract, and the penis becomes flaccid. Sperm can reach the woman's fallopian tube within 5 minutes and can remain viable in the female reproductive tract for 4 to 5 days. Of the millions of sperm contained in the ejaculate, a few thousand reach each fallopian tube, but only one fertilizes the ovum. The sphincter at the base of the bladder closes during ejaculation so that sperm does not enter the bladder and urine cannot be expelled.

PHYSIOLOGY OF THE FEMALE SEX ACT

The female psyche can initiate or inhibit the sexual responses. Local stimulation to the breasts, vulva, vagina, and perineum creates sexual sensations. The sensitive nerves in the glans of the clitoris send signals to the sacral areas of the spinal cord, and these signals are transmitted to the brain. Parasympathetic nerves from the sacral plexus return signals to the erectile tissue around the vaginal introitus, dilating and filling the arteries and resulting in a tightening of the vagina around the penis. These signals stimulate the Bartholin glands at the vaginal introitus to secrete mucus that aids in vaginal lubrication. The parasympathetic nervous system causes the perineal muscles and other muscles in the body to contract. The posterior pituitary gland secretes **oxytocin**, which stimulates contraction of the uterus and dilation of the cervical canal. This process (orgasm) is believed to aid in the transport of the sperm to the fallopian tubes. (This process is also the reason why sexual abstention is advised when there is a high risk for miscarriage or preterm labor.)

Following orgasm, the muscles relax (resolution), and this is usually accompanied by a sense of relaxed satisfaction. The egg lives for only 24 hours after ovulation; sperm must be available during that time if fertilization is to occur.

Get Ready for the NCLEX® Examination!

Key Points

- Puberty is the time when the reproductive organs mature to become capable of reproduction, and secondary sex characteristics develop.
- A sexually active girl can become pregnant before her first menstrual period, because ovulation occurs *before* menstruation.
- At birth, every female has all the ova that will be available during her reproductive years.
- Testosterone is the principal male hormone. Estrogen and progesterone are the principal female hormones. Testosterone secretion continues throughout a man's life, but estrogen and progesterone secretions are very low after a woman reaches the climacteric.
- The penis and scrotum are the male external genitalia. The scrotum keeps the testes cooler than the rest of the body, promoting normal sperm production.
- The two main functions of the testes are to manufacture sperm and to secrete male hormones (androgens), primarily testosterone.
- The myometrium (middle muscular uterine layer) is functional in pregnancy and labor. The endometrium (inner uterine layer) is functional in menstruation and implantation of a fertilized ovum.
- The female breasts are composed of fatty and fibrous tissue and of glands that can secrete milk. The size of a woman's breasts is determined by the amount of fatty tissue and does not influence her ability to secrete milk.
- The female reproductive cycle consists of regular changes in hormone secretions from the anterior pituitary gland and the ovary, maturation and release of an ovum, and buildup and breakdown of the uterine lining.
- There are four basic pelvic shapes, but women often have a combination of characteristics. The gynecoid pelvis is the most favorable for vaginal birth.
- The pelvis is divided into a false pelvis above the linea terminalis and the true pelvis below this line. The true pelvis is most important in the childbirth process. The true pelvis is further divided into the pelvic inlet, the pelvic cavity, and the pelvic outlet.

Additional Learning Resources

SG Go to your Study Guide for additional learning activities to help you master this chapter content.

evolve Go to your Evolve website (http://evolve.elsevier.com/Leifer) for the following learning resources:

- Animations
- Answer Guidelines for Critical Thinking Questions
- Answers and Rationales for Review Questions for the NCLEX® Examination
- Glossary with English and Spanish pronunciations
- Interactive Review Questions for the NCLEX® Examination
- Patient Teaching Plans in English and Spanish
- Skills Performance Checklists
- Video clips and more!

 Online Resources
- Family Support Group: www.4parents.org
- Fetal Diagnostic Centers: www.fetal.com

Review Questions for the NCLEX® Examination

1. Spermatozoa are produced in the:
   1. vas deferens.
   2. seminiferous tubules.
   3. prostate gland.
   4. Leydig cells.

2. A woman can keep a diary of her menstrual cycles to help determine her fertile period. She understands that after ovulation she will remain fertile for:
   1. 2 hours.
   2. 24 hours.
   3. 3 to 5 days.
   4. 7 to 14 days.

3. Which data indicate that the woman may have pelvic dimensions that would be inadequate for a normal vaginal delivery? A woman with a(n):
   1. anthropoid-shaped pelvis with a history of pelvic inflammatory disease
   2. gynecoid-shaped pelvis with a history of rickets
   3. anthropoid-shaped pelvis that previously delivered a 9-lb infant
   4. gynecoid-shaped pelvis with a history of poor nutrition

4. The muscular layer of the uterus that is the functional unit in pregnancy and labor is the:
   1. perimetrium.
   2. myometrium.
   3. endometrium.
   4. cervix.

5. During a prenatal clinic visit, a woman states that she probably will not plan to breastfeed her infant because she has very small breasts and believes she cannot provide adequate milk for a full-term infant. The best response of the nurse would be:
   1. "Ask the physician if he or she will prescribe hormones to build up the breasts."
   2. "I can provide you with exercises that will build up your breast tissue."
   3. "The fluid intake of the mother will determine the milk output."
   4. "The size of the breast has no relationship to the ability to produce adequate milk."

Critical Thinking Questions

1. A patient is admitted to the labor unit and has not had any prenatal care. Her history shows that she sustained a fractured pelvis from an automobile accident several years previously. The patient states she is interested in natural childbirth. What is the nurse's best response?
2. A male adolescent fears he is becoming incontinent because he notices his pajama pants are wet on occasion when he awakes in the morning. He asks if there is medicine to stop this problem. What is the best response from the nurse?

Fetal Development

Objectives

1. Define each key term listed.
2. Describe the process of gametogenesis in human reproduction.
3. Explain human fertilization and implantation.
4. Describe embryonic development.
5. Describe fetal development and the maturation of body systems.
6. Describe the development and functions of the placenta, the umbilical cord, and the amniotic fluid.
7. Compare fetal circulation to circulation after birth.
8. Explain the similarities and differences in the two types of twins.

Key Terms

age of viability (p. 38)
amniotic sac (ăm-nē-Ŏ-tĭk SĂK, p. 35)
autosomes (p. 31)
chorion (KŌ-rē-ŏn, p. 35)
decidua (dĕ-SĬD-yū-ă, p. 35)
diploid (DĬP-loid, p. 31)
dizygotic (DZ) (dī-zī-GŎT-ĭk, p. 41)
fertilization (p. 32)
gametogenesis (găm-ĕ-tō-JĔN-ĕ-ĭs, p. 32)

germ layers (p. 35)
haploid (HĂP-loid, p. 32)
monozygotic (MZ) (mŏn-ō-zī-GŎT-ĭk, p. 41)
oogenesis (ō-ō-JĔN-ĕ-sĭs, p. 31)
placenta (plă-SĔN-tă, p. 39)
spermatogenesis (spŭr-mă-tō-JĔN-ĕ-sĭs, p. 31)
teratogens (TĔR-ă-tō-jĕnz, p. 31)
Wharton's jelly (p. 39)

The human body contains many millions of cells at birth, but life begins with a single cell created by the fusion of a sperm with an ovum. Deoxyribonucleic acid (DNA) programs a genetic code into the nucleus of the cell; the nucleus controls the development and function of the cell. Defects in the DNA code can result in inherited disorders. The genes and chromosomes contained within the DNA determine the uniqueness of the traits and features of the developing person.

Normal human chromosomes begin in pairs, one supplied by the mother and the other by the father. Each body cell contains 46 chromosomes, made up of 22 pairs of **autosomes** (body chromosomes) and 1 pair of sex chromosomes that determine the sex of the fetus. Each chromosome contains genes that involve heredity. Cell division then occurs, which is the basis of human growth and regeneration.

Biological development is not isolated. It is influenced by the external environment, such as maternal drug use (**teratogens** that cause damage to growing cells include some prescribed medications), maternal undernutrition, or smoking by the mother, and it is now known that sounds such as music are heard by the fetus and are recognized by the newborn. All these factors influence prenatal growth and development.

The experience of the fetus during prenatal life influences the healthy outcome of the newborn and also influences susceptibility to diseases that may occur when the fetus reaches adulthood. Early prenatal care is essential to the optimum outcome of the pregnancy (see Chapter 4). The experience of the fetus during prenatal life influences the healthy outcome of the newborn and also influences the susceptibility to diseases that may occur when the newborn reaches adulthood.

CELL DIVISION AND GAMETOGENESIS

The division of a cell begins in its nucleus, which contains the gene-bearing chromosomes. The two types of cell division are mitosis and meiosis. *Mitosis* is a continuous process by which the body grows and develops and dead body cells are replaced. In this type of cell division, *each daughter cell contains the same number* of chromosomes as the parent cell. The 46 chromosomes in a body cell are called the **diploid** number of chromosomes. The process of mitosis in the sperm is called **spermatogenesis**, and in the ovum it is called **oogenesis**.

Meiosis is a different type of cell division in which the reproductive cells undergo two sequential divisions.

During meiosis, the number of chromosomes in each cell is reduced by half, to 23 chromosomes per cell, each including only one sex chromosome. This is called the **haploid** number of chromosomes. This process is completed in the sperm before it travels toward the fallopian tube and in the ovum if it is fertilized after ovulation. At the moment of **fertilization** (when the sperm and the ovum unite), the new cell contains 23 chromosomes from the sperm and 23 chromosomes from the ovum, thus returning to the diploid number of chromosomes (46); traits are therefore inherited from both the mother and the father. The formation of gametes by this type of cell division is called **gametogenesis** (Figure 3-1).

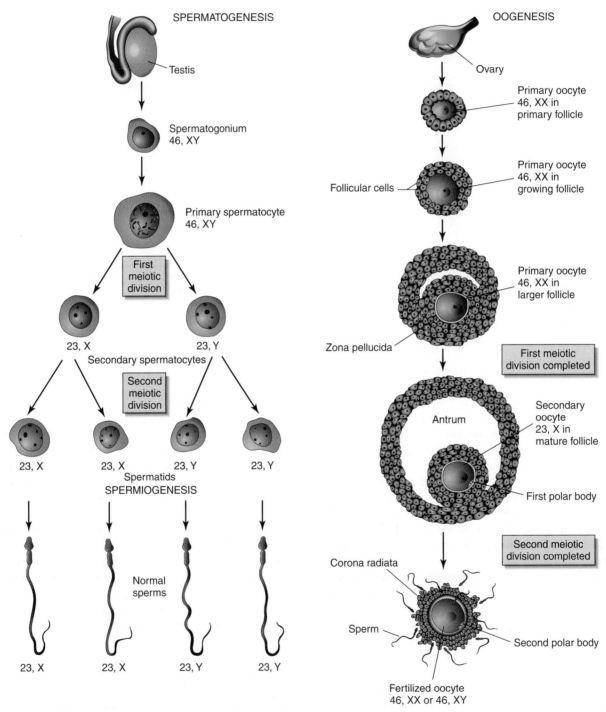

FIGURE 3-1 Normal gametogenesis. Four sperm develop from one spermatocyte, each with 23 chromosomes—including one sex chromosome, either an X or a Y. In oogenesis, one ovum develops with 23 chromosomes—including one sex chromosome, always an X. An XY combination produces a boy, and an XX combination produces a girl. (From Moore KL, Persaud TVN, Torchia MG: *The developing human: clinically oriented embryology*, ed 9, Philadelphia, 2012, Saunders.)

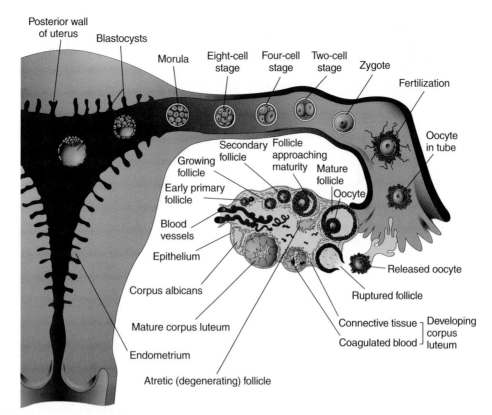

FIGURE 3-2 Ovulation and fertilization. Ovulation occurs; the egg is caught by the fimbriae (fingerlike projections of the fallopian tube) and is guided into the fallopian tube where fertilization occurs. The zygote continues to multiply (but not grow in size) as it passes through the fallopian tube and implants into the posterior wall of the uterus. (From Moore KL, Persaud TVN, Torchia MG: *The developing human: clinically oriented embryology,* ed 9, Philadelphia, 2012, Saunders.)

FERTILIZATION

Fertilization occurs when a sperm penetrates an ovum and unites with it, restoring the total number of chromosomes to 46. It normally occurs in the outer third of the fallopian tube, near the ovary (Figure 3-2). The sperm pass through the cervix and the uterus and into the fallopian tubes by means of the flagellar (whiplike) activity of their tails and can reach the fallopian tubes within 5 minutes after coitus. As soon as fertilization occurs, a chemical change in the membrane around the fertilized ovum prevents penetration by another sperm.

The time during which fertilization can occur is brief because of the short life span of mature gametes. The ovum is estimated to survive for up to 24 hours after ovulation. The sperm remains capable of fertilizing the ovum for up to 5 days after being ejaculated into the area of the cervix.

> **Nursing Tip**
>
> During sexual counseling the nurse should emphasize that the survival time of sperm ejaculated into the area of the cervix may be up to 5 days and that pregnancy can occur with intercourse as long as 5 days before ovulation.

SEX DETERMINATION

The sex of human offspring is determined at fertilization. The ovum always contributes an X chromosome (gamete), whereas the sperm can carry an X or a Y chromosome (gamete). When a sperm carrying the X chromosome fertilizes the X-bearing ovum, a female child (XX) results. When a Y-bearing sperm fertilizes the ovum, a male child (XY) is produced (Figure 3-3).

Because sperm can carry either an X or a Y chromosome, the male partner determines the sex of the child. However, the pH of the female reproductive tract and the estrogen levels of the woman's body affect the survival rate of the X- and Y-bearing sperm as well as the speed of their movement through the cervix and the fallopian tubes. Thus the female physiology has some influence on which sperm fertilizes the mature ovum.

> **Nursing Tip**
>
> Both mother and father influence the sex of their offspring, although the father contributes the actual sex chromosome. This fact may reduce blame in some cultures when the child is not of the desired sex.

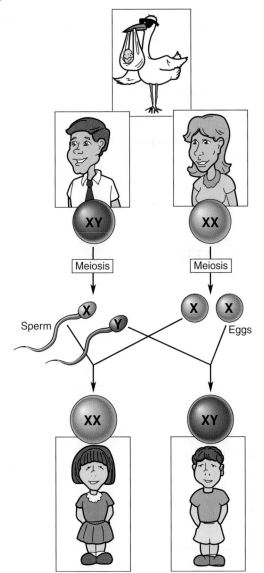

FIGURE 3-3 Sex determination. If an X chromosome from the male unites with an X chromosome from the female, the child will be a female (XX). If a Y chromosome from the male unites with an X chromosome from the female, the child will be a male (XY). (From Herlihy B, Maebius NK: *The human body in health and illness*, ed 4, Philadelphia, 2011, Saunders.)

INHERITANCE

Each gene (a segment of the DNA chain) is coded for inheritance. The coded information carried by the DNA in the gene is responsible for individual traits, such as eye and hair color, facial features, and body shape. Genes carry instructions for *dominant* and *recessive* traits. Dominant traits usually overpower recessive traits and are passed on to the offspring. If only one parent carries a dominant trait, an average of 50% of the offspring will have (and thus display) that dominant trait. If *each* parent carries a recessive trait, there is a higher chance that one of the offspring will display that trait (Figure 3-4).

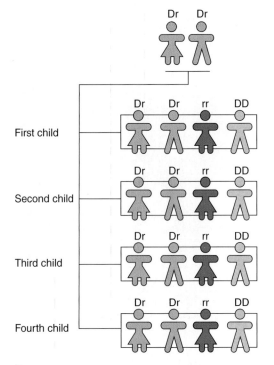

Key

■ Person has disorder
■ Person carries one gene for disorder but does not have disorder
■ Person has no disorder and does not carry one gene for disorder

FIGURE 3-4 Inheritance. This figure shows how a disorder carried as a recessive trait can be passed along to an offspring when each parent is a carrier of that recessive trait. *D* represents a dominant gene; *r* represents a recessive gene.

TUBAL TRANSPORT OF THE ZYGOTE

The zygote is the cell formed by the union of the sperm and the ovum, and it is transported through the fallopian tube and into the uterus. Fertilization normally occurs in the outer third of the fallopian tube. During transport through the fallopian tube, the zygote undergoes rapid mitotic division, or cleavage. Cleavage begins with two cells, which subdivide into four and then eight cells to form the blastomere. The size of the zygote does not increase; rather, the individual cells become smaller as they divide and eventually form a solid ball called the *morula* (see Figure 3-2).

The morula enters the uterus on the third day and floats there for another 2 to 4 days. The cells form a cavity, and two distinct layers evolve. The inner layer is a solid mass of cells called the *blastocyst* (see Figure 3-2), which develops into the embryo and the embryonic membranes. The outer layer of cells, called the *trophoblast*, develops into an embryonic membrane, the chorion. Occasionally the zygote does not move through the fallopian tube and instead becomes implanted in the lining of the tube, resulting in a tubal ectopic pregnancy (see Chapter 5).

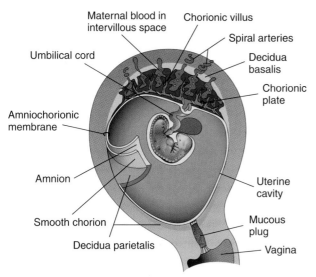

FIGURE 3-5 The pregnant uterus at 4 weeks showing the relationship of the fetal membranes to the decidua of the uterus and the embryo. (From Moore KL, Persaud TVN, Torchia MG: *The developing human: clinically oriented embryology,* ed 9, Philadelphia, 2012, Saunders.)

Box 3-1	Body Parts That Develop from the Primary Germ Layers

ECTODERM
Outer layer of skin
Oil glands and hair follicles of skin
Nails and hair
External sense organs
Mucous membrane of mouth and anus

MESODERM
True skin
Skeleton
Bone and cartilage
Connective tissue
Muscles
Blood and blood vessels
Kidneys and gonads

ENDODERM
Lining of trachea, pharynx, and bronchi
Lining of digestive tract
Lining of bladder and urethra

IMPLANTATION OF THE ZYGOTE

The zygote usually implants in the upper section of the posterior uterine wall. The cells burrow into the prepared lining of the uterus, called the endometrium. The endometrium is now called the **decidua**; the area under the blastocyst is called the *decidua basalis* and gives rise to the maternal part of the placenta (Figure 3-5).

DEVELOPMENT

CELL DIFFERENTIATION

During the week between fertilization and implantation, the cells within a zygote are identical to one another. After implantation, the cells begin to differentiate and develop special functions. The chorion, the amnion, the yolk sac, and the primary **germ layers** appear.

Chorion

The **chorion** develops from the trophoblast (outer layer of embryonic cells) and envelops the amnion, embryo, and yolk sac. It is a thick membrane with fingerlike projections called villi on its outermost surface. The villi immediately below the embryo extend into the decidua basalis on the uterine wall and form the embryonic or fetal portion of the placenta (see Figure 3-6).

Amnion

The amnion is the second membrane; it is a thin structure that envelops and protects the embryo. It forms the boundaries of the amniotic cavity, and its outer aspect meets the inner aspect of the chorion.

The chorion and the amnion together form an **amniotic sac** filled with fluid (bag of waters) that permits the embryo to float freely. Amniotic fluid is clear, has a mild odor, and often contains bits of vernix (fetal skin covering) or lanugo (fetal hair on the skin). The volume of amniotic fluid steadily increases from about 30 mL at 10 weeks of pregnancy to 350 mL at 20 weeks. The volume of fluid is about 1000 mL at 37 weeks. In the latter part of pregnancy, the fetus may swallow up to 400 mL of amniotic fluid per day and normally excretes urine into the fluid. The following are functions of amniotic fluid:

- Maintains an even temperature
- Prevents the amniotic sac from adhering to the fetal skin
- Allows symmetrical growth
- Allows buoyancy and fetal movement
- Acts as a cushion to protect the fetus and the umbilical cord from injury

Yolk Sac

On the ninth day after fertilization, a cavity called the yolk sac forms in the blastocyst. It functions only during embryonic life and initiates the production of red blood cells. This function continues for about 6 weeks until the embryonic liver takes over. The umbilical cord then encompasses the yolk sac, and the yolk sac degenerates.

Germ Layers

After implantation, the zygote in the blastocyst stage transforms its embryonic disc into three primary germ layers known as ectoderm, mesoderm, and endoderm. Each germ layer develops into a different part of the growing embryo. The specific body parts that develop from each layer are listed in Box 3-1.

PRENATAL DEVELOPMENTAL MILESTONES

Table 3-1 follows the developmental milestones during intrauterine development. Developmental milestones exist in fetal growth and development, as they do in

Table 3-1   Embryonic and Fetal Development

AGE	LENGTH AND WEIGHT	DEVELOPMENT
Week 3	1.5-2.5 mm	*Cardiovascular:* Single tubular heart is formed. *Nervous:* Neural tube forms; primitive spinal cord and brain appear.

Neural groove
Cut surface of amnion
Neural groove
Neural fold in region of developing spinal cord
Location of primitive streak
Neural fold in region of developing brain
Yolk sac
First pairs of somites
Connecting stalk
Part of chorionic sac

Actual size 2.5 mm

| Week 4 | 3.5-4 mm | *Gastrointestinal (GI):* Esophagus and trachea separate; stomach forms.
Nervous: Neural tube closes; forebrain forms.
Musculoskeletal: Upper and lower limb buds appear.
Senses: Ears and eyes begin to form. |

Forebrain
Heart
Upper limb bud

| Week 6 | 11-13 mm | *Senses:* Auditory canal forms; eye is obvious.
Cardiovascular: Heart has all four chambers.
GI: Nasal cavity and upper lip form. |

External acoustic meatus
Auricular hillocks forming auricle of external ear
Eyelid
Pigmented eye
Nasolacrimal groove
Nasal pit
Umbilical cord
Heart prominence
Foot plate
Digital rays of hand plate

Actual size 11.0 mm

Continued

growth and development after birth. Three basic stages characterize prenatal development: zygote, embryo, and fetus. The zygote continues to grow and develop as it passes through the fallopian tube and implants into the wall of the uterus. The second to the eighth week of development is known as the embryonic stage; the developing infant is called an *embryo.* From the ninth week of development until birth, the developing infant is called a *fetus.* By the second week after fertilization, the ectoderm, the endoderm, and the amnion begin to develop.

By the third week the mesoderm and neural tube form, and the primitive heart begins to pump. It is at this time that some mothers first realize they have "missed" their menstrual period and suspect they are pregnant (therefore the fetus is affected by maternal influences even before the pregnancy becomes known).

Table **3-1**   Embryonic and Fetal Development—cont'd

AGE	LENGTH AND WEIGHT	DEVELOPMENT
Week 8 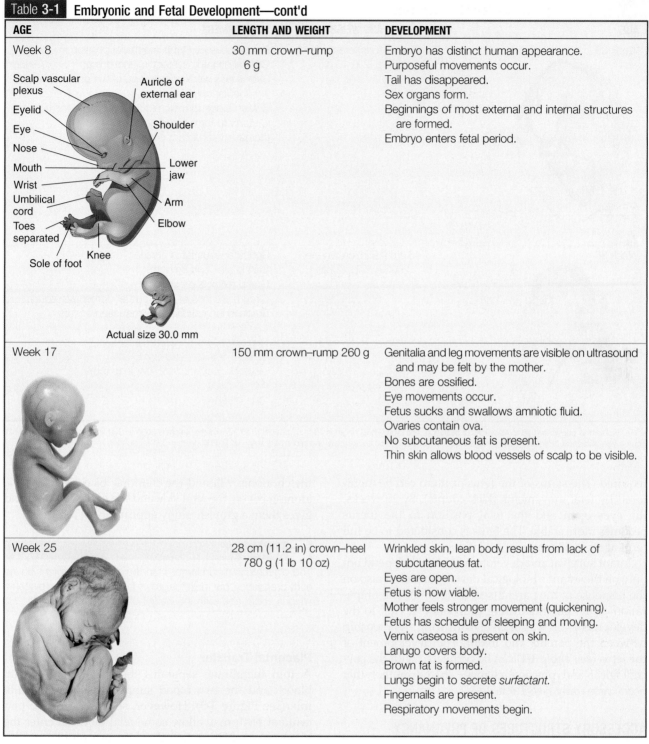 Scalp vascular plexus, Eyelid, Eye, Nose, Mouth, Wrist, Umbilical cord, Toes separated, Sole of foot, Knee, Auricle of external ear, Shoulder, Lower jaw, Arm, Elbow — Actual size 30.0 mm	30 mm crown–rump 6 g	Embryo has distinct human appearance. Purposeful movements occur. Tail has disappeared. Sex organs form. Beginnings of most external and internal structures are formed. Embryo enters fetal period.
Week 17	150 mm crown–rump 260 g	Genitalia and leg movements are visible on ultrasound and may be felt by the mother. Bones are ossified. Eye movements occur. Fetus sucks and swallows amniotic fluid. Ovaries contain ova. No subcutaneous fat is present. Thin skin allows blood vessels of scalp to be visible.
Week 25	28 cm (11.2 in) crown–heel 780 g (1 lb 10 oz)	Wrinkled skin, lean body results from lack of subcutaneous fat. Eyes are open. Fetus is now viable. Mother feels stronger movement (quickening). Fetus has schedule of sleeping and moving. Vernix caseosa is present on skin. Lanugo covers body. Brown fat is formed. Lungs begin to secrete *surfactant*. Fingernails are present. Respiratory movements begin.

Continued

Nutrition Considerations

Folic Acid and Neural Tube Defects

It is now known that folic acid supplements can prevent most neural tube defects such as spina bifida. However, in an unplanned pregnancy, it is possible for a neural tube defect to occur before the mother confirms her pregnancy state. Early prenatal care with good nutrition and folic acid supplements are desirable so the embryo is protected in the very first days and weeks of development.

By 8 weeks of gestation the ovaries or testes are present, the beginnings of all systems have developed, and there is movement in the extremities. The fetal period begins at the ninth week, and by the tenth week the external genitalia are visible to ultrasound examination. At the fourteenth week, the fetus moves in response to external stimuli. By 20 weeks of gestation the lungs have matured functionally enough for the fetus to survive outside the uterus (**age of viability**), but special care in the neonatal intensive care unit (NICU) would be

Table 3-1	Embryonic and Fetal Development—cont'd	
AGE	**LENGTH AND WEIGHT**	**DEVELOPMENT**
Week 29	38 cm (15 in) crown–heel 1260 g (2 lb 10 oz)	Fetus assumes stable (cephalic) position in utero. Central nervous system is functioning. Skin is less wrinkled because of the presence of subcutaneous fat. Spleen stops forming blood cells, and bone marrow starts to form blood cells. Increased surfactant is present in lungs.
Week 36	48 cm (19 in) crown–heel 2500 g (5 lb 12 oz)	Subcutaneous fat is present. Skin is pink and smooth. Grasp reflex is present. Circumferences of head and abdomen are equal. Surge in lung surfactant production occurs.

NOTE: Full term is considered 38 to 40 weeks of gestation. The crown–heel length is 48 to 52 cm (18 to 21 in), and the weight is 3000 to 3600 g (6 lb 1 oz to 7 lb 15 oz).
Figures from Moore KL, Persaud TVN, Torchia MG: *The developing human: clinically oriented embryology,* ed 9, Philadelphia, 2012, Saunders.

required. The status of the fetus in utero can be monitored by fetal movements (kick counts). By 28 weeks, the eyes open and the fetal position in the uterus becomes more stable. The fetus is considered to be full term at 38 to 40 weeks of gestation.

Infant survival and development at birth depend not only on the infant's biological development but also on the response of the parent (see Table 15-5). The preparation of the parents during pregnancy is vital to the development of a positive, nurturing relationship between the parents and infant. The development of the fetus (see Table 3-1) can be correlated with the psychological and physical changes in the mother that occur prenatally (see Table 4-6).

ACCESSORY STRUCTURES OF PREGNANCY

The placenta, the umbilical cord, and the fetal circulation support the fetus as it completes prenatal life and prepares for birth.

PLACENTA

The **placenta** (afterbirth) is a temporary organ for fetal respiration, nutrition, and excretion. It also functions as an endocrine gland. The placenta forms when the chorionic villi of the embryo extend into the blood-filled spaces of the mother's decidua basalis. The maternal part of the placenta arises from the decidua basalis and has a beefy, red appearance. The fetal side of the placenta develops from

the chorionic villi and the chorionic blood vessels. The amnion covers the fetal side and the umbilical cord and gives them a grayish, shiny appearance at term.

 Nursing Tip

The placenta is much larger than the developing infant during early pregnancy, but the fetus grows faster. At term, the placenta weighs about one sixth the weight of the infant.

Placental Transfer

A thin membrane separates the maternal and fetal blood, and the two blood supplies do not normally mix (see Figure 3-5). However, separation of the placenta at birth may allow some fetal blood to enter the maternal circulation, which can cause problems with fetuses in subsequent pregnancies if the blood types are not compatible (see Chapter 5).

Fetal deoxygenated blood and waste products leave the fetus through the two umbilical arteries and enter the placenta through the branch of a main stem villus, which extends into the intervillus space (lacuna). Oxygenated, nutrient-rich blood from the mother spurts into the intervillus space from the spiral arteries in the decidua (see Figures 3-5 and 3-6). The fetal blood releases carbon dioxide and waste products and takes in oxygen and nutrients before returning to the fetus through the umbilical vein.

The thin placental membrane provides some protection but is not a barrier to most substances ingested by the mother. Many harmful substances such as drugs (therapeutic and abused), nicotine, and viral infectious agents are transferred to the fetus and may cause fetal drug addiction, congenital anomalies, and fetal infection.

Placental Hormones

Four hormones are produced by the placenta: progesterone, estrogen, human chorionic gonadotropin (hCG), and human placental lactogen (hPL).

Progesterone. Progesterone is first produced by the corpus luteum and later by the placenta. It has the following functions during pregnancy:
- Maintains uterine lining for implantation of the zygote
- Reduces uterine contractions to prevent spontaneous abortion
- Prepares the glands of the breasts for lactation
- Stimulates testes to produce testosterone, which aids the male fetus in developing the reproductive tract

Estrogen. Estrogen has three important functions during pregnancy:
1. Stimulates uterine growth
2. Increases the blood flow to uterine vessels
3. Stimulates development of the breast ducts to prepare for lactation

The effects of estrogen not directly related to pregnancy include the following:
- Increased skin pigmentation (such as the "mask of pregnancy")
- Vascular changes in the skin and the mucous membranes of the nose and mouth
- Increased salivation

Human Chorionic Gonadotropin. hCG is the hormone "signal" sent to the corpus luteum that conception has occurred. The hCG causes the corpus luteum to persist and to continue the production of estrogen and progesterone to sustain pregnancy. hCG is detectable in maternal blood as soon as implantation occurs—usually 7 to 9 days after fertilization—and is the basis for most pregnancy tests.

Human Placental Lactogen. hPL is also known as human chorionic somatomammotropin (hCS). hPL causes decreased insulin sensitivity and utilization of glucose by the mother, making more glucose available to the fetus to meet growth needs.

UMBILICAL CORD

The umbilical cord develops with the placenta and fetal blood vessels and is the lifeline between mother and fetus. Two arteries carry blood away from the fetus, and one vein returns blood to the fetus. **Wharton's jelly** covers and cushions the cord vessels and keeps the three vessels separated. The vessels are coiled within the cord to allow movement and stretching without restricting circulation. The normal length of the cord is about 55 cm (22 inches). The umbilical cord usually protrudes from the center of the placenta.

 Memory Jogger

An easy way to remember the number and type of umbilical cord vessels is the woman's name *AVA:* **A**rtery, **V**ein, **A**rtery.

FETAL CIRCULATION

After the fourth week of gestation, circulation of blood through the placenta to the fetus is well established (see Figure 3-6). Because the fetus does not breathe and the liver does not have to process most waste products, several physiological diversions in the prebirth circulatory route are needed. There are three fetal circulatory shunts:
1. *Ductus venosus:* diverts some blood away from the liver as it returns from the placenta
2. *Foramen ovale:* diverts most blood from the right atrium directly to the left atrium, rather than circulating it to the lungs
3. *Ductus arteriosus:* diverts most blood from the pulmonary artery into the aorta

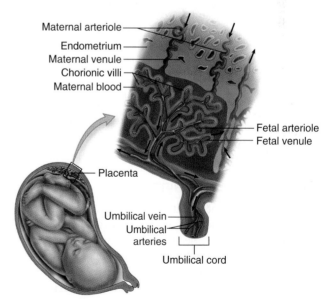

FIGURE 3-6 Maternal–fetal circulation showing the relationship of the fetus and the placenta in the uterus. Close placement of the fetal blood supply to the maternal blood in the placenta is shown. The maternal blood in the lacuna permits the diffusion of nutrients and other substances; some harmful substances are prevented from passing through by a thin placental barrier. No mixing of fetal or maternal blood occurs. (From Patton KT, Thibodeau GA: *Anatomy & physiology*, ed 8, St Louis, 2013, Mosby.)

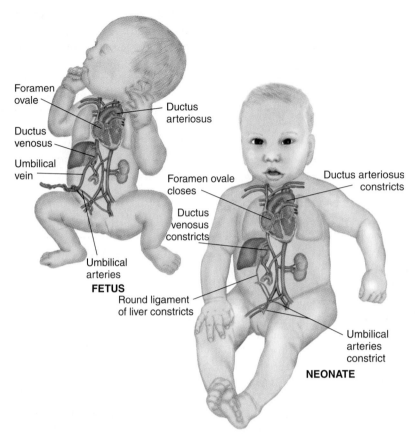

Foramen ovale

Ductus arteriosus

Ductus venosus

Umbilical vein

Foramen ovale closes

Ductus arteriosus constricts

Ductus venosus constricts

Umbilical arteries

FETUS

Round ligament of liver constricts

Umbilical arteries constrict

NEONATE

FIGURE 3-7 Changes in fetal–newborn circulation at birth. The changes in the circulation of the fetus and the neonate are shown. The ductus arteriosus, the ductus venosus, and the foramen ovale are shunts that close because of the expansion of the lungs and pressure changes within the heart. (From McKinney ES et al: *Maternal-child nursing*, ed 3, St Louis, 2009, Saunders.)

CIRCULATION BEFORE BIRTH

Oxygenated blood enters the fetal body through the umbilical vein. About half of the blood goes to the liver through the portal sinus, with the remainder entering the inferior vena cava through the *ductus venosus*. Blood in the inferior vena cava enters the right atrium, where most passes directly into the left atrium through the *foramen ovale*. A small amount of blood is pumped to the lungs by the right ventricle. The rest of the blood from the right ventricle joins that from the left ventricle through the *ductus arteriosus*. After circulating through the fetal body, blood containing waste products is returned to the placenta through the umbilical arteries.

CIRCULATION AFTER BIRTH

Fetal shunts are not needed after birth after the infant breathes and blood is circulated to the lungs. The foramen ovale closes, because pressure in the right side of the heart falls as the lungs become fully inflated and there is now little resistance to blood flow. The infant's blood oxygen level rises, causing the ductus arteriosus to constrict. The ductus venosus closes when the flow from the umbilical cord stops (Figure 3-7).

Closure of Fetal Circulatory Shunts

The foramen ovale closes functionally (temporarily) within 2 hours after birth and permanently by age 3 months. The ductus arteriosus closes functionally

within 15 hours and permanently in about 3 weeks. The ductus venosus closes functionally when the cord is cut and permanently in about 1 week. After permanent closure, the ductus arteriosus and the ductus venosus become ligaments.

Because the foramen ovale and ductus arteriosus are initially closed functionally, some conditions may cause one or the other to reopen after birth. A condition that impedes full lung expansion (e.g., respiratory distress syndrome) can increase resistance to blood flow from the heart to the lungs, causing the foramen ovale to reopen. Similar conditions often reduce the blood oxygen levels and can cause the ductus arteriosus to remain open. See Chapter 26 for further discussion of newborn congenital cardiac problems.

IMPAIRED PRENATAL DEVELOPMENT AND SUBSEQUENT ILLNESS

Research has shown that undernutrition in utero can result in permanent changes in fetal structure, physiology, and metabolism and can influence the development of conditions such as heart disease and stroke in adult life (Health Promotion box). Other factors that influence health in later life can be the exposure to toxins in utero or factors that occur in the first 3 years of growth and development.

During the first 3 months of fetal life, the fetus is most susceptible to external influences such as undernutrition. However, different organs and tissues undergo rapid development at specific times during gestational life and are therefore very sensitive to undernourishment or viral and/or toxic influences during these periods.

Infants with intrauterine growth restriction may have a reduced number of cells in their organs and can therefore be predisposed to the development of specific diseases later in life. For example, a reduced number of pancreatic beta cells can impair insulin secretion and result in a health problem in the adult. Obesity, inactivity, and other factors during the life span influence the timing and severity of adult-onset diseases.

It is also possible that in utero changes in vascular or renal structures or in hormonal systems resulting from in utero malnourishment can influence the development of hypertension later in life. Studies have also shown that impaired fetal liver growth in late gestation can permanently impair lipid metabolism and predispose to increased cholesterol levels in adult life. A reduced liver size can be identified by measuring abdominal circumference at birth.

Nursing Tip

The best assessment of fetal growth takes weight, length of gestation, placental size, and newborn head and abdominal circumference into consideration.

MULTIFETAL PREGNANCY

Twins occur once in every 90 pregnancies in North America. When hormones are given to assist with ovulation, twinning and other multifetal births (triplets, quadruplets, and quintuplets) are more likely to occur. The first set of septuplets (seven fetuses) to survive was born in the United States in 1997. In 2009, the first set of octuplets was born, all of whom survived.

Monozygotic (MZ) twins (Figure 3-8, *A*), often called identical twins, are genetically identical, are of the same sex, and look alike, because they develop from

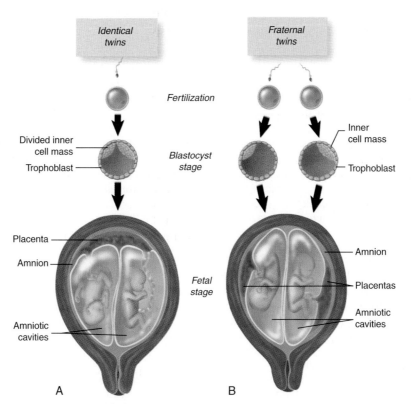

FIGURE 3-8 Multiple births. **A,** Identical (monozygotic) twins develop when the embryonic tissue from a single egg splits to form two individuals. The twins share the placenta. **B,** Fraternal (dizygotic) twins develop when two different ova are fertilized at the same time by two different sperm, producing separate zygotes. Each twin has its own placenta, amnion, and chorion. (From Thibodeau GA, Patton KT: *Anatomy & physiology,* ed 7, St Louis, 2012, Mosby.)

a single fertilized ovum. Physical differences between monozygotic twins are caused by prenatal environmental factors involving variations in the blood supply from the placenta. Most monozygotic twins begin to develop at the end of the first week after fertilization. The result is two identical embryos, each with its own amnion but with a common chorion and placenta and some common placental vessels. If the embryonic disc does not divide completely, various types of conjoined (formerly called Siamese) twins may form. They are named according to the regions that are joined (e.g., *thoracopagus* indicates an anterior connection of the thoracic regions). Conjoined twins have a single amnion.

Dizygotic (DZ) twins (see Figure 3-8, *B*), also called fraternal twins, may or may not be of the same sex, and they develop from two separate ova fertilized by two separate sperm. Dizygotic twins always have two amnions, two chorions, and two placentas, although their chorions and placentas sometimes fuse. Dizygotic twin pregnancies tend to repeat in families, and the incidence increases with maternal age. The twins are about as much alike as any other siblings.

Many twin or higher multiples are born prematurely, because the uterus becomes overly distended. The placenta may not be able to supply sufficient nutrition to both fetuses, with the result that one or both twins is smaller than average.

Get Ready for the NCLEX® Examination!

Key Points

- The uniqueness of each individual results from the blending of genes on the 46 chromosomes contained in each body cell and the environment of the embryo and fetus during development.
- Gametogenesis in the male is called spermatogenesis. Each mature sperm has 22 autosomes, plus either an X or a Y sex chromosome, for a total of 23. Gametogenesis in the female is called oogenesis. It begins at ovulation and is not completed until fertilization occurs. The mature ovum has 22 autosomes plus the X sex chromosome, for a total of 23. At conception, the total number of chromosomes is restored to 46.
- When the ovum is fertilized by an X-bearing sperm, a female offspring results; when it is fertilized by a Y-bearing sperm, the child will be male.
- After fertilization in the fallopian tube, the zygote enters the uterus, where implantation is complete by 7 days after fertilization. If the zygote fails to move through the tube, implantation occurs there, and a tubal ectopic pregnancy results.
- When implantation occurs in the uterine lining, the cells of the zygote differentiate and develop into the following structures: chorion, amnion, yolk sac, and primary germ layers. The chorion develops into the embryonic or fetal portion of the placenta; the amnion encloses the embryo and the amniotic fluid; the primary germ layers develop into different parts of the growing fetus; and the yolk sac, which functions only during embryonic life, begins to form red blood cells.
- The three germ layers of the embryo are the ectoderm, the mesoderm, and the endoderm. All structures of the individual develop from these layers.
- All body systems are formed and functioning in a simple way by the end of the eighth week.
- The accessory structures of pregnancy are the placenta, the umbilical cord, and the fetal circulation.
- These structures continuously support the fetus throughout prenatal life in preparation for birth.
- The amniotic fluid maintains an even temperature around the fetus, allows free floating and symmetrical growth, and acts as a cushion to protect the fetus and the umbilical cord.
- The placenta is an organ for fetal respiration, nutrition, and excretion. It is also a temporary endocrine gland that produces progesterone, estrogen, human chorionic gonadotropin (hCG), and human placental lactogen (hPL).
- The umbilical cord contains 2 arteries that carry blood *away* from the fetus and one vein that carries blood *to* the fetus.
- Fetal circulation transports oxygen and nutrients to the fetus and disposes of carbon dioxide and other waste products from the fetus. The temporary fetal circulatory structures are the *foramen ovale,* the *ductus arteriosus*, and the *ductus venosus*. They divert most blood from the fetal liver and lungs, because these organs do not fully function during prenatal life.
- *Monozygotic twins* develop from a single ovum and are identical. *Dizygotic twins* develop from 2 separate ova and 2 separate sperm and have a separate amnion and placenta.

Additional Learning Resources

SG Go to your Study Guide for additional learning activities to help you master this chapter content.

evolve Go to your Evolve website (http://evolve.elsevier.com/Leifer) for the following learning resources:
- Animations
- Answer Guidelines for Critical Thinking Questions
- Answers and Rationales for Review Questions for the NCLEX® Examination
- Glossary with English and Spanish pronunciations
- Interactive Review Questions for the NCLEX® Examination
- Patient Teaching Plans in English and Spanish
- Skills Performance Checklists
- Video clips and more!

 Online Resources
- Female reproductive system: www.nlm.nih.gov/medlineplus/femalereproductivesystem.html
- Fetal Diagnostic Centers: www.fetal.com

- Intrauterine growth restriction: http://familydoctor.org/online/famdocen/home/women/pregnancy/fetal/313.html
- Male reproductive system: www.nlm.nih.gov/medlineplus/malereproductivesystem.html

Review Questions for the NCLEX® Examination

1. The child's sex is determined by the:
   1. dominance of either the X or the Y chromosome.
   2. number of X chromosomes in the ovum.
   3. ovum, which contributes either an X or a Y chromosome.
   4. sperm, which contains either an X or a Y chromosome.

2. A woman who wants to become pregnant should avoid all medications unless they are prescribed by a physician who knows she is pregnant, because:
   1. the placenta allows most medications to cross into the fetus.
   2. medications often have adverse effects when taken during pregnancy.
   3. fetal growth is likely to be slowed by many medications.
   4. the pregnancy is likely to be prolonged by some medications.

3. When a couple has unprotected sexual intercourse 4 days before the woman ovulates, the risk of the woman becoming pregnant is:
   1. limited, because the ova only lives for 24 hours.
   2. very high, because both the ova and the sperm are capable of fertilizing at that time.
   3. unknown.
   4. very low, because that is not the woman's "fertile period."

4. The purpose of the foramen ovale is to:
   1. increase fetal blood flow to the lungs.
   2. limit blood flow to the liver.
   3. raise the oxygen content of fetal blood.
   4. reduce blood flow to the lungs.

5. Why are twins often born early?
   1. The uterus becomes overdistended.
   2. The placenta becomes distended.
   3. The woman's body cannot tolerate the weight.
   4. The fetuses become too large to deliver vaginally.

Critical Thinking Questions

1. A patient discusses her family planning decisions. She states that she will come to the clinic for prenatal care and will begin to take prenatal vitamins as soon as she knows she is pregnant. What would be the best response from the nurse?

2. A patient in the thirty-second week of gestation states that she wants to deliver her infant now, because she feels so "big and uncomfortable." She states that she knows the infant has been fully formed since the first trimester and does not mind if it is a little small at birth. What would be the best response from the nurse?

Prenatal Care and Adaptations to Pregnancy

Objectives

1. Define each key term listed.
2. List the goals of prenatal care.
3. Discuss prenatal care for a normal pregnancy.
4. Explain the nurse's role in prenatal care.
5. Calculate the expected date of delivery and duration of pregnancy.
6. Differentiate among the presumptive, probable, and positive signs of pregnancy.
7. Describe the physiological changes that occur during pregnancy.
8. Identify nutritional needs for pregnancy and lactation.
9. Discuss the importance and limitations of exercise in pregnancy.
10. Describe patient education related to travel and common discomforts of pregnancy.
11. Discuss nursing support for emotional changes that occur in a family during pregnancy.
12. Identify special needs of the pregnant adolescent, the single parent, and the older couple.
13. Apply the nursing process in developing a prenatal teaching plan.
14. Identify the effects of medication ingestion on pregnancy and lactation.
15. Review immunization administration during pregnancy.

Key Terms

abortion (p. 47)

antepartum (p. 44)

aortocaval compression (a-ŏr-tō-KĀ-văl kŏm-PRĔSH-ŭn, p. 53)

birth plan (p. 73)

Braxton Hicks contractions (p. 49)

Chadwick's sign (p. 49)

chloasma (p. 49)

colostrum (kŏ-LŎS-trŭm, p. 52)

estimated date of delivery (EDD) (p. 45)

gestational age (p. 47)

Goodell's sign (p. 49)

gravida (GRĂV-ĭ-dă, p. 47)

Hegar's sign (p. 49)

intrapartum (p. 44)

lactation (lăk-TĀ-shŭn, p. 51)

last normal menstrual period (LNMP) (p. 45)

lightening (p. 52)

McDonald's sign (p. 49)

Multipara (mŭl-TĬP-ă-ră, p. 47)

Nägele's rule (NĀ-gĕ-lēz rūl, p. 47)

para (PĂR-ă, p. 47)

postpartum (p. 44)

primigravida (prĭ-mĭ-GRĂV-ĭ-dă, p. 47)

primipara (prĭ-MĬP-ă-ră, p. 47)

pseudoanemia (sū-dō-ă-NĒ-mē-ă, p. 53)

quickening (p. 49)

supine hypotension syndrome (p. 53)

trimesters (p. 48)

Pregnancy is a temporary, physiological (that is, normal) process that affects the woman physically and emotionally. All systems of her body adapt to support the developing fetus. There are three phases of pregnancy: **antepartum** or prenatal (before birth), **intrapartum** (during birth), and **postpartum** (after birth). The focus of nursing care during pregnancy is to teach the mother how to maintain good health or, in the case of a mother with a condition that places her or her fetus at risk, to improve her health as much as possible to promote a healthy outcome for both mother and fetus. Good prenatal care can also help prevent adult-onset diseases in the infant. This chapter reviews prenatal care, the physiological and psychological changes of pregnancy, and nursing care to meet the needs of women and families.

GOALS OF PRENATAL CARE

Prenatal care is a primary example of preventive medicine.

Early and regular prenatal care is the best way to ensure a healthy outcome for both mother and child. Obstetricians, family practice physicians, certified nurse-midwives (CNMs), and nurse practitioners provide prenatal care. The nurse assists the health care provider in evaluating the expectant family's physical, psychological, and social needs and teaches the woman self-care. These are the major goals of prenatal care:

- Promote the health of the mother, fetus, newborn, and family.
- Ensure a safe birth for mother and child by promoting good health habits and reducing risk factors.
- Teach health habits that may be continued after pregnancy.
- Educate in self-care for pregnancy.
- Develop a partnership with parents and family to provide continuous and coordinated health care.
- Provide physical care.
- Prepare parents for the responsibilities of parenthood.

To achieve these goals, health care providers must do more than offer physical care. Health care providers must work as a team to create an environment that allows for cultural and individual differences while also being supportive of the entire family.

Nursing Tip

The major roles of the nurse during prenatal care include collecting data from the pregnant woman, identifying and reevaluating risk factors, educating in self-care, providing nutrition counseling, and promoting the family's adaptation to pregnancy.

Legal & Ethical Considerations

Documenting abnormal data such as high blood pressure *must* be followed by documentation of intervention or referral for follow-up care.

PRENATAL VISITS

Ideally, health care for childbearing begins before conception. Preconception care identifies risk factors that may be changed before conception to reduce their negative impact on the outcome of pregnancy. For example, the woman may be counseled about how to improve her nutritional state before pregnancy or may receive immunizations to prevent infections that would be harmful to the developing fetus. *An adequate folic acid intake before conception can reduce the incidence of congenital anomalies* (see Chapter 14). Some risk factors cannot be eliminated, such as preexisting diabetes, but preconception care helps the woman to begin pregnancy in the best possible state of health.

Prenatal care should begin, if not before conception, then as soon as a woman suspects that she is pregnant. A complete history and physical examination will help identify problems that may affect the woman or her fetus. The history should include the following:

- *Obstetric history:* Number and outcomes of past pregnancies; problems in the mother or infant
- *Menstrual history:* Usual frequency of menstrual cycles and duration of flow; first day of the **last normal menstrual period (LNMP)**; any "spotting" since the LNMP

- *Contraceptive history:* Type used; whether an oral contraceptive was taken before the woman realized she might be pregnant; whether an intrauterine device is still in place
- *Medical and surgical history:* Infections such as hepatitis or pyelonephritis; surgical procedures; trauma that involved the pelvis or reproductive organs
- *Family history of the woman and her partner:* To identify genetic or other factors that may pose a risk for the pregnancy
- *Health history of the woman and her partner:* To identify risk factors (e.g., genetic defects or the use of alcohol, drugs, or tobacco) and possible blood incompatibility between the mother and the fetus
- *Psychosocial history of the woman and her partner:* To identify stability of lifestyle and ability to parent a child; significant cultural practices or health beliefs that may affect the pregnancy

The woman has a complete physical examination on her first visit to evaluate her general health, determine her baseline weight and vital signs, evaluate her nutritional status, and identify current physical or social problems. A pelvic examination is performed to evaluate the size, adequacy, and condition of the pelvis and reproductive organs and to assess for signs of pregnancy (see Box 4-3).

Health Promotion

Optimal prenatal care uses a "teachable moment" to introduce knowledge and lifelong skills in self-care and wellness that includes continuing health care screening, immunizations, and regular follow-up of all risk factors throughout life for each member of the family.

Her **estimated date of delivery (EDD)** is calculated based on the LNMP. An ultrasound examination may be done at this visit or at a later visit to confirm the EDD. An assessment for risk factors that may affect the pregnancy is performed during the first visit and is updated at subsequent visits.

Several routine laboratory tests are performed on the first or the second prenatal visit. Others are done at specific times during pregnancy and may be repeated at certain intervals. Several tests are done for all pregnant women; others are based on the presence of various risk factors. The U.S. Preventive Services Task Force (USPSTF) has updated its recommendations concerning obtaining urine cultures at 12 to 16 weeks of gestation to screen for asymptomatic bacteriuria. Early treatment of this condition can prevent preterm births. The 2011 ACOG guidelines recommend a vaginal and rectal swab be done to detect Group B streptococcus (GBS) at 35 to 37 weeks gestation to protect mother and infant from infection during labor and birth (Brown, 2013). Table 4-1 lists prenatal laboratory tests. To prevent unnecessary fears or stress, it is important that the nurse explain that most tests are used to establish a baseline normal for comparison throughout pregnancy.

Table 4-1 Prenatal Laboratory Tests*

TEST	PURPOSE
First Trimester (Routine)	
Blood type and Rh factor and antibody screen	Determines risk for maternal–fetal blood incompatibility
Complete blood count (CBC)	Detects anemia, infection, or cell abnormalities
Hemoglobin or hematocrit	Detects anemia
VDRL or rapid plasma reagin (RPR)	Syphilis screen mandated by law
Rubella titer	Determines immunity to rubella
Tuberculosis screening PPD skin test or serum blood test (QuantiFERON-TB Gold)*	Screening test for exposure to tuberculosis
Hepatitis B screen	Identifies carriers of hepatitis B (recommended by American College of Obstetricians and Gynecologists)
Human immunodeficiency virus (HIV) screen	Detects HIV infection; required by some states (counseling concerning prevention and risks should be provided to all prenatal patients)
Urinalysis and culture	Detects infection, renal disease, or diabetes Recommended to screen for asymptomatic bacteriuria
Papanicolaou (Pap) test	Screens for cervical cancer (if not done within 6 months before conception)
Vaginal culture	Detects group B streptococci or sexually transmitted infections (STIs) such as gonorrhea, *Chlamydia*
First Trimester (If Indicated)	
Hemoglobin electrophoresis	Identifies presence of sickle cell trait or disease (in women of African or Mediterranean descent)
Endovaginal ultrasound	Performed when high risk of fetal loss is suspected
Second Trimester (Routine)	
Blood glucose screen: sample drawn 1 hour after 50 g of liquid glucose is ingested	Routine test done at 24-28 weeks of gestation to identify gestational diabetes; results above 135 mg/dL necessitate medical follow-up
Serum alpha-fetoprotein	Optional routine test to identify neural tube or chromosomal defect in fetus
Ultrasonography	Optional noninvasive routine test to identify some anomalies and confirm estimated date of delivery (EDD)
Second Trimester (If Indicated)	
Amniocentesis	Performed at 16-20 weeks of gestation when high-risk problem is suspected
Third Trimester (If Indicated)	
Real-time ultrasonography	Performed when problem is suspected: • Detects reduced amniotic fluid, which can result in fetal problem • Detects excess amniotic fluid, which would indicate fetal anomaly or maternal problem • Confirms gestational age or cephalopelvic disproportion • In tandem with amniocentesis, determines fetal lung maturity (lecithin and sphingomyelin ratio) • Confirms presence of anomaly that may necessitate fetal or neonatal surgery
Cervical fibronectin assay	Determines risk of preterm labor when problem is suspected

EDD, Estimated date of delivery; *VDRL*, Venereal Disease Research Laboratory (test).
*Additional optional prenatal diagnostic tests are described in Table 5-1.
Data from American Congress of Obstetricians and Gynecologists. (2012). Guidelines for Perinatal Care, Washington DC.

The development of human genome mapping has expanded the prenatal detection of genetic disorders and provides the basis for future therapeutic interventions. The future direction of prenatal testing is to provide early, accurate, noninvasive screening tests.

The recommended schedule for prenatal visits in an uncomplicated pregnancy is as follows:

- Conception to 28 weeks—every 4 weeks
- 29 to 36 weeks—every 2 weeks
- 37 weeks to birth—weekly

⚠ Safety Alert!

Early and regular prenatal care is important for reducing the number of low-birth-weight infants born and for reducing morbidity and mortality for mothers and newborns.

The pregnant woman is seen more often if complications arise. Routine assessments made at each prenatal visit include the following:

- Review of known risk factors and assessment for new ones

- Vital signs: The woman's blood pressure should be taken in the same arm and in the same position each time for accurate comparison with her baseline value.
- Weight to determine if the pattern of gain is normal: Low prepregnancy weight or inadequate gains are risk factors for preterm birth, a low-birth-weight infant, and other problems. A sudden, rapid weight gain is often associated with gestational hypertension.
- Urinalysis for protein, glucose, and ketone levels.
- Blood glucose screening between 24 and 28 weeks of gestation: Additional testing is done if the result of this screening test is 135 mg/dl or higher.
- Fundal height to determine if the fetus is growing as expected and the volume of amniotic fluid is appropriate (see Figure 4-3).
- Leopold's maneuvers to assess the presentation and position of the fetus by abdominal palpation (usually at about 36 weeks gestation).
- Fetal heart rate: During very early pregnancy, the fetal heart rate is measured with a Doppler transducer; in later pregnancy, it may also be heard with a fetoscope. Beating of the fetal heart can be seen on ultrasound examination as early as 8 weeks after the LNMP.
- Review of nutrition for adequacy of calorie intake and specific nutrients.
- Discomforts or problems that have arisen since the last visit.

⌂ Nursing Tip

The nurse listens to concerns and answers questions from the expectant family during each prenatal visit. This is a prime time for teaching good health habits, because most women are highly motivated to improve their health.

The nurse establishes rapport with the expectant family by conveying interest in their needs, listening to their concerns, and directing them to appropriate resources. The health care team must show sensitivity to the family's cultural and health beliefs and incorporate as many as possible into care. For example, Muslim laws of modesty dictate that a woman be covered (hair, body, arms, and legs) when in the presence of an unrelated male, and therefore a female health care provider is often preferred. Latino families expect a brief period of conversation during which pleasantries are exchanged before "getting to the point" of the visit. An Asian woman may nod her head when the nurse teaches her, leading the nurse to believe that she understands and will use the teaching. However, the woman may be showing respect to the nurse rather than agreement with what is taught. Eye contact, which is valued by many Americans, is seen as confrontational in some cultures.

DEFINITION OF TERMS

The following terms are used to describe a woman's obstetric history:

- *Gravida:* Any pregnancy, regardless of duration; also, the number of pregnancies, including the one in progress, if applicable.
- *Nulligravida:* A woman who has never been pregnant.
- *Primigravida:* A woman who is pregnant for the first time.
- *Multigravida:* A woman who has been pregnant before, regardless of the duration of the pregnancy.
- *Para:* A woman who has given birth to one or more children who reached the age of viability (20 weeks of gestation), regardless of the number of fetuses delivered and regardless of whether those children are now living.
- *Primipara:* A woman who has given birth to her first child (past the point of viability), regardless of whether the child was alive at birth or is now living. The term is also used informally to describe a woman before the birth of her first child.
- *Multipara:* A woman who has given birth to two or more children (past the point of viability), regardless of whether the children were alive at birth or are presently alive. The term is also used informally to describe a woman before the birth of her second child.
- *Nullipara:* A woman who has not given birth to a child who reached the point of viability.
- *Abortion:* Termination of pregnancy before viability (20 weeks of gestation), either spontaneous or induced.
- *Gestational age:* Prenatal age of the developing fetus calculated from the first day of the woman's LNMP.
- *Fertilization age:* Prenatal age of the developing fetus as calculated from the date of conception; approximately 2 weeks less than the gestational age.
- *Age of viability:* A fetus that has reached the stage (usually at 20 weeks) where it is capable of living outside of the uterus.

The word *gravida* indicates the number of pregnancies. The word *para* indicates the outcome of the pregnancies. The gravida number increases by 1 each time a woman is pregnant, whereas the para number increases *only* when a woman delivers a fetus of at least 20 weeks of gestation. For example, a woman who has had two spontaneous abortions (miscarriages) at 12 weeks of gestation, has a 3-year-old son, and is now 32 weeks pregnant would be described as gravida 4, para 1, abortions 2. The TPALM system (Box 4-1) is a standardized way to describe the detailed outcomes of a woman's pregnancies on her prenatal record.

DETERMINING THE ESTIMATED DATE OF DELIVERY

The average duration of a term pregnancy is 40 weeks (280 days) after the first day of the LNMP. **Nägele's rule** is used to determine the EDD. To calculate the EDD,

Box 4-1	TPALM System to Describe Parity					

T   Number of *term* infants born (infants born after at least 37 weeks of gestation)
P   Number of *preterm* infants born (infants born after 20 weeks or before 37 weeks of gestation)
A   Number of pregnancies *aborted before 20 weeks of gestation* (spontaneously or induced)
L   Number of children now *living*
M   *Multiple* birth number of multiple gestations (optional)

EXAMPLE

Name	Gravida	Term	Preterm	Abortions	Living	Multiple
Katie Field	3	1	0	1	1	0
Anna Luz	4	1	1	1	2	0

Katie Field: Gravida 3, TPALM (para) 10110.
Anna Luz: Gravida 4, TPALM (para) 11120.

Box 4-2	Nägele's Rule to Determine the Estimated Date of Delivery (EDD)

1. Determine first day of the last normal menstrual period (LNMP)
2. Count backward 3 months
3. Add 7 days
4. Correct the year if necessary

EXAMPLE
1. First day of last normal menstrual period: January 27
2. Count backward 3 months: October 27
3. Add 7 days: November 3 is EDD

Box 4-3	Signs of Pregnancy

PRESUMPTIVE
Amenorrhea
Nausea
Breast tenderness
Deepening pigmentation
Urinary frequency
Quickening

PROBABLE
Goodell's sign
Chadwick's sign
Hegar's sign
McDonald's sign
Abdominal enlargement
Braxton Hicks contractions
Ballottement
Striae
Positive pregnancy test

POSITIVE
Audible fetal heartbeat
Fetal movement felt by examiner
Ultrasound visualization of fetus

one identifies the first day of the LNMP, counts backward 3 months, and then adds 7 days (Box 4-2). The year is updated if applicable. The EDD is an *estimated* date, and many normal births occur before or after this date. The EDD may also be determined with a gestation wheel, an electronic calculator designed for this purpose, a physical examination, an ultrasound, or a combination of these methods.

Pregnancy is divided into three 13-week parts called **trimesters**. Predictable changes occur in the woman and the fetus in each trimester. Understanding these developments helps to better provide anticipatory guidance and identify deviations from the expected pattern of development.

DIAGNOSIS OF PREGNANCY

The signs of pregnancy are divided into three general groups: presumptive, probable, and positive, depending on how likely they are to be caused by factors other than pregnancy (Box 4-3).

PRESUMPTIVE SIGNS OF PREGNANCY

The presumptive indications of pregnancy are those from which a definite diagnosis of pregnancy cannot be made. These signs and symptoms are common during pregnancy but can often be caused by other conditions.

Amenorrhea, the cessation of menses, in a healthy and sexually active woman is often the first sign of pregnancy. However, strenuous exercise, changes in metabolism and endocrine dysfunction, chronic disease, certain medications, anorexia nervosa, early menopause, or serious psychological disturbances may also be the cause.

Nausea and sometimes *vomiting* occur in at least half of all pregnancies and may be the result of an increase of human chorionic gonadotropin (hCG) levels in early pregnancy and is not associated with unfavorable outcomes for mother or infant (Gabbe, 2012). "Morning sickness" describes the symptoms, but they may occur at any time of day. Distaste for certain foods or even their odors may be the main complaint. The nausea begins about 4 weeks after the LNMP and usually improves by the end of the twentieth week (Kramer, 2013). By screening the woman for nausea and vomiting during prenatal visits, the nurse can offer interventions and supportive care that can increase the quality of the pregnancy experience. Emotional problems or gastrointestinal upsets may also cause nausea and vomiting.

Breast changes include tenderness and tingling as hormones from the placenta stimulate growth of the ductal system in preparation for breastfeeding. Similar breast changes also occur premenstrually in many women. Striae are pink to brown lines that may develop as the breasts enlarge (Figure 4-1).

Pigmentation changes occur primarily in dark-skinned women. They include increased pigmentation of the face (**chloasma**, or "mask of pregnancy"), breasts (darkening of the areolae), and abdomen (linea nigra, a line extending in the midline of the abdomen from just above the umbilicus to the symphysis pubis). See Figure 4-2 for common skin changes of pregnancy.

Frequency and *urgency of urination* are common in the early months of pregnancy. The enlarging uterus, along with the increased blood supply to the pelvic area, exerts pressure on the bladder. Urinary frequency occurs in the first trimester until the uterus expands and becomes an abdominal organ in the second trimester. The pregnant woman experiences frequency of urination again in the third trimester when the presenting part descends in the pelvis in preparation for birth. Causes of urinary disturbances other than pregnancy are urinary tract infections and pelvic masses.

Fatigue and *drowsiness* are early symptoms of pregnancy. It is believed that fatigue is caused by increased metabolic needs of the woman and fetus. In an otherwise healthy young woman, it is a significant sign of pregnancy. However, illness, stress, or sudden changes in lifestyle may also cause fatigue.

Quickening, fetal movement felt by the mother, is first perceived at 16 to 20 weeks of gestation as a faint fluttering in the lower abdomen. Women who have previously given birth often report quickening at an earlier stage, because they know how to identify it. This is an important event to record, because it marks the approximate midpoint of the pregnancy and is another reference point to verify gestational age. Abdominal gas, normal bowel activity, or false pregnancy (pseudocyesis) are other possible causes of this fluttering in the lower abdomen.

PROBABLE SIGNS OF PREGNANCY

The probable indications of pregnancy provide stronger evidence of pregnancy. However, these also may be caused by other conditions.

Goodell's sign is the softening of the cervix and the vagina caused by increased vascular congestion. **Chadwick's sign** is the purplish or bluish discoloration of the cervix, vagina, and vulva caused by increased vascular congestion. Hormonal imbalance or infection may also cause both Goodell's and Chadwick's signs. **Hegar's sign** is a softening of the lower uterine segment. Because of the softening, it is easy to flex the body of the uterus against the cervix, which is known as **McDonald's sign**.

Abdominal and uterine enlargement occurs rather irregularly at the onset of pregnancy. By the end of the twelfth week, the uterine fundus may be felt just above the symphysis pubis, and it extends to the umbilicus between the twentieth and twenty-second weeks (Figure 4-3). Uterine or abdominal tumors may also cause enlargement.

Braxton Hicks contractions are irregular, painless uterine contractions that begin in the second trimester. These contractions give the sensation of the abdomen being hard and tense. They become progressively more noticeable as term approaches and are more pronounced in multiparas. They may become strong enough to be mistaken for true labor. Uterine fibroids (benign tumors) may also cause these contractions.

Ballottement is a maneuver by which the fetal part is displaced by a light tap of the examining finger on the

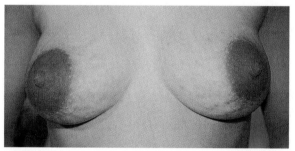

FIGURE 4-1 Striae and pigmentation of breasts. Note the darkened pigmentation of areolae and the pink-white lines at the base of the breasts that are caused by stretching of the elastic tissue as the breasts enlarge. Pigmentation will disappear after pregnancy, and striae will fade into silvery strands. (From Swartz MH: *Textbook of physical diagnosis: history and examination,* ed 6, Philadelphia, 2009, Saunders.)

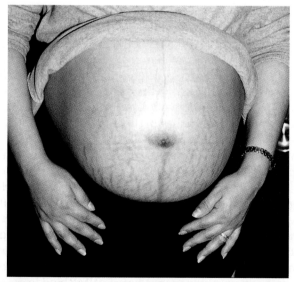

FIGURE 4-2 Abdominal striae are pinkish white or purple-gray lines that may occur in pregnancy. They may be found on the breasts, abdomen, and thighs. The dark line at the midline is the linea nigra, an area of increased pigmentation most noticeable in dark-skinned women.

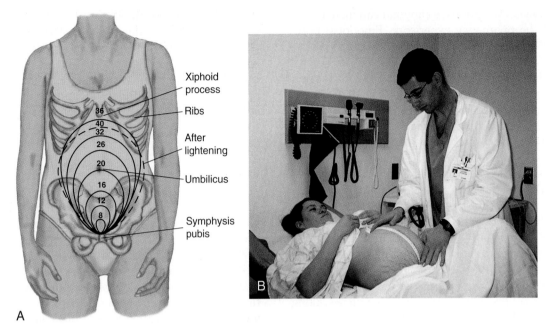

FIGURE 4-3 Height of fundus during gestation. **A,** The numbers represent the weeks of gestation, and the circles represent the height of the fundus expected at that stage of gestation. Note: The fortieth week is represented by a dotted line to indicate lightening has occurred. **B,** A health care provider measures the height of the fundus during a clinic visit. (**A** from Murray SS, McKinney ES, Gorrie TM: *Foundations of maternal-newborn nursing*, ed 2, Philadelphia, 1998, Saunders. **B** courtesy Pat Spier, RN-C.)

cervix, and then the part rebounds quickly. Uterine or cervical polyps (small tumors) may cause the sensation of ballottement on the examiner's finger.

Fetal outline may be identified by palpation after the twenty-fourth week. It is possible to mistake a tumor for a fetus.

Abdominal striae (stretch marks) are fine, pinkish white or purplish gray lines that some women develop when the elastic tissue of the skin has been stretched to its capacity (see Figure 4-2). Increased amounts of estrogen cause a rise in adrenal gland activity. This change, in addition to the stretching, is believed to cause breakdown and atrophy of the underlying connective tissue in the skin. Striae are seen on the breasts, thighs, abdomen, and buttocks. After pregnancy, the striae lose their bright color, and they become thin, silvery lines. Striae may occur with skin stretching from any cause, such as weight gain.

Pregnancy tests use maternal urine or blood to determine the presence of human chorionic gonadotropin (hCG), a hormone produced by the chorionic villi of the placenta. Home pregnancy tests based on the presence of hCG in the urine are capable of greater than 97% accuracy, but the instructions must be followed *precisely* to obtain this accuracy. Professional pregnancy tests are based on urine or blood serum levels of hCG, and they are more accurate. A highly reliable pregnancy test is the *radioimmunoassay* (RIA). The RIA is a blood test that accurately identifies pregnancy as early as 1 week after ovulation. Pregnancy tests of all types are probable indicators, because several factors may interfere with their accuracy: medications such as antianxiety or anticonvulsant drugs, blood in the urine, malignant tumors, or premature menopause.

POSITIVE SIGNS OF PREGNANCY

Only a developing fetus causes positive signs of pregnancy. They include demonstration of fetal heart activity, fetal movements felt by an examiner, and visualization of the fetus with ultrasound.

Fetal heartbeat may be detected as early as 10 weeks of pregnancy by using a Doppler device. The examiner can detect the fetal heartbeat using a fetoscope between the eighteenth and twentieth weeks of pregnancy. When the fetal heartbeat is heard with a fetoscope, it is important because it provides another marker of the approximate midpoint of gestation. When assessing the fetal heartbeat with a Doppler device or fetoscope, the woman's pulse rate must be assessed at the same time to be certain that the fetal heart is what is actually heard. The fetal heart rate at term ranges between a low of 110 to 120 beats/min and a high of 150 to 160 beats/min. The rate is higher in early gestation and slows as term approaches.

Additional sounds that may be heard while assessing the fetal heartbeat are the uterine and funic souffles. *Uterine souffle* is a soft blowing sound heard over the uterus during auscultation. The sound is synchronous with the mother's pulse and is caused by blood entering the dilated arteries of the uterus. The *funic souffle* is a soft swishing sound heard as the blood passes through the umbilical cord vessels.

A trained examiner can feel fetal movements in the second trimester. The examiner must distinguish fetal

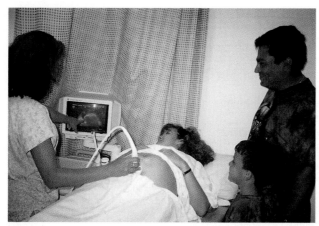

FIGURE 4-4 The pregnant woman's family may be present during an ultrasound.

activity, because, to a prospective mother, normal intestinal movements can appear similar to the faint fetal movements typical of early pregnancy. Fetal movements can be seen with ultrasonography.

Identification of the embryo or fetus by means of ultrasound photography of the gestational sac is possible as early as 4 to 5 weeks of gestation with 100% reliability. This noninvasive method is the earliest positive sign of a pregnancy. An ultrasound is often routinely performed around the twentieth week of gestation (Figure 4-4).

PHYSIOLOGICAL CHANGES IN PREGNANCY

The woman's body undergoes dramatic changes as she houses and nourishes her growing child. Most of these changes reverse shortly after birth.

ENDOCRINE SYSTEM

Hormones are essential to maintain pregnancy, and the dramatic increase in hormones during pregnancy affects all body systems. Most hormones are produced by the corpus luteum initially and later by the placenta. The most striking change in the endocrine system during pregnancy is the addition of the placenta as a temporary endocrine organ that produces large amounts of estrogen and progesterone to maintain the pregnancy (as well as hCG and human placental lactogen [hPL]). hPL increases maternal insulin resistance during pregnancy, providing the fetus with glucose needed for growth (Table 4-2).

REPRODUCTIVE SYSTEM

Uterus

The uterus undergoes the most obvious changes in pregnancy. Before pregnancy, the uterus is a small, muscular, pear-shaped pelvic organ that weighs about 60 g (2 oz), measures 7.5 cm (3 inches) × 5 cm (2 inches) × 2.5 cm (1 inch), and has a capacity of about 10 mL (⅓ oz). The uterus expands gradually during pregnancy by increasing both the number of myometrial (muscle)

cells during the first trimester and the size of individual cells during the second and third trimesters. The uterus becomes a temporary abdominal organ at the end of the first trimester. At term, the uterus reaches the woman's xiphoid process and weighs about 1000 g (2.2 lb). Its capacity is about 5000 mL (5 quarts), enough to house the term fetus, the placenta, and amniotic fluid.

Cervix

Soon after conception, the cervix changes in color and consistency. Chadwick's and Goodell's signs appear. The glands of the cervical mucosa increase in number and activity. Secretion of thick mucus leads to the formation of a *mucous plug* that seals the cervical canal. The mucous plug prevents the ascent of vaginal organisms into the uterus. With the beginning of cervical thinning (*effacement*) and opening (*dilation*) near the onset of labor, the plug is loosened and expelled.

Ovaries

The ovaries do not produce ova (eggs) during pregnancy. The *corpus luteum* (empty graafian follicle; see Chapter 2) remains on the ovary and produces progesterone to maintain the *decidua* (uterine lining) during the first 6 to 7 weeks of the pregnancy until the placenta can perform this function.

Vagina

The vaginal blood supply increases, causing the bluish color of Chadwick's sign. The vaginal mucosa thickens, and rugae (ridges) become prominent. The connective tissue softens to prepare for distention as the child is born. Secretions of the vagina increase. In addition, the vaginal pH becomes more acidic to protect the vagina and uterus from pathogenic microorganisms. However, the vaginal secretions also have higher levels of glycogen, a substance that promotes the growth of *Candida albicans*, the organism that causes yeast infections.

The most common cause of vaginal discharge is *bacterial vaginosis* (BV), in which there is a decrease in normal lactobacilli and an increase in bacteroids and other anaerobic microorganisms. There may be a milky-white vaginal discharge, but often there are no other clinical symptoms. Bacterial vaginosis has been associated with preterm labor, and many obstetricians routinely screen pregnant women for BV early in pregnancy. Treatment with antimicrobials between 12 and 20 weeks of gestation is common.

Breasts

Hormone-induced breast changes occur early in pregnancy. High levels of estrogen and progesterone prepare the breasts for **lactation**. The areolae of the breasts usually become deeply pigmented, and sebaceous glands in the nipples (tubercles of Montgomery) become prominent. The tubercles secrete a substance that lubricates the nipples.

Table 4-2	Hormones Essential in Pregnancy
HORMONE	**SOURCE AND SIGNIFICANCE**
Estrogen	Produced by ovaries and placenta Responsible for enlargement of uterus, breasts, and genitals Promotes fat deposit changes Stimulates melanocyte-stimulating hormone in hyperpigmentation of skin Promotes vascular changes Promotes development of striae gravidarum Alters sodium and water retention
Progesterone	Produced by corpus luteum and ovary and later by placenta Maintains endometrium for implantation Inhibits uterine contractility, preventing abortion Promotes development of secretory ducts of breasts for lactation Stimulates sodium secretion Reduces smooth muscle tone (causing constipation, heartburn, varicosities)
Thyroxine (T₄)	Influences thyroid gland's size and activity and increases heart rate Increases basal metabolic rate 23% during pregnancy
Human chorionic gonadotropin (hCG)	Produced early in pregnancy by trophoblastic tissue Stimulates progesterone and estrogen by corpus luteum to maintain pregnancy until placenta takes over Used in pregnancy tests to determine pregnancy state
Human placental lactogen (hPL), also called chorionic somatomammotropin	Produced by placenta Affects glucose and protein metabolism Has a diabetogenic effect—allows increased glucose to stimulate pancreas and increase insulin level
Melanocyte-stimulating hormone (MSH)	Produced by anterior pituitary gland Causes pigmentation of skin to darken, resulting in brown patches on face (chloasma [melasma gravidarum]), dark line on abdomen (linea nigra), darkening of moles and freckles, and darkening of nipples and areolae
Relaxin	Produced by corpus luteum and placenta Remodels collagen, causing connective tissue of symphysis pubis to be more movable and cervix to soften Inhibits uterine activity
Prolactin	Prepares breasts for lactation
Oxytocin	Produced by posterior pituitary gland Stimulates uterine contraction Is inhibited by progesterone during pregnancy After birth, helps keep uterus contracted Stimulates milk ejection reflex during breastfeeding

In the last few months of pregnancy, a thin yellow fluid called **colostrum** may be expressed from the breasts. This "premilk" is high in protein, fat-soluble vitamins, and minerals, but it is low in calories, fat, and sugar. Colostrum contains the mother's antibodies to diseases and is secreted for the first 2 to 3 days after birth in the breastfeeding woman.

RESPIRATORY SYSTEM

The pregnant woman breathes more deeply, but her respiratory rate increases only slightly, if at all. These changes increase oxygen and carbon dioxide exchange, because she moves more air in and out with each breath. Oxygen consumption increases by 15% during pregnancy. The expanding uterus exerts upward pressure on her diaphragm, causing it to rise about 4 cm (1.6 inch).

To compensate, her rib cage flares, increasing the circumference of the chest about 6 cm (2.4 inches). Dyspnea may occur until the fetus descends into the pelvis (**lightening**), relieving upward pressure on the diaphragm.

Increased estrogen levels during pregnancy cause edema or swelling of the mucous membranes of the nose, pharynx, mouth, and trachea. The woman may have nasal stuffiness, epistaxis (nosebleeds), and changes in her voice. A similar process occurs in the ears, causing a sense of fullness or earaches.

CARDIOVASCULAR SYSTEM

The growing uterus displaces the heart upward and to the left. The blood volume gradually increases (*hypervolemia*) to about 45% greater than that of the prepregnant state by 32 to 34 weeks of gestation, at which time it

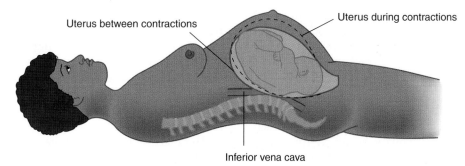

Uterus between contractions   Uterus during contractions

Inferior vena cava

FIGURE 4-5 Supine hypotension syndrome. When a pregnant woman lies on her back (supine), the weight of the uterus with its fetal contents presses on the vena cava and the abdominal aorta. Placing a wedge pillow under the woman's right hip helps to relieve compression of these vessels. (From Matteson PS: *Women's health during the childbearing years: a community-based approach*, St Louis, 2001, Mosby.)

levels off or declines slightly. This increase provides added blood for these purposes:

- Exchange of nutrients, oxygen, and waste products within the placenta
- Needs of expanded maternal tissue
- Reserve for blood loss at birth

Cardiac output increases, because more blood is pumped from the heart with each contraction, the pulse rate increases by 10 to 15 beats/min, and the basal metabolic rate (BMR) may increase 20% during pregnancy.

Blood pressure does not increase with the higher blood volume, because resistance to blood flow through the vessels decreases. A blood pressure of 140/90 mm Hg or a significant elevation above the woman's baseline measurement calls for attention. **Supine hypotension syndrome**, also called **aortocaval compression** or vena cava syndrome, may occur if the woman lies on her back (Figure 4-5). The supine position allows the heavy uterus to compress her inferior vena cava, reducing the amount of blood returned to her heart. Circulation to the placenta may also be reduced by increased pressure on the woman's aorta, resulting in fetal hypoxia. Symptoms of supine hypotension syndrome include faintness, lightheadedness, dizziness, and agitation. Displacing the uterus to one side by turning the patient (preferably to the left) is all that is needed to relieve the pressure. If the woman must remain flat for any reason, a small towel roll placed under one hip will also help to prevent supine hypotension syndrome.

Orthostatic hypotension may occur whenever a woman rises from a recumbent position, resulting in faintness or lightheadedness. Cardiac output decreases, because venous return from the lower body suddenly drops. *Palpitations* (sudden increase in heart rate) may occur from increases in thoracic pressure, particularly if the woman moves suddenly.

Although both plasma (fluid) and red blood cells (erythrocytes) increase during pregnancy, they do not increase by the same amount. The fluid part of the blood increases more than the erythrocyte component. This leads to a *dilutional anemia* or **pseudoanemia** (false anemia). As a result, the normal prepregnant

hematocrit level of 36% to 48% may fall to 33% to 46%. Although this is not true anemia, the hematocrit count is reevaluated to determine patient status and needs. The white blood cell (leukocyte) count also increases about 8% (mostly neutrophils) and returns to prepregnant levels by the sixth day postpartum (Table 4-3).

There are increased levels of clotting factors VII, VIII, and X and plasma fibrinogen during the second and third trimesters of pregnancy. This hypercoagulability state helps prevent excessive bleeding after delivery when the placenta separates from the uterine wall. However, these changes increase the possibility of thrombophlebitis during pregnancy and are the reason that the pregnant patient requires careful assessment for this risk and specific teaching to prevent the venous stasis that can lead to thrombophlebitis.

The current increased interest in physical fitness has resulted in many pregnant women continuing to exercise during pregnancy. The effects of exercise on the cardiovascular system that already has an increased blood volume, increased cardiac output, and increased coagulability during pregnancy must be reviewed before an

Table **4-3**	Normal Blood Values in Nonpregnant and Pregnant Women	
VALUE	**NONPREGNANT**	**PREGNANT**
Hemoglobin (g/dL)	12-16	11-12 (10.5 in second trimester)
Hematocrit (%)	36-48	33-46 (33 in second trimester)
Red blood cells (million/mm³)	3.8-5.1	4.5-6.5
White blood cells (increase during labor and postpartum up to 25,000/mm³)	5000-10,000/ mm³	5000-15,000/mm³
Fibrinogen (mg/dl)	200-400	300-600

Data from Blackburn S: *Maternal, fetal and neonatal physiology: a clinical perspective*, ed 4, Philadelphia, 2013, Saunders.

exercise plan is implemented. Venous pressure may increase in the femoral veins as the size and weight of the uterus increase, resulting in varicose veins in the legs of some women.

GASTROINTESTINAL SYSTEM

The growing uterus displaces the stomach and intestines toward the back and sides of the abdomen (Figure 4-6). Increased salivary secretion (ptyalism) sometimes affects taste and smell. The mouth tissues may become tender and bleed more easily because of increased blood vessel development caused by high estrogen levels. Contrary to popular belief, teeth are not affected by pregnancy.

The demands of the growing fetus increase the woman's appetite and thirst. The acidity of gastric secretions is decreased; emptying of the stomach and motility (movement) of the intestines are slower. Women often feel bloated and may experience constipation and hemorrhoids. *Pyrosis* (heartburn) is caused by the relaxation of the cardiac sphincter of the stomach, which permits reflux (backward flow) of the acid secretions into the lower esophagus.

Glucose metabolism is altered because of increased insulin resistance during pregnancy. This allows more glucose use by the fetus but also places the woman at risk for the development of gestational diabetes mellitus. Progesterone and estrogen relax the muscle tone of the gallbladder, resulting in the retention of bile salts, and this can lead to pruritus (itching of the skin) during pregnancy.

URINARY SYSTEM

The urinary system excretes waste products for both the mother and the fetus during pregnancy. The glomerular filtration rate of the kidneys increases. The renal tubules increase the reabsorption of substances that the body needs to conserve, but the tubules may not be able to keep up with the high load of some substances filtered by the glomeruli (e.g., glucose). Therefore glycosuria and proteinuria are more common during pregnancy. Water is retained, because it is needed for increased blood volume and for dissolving nutrients that are provided for the fetus.

The relaxing effects of progesterone cause the renal pelvis and ureters to lose tone, resulting in decreased peristalsis to the bladder. The diameter of the ureters and the bladder capacity increase because of the relaxing effects of progesterone, causing urine stasis. The combination of urine stasis and nutrient-rich urine makes the pregnant woman more susceptible to urinary tract infection. Consuming at least eight glasses of water each day reduces the risk for urinary tract infection. Although the bladder can hold up to 1500 mL of urine, the pressure of the enlarging uterus causes increasing frequency of urination, especially in the first and third trimesters. Changes in the renal system may take 6 to 12 weeks after delivery to return to the prepregnant state.

Fluid and Electrolyte Balance

The increased glomerular filtration rate in the kidneys increases sodium filtration by 50%, but the increase in the tubular resorption rate results in 99% reabsorption of the sodium. Sodium retention is influenced by many factors, including elevated levels of the hormones of pregnancy. Although the fetus uses much of the sodium, the remainder is in the maternal circulation and can cause a maternal accumulation of water (edema). This fluid retention may cause a problem if the woman in labor is given intravenous fluids containing oxytocin (Pitocin), which has an *antidiuretic* effect

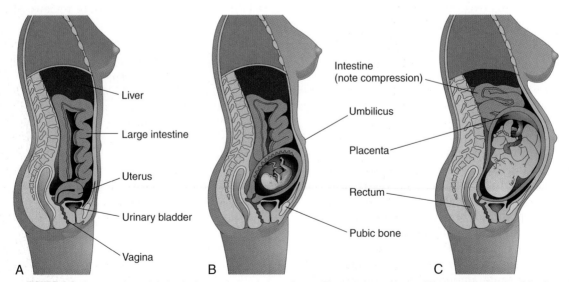

Liver

Large intestine

Uterus

Urinary bladder

Vagina

A

Intestine (note compression)

Umbilicus

Placenta

Rectum

Pubic bone

B   C

FIGURE 4-6 Compression of abdominal contents as uterus enlarges. The nonpregnant state **(A)** shows the relationship of the uterus to the abdominal contents. As the uterus enlarges at 20 weeks of gestation **(B)** and 30 weeks of gestation **(C)**, the abdominal contents are displaced and compressed. (From Moore KL, Persaud TVN, Torchia MG: *The developing human: clinically oriented embryology*, ed 9, Philadelphia, 2012, Saunders.)

and can result in water intoxication. Agitation and delirium—possible signs of water intoxication—should be recorded and reported, and an accurate intake and output record should be kept during labor and the immediate postpartum phase.

In pregnancy, blood is slightly more alkaline than in the nonpregnant state, and this mild alkalemia is enhanced by the hyperventilation that often occurs during pregnancy. This status does not affect a normal pregnancy.

INTEGUMENTARY AND SKELETAL SYSTEMS

The high levels of hormones produced during pregnancy cause a variety of temporary changes in the integument (skin) of the pregnant woman. In addition to the pigmentary changes discussed under the presumptive signs of pregnancy, the sweat and sebaceous glands of the skin become more active to dissipate heat from the woman and fetus. Small red elevations of skin with lines radiating from the center, called spider nevi, may occur. The palms of the hands may become deeper red. Most skin changes are reversed shortly after giving birth.

The woman's posture changes as her child grows within the uterus. The anterior part of her body becomes heavier with the expanding uterus, and the lordotic curve in her lumbar spine becomes more pronounced. The woman often experiences low backaches, and, in the last few months of pregnancy, rounding of the shoulders may occur along with aching in the cervical spine and upper extremities.

The pelvic joints relax with hormonal changes during late pregnancy and entry of the fetal presenting part into the pelvic brim in the last trimester. A woman often has a "waddling" gait in the last few weeks of pregnancy because of a slight separation of the symphysis pubis.

> ### ! Safety Alert!
> A change in the center of gravity and joint instability because of the softening of the ligaments predispose the pregnant woman to problems with balance. Interventions concerning safety should be part of prenatal education.

NUTRITION FOR PREGNANCY AND LACTATION

Good nutrition is vital to good health and essential for normal growth and development. It is also essential to establish and maintain a healthy pregnancy and give birth to a healthy child. Good nutritional habits begun before conception and continued during pregnancy, promote adaptation to the maternal and fetal needs. In a joint effort, the U.S. Department of Agriculture (USDA) and the U.S. Department of Health and Human Services created MyPlate, which offers dietary guidelines for Americans (Figure 4-7). An example of how a food pyramid can be modified to fit Latin American dietary preferences is shown in Figure 4-8.

> ### Nutrition Considerations
> **Maternal Diet and Fetal Health**
> There is a high correlation between maternal diet and fetal health. To ensure that deficiencies do not occur during the critical first weeks of pregnancy, the nurse explains to women of childbearing age the value of eating well-balanced meals so they may start pregnancy in a good nutritional state.

A healthy, balanced, nutrient-dense diet combined with adequate physical activity is the core of the revised dietary guidelines. A personalized portion-sized diet plan that includes individualized activity level advice is available online at www.MyPyramid.gov. Additional recommendations for specific populations can be found at www.healthierus.gov/dietaryguidelines. Women who follow this guide before pregnancy will be well nourished at the time of conception. Before and during pregnancy, women should read food labels carefully to promote the intake of calories that are nutrient dense rather than empty.

During pregnancy and lactation, an adequate dietary intake of docosahexaenoic acid–omega 3 fatty acid (DHA) is essential for optimal brain development of the fetus and infant. The World Health Organization (WHO) recommends that a full-term infant receives 20 mg of DHA per kilogram per day. Maternal dietary sources of DHA include fish such as mackerel, Atlantic and sockeye salmon, halibut, tuna, flounder, egg yolk, red meat, poultry, canola oil, and soybean oil; two to three servings per week are recommended. Frying these foods detracts from DHA content. Refer to Table 15-6 for culturally diverse food patterns.

Nursing Care Plan 4-1 on p. 58 lists common nursing diagnoses and interventions related to nutrition during pregnancy and lactation.

RECOMMENDED DIETARY ALLOWANCES AND RECOMMENDED DIETARY INTAKES

In the United States, the Food and Nutrition Board of the Institute of Medicine (IOM), the National Academy of Science in cooperation with the USDA, and the U.S. Department of Health and Human Services developed recommended dietary allowances (RDAs) of nutrient intake required to maintain optimal health. In the past, RDAs reflected the fact that nutrients were primarily supplied by foods, in particular, nonfortified ones. Research by the Food and Nutrition Board showed an increasing use of dietary supplements and fortified foods, resulting in the need to describe upper limits of intake levels to prevent toxicity. Adverse responses (toxicity) can occur if the combination of intake in the form of supplements and food, whether fortified or not, exceeds the present upper limits of safety. When scientific evidence is insufficient to determine RDA, an adequate intake is likely provided by an adequate diet. Consuming dietary supplements of trace elements can result in toxicity if upper limits of intake are consistently exceeded.

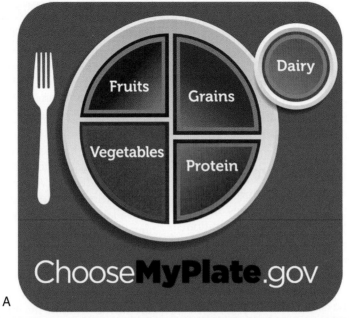

A

Food Group	1st Trimester	2nd and 3rd Trimesters	What counts as 1 cup or 1 ounce?	Remember to...
	Eat this amount from each group daily.*			
Fruits	2 cups	2 cups	1 cup fruit or juice ½ cup dried fruit	*Focus on fruits—* Eat a variety of fruits.
Vegetables	2½ cups	3 cups	1 cup raw or cooked vegetables or juice 2 cups raw leafy vegetables	*Vary your veggies—* Eat more dark-green and orange vegetables and cooked dry beans.
Grains	6 ounces	8 ounces	1 slice bread 1 ounce ready-to-eat cereal ½ cup cooked pasta, rice, or cereal	*Make half your grains whole*—Choose whole instead of refined grains.
Meat & Beans	5½ ounces	6½ ounces	1 ounce lean meat, poultry, or fish ¼ cup cooked dry beans ½ ounce nuts or 1 egg 1 tablespoon peanut butter	*Go lean with protein—* Choose low-fat or lean meats and poultry.
Milk	3 cups	3 cups	1 cup milk 8 ounces yogurt 1½ ounces cheese 2 ounces processed cheese	*Get your calcium-rich foods*—Go low-fat or fat-free when you choose milk, yogurt, and cheese.

*These amounts are for an average pregnant woman. You may need more or less than the average. Check with your doctor to make sure you are gaining weight as you should.

In each food group, choose foods that are low in "extras"—solid fats and added sugars.

Pregnant women and women who may become pregnant should not drink alcohol. Any amount of alcohol during pregnancy could cause problems for your baby.

Most doctors recommend that pregnant women take a prenatal vitamin and mineral supplement every day **in addition to** eating a healthy diet. This is so you and your baby get enough folic acid, iron, and other nutrients. But don't overdo it. Taking too much can be harmful.

B

FIGURE 4-7 A, MyPlate is based on the 2010 dietary guidelines for Americans to encourage healthful eating for all people. The colors on the plate illustrate the five food groups as a placesetting for a meal, showing approximate portion size recommended for proteins, vegetables, fruits, grains, and dairy. Consumers can access the website www.Choosemyplate. gov to find printable references, sample menus, and recommended foods for each food group. **B,** The USDA site provides specific recommendations for pregnant women. (Courtesy U.S. Department of Agriculture.)

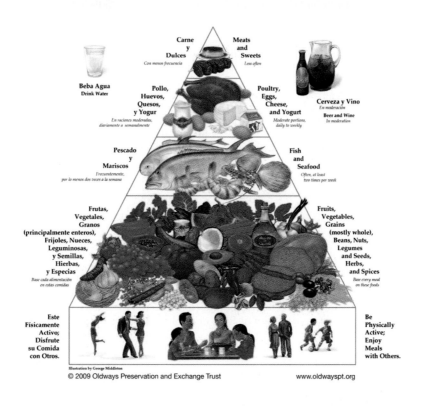

FIGURE 4-8   The Traditional Healthy Latin American Diet Pyramid. This diet pyramid is a modification of the North American diet and has daily physical activity as its base. It contains foods common to the Latin American diet. (© Oldways Preservation and Exchange Trust, 2009.)

The Committee of the USDA Human Nutrition and Research Center published recommended dietary intakes (RDIs) focusing on specific nutrients (see http://fnic.nal.usda.gov). Research is ongoing. Future nutrient recommendations will be expressed as dietary reference intakes (DRIs). DRI is an umbrella term that includes the RDA and tolerable upper levels of intake. The RDA will be retained for any nutrient for which revision to the new DRI has not been made, and both RDAs and RDIs will be used until research is completed. Current RDAs and RDIs of nutrients for various age groups, including those for pregnant and lactating women, can be found on the Evolve website or in a nutrition textbook.

! Safety Alert!

Avoid exceeding recommended dosages of vitamins and minerals, because a balance is needed for health. For example, excess intake of vitamin C can inhibit the use of vitamin B_{12}.

WEIGHT GAIN

In the past a woman's weight gain was restricted during pregnancy. It was thought that minimal weight gain would keep the fetus small and therefore easier to deliver. Evidence shows that low maternal weight gain is associated with complications such as preterm labor, and recommendations for weight gain during pregnancy have gradually increased. Guidelines for weight gain during pregnancy are based on the woman's prepregnant weight and BMI. (The BMI considers the height and weight of the average American adult.) Women with a BMI of 18.5 to 24.9 are considered normal weight; women with a BMI of less than 18.5 are considered underweight; women with a BMI of 25 to 25.9 are considered overweight; and women with a BMI greater than 30 are considered obese. A BMI calculator is available at www.nhlbisupport.com/bmi. Current IOM (2009) recommended weight gains during pregnancy with a *single* fetus are as follows:

- Normal-weight women: 25 to 35 lb (11.5 to 16 kg)
- Underweight women: 28 to 40 lb (12.5 to 18 kg)

Nursing Care Plan 4-1   **Nutrition During Pregnancy and Lactation**

PATIENT DATA Mrs. Switzer is seen in the clinic. She is 35 years old, in the first trimester of her first pregnancy, and appears interested in learning how to "start a healthy diet" in order to have a healthy pregnancy outcome.

Selected Nursing Diagnosis Deficient knowledge related to importance of nutrition in pregnancy and lactation

Goals	Nursing Interventions	Rationales
Patient will verbalize the need for good nutrition during pregnancy and lactation.	Determine age, parity, present weight, prepregnant nutritional status, food preferences and dislikes, food intolerances, and general health of pregnant patient. Determine socioeconomic and cultural factors that may influence food choices. Make recommendations to fit specific needs. Consult with a dietitian if the patient's nutritional needs are complex.	Many factors influence nutritional status of patient during pregnancy and lactation; nutrition teaching must be individualized to best meet her pregnancy nutritional needs. Socioeconomic and cultural factors affect the patient's food choices. These factors must be considered to increase the chance that a patient will adhere to dietary recommendations. The assessment may identify the need for referral to programs such as the Women, Infants, and Children (WIC) nutrition program.
	Review specific nutritional needs and food sources for optimal outcome of pregnancy and successful lactation.	If patient understands specific nutritional needs of pregnancy and food sources, she is more likely to choose foods that meet these needs.
	Provide written information in the patient's primary language regarding nutrition and food preparation. Modify the information to incorporate cultural practices or food dislikes or intolerances.	Written information reinforces verbal teaching and helps patient to recall forgotten information. Recommendations must fit within a patient's individualized needs to increase the chance that she will adhere to them.
	Encourage questions and provide appropriate answers.	Encouraging the patient's questions allows the nurse to identify and correct areas of inadequate knowledge or misunderstanding.
Patient will implement good nutrition during pregnancy and lactation, as evidenced by a 24-hour diary.	Teach the patient the purpose of and how to maintain a 24-hour food diary. Teach the patient to eat normally and to write down everything she eats and drinks, including approximate amounts, for 1 day. Review the 24-hour intake from the diary and make appropriate recommendations for improvement. Refer to a dietitian if nutritional assessment shows complex needs.	A 24-hour food diary helps the nurse to evaluate a patient's usual diet and her likes and dislikes, as well as how to improve her diet. It may help identify the need for a dietitian referral. Analysis of usual meals and snacks enables the nurse to identify adequate and inadequate intake of specific nutrients. The 24-hour diary allows the nurse to reinforce areas of adequate intake and concentrate on areas of deficient nutrients.
	Teach the patient about the Food Guide MyPlate and how to read food labels.	Choices on the Food Guide MyPlate provide essential nutrients on a daily basis. Reading labels helps the patient to select more nutritious items from those that are available.
Patient will demonstrate a gradual weight gain appropriate for her pregnancy (25 to 35 lb for most women).	Maintain a chart to show the patient's actual weight at each visit. Review progress of weight with patient at each visit and compare it with the recommended amount of gain for that point in pregnancy.	Weight chart identifies both the amount and the pattern of weight gain to identify inadequate or excessive gain. Reviewing the patient's weight identifies whether the patient's weight gain is normal and whether additional teaching or exploration of needs is required.

Critical Thinking Questions

1. Mrs. Switzer says she is anxious to complete the clinic appointment, because she wants to "light up a cigarette." What is your major concern about her smoking? What interventions would be appropriate?
2. Mrs. Switzer states that her dietary pattern is heavily influenced by her perceived "food cravings," which have occurred increasingly in the past month. What would be your approach to this problem?

- Overweight women: 11 to 25 lb (5 to 11.5 kg)
- Obese women: 11 to 15 lb (5 to 6.8 kg)

Women carrying *twins* should gain more weight:
- Normal-weight women: 37 to 54 lb (16.5 to 24.5 kg).
- Overweight women: 31 to 50 lb (14 to 23 kg)
- Obese women: 25 to 42 lb (11.5 to 19 kg)

The adolescent should gain in the upper part of the range currently recommended for adult women.

The pattern of weight gain is also important. The general recommendation is that women gain up to 4.4 lb (2 kg) during the first trimester and approximately 1 lb (0.44 kg) per week during the rest of pregnancy. Nausea and vomiting and some transient food dislikes often limit weight gain or cause weight loss during the first trimester, but the weight is usually regained when the gastrointestinal upsets subside.

Women often want to know why they should gain so much weight when their infant weighs only 7 or 8 lb. The nurse can use the distribution of weight gain during pregnancy shown in Table 4-4 to teach women about all the factors that contribute to weight gain.

Table **4-4** Distribution of Weight Gain in Pregnancy

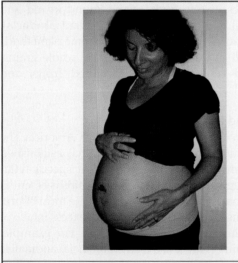

SOURCE OF WEIGHT GAIN	WEIGHT GAIN IN LB (kg)
Uterus	2.5 (1.1)
Fetus	7.0-7.5 (3.2-3.4)
Placenta	1.0-1.5 (0.5-0.7)
Amniotic fluid	2.0 (0.9)
Breasts	1.5-3.0 (0.7-1.4)
Blood volume	3.5-4.0 (1.6-1.8)
Extravascular fluids	3.5-5.0 (1.6-2.3)
Maternal reserves	4.0-9.5 (1.8-4.3)
Total	**25.0-35.0 (11.4-15.9)**

Data from Gabbe SG et al: *Obstetrics: normal and problem pregnancies*, ed 6, Philadelphia, 2012, Saunders.

NUTRITIONAL REQUIREMENTS DURING PREGNANCY

A calorie increase of about 300 kcal/day is recommended to provide for the growth of the fetus, the placenta, amniotic fluid, and maternal tissues; 300 kcal is not a large increase. A banana, a carrot, a piece of whole wheat bread, and a glass of low-fat milk total about 300 kcal. A half of a roast beef sandwich on whole wheat bread and a fresh green salad added to a healthy diet would also meet the added caloric requirement. Caloric intake must be nutritious to have beneficial effects on pregnancy. Four nutrients are especially important in pregnancy: protein, calcium, iron, and folic acid. The amounts required are specified in Table 4-5.

The pregnant woman should use MyPlate to choose her daily diet. Servings that will supply enough of the additional nutrients needed are presented in Table 4-5.

🍎 Nutrition Considerations

Sample Menu for a Pregnant Woman*

BREAKFAST
Orange juice ($^1/_2$ cup)
Oatmeal ($^1/_2$ cup)
Whole-grain or enriched toast (1 slice)
Peanut butter (2 teaspoons)
Decaffeinated coffee or tea

MIDMORNING SNACK
Apple
High-bran cereal ($^1/_4$ cup)
Nonfat or reduced-fat milk ($^1/_2$ cup)

LUNCH
Turkey (2 oz) sandwich on rye or whole-grain bread with lettuce and tomato and 1 teaspoon of mayonnaise
Green salad
Salad dressing (2 teaspoons)
Fresh peach
Nonfat or low-fat milk (1 cup)

MIDAFTERNOON SNACK
Nonfat or low-fat milk (1 cup)
Graham crackers (4 squares)

DINNER
Baked chicken breast (3 oz)
Baked potato with 2 tablespoons of sour cream
Peas and carrots (½ cup)
Green salad
Salad dressing (2 teaspoons)

EVENING SNACK
Nonfat frozen yogurt (1 cup)
Fresh strawberries

*This menu assumes that the woman is of normal prepregnancy weight, that her weight gain is appropriate, that her activity is moderate, and that she is carrying only one fetus. Changes would be needed for the underweight or overweight woman, the adolescent, or a woman with a multifetal pregnancy.
Modified from Mahan LK, Escott-Stump S, Raymond J: *Krause's food, nutrition, and diet therapy*, ed 13, Philadelphia, 2012, Saunders.

Table 4-5	Daily Food Pattern for Pregnancy
FOOD	**AMOUNT**
Milk, nonfat or low-fat, yogurt, cheese	3-4 cups
Meat (lean), poultry, fish, eggs	2 servings (total 4-6 oz)
Vegetables, cooked or raw: dark green or deep yellow; starchy, including potatoes, dried peas, and beans; all others	3-5 servings, all types, often
Fruits, fresh or canned, dark orange, including apricots, peaches, cantaloupe	2-4 servings, all types, often
Whole-grain and enriched breads and cereals	7 or more servings
Fats and sweets	In moderate amounts
Fluids	8-10 glasses (8 oz)

Modified from Mahan LK, Escott-Stump S, Raymond J: *Krause's food, nutrition, and diet therapy,* ed 13, Philadelphia, 2012, Saunders.

Protein

Added protein is needed for metabolism and to support the growth and repair of maternal and fetal tissues. An intake of 60 g/day is recommended during pregnancy. The best sources of protein are meat, fish, poultry, and dairy products. Beans, lentils, and other legumes; breads and cereals; and seeds and nuts in combination with another plant or animal protein can provide all the amino acids (components of protein) needed.

Examples of complementary plant protein combinations are corn and beans, lentils and rice, and peanut butter and bread. Plant proteins are also complemented with animal proteins, such as in grilled cheese sandwiches, cereal with milk, and chili made of meat and beans. The complementary foods must be eaten together, because all the amino acids necessary for building tissues (essential amino acids) must be present at the same time.

Information about nonmeat sources of protein should be provided to women who are vegetarians to ensure that their protein needs are met. The information can also help reduce the family's food budget, because many plant protein sources are less expensive than animal sources. Fish containing high mercury levels such as albacore tuna and mackerel should be eaten with caution. Raw meat and raw eggs can be contaminated and should be avoided during pregnancy and lactation.

Calcium

Pregnancy and lactation increase calcium requirements by nearly 50%. The dietary reference intake (DRI) of calcium for pregnant women is 1200 mg. Dairy products are the single most plentiful source of this nutrient. Other sources of calcium include enriched cereals, legumes, nuts, dried fruits, broccoli, green leafy vegetables, and canned salmon and sardines that contain bones. Calcium supplements are necessary for women who do not drink milk (or do not eat sufficient amounts of equivalent products). Supplements are also necessary for women younger than 25 years of age, because their bone density is not complete. Calcium supplements should be taken separately from iron supplements for best absorption. An adequate intake of vitamin D is required to enhance calcium absorption.

Iron

Pregnancy causes a heavy demand for iron, because the fetus must store an adequate supply to meet the needs in the first 3 to 6 months after birth. In addition, the pregnant woman increases her production of erythrocytes. The DRI is 15 mg/day for nonpregnant adult women and 30 mg/day for pregnant women. Women who have a known iron deficiency may need more.

It is difficult to obtain this much iron from the diet alone, and most health care providers prescribe iron supplements of 30 mg/day beginning in the second trimester, after morning sickness decreases. Taking the iron on an empty stomach improves absorption, but many women find it difficult to tolerate without food. It should not be taken with coffee or tea or with high-calcium foods such as milk. Vitamin C (ascorbic acid) may enhance iron absorption (Mahan and Escott-Stump, 2012).

Iron comes in two forms, *heme* (found in red and organ meats) and *nonheme* (found in plant products). The body absorbs heme iron best. Nonheme plant foods that are high in iron include molasses, whole grains, iron-fortified cereals and breads, dried fruits, and dark-green, leafy vegetables.

Vitamins and Minerals

True vitamin deficiency is rare in North America. The Food and Nutrition Board of the IOM has established dietary recommended intakes (DRIs) of specific vitamins. Although adequate intake of vitamins is essential during pregnancy, and supplements in the form of prenatal vitamins are routinely prescribed, excess intake of some vitamins can result in problems. For example, excess vitamin A can cause fetal craniofacial anomalies and cardiac defects, and intake should not exceed 3000 mcg/day. Vitamin B[6] (pyridoxine) is often prescribed to reduce the nausea of pregnancy, but excess intake can cause numbness and nerve damage. An adequate intake of zinc is required during pregnancy especially in vegetarians and vegan diets, because whole grains decrease zinc absorption. Copper and zinc are part of the prenatal vitamin formula. Most vitamins essential during pregnancy are part of the prenatal vitamin supplement prescribed for pregnant women. Folates are essential in early pregnancy to prevent neural tube defects but are prescribed separately from the prenatal vitamin, because the amount needed cannot be achieved in the prenatal formula. Iron should be taken between meals if possible and with orange juice or a source of vitamin C to enhance absorption. Iron and calcium should not be taken together at the same time. Women should be referred for guidance from a Registered Dietician if they have multiple gestations, an eating disorder, or a restricted diet such as vegan or vegetarian.

 Nutrition Considerations

Vitamin B$_6$ and ginger are often recommended to relieve the common discomfort of nausea during pregnancy.

Folic Acid

Folic acid (folacin or folate) is a water-soluble B vitamin essential for the formation and maturation of both red and white blood cells in bone marrow. This vitamin can also reduce the incidence of neural tube defects such as spina bifida and anencephaly *when taken at conception,* and supplementation for 3 months before pregnancy may prevent autism (Lockwood, 2013). The DRI for a pregnant woman is 400 mcg (0.4 mg) per day. Food sources of folic acid are liver, lean beef, kidney and lima beans, dried beans, potatoes, whole-wheat bread, peanuts, and fresh, dark-green, leafy vegetables. Folic acid supplements in nonpregnant women have shown to be of value in decreasing cervical dysplasia and bacterial vaginosis. However, supplementation beyond 1000 mcg per day is associated with the development of insulin resistance, obesity, and allergic asthma (Simmons, 2013). Folic acid can also negatively interact with drugs such as methotrexate and antimalarial drugs (Lucock, 2009). Folic acid supplements, although essential during pregnancy, should be used with care to prevent negative effects in nonpregnant women.

Fluids

The pregnant woman should drink 8 to 10 8-oz glasses of fluid each day, most of which should be water. Caffeinated drinks and drinks high in sugar should be limited. Caffeine acts as a diuretic, which counteracts some of the benefit of the fluid intake. The woman should limit her daily caffeine consumption to two cups of coffee or their equivalent. Women at risk for insufficient amniotic fluid (oligohydramnios) have had successful outcomes by increasing their daily fluid intake (Gabbe, 2012).

Sodium

In the past, sodium intake of pregnant women was restricted in an attempt to prevent edema and gestational hypertension. However, sodium intake is essential for maintaining normal sodium levels in plasma, bone, brain, and muscle, because both tissue and fluid expand during the prenatal period. Sodium should not be restricted during pregnancy, but foods high in sodium, such as lunchmeats and chips, should be avoided during pregnancy.

Diuretics to rid the body of excess fluids are not recommended for the healthy pregnant woman, because they reduce fluids necessary for the fetus. The added fluid during pregnancy supports the mother's increased blood volume.

Special Nutrition Considerations

Pregnant Adolescent. *Gynecological age* is the number of years between the onset of menses and the date of conception. The adolescent who conceives soon after having her first period has greater nutritional needs than one who is more sexually mature. The nurse must consider the adolescent's characteristics of resistance, ambivalence, and inconsistency when planning nutritional interventions (see Chapter 20). The nurse must also remember that the girl's peer group is of utmost importance to her and should help the adolescent find nutritious foods that allow her to fit in with her friends.

Inadequate weight gain and nutrient deficits are more likely to occur in the pregnant adolescent. The girl's continuing growth plus the growth of the fetus may make it difficult for her to meet her nutritional needs. In addition, a body image in which she sees herself as "fat" at a time when appearance is a high priority, combined with peer pressure to eat "junk" foods, places the pregnant adolescent at special risk.

Even a moderate positive change in diet helps, and the nurse should give the girl positive reinforcement for her efforts. Fast foods with poor nutritional content are often the adolescent's foods of choice. However, the nurse can point out to the adolescent that many fast food restaurants offer salads, chicken, tacos, baked potatoes, and pizza. These foods provide many important nutrients and still allow her to socialize with her peers at mealtimes.

Nutritional intervention is necessary early in prenatal care to ensure a healthy mother and child. The younger and smaller teenage adolescent may need an additional 200 kcal/day in addition to the recommended increase of about 300 kcal/day for a normal pregnancy to meet her own growth needs and those of the developing fetus. Many communities offer programs for adolescents that provide social support, education about prenatal care, and nutritional advice. Adolescents often respond well in these peer groups. The nurse often refers these young women to programs such as Women, Infants, and Children (WIC) and food-stamp programs if needed.

Vegetarian or Vegan Diets. Women who follow vegetarian or vegan diets should focus on protein-rich foods such as soy milk, tofu, tempeh, and beans, and they should supplement the diet with prenatal vitamins to meet the dietary needs of pregnancy. See www.fda.gov concerning dietary guidelines for vegetarian/vegan diets.

Pica. The craving for and ingestion of nonfood substances such as clay, starch, raw flour, and cracked ice is called *pica.* Ingestion of small amounts of these substances may be harmless, but frequent ingestion in large amounts may cause significant health problems. Starch can interfere with iron absorption, and large amounts of clay may cause fecal impaction. Any other nonfood substance ingested in large quantities may be harmful, because the necessary nutrients for healthy fetal development will not be available.

Pica is a difficult habit to break, and the nurse often becomes aware of the practice when discussing nutrition, food cravings, and myths with the pregnant woman. The nurse should educate the pregnant woman in a nonjudgmental way about the importance of good nutrition so the pica habit can be eliminated or at least decreased.

Lactose Intolerance. Intolerance to lactose is caused by a deficiency of lactase, the enzyme that digests the sugar in milk. Some women cannot digest milk or milk products, which increases their risk for calcium deficiency. Native Americans, Latinos, and persons of African, Middle Eastern, and Asian descent have a higher incidence of lactose intolerance than Caucasians. Signs and symptoms of lactose intolerance include abdominal distention, flatulence, nausea, vomiting, and loose stools after ingestion of dairy products. In such cases, a daily calcium supplement can be taken.

Substitutes for dairy products are listed in the section on calcium. Lactose-intolerant women may tolerate cultured or fermented milk products such as aged cheese, buttermilk, and yogurt. The enzyme lactase (LactAid) is available in tablet form or as a liquid to add to milk. Lactase-treated milk is also available commercially and can be used under a physician's direction.

Cultural Preferences. People of varied cultures believe that specific foods include a dominant trait that affects the "humoral balance" in the body when ingested. Classification of food as "hot" or "cold" has nothing to do with the actual temperature. Examples of hot foods include peanuts, mangoes, ice cream, tea, cereal grains, and hard liquor. Examples of cold foods include milk, green leafy vegetables, freshwater fish, chicken, bananas, and citrus fruits. In this belief framework, several health problems are classified as hot or cold, requiring a cold or hot food for balance.

To support the nutritional needs of patients from various cultures, teachings must include these cultural beliefs and practices. See Chapter 15 for more details concerning food and culture.

Gestational Diabetes Mellitus. Gestational diabetes mellitus is first diagnosed during pregnancy rather than being present before pregnancy (see Chapter 5). Calories should be evenly distributed during the day among three meals and three snacks to maintain adequate and stable blood glucose levels. Pregnant diabetic women are susceptible to hypoglycemia (low blood glucose level) during the night, because the fetus continues to use glucose while the mother sleeps. It is suggested that the final bedtime snack be one of protein and a complex carbohydrate to provide more blood glucose stability. A registered dietitian may supervise

dietary management. Glycemic control during the first and second trimesters is most important in preventing complications such as macrosomia (abnormally large newborn). Women with uncontrolled diabetes and fasting blood glucose levels greater than 500 mg/dL in the last trimester have an increased risk of stillbirth.

NUTRITIONAL REQUIREMENTS DURING LACTATION

The caloric intake during lactation should be about 500 calories more than the nonpregnant woman's RDA. An indicator of adequate caloric intake is a stable maternal weight and a gradually increasing infant weight. The maternal protein intake should be 65 mg/day so the growing infant has adequate protein. Calcium intake and iron intake are the same as during pregnancy to allow for the infant's demand on the mother's supply. Vitamin supplements are often continued during lactation. Fluids sufficient to relieve thirst and replace fluids lost via breastfeeding should be taken. Drinking 8 to 10 glasses of liquids other than those containing caffeine is adequate.

Some foods should be omitted during lactation if they cause gastric upset in the mother or child. The mother will often identify foods that seem to upset her child. Caffeine should be restricted to the equivalent of two cups of coffee each day. Lactating mothers should be instructed that many types of drugs she may take can be secreted in varying amounts in the breast milk. Drugs should be taken only with the health care provider's advice. Alcohol intake should be restricted to an occasional single serving for breastfeeding women.

EXERCISE DURING PREGNANCY

There is evidence that mild to moderate exercise is beneficial during normal pregnancy, but vigorous exercise should be avoided. The nurse should guide the patient concerning exercise during pregnancy based on the understanding that the maternal circulatory system is the lifeline to the fetus, and any alteration can affect the growth and survival of the fetus. The maternal cardiac status and fetoplacental reserve should be the basis for determining exercise levels during all trimesters of pregnancy. Current health and fitness lifestyles mandate the inclusion of information concerning exercise during pregnancy in prenatal education programs (Lewis et al, 2008).

A history of the exercise practices of the patient is important, and gathering such data is the first step in the nursing process. Women who have had previous training may have a higher tolerance for exercise than women who have led a sedentary lifestyle. The goal of exercise during pregnancy should be *maintenance* of fitness, not improvement of fitness or weight loss (Figure 4-9). The following are some basic factors that should be evaluated and discussed.

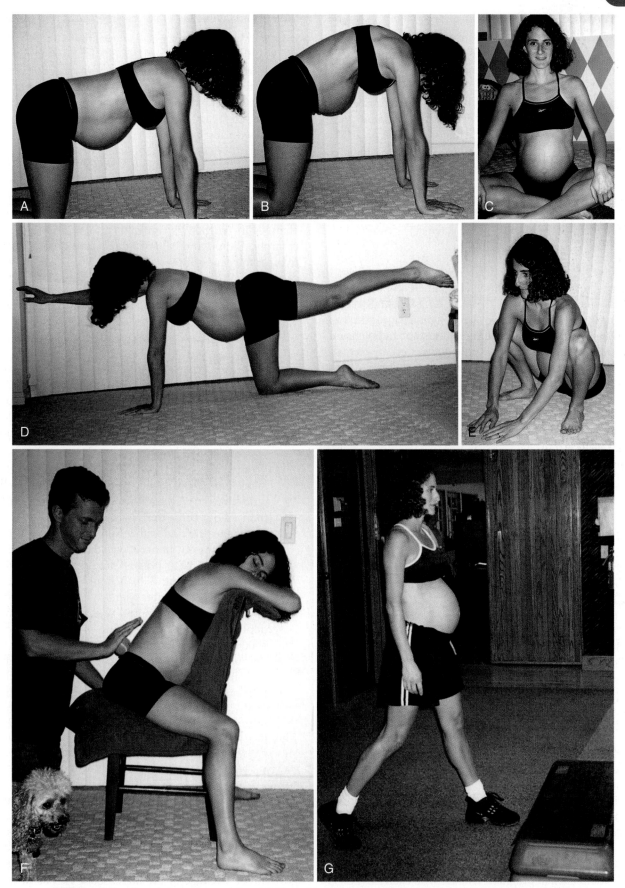

FIGURE 4-9 Exercises during pregnancy. **A** and **B,** The pelvic tilt. **C,** Tailor sitting position. **D,** Proper stretch position. **E,** Proper squat position. **F,** Back massage with a tennis ball used as pressure. **G,** A pregnant woman participating in step aerobics class for moderate exercise.

ELEVATED TEMPERATURE

Exercise can elevate the maternal temperature and result in decreased fetal circulation and cardiac function. Maternal body temperature should not exceed 38° C (100.4° F), which rules out the use of hot tubs and saunas during pregnancy. Maternal heat exposure during the first trimester of pregnancy has been associated with neural tube defects and miscarriage (Lewis et al, 2008). Exercise-related increases in body temperature are somewhat more easily tolerated because of the normal physiology of pregnancy as it pertains to increased peripheral blood flow, thermal inertia from weight gain, and peripheral venous pooling. Monitoring the body temperature in addition to the exercise intensity is essential.

HYPOTENSION

When the flat supine position is assumed and the uterus presses on the vena cava, the increasing size and weight of the uterus can cause poor venous return and result in supine hypotension syndrome. Orthostatic hypotension can also reduce blood flow to the fetus. Certain exercise positions may need to be modified during pregnancy to avoid these problems, which can cause fetal hypoxia.

CARDIAC OUTPUT

Pregnancy increases the workload of the heart. The increase in peripheral pooling during pregnancy results in a decrease in cardiac output reserves for exercise. When exercise is allowed to exceed the ability of the cardiovascular system to respond, blood may be diverted from the uterus, causing fetal hypoxia. Exercise increases catecholamine levels, which the placenta may not be able to filter, resulting in fetal bradycardia and hypoxia. Strenuous and prolonged exercise causes blood flow to be distributed to the skeletal muscles and skin and away from the viscera, uterus, and placenta. If the reduction in uterine blood flow exceeds 50%, serious adverse effects to the fetus may occur. For this reason, moderate exercise is preferred for pregnant women as opposed to strenuous or prolonged exercise. Exercise increases maternal hematocrit levels and uterine oxygen uptake, so moderate exercise will not cause decreased oxygen supplies to the fetus.

HORMONES

Exercise can cause changes in oxygen consumption and epinephrine, glucagon, cortisol, prolactin, and endorphin levels. In early pregnancy these hormonal changes can negatively affect implantation of the zygote and vascularization of the uterus. In late pregnancy the increases in catecholamines during exercise can trigger labor. However, studies have not shown increased rates of preterm deliveries in pregnant women who exercise (Lewis et al, 2008). Joint instability caused by hormonal changes can result in injury if the woman engages in deep flexion or extension of joints. Range of motion (ROM) should not extend beyond prepregnancy abilities.

OTHER FACTORS

In general, moderate exercise several times a week from the eighth week through delivery is advised during pregnancy, with avoidance of vigorous activity and competitive sports. Moderate exercise during pregnancy has many beneficial effects including a more positive self-image, a decrease in musculoskeletal discomforts during pregnancy, and a more rapid return to prepregnant weight after delivery (Lewis et al, 2008). The American Diabetes Association supports moderate exercise during pregnancy. Even the trained woman should avoid vigorous exercise in hot, humid weather. Safety measures are advisable because of the changes in the body's center of gravity as the uterus enlarges. Liquid and calorie intake should be adjusted to meet the needs of pregnancy as well as the demands of exercise. Women who have complications or medical conditions such as hypertension or multiple gestations should consult a health care provider before engaging in any exercise program during pregnancy.

Nursing guidance should include the following:

- The woman should start with a warm-up and end with a cool-down period.
- Women who are beginning an exercise program should not exceed the American Congress of Obstetricians and Gynecologists (ACOG, 2007) recommendations for moderate exercise, which was reaffirmed in 2011.
- Women who have exercised regularly at higher levels before pregnancy may follow more liberal guidelines of weight-bearing exercise for no more than 1 hour three to five times a week.
- Exercise combined with a balanced diet that is rich in unprocessed, nonroot vegetables, nuts, fruits, and whole-grain breads are beneficial during pregnancy. Eating 2 to 3 hours before exercise and immediately after exercise is recommended.
- The woman should avoid scuba diving below a depth of 30 feet or exercising in altitudes above 8000 feet during pregnancy.
- The woman should avoid becoming overheated and should drink plenty of water during exercise.
- Intensity of exercise should be modified according to the "talk test" (should be able to complete a conversational sentence without taking an extra breath).

TRAVEL DURING PREGNANCY

Many women choose to maintain a normal lifestyle and travel during a normal pregnancy. Air travel is generally safe for the pregnant woman up to 36 weeks gestation, but the availability of medical care at the destination should be checked online at www.cdc. gov/travel. Because of the increased levels of clotting factors and plasma fibrinogen that normally occur during pregnancy, the woman should be counseled to avoid long periods of sitting, because there is an increased risk of developing thromboembolism

(Gabbe, 2012). She should also avoid locations that pose a high risk for exposure to infectious diseases. A copy of obstetric records should be taken, and the location of medical facilities in the area to be visited should be identified. For more information concerning air travel during pregnancy, consult www.ACOG.org/Resources_And_Publications/Committee_opinions/committee-on-obstetric-practice/air-travel-during-pregnancy.

Guidance concerning hand hygiene and dietary precautions to prevent diarrhea are essential. If needed, special oral rehydration solutions may be available, or bottled drinks may provide the fluid, sugar, and electrolytes needed. Until medical attention is available, the WHO recommends an oral rehydration drink formula combining 1 L of water, 1 teaspoon of salt, 4 teaspoons of cream of tartar, $^1/_2$ teaspoon of baking soda, and 4 tablespoons of sugar (CDC, 2010). The woman should be advised to wear comfortable shoes and long-sleeved clothing and use mosquito nets around the bed in insect-prone areas. Insect repellants that contain the chemical abbreviated as *DEET* are usually safe after the first trimester. Sunblock should be applied as appropriate.

COMMON DISCOMFORTS IN PREGNANCY

Various discomforts occur during normal pregnancy as a result of physiological changes. The nurse should teach the woman measures to relieve these discomforts (Table 4-6). The nurse should also explain signs of problems that can be confused with the normal discomforts

Table 4-6   Self-Care for Common Discomforts of Pregnancy

DISCOMFORT	INFLUENCING FACTORS	SELF-CARE MEASURES
First Trimester		
Nausea with or without vomiting	Elevation in hormones, decrease in gastric motility, fatigue, emotional factors; usually does not last beyond 16 weeks; if vomiting persists, may lead to hyperemesis gravidarum	Avoid an empty stomach. Eat dry crackers or toast ½ to 1 hour before rising in the morning. Eat small, frequent meals. Drink fluids between meals. Avoid greasy, odorous, spicy, or gas-forming foods. Increase vitamin B_6.
Breast tenderness	Increased vascular supply and hypertrophy of breast tissue caused by estrogen and progesterone. Results in tingling, fullness, and tenderness	Wear a supportive bra (to alleviate tingling and tenderness). Avoid soap to the nipples (to prevent cracking).
Urinary frequency	Pressure of growing uterus on bladder in both first and third trimesters. Progesterone relaxes smooth muscles of bladder	Void when urge is felt (to prevent urinary stasis); increase fluid intake during day. Decrease fluid in late evening to lessen nocturia; limit caffeine. Practice Kegel exercises.
Vaginal discharge (leukorrhea)	Increased production of mucus by endocervical glands in response to elevated estrogen levels and increased blood supply to the pelvic area, causing white, viscid vaginal discharge	Bathe or shower daily. Wear cotton underwear. Avoid tight undergarments and pantyhose. Keep the perineal area clean and dry. Avoid douching and using tampons. Wipe the perineal area from front to back after toileting. Contact health care provider if there is a change in color, odor, or character of discharge.
Second and Third Trimesters		
Heartburn (pyrosis)	Increased production of progesterone, causing relaxation of esophageal sphincter. Regurgitation or backflow of gastric contents into the esophagus, causing burning sensation behind the sternum, burping, and sour tastes in mouth	Sit up for 30 min after eating a meal. Avoid gas-forming and greasy foods. Avoid overeating. Use low-sodium liquid antacids such as Gelusil or Maalox (liquid will coat lining better than tablets); avoid sodium bicarbonate and Alka Seltzer.
Constipation and flatulence (gas)	Increased levels of progesterone, causing bowel sluggishness with increased water absorption (results in hardened stool). Pressure of enlarging uterus on intestine. Diet, lack of exercise, and decreased fluids. Iron supplements contributing to hardening of stools	Increase fluid intake (a minimum of 8 glasses per day, not including carbonated or caffeinated beverages because of their diuretic effect), roughage in diet, and exercise. Exercise to stimulate peristalsis. Establish regular schedule for bowel movement. Do not take mineral oil or enemas. Consult health care provider about taking a stool softener (docusate).

Continued

Table 4-6	Self-Care for Common Discomforts of Pregnancy—cont'd

DISCOMFORT	INFLUENCING FACTORS	SELF-CARE MEASURES
Second and Third Trimesters—cont'd		
Hemorrhoids	Varicosities (distended veins) of rectum caused by vascular enlargement of pelvis, straining from constipation, and descent of fetal head into pelvis May disappear after birth, when pressure is relieved	Use anesthetic ointment, cool witch hazel pads, or rectal suppositories. May disappear after birth, when pressure is relieved Take sitz baths, increase fiber in diet, and have regular bowel habits to avoid constipation.
Backaches	Result of the spine's adaptation to posture changes as the uterus enlarges Enlarging uterus altering center of gravity, resulting in lordosis (exaggeration of lumbosacral curve) and muscle strain	Maintain correct posture with head up and shoulders back; use good body mechanics. Avoid exaggerating lumbar curve. Squat rather than bending over when picking up objects (bend at knees, not waist). Wear low-heeled shoes to help maintain better posture. Do exercises such as tailor sitting (cross-legged), shoulder circling, and pelvic rocking. Rest; applying localized heat may help.
Round ligament pain	Abdominal ligaments stretched by enlarging uterus, causing pain in lower abdomen after sudden movements	Avoid jerky or quick movements. Use pillow support for abdomen. Use good body mechanics.
Leg cramps	Pressure of uterus on blood vessels that impairs circulation to legs, causing muscle strain and fatigue Imbalance in the calcium/phosphorus ratio	Dorsiflex foot and straighten leg with downward pressure on knee or stand with feet flat on floor when cramps occur (see Figure 5-7). Evaluate diet and calcium intake.
Headache	Emotional tension and fatigue Increased circulatory blood volume and heart rate causing dilation and distention of cerebral vessels	Obtain emotional support. Practice relaxation exercises. Eat regular meals. If headaches continue, report to caregiver (potential gestational hypertension).
Varicose veins	Relaxation of smooth muscle in walls of veins caused by elevated progesterone Pressure of enlarging uterus causing pressure on veins, resulting in development of varicosities in vulva, rectum, and legs	Avoid lengthy standing or sitting, constrictive clothing, and bearing down during bowel movements. Walk frequently. Rest with legs elevated. Wear support stockings; avoid tight knee-highs. Exercise (to stimulate venous return). Relieve hemorrhoid swelling with warm sitz baths, local application of astringent compresses, or analgesic ointment.
Edema of feet and ankles	Circulatory congestion of lower extremities	Elevate legs when sitting. Increase rest periods. Avoid constrictive clothing and prolonged standing or sitting.
Faintness and dizziness	Vasomotor instability or postural hypotension Standing for long periods with venous stasis in lower extremities	Avoid sudden changes in position, prolonged standing, and warm crowded areas. Move slowly from rest position. Avoid hypoglycemia by eating 4-5 small meals daily. Lie on left side when resting to avoid supine hypotensive syndrome (pressure of uterus on vena cava). If symptoms do not lessen, report to caregiver.
Fatigue	Hormonal changes in early pregnancy and periodic hypoglycemia as glucose is used by embryo for rapid growth More prominent in early months of pregnancy	Try to get 8-10 hours of sleep. Take naps during the day if possible. Use relaxation techniques, meditation, or change of scenery.
Dyspnea	Later in pregnancy, caused by uterus rising into abdomen and pressing on diaphragm	Sleep with several pillows under head. Use deep chest breathing before going to sleep. Use proper posture while sitting or standing. Avoid exertion.

of pregnancy. Providing information written in the woman's primary language gives her a reference if she has questions later.

Water aerobics in healthy women can relieve edema, because the hydrostatic pressure forces fluid into the circulation, stimulating glomerular filtration and excretion of water. Care should be taken to avoid excessive water temperatures during water aerobics (see Exercise during Pregnancy on p. 64). Using saline nasal drops or room humidifiers can relieve nasal stuffiness caused by edema of nasal tissues as a result of the high level of estrogen.

PSYCHOSOCIAL ADAPTATION TO PREGNANCY

Pregnancy creates a variety of confusing feelings for all members of the family, whether or not the pregnancy was planned. Both parents may feel ambivalence about the pregnancy and being a parent. First-time parents may be anxious about how the infant will affect their relationship as a couple. Parents who already have a child may wonder how they can stretch their energies, love, and finances to another infant and how the infant will affect their older child or children. The nurse who provides prenatal care helps families to work through this phase in their lives. Identifying and managing psychosocial problems is essential to the positive outcome of pregnancy.

Identifying barriers to accessing care is a primary nursing responsibility. Inadequate health insurance coverage, financial problems, knowledge deficit concerning community resources, lack of transportation, and the need for day care for other children or older adult parents are examples of problems that can be referred to a social service worker. Frequent housing relocation may indicate domestic violence, legal problems, or financial difficulties that may need attention to ensure compliance with regular prenatal care. Nutritional needs and patterns relating to age, ethnicity, or financial constraints should be discussed. Tobacco or substance abuse should be assessed. Stress in the life of the mother should be reviewed, and appropriate referrals to mental health professionals or educational programs should be made to reduce the levels of stress that can affect pregnancy outcome.

IMPACT ON THE MOTHER

In 1984, researcher Reva Rubin noted four maternal tasks that the woman accomplishes during pregnancy as she becomes a mother:

1. Seeking safe passage for herself and her fetus: This involves both obtaining health care by a professional and adhering to important cultural practices.
2. Securing acceptance of herself as a mother and for her fetus: Will her partner accept the infant? Does her partner or family have strong preferences for a child of a particular sex? Will the child be accepted even if he or she does not fit the ideal?
3. Learning to give of self and to receive the care and concern of others: The woman will never again be the same carefree girl she was before her infant's arrival. She depends on others in ways she has not experienced before.
4. Committing herself to the child as she progresses through pregnancy: Much of the emotional work of pregnancy involves protecting and nurturing the fetus.

Pregnancy is more than a physical event in a woman's life. During the months of pregnancy, she first accepts the fetus as part of herself and gradually moves to acceptance of the child as an independent person. She evolves from being a pregnant woman to being a mother. The woman's responses change as pregnancy progresses. These changes will be discussed here within the framework of the three trimesters of pregnancy.

First Trimester

The woman may have difficulty believing that she is pregnant during early pregnancy, because she may not feel different. If a home pregnancy test was positive, the woman often feels "more pregnant" after a professional confirms it. An early sonography examination helps the woman to see the reality of the developing fetus within her. Women (and their partners) often show off their sonogram photos just as they will show their infant pictures later.

Most women have conflicting feelings about being pregnant (*ambivalence*) during the early weeks. Many, if not most, pregnancies are unplanned. The parents may have wanted to wait longer so they could achieve career or educational goals or to have longer spacing between children. Women who planned their pregnancies, or even worked hard to overcome infertility, also feel ambivalence. They wonder if they have done the right thing and at the right time. Moreover, the woman often feels that she should not have these conflicting feelings. The nurse can help the woman to express these feelings of ambivalence and reassure her that they are normal.

The woman focuses on herself during this time. She feels many new physical sensations, but none of them seem related to a child. These physical changes and the higher hormone levels cause her emotions to be more unstable (*labile*). The nurse can reassure the woman and her partner (who is often confused by her moods) about the cause of these fluctuations, that they are normal, and that they will stabilize after pregnancy.

Second Trimester

The fetus becomes real to the woman during the second trimester. Her weight increases, and the uterus becomes obvious as it ascends into the abdomen. If she has not already heard the fetal heartbeat or seen it beating on a sonogram, the woman usually will have an opportunity to hear it early in the second trimester. She feels fetal movement, and this is a powerful aid in helping her to distinguish the fetus as a separate person from herself.

The second trimester is a more stable time of pregnancy during which most women have resolved many of their earlier feelings of ambivalence and begin to take on the role of an expectant mother. The woman becomes totally involved with her developing child and her changing body image *(narcissism)*. She often devotes a great deal of time to selecting just the right foods and the best environment to promote her health and that of her infant. She welcomes the solicitous concern of others when they caution her not to pick up a heavy package or work too hard. She may lose interest in work or other activities as she devotes herself to the project of nurturing her fetus. The nurse can take advantage of her heightened interest in healthful living to teach good nutrition and other habits that can benefit the woman and her family long after the child is born.

The woman "tries on" the role of mother by learning what infants are like. She wants to hear stories of what she and her mate were like when they were infants. She often fantasizes about how her child will look and behave or what sex the child will be. She may or may not want to know the sex of the infant if it is apparent on a sonogram, sometimes preferring to be surprised at the birth. The woman who previously has had a child undergoes a similar transition as she imagines what this specific child will be like and how he or she will compare to any siblings.

The body changes resulting from pregnancy become evident during the second trimester. The woman may welcome them as a sign to all that her fetus is well protected and thriving (Figure 4-10). However, these same changes may be unwelcome to her, because they can be perceived as unattractive and can cause discomfort.

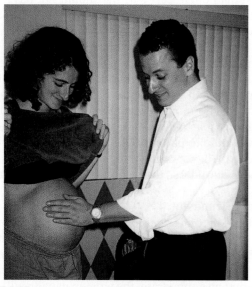

FIGURE 4-10 The body changes during pregnancy are evident, and the woman may welcome them as a sign to all that her pregnancy is real and her fetus is thriving.

The body changes may alter her sexual relationship with her partner as well. Both partners may fear harming the developing fetus, particularly if there has been a previous miscarriage. Her increasing size, discomforts, and the other changes of pregnancy may make one or both partners have less interest in intercourse. The nurse can assure them that these changes are temporary and can help them explore other expressions of love and caring.

Third Trimester

As her body changes even more dramatically, a woman alternates between feeling "absolutely beautiful and productive" and feeling "as big as a house and totally unloved" by her partner. These mood swings reflect her sense of increased vulnerability and dependence on her partner. She becomes introspective about the challenge of labor that is ahead and its outcome. Her moods may again be more labile.

The woman begins to separate herself from the pregnancy and to commit herself to the care of an infant. She and her partner begin making concrete preparations for the infant's arrival. They buy clothes and equipment the infant will need. Many take childbirth preparation classes. The woman's thinking gradually shifts from "I am pregnant" to "I am going to be a mother."

The minor discomforts of pregnancy become tiresome during the last weeks before delivery, and the woman may feel that the pregnancy will never end. With the understanding and support of her family and health care professionals, she can develop inner strength to accomplish the tasks of birth.

IMPACT ON THE FATHER

Responses of fathers vary widely. Some want to be fully involved in the physical and emotional aspects of pregnancy. Others prefer a management role, helping the woman adhere to recommendations of her physician or nurse-midwife. Some fathers want to "be there" for the woman, but prefer not to take an active role during pregnancy or birth. Cultural values influence the role of fathers, because pregnancy and birth are viewed exclusively as women's work in some cultures. The nurse should not assume that a father is disinterested if he takes a less active role in pregnancy and birth.

Fathers go through phases similar to those of expectant mothers. Pregnancy is considered the beginning of a separate developmental stage called "Growth and Development of a Parent" (see Table 15-5). Fathers who do not anticipate changes specific to the normal event of pregnancy may be confused or concerned by new feelings or behaviors and the changes that occur in family dynamics.

For fathers, the announcement phase begins when pregnancy is confirmed. Initially they may also have difficulty perceiving the fetus as real. Ambivalence and self-questioning about their readiness for fatherhood are typical. Fathers who attend prenatal appointments

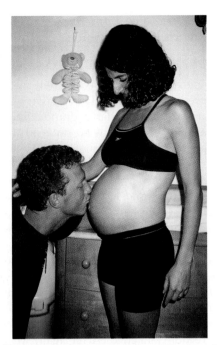

FIGURE 4-11 The father begins to develop a relationship with the fetus as he hears the fetal heartbeat and feels fetal movement.

Box 4-4	Developmental Stages of Fatherhood

- Announcement
- Adjustment
- Focus

with the woman can see the fetus on ultrasound or hear the fetal heartbeat, making the child seem more like a real person (Figure 4-11). Acceptance of the pregnancy results in strengthening of the family support system and expansion of the social network. Rejection of the pregnancy may result in lack of communication and resentment.

The second phase of the father's response is the adjustment phase. The father may revise financial plans, become involved in planning the child's room or furniture, and actively listen to the fetal heartbeat and feel fetal movement (see Figure 4-11). Lack of adjustment may result in an increase in outside interests or the development of various symptoms in a struggle to regain the attention he may feel he has lost to the fetus.

The third phase of the father's response is the focus phase, where active plans for participation in the labor process, birth, and change in lifestyle result in the partner "feeling like a father" (Box 4-4). The nurse's role is to help the father achieve positive outcomes in each phase (see Table 4-7 on pp. 73–75).

The father is often asked to provide emotional support to his partner while struggling himself with the issue of fatherhood. Too often, he receives the message that his only job is to support the pregnant woman rather than to be a parent who is also important and who has needs. The nurse should explore the father's feelings and encourage him during prenatal appointments, childbirth preparation classes, and labor and birth. He is trying to learn the role of father, just as the woman is trying to learn the role of mother. Documenting the health history of the father is important, because health problems such as genetic disorders, chronic illness, or lifestyle practices such as drug abuse, tobacco use, etc., can adversely affect the health of the mother, infant, or family. The father's blood type and Rh is also important when the mother is Rh negative.

IMPACT ON THE PREGNANT ADOLESCENT

Pregnant adolescents often have to struggle with feelings they find difficult to express. They are fraught with conflict about how to handle an unplanned pregnancy. Initially, they must face the anxiety of breaking the news to their parents and to the father of the child. Denial of the pregnancy until late in gestation is not uncommon. There may be financial problems, shame, guilt, relationship problems with the infant's father, and feelings of low self-esteem. Alcoholism and substance abuse may be a part of the complex picture.

The nurse must assess the girl's developmental and educational level and her support system to best provide care for her. A critical variable is the girl's age. Young adolescents have difficulty considering the needs of others, such as the fetus. The nurse helps the adolescent girl to complete the developmental tasks of adolescence while assuming the new role of motherhood. Ideally, separate prenatal classes tailored to their needs help adolescent girls learn to care for themselves and assume the role of mother.

The nurse must anticipate resistive behavior, ambivalence, and inconsistency in the adolescent. The nurse must consider the girl's developmental level and the priorities typical of her age, such as the importance of her peer group, focus on appearance, and difficulty considering the needs of others. The pregnant adolescent must cope with two of life's most stress-laden transitions simultaneously: adolescence and parenthood.

IMPACT ON THE OLDER COUPLE

Women who become pregnant for the first time after age 35 years are described as "elderly primips" or "advanced maternal age," because they are at a later stage in their childbearing cycle, and they may face special problems during pregnancy and labor. Many factors contribute to the trend of postponing pregnancy until after age 35 years:

- Effective birth control alternatives
- Increasing career options for women
- High cost of living (delays childbearing until financial status is secure)
- Development of fertilization techniques to enable later pregnancy

The "older couple" usually adjusts readily to pregnancy, because they are often well educated, have achieved life experiences that enable them to cope with the realities of parenthood, and are ready for the lifestyle change. Although the older couple may adjust to the process of pregnancy and parenthood, they may find themselves "different" from their peers, and this can result in impaired social interaction. Concerns of the older parent relate to age and energy level as the child grows, confronting the issues of their own mortality, and child care requirements. Meeting financial needs of a college-age child at retirement is a special issue that may require discussion and planning. Many older parents are placed in a "high-risk" prenatal group that may limit their options for selecting a birth center. However, the pregnancy should be treated as normal unless problems are identified.

Advances in maternal care and delivery practices have decreased the risk of unfavorable pregnancy outcomes, although special problems exist. Women greater than 35 years of age may have a decreased ability to adjust their uterine blood flow to meet the needs of the fetus (Creasy et al, 2009). There also may be an increase in multiple pregnancies if fertility drugs were used, which increases fetal risk. The increased risk of a congenital anomaly usually results in the offering of special tests during pregnancy (chorionic villi sampling, amniocentesis), which increases the cost factor of prenatal care.

IMPACT ON THE SINGLE MOTHER

Whether an adolescent or a mature woman, the single mother has special emotional needs. Some single mothers can turn to their parents, siblings, or close friends for support. Women who do not have emotional support from significant others will have more difficulty completing the tasks of pregnancy. Their uncertainty in day-to-day living competes with mastering the emotional tasks of pregnancy.

Some single mothers may have conceived by in vitro fertilization because of a strong desire to have a child even in the absence of a stable relationship. These women often are nearing the end of their childbearing years and perceive a "now or never" view of motherhood. Single women who plan pregnancies often prepare for the financial and lifestyle changes. Achieving social acceptance is not as difficult today as it was many years ago when single motherhood was taboo and was considered a distinct disgrace to the maternal family. The nurse should maintain a nonjudgmental attitude and assist the single mother to successfully achieve the psychological tasks of pregnancy.

IMPACT ON THE SINGLE FATHER

The single father may take an active interest in and financial responsibility for the child. The couple may plan marriage eventually, but it is often delayed. A single father may provide emotional support for the mother during the pregnancy and birth. He often has strong feelings of surprise and accomplishment when he becomes aware of his partner's pregnancy. He may want to participate in plans for the child and take part in infant care after birth. However, the woman sometimes rejects his participation.

IMPACT ON GRANDPARENTS

Prospective grandparents have different reactions to a woman's pregnancy as well. They may eagerly anticipate the announcement that a grandchild is on the way, or they may feel that they are not ready for the role of grandparent, which they equate with being old. The first grandchild often causes the most excitement in grandparents. Their reaction may be more subdued if they have several grandchildren, which may hurt the excited pregnant couple.

Grandparents have different ideas of how they will be involved with their grandchildren. Distance from the younger family dictates the degree of involvement for some. They may want to be involved fully in the plans for the infant and to help with child care, and they often travel a great distance to be there for the big event. Other grandparents want less involvement, because they welcome the freedom of a childless life again. Many grandparents are in their 40s and 50s, a time when their own career demands and care of their aging parents compete with their ability to be involved with grandchildren.

If grandparents and the expectant couple have similar views of their roles, little conflict is likely. However, disappointment and conflict may occur if the pregnant couple and the grandparents have significantly different expectations of their role and involvement. The nurse can help the young couple understand their parents' reactions and help them to negotiate solutions to conflicts that are satisfactory to both generations.

IMPACT ON SIBLINGS

Preparation for the arrival of a new baby in the family should start before the arrival of the newborn and before the sibling feels the change that a new family member brings. All siblings will be affected by the arrival of a new baby into the family. Young children may lack resources to cope with their feelings of being displaced, and some behavior changes may be expected. Special time and effort is needed to make the siblings feel that they are loved as they were before.

PRENATAL EDUCATION

Prenatal education is an interactive process that requires input from the patient concerning individual needs and assessment of outcome: a healthy mother and child and an intact family unit. A plan for prenatal education is based on the desired outcome and includes the development of positive attitudes and perceptions, achievement of knowledge of facts, and the learning of skills to cope with pregnancy, labor, and the transition into parenthood. Examples include the *perception* that pregnancy is a normal process that is enhanced by good nutrition and a healthy lifestyle; the *knowledge* to select the proper diet; and the learning of *skills* to perform exercises, breathing, and relaxation techniques to prepare the woman for labor.

Prenatal education should progress according to the nursing process, as follows:

- *Assess* the history and cultural needs.
- *Diagnose* the knowledge deficit.
- *Plan* the goals and priorities.

- *Outcomes identification* clarifies expected outcomes.
- *Teach* (implement) the facts and rationales.
- *Evaluate* the knowledge gained and the goals achieved.

Collecting data to assess cultural needs can be individualized to the patient with the use of a **birth plan** (Figure 4-12). The birth plan can be presented in

---

Cultural Assessment Data Collection Tool to Assist in Developing an Individualized Plan of Care

(This tool can be translated into multiple languages and allows the nurse to compare the client's answers to those on an identical tool written in the nurse's dominant language. This data collection will enable the nurse to provide care to clients in a way that is culturally satisfying to them.)

Birth Plan

Providing answers to the following questions will give us information that will enable us to make your birthing experience a more positive experience.

Whom do you plan on having present to support you while you are in labor?
- ❏ Husband
- ❏ Female family member
- ❏ Friend
- ❏ No one

Have you attended a childbirth class?
- ❏ Yes
- ❏ No

If yes, what method of childbirth preparation?
- ❏ Lamaze
- ❏ Bradley
- ❏ Other

Which gender of health care provider do you prefer?
- ❏ Male
- ❏ Female
- ❏ No preference

During pelvic examinations does your husband wish to be present if done by a male physician?
- ❏ Yes
- ❏ No

During labor will you:
- ❏ Prefer to be involved in decision making
- ❏ Prefer to have someone tell you what to do

When you are in pain do you:
- ❏ Become quiet
- ❏ Verbally express your pain
- ❏ Yell and/or cry

Regarding pain medicine do you:
- ❏ Prefer to ask for it when you want it
- ❏ Have the nurse offer it to you

Do you feel comfortable in freely making requests to MD/CNM/nurse?
- ❏ Yes
- ❏ No

Do you prefer to be addressed by:
- ❏ Your first name
- ❏ Your last name

What type of infant feeding are you planning?
- ❏ Breastfeeding
- ❏ Bottle feeding
- ❏ Both
- ❏ Breastfeeding after colostrum changes to milk

Do you prefer to drink water:
- ❏ At room temperature
- ❏ With ice

After delivery do you prefer:
- ❏ Hot beverages
- ❏ Cold beverages

Do you want to know the sex of the baby:
- ❏ When an ultrasound is done
- ❏ Immediately after birth
- ❏ After the placenta is delivered

While in the hospital after having your baby do you prefer:
- ❏ Showers
- ❏ Baths
- ❏ Sponge baths
- ❏ None

Do you believe it is okay to wash your hair in the first few days after delivery?
- ❏ Yes
- ❏ No

According to your cultural practices when do women who have had a baby usually get up to walk around?
- ❏ Within the first few hours after delivery
- ❏ The day after delivery
- ❏ Prefer to stay in bed

According to your cultural practices who usually provides most of the infant care in the first few days of life?
- ❏ Mother of infant
- ❏ Both parents of infant
- ❏ Nurse and/or family members

If infant is a male, do you plan to have him circumcised?
- ❏ Yes
- ❏ No

If yes, when do you prefer it should be done?
- ❏ During hospitalization
- ❏ Day eight
- ❏ After discharge

According to your cultural practices when is it acceptable for others to praise your baby?
- ❏ Anytime
- ❏ Only if they are touching infant
- ❏ Never

After delivery how long will it be before you resume normal activities outside the home?
- ❏ At least 1 week
- ❏ Two weeks
- ❏ One month
- ❏ 45 days
- ❏ Over 45 days
- ❏ No specific amount of time

FIGURE 4-12 A birth plan is a cultural assessment data collection tool that is used to assist in developing an individualized plan of care. This tool can be translated into multiple languages and allows the nurse to compare the patient's answers to an identical tool in the nurse's dominant language, thus enabling the nurse to provide care that is culturally sensitive. (From Leifer G: *Maternity nursing*, ed 11, Philadelphia, 2012, Saunders.)

multiple languages, and the nurse can compare answers to the tool written in the nurse's primary language. Prenatal teaching can be planned according to the nursing process. Teaching can occur in formal childbirth education classes or informally during a clinic visit. Every contact a nurse has with a pregnant patient is an opportunity for teaching.

THE EFFECT OF PREGNANCY AND LACTATION ON MEDICATION METABOLISM

The physiological changes in pregnancy affect the metabolism of medications administered to the mother. Subtherapeutic drug levels may occur because of the increased plasma volume, cardiac output, and glomerular filtration that occur during pregnancy. A decreased gastric emptying time during pregnancy changes absorption of drugs and can delay onset of action. Parenteral medication may be absorbed more rapidly because of increased blood flow and may have a faster onset of action than in the nonpregnant state. The increased levels of estrogen and progesterone may alter hepatic (liver) function, resulting in drug accumulation in the body.

Drugs can cross the placenta and have an impact on fetal development, especially in the first trimester, and have increased absorption levels in the developing fetus in the third trimester. The mother should be instructed to check with her health care provider before taking over-the-counter medications. Taking ibuprofen in the third trimester can cause early closure of the ductus arteriosus, resulting in fetal distress.

Drugs can pass into breast milk by diffusion and be can be ingested by the neonate during breastfeeding. If the lactating mother must take a medication, it should be administered *immediately after* the infant breastfeeds to minimize passage to the infant. The U.S. Food and Drug Administration (FDA) has established a series of risk categories for medication use during pregnancy, and it is published in most drug books that nurses can use as references. All women of childbearing age should be counseled about the risk of ingesting drugs during pregnancy and lactation. Pregnancy risk categories allow for some assessment of risk to the fetus when a drug is prescribed in a pregnant woman (Box 4-5).

IMMUNIZATIONS DURING PREGNANCY

Live-virus vaccines are contraindicated during pregnancy because of possible adverse effects on the fetus. The Immunization Action Coalition (2010) has developed a screening questionnaire to determine if a vaccination is contraindicated or appropriate for a patient. Products containing thimerosal should not

Box 4-5	U.S. Food and Drug Administration (FDA) Pregnancy Risk Categories for Drugs

Category A: No risk demonstrated to the fetus in any trimester
Category B: No adverse effects in animals; no human studies available
Category C: Only prescribed after risks to the fetus are considered. Animal studies have shown adverse reaction; no human studies available
Category D: Definite fetal risks, but may be given in spite of risks in life-threatening situations
Category X: Absolute fetal abnormalities. Not to be used anytime during pregnancy

Data from Hodgson B, Kizior R: *Nursing drug handbook*, Philadelphia, 2013, Saunders.

be given to pregnant women because of the risk of mercury poisoning. Most vaccines are available in an alternative thimerosal-free form to be used for women who are pregnant. Vaccines contraindicated during pregnancy include *bacille Calmette-Guerin* (BCG), human papillomavirus (HPV), live attenuated influenza vaccine (LAIV) in nasal spray form because it is a live virus (CDC, 2008), and measles, mumps, and rubella (MMR). A woman is advised to avoid pregnancy for at least 1 month following an MMR immunization.

When exposure to or high risk of infection is present, vaccinations allowable during pregnancy include hepatitis A and B; inactivated influenza; meningococcal (MCV-4), only if the patient is at high risk for disease; pneumococcal polysaccharide vaccine (PPV) in high-risk women; inactivated polio vaccine when immediate protection is required; rabies if risk for infection is high; and tetanus-diphtheria (Td) after 29 weeks of gestation. Pregnant women at high risk of infection can also be given the vaccine for Japanese encephalitis and anthrax (CDC, 2008). The flu vaccination is also recommended to protect pregnant women. Vaccines in vials with natural rubber tops should not be administered to women who are allergic to latex.

NURSING CARE DURING PREGNANCY

Table 4-7 describes the physiological and psychological changes that occur during pregnancy, the related signs and symptoms noted in the patient, and some suggested nursing interventions or teaching points appropriate to that phase. The rationales for a nursing care plan can be based on the information within this table. Teaching for the prenatal patient should include the risks of smoking, alcohol use, and illicit drug use as well as the advantages of breastfeeding and good nutrition during pregnancy.

Table 4-7	Physiological and Psychological Changes in Pregnancy, Nursing Interventions, and Teaching	
MATERNAL CHANGES	**SIGNS AND SYMPTOMS**	**NURSING INTERVENTIONS AND TEACHING**
First Trimester		
Fertilization occurs. Increased progesterone levels result in amenorrhea. Sodium (Na) retention increases. Nitrogen (N) stores decrease.	Pregnancy test is positive.	Guide patient regarding nutritional needs and folic acid requirements. Encourage patient to seek early prenatal care. Assess attitude toward this pregnancy and how it affects family.
Blood volume increases. Levels of relaxin hormone increase. Levels of human chorionic gonadotropin (hCG) hormone increase.	Fainting is possible. Morning nausea can occur. Relaxation of gastrointestinal (GI) muscles can cause "heartburn." Sensitivity to odors increases.	Teach patient how to rise slowly from prone position. Teach patient how to cope with nausea without medication: • Eat dry crackers before arising. • Use acupressure.
Pituitary gland releases melanin-stimulating hormone.	Pigmentation deepens on face (chloasma) and on abdomen (linea nigra).	Discuss body changes and assure patient that pigmentation will fade after puerperium.
Fetus grows. Uterus begins to enlarge.	Abdomen enlarges at end of first trimester when uterus rises out of pelvis. Small weight gain occurs. Enlarged uterus presses on bladder.	Teach methods to minimize fetal problems: • Avoid high temperatures around abdomen (baths and spas). • Discuss effects of medications and herbs on fetal development. Discuss impact of frequency of urination on lifestyle and activities. Facilitate communication with partner concerning sexual relationships during pregnancy. Discuss nutritional and folic acid needs, control of caffeine intake in second and third trimesters, and omega–fatty acid intake.
For fathers, announcement phase begins when pregnancy is confirmed, followed by adjustment phase and, finally, focus phase in third trimester and during labor, when "feeling like a father" develops.	Parents adjust to reality of pregnancy.	Review father's role as well as mother's responses. Refer to community agencies as needed. Assess for misinformation and knowledge deficit. Help parents identify concerns. Answer questions. Discuss relevant topics such as care of siblings and role of grandparents.
Second Trimester		
Corpus luteum is absorbed, and placenta takes over fetal support (between third and fourth months).	Blood volume increases in placental bed.	Teach patient how to minimize risk of habitual abortion between third and fourth month when placenta begins to take over.
Broad ligament stretches as uterus enlarges.	Occasional pain in groin area occurs.	Teach patient Kegel exercises to strengthen pelvic muscles.
Vascularity of pelvis increases.	Sexual pleasure and desire increases. White discharge may occur.	Discuss modifications of positions for sexual comfort and pleasure. Teach patient to avoid routine douches. Teach patient perineal skin hygiene.
Blood volume and vasomotor lability increase.	Orthostatic hypotension can occur.	Teach patient to change positions slowly and to avoid warm, crowded areas.
Cardiac output increases.	Physiological anemia may occur.	Iron supplements may be prescribed for anemia. Teach patient how to prevent constipation, and teach about change in stool color during iron therapy.
Renal threshold decreases.	Perineal itching may occur.	Test for glucose in urine and require glucose tolerance test in second trimester to rule out gestational diabetes. Teach patient hygienic measures when high glucose level is present (front to back wiping; wearing cotton panties).

Continued

MATERNAL CHANGES	SIGNS AND SYMPTOMS	NURSING INTERVENTIONS AND TEACHING
Second Trimester—cont'd		
Uterus rises out of pelvis. Estrogen relaxes sacroiliac joint.	Body's center of gravity changes.	Teach patient proper shoe and heel height to prevent falling. Teach placement of automobile restraints across hips rather than across abdomen. Teach patient to avoid lying supine in bed after fourth month of pregnancy to prevent supine hypotension syndrome. Teach posture and pelvic rocking exercises. Instruct that clothes should hang from shoulders.
	Pressure on bladder and rectum increases.	Instruct patient to anticipate urinary frequency during long trips. Teach patient Kegel exercises to strengthen pelvic floor.
Enlarging uterus compresses nerves supplying lower extremities.	Leg muscle spasms occur, especially when reclining.	Check for Homans' sign (see Figure 10-2). Teach patient how to dorsiflex the foot to help relieve spasms. Massage foot.
Decreased calcium levels and increased phosphorus levels are possible.		Teach patient to use oral aluminum hydroxide gel to reduce phosphorus levels if elevated (when recommended by health care provider).
Late in second trimester cardiac reserve begins to decrease and respiratory effort to increase.	Physiological stress is possible if exercise levels are not decreased.	Teach patient to monitor pulse rate (maximum 90 beats/min), and teach patient that inability to converse without taking frequent breaths is a sign of physiological stress. Teach patient to stop exercising if numbness, pain, or dizziness occurs.
Hormonal influence causes "id" to come to surface.	Mood swings occur.	Prepare spouse or significant other and family for mood swings, outspoken behavior, and labile emotions ("speaks before she thinks").
Levels of relaxin hormone increase.	Sphincter of stomach relaxes, and gastrointestinal motility is slowed.	Teach patient how to prevent constipation. Instruct patient to increase fluid intake and avoid gas-forming foods.
Increase in estrogen levels causes increased excretory function of skin.	Skin itches.	Teach patient to wear loose clothing, shower frequently, and use bland soaps and oils for comfort.
Anterior pituitary secretes melanin-stimulating hormone.	Skin pigmentation deepens.	Prepare patient to anticipate development of spider nevi and skin pigmentation. Reassure patient that most fade after puerperium.
Estrogen levels increase.	Increased estrogen levels develop increased vascularity of oral tissues, resulting in gingivitis and stuffy nose. Estrogen levels develop network of increased arterioles.	Teach proper oral hygiene techniques. Edema can occur. Assess blood pressure, and report proteinuria.
Pituitary gland secretes prolactin.	Colostrum leaks from nipples and sometimes cakes. Breasts enlarge.	Teach patient to cleanse nipples to keep ducts from being blocked by colostrum. Avoid soaps, ointments, and alcohol that dry skin. Teach patient not to stimulate nipples by massage or exercise, because doing so may increase risk for preterm labor.
As breast size increases, drooping of shoulders causes traction on brachial plexus.	Fingers tingle.	Teach patient proper posture. Encourage use of a supportive maternity bra.
Placental barrier allows certain elements and organisms to pass through to fetus.	Some medications can pass through placental barrier and cause fetal defects.	Advise patient not to smoke and not to self-treat with medications. Teach patients that certain jobs should be avoided during pregnancy (e.g., working as parking attendant, in a dry cleaning plant, and in a chemistry laboratory).
Travel becomes more difficult.	Because of placental permeability, traveling to countries that have endemic diseases can have negative effect on fetus; active, live viral immunization should be avoided.	Advise patient regarding travel.

Continued

Table 4-7 Physiological and Psychological Changes in Pregnancy, Nursing Interventions, and Teaching—cont'd

MATERNAL CHANGES	SIGNS AND SYMPTOMS	NURSING INTERVENTIONS AND TEACHING
Second Trimester—cont'd		
	Lowered oxygen levels can cause fetal hypoxia.	Most commercial airlines have cabin pressure controlled at or below 5000-ft level and therefore do not pose risk to fetus.
Increased levels of platelets occur.	Women are prone to thrombophlebitis if they are inactive for long periods.	Encourage patient to keep hydrated because of low cabin humidity in airplanes and to move around to help prevent thrombophlebitis.
Fetal growth continues.	Mother feels signs of life; fetus moves and kicks.	Teach proper nutrition to foster fetal growth without adding extra "empty" calories. Encourage patient to attend child care and parenting classes.
Third Trimester		
Weight gain typically approaches 20-25 lb.	Patient tires easily.	Teach patient need for rest periods and organization of work.
Colostrum forms.	Colostrum may leak from breasts.	Teach patient care of nipples. Introduce nipple pads. Avoid nipple stimulation to prevent preterm labor.
Increased estrogen levels cause edema of larynx.	Voice changes.	Singers may note loss of vocal quality.
Maximum increase in cardiac output (increase in stroke volume) occurs.	Patient tires easily.	Teach patient of need for rest periods.
Edema of hands and wrists is possible.	Risk for carpal tunnel syndrome increases.	Teach patient signs of gestational hypertension (GH) and assess water retention.
Uterus increases in size.	Pressure on stomach occurs. Pressure on diaphragm occurs. Venous congestion increases.	Discuss how to cope with decrease in appetite and shortness of breath. Teach patient how to avoid constipation and leg varicosities. Teach "talk test" for self-evaluation of exercise tolerance to prevent fetal hypoxia (must be able to finish a sentence before taking a breath).
Awareness of Braxton Hicks contractions increases.	Fetal head may engage (uterus drops) (lightening).	Teach patient signs of labor and when to come to hospital. Offer tour of labor and delivery unit.
Hormone levels increase.	"Id" is at the surface. Woman becomes self-centered and worries how she will manage labor.	Review labor management learned in prenatal classes. Discuss sibling care and support system.

Unfolding Case Study

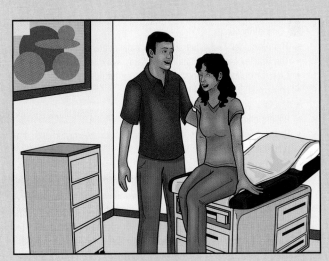

Tess is a 22-year-old woman who comes to the clinic with her husband Luis for a prenatal checkup on May 10, 2014. This is her first pregnancy, and they are both very excited about starting a family. Her physical exam is within normal limits, but she does complain of nausea in the mornings. Her LNMP was March 1, 2014.

QUESTIONS

1. What is Tess's GTPAL?
2. When is her due date?
3. How many weeks pregnant is she today?
4. What advice would the nurse give Tess concerning her complaint of nausea?
5. Describe the probable signs of pregnancy that the health care provider will assess for during this first visit.
6. Tess says that she and her husband Luis want to take a last vacation together before starting their family responsibilities. They plan to leave on a 2-week trip to Europe starting November 30. What advice would the nurse give to them?

Get Ready for the NCLEX® Examination!

Key Points

- Early and regular prenatal care promotes the healthiest possible outcome for mother and infant.
- The woman's estimated date of delivery is calculated from her last normal menstrual period.
- The length of a pregnancy is 40 weeks after the last normal menstrual period. The expected date of delivery is determined by using Nägele's rule.
- Presumptive signs of pregnancy often have other causes. Probable signs more strongly suggest pregnancy but can still be caused by other conditions. Positive signs have no other cause except pregnancy. The three positive signs of pregnancy include detection of a fetal heartbeat, recognition of fetal movements by a trained examiner, and visualization of the embryo or fetus on ultrasound.
- The optimal weight gain during pregnancy is 25 to 35 lb (11.4 to 15.9 kg).
- The uterus undergoes the most obvious changes in pregnancy: it increases in weight from approximately 60 g (2 oz) to 1000 g (2.2 lb); it increases in capacity from about 10 mL (⅓ oz) to 5000 mL (5 quarts). Pregnancy affects all body systems.
- The mother's blood volume is about 45% greater than her prepregnant volume to enable perfusion of the placenta and extramaternal tissues. Her blood pressure does not increase, because resistance to blood flow in her arteries decreases. The fluid portion of her blood increases more than the cellular portion, resulting in a pseudoanemia.
- The common discomforts of pregnancy occur as a result of hormonal, physiological, and anatomical changes normally occurring during pregnancy. The nurse should teach relief measures and explain abnormal signs to report to the health care provider.
- Supine hypotension syndrome, also known as aortocaval compression or vena cava syndrome, may occur if the pregnant woman lies flat on her back. Turning to one side or placing a small pillow under one hip can help relieve this hypotension.
- To provide for the growth of the fetus and maternal tissues, the mother needs 300 extra, high-quality calories daily. Important nutrients that must be increased are protein, calcium, iron, and folic acid. Five hundred extra calories a day are needed for lactation.
- Adequate folic acid intake before conception of 400 mg or 0.4 mcg can reduce the incidence of neural tube defects such as anencephaly or spina bifida in the newborn. Supplementation for 3 months before conception may prevent autism. However intake should not exceed 1000 mcg per day and folic acid supplements for nonpregnant women should be used with care.
- Adequate vitamin intake is essential for optimum fetal development. However, excess vitamin intake can be toxic.
- Fathers should be included in prenatal care to the extent they and the woman desire.
- The health history of the father is important, because genetics, illness or lifestyle practices may affect the health of all members of the family.
- Adaptation to pregnancy occurs in the mother, the father, and other family members. Prenatal care involves physical and psychological aspects and should be family centered.
- Childbirth education includes formal classes and informal counseling. Education should include nutrition, prenatal visits, exercise, breathing and relaxation techniques, the birth process, safety issues, and beginning parenting skills.
- Live virus vaccines are contraindicated during pregnancy.
- Specific laboratory screening tests are performed during pregnancy to assure a positive outcome for both mother and infant.
- The physiological changes during pregnancy influence the metabolism of ingested medications.
- Medications ingested during pregnancy can affect fetal development.

Additional Learning Resources

SG Go to your Study Guide for additional learning activities to help you master this chapter content.

evolve Go to your Evolve website (http://evolve.elsevier.com/Leifer) for the following learning resources:
- Animations
- Answer Guidelines for Critical Thinking Questions
- Answers and Rationales for Review Questions for the NCLEX® Examination
- Glossary with English and Spanish translations
- Interactive Review Questions for the NCLEX® Examination
- Patient Teaching Plans in English and Spanish
- Skills Performance Checklists
- Video clips and more!

 Online Resources
- The Alexander Technique: www.alexandertechnique.com/articles
- The Bradley Method of natural childbirth: www.bradleybirth.com/cc.htm
- Exercise during pregnancy: http://csep.ca/forms.asp
- Lamaze International: www.lamaze.org
- MyPlate: www.choosemyPlate.gov
- Patient care updates: www.patientcareonline.com
- Pregnancy and childbirth prenatal care: www.makewayforbaby.com/prenatalcare.htm

Review Questions for the NCLEX® Examination

1. A woman arrives in the clinic for her prenatal visit. She states that she is currently 28 weeks pregnant with twins; has a 5-year-old son who was delivered at 39 weeks gestation; and a 3-year-old daughter delivered at

34 weeks gestation; and her last pregnancy terminated at 16 weeks gestation. The nurse will interpret her obstetrical history as:

1. G4 T2 P2 A1 L4.
2. G3 T2 P0 A1 L2.
3. G3 T1 P1 A1 L2.
4. G4 T1 P1 A1 L2.

2. Exercise during pregnancy should be practiced to achieve which of the following goals?

   1. Maintaining physical fitness.
   2. Minimizing weight gain.
   3. Achieving weight loss.
   4. Improving physical fitness.

3. During a prenatal examination at 30 weeks of gestation, a woman is lying on her back on the examining table. She suddenly complains of dizziness and feeling faint. The most appropriate response of the nurse would be to:

   1. reassure the woman and take measures to reduce her anxiety level.
   2. offer the woman some orange juice or other rapidly absorbed form of glucose.
   3. place a pillow under the woman's head.
   4. turn the woman onto her side.

4. A woman being seen for her first prenatal care appointment has a positive home pregnancy test, and her chart shows a TPALM recording of 40120. The nurse would anticipate that:

   1. minimal prenatal teaching will be required because this is her fourth pregnancy.
   2. the woman will need help in planning the care of her other children at home during her labor and delivery.
   3. the woman should experience minimal anxiety because she is familiar with the progress of pregnancy.

   4. this pregnancy will be considered high risk, and measures to reduce anxiety will be needed.

5. A woman's LNMP was on April 1, 2013. She has been keeping her prenatal clinic appointments regularly but states she needs to alter the dates of a future appointment, because she and her husband are going on an ocean cruise vacation for the New Year's celebration from December 30 through January 7, 2014. The best response of the nurse would be:

   1. "Prenatal visits can never be altered. Every visit is important."
   2. "Be sure to take antinausea medication when going on an ocean cruise."
   3. "Perhaps you might consider rescheduling your vacation around the Thanksgiving holiday rather than the New Year's dates."
   4. "I will reschedule your clinic appointment to accommodate your vacation plans."

Critical Thinking Questions

1. A 35-year-old primipara woman in her twentieth week of pregnancy states that she does not want to drink the liquid glucose for the routine blood glucose screen, because it does not taste good. She states that she is not a diabetic and does not think the test is necessary for her. What is the best response by the nurse?

2. A woman entering her second trimester of pregnancy states that she is noticing increasing stretch marks on her abdomen. She is afraid these marks will remain prominent after pregnancy, and she wants to go on a low-calorie diet to prevent her abdomen from becoming too large. What information should the nurse include in her teaching plan for this patient?

Objectives

1. Define each key term listed.
2. Explain the use of fetal diagnostic tests in women with complicated pregnancies.
3. Identify methods to reduce a woman's risk for antepartum complications.
4. Describe antepartum complications, their treatment, and their nursing care.
5. Discuss the management of concurrent medical conditions during pregnancy.
6. Describe environmental hazards that may adversely affect the outcome of pregnancy.
7. Describe how pregnancy affects care of the trauma victim.
8. Describe psychosocial nursing interventions for the woman who has a high-risk pregnancy and for her family.

Key Terms

abortion (p. 82)
age of viability (p. 83)
cerclage (sĕr-KLĂHZH, p. 83)
disseminated intravascular coagulation (DIC) (p. 90)
eclampsia (ĕ-KLĂMP-sē-ă, p. 90)
erythroblastosis fetalis (ĕ-rĭth-rō-blăs-Ō-sĭs fĕ-TĂ-lĭs, p. 95)
gestational diabetes mellitus (GDM) (p. 96)
hydramnios (hī-DRĂM-nē-ŏs, p. 97)

incompetent cervix (ĭn-KŎM-pă-tănt SŬR-vĭkz, p. 83)
isoimmunization (ī-sō-ĭm-myū-nĭ-ZĀ-shŭn, p. 95)
macrosomia (măk-rō-SŌ-mē-ă, p. 97)
preeclampsia (prē-ĕ-KLĂMP-sē-ă, p. 90)
preterm labor (p. 83)
products of conception (POC) (p. 87)
teratogen (TĚR-ă-tō-jĕn, p. 107)
tonic-clonic seizures (p. 92)

Most women have uneventful pregnancies that are free of complications. Some, however, have complications that threaten their well-being and that of their babies. Many problems can be anticipated in the course of prenatal care and thus prevented or made less severe. Others occur without warning.

Women who have no prenatal care or begin care late in pregnancy may have complications that are severe, because the problems were not identified early. Danger signs that should be taught to every pregnant woman and reinforced at each prenatal visit are listed in the Patient Teaching box. The woman should be taught to notify her health care provider if any of these danger signs occur. A high-risk pregnancy is defined as one in which the health of the mother or fetus is in jeopardy.

The causes of high-risk pregnancies usually include the following characteristics:

- Relate to the pregnancy itself
- Occur because the woman has a medical condition or injury that complicates the pregnancy
- Result from environmental hazards that affect the mother or her fetus
- Arise from maternal behaviors or lifestyles that have a negative effect on the mother or fetus

Early and consistent assessment for risk factors during prenatal visits is essential for a positive outcome for the mother and the fetus.

ASSESSMENT OF FETAL HEALTH

Extraordinary technical advances have enabled the management of high-risk pregnancies so that both the mother and the fetus have positive outcomes. Various tests can be used prenatally to assess the well-being of the fetus. Nursing responsibilities during the assessment of fetal health include preparing the patient properly, explaining the reason for the test, and clarifying and interpreting results in collaboration with other health care providers. The nurse can provide the psychosocial support that will allay or reduce parental anxiety. Figure 5-1 shows amniocentesis, and Table 5-1 reviews common diagnostic tests that assess the status of the fetus. Fetal assessment techniques used during labor are discussed in Chapter 6.

The future of fetal assessment lies in the continued development of new ultrasound technologies and hand-held receivers. Ultrasound pictures taken by a portable instrument can be transmitted via the Internet to be interpreted by experts in medical centers.

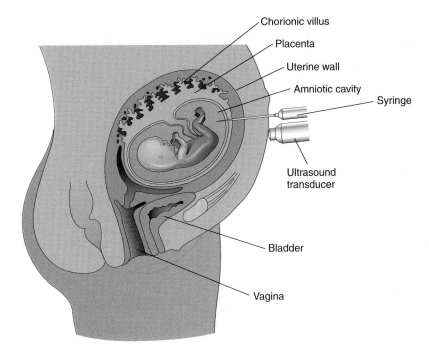

FIGURE 5-1 Amniocentesis. An ultrasound transducer on the abdomen ensures needle placement away from the body of the fetus and the placenta. A needle is inserted into the amniotic cavity, and a sample of amniotic fluid is collected for laboratory examination and fetal assessment. (From Moore KL, Persaud TVN, Torchia MG: *The developing human: clinically oriented embryology,* ed 9, Philadelphia, 2012, Saunders.)

Telemedicine, a growing field, is a specialized technology in prenatal care. Newer and noninvasive prenatal assessment technologies are reviewed in Table 5-10 at the end of the chapter.

Patient Teaching

Danger Signs in Pregnancy

The nurse should teach the woman to report promptly any danger signs that occur during pregnancy, including the following:
- A sudden gush of fluid from vagina
- Vaginal bleeding
- Abdominal pain
- Persistent vomiting
- Epigastric pain
- Edema of face and hands
- Severe, persistent headache
- Blurred vision or dizziness
- Chills with fever greater than 38.0° C (100.4° F)
- Painful urination or reduced urine output

PREGNANCY-RELATED COMPLICATIONS

HYPEREMESIS GRAVIDARUM

Mild nausea and vomiting are easily managed during pregnancy (see Chapter 4). In contrast, the woman with hyperemesis gravidarum has excessive nausea and vomiting that can significantly interfere with her food intake and fluid balance. Fetal growth may be restricted, resulting in a low-birth-weight infant. Dehydration impairs perfusion of the placenta, reducing the delivery of blood oxygen and nutrients to the fetus.

Manifestations. Hyperemesis gravidarum differs from "morning sickness" of pregnancy in one or more of the following ways:
- Persistent nausea and vomiting, often with complete inability to retain food and fluids
- Significant weight loss (more than 5% of prepregnant weight)
- Dehydration as evidenced by a dry tongue and mucous membranes, decreased turgor (elasticity) of the skin, scant and concentrated urine, and a high serum hematocrit level
- Electrolyte and acid-base imbalances
- Ketonuria
- Psychological factors such as unusual stress, emotional immaturity, passivity, or ambivalence about the pregnancy

Treatment. The health care provider will rule out other causes for the excessive nausea and vomiting, such as gastroenteritis or liver, gallbladder, or pancreatic disorders, before making this diagnosis. The medical treatment for hyperemesis gravidarum is to correct dehydration and electrolyte or acid-base imbalances with oral or intravenous fluids. Antiemetic drugs may be prescribed. Dopamine antagonists such as promethazine or selective serotonin antagonists such as ondansetron are commonly prescribed to treat nausea and vomiting. Ginger, methylprednisone, and erythromycin are experimental therapies that show promise in the near future for treatment of hyperemesis gravidarum (Gabbe, 2012). Occasionally, severe cases

Table 5-1 Fetal Diagnostic Tests

TEST	DESCRIPTION	USE(S) DURING PREGNANCY
Ultrasound examination	Uses high-frequency sound waves to visualize structures within the body; the examination may use a transvaginal probe or an abdominal transducer; abdominal ultrasound during early pregnancy requires a full bladder for proper visualization (have the woman drink 1-2 quarts of water before the examination). A targeted comprehensive ultrasound detects specific anomalies. Echo or Doppler scan detects fetal heart activity at 6-10 weeks. Three-dimensional (3-D) imaging produces clear detail and features.	Visualize a gestational sac in early pregnancy to confirm the pregnancy. Identify site of implantation (uterine or ectopic). Verify fetal viability or death. Identify a multifetal pregnancy, such as twins or triplets. Diagnose some fetal structural abnormalities. Guide procedures, such as chorionic villus sampling, amniocentesis, or percutaneous umbilical blood sampling. Determine gestational age of the embryo or fetus. Locate the placenta. Determine the amount of amniotic fluid. Observe fetal movements. Nonmedical use of ultrasound during pregnancy is discouraged (ACOG, 2009; Aium, 2012).
Amniotic fluid volume (AFV)	This ultrasound scan measures the amniotic fluid pockets in all four quadrants surrounding the mother's umbilicus and produces an amniotic fluid index (AFI).	From 5-19 cm is considered normal; <5 cm is known as *oligohydramnios* (insufficient amniotic fluid) and is associated with growth restriction and fetal distress during labor because of "kinking" of the cord. A measurement >30 cm is *polyhydramnios* (excess amniotic fluid) and is associated with neural tube defects, gastrointestinal obstruction, and fetal hydrops.
Estimation of gestational age	This ultrasound examination at 8 weeks of gestation can measure the gestational sac. Ultrasound is more accurate than the LMP if used before 22 weeks gestation in determining fetal age (Gabbe, 2012).	Between 7 and 14 weeks the crown–rump length can indicate fetal age. After 12 weeks the biparietal diameter of the fetus and the femur length provide an accurate estimation of fetal age. The biparietal diameter of the fetus at 36 weeks is 8.7 cm, and at term it is 9.8 cm.
Magnetic resonance imaging (MRI)	This imaging technique provides a noninvasive radiological view of fetal structures, including the placenta.	Used when there is a high suspicion of an anomaly.
Kick count	Maternal assessment of fetal movement	Fewer than three fetal kicks within 1 hour or fewer than 10 kicks or cessation of fetal movement for 12 hours indicates the need for evaluation. A daily fetal movement record is kept at home once a day, and the findings are evaluated during prenatal visits to ensure fetal health. The sleep cycle of the fetus should be considered when selecting a time to evaluate fetal movement.
Doppler ultrasound blood flow assessment	This assessment uses high-frequency sound waves to study the flow of blood through vessels. Color Doppler can detect the speed and direction of blood flow within fetal vessels.	Determine adequacy of blood flow through the placenta and umbilical cord vessels in women in whom it is likely to be impaired (such as those with pregnancy-induced hypertension or diabetes mellitus).
Alpha-fetoprotein testing (AFP)	Test determines the level of this fetal protein in the pregnant woman's serum or in a sample of amniotic fluid; correct interpretation requires an accurate gestational age. AFP measurement of high hCG and low unconjugated estriol in maternal blood at 18 weeks gestation is a marker for trisomy 18 and 21 and indicated need for follow-up.	Identify high levels, which are associated with open defects, such as spina bifida (open spine), anencephaly (incomplete development of the skull and brain), or gastroschisis (open abdominal cavity). Identify low levels, which are associated with chromosome abnormalities or gestational trophoblastic disease (hydatidiform mole).
Chorionic villus sampling	Sampling consists of obtaining a small part of the developing placenta to analyze fetal cells at 10-12 weeks of gestation.	Identify chromosome abnormalities or other defects that can be determined by analysis of cells. Results of chromosome studies are available 24-48 hours later. Cannot be used to determine spina bifida or anencephaly (see AFP testing). Higher rate of spontaneous abortion after procedure than after amniocentesis. Reports of limb reduction defects in newborns. $Rh_0(D)$ immune globulin (RhoGAM) is given to the Rh-negative woman.

Table 5-1   Fetal Diagnostic Tests—cont'd

TEST	DESCRIPTION	USE(S) DURING PREGNANCY
Amniocentesis	This procedure consists of insertion of a thin needle through the abdominal and uterine walls to obtain a sample of amniotic fluid, which contains cast-off fetal cells and various other fetal products (see Figure 5-1). Standard genetic amniocentesis is done at 15-17 weeks of gestation. Amniocentesis before 15 weeks gestation is not recommended because of risk of clubfoot (Gabbe, 2012).	*Early pregnancy:* Identify chromosome abnormalities, biochemical disorders (such as Tay-Sachs disease), and level of AFP. A fetus cannot be tested for every possible disorder. Amniocentesis after 15 weeks gestation carries a 1:400 risk of complication (Gabbe, 2012). *Late pregnancy:* Identify severity of maternal–fetal blood incompatibility and assess fetal lung maturity. $Rh_o(D)$ immune globulin is given to the Rh-negative woman.
Non–stress test (NST)	Test comprises evaluation with an electronic fetal monitor of the fetal heart rate (FHR) for accelerations of at least 15 beats/min lasting 15 seconds in a 20-minute period. Fetal movements do not have to accompany the accelerations.	Identify fetal compromise in conditions associated with poor placenta function, such as hypertension, diabetes mellitus, or postterm gestation. Adequate accelerations of the FHR are reassuring that the placenta is functioning properly and the fetus is well oxygenated.
Vibroacoustic stimulation test	This procedure is similar to the NST; in addition, an artificial larynx device is used to stimulate the fetus with sound. Expected response is acceleration of the FHR, as in the NST.	Clarify (if the NST is questionable) whether the fetus is well oxygenated, thereby reducing the need for more complex testing. Clarify (during labor) questionable FHR patterns.
Contraction stress test (CST)	Test is an evaluation of the FHR response to mild uterine contractions by using an electronic fetal monitor; contractions may be induced by self-stimulation of the nipples, which causes the woman's pituitary gland to release oxytocin, or by intravenous oxytocin (Pitocin) infusion. The woman must have at least three contractions at least 40 seconds in duration in a 10-minute period for interpretation of the CST.	Purposes are the same as for the NST; the CST may be done if the NST results are nonreassuring (the fetal heart does not accelerate) or if they are questionable. Late decelerations after a contraction can indicate that fetus may not tolerate labor. Normal CST results mean there are no late decelerations and the fetus can probably tolerate labor.
Biophysical profile (BPP)	Profile consists of a group of five fetal assessments: fetal heart rate and reactivity (the NST), fetal breathing movements, fetal body movements, fetal tone (closure of the hand), and the volume of amniotic fluid (AFI). Some centers omit the NST, and others assess only the NST and AFI.	Identify reduced fetal oxygenation in conditions associated with poor placental function, but with greater precision than the NST alone. As fetal hypoxia gradually increases, FHR changes occur first, followed by cessation of fetal breathing movement, gross body movements, and finally loss of fetal tone. Amniotic fluid volume is reduced when placental function is poor (shows pockets of low or absent amniotic fluid).
Percutaneous umbilical blood sampling	Procedure serves to obtain a fetal blood sample from a placental vessel or from the umbilical cord; this may be used to give a blood transfusion to an anemic fetus.	Identify fetal conditions that can be diagnosed only with a blood sample. Blood transfusion may be necessary for fetal anemia caused by maternal–fetal blood incompatibility, placenta previa, or abruptio placentae.
Tests of fetal lung maturity: Lecithin/ sphingomyelin (L/S) ratio Foam stability index (FSI, or "shake test")	These tests use a sample of amniotic fluid (obtained by amniocentesis or from the pool of fluid in the vagina) to determine substances that indicate fetal lungs are mature enough to adapt to extrauterine life. A 2:1 ratio indicates fetal lung maturity (3:1 ratio desirable for diabetic mother); fluid usually obtained by amniocentesis. Presence of phosphatidylglycerol (PG) Presence of phosphatidylinositol (PI) Persistence of a ring of bubbles for 15 minutes after shaking together equal amounts of 95% ethanol, isotonic saline, and amniotic fluid	Evaluate whether the fetus is likely to have respiratory complications in adapting to extrauterine life. May be done to determine whether the fetal lungs are mature before performing an elective cesarean birth or inducing labor if the gestational age is questionable. Also used to evaluate whether the fetus should be promptly delivered or allowed to mature further when the membranes rupture and the gestation is at <37 weeks or if the gestation is questionable.

necessitate total parenteral nutrition. The woman may need hospital admission to correct dehydration and inadequate nutrition if home measures are not successful. Thiamine is often administered before IV dextrose to prevent Wernicke's syndrome that is characterized by double vision and ataxia (Gabbe, 2012). The condition is self-limiting in most women, although it is quite distressing to the woman and her family.

Nursing Care. Nursing care focuses on patient teaching, because most care occurs in the home. The woman should be taught how to reduce factors that trigger nausea and vomiting. She should avoid food odors, which may abound in meal preparation areas and tray carts if she is hospitalized. If she becomes nauseated when her food is served, the tray should be removed promptly and offered again later.

Accurate intake and output and daily weight records are kept to assess fluid balance. Frequent, small amounts of food and fluid keep the stomach from becoming too full, which can trigger vomiting. Easily digested carbohydrates, such as crackers or baked potatoes, are tolerated best. Foods with strong odors should be eliminated from the diet. Taking liquids between solid meals helps to reduce gastric distention. Sitting upright after meals reduces gastric reflux (backflow) into the esophagus.

The emesis basin is kept out of sight so that it is not a visual reminder of vomiting. It should be emptied at once if the woman vomits, and the amount should be documented on the intake and output record.

Stress may contribute to hyperemesis gravidarum; stress may also result from this complication. The nurse should provide support by listening to the woman's feelings about pregnancy, child rearing, and living with constant nausea. Although psychological factors may play a role in some cases of hyperemesis gravidarum, the nurse should not assume that every woman with this complication is adjusting poorly to her pregnancy.

BLEEDING DISORDERS OF EARLY PREGNANCY

Several bleeding disorders can complicate early pregnancy, such as spontaneous abortion (miscarriage) (Figure 5-2), ectopic pregnancy (see Figure 5-3), or hydatidiform mole (see Figure 5-4). Maternal blood loss decreases the oxygen-carrying capacity of the blood, resulting in fetal hypoxia, and places the fetus at risk.

Abortion

Abortion is the spontaneous (miscarriage) or intentional termination of a pregnancy before the age of viability (20 weeks of gestation). Table 5-2 differentiates types of abortions.

Treatment. When a *threatened* abortion occurs, efforts are made to keep the fetus in utero until the age of viability. In recurrent pregnancy loss, causes are

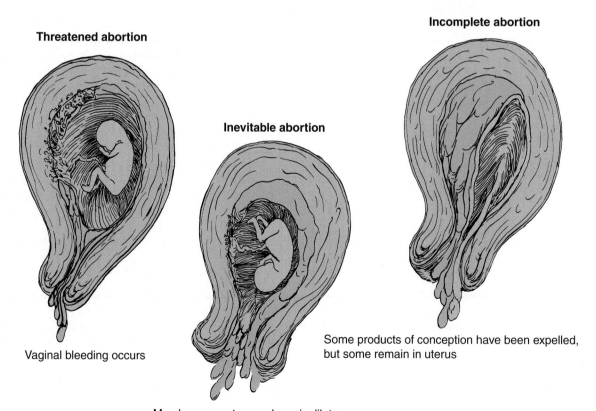

Threatened abortion

Vaginal bleeding occurs

Inevitable abortion

Membranes rupture and cervix dilates

Incomplete abortion

Some products of conception have been expelled, but some remain in uterus

FIGURE 5-2 Three types of spontaneous abortion.

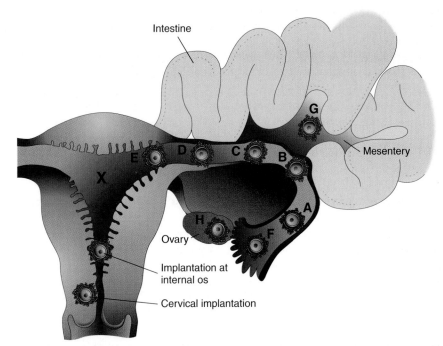

FIGURE 5-3 The ovary *(H)*, uterus and fallopian tubes, illustrating various abnormal implantation sites. *A* to *F* are tubal pregnancies (the most common); *G* is an abdominal pregnancy; and *X* indicates the wall of the uterus where normal implantation should occur. (From Moore KL, Persaud TVN, Torchia MG: *The developing human: clinically oriented embryology,* ed 9, Philadelphia, 2012, Saunders.)

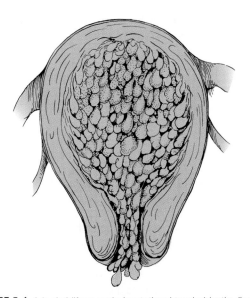

FIGURE 5-4 A hydatidiform mole (gestational trophoblastic disease).

investigated that could include genetic, immunological, anatomical, endocrine, or infectious factors. **Cerclage,** or suturing an **incompetent cervix** that opens when the growing fetus presses against it, is successful in most cases. A low human chorionic gonadotropin (hCG) level or low fetal heart rate by 8 weeks of gestation may be an ominous sign.

Termination of pregnancy after 20 weeks of gestation **(age of viability)** is called **preterm labor** and is discussed in Chapter 8. Table 5-3 describes procedures used in pregnancy termination. In all cases of pregnancy loss,

counseling of the parent(s) is essential. Even when the mother elects to terminate pregnancy, there are emotional responses that should be recognized and addressed.

Oxytocin (Pitocin) controls blood loss before and after curettage, much as the drugs do after term birth. $Rh_0(D)$ immune globulin (RhoGAM [300 mcg] or the lower-dose MICRhoGAM [50 mcg]) is given to Rh-negative women after any abortion to prevent the development of antibodies that might harm the fetus during a subsequent pregnancy.

Nursing Care

Physical care. The nurse documents the amount and character of bleeding and saves anything that looks like clots or tissue for evaluation by a pathologist. A pad count and an estimate of how saturated each is (e.g., 50%, 75%) documents blood loss most accurately. The woman with threatened abortion who remains at home is taught to report increased bleeding or passage of tissue.

The nurse should check the hospitalized woman's bleeding and vital signs to identify hypovolemic shock resulting from blood loss. She should not eat (remain NPO) if she has active bleeding to prevent aspiration if anesthesia is required for dilation and evacuation (D&E) treatment. Laboratory tests, such as a hemoglobin level and hematocrit, are ordered.

After vacuum aspiration or curettage, the amount of vaginal bleeding is observed. The blood pressure, pulse, and respirations are checked every 15 minutes

Table 5-2 Types of Abortions

TYPE	DESCRIPTION	TREATMENT OR INTERVENTION
Spontaneous (Nonintentional) Abortion: Unintentional Termination of Pregnancy Before Viability (20 Weeks of gestation)		
Threatened abortion	Cramping and backache with light spotting; cervix is closed, and no tissue is passed	Ultrasound is used to determine if fetus is living; bed rest is prescribed; avoid coitus.
Inevitable abortion	Increased bleeding, cramping; cervix dilates	Patient is placed on bed rest and monitored; awaits natural evacuation of uterus. Save peripads.
Incomplete abortion	Bleeding, cramping, dilation of cervix, passage of tissue	Uterus may be emptied of remaining tissue by dilation and evacuation (D&E) or vacuum extraction (see Table 5-3). Save peripads.
Complete abortion	Passage of all products of conception (POC); cervix closes; bleeding stops	Patient is monitored, and emotional support is given. Give RhoGAM if indicated.
Missed abortion	Fetus dies in utero but is not expelled; uterine growth stops; sepsis can occur	If fetus is not expelled, uterus is evacuated by D&E (see Table 5-3).
Recurrent abortion	Two or more consecutive spontaneous abortions (habitual abortion), usually caused by incompetent cervix or progesterone levels inadequate to maintain pregnancy	Incompetent cervix is treated with cerclage, a reinforcement of the cervix with a surgical suture; the patient is then monitored for early signs of labor at term to prevent uterine rupture.
Induced Abortion: Intentional Termination of Pregnancy Before Age of Viability		
Therapeutic abortion	Intentional termination of pregnancy to preserve the health of the mother	Induced abortion is currently legal in the United States when performed by a qualified health care provider. Supportive counseling must be part of the plan of care.
Elective abortion	Intentional termination of pregnancy for reasons other than the health of the mother (such as fetal anomaly)	Septic abortion (hemorrhage and infection) is a risk to the mother; counseling is advised even if the mother elects to abort.

Table 5-3 Procedures Used in Early Pregnancy Termination

PROCEDURE AND DESCRIPTION	COMMENTS
Vacuum aspiration (vacuum curettage): Cervical dilation with metal rods or laminaria (a substance that absorbs water and swells, thus enlarging the cervical opening) followed by controlled suction through a plastic cannula to remove all products of conception (POC)	Used up to 12 weeks gestation; also used to remove remaining POC after spontaneous abortion; may be followed by curettage (see *Dilation and evacuation);* paracervical block (local anesthesia of the cervix) or general anesthesia needed; conscious sedation with midazolam (Versed) may be used.
Dilation and evacuation (D&E): Dilation of the cervix as in vacuum curettage followed by gentle scraping of the uterine walls to remove POC	Used for first-trimester or early second trimester abortions and to remove all POC after a spontaneous abortion; greater risk of cervical or uterine trauma and excessive blood loss than with vacuum curettage; paracervical block or general anesthesia can be used.
Mifepristone (RU486) (Mifeprex) followed by misoprostol (Cytotec)	An oral medication that may be taken until up to 5 weeks of gestation; often used with a prostaglandin agent that causes bleeding and termination of pregnancy within 5 days.
Methotrexate (Folex) (Mexate)	Used up to 7 weeks gestation. An oral or intramuscular medication given with misoprostol, a prostaglandin analog; applied intravaginally, causes termination of pregnancy within 1 or 2 days.
Laminara causes cervical dilation followed by dilation and evacuation of uterine contents (D & E).	Used in second trimester abortions or fetal death.

for 1 hour, then every 30 minutes until discharge from the postanesthesia care unit. The mother's temperature is checked on admission to the recovery area and every 4 hours until discharge to monitor for infection.

Most women are discharged directly from the recovery unit to their home after curettage. Guidelines for self-care at home include the following:

- Report increased bleeding. Do not use tampons, which may cause infection.
- Take temperature every 8 hours for 3 days. Report signs of infection (temperature of 38° C [100.4° F] or higher; foul odor or brownish color of vaginal drainage).
- Take an oral iron supplement if prescribed.
- Resume sexual activity as recommended by the health care provider (usually after the bleeding has stopped).

- Return to the health care provider at the recommended time for a checkup and contraception information.
- Pregnancy can occur before the first menstrual period returns after the abortion procedure.

Emotional care. Society often underestimates the emotional distress spontaneous abortion causes the woman and her family. Even if the pregnancy was not planned or not suspected, they often grieve for what might have been. Their grief may last longer and be deeper than they or other people expect. The nurse listens to the woman and acknowledges the grief she and her partner feel. The Communication box gives examples of effective and ineffective techniques for communicating with the family experiencing pregnancy loss. Spiritual support of the family's choice and community support groups may help the family work through the grief of any pregnancy loss. Nursing Care Plan 5-1 suggests interventions for families experiencing early pregnancy loss.

★ Nursing Care Plan 5-1   The Family Experiencing Early Pregnancy Loss

PATIENT DATA A woman is admitted at 18 weeks of gestation and within a few hours delivers a fetus that does not survive. The woman asks what she has done wrong to cause this loss.

Selected Nursing Diagnosis: Grieving related to loss of anticipated infant

Goals	Nursing Interventions	Rationales
The woman and family will express grief to significant others. The woman and family will complete each stage of the grieving process within individual time frames.	Promote expression of grief by providing privacy, eliminating time restrictions, allowing support persons of choice to visit, and recognizing individualized grief expressions and cultural norms. Use the four stages of grief as a basis for nursing interventions: • *Stage 1:* Shock and disbelief at loss; characterized by numbness, apathy, and impaired decision making • *Stage 2:* Seeking answers for why loss happened; characterized by crying, tears, guilt, loss of appetite, insomnia, and blame placing • *Stage 3:* Disorganization; characterized by feelings of purposelessness and malaise; gradual resumption of normal activities • *Stage 4:* Reorganization; characterized by sad memories but return of daily functioning Use open communication techniques: • Quiet presence • Expression of sympathy ("I'm sorry this happened") • Open-ended statements ("This must be really sad for you") • Reflection of patient's expressed feelings ("You feel guilty because you didn't stay in bed constantly?") Reinforce explanations given by the health care provider or others (e.g., what the problem was, why it occurred); use simple language.	Grief is an individual process, and people react to it in different ways; these measures encourage woman and family to express grief and begin resolving it. Knowledge of normal stages of grieving helps the nurse identify whether it is progressing normally or if there is dysfunctional grieving in any family member. Stages help the nurse better interpret patients' behavior—for example, blame placing is a normal part of grieving and is not necessarily directed at the nurse or caregivers. This allows the nurse to reassure the patient that feelings are normal without diminishing the intensity of the feelings. Presence, empathy, and open communication encourage the family to express feelings about the loss, which is the first step in resolving them. Refer as needed to community agency or multidisciplinary health care team. Grieving people often do not hear or understand explanations the first time they are given because their concentration is impaired.

Critical Thinking Questions
1. What steps should the nurse take to assist the woman in coping with the loss of her pregnancy?
2. How should questions be formulated to foster communication with the patient?

Communication

The Family Experiencing Pregnancy Loss

EXAMPLES OF EFFECTIVE COMMUNICATION TECHNIQUES

Keep the family together.

Wait quietly with family: "Be there."

Say, "I'm sorry" or "I'm here if you need to talk."

Touch (may not be appreciated by some people or in some cultures).

Refer to spontaneous abortion as "miscarriage" rather than the harsher-sounding "abortion."

Provide mementos as appropriate (lock of hair, photograph, footprint); save keepsakes for later retrieval if the family does not want them immediately.

Alert other hospital personnel to the family's loss to prevent hurtful comments or questions.

Allow the family to see the fetus if they wish; prepare them for the appearance of the fetus.

Reduce the number of staff with whom the family must interact.

Summon a hospital chaplain such as a minister or rabbi.

Make referrals to support groups in the area.

EXAMPLES OF INEFFECTIVE COMMUNICATION TECHNIQUES

Do not give the woman or family any information.

Separate family members.

Discourage expressions of sadness; for example, expect the father to be strong for the mother's sake.

Avoid interacting with the family and talking about their loss.

Act uncomfortable with the family's expressions of grief.

Minimize the importance of the pregnancy by comments such as "You're young—you can always have more children"; "At least you didn't lose a real baby"; "It was for the best; the baby was abnormal"; or "You have another healthy child at home."

Say, "I know how you feel"; self-disclosure of your similar experience must be used carefully and only if it is likely to be therapeutic to the patient.

Encourage the family not to cry.

Ectopic Pregnancy

Ectopic pregnancy occurs when the fertilized ovum (zygote) is implanted outside the uterine cavity (see Figure 5-3). Of all ectopic pregnancies, 95% occur in the fallopian tube (tubal pregnancy). An obstruction or other abnormality of the tube prevents the zygote from being transported into the uterus. Scarring from a previous pelvic infection or deformity of the fallopian tubes or inhibition of normal tubal motion to propel the zygote into the uterus may result from the following:

- Hormonal abnormalities
- Inflammation
- Infection
- Adhesions
- Congenital defects
- Endometriosis (uterine lining occurring outside the uterus)

Use of an intrauterine device for contraception may contribute to ectopic pregnancy, because these devices promote inflammation within the uterus. A woman who has had a previous tubal pregnancy or a failed tubal ligation is also more likely to have an ectopic pregnancy.

A zygote that is implanted in a fallopian tube cannot survive for long, because the blood supply and size of the tube are inadequate. The zygote or embryo may die and be resorbed by the woman's body, or the tube may rupture with bleeding into the abdominal cavity, creating a surgical emergency.

Manifestations. The woman has a history of a missed menstrual period and often complains of lower abdominal pain, sometimes accompanied by light vaginal bleeding. If the tube ruptures, she may have sudden severe lower abdominal pain, vaginal bleeding, and signs of hypovolemic shock (Box 5-1). The amount of vaginal bleeding may be minimal, because most blood is lost into the abdomen rather than externally through the vagina. Shoulder pain is a symptom that often accompanies bleeding into the abdomen (referred pain).

Treatment. A sensitive pregnancy test for hCG is done to determine if the woman is pregnant. Transvaginal ultrasound examination determines whether the embryo is growing within the uterine cavity. Culdocentesis (puncture of the upper posterior vaginal wall with removal of peritoneal fluid) may occasionally be performed to identify blood in the woman's pelvis, which suggests tubal rupture. A laparoscopic examination may be done to view the damaged tube with an endoscope (lighted instrument for viewing internal organs).

The physician attempts to preserve the tube if the woman wants other children, but this is not always possible. The priority medical treatment is to control blood loss. Blood transfusion may be required for massive hemorrhage. One of the following three courses of treatment is chosen, depending on the gestation and the amount of damage to the fallopian tube:

1. No action is taken if the woman's body is resorbing the pregnancy.

Box 5-1   Signs and Symptoms of Hypovolemic Shock

- Fetal heart rate changes (increased, decreased, less fluctuation)
- Rising, weak pulse (tachycardia)
- Rising respiratory rate (tachypnea)
- Shallow, irregular respirations; air hunger
- Falling blood pressure (hypotension)
- Decreased (usually less than 30 mL/hr) or absent urine output
- Pale skin or mucous membranes
- Cold, clammy skin
- Faintness
- Thirst

2. Medical therapy with methotrexate (if the tube is not ruptured) inhibits cell division in the embryo and allows it to be resorbed.
3. Surgery to remove the **products of conception (POC)** from the tube is performed if damage is minimal; severe damage requires removal of the entire tube and occasionally the uterus.

Nursing Care. Nursing care includes observing for hypovolemic shock as in spontaneous abortion. Vaginal bleeding is assessed, although most lost blood may remain in the abdomen. The nurse should report increasing pain, particularly shoulder pain, to the physician.

If the woman has surgery, preoperative and postoperative care is similar to that for other abdominal surgery, as follows:

- Measurement of vital signs to identify hypovolemic shock; of temperature to identify infection
- Assessment of lung and bowel sounds
- Intravenous fluid; blood replacement may be ordered if the loss was substantial
- Antibiotics as ordered
- Pain medication, often with patient-controlled analgesia (PCA) after surgery
- NPO status preoperatively; oral intake usually resumes after surgery, beginning with ice chips and then clear liquids, and it is advanced as bowel sounds resume
- Indwelling Foley catheter as ordered. Urine output is a significant indicator of fluid balance and will fall or stop if the woman hemorrhages; minimum acceptable urine output is 30 mL/hr
- Bed rest before surgery; progressive ambulation postoperatively; the nurse should have adequate assistance when the woman first ambulates, because she is more likely to faint if she lost a significant amount of blood

In addition to physical preoperative and postoperative care, the nurse provides emotional support, because the woman and her family may experience grieving similar to that accompanying spontaneous abortion. Loss of a fallopian tube threatens future fertility and is another source of grief. However, future pregnancies are possible if the remaining fallopian tube is normal.

Nursing Tip

Supporting and encouraging the grieving process in families who suffer a pregnancy loss, such as a spontaneous abortion or ectopic pregnancy, allow them to resolve their grief.

Hydatidiform Mole

Hydatidiform mole (*gestational trophoblastic disease*; also known as a *molar pregnancy*) occurs when the chorionic villi (fringelike structures that form the placenta) increase abnormally and develop vesicles (small sacs) that resemble tiny grapes (see Figure 5-4). The mole may be complete, with no fetus present, or partial, in which only part of the placenta has the characteristic vesicles. Hydatidiform mole may cause hemorrhage, clotting abnormalities, hypertension, and later development of cancer (choriocarcinoma). Chromosome abnormalities are found in many cases of hydatidiform mole. It is more likely to occur in women at the age extremes of reproductive life, and a woman who has had one molar pregnancy has a 1% chance of another molar pregnancy in the future.

Manifestations. Signs associated with hydatidiform mole appear early in pregnancy and can include the following:

- Bleeding, which may range from spotting to profuse hemorrhage; cramping may be present
- Rapid uterine growth and a uterine size that is larger than expected for the gestation
- Failure to detect fetal heart activity
- Signs of hyperemesis gravidarum (see p. 79)
- Unusually early development of gestational hypertension (see p. 90)
- Higher than expected levels of hCG
- A distinctive "snowstorm" pattern on ultrasound but no evidence of a developing fetus in the uterus

Nursing Tip

The nurse should teach the woman to report promptly any danger signs that occur during pregnancy.

Treatment. The uterus is evacuated by vacuum aspiration and D&E. The level of hCG is tested and retested until it is undetectable, and the levels are followed for at least 1 year. Persistent or rising levels suggest that vesicles remain or that malignant change has occurred. The woman should delay conceiving until follow-up care is complete, because a new pregnancy would confuse tests for hCG. $Rh_o(D)$ immune globulin is prescribed for the Rh-negative woman.

Nursing Care. The nurse observes for bleeding and shock; care is similar to that given in spontaneous abortion and ectopic pregnancy. If the woman also experiences hyperemesis or preeclampsia, the nurse incorporates care related to those conditions as well. The woman has also lost a pregnancy, so the nurse should provide care related to grieving, similar to that for a spontaneous abortion. The need to delay another pregnancy may be a concern if the woman is nearing the end of her reproductive life and wants a child; therefore the need for follow-up examinations is reinforced. The woman is encouraged and taught how to use contraception (see Chapter 11).

BLEEDING DISORDERS OF LATE PREGNANCY

Placenta previa or abruptio placentae often cause bleeding in late pregnancy (Table 5-4).

Table 5-4   Comparison of Placenta Previa and Abruptio Placentae

	PLACENTA PREVIA	ABRUPTIO PLACENTAE
Presenting signs and symptoms	Abnormal implantation of the placenta in the lower uterus *Marginal:* Approaches, but does not reach, the cervical opening (≤3 cm) *Partial:* Partially covers the cervical opening *Total:* Completely covers the cervical opening	Premature separation of the normally implanted placenta *Partial:* Detachment of part of the placenta *Marginal:* Detachment at the edge of the placenta *Central:* Detachment of the center surface of the placenta; edges stay attached *Total:* Complete detachment of the placenta
Bleeding	Obvious vaginal bleeding, usually bright; may be profuse	Visible dark vaginal bleeding or concealed bleeding within the uterus; enlargement of uterus suggests that blood is accumulating within the cavity
Pain	None, other than from normal uterine contractions if in labor	Gradual or abrupt onset of pain and uterine tenderness; possibly low back pain
Uterine consistency	Uterus soft; no abnormal contractions or irritability	Uterus firm and boardlike; may be irritable, with frequent, brief contractions
Fetus	Fetus may be in an abnormal presentation, such as breech or transverse lie (see Chapter 8)	Fetal presentation usually normal
Blood clotting	Normal	Often accompanied by impaired blood clotting More likely to occur if the woman recently ingested cocaine
Postpartum complications	*Infection:* Placental site is near the nonsterile vagina *Hemorrhage:* Lower uterine segment does not contract as effectively to compress bleeding vessels Signs of fetal compromise if maternal shock or extensive placental detachment occur Fetal or neonatal anemia may occur because of blood loss	*Infection:* Bleeding into uterine muscle fibers predisposes to bacterial invasion *Hemorrhage:* Bleeding into uterine muscle fibers damages them, inhibiting uterine contraction after birth Signs of fetal compromise, depending on amount and location of the placental surface that is disrupted Fetal or neonatal anemia may occur because of blood loss

Placenta Previa

Placenta previa occurs when the placenta develops in the lower part of the uterus rather than the upper. There are three degrees of placenta previa, depending on the location of the placenta in relation to the cervix (Figure 5-5, *A*), as follows:

Marginal: Placenta reaches within 2 to 3 cm of the cervical opening

Partial: Placenta partly covers the cervical opening

Total: Placenta completely covers the cervical opening

A low-lying placenta is implanted near the cervix but does not cover any of the opening. This variation is not a true placenta previa and may or may not be accompanied by bleeding. The low-lying placenta may be discovered during a routine ultrasound examination in early pregnancy. It also may be diagnosed during late pregnancy, because the woman has signs similar to those of a true placenta previa.

Manifestations. Painless vaginal bleeding, usually bright red, is the main characteristic of placenta previa. The woman's risk of hemorrhage increases as term approaches and the cervix begins to efface (thin) and

dilate (open). These normal prelabor changes disrupt the placental attachment. The fetus is often in an abnormal presentation (e.g., breech or transverse lie), because the placenta occupies the lower uterus, which often prevents the fetus from assuming the normal head-down presentation.

The fetus or neonate may have anemia or hypovolemic shock, because some of the blood lost may be fetal blood. Fetal hypoxia may occur if a large disruption of the placental surface reduces the transfer of oxygen and nutrients.

The woman with placenta previa is more likely than others to experience an infection or hemorrhage after birth for the following reasons:

• Infection is more likely to occur because vaginal organisms can easily reach the placental site, which is a good growth medium for microorganisms.

• Postpartum hemorrhage may occur because the lower segment of the uterus, where the placenta was attached, has fewer muscle fibers than the upper uterus. The resulting weak contraction of the lower uterus does not compress the open blood vessels at the placental site as effectively as would the upper segment of the uterus.

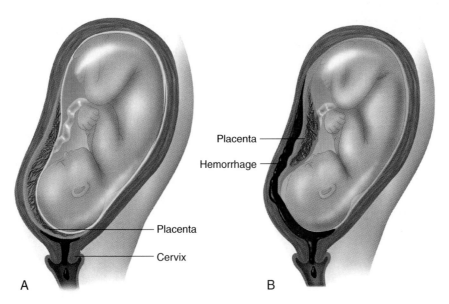

A   B

FIGURE 5-5 Placenta previa and abruptio placentae. **A,** Placenta previa. The placenta *(purple in this illustration)* is implanted low in the uterus. Detachment of the placenta from the uterine wall occurs as the cervix dilates, resulting in bleeding. **B,** Abruptio placentae. The placenta *(purple)* is implanted normally in the uterus but separates from the uterine wall. If the fetal head is engaged, bleeding *(red in this illustration)* may accumulate in the uterus instead of being expelled externally. (From Patton KT, Thibodeau GA: *Anatomy & physiology,* ed 8, St Louis, 2013, Mosby.)

Treatment. Medical care depends on the length of gestation and the amount of bleeding. The goal is to maintain the pregnancy until the fetal lungs are mature enough that respiratory distress is less likely. Delivery will be done if bleeding is sufficient to jeopardize the mother or fetus, regardless of gestational age.

The woman should lie on her side or have a pillow under one hip to avoid supine hypotension. If bleeding is extensive or the gestation is near term, a cesarean section is performed for partial or total placenta previa. The woman with a low-lying placenta or marginal placenta previa may be able to deliver vaginally unless the blood loss is excessive.

Nursing Care. The priorities of nursing care include monitoring the fetal heart and the character of contractions. Documenting and reporting vaginal blood loss and signs and symptoms of shock are important. Vital signs are taken every 15 minutes if the woman is actively bleeding, and oxygen is often given to increase the amount delivered to the fetus. Vaginal examination is not done, because it may precipitate bleeding if the placental attachment is disrupted. The fetal heart rate is monitored continuously. As needed, the nurse implements care for a cesarean delivery (see Chapter 8). The parents of the infant are often fearful for their child, particularly if a preterm delivery is required. Supportive care should be provided.

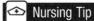 **Nursing Tip**

If placenta previa is suspected, the physician will perform a vaginal examination with preparations for both vaginal and cesarean delivery (a double setup) in place.

Abruptio Placentae

An abruptio placenta is the premature separation of a placenta that is normally implanted. Predisposing factors include the following:

- Hypertension
- Cocaine (which causes vasoconstriction)
- Cigarette smoking and poor nutrition
- Blows to the abdomen, such as might occur in battering or accidental trauma
- Previous history of abruptio placentae
- Folate deficiency

Abruptio placentae may be partial or total (see Figure 5-5, *B*); it may be marginal (separating at the edges) or central (separating in the middle). Bleeding may be visible or concealed behind the partially attached placenta.

Nursing Tip

Pain is an important symptom that distinguishes abruptio placentae from placenta previa.

Manifestations. Bleeding accompanied by abdominal or low back pain is the typical characteristic of abruptio placentae. Unlike the bleeding in placenta previa, most or all of the bleeding may be concealed behind the placenta. Obvious dark-red vaginal bleeding occurs when blood leaks past the edge of the placenta. The woman's uterus is tender and unusually firm (boardlike), because blood leaks into its muscle fibers. Frequent, cramplike uterine contractions often occur (uterine irritability).

The fetus may or may not have problems, depending on how much placental surface is disrupted. As in placenta previa, some of the blood lost may be fetal, and the fetus or neonate may have anemia or hypovolemic shock.

Disseminated intravascular coagulation (DIC) is a complex disorder that may complicate abruptio placentae. The large blood clot that forms behind the placenta consumes clotting factors, which leaves the rest of the mother's body deficient in these factors. Clot formation and anticoagulation (destruction of clots) occur simultaneously throughout the body in the woman with DIC. She may bleed from her mouth, nose, incisions, or venipuncture sites because the clotting factors are depleted.

Postpartum hemorrhage may also occur, because the injured uterine muscle does not contract effectively to control blood loss. Infection is more likely to occur, because the damaged tissue is susceptible to microbial invasion.

Treatment. The treatment of choice, immediate cesarean delivery, is performed because of the risk for maternal shock, clotting disorders, and fetal death. Blood and clotting factor replacement may be needed because of DIC. The mother's clotting action quickly returns to normal after birth, because the source of the abnormality is removed.

Nursing Care. Preparation for cesarean section and close monitoring of vital signs and fetal heart are essential. Signs of shock and bleeding from the nose, the gums, or other unexpected sites should be promptly reported. Rapid increase in the size of the uterus suggests that blood is accumulating within it. The uterus is usually very tender and hard. Nursing care after delivery is similar to that with placenta previa.

The fetus sometimes dies before delivery. See Nursing Care Plan 5-1 for nursing care related to fetal death (stillbirth) and support of the grieving family. Many therapeutic communication techniques outlined in the Communication box on p. 86 are appropriate. The care of a pregnant woman with excessive bleeding is summarized in Box 5-2.

Box 5-2 | Care of the Pregnant Woman with Excessive Bleeding

Document blood loss.
Closely monitor vital signs, including intake and output.
Observe for:
• Pain
• Uterine rigidity or tenderness
Verify that orders for blood typing and cross-match have been implemented.
Monitor intravenous infusion.
Prepare for surgery, if indicated.
Monitor fetal heart rate and contractions.
Monitor laboratory results, including coagulation studies.
Administer oxygen by mask.
Prepare for newborn resuscitation.

HYPERTENSION DURING PREGNANCY

Hypertension may exist before pregnancy (chronic hypertension), but often it develops as a pregnancy complication (gestational hypertension [GH], formerly known as pregnancy-induced hypertension [PIH]). Table 5-5 compares the different types of hypertension during pregnancy. The term **preeclampsia** may be used when GH includes proteinuria. Preeclampsia progresses to **eclampsia** when convulsions occur. One sometimes hears the term *toxemia,* an old term for GH.

The cause of GH is unknown, but birth is its cure. It usually develops after the twentieth week of gestation. Vasospasm (spasm of the arteries) is the main characteristic of GH. Although the cause is unknown, any of several risk factors increases a woman's chance of developing GH (Box 5-3).

There has been a gradual increase in the number of women delaying pregnancy until beyond the age of 30 years, and the chances of chronic hypertension complicating pregnancy has increased. Chronic hypertension is considered moderate if the systolic reading is between 140 and 160 mm Hg and the diastolic reading is below 110 mm Hg. However, an increase over baseline blood pressure of 30 mm Hg or more systolic and 15 mm Hg diastolic will place the woman in a high-risk category. Therefore a woman with a baseline blood

---

Table 5-5 | Hypertensive Disorders of Pregnancy

DISORDER	CHARACTERISTICS
Gestational hypertension (GH)	Development of hypertension (blood pressure >140/90 mm Hg) in a previously normotensive woman after 20 weeks of gestation Does not include proteinuria; blood pressure usually returns to normal 6 weeks postpartum
Preeclampsia	As above, with renal involvement leading to proteinuria
Eclampsia	As above, with central nervous system (CNS) involvement causing seizures Liver and coagulation abnormalities dominate the clinical picture
Chronic hypertension	Presence of hypertension before 20 weeks of gestation; usually, hypertension lasting >42 days postpartum
Preeclampsia with superimposed chronic hypertension	Chronic hypertension that has new occurrence of proteinuria or occurrence of thrombocytopenia and increased liver enzymes (formerly known as HELLP syndrome (**h**emolysis, **e**levated **l**iver enzymes, **l**ow **p**latelets)

Data from Gabbe S, Niebyl J, Simpson J et al: *Obstetrics: normal and problem pregnancies,* Philadelphia, 2012, Saunders; ACOG: *Chronic hypertension in pregnancy: practice bulletin #29,* Washington, D.C., 2010, ACOG; ACOG: *Diagnosis and management of preeclampsia and eclampsia: practice bulletin #33,* Washington D.C., 2010, ACOG.

Box 5-3	Risk Factors for Gestational Hypertension

- First pregnancy
- Obesity
- Family history of gestational hypertension (GH)
- Age more than 35 years or less than 19 years
- Multifetal pregnancy (e.g., twins)
- Chronic hypertension
- Chronic renal disease
- Diabetes mellitus

Modified from Creasy R et al: *Maternal-fetal medicine*, ed 6, Philadelphia, 2009, Saunders; Gabbe S et al: *Obstetrics: normal and problem pregnancies*, Philadelphia, 2012, Elsevier.

pressure that is normally low, such as 90/60 mm Hg, may be at risk for GH if her blood pressure rises to 120/80 mm Hg (Creasy, 2009) especially if proteinuria occurs. Blood pressure normally decreases during the first two trimesters.

Hypertension is closely related to the development of complications, such as abruptio placentae, fetal growth restriction, preeclampsia, prematurity, and stillbirth, so special care of the pregnant woman with hypertension is essential. The approach to chronic hypertension during pregnancy is complex, because many drugs used to treat hypertension, such as atenolol, cause a drop in mean arterial blood pressure and can result in restricted fetal growth and other problems. For this reason, antihypertensive medication is not administered for mild to moderate levels of high blood pressure. Instead, frequent prenatal visits, urinalysis to detect proteinuria, and fetal assessments are the standards of care, and medication is started if the blood pressure exceeds the moderate range. Drugs of choice include methyldopa (Aldomet), alpha-adrenergic and beta-adrenergic blockers (labetalol), and calcium channel blockers (nifedipine) in some cases of hypertensive crisis.

Manifestations of Gestational Hypertension.
Vasospasm impedes blood flow to the mother's organs and placenta, resulting in one or more of these signs: (1) hypertension, (2) edema, and (3) proteinuria (protein in the urine). Severe GH can also affect the central nervous system, eyes, urinary tract, liver, gastrointestinal system, and blood clotting function. Table 5-6 summarizes laboratory tests that aid in diagnosis.

Hypertension. Despite an increase in blood volume and cardiac output, most pregnant women do not experience a rise in blood pressure, because they have a resistance to factors that cause vasoconstriction. In addition, the resistance to blood flow in their vessels (peripheral vascular resistance) decreases because of the effects of hormonal changes. A blood pressure of 140/90 mm Hg or above is considered to constitute hypertension in pregnancy.

Edema. Edema can occur because fluid leaves the blood vessels and enters the tissues. Although total body fluid is increased, the amount within the blood

Table 5-6	Laboratory Tests for Patients with Gestational Hypertension

TEST	RATIONALE
Hemoglobin and hematocrit	Detects hemoconcentration for indication of severity of gestational hypertension (GH)
Platelets	Thrombocytopenia suggests GH
Urine for protein	Proteinuria confirms GH when hypotension is present
Serum creatinine	Elevated creatinine and oliguria suggest GH
Serum uric acid	Elevated uric acid suggests GH
Serum transaminase	Elevated transaminase confirms liver involvement in GH

Data from Gabbe S et al: *Obstetrics: normal and problem pregnancies*, Philadelphia, 2012, Saunders.

vessels is reduced (hypovolemia), further decreasing blood flow to the maternal organs and placenta. It is likely to be the first sign the woman notices but is not essential to the diagnosis.

Sudden excessive weight gain is the first sign of fluid retention. Visible edema follows the weight gain. Edema of the feet and legs is common during pregnancy, but edema above the waist suggests GH. The woman may notice facial swelling or may stop wearing rings because they are hard to remove. Edema is severe if a depression remains after the tissue is compressed briefly with the finger ("pitting" edema).

Edema resolves quickly after birth as excess tissue fluid returns to the circulation and is excreted in the urine. Urine output may reach 6 L/day and often exceeds fluid intake.

Proteinuria. Proteinuria develops as reduced blood flow damages the kidneys. This damage allows protein to leak into the urine. A clean-catch (midstream) or catheterized urine specimen is used to check for proteinuria, because vaginal secretions might lead to a false-positive result.

Other Manifestations of Preeclampsia. Other signs and symptoms occur with severe preeclampsia. All are related to decreased blood flow and edema of the organs involved.

Central nervous system. A severe, unrelenting headache may occur because of brain edema and small cerebral hemorrhages. The severe headache often precedes a convulsion. Deep tendon reflexes become hyperactive because of central nervous system irritability.

Eyes. Visual disturbances such as blurred or double vision or "spots before the eyes" occur because of arterial spasm and edema surrounding the retina. Visual disturbances often precede a convulsion.

Urinary tract. Decreased blood flow to the kidneys reduces urine production and worsens hypertension.

Respiratory system. Pulmonary edema (accumulation of fluid in the lungs) may occur with severe GH.

Gastrointestinal system and liver. Epigastric pain or nausea occurs because of liver edema, ischemia, and necrosis and often precedes a convulsion. Liver enzyme levels are elevated because of reduced circulation, edema, and small hemorrhages.

Blood clotting. HELLP syndrome is a variant of GH that involves **h**emolysis (breakage of erythrocytes), **e**levated **l**iver enzymes, and **l**ow **p**latelets. Hemolysis occurs as erythrocytes break up when passing through small blood vessels damaged by the hypertension. Obstruction of hepatic blood flow causes the liver enzyme levels to become elevated. Low platelet levels occur when the platelets gather at the site of blood vessel damage, reducing the number available in the general circulation. Low platelet levels cause abnormal blood clotting.

Eclampsia. Progression to eclampsia occurs when the woman has one or more generalized **tonic-clonic seizures.** Facial muscles twitch; this sign is followed by generalized contraction of all muscles (tonic phase), then alternate contraction and relaxation of the muscles (clonic phase). An eclamptic seizure may result in cerebral hemorrhage, abruptio placentae, fetal compromise, or death of the mother or fetus. Magnesium is administered to control seizures; close fetal monitoring is essential as well as monitoring the uterine contractions; and measures to prevent aspiration are responsibilities of the nurse. Delivery may be expedited.

Effects on the Fetus. GH reduces maternal blood and nutrition flow through the placenta and decreases the oxygen available to the fetus. Fetal hypoxia may result in meconium (first stool) passage into the amniotic fluid or in fetal distress. The fetus may have intrauterine growth restriction and at birth may be long and thin with peeling skin if the reduced placental blood flow has been prolonged. Fetal death sometimes occurs.

Treatment. Medical care focuses on prevention and early detection of GH. Drugs are sometimes needed to prevent convulsions and to reduce blood pressure that is dangerously high.

Prevention. Correction of some risk factors reduces the risk for GH. For example, improving the diet, particularly of the pregnant adolescent, may prevent GH and promote normal fetal growth. Other risk factors, such as family history, cannot be changed. Early and regular prenatal care allows GH to be diagnosed promptly so that it is more effectively managed.

Management. Treatment of GH depends on the severity of the hypertension and on the maturity of the fetus. Treatment focuses on (1) maintaining blood flow to the woman's vital organs and the placenta, and (2) preventing convulsions. Birth is the cure for GH. If the fetus is mature, pregnancy is ended by labor induction or cesarean birth. If GH is severe, the fetus is often in greater danger from being in the uterus than from being born prematurely.

Some women with mild GH can be managed at home if they can comply with treatment and if home nursing visits are possible. If the woman has severe GH or cannot comply with treatment, or if home nursing visits are not available, she is usually admitted to the hospital. Conservative treatment, whether at home or in the hospital, includes the following:

- Activity restriction to allow blood that would be circulated to skeletal muscles to be conserved for circulation to the mother's vital organs and the placenta. The woman should remain on reduced activity with frequent rest periods lying on her side to improve blood flow to the placenta.
- Maternal assessment of fetal activity ("kick counts"). She should report a decrease in movements or if none occur during a 4-hour period.
- Blood pressure monitoring two to four times per day in the same arm and in the same position. A family member must be taught the technique if the woman can safely remain at home.
- Daily weight measurement on the same scale, in the same type of clothing, and at the same time of day to observe for sudden weight gain.
- Checking urine for protein with a dipstick using a first-voided, clean-catch specimen.

🏠 **Home Care Considerations**

Hypertension in Pregnancy

Patient teaching for home care should include the following:
- Exercise may have to be curtailed
- Avoid weight loss programs
- Discontinue smoking and alcohol use
- Primary management is without drugs, because blood pressure normally falls in the first two trimesters of pregnancy
- Daily blood pressure measurement
- Daily weight
- Daily urine dipstick for protein
- Monitor fetal kicks and uterine activity
- Balanced diet with sufficient protein to replace loss
- Teach signs and symptoms of problems to report
- Encourage side lying during rest periods

Diuretics and sodium restriction are not prescribed for GH. They are not effective for the treatment of GH and may aggravate it, because they further deplete the woman's blood volume. Aspirin therapy or dietary supplements such as calcium have not proved helpful in managing GH. The intake of high-salt foods is discouraged. The woman's diet should have adequate calories and protein (see Chapter 4 for prenatal dietary guidelines). See Table 5-1 for fetal assessment tests that may be done.

Drug Therapy. Several drugs may also be used to treat GH, as described in the sections that follow. *Magnesium sulfate* is an anticonvulsant administered to prevent seizures. It also may slightly reduce the blood pressure, but its main purpose is as an anticonvulsant. It is usually given by intravenous infusion (controlled with an infusion pump). Administration continues for at least 12 to 24 hours after birth, because the woman remains at risk for seizures.

The kidneys excrete magnesium. Poor urine output (less than 30 mL/h) may allow serum levels of magnesium to reach toxic levels. Excess magnesium first causes loss of the deep tendon reflexes, which is followed by depression of respirations; if levels continue to rise, collapse and death can occur. Close monitoring of the respiratory rate is essential in women who receive magnesium sulfate. Calcium gluconate reverses the effects of magnesium and should be available for immediate use when a woman receives magnesium sulfate.

The therapeutic serum level of magnesium is 4 to 8 mg/dL, which would be an abnormal level in a person not receiving this therapy. The woman with this serum level is slightly drowsy but retains all her reflexes and has normal respiratory function; the level is high enough to prevent convulsions.

Magnesium inhibits uterine contractions. Most women receiving the drug during labor must also receive oxytocin to strengthen labor contractions (see Chapter 8). They are at increased risk for postpartum hemorrhage, because the uterus does not contract firmly on bleeding vessels after birth. This contraction-inhibiting effect of magnesium makes it useful to stop preterm labor. An essential nursing responsibility when caring for women receiving magnesium sulfate is to monitor contractions during labor and to take measures to maintain a firm uterine fundus postpartum. The nurse should alert the newborn nursery staff when magnesium sulfate has been administered during labor, because if the newborn is treated with aminoglycosides (such as kanamycin [Kantrex] or neomycin), an interaction can occur and can result in toxic responses in the newborn.

Antihypertensive drugs are used to reduce blood pressure when it reaches a level that might cause intracranial bleeding, usually higher than 160/100 mm Hg. Severe hypertension can harm the fetus by causing abruptio placentae or placental infarcts (death of placental tissue). The goal of antihypertensive therapy is a gradual reduction of blood pressure to normal levels. The nurse should observe for untoward signs such as sudden hypotension. Hydralazine and labetalol are the drugs most often used.

Nursing Care. Nursing care focuses on (1) assisting women to obtain prenatal care, (2) helping them cope with therapy, (3) caring for acutely ill women, and (4) administering medications. Nursing Care Plan 5-2 presents common interventions for women with GH.

Promoting prenatal care. Nurses can promote awareness of how prenatal care allows risk identification and early intervention if complications arise. Nurses can help the woman to feel like an individual—especially in busy clinics, which often seem impersonal—thus encouraging her to return regularly.

Helping to cope with therapy. Daily weight measurements identify sudden weight gain that precedes visible edema. The weight should be checked early in the morning, after urination, with the woman wearing similar clothes each day. The nurse helps the woman to understand the importance of reduced activity and frequent rest periods and to plan ways to manage them. Activity diverts blood from the placenta, reducing the infant's oxygen supply, so the nurse must impress on the woman how important rest is to her child's well-being. Positioning the patient on her side during bed rest helps to improve blood flow to the placenta and more effectively provides oxygen and nutrients to the fetus. See the discussion of preterm labor (Chapter 8) for more information about care related to bed rest.

Caring for the acutely ill woman. The acutely ill woman requires intensive nursing care directed by an experienced registered nurse. A quiet, low-light environment reduces the risk of seizures. The woman should remain on bed rest on her side, often the left side, to promote maximum fetal oxygenation. Side rails should be padded and raised to prevent injury if a convulsion occurs. Stimulation such as loud noises or bumping of the bed should be avoided. Visitors are usually limited to one or two support persons. Suction equipment is available for immediate use.

If a seizure occurs, the nursing focus is to prevent injury and restore oxygenation to the mother and fetus. If the woman is not already on her side, the nurse should try to turn her before the seizure begins. The nurse does not forcibly hold the woman's body but protects her from injury caused by striking hard surfaces.

Breathing can stop during a seizure. An oral airway, inserted after the seizure, facilitates breathing and suctioning of secretions. Aspiration of secretions can occur during a seizure, so the health care provider may order chest radiographs and arterial blood gas measurements. Oxygen by face mask improves fetal oxygenation. The woman is reoriented to the environment when she regains consciousness. Labor may progress rapidly after a seizure, often while the woman is still drowsy, and the fetus is monitored continuously (see Chapter 6 for signs of impending birth).

Administering medications. An experienced registered nurse administers magnesium sulfate. A licensed practical nurse or licensed vocational nurse (LPN/LVN) may assist. Hospital protocols provide specific guidelines for care when magnesium sulfate is given. Common protocols include the following:

- Blood pressure, pulse, respirations recorded hourly
- Temperature recorded every 4 hours
- Deep tendon reflexes checked every 1 to 4 hours
- Intake and output recorded (often hourly); an indwelling Foley catheter may be ordered
- Urine protein checked with a reagent strip (dipstick) at each voiding

★ Nursing Care Plan 5-2   The Woman with Gestational Hypertension

PATIENT DATA A woman is admitted with signs of mild gestational hypertension (GH), and plans are made for discharge to the home with careful follow-up. The woman asks what she can do to avoid further complications and problems.

Selected Nursing Diagnosis: Deficient knowledge related to home care of mild GH

Goals	Nursing Interventions	Rationales
The woman will restate correct home care measures related to GH. The woman will keep prescribed prenatal appointments.	Ask the woman what she knows about hypertension during pregnancy; include family members if present. Teach the woman the importance of keeping prenatal appointments, which will be more frequent because she has mild GH. Reinforce to the woman the prescribed measures to care for herself at home: • Remain on bed rest, spending most of the time on her side (may walk to the bathroom and eat meals at table in most cases) • Eat a well-balanced, high-protein diet; limit high-sodium foods such as potato chips, salted nuts, pickles, and many snack foods; include high-fiber foods and at least eight glasses of noncaffeinated drinks each day. Consider food preferences and economic restraints when helping the woman choose appropriate foods. • Discuss quiet activities the woman enjoys that can be done while she is on bed rest. Teach the woman to report signs promptly that indicate worsening GH: headache; visual disturbances (blurring, flashes of light, "spots before the eyes"); gastrointestinal symptoms (nausea, pain); worsening edema, especially of the face and fingers; noticeable drop in urine output.	Allows the nurse to build on woman's existing knowledge, reinforcing it and correcting any misunderstandings of the woman or family. GH can quickly become more severe between prenatal care visits. If the woman understands why she should keep appointments, she is more likely to do so. If woman understands these measures to limit the severity of GH, she may be more motivated to maintain them: • Bed rest reduces the flow of blood to the skeletal muscles, thus making more available to placenta; this enhances fetal oxygenation. • Women with GH lose protein in their urine, which must be replaced to maintain nutrition and fluid balance; severe sodium restriction may increase severity of GH, but a high sodium intake may worsen hypertension and decrease the woman's blood volume; fiber and fluids help to reduce constipation, which is more likely when activity is restricted. • Bed rest can lead to boredom, and the woman may not maintain the prescribed activity if she is unaware of which activities she can do. GH can worsen despite careful home management and patient compliance; if the woman has these symptoms, she needs to be evaluated and possibly hospitalized to prevent progression to eclampsia.

Selected Nursing Diagnosis: Effective therapeutic regimen management related to GH

Goals	Nursing Interventions	Rationales
Blood pressure will remain within normal limits. Fetal heart rate will remain in a reassuring pattern. There will be an absence of peripheral facial and abdominal edema. Weight gain will be within normal limits. Seizures will not occur.	Monitor and record baseline vital signs. Monitor changes in fetal heart rate (FHR). Monitor urine protein (proteinuria). With severe preeclampsia, keep the room quiet with minimal stimulation in environment. Monitor weight gain, fluid intake and output, and edema above the waist.	Compare baseline data to changes that occur that may indicate fetus is in jeopardy. FHR reflects fetal status. Protein of 3+ or more may be a sign of impending eclampsia. Environmental stimulants can precipitate seizure. Weight gain exceeding 0.5 kg/week is indicative of GH. Urine output of less than 30 mL/hr may indicate renal shutdown. Edema may indicate increasing complications.

Critical Thinking Questions

1. A woman in the prenatal clinic states that high blood pressure runs in her family, and she has been taking medication for a slightly elevated blood pressure for many years. She states she has had most success with the medication she is currently taking (atenolol) and would like to continue this regimen during her pregnancy. What is the best response from the nurse?
2. In developing a teaching plan for a woman with GH, what factors must be considered and included in the plan?

- Laboratory blood levels of magnesium ordered every 4 hours

Deterioration of the maternal or fetal condition is promptly reported. Signs and symptoms of deterioration include the following:

- Increasing hypertension, particularly if blood pressure is 160/100 mm Hg or higher
- Signs of central nervous system irritability, such as facial twitching or hyperactive deep tendon reflexes
- Decreased urine output, especially if less than 25 mL/hr
- Abnormal fetal heart rates
- Symptoms such as severe headache, visual disturbances, or epigastric pain, which often immediately precede a convulsion

The registered nurse reports the following signs of possible magnesium toxicity, or factors that may cause magnesium toxicity, to the physician and prepares calcium gluconate to reverse this toxicity:

- Absent deep tendon reflexes
- Respiration rate under 12 breaths/min
- Urine output less than 30 mL/hr (allows accumulation of excess magnesium in the blood)
- Serum magnesium levels above 8 mg/dL

Providing postpartum care. GH is of concern to the prenatal patient and the fetus and continues to be a threat in the postpartum period. Women with chronic hypertension are at risk for pulmonary edema, renal failure, and convulsions. Close monitoring for 48 hours after delivery is essential. Patients requiring antihypertensive drugs postpartum who are breastfeeding are usually given methyldopa or labetalol. Other antihypertensive drugs may have adverse effects on the breastfeeding infant. Diuretics decrease milk production and are generally not administered.

BLOOD INCOMPATIBILITY BETWEEN THE PREGNANT WOMAN AND THE FETUS

The placenta allows maternal and fetal blood to be close enough to exchange oxygen and waste products without actually mixing (see Chapter 3). However, small leaks that allow fetal blood to enter the mother's circulation may occur during pregnancy or when the placenta detaches at birth. No problem occurs if maternal and fetal blood types are compatible. However, if the maternal and fetal blood factors differ, the mother's body will produce antibodies to destroy the foreign fetal red blood cells (RBCs, or erythrocytes). These antibodies will pass through the placenta to the fetus and destroy the Rh-positive blood cells in the fetus.

Rh and ABO Incompatibility

The Rh-negative blood type is an autosomal recessive trait, which means that a person must receive a gene for this characteristic from both parents. The Rh-positive blood type is a dominant trait. The Rh-positive person may have inherited two Rh-positive genes or may have one Rh-positive and one Rh-negative gene.

This explains why two Rh-positive parents can conceive a child who is Rh-negative.

People either have the Rh blood factor on their erythrocytes or they do not. If they have the factor, they are Rh positive; if not, they are Rh negative. An Rh-positive person can receive Rh-negative blood with no untoward effects (if all other factors are compatible), because in Rh-negative blood this factor is absent. However, the reverse is not true—Rh incompatibility between the woman and fetus can occur only if the woman is Rh negative and the fetus is Rh positive.

A person with Rh-negative blood is not born with antibodies against the Rh factor. However, exposure to Rh-positive blood causes the person to make antibodies to destroy Rh-positive erythrocytes. The antibodies remain ready to destroy any future Rh-positive erythrocytes that enter the circulation (sensitization).

If fetal Rh-positive blood leaks into the Rh-negative mother's circulation, her body may respond by making antibodies to destroy the Rh-positive erythrocytes. This process is called **isoimmunization**. Because this leakage usually occurs at birth, the first Rh-positive child is rarely seriously affected. However, the woman's blood levels of antibodies increase rapidly each time she is exposed to more Rh-positive blood (in subsequent pregnancies with Rh-positive fetuses). Antibodies against Rh-positive blood cross the placenta and destroy the fetal Rh-positive erythrocytes before the infant is born. A similar response occurs with ABO incompatibility when the mother is type O and the infant's blood type is type A or type B.

Manifestations. The woman has no obvious effects if her body produces anti-Rh antibodies. Rising antibody titers in laboratory tests evidence increased levels of these antibodies in her blood. Noninvasive DNA testing of maternal plasma can now also determine fetal Rh status (Moise, 2005a). When these maternal anti-Rh antibodies cross the placenta and destroy fetal erythrocytes, **erythroblastosis fetalis** results (Figure 5-6). The effect on the newborn is discussed in Chapter 14.

Treatment and Nursing Care. The primary management to prevent the manufacture of anti-Rh antibodies is by giving $Rh_o(D)$ immune globulin (RhoGAM) to the Rh-negative woman at 28 weeks of gestation and within 72 hours after birth of an Rh-positive infant or abortion (see Chapter 14). It is also given after amniocentesis and to women who experience bleeding during pregnancy, because fetal blood may leak into the mother's circulation at these times. If the fetal blood type is unknown (as with abortion), $Rh_o(D)$ immune globulin is given to the Rh-negative mother. $Rh_o(D)$ immune globulin has greatly decreased the incidence of infants with Rh-incompatibility problems. However, some women are still sensitized, usually because they did not receive $Rh_o(D)$ immune globulin after childbirth

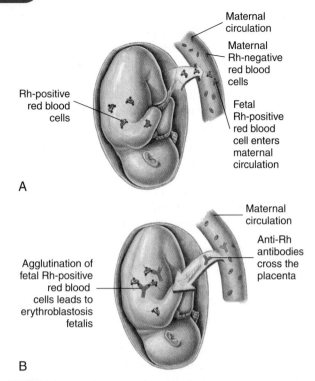

A

B

FIGURE 5-6 Erythroblastosis fetalis. **A,** A few fetal Rh-positive red blood cells enter the circulation of the Rh-negative mother during pregnancy or at birth, causing the mother to produce antibodies against Rh-positive blood cells. **B,** The Rh-positive antibodies from the maternal circulation cross the placenta, enter the fetal circulation, and destroy fetal Rh-positive blood cells. (From Thibodeau GA, Patton KT: *Structure and function of the body*, ed 12, St Louis, 2004, Mosby.)

or abortion. Rh₀(D) immune globulin will not be effective if sensitization has already occurred.

Nursing Tip

Most cases of Rh incompatibility between an Rh-negative mother and an Rh-positive fetus can be prevented with the administration of Rh₀(D) immune globulin (RhoGAM) in every case in which incompatibility is indicated.

The woman who is sensitized to destroy Rh-positive blood cells is carefully monitored during pregnancy to determine if too many fetal erythrocytes are being destroyed. Several fetal assessment tests may be used, including the Coombs' test, amniocentesis, or percutaneous umbilical blood sampling (see Table 5-1).

An intrauterine transfusion may be performed for the severely anemic fetus. The Rh factor should be documented on the chart and the health care provider notified if the woman is Rh negative. See Chapter 14 for the effect of Rh and ABO incompatibility on the newborn.

PREGNANCY COMPLICATED BY MEDICAL CONDITIONS

Health problems that are present before pregnancy can influence the outcome of pregnancy and necessitate special management. Chronic health problems discussed in this section include diabetes mellitus, heart disease, anemia, and infections.

DIABETES MELLITUS

Diabetes mellitus (DM) can be classified according to whether it preceded pregnancy or had its onset during pregnancy. Types of DM include the following (ADA, 2011):

- *Type 1 diabetes mellitus:* Usually caused by an autoimmune destruction of the beta cells of the pancreas resulting in an insulin deficiency.
- *Type 2 diabetes mellitus:* Usually caused by insulin resistance; usually has a strong genetic predisposition and is associated with obesity.
- *Pregestational diabetes mellitus:* Type 1 or 2 diabetes that existed before pregnancy occurred.
- **Gestational diabetes mellitus (GDM):** Glucose intolerance with onset during pregnancy. In true GDM, glucose usually returns to normal by 6 weeks postpartum.

Consult a medical-surgical nursing text for a more detailed discussion of diabetes mellitus in the nonpregnant person.

Pathophysiology

Diabetes mellitus is a disorder in which there is inadequate insulin to move glucose from the blood into body cells. It occurs because the pancreas produces no insulin or insufficient insulin, or because cells resist the effects of insulin. Essentially, cells starve because they cannot obtain glucose. To compensate, the body metabolizes protein and fat for energy, which causes ketones and acids to accumulate (ketoacidosis). The person loses weight despite eating large amounts of food (polyphagia). Fatigue and lethargy accompany cell starvation. To dilute excess glucose in the blood, thirst increases (polydipsia), and fluid moves from the tissues into the blood. This results in tissue dehydration and the excretion of large amounts (polyuria) of glucose-bearing urine (glycosuria).

Effect of Pregnancy on Glucose Metabolism

Pregnancy affects a woman's metabolism (whether or not she has DM) to make ample glucose available to the growing fetus. Hormones (estrogen and progesterone), an enzyme (insulinase) produced by the placenta, and increased prolactin levels have two effects:

- Increased resistance of cells to insulin
- Increased speed of insulin breakdown

Most women respond to these changes by secreting extra insulin to maintain normal carbohydrate metabolism while still providing plenty of glucose for the fetus. If the woman cannot increase her insulin production, she will have periods of *hyperglycemia* (increased blood glucose levels) as glucose accumulates in the blood. Because the fetus continuously draws glucose from the mother, maternal *hypoglycemia* (low blood glucose) can occur between meals and during the night. There is also a normally increased tissue resistance to maternal insulin action in the second and third trimesters, and the fetus is then at risk for organ damage resulting from hyperglycemia.

Preexisting Diabetes Mellitus

Women who are diabetic before pregnancy must alter the management of their condition. The time of major risk for congenital anomalies to occur from maternal hyperglycemia is during the embryonic period of development in the first trimester. Therefore, women who are diabetic **before** pregnancy have a greater risk of having a newborn with a congenital anomaly than a woman who develops gestational diabetes, which is usually manifested after the first trimester. With careful management, most diabetic women can have successful pregnancies and healthy babies. Nevertheless, there are many potential complications of diabetes (Box 5-4).

Gestational Diabetes Mellitus

Gestational diabetes mellitus (GDM) is common and resolves quickly after birth; however, some women who experience GDM develop overt diabetes later in life. The following factors in a woman's history are linked to gestational diabetes (ACOG, 2011):

- Maternal obesity (>90 kg or 198 lb)
- Large infant (>4000 g or about 9 lb [Figure 5-7], **macrosomia**)
- Maternal age older than 25 years
- Previous unexplained stillbirth or infant having congenital abnormalities

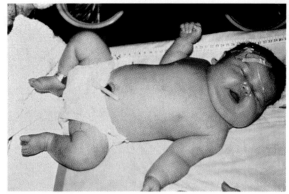

FIGURE 5-7 Macrosomic infant. A newborn with macrosomia caused by maternal diabetes mellitus during pregnancy. This infant weighed 5 kg (11 lb) at birth. Newborns with macrosomia often have respiratory and other problems. (From Zitelli BJ, Davis HW, ed: *Atlas of pediatric physical diagnosis*, ed 6, St Louis, 2012, Mosby.)

- History of GDM in a previous pregnancy
- Family history of DM
- Fasting glucose more than 126 mg/dL or post-meal glucose more than 200 mg/dL

Nursing Care Plan 5-3 lists specific interventions for the pregnant woman with GDM.

Treatment. The nonpregnant woman with diabetes is treated with a balance of insulin or an oral hypoglycemic drug (agent that reduces blood glucose level), diet, and exercise. Some people with mild diabetes do not need drugs and control their condition by diet and exercise alone. Medical therapy during pregnancy includes identification of gestational diabetes, diet modifications, monitoring of blood glucose levels, insulin, exercise, and selected fetal assessments.

Identification of GDM. If the woman does not have preexisting diabetes, a prenatal screening test to identify GDM is routinely performed between 24 and 28 weeks of gestation but may be done earlier if risk factors are present (Gabbe, 2012). The woman drinks 50 g of an oral glucose solution (fasting is not necessary), and a blood sample is taken 1 hour later and is analyzed for glucose. If the blood glucose level is 140 mg/dL or higher, a more complex, 3-hour glucose tolerance test is done.

Diet modifications. The woman is counseled to avoid single large meals with high amounts of simple carbohydrates. A balanced food intake is divided among three meals and at least two snacks throughout the day to maintain stable blood glucose levels. The timing and content of meals and snacks may require adjustment to prevent early-morning hypoglycemia. Foods that release glucose slowly are preferred to avoid rapid changes in blood glucose.

Monitoring of blood glucose levels. To ensure a successful pregnancy, the woman must keep her blood glucose levels as close to normal as possible and be taught the signs and symptoms of both hypoglycemia and hyperglycemia (Table 5-7). The pregnant diabetic woman

---

| Box 5-4 | Effects of Diabetes in Pregnancy |

MATERNAL EFFECTS
Spontaneous abortion
Gestational hypertension
Preterm labor and premature rupture of the membranes
Hydramnios (excessive amniotic fluid; also called polyhydramnios)
Infections:
- Vaginitis
- Urinary tract infections

Complications of large fetal size:
- Birth canal injuries
- Forceps-assisted or cesarean birth

Ketoacidosis

FETAL AND NEONATAL EFFECTS
Congenital abnormalities
Macrosomia (large size)
Intrauterine growth restriction
Birth injury
Delayed lung maturation; respiratory distress syndrome
Neonatal hypoglycemia
Neonatal hypocalcemia
Neonatal hyperbilirubinemia and jaundice
Neonatal polycythemia (excess erythrocytes) caused by hypoxia
Perinatal death

★ Nursing Care Plan 5-3   The Pregnant Woman with Gestational Diabetes Mellitus

PATIENT DATA A woman, para 0, gravida 1, is diagnosed with gestational diabetes mellitus (GDM). She states that she has no diabetes in her family history and has never been on any type of restricted diet. She is discharged to receive home care and close follow-up.

Selected Nursing Diagnosis: Ineffective therapeutic regimen management related to lack of knowledge about new diagnosis

Goals	Nursing Interventions	Rationales
The woman will identify appropriate and inappropriate food choices. The woman will demonstrate correct self-care techniques for assessing blood glucose and administering insulin. The woman will verbalize symptoms of hypoglycemia and hyperglycemia, including correct self-care.	Determine knowledge of diabetes and its management, including family members if appropriate.	Allows nurse to identify correct and incorrect information and relate new knowledge to what the woman already knows, thus promoting individualized teaching.
	Assist the registered nurse to teach prescribed diet; provide written information; and have the woman identify appropriate foods and the best time to eat them. General guidelines are as follows: • Avoid simple sugars, such as cakes, candies, and ice creams, because they are quickly converted to glucose, causing wide fluctuations in blood glucose levels. • Eat complex, high-fiber carbohydrates such as grains, breads, and pasta; these foods are converted to glucose slowly, thus helping maintain stable blood glucose levels. • Eat three meals a day plus at least two snacks to balance insulin and provide sustained release of glucose to prevent hypoglycemia during late afternoon and evening.	A woman who understands dietary requirements is more likely to follow them carefully; written information helps to refresh her memory if she forgets verbal teaching. Her verbalizing of food choices allows the nurse to determine if the woman has correctly learned the information.
	Consult with a dietitian to help maintain cultural food patterns.	A dietitian specializes in foods and nutrition and can help the woman to select foods that are acceptable within her dietary limits and that meet her preferences and cultural needs.
	Assist the registered nurse to teach the woman how to perform blood glucose monitoring; have her perform a return demonstration and/or verbalize the regimen. Common teaching includes testing frequency, accurate technique, and responses to low or high levels.	Insulin requirements fluctuate during pregnancy, generally increasing as pregnancy progresses. Frequent blood glucose monitoring allows adjustment of insulin, thus maintaining stable blood glucose levels; and stable blood glucose levels are associated with better outcomes for mother and infant. Return demonstration of skills or verbalizing of information helps the nurse determine if the woman has learned the information.
	Assist the registered nurse to teach insulin self-administration (see Chapter 31 for additional information); and have woman give a return demonstration and/or verbalization of each step. Teaching includes when to take insulin and how to administer it.	Correct insulin administration helps maintain the most stable blood glucose levels; see previous point for rationale for return demonstration and verbalization.
	Teach signs and symptoms of hypoglycemia and hyperglycemia (see Table 5-7); teach appropriate responses to these signs and symptoms.	Persistence of low or high blood glucose levels requires adjustment of insulin dose and/or food intake; in addition, hyperglycemia may be an early sign of infection in the diabetic woman. A woman who understands the signs and symptoms and the corrective actions is likely to seek the care needed to maintain optimal blood glucose levels.
	Explain that gestational diabetes usually resolves quickly after birth but may recur in future pregnancies or in midlife.	Advance information about possible future diabetes improves ongoing health monitoring.

⭐ Nursing Care Plan 5-3   The Pregnant Woman with Gestational Diabetes Mellitus—cont'd

Selected Nursing Diagnosis: Deficient knowledge related to complications of diabetes during pregnancy

Goals	Nursing Interventions	Rationales
The woman will verbalize correct responses to potential complications of gestational diabetes.	Teach danger signs in pregnancy (see Patient Teaching box on p. 79) and reinforce them at each prenatal visit.	Increases likelihood that woman will seek prompt treatment for all pregnancy complications, including those relating to diabetes.
	Teach the signs and symptoms of urinary tract infection and vaginal infection, especially candidiasis or yeast infection (see Chapter 11).	Candidiasis is common in women with diabetes mellitus; urinary tract infections are common and can also lead to maternal sepsis or preterm labor.
	Explain the importance of keeping prenatal appointments.	Prenatal visits at prescribed intervals can prevent or allow early intervention for complications.
	Teach about fetal diagnostic tests done; for example, biophysical profile evaluates how well placenta is delivering oxygen and nutrients to fetus.	Fetal diagnostic tests allow for early identification and prompt intervention for problems; knowledge decreases woman's anxiety related to the unknown. If the woman does not understand the reason for routinely required diagnostic tests, she may incorrectly assume that she or her infant is in danger.

Critical Thinking Questions

1. A 25-year-old primigravida has been diagnosed with gestational diabetes mellitus at 25 weeks of gestation and has been managing her condition at home with diet, exercise, and insulin. During a clinic visit early in her third trimester, she states that her mother had large infants and "everything was just fine," and she does not feel any extra tests or monitoring or changes in her insulin regimen are necessary. What would the best response of the nurse be to ensure patient compliance with the prescribed regimen?
2. A woman with GDM seeks care for complaints of dysuria and pruritus in the perineal area and difficulty in controlling her blood sugar during the past few weeks. What questions should the nurse ask, and what actions should be anticipated?

Table 5-7   Comparison of Hypoglycemia and Hyperglycemia in the Diabetic Woman

HYPOGLYCEMIA	HYPERGLYCEMIA
Cause	
Excess insulin, excess exercise, and/or inadequate food intake	Inadequate insulin, reduced activity, and/or excessive food intake; more likely if the woman has an infection, because this increases her need for insulin
Blood Glucose Level	
Below normal (usually <60 mg/dL)	Above normal (>120 mg/dL)
Urine	
Urine glucose absent	Glycosuria (glucose in the urine); possibly ketonuria (ketones in the urine)
Behavioral and Physiological Manifestations	
Hunger; trembling; weakness; faintness; lethargy; headache; irritability; sweating; pale, cool, moist skin; blurred vision; loss of consciousness	Fatigue; headache; flushed, hot skin; dry mouth; thirst; dehydration; frequent urination; weight loss; nausea and vomiting; rapid, deep respirations (Kussmaul's respirations); acetone odor to the breath; depressed reflexes
Corrective Measures	
Drink a glass of milk or juice; eat a piece of fruit or two crackers; recurrent hypoglycemia necessitates adjustment of insulin or food intake	Evaluate food intake; emphasize importance of patient being honest if she "cheats" to prevent inappropriately adjusting insulin dose; identify and treat infections; insulin dose often adjusted throughout pregnancy to maintain normal glucose levels

monitors her blood glucose levels several times a day as directed by the health care provider. Blood glucose self-monitoring is discussed in Chapter 31. Glycosylated hemoglobin (HgbA$_{1C}$) is performed every 3 months to provide an indication of long-term (4- to 6-week) glucose control, and lower values can indicate successful glucose management of the pregnant diabetic. However, HgbA$_{1C}$ monitoring cannot be used as a guide to adjust daily insulin needs during pregnancy.

Monitoring of ketones. Urine ketones may be checked to identify the need for more carbohydrates. If the woman's carbohydrate intake is insufficient, she may metabolize fat and protein to produce glucose, resulting in ketonuria. However, ketonuria that is accompanied by hyperglycemia requires prompt evaluation for diabetic ketoacidosis. Ketoacidosis can be rapidly fatal to the fetus. It is more likely to occur if the woman has preexisting diabetes or if she has an infection.

Insulin administration. Most oral hypoglycemic agents have not been used during pregnancy in the past because they can cross the placenta, possibly resulting in fetal birth defects or neonatal hypoglycemia. However, oral hypoglycemic drugs have been used in the last decade to treat GDM with success (Gabbe, 2012). Glyburide, which does not cross the placenta, has been considered superior to metformin, which does cross the placenta but has not been shown to be teratogenic to the fetus. However, because both oral agents often require supplemental injectable insulin to maintain adequate glucose control, injectable insulin is the preferred drug to lower blood glucose levels during pregnancy. GDM may be controlled by diet and exercise alone, or the woman may require insulin injections. The dose and frequency of insulin injections are tailored to a woman's individual needs. Insulin is often administered on a sliding scale, in which the woman varies her dose of insulin based on each blood glucose level.

The insulin regimen of a diabetic woman is different during pregnancy than in the nonpregnant state. Typically, insulin dosage may have to be reduced to avoid hypoglycemia in the first trimester, when nausea decreases appetite and physical activity may be reduced. In the second trimester, increasing placental hormones increases insulin resistance (see Chapter 4), and the dosage of insulin may have to be increased. Insulin requirements may drop again at 38 weeks of gestation. GDM resolves promptly after birth, when the insulin-antagonistic (diabetogenic) effects of pregnancy cease.

Neutral protamine Hagedorn (NPH) or Lente insulin is not given at dinnertime, because hypoglycemia during the night can occur. Humalog or insulin lispro is a fast-acting insulin that is highly effective if given before meals. Glargine insulin is not recommended for use during pregnancy because of variations in the basal insulin needs during pregnancy (Gabbe, 2012). The use of an insulin pump has proved of great value for glucose control in pregnant and nonpregnant patients with DM. (See Chapter 31 for the discussion of insulin administration and insulin pumps.)

Exercise. A pregnant woman with preexisting diabetes may have vascular damage, and exercise may then result in ischemia (decreased circulation) to the placenta and result in hypoxia (decreased oxygen) to the fetus. The health care provider should prescribe the level of exercise, and blood glucose levels should be monitored closely. In GDM, however, exercise can help control blood glucose levels, and diet and exercise can minimize the need for insulin. The woman with GDM should be counseled that exercise after meals is preferred, because glucose levels are higher at that time. Hypoglycemia can occur if the woman exercises when the effects of the last insulin dose are at peak. Hyperglycemia can occur if the woman exercises when the effects of the last dose of insulin have decreased. Therefore blood glucose levels should be monitored before, during, and after exercise (see Table 5-7).

Fetal assessments. Assessments (see Table 5-1) may identify fetal growth and the placenta's ability to provide oxygen and nutrients. Ultrasound examinations are used to identify intrauterine growth restriction, macrosomia, excess amniotic fluid (polyhydramnios) in the woman with poorly controlled diabetes, or decreased amniotic fluid (oligohydramnios) in placental failure.

Diabetes can affect the blood vessels that supply the placenta, impairing the transport of oxygen and nutrients to the fetus and the removal of fetal wastes. The non–stress test, the contraction stress test, and the biophysical profile provide information about how the placenta is functioning. Tests of fetal lung maturity are common if early delivery is considered.

Care during labor. Labor is work (exercise) that affects the amount of insulin and glucose needed. Some women receive an intravenous infusion of a dextrose solution plus regular insulin as needed. Regular insulin is the *only* type given intravenously. Blood glucose levels are assessed hourly, and the insulin dose is adjusted accordingly. Because macrosomia (large fetal size) is a common complication of GDM, close monitoring of the fetus during labor is essential, and cesarean delivery may be indicated. (See Chapter 8 for care of a woman requiring cesarean section.)

Care of the neonate. Infant complications after birth may include hypoglycemia, respiratory distress, and injury caused by macrosomia. Some infants experience growth restriction because the placenta functions poorly. Neonatal nurses and a neonatologist (a physician specializing in care of newborns) are often present at the birth. (See Chapter 14 for a discussion of these neonatal problems.)

Nursing Care. Nursing care of the pregnant woman with diabetes mellitus involves helping her to learn to care for herself and providing emotional care to meet the demands imposed by this complication. Care during labor primarily involves careful monitoring for signs of fetal distress.

Teaching self-care. Most women with preexisting diabetes already know how to check their blood glucose level and administer insulin. They should be taught why diabetes management changes during pregnancy. The woman with newly diagnosed GDM must be taught these self-care skills.

The woman is taught how to select appropriate foods for the prescribed diet. She is more likely to maintain the diet if her caregivers are sensitive to her food preferences and cultural needs. A dietitian can determine foods to meet her needs and help find solutions to problems in adhering to the diet.

The woman who takes insulin may experience episodes of hypoglycemia (low blood glucose) or hyperglycemia (high blood glucose) (see Table 5-7). The woman is taught to recognize and respond to each condition, and family members are included in the teaching. Maintaining glycemic control during pregnancy is essential to prevent later complications such as macrosomia.

Providing emotional support. Pregnant women with diabetes often find that living with the glucose monitoring, diet control, and frequent insulin administration is bothersome. The expectant mother may be anxious about the outcome for herself and her child. Therapeutic communication helps her to express her frustrations and fears. For example, to elicit her feelings about her condition the nurse might say, "Many women find that all the changes they have to make are demanding. How has it been for you?" It may help to emphasize that the close management is usually temporary, especially if she has GDM.

A woman who is actively involved in her care is more likely to maintain the prescribed therapy. Referral to a diabetes management center is often helpful. As she learns to manage her care, liberal praise motivates the woman to maintain her therapy.

Encouraging breastfeeding. Studies have shown that newborns who have been exclusively breastfed have a lower incidence of developing diabetes later in life. Breastfeeding should be encouraged if the newborn does not have perinatal complications related to maternal diabetes, such as macrosomia, respiratory problems, or anomalies. Blood glucose levels of newborns are monitored closely in the first 24 hours of life. Breastfeeding uses glucose reserves in the mother, and glucose monitoring of the mother after breastfeeding is important. Taking in fluids or food during breastfeeding may be desirable.

HEART DISEASE

Heart disease affects a small percentage of pregnant women. During a normal pregnancy, an increase in heart rate, blood volume, and cardiac output places a physiological strain on the heart that may not be tolerated in a woman with preexisting heart disease. Cardiac failure can occur prenatally, during labor, or in the postpartum period.

Manifestations. Increased levels of clotting factors predispose a woman to thrombosis (formation of clots in the veins). If her heart cannot meet these increased demands of pregnancy, congestive heart failure (CHF) results, and the fetus suffers from reduced placental blood flow. Box 5-5 lists signs and symptoms of CHF.

During labor, each contraction temporarily shifts 300 to 500 mL of blood from the uterus and placenta into the woman's circulation, possibly overloading her weakened heart. Excess interstitial fluid rapidly returns to the circulation after birth, predisposing the woman to circulatory overload during the postpartum period. She remains at an increased risk for CHF after birth until her circulating blood volume returns to normal levels in the postpartum period.

> ⚠ **Safety Alert!**
>
> The nurse should observe the woman with heart disease for signs of congestive heart failure, which can occur before, during, or after birth.

Treatment. The pregnant woman with heart disease is usually under the care of both a cardiologist and an obstetrician. She needs more frequent antepartum visits to determine how her heart is coping with the increased demands of pregnancy. Excessive weight gain must be avoided, because it adds to the demands on her heart. Preventing anemia with adequate diet and supplemental iron prevents a compensatory rise in the heart rate, which would add to the strain on the woman's heart. The priority of care is to limit physical activity to decrease the demands made on the heart. The limitation of activity can range from frequent rest periods to strict bed rest, depending on the degree of heart impairment. A woman on prolonged bed rest for any reason has a greater risk for forming venous thrombi (blood clots).

Drug therapy may include heparin to prevent clot formation. Anticoagulants such as warfarin (Coumadin) may cause birth defects and are not given during

---

Box 5-5   Signs of Congestive Heart Failure During Pregnancy

- Orthopnea (having to sit upright to breathe more easily)
- Persistent cough, often with expectoration of mucus that may be blood-tinged
- Moist lung sounds because of fluid within lungs
- Difficulty breathing on exertion
- Palpitations
- Fatigue or fainting on exertion
- Severe pitting edema of the lower extremities or generalized edema
- Changes in fetal heart rate indicating hypoxia or growth restriction if placental blood flow is reduced

pregnancy. Beta-adrenergic blocking drugs used to treat hypertension and dysrhythmias can cause fetal bradycardia (slow heartbeat), respiratory depression, and hypoglycemia. Thiazide diuretics can cause harmful effects on the fetus, especially if administered in the third trimester. Angiotensin-converting enzyme (ACE) inhibitors are contraindicated for use during pregnancy.

A vaginal birth is preferred over cesarean delivery because it carries less risk for infection or respiratory complications that would further tax the impaired heart. Forceps or a vacuum extractor may be used to decrease the need for maternal pushing (see Chapter 8).

Nursing Care. A woman with heart disease may already be familiar with its management. She should be taught about any necessary changes, such as the change from warfarin anticoagulants to subcutaneous heparin, and should be instructed in how to inject the drug. Laboratory tests include partial thromboplastin time (PTT), activated partial thromboplastin time (aPTT), and platelet counts. She should promptly report signs of excess anticoagulation, such as bruising without reason, petechiae (tiny red spots on the skin), nosebleeds, or bleeding from the gums when brushing her teeth.

The woman is taught signs that may indicate CHF so she can promptly report them. The nurse helps her to identify how she can obtain rest to minimize the demands on her heart. She should avoid exercise in extreme temperatures. She should be taught to stop an activity if she experiences dyspnea, chest pain, or tachycardia.

The woman may need help to plan her diet so that she has enough calories to meet her needs during pregnancy while not gaining too much weight. She should be taught about foods that are high in iron and folic acid to prevent anemia. She should avoid foods high in sodium, such as smoked meats and potato chips. Patients receiving heparin therapy should avoid foods high in vitamin K.

Stress can also increase demands on the heart. The nurse should discuss stressors in the woman's life and help her to identify ways to reduce them. During hospitalization the health care provider should be notified if the pulse exceeds 100 beats/min or respirations are greater than 25 breaths/min at rest. Signs of dyspnea (difficulty in breathing), coughing, and abnormal breath sounds should be recorded and reported. Postpartum bradycardia (slowed heart rate) should be reported to the health care provider, because the heart may fail as a result of the increased blood volume that occurs after delivery.

ANEMIA

Anemia is the reduced ability of the blood to carry oxygen to the cells. Hemoglobin levels that are lower than 10.5 g/dL in the second trimester and that are below 11 g/dL in the first and third trimesters indicate anemia during pregnancy (Creasy et al, 2009). Four anemias are significant during pregnancy: two nutritional anemias (iron-deficiency anemia and folic acid–deficiency anemia), and two anemias resulting from genetic disorders (sickle cell disease and thalassemia).

Nutritional Anemias

Most women with anemia have vague symptoms, if any. The anemic woman may fatigue easily and have little energy. Her skin and mucous membranes are pale. Shortness of breath, a pounding heart, and a rapid pulse may occur with severe anemia. The woman who develops anemia gradually has fewer symptoms than the woman who becomes anemic abruptly, such as through blood loss.

Iron-Deficiency Anemia. Pregnant women need additional iron for their own increased blood volume, for transfer to the fetus, and for a cushion against the blood loss expected at birth. The RBCs are small (microcytic) and pale (hypochromic) in iron-deficiency anemia. The tannic acid in tea and bran may decrease absorption of iron from foods eaten at the same meal.

Prevention. Iron supplements are commonly used to meet the needs of pregnancy and maintain iron stores. Vitamin C may enhance the absorption of iron. Iron should not be taken with milk or antacids, because calcium impairs absorption.

Treatment. The woman with iron-deficiency anemia needs extra iron to correct the anemia and replenish her stores. She is treated with oral doses of *elemental iron* and continues this therapy for about 3 months after the anemia has been corrected.

Folic Acid–Deficiency Anemia. Folic acid (also called folate or folacin) deficiency is characterized by large, immature RBCs (megaloblastic anemia). Iron-deficiency anemia is often present at the same time. Anticonvulsants, oral contraceptives, sulfa drugs, and alcohol can decrease the absorption of folate from food.

Prevention. Folic acid is essential for normal growth and development of the fetus. Folic acid deficiency has been associated with neural tube defects in the newborn. A daily supplement of 400 mcg (0.4 mg) ensures adequate folic acid and is now recommended for all women of childbearing age.

Treatment. Treatment of folate deficiency is with folic acid supplementation, 1 mg/day (over twice the amount of the preventive supplement). The preventive dosage of supplementary folic acid may be higher for women who have previously had a child who had a neural tube defect.

Genetic Anemias

Sickle Cell Disease. Unlike those with nutritional anemias, people with sickle cell disease have abnormal hemoglobin that causes their erythrocytes to become distorted into a sickle (crescent) shape during episodes of hypoxia or acidosis. It is an autosomal recessive disorder, meaning that the affected person receives an abnormal gene from each parent. The abnormally shaped blood cells do not flow smoothly, and they clog small blood vessels. The sickle cells are destroyed more rapidly, resulting in chronic anemia. Approximately 1 of 12 African Americans has the trait (HgbAS). (See Chapter 27 for further discussion of sickle cell disease.)

Pregnancy may cause a sickle cell crisis, with massive erythrocyte destruction and occlusion of blood vessels. The main risk to the fetus is occlusion of vessels that supply the placenta, leading to preterm birth, growth restriction, and fetal death.

The woman should have frequent evaluation and treatment for anemia during prenatal care. Fetal evaluations concentrate on fetal growth and placental function. Oxygen and fluids are provided continuously during labor to prevent sickle cell crisis. Genetic counseling should be offered.

Thalassemia. Thalassemia is a genetic trait that causes an abnormality in one of two chains of hemoglobin, the alpha (α) or beta (β) chain. The β chain variety is most often encountered in the United States. The person can inherit an abnormal gene from each parent, causing β-thalassemia major, or Cooley's anemia. If only one abnormal gene is inherited, the person will have β-thalassemia minor.

The woman with β-thalassemia minor usually has few problems other than mild anemia, and the fetus does not appear to be affected. However, administration of iron supplements may cause iron overload in a woman with β-thalassemia, because the body absorbs and stores iron in higher-than-usual amounts.

Nursing Care for Anemias During Pregnancy

The woman is taught which foods are high in iron and folic acid to help her prevent or treat anemia. She is taught how to take the supplements so that they are optimally effective. For example, the nurse explains that although milk is good to drink during pregnancy, it should not be taken at the same time as the iron supplement, or the iron will not be absorbed as easily. Foods high in vitamin C may enhance absorption.

 Nutrition Considerations

Foods Recommended in Pregnancy

FOODS HIGH IN IRON

Meats, chicken, fish, liver, legumes, green leafy vegetables, whole or enriched grain products, nuts, blackstrap molasses, tofu, eggs, dried fruits

FOODS HIGH IN FOLIC ACID

Green leafy vegetables, asparagus, green beans, fruits, whole grains, liver, legumes, yeast

FOODS HIGH IN VITAMIN C (MAY ENHANCE ABSORPTION OF IRON)

Citrus fruits and juices, strawberries, cantaloupe, cabbage, green and red peppers, tomatoes, potatoes, green leafy vegetables

To prevent or correct nutritional anemias, such as iron and folic acid deficiencies, the nurse should teach all women appropriate food sources for those nutrients.

The woman is taught that when she takes iron, her stools will be dark green to black and that mild gastrointestinal discomfort may occur. She should contact her physician or nurse-midwife if these side effects trouble her; another iron preparation may be better tolerated. She should not take antacids with iron.

The woman with sickle cell disease requires close medical and nursing care. She should be taught to prevent dehydration and activities that cause hypoxia. The woman with β-thalassemia is taught to avoid situations in which exposure to infection is more likely (e.g., crowds during flu season) and to report any symptoms of infection promptly. (See Chapter 27 for a discussion of sickle cell anemia and thalassemia.)

Obesity, Bariatric Surgery, and Pregnancy

The obese woman who is pregnant has a high risk for developing complications during pregnancy such as gestational diabetes, hypertension, cardiac problems, preeclampsia, and respiratory problems. The obese patient is often placed in a high-risk category for prenatal care to receive special assessments, guidance, and close follow-up care.

When gastric bypass surgery is performed, women are cautioned to delay pregnancy for 1 to 2 years to avoid weight loss during pregnancy. However, the reduced absorption in the stomach and small bowel may result in a deficiency of essential nutrients during pregnancy. Professional nutritional guidance during pregnancy is essential. In some patients following bariatric surgery, consumption of simple sugars can lead to a condition known as "dumping syndrome," which is manifested by nausea, vomiting, cramping, and diarrhea. Blood glucose levels should be monitored. Abdominal complaints during pregnancy should be monitored closely to determine whether they are related to the gastric bypass surgery. When bariatric surgery via gastric band placement is undertaken, the band can be adjusted during pregnancy to allow adequate nutrient intake during pregnancy.

INFECTIONS

The acronym *TORCH* has been used to describe infections that can be devastating for the fetus or newborn. The letters stand for the first letters of four infections or infectious agents: **T**oxoplasmosis, **R**ubella, **C**ytomegalovirus, and **H**erpes simplex virus; the *O* is sometimes used to designate "**O**ther" infections. However, there are many more infections that can be devastating for the mother, fetus, or newborn. Some of these are damaging any time they are acquired, whereas others are relatively harmless except when acquired during pregnancy. See Chapter 4, Table 4-1, for routine prenatal laboratory testing.

Viral Infections

Viral infections often have no effective therapy and may cause serious problems in the mother and/or the fetus or newborn. However, immunizations can prevent some of these infections. An infant born to a mother with an active viral infection, such as rubeola or varicella, must be placed on airborne and contact isolation. Refer to Appendix A for isolation precautions.

Cytomegalovirus. Cytomegalovirus (CMV) infection is widespread and commonly occurs during the childbearing years. The infection is often asymptomatic in the mother. However, an infected infant may have some of the following serious problems:

- Mental retardation
- Seizures
- Blindness
- Deafness
- Dental abnormalities
- Petechiae (often called a "blueberry muffin" rash)

Treatment and nursing care. There is no effective treatment for CMV infection. Primary prevention via hand washing is essential. Antiviral drugs may prevent shedding of the virus but are toxic. Therapeutic pregnancy termination may be offered if CMV infection is discovered during early pregnancy.

Rubella. Rubella is a mild viral disease with a low fever and rash. However, its effects on the developing fetus can be destructive. Rubella occurring in very early pregnancy can disrupt the formation of major body systems, whereas rubella acquired later is more likely to damage organs that are already formed. Some effects of rubella on the embryo or fetus include the following:

- Microcephaly (small head size)
- Mental retardation
- Congenital cataracts
- Deafness
- Cardiac defects
- Intrauterine growth restriction (IUGR)

Treatment and nursing care. Immunization against rubella infection has been available for some time, but some women of childbearing age are still susceptible. When a woman of childbearing age is immunized, she should not get pregnant for at least 1 month after the immunization. The vaccine is offered during the postpartum period to nonimmune women. It is *not* given during pregnancy, because it is a live attenuated (weakened) form of the virus.

⌂ Nursing Tip

Rubella is a cause of birth defects that is almost completely preventable by immunization before childbearing age. The nurse should check each postpartum woman's chart for rubella immunity and notify her physician or nurse-midwife if she is not immune.

Herpesvirus. There are two types of herpes viruses. Type 1 is more likely to cause fever blisters or cold sores. Type 2 is more likely to cause genital herpes. After the primary infection occurs, the virus becomes dormant in the nerves and may be reactivated later as a recurrent (secondary) infection. Initial infection during the first half of pregnancy may cause spontaneous abortion, IUGR, and preterm labor. Most pregnancies are affected by recurrent infections rather than primary infections. The infant is infected in one of the following ways:

- The virus ascends into the uterus after the membranes rupture.
- The infant has direct contact with infectious lesions during vaginal delivery.

Neonatal herpes infection can be either localized or disseminated (widespread). Disseminated neonatal infection has a high mortality rate, and survivors may have neurological complications.

Treatment and nursing care. Avoiding contact with the lesions can prevent neonatal herpes infection. If the woman has active genital herpes lesions when the membranes rupture or labor begins, a cesarean delivery may be required to prevent fetal contact during birth or the development of an ascending infection. Cesarean birth is not necessary if there are no active genital lesions. The mother and infant do not need to be isolated as long as direct contact with lesions is prevented (see Appendix A). Breastfeeding is safe if there are no lesions on the breasts. Antiviral drugs such as Acyclovir may be given orally during pregnancy to reduce the occurrence of active lesions at the time of birth (Gabbe, 2012).

Hepatitis B. Blood, saliva, vaginal secretions, semen, and breast milk can transmit the virus that causes hepatitis B infection; the infection can also cross the placenta. The woman may be asymptomatic or acutely ill with chronic low-grade fever, anorexia, nausea, and vomiting. Some become chronic carriers of the virus. The fetus may be infected transplacentally or by contact at birth with blood or vaginal secretions. The infant may become a chronic carrier and a continuing source of infection. Box 5-6 lists those who are at greater risk of having hepatitis B infection.

Treatment and nursing care. All women should be screened for hepatitis B during the course of prenatal care, and the screening should be repeated during the third trimester for women in high-risk groups. Infants born to women who are positive for hepatitis B should receive a single dose of hepatitis B immune globulin (for temporary immunity right after birth) followed by hepatitis B vaccine (for long-term immunity). The Centers for Disease Control and Prevention (CDC) recommends routine immunization with hepatitis B vaccine for all newborns (those born to carrier mothers and to noncarrier mothers) at birth and at ages 1 to 2 months and 6 to 18 months (CDC, 2008). Immunization during

| Box 5-6 | Persons at Higher Risk for Hepatitis B Infection |

- Intravenous drug users
- Persons with multiple sexual partners
- Persons with repeated infection with sexually transmitted infections
- Health care workers with occupational exposure to blood products and needle sticks
- Hemodialysis patients
- Recipients of multiple blood transfusions or other blood products
- Household contact with hepatitis carrier or hemodialysis patient
- Persons arriving from countries where there is a higher incidence of the disease

pregnancy is not contraindicated. If possible, injections should be delayed until after the infant's first bath, so that blood and other potentially infectious secretions are removed to avoid introducing them under the skin. Because they have occupational exposure to blood and other infectious secretions, health care staff should be immunized against hepatitis B.

Sexually Transmitted Infections

Sexually transmitted infections (STIs), formerly known as sexually transmitted diseases (STDs), are those for which a common mode of transmission is sexual intercourse, although several can also be transmitted in other ways. Herpesvirus has been discussed. Other infections that are typically transmitted sexually are syphilis, gonorrhea, chlamydia, trichomoniasis, and condylomata acuminata (genital warts).

Changes in the vaginal secretions that occur during pregnancy can increase the risk of developing a vaginal infection. The high estrogen levels present during pregnancy thicken the vaginal mucosa and increase secretions that have a high glycogen content. This makes the woman susceptible to yeast infections and other microorganisms. Later in pregnancy the pH of the vagina decreases, resulting in a protective effect.

All sexual contacts of persons infected with a disease that can be sexually transmitted should be informed and treated; otherwise the cycle of infection and reinfection will continue. Consistent use of a latex condom, including the female condom, helps to reduce the sexual spread of STIs. STIs and vaginal infections are discussed in detail in Chapter 11.

Human Immunodeficiency Virus. Human immunodeficiency virus (HIV) is the causative organism of acquired immunodeficiency syndrome (AIDS). The virus eventually cripples the immune system, making the person susceptible to infections that eventually can result in death. There is no known immunization or curative treatment, but control of opportunistic infections has increased the life expectancy of treated adults.

See Chapter 11 and a medical-surgical text for further discussion of HIV, infections associated with the syndrome, and treatment.

Although first identified in homosexual males, the incidence of HIV infection and AIDS continues to rise in women. HIV infection is acquired in one of the following four ways:

1. Unprotected (through condom nonuse, breakage, or slippage) sexual contact (anal, vaginal, or oral) with an infected person
2. Sharing a needle with an infected person
3. Mucous membrane exposure to infected body fluids
4. Perinatal exposure (infants)

The infant may be infected in one of the following three ways:

1. Transplacentally
2. Through contact with infected maternal secretions at birth
3. Through breast milk

The infected woman has a 20% to 40% chance of transmitting the virus to her fetus perinatally. Infants born to HIV-positive women will be HIV positive at birth, because maternal antibodies to the virus pass through the placenta to the infant. A period of 3 to 6 months is needed to identify the infants who are truly infected.

Nursing care. Counseling should be provided to all women concerning behaviors that place them at risk for contracting HIV (Box 5-7). HIV testing is recommended for all prenatal patients. HIV-positive women should be educated that the transmission of HIV infection to the newborn can be greatly reduced by appropriate drug therapy. Pregnant women with AIDS are more susceptible to infection, and the fetus may develop an impaired immune system that increases the risk of opportunistic infections after birth. Breastfeeding is contraindicated for mothers who are HIV positive.

The fetus and the woman are monitored closely during the antepartum period. All infants born to HIV-positive women are presumed to be HIV positive, and standard precautions (see Appendix A) are initiated for both mother and infant. The infant may receive drug therapy with zidovudine starting 6 to 12 hours after birth and continuing during the first 6 weeks of

| Box 5-7 | High-Risk Factors for Human Immunodeficiency Virus (HIV) |

- Intravenous drug abuse and needle sharing
- Multiple sexual partners
- Prostitution
- Blood transfusion before 1985
- History of sexually transmitted diseases
- Immigration from area where infection is endemic, such as Haiti or Central Africa
- Sexual partner in a high-risk group
- Sexual partner with HIV infection

life. The nurse should anticipate and help the mother cope with the anxiety that is almost certain to occur about whether the neonate is infected. Social services can help the family with the care of the child at home. Women should be taught about the risks of sharing needles, the importance of using condoms, and the need to avoid oral sex.

 Safety Alert!

The nurse should wear protective equipment, such as gloves, with *every* potential exposure to a patient's body secretions. This practice protects the nurse from direct exposure to many pathogenic organisms.

Nonviral Infections

Toxoplasmosis. Toxoplasmosis is caused by *Toxoplasma gondii,* a parasite that may be acquired by contact with cat feces or raw meat and transmitted through the placenta. The woman is usually asymptomatic or has mild symptoms. Congenital toxoplasmosis includes the following possible signs in the newborn:

- Low birth weight
- Enlarged liver and spleen
- Jaundice
- Anemia
- Inflammation of eye structures
- Neurological damage

Treatment and nursing care. Treatment of the mother reduces the risk of congenital infection. Pyrimethamine and sulfonamide drugs are used after the first trimester. Spiramycin, used successfully in Europe, may be available for use in the United States via the CDC. Treatment of infants involves pyrimethamine, sulfadiazine, and leucovorin for 1 year, which may reduce the severity of the congenital effects of the disease (Gabbe, 2012). Therapeutic abortion may be offered to the woman who contracts the infection during the first half of pregnancy. Nurses can teach women the following measures to reduce the likelihood of acquiring the infection:

- Cook all meat thoroughly.
- Wash hands and all kitchen surfaces after handling raw meat.
- Avoid touching the mucous membranes of the eyes or mouth while handling raw meat.
- Avoid uncooked eggs and unpasteurized milk.
- Wash fresh fruits and vegetables well.
- Avoid materials contaminated with cat feces, such as litter boxes, sand boxes, and garden soil.

Group B Streptococcus Infection. Group B streptococcus (GBS) is a leading cause of perinatal infections that result in a high neonatal mortality rate. The organism can be found in the woman's rectum, vagina, cervix, throat, or skin. Although she is colonized with the organism, the woman is usually asymptomatic, but the infant may be infected through contact at birth with vaginal secretions. The risk is greater if the woman has a long labor or premature rupture of membranes. GBS is a significant cause of maternal postpartum infection (endometritis, or infection of the uterine interior), especially after cesarean birth. Symptoms include an elevated temperature within 12 hours after delivery, rapid heart rate (tachycardia), and abdominal distention. Diagnosis of GBS is confirmed by vaginal and rectal culture.

GBS infection can be deadly for the infant. A newborn may have either early-onset (before 7 days) or late-onset (after 7 days) GBS infection.

Prevention and treatment. A culture of the woman's rectum and lower vagina for the presence of GBS is routinely taken at 35 to 37 weeks of gestation. The test can be done during labor if the woman did not have prenatal care. With rapid testing techniques, the results can be available within an hour (Brown, 2013). All positive cultures require antibiotic treatment during labor. High-risk factors such as previous history of GBS infection, prolonged rupture of the membranes, or fever above 37.7° C (100° F) during labor necessitate antibiotic treatment to prevent GBS infection. Any GBS-positive urine culture is considered a cause for antibiotic treatment during pregnancy, and the newborn is treated with antibiotics at birth (Verani, 2010).

Tuberculosis. The incidence of tuberculosis is rising in the United States, and drug-resistant strains of the bacterium are emerging. Pregnant women are screened for pulmonary tuberculosis by either a tuberculin skin test or a serum QuantiFERON-TB Gold (QFT-G) test, as would be the case for any other patient (refer to a medical-surgical nursing text). If the screening test is positive, the woman should have a chest radiograph (x-ray film) with the pregnant abdomen shielded by a lead apron. If required, sputum cultures that are positive for the bacterium confirm the diagnosis.

The adult with tuberculosis experiences fatigue, weakness, loss of appetite and weight, fever, and night sweats. The newborn may acquire the disease by contact with an untreated mother after birth.

Treatment and nursing care. The local public health department is notified of positive cultures and/or chest radiograph results, and isoniazid and rifampin are usually prescribed for 9 months. Pregnant women who are taking isoniazid should also take pyridoxine to reduce the risk of peripheral neuritis. Ethambutol may be prescribed if drug-resistant tuberculosis is suspected. If the mother has active pulmonary tuberculosis, the infant must be kept in a separate area away from the mother. The local health department must be notified, and the discharge plan of the mother and infant must be approved before they are allowed to leave the hospital. The infant may receive preventive therapy with isoniazid for 3 months after birth. The health care staff, including nurses, must teach the family how the organism is transmitted and the importance of continuing the antitubercular drugs consistently for the full course of therapy. Incompletely treated tuberculosis is a significant cause in the development of drug-resistant organisms. Modern antitubercular drugs usually render the sputum culture negative within 2 weeks; thus home care is the protocol, with health department follow-up.

Urinary Tract Infections

Bacteruria involving the Group B streptococcus was discussed previously. Urinary tract infections (UTIs) are common in females because of the short urethra and the ease of contamination of the urethra from the rectum and because of contamination from the vagina during sexual activity.

The urinary tract is normally self-cleaning, because acidic urine inhibits the growth of microorganisms and flushes them out of the body with each voiding. Pregnancy alters this self-cleaning action, because pressure on urinary structures keeps the bladder from emptying completely and because the ureters dilate and lose motility under the relaxing effects of the hormone progesterone. Urine that is retained in the bladder becomes more alkaline, providing a favorable environment for the growth of microorganisms.

Some women have excessive microorganisms in their urine but no symptoms (asymptomatic bacteruria). The asymptomatic infection may eventually cause cystitis (bladder infection) or pyelonephritis (kidney infection). The woman with cystitis has the following signs and symptoms:

- Burning with urination
- Increased frequency and urgency of urination
- A normal or slightly elevated temperature

If not treated, cystitis can ascend in the urinary tract and cause pyelonephritis. Pyelonephritis is a particularly serious infection in pregnancy and is accompanied by these signs and symptoms:

- High fever
- Chills
- Flank pain or tenderness
- Nausea and vomiting

Maternal hypertension, chronic renal disease, and preterm birth may occur with pyelonephritis during pregnancy. The high maternal fever is dangerous for the fetus, because it increases the fetal metabolic rate, which in turn increases fetal oxygen needs to levels that the mother cannot readily supply.

Treatment. UTIs are treated with antibiotics, often ampicillin. Asymptomatic bacteruria is treated with oral antibiotics for 10 days, cystitis for 1 to 2 weeks. Pyelonephritis is treated with multiple antibiotics, initially administered intravenously. Cystitis in pregnant women is treated with a full 7 days of antibiotic therapy.

⬛ Nursing Tip

The nurse should teach all females measures to reduce their risk for urinary tract infections.

Nursing Care. All females should be taught how to reduce the introduction of rectal microorganisms into the bladder. For example, a front-to-back direction should be used when wiping after urination or a bowel movement, when doing perineal cleansing, or when applying and removing perineal pads. The nurse can begin teaching during the woman's prenatal visits and reinforce the training during the postpartum stay. The mother should be taught how to clean and diaper an infant girl to avoid fecal contamination of her urethra.

Adequate fluid intake promotes frequent voiding. Drinking at least eight glasses of liquid per day and excluding caffeine-containing beverages help to flush urine through the urinary tract regularly. Cranberry juice may make the urine more acidic and therefore less conducive to the growth of infectious organisms.

Sexual intercourse mildly irritates the bladder and urethra, which can promote a UTI. Urinating before intercourse reduces irritation; urinating afterward flushes urine from the bladder. Using water-soluble lubricant during intercourse can also reduce periurethral irritation.

Pregnant women should be taught the signs and symptoms of cystitis and pyelonephritis so that they will know to seek treatment at once.

ENVIRONMENTAL HAZARDS DURING PREGNANCY

A **teratogen** is a substance that causes an adverse effect on the developing embryo or fetus. Some birth defects are caused by a combination of genetic and environmental factors. The specific anomaly that develops depends on the time of exposure to the environmental teratogen in relation to the stage of development of the embryo. In the first weeks of life, the vital organs are developing, and exposure to an environmental teratogen may cause miscarriage. Exposure to a teratogen in later pregnancy might result in growth restriction. The four main teratogens of concern during pregnancy are drugs, chemicals, infectious agents, and radiation.

BIOTERRORISM AND THE PREGNANT PATIENT

The concepts learned in a microbiology class come to life when nurses discuss the current threat of bioterrorism. In general, there are three basic categories of biological agents:

- *Category A:* Easily transmitted from person to person (such as smallpox, anthrax, or tularemia)
- *Category B:* Spread via food and water (such as Q fever, brucellosis, and *Staphylococcus* enterotoxin B [SEB])
- *Category C:* Spread via manufactured weapons designed to spread disease (such as hantavirus and tick-borne encephalitis)

Even diseases not normally transmitted by airborne means can be altered to make them transmissible by air. Therefore routine knowledge of an illness related to bioterrorist attacks does not always indicate all possible methods of transmission.

The obstetrical nurse must be observant for unusual symptoms present in large numbers of young, healthy pregnant patients who come to the clinic or emergency department. Such an unusual increase should trigger suspicion of a bioterrorism-related illness and be reported to the charge nurse or unit manager. These suspicions should then be promptly reported to the infection control department of the facility, which will then contact the local health department and the CDC to ensure that appropriate protocols are activated. A laboratory test, rapid antigen detection for influenza, can be performed on these patients. A positive result on this test rules out symptoms that mimic influenza but may be an early sign of a bioterrorism-related infection.

The approach to the care of a pregnant patient who is a victim of a bioterrorist attack may follow protocols similar to those presented in this section of general trauma during pregnancy. Other general protocols relate to the use of standard precautions (see Appendix A), the maintenance of a safe food and water supply to ensure adequate nutrition and hydration, and the maintenance of a safe air supply to prevent further transmission of disease (Table 5-8). The use of available vaccines for the pregnant patient can adversely affect the fetus and must be carefully evaluated, and informed consent must be obtained. Administration of the measles, mumps, and rubella (MMR) vaccine is contraindicated, but most other vaccines may be given if the risk of the disease is truly significant (CDC, 2008). Whenever possible, the choice of antimicrobial treatment must also be weighed according to the risks to the fetus and the mother.

Nurses should participate in community emergency preparedness programs that set up response protocols for patients of all ages and provide shelters, supportive services, intensive care units, emergency supplies, and communication services. The Association for Women's Health and Neonatal Nurses (AWHONN) recommends that families who are pregnant keep on hand an emergency birth kit that includes ready-to-feed formula and a basic disaster supply kit. Advice concerning suggested contents can be accessed at www. AWHONN.org. Continuing education units (CEUs) are now available to help the nurse stay current in this area of nursing. *Morbidity and Mortality Weekly Report (MMWR)*, published by the CDC, is available to health care professionals via the Internet and reports on any unusual biological or chemical outbreaks across the nation and worldwide (www.cdc.gov/mmwr). The role of the nurse in the care of the maternal–child patient during a natural or man-made disaster is discussed in detail in Chapter 32.

SUBSTANCE ABUSE

The use of illicit or recreational drugs during pregnancy has an adverse effect on both the mother and the fetus. Often multiple drugs are used, and lifestyle factors such as malnutrition, poor prenatal care, and STIs may also exist concurrently. Prescribed drugs are assigned "pregnancy risk categories" by the U.S. Food and Drug Administration (FDA), which are published in most drug reference books. Classifications range from A (no risk) to D (positive evidence of risk) and X (contraindicated for use in pregnancy). See Chapter 4 for a detailed review of the drug classifications.

It is well established that several legal and illicit substances are harmful to the developing fetus (Figure 5-8). The fetus of the woman who takes drugs (legal or illicit) or drinks alcohol is exposed to higher levels of the substance for a longer time, because the substances become concentrated in the amniotic fluid, and the fetus ingests the fluid. Many environmental substances are most harmful to the fetus early in pregnancy, perhaps before the woman realizes she is pregnant. Table 5-9 reviews some substances that are harmful to the fetus.

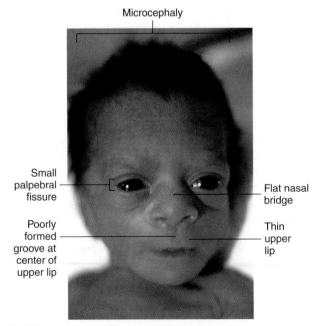

FIGURE 5-8 Fetal alcohol syndrome (FAS). The facial features of an infant with FAS include short palpebral (eye) fissures; a flat nasal bridge; a thin, flat upper lip; a poorly formed groove at the center of the upper lip; and a small head (microcephaly). (From Clark DA: *Atlas of neonatology: a companion to Avery's diseases of the newborn,* ed 7, Philadelphia, 2000, Saunders.)

Table 5-8	Precautions Required for Common Bioterrorism Agents
AGENT	**PRECAUTION**
Botulism, anthrax, tularemia	Standard precautions
Smallpox	Airborne and contact precautions
Pneumonic plague	Droplet precautions
Hemorrhagic fever	Airborne, droplet, and contact precautions

Table 5-9   Substances Harmful to the Fetus

SUBSTANCE	EFFECTS
Alcohol	Alcohol is the most commonly abused substance by women of childbearing age. Fetal alcohol syndrome (FAS) is well documented (see Figure 5-8) and includes growth restriction, mental retardation, and facial abnormalities. No "safe" level of alcohol ingestion during pregnancy is known.
Cocaine	Cocaine is a powerful central nervous system (CNS) stimulant that causes vasoconstriction that may precipitate preterm labor. It can cause hypertension, seizures, and stroke in the mother; fetal anomalies; and addiction in the newborn.
Marijuana	Harmful effects of marijuana use during pregnancy are not clearly identified but cannot be ruled out. Marijuana users may ingest or use other substances listed in this table, and this lifestyle may be harmful to the fetus.
Tobacco	Smoking can cause fetal growth restriction. Nicotine causes vasoconstriction that reduces blood flow to the placenta. Nicotine patches also expose the fetus to this substance. Poor pregnancy outcome has been linked to smoking.
Heroin	The heroin-addicted woman is likely to be exposed to human immunodeficiency virus (HIV) because the drug is taken intravenously and may include the use of dirty needles and a lifestyle of high-risk behaviors. Withdrawal syndrome (agitation, cramps, diarrhea, rhinorrhea [runny nose]) occurs if drug is stopped suddenly. Neonatal abstinence syndrome occurs within 24 hours of birth (high-pitched cry, tremors, seizures, and disrupted sleep–wake cycles). Serious maternal and fetal effects occur.
Amphetamines	Often associated with maternal malnutrition and tachycardia. Can cause fetal anomalies, intrauterine growth restriction, and withdrawal symptoms in the newborn, or can cause fetal death.
Anticoagulants	Warfarin (Coumadin) can cross the placenta and cause spontaneous abortion, growth restriction, central nervous system (CNS) problems, and facial defects (fetal warfarin syndrome). Heparin does not cross the placenta and is the drug of choice when an anticoagulant is required; however, heparin can cause premature labor.
Antibiotics	A few antibiotics have an adverse effect on the fetus, although no anomalies have been reported. Tetracycline exposure after the fourth month of gestation can cause yellowing of the deciduous teeth and hyperplasia of the enamel. To prevent tooth discoloration, tetracycline is not advised for children under age 7 years. Drugs such as streptomycin and kanamycin are associated with damage to the eighth cranial nerve and hearing loss in the newborn.
Anticonvulsants	Dilantin (diphenylhydantoin) can cause craniofacial abnormalities and mental retardation in the fetus and may be carcinogenic. The woman must be counseled concerning the risk of medication and the benefits of seizure control during pregnancy. Trimethadione (Tridione) and paramethadione (Paradione) are used to treat petit mal epilepsy and are contraindicated for use in pregnancy because of the high risk for major anomalies. Pregnant women who must take valproic acid (Depakene) or carbamazepine (Tegretol) should have fetal assessments for skeletal anomalies and neural tube defects. The use of phenobarbital has not been associated with the development of anomalies, but neonatal withdrawal may occur.
Isotretinoin (Accutane) and vitamin A derivatives	Isotretinoin and etretinate are used for skin disorders; they are clearly associated with fetal anomalies and are contraindicated for use in pregnancy. Birth control is advised for a minimum of 3 months after isotretinoin therapy.
Diethylstilbestrol (DES)	DES can cause uterine malformation, vaginal carcinoma, and testicular abnormalities in the newborn.
Angiotensin-converting enzyme (ACE) inhibitors (captopril, enalapril)	ACE inhibitors can cause fetal kidney anomalies, growth restriction, and oligohydramnios (decreased amniotic fluid).
Folic acid antagonists (methotrexate, amethopterin)	Folic acid antagonists cause spontaneous abortion and serious fetal anomalies.
Lithium	Lithium is associated with the development of congenital heart disease. It can also be toxic to the thyroid and the kidneys of the fetus.
Radiation	Radiation exposure before 6 weeks of gestation can cause serious fetal damage that includes leukemia, eye and CNS anomalies, and fetal loss. Doses for diagnostic tests are small, and the risk to the fetus is small; however, abdominal protection with lead aprons is advised. Therapeutic radiation is contraindicated during pregnancy.

> **Nursing Tip**
>
> When asking questions about substance use during pregnancy, the nurse should focus on how the information will help nurses and physicians provide the safest and most appropriate care to the pregnant woman and her infant.

Treatment and Nursing Care. Care focuses on identifying the substance-abusing woman early in pregnancy, educating her about the effects of substance abuse, and encouraging her to reduce or eliminate use. Appropriate referrals should be made.

> **Nursing Tip**
>
> A single episode of consuming two alcoholic drinks during pregnancy can lead to the loss of some fetal brain cells. One drink is defined as 12 oz of beer, 5 oz of wine, or 1.5 oz of hard liquor (Wittendorf and Muenke, 2005).

A partnership should be created with the woman, and a plan for compromises and treatment should be developed. Dietary support, monitoring of the woman's weight gain, and fetal assessment promote better pregnancy outcomes.

In the case of therapeutic drugs, the woman's need for the drug is weighed against the potential for fetal harm it may cause and the fetal or maternal harm that may occur if the woman is not treated. In general, the health care provider will choose the least teratogenic drug that is effective and prescribe it in the lowest effective dose.

Educating females about the effect of drugs on a developing fetus is best done before pregnancy. Because drug use is prevalent in schools, preadolescence is not too soon to begin this education. Women should be taught to eliminate the use of any unnecessary substance before becoming pregnant. A woman is encouraged to tell her health care provider if she thinks she is pregnant (or is trying to conceive) before having a nonemergency radiograph, being prescribed a drug, or taking herbal or food supplements.

A trusting, therapeutic nurse–patient relationship makes it more likely that a woman will be truthful about the use of substances, both legal and illicit. The nurse who collects data must use a nonjudgmental approach and treat the issue as a health problem rather than a moral problem. The nurse should support the woman who is trying to reduce her drug use. The nurse should praise her efforts to improve her overall health and to have a successful pregnancy.

A multidisciplinary approach is needed to plan for the care of a mother and newborn that includes referral to community agencies after discharge or child protective services if needed. Drugs that are contraindicated for use in women who are breastfeeding are identified in various drug references. These references should be used as a guide in counseling mothers concerning breastfeeding. See Chapter 14 for discussion of neonatal abstinence syndrome.

TRAUMA DURING PREGNANCY

There is a high incidence of trauma during the childbearing years. The incidence of trauma during pregnancy may continue to rise, because women are increasingly employed during their pregnancy, and there is a trend toward a more violent society. Automobile accidents, homicide, and suicide are the three leading causes of traumatic death (Hoyert, 2012). Although pregnant women usually are more careful to protect themselves from harm, increased stress from pregnancy may lead to injury both in and out of the home.

Falls are not uncommon because of the woman's altered sense of balance. The pregnant woman also needs to be especially careful when stepping in and out of the bathtub or when using a ladder or stepstool.

The *automobile* is another hazard. The woman needs to wear a seat belt every time she is in a car, both as a driver and as a passenger. The lap portion of the belt is placed low, just below her protruding abdomen. The pregnant woman and her fetus are more likely to suffer severe injury or death because of not being restrained during a crash than they are to be injured by the restraint itself. Air bags are a supplemental restraint and are intended for use in addition to seat belts. No one should ride with anyone who has been drinking alcohol or whose judgment is impaired for other reasons.

Terrorist acts that involve bombs or blasts usually cause significant bodily injury in gas-filled parts of the body, such as the lungs, gastrointestinal tract, and middle ear. Symptoms of "blast lung" can develop as late as 48 hours after the blast and can include bradycardia, low blood pressure, dyspnea, cough, and bloody sputum (hemoptysis). Bomb fragments can contain contaminated or infectious materials and can penetrate the skin, which may necessitate special isolation precautions (see Appendix A).

Physical trauma is usually blunt trauma (falls or blows to the body) but may be penetrating trauma (knife or gunshot wounds). Physical abuse against women (battering) is a significant cause of trauma, and violence often escalates during pregnancy. Battering occurs in all ethnic groups and all social strata. It often begins or becomes worse during pregnancy. The abuser is usually her male partner, but he may be another male, such as the father of a pregnant adolescent. Men who abuse women are also likely to abuse children in the relationship.

Women abused during pregnancy are more likely to have miscarriages, stillbirths, and low-birth-weight babies. They often enter prenatal care late, if at all. The risk of homicide escalates during pregnancy.

Abuse during pregnancy, as at other times, may take many forms. It is not always physical abuse; many women are abused emotionally. Emotional abuse makes leaving the relationship especially difficult, because it lowers the woman's self-esteem and isolates her from sources of help. The time of greatest danger to the abused woman occurs when she leaves her abuser.

Manifestations of Battering. In addition to having late or erratic prenatal care, the battered woman may have bruises or lacerations in various stages of healing. A radiograph may show old fractures. The woman tends to minimize injury or "forget" its severity. She may assume responsibility for the trauma, as evidenced by remarks such as, "If I had only kept the children quiet, he wouldn't have gotten so mad." Her abuser is often particularly attentive after the battering episode.

Treatment and Nursing Care of the Pregnant Woman Experiencing Trauma. Nurses must be aware that any woman may be in an abusive relationship. Therapeutic, nonjudgmental communication helps establish a trusting nurse–patient relationship. Nonabused women, including nurses, often cannot understand why a woman would stay in a harmful relationship. The abuser has usually isolated the woman by controlling who she sees, where she goes, and how she spends money. Emotional abuse often supplements physical abuse, making the woman feel that she is "stupid" or "no good" and that she is "lucky that he loves her, because no one else would ever love her." She usually feels that she has no choice but to stay in the abusive relationship. She may assume part of the blame, believing that her abuser will stop hurting her if she tries harder.

The woman being assessed for abuse is taken to a private area. The nurse determines whether there are factors that increase the risk for severe injuries or homicide, such as drug use by the abuser, a gun in the house, previous use of a weapon, or violent behavior by the abuser outside the home. The nurse also determines whether the children are being hurt. It is vital that the abuser does not discover that the woman has reported the abuse or that she intends to leave.

⛔ Safety Alert!

If a woman confides that she is being abused during pregnancy, this information must be kept absolutely confidential. Her life may be in danger if her abuser learns that she has told anyone. She should be referred to local shelters, but the decision to leave her abuser is hers alone.

Nurses can refer women to shelters and other services if they wish to leave the abuser. However, the decision about whether to end the relationship rests with the woman. Abuse of children must be reported to appropriate authorities.

In addition to a routine comprehensive assessment, the pregnant woman should have fetal monitoring for 4 to 6 hours after any trauma. The nurse should understand the changes in anatomy and physiology that normally occur during pregnancy and should ensure that the pregnant woman is not positioned on her back to prevent supine hypotensive syndrome (see Chapter 4). Modifications in the technique of performing cardiopulmonary resuscitation (CPR) on a pregnant woman are described in Box 5-8.

Box 5-8   Modification of Standard Cardiopulmonary Resuscitation (CPR) for Pregnant Women

- Displace uterus laterally by placing a wedge or rolled blanket under one hip (prevents supine hypotensive syndrome) (Stapleton et al, 2001).
- If defibrillation is used, place the paddles one rib interspace higher than usual (because of the normal heart displacement caused by the enlarged term uterus).
- Chest compressions may be administered at a point slightly higher on the sternum (the term uterus displaces the diaphragm to a higher position). Do NOT use abdominal thrusts.
- Determine resting uterine tone after CPR of a pregnant woman.
- Provide hemodynamic monitoring for the woman after CPR.
- Maintain continuous electronic fetal monitoring (EFM) of the fetus.

Nursing care for the acutely injured pregnant woman supplements medical management: the focus is on stabilizing the mother's condition when life-threatening injuries occur. Placing a small pillow under one hip tilts the heavy uterus off the inferior vena cava to improve blood flow throughout the woman's body and to the placenta. An assessment of vital signs and urine output reflects blood circulation to the kidneys. Urine output should average at least 30 mL/hr. Bloody urine may indicate damage to the kidneys or the bladder.

The nurse assesses for uterine contractions or tenderness, which may indicate onset of labor or abruptio placentae. Continuous electronic fetal monitoring (see Chapter 6) is usually instituted if the fetus is viable, even in cases of mild abdominal trauma.

In cases of severe trauma and blood loss, the nurse must relate the increased blood volume of pregnancy to the probable need for increased fluid and blood intake to stabilize the pregnant trauma patient. Peripheral vasoconstriction that normally occurs as a response to shock will cause a decreased flow of oxygen to the fetus. Placing a pillow under one hip to prevent pressure of the uterus on the vena cava is essential. Because of the increased coagulability of the pregnant woman, the aftermath of trauma can result in a high risk for blood-clotting problems such as thrombophlebitis. Values of fibrinogen of 200 to 400 mg/100 mL may be normal for a nonpregnant patient but are indicative of the development of DIC in the pregnant woman, who normally has a fibrinogen level of 400 to 650 mg/100 mL. A fractured pelvis may result in cephalopelvic disproportion (CPD) and necessitate cesarean delivery. Dopamine, a drug routinely used to achieve hemodynamic stability in trauma patients, causes uteroplacental vasoconstriction and may lead to fetal death.

The use of tocolytics to delay labor may be contraindicated in some types of trauma, such as burns. Magnesium sulfate is a vasodilator and also may be contraindicated for use in some types of trauma and shock. Electrical shock injuries can be more serious to the fetus even though the mother does not seem to be seriously injured, because amniotic fluid offers low resistance to the passage of the electrical current to the fetus. In general, it is important for the nurse to understand and correlate the physiology of pregnancy to help the mother and fetus who are victims of trauma. See Box 5-8 for CPR modification during pregnancy.

> ⓘ **Safety Alert!**
>
> Even minor motor vehicle accidents can cause increased abdominal pressure on the pregnant abdomen via flexion of the body or seatbelt pressure and can result in stretching or tearing vessels within the uterus. Therefore every pregnant woman in the ER following trauma should receive close uterine and fetal monitoring.

EFFECTS OF A HIGH-RISK PREGNANCY ON THE FAMILY

Normal pregnancy can be a crisis, because it is a time of significant change and growth. The woman with a complicated pregnancy has stressors even beyond those of the normal pregnancy. Her family is also affected by the pregnancy and the impending birth.

DISRUPTION OF USUAL ROLES

The woman who experiences a difficult pregnancy must often remain on bed rest at home or in the hospital, sometimes for several weeks. Others must assume her usual roles in the family, in addition to their own obligations. Finding caregivers for young children in the family may be difficult if extended family lives far away. Placing the children in day care may not be an option if financial problems exist.

Nurses can help families adjust to these disruptions by identifying sources of support to help maintain reasonably normal household function.

FINANCIAL DIFFICULTIES

Many women work outside the home, and their salary may stop if they cannot work for an extended period. At the same time, their medical costs are rising. Social service referrals may help the family cope with their expenses.

DELAYED ATTACHMENT TO THE INFANT

Pregnancy normally involves gradual acceptance of and emotional attachment to the fetus, especially after the woman feels fetal movement. Fathers feel a similar attachment, although at a slower pace. The woman who has a high-risk pregnancy often halts planning for the child and may withdraw emotionally to protect herself from pain and loss if the outcome is poor.

LOSS OF EXPECTED BIRTH EXPERIENCE

Couples rarely anticipate problems when they begin a pregnancy. Most have specific expectations about how their pregnancy, particularly the birth, will proceed. A high-risk pregnancy may result in the loss of their expected experience. If the loss is during early pregnancy, they may be unable to attend childbirth preparation classes or to have a vaginal birth. Perinatal loss shatters the hopes of human life and severs a unique attachment between mother and fetus (Figure 5-9). Parents exhibit mourning behaviors associated with the various stages of the grieving process. Health care providers must address these aspects of the grieving process as they work with the parents through interventions, including the following:

- Allowing parents to remain together in privacy
- Accepting behaviors related to grieving
- Developing a plan of care to provide support to the family
- Offering a memento such as a footprint, ID band, lock of hair, and so forth (see Figure 5-9)
- Offering parents an opportunity to hold the infant, if they choose
- Preparing parents for the appearance of the infant
- Providing parents with educational materials and referrals to support groups
- Discussing wishes concerning religious and cultural rituals

Many new noninvasive technologies are on the horizon to detect problem pregnancies and to enable early diagnosis and treatment (Table 5-10). The most promising development is the noninvasive examination of maternal blood (DNA) and paternal saliva to provide a genome-wide prenatal diagnosis of both dominant and recessive fetal anomalies (Kitzman, 2012). At present, cell-free DNA in the maternal blood is used for the prenatal detection of trisomy 13, 18 and 21 (Simpson, 2013).

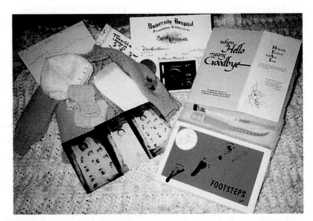

FIGURE 5-9 Memory kit. This "memory kit" includes pictures of the newborn, clothing, death certificate, footprints, ID band, fetal monitor printout, and ultrasound picture.

Table 5-10	Some Noninvasive Technologies in Prenatal Assessment
TECHNIQUE	**OUTCOME**
AmniSure	Identifies a placental protein that is present in amniotic fluid to help diagnose premature rupture of the membranes.
Three-dimensional (3-D) ultrasound	Enables clear in utero identification of malformations, such as cleft lip or palate, abdominal wall defects, and spinal anomalies. Early tests can measure gestational sac and cervical volume to enable early treatment of incompetent cervix and intrauterine growth restriction (IUGR).
Fetal DNA	Cell-free DNA in the maternal blood can detect prenatal occurrence of trisomy 13, 18, and 21 in the fetus with high reliability.
Fetal trophoblast cells	Cells isolated from the maternal external cervical opening at 12-15 weeks of gestation can provide identification of genetic disorders. The test is safer than amniocentesis for this purpose.
Proteomic technology	Amniotic fluid protein studied by proteomic technology, referred to as SELDI-TOF-MS, enables identification of biomarkers of diseases that may lead to preterm birth or fetal injury. Early diagnosis and treatment can prevent premature birth.

Data from Cousins L et al: AmniSure placental alpha microglobulin-1 rapid immunoassay versus standard diagnostic methods for detection of ruptured membranes, *Am J Perinatal* 22:317-320, 2005; Buhimschi I, Cristner B, Buhimschi C: Proteomic biomarker analysis of amniotic fluid for identification of intraamniotic inflammation, *BJOG* 112:173-181, 2005; Gabbe S et al: *Obstetrics: normal and problem pregnancies*, ed 6, St Louis, 2012, Elsevier; Manning F: Antepartal fetal testing: a clinical appraisal, *Curr Opin Obstet Gynecol* 21:348, 2009.

Unfolding Case Study

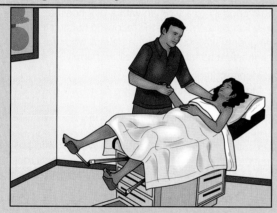

Tess and her husband Luis were introduced to the reader in Chapter 4 and will be followed throughout the Maternity section of this text as her birth story unfolds.

Tess, P1G0, returns to the prenatal clinic before her scheduled appointment, and she is now 10-weeks pregnant and complaining of spotting and a worsening of her nausea with some vomiting. An examination shows that her cervix is closed and Chadwick's sign is positive, but no fetal heart tones are heard.

QUESTIONS

1. What is the significance of a positive Chadwick's sign?
2. What are the causes of bleeding early in pregnancy?
3. What data concerning history will the nurse obtain from Tess?
4. When would nausea and vomiting during pregnancy not be considered a normal occurrence?
5. How is excessive nausea and vomiting during pregnancy treated?
6. What is the significance of the fact that the health care provider cannot hear fetal heart tones at this visit?

Get Ready for the NCLEX® Examination!

Key Points

- Hyperemesis gravidarum is persistent nausea and vomiting of pregnancy and often interferes with nutrition and fluid balance.
- The most common reason for early spontaneous abortion is abnormality of the developing fetus or the placenta.
- If a woman has a tubal rupture from an ectopic pregnancy, the nurse should observe for shock.
- Because of hemorrhage into the abdomen in the case of a tubal rupture, vaginal blood loss may be minimal, even though intraabdominal blood loss can be massive.

- The woman who has gestational trophoblastic disease (hydatidiform mole) should have follow-up medical care for 1 year to detect the possible development of choriocarcinoma. She should not become pregnant during this time.
- Placenta previa is the abnormal implantation of the placenta in the lower part of the uterus.
- Abruptio placentae is the premature separation of the placenta that is normally implanted.
- The three main manifestations of preeclampsia are hypertension, edema, and proteinuria.
- Eclampsia occurs when the woman has a seizure.
- A positive non–stress test (NST) indicates heart accelerations and is reassuring of fetal health.

- A negative contraction stress test (CST) indicates there are no late decelerations after a uterine contraction and denotes fetal health.
- An abortion is the termination of pregnancy before the fetus is viable.
- Positioning the mother on her left side during bed rest helps improve blood flow to the placenta and prevent pressure on the vena cava.
- A blood pressure of 140/90 mm Hg or above is considered hypertension in the pregnant patient.
- A routine, noninvasive ultrasound examination can confirm pregnancy, detect some anomalies, and show the sex of the fetus.
- Rh$_o$(D) immune globulin (RhoGAM) can be administered to an Rh-negative mother to prevent blood incompatibilities between the mother and an Rh-positive fetus (erythroblastosis fetalis).
- GDM first occurs during pregnancy and resolves after pregnancy. The newborn may be excessively large (macrosomia), and the mother may develop DM later in life. Control of blood glucose level is essential to protect the fetus.
- TORCH diseases of pregnancy include **to**xoplasmosis, **r**ubella, **c**ytomegalovirus, and **h**erpes, with the **o** also denoting *others*.
- The nurse must consider the physiological changes that occur during pregnancy to understand and care for the pregnant trauma victim. Both the mother and the fetus must be monitored closely.
- Urinary tract infections are more common during pregnancy, because compression and dilation of the ureters result in urine stasis. Preterm labor is more likely to occur if a woman has pyelonephritis.
- The fetus of the woman who takes drugs (legal or illicit) or drinks alcohol is exposed to higher levels of the substance for a longer time, because the substances become concentrated in the amniotic fluid and the fetus ingests the fluid.
- Drugs and alcohol consumed by the mother can cross the placenta and adversely affect the developing fetus.
- The nurse must be prepared to recognize the effects of adverse environmental factors on the maternal–child patient.

Additional Learning Resources

SG Go to your Study Guide for additional learning activities to help you master this chapter content.

evolve Go to your Evolve website (http://evolve.elsevier.com/Leifer) for the following learning resources:
- Animations
- Answer Guidelines for Critical Thinking Questions
- Answers and Rationales for Review Questions for the NCLEX® Examination
- Glossary with English and Spanish pronunciations
- Interactive Review Questions for the NCLEX® Examination
- Patient Teaching Plans in English and Spanish
- Skills Performance Checklists
- Video clips and more!

 Online Resources
- Office on Violence Against Women: www.ovw.usdoj.gov
- Pregnancy and exercise: www.familydoctor.org/handouts/305.html
- AIDS info (2012) HIV and Pregnancy www.AIDSinfo.NIH.GOV

Review Questions for the NCLEX® Examination

1. A woman has an incomplete abortion followed by vacuum aspiration. She is now in the recovery room with her husband and is crying softly. Select the most appropriate nursing action.
   1. Leave the couple alone, except for necessary recovery-room care.
   2. Tell the couple that most abortions are for the best, because the infant would have been abnormal.
   3. Tell the couple that spontaneous abortion is very common and does not mean that they cannot have other children.
   4. Express your regret at their loss and remain nearby if they want to talk about it.

2. Her health care provider gives magnesium sulfate intravenously to a woman with a diagnosis of preeclampsia. Which of the following nursing interventions are priority when caring for a patient who has received magnesium sulfate? (Select all that apply.)
   1. Monitor uterine tone.
   2. Monitor urine output.
   3. Keep patient NPO.
   4. Monitor respiratory rate.

3. It is important to emphasize that a woman who has gestational trophoblastic disease (hydatidiform mole) should continue to receive follow-up medical care after initial treatment, because:
   1. choriocarcinoma sometimes occurs after the initial treatment.
   2. she has lower levels of immune factors and is vulnerable to infection.
   3. anemia complicates most cases of hydatidiform mole.
   4. permanent elevation of her blood pressure is more likely.

4. Select the primary difference between the symptoms of placenta previa and abruptio placentae.
   1. Fetal presentation
   2. Presence of pain
   3. Abnormal blood clotting
   4. Presence of bleeding

5. During the prenatal clinic visit, your intervention with an abused woman is successful if you have assessed the status of the woman and:
   1. persuaded her to leave her abusive partner.
   2. informed her of her safety options.
   3. convinced her to notify the police.
   4. placed her in a shelter for abused women.

Objectives

1. Define each key term listed.
2. Discuss specific cultural beliefs the nurse may encounter when providing care to a woman in labor.
3. Compare the advantages and disadvantages for each type of childbearing setting: hospital, freestanding birth center, and home.
4. Describe the four components ("four Ps") of the birth process: **p**owers, **p**assage, **p**assenger, and **p**syche.
5. Describe how the four Ps of labor interrelate to result in the birth of an infant.
6. Explain the normal processes of childbirth: premonitory signs, mechanisms of birth, and stages and phases of labor.
7. Explain how false labor differs from true labor.
8. Determine appropriate nursing care for the intrapartum patient, including the woman in false labor and the woman having a vaginal birth after cesarean (VBAC).
9. Explain common nursing responsibilities during the labor and birth.
10. Describe the care of the newborn immediately after birth.

Key Terms

accelerations (p. 135)
absent variability (p. 135)
acrocyanosis (ăk-rō-sī-ă-NŌ-sĭs, p. 151)
adjustment (p. 139)
amnioinfusion (ăm-nē-ō-ĭn-FYŪ-zhŭn, p. 137)
amniotomy (ăm-nēŎT-ŏ-mē, p. 137)
baseline fetal heart rate (p. 133)
baseline variability (p. 134)
bloody show (p. 126)
cold stress (p. 150)
coping (p. 139)
crowning (p. 145)
decelerations (p. 135)
dilate (p. 120)
doula (DŪ-lă, p. 142)
efface (ĕ-FĀS, p. 120)
episodic changes (p. 135)
fetal bradycardia (p. 133)
fetal tachycardia (p. 134)
fontanelle (FŎN-tă-nĕl, p. 122)

laboring down (p. 142)
late decelerations (p. 135)
Leopold's maneuver (p. 130)
lie (p. 122)
marked variability (p. 135)
moderate variability (p. 135)
molding (p. 122)
neutral thermal environment (p. 150)
nitrazine test (p. 137)
nuchal cord (NŪ-kăl kŏrd, p. 135)
ophthalmia neonatorum (ŏf-THĂL-mē-ă nē-ō-nă-TŎR-ăm, p. 152)
periodic changes (p. 135)
prolonged decelerations (p. 136)
station (p. 126)
sutures (p. 122)
Trial of Labor After Cesarean (TOLAC) (p. 143)
uteroplacental insufficiency (yū-tăr-ō-plă-SĔN-tăl ĭn-sŭ-FĬSH-ăn-sē, p. 135)
vaginal birth after cesarean (VBAC) (p. 143)

Childbirth is a normal physiological process that involves the health of the mother and a fetus who will become part of our next generation. The nursing care is unique, because every nursing intervention involves the welfare of two patients and the use of skills from medical-surgical and pediatric nursing, psychosocial and communication skills, and specific skills involved in obstetric care. In addition, labor and delivery are often a family affair, with fathers, grandparents, and others closely involved. Each family participant often remembers the details of this experience for a long time.

 Nursing Tip

The bedside nurse in the labor and delivery unit bridges the gap between sophisticated technology and the individual patient's needs, providing a positive outcome both physically and psychologically.

The privacy and rights of the mother must be protected, the policies and procedures of the institution must be considered, and the nurse must be familiar with the scope of practice set out by the state board of nursing. Recent changes in the management of labor and delivery include practices related to induction and augmentation of labor, fetal monitoring techniques, maternal positions, types of analgesia offered, and assistive devices such as vacuum extraction.

This chapter provides information concerning the birth process and the nursing responsibilities during labor and delivery.

CULTURAL INFLUENCE ON BIRTH PRACTICES

The needs of the woman giving birth may be influenced by her cultural background, which may be very different from that of the nurse but must be understood and respected. In a multicultural environment, nothing is routine. Patient and cultural preferences require flexibility on the part of the nurse. Women of most cultures prefer the presence of a support person at all times during labor and delivery, and that can include the father or family as well as professional staff. The United States is a multicultural society. Table 6-1 lists common traditional birth practices of selected cultures. The practices of these cultural groups may vary depending on the amount of time they have been in the United States and the degree to which they have assimilated into the culture.

SETTINGS FOR CHILDBIRTH

Depending on facilities available in the area and the risks for complications, a woman can choose among three settings in which to deliver her child. Most women give birth in the hospital, whereas others choose freestanding birth facilities or their own home with a nurse-midwife or lay midwife in attendance.

HOSPITALS

The woman who chooses a hospital birth may have a "traditional" setting, in which she labors, delivers, and recovers in separate rooms. After the recovery period, she is transferred to the postpartum unit. A more common setting for hospital maternity care is the birthing room, often called a labor, delivery, and recovery (LDR) room. The woman labors, delivers, and recovers all in the same room. She is then transferred to the postpartum unit for continuing care. The appearance of the birthing room is more homelike than institutional. The fully functional birthing bed has wood trim that hides its utilitarian purpose (Figure 6-1). The beds have receptacles for various fittings, such as a "squat bar," which facilitates squatting during second-stage labor. The foot of the bed can be detached or rolled away to reveal foot supports or stirrups.

Another hospital birth setting is a single-room maternity care arrangement, often called a labor, delivery, recovery, and postpartum (LDRP) room. It is similar to the LDR room, but the mother and infant remain in the same room until discharge.

Advantages of hospital-based birth settings include the following:

- Preregistration, which allows important information to be available on admission
- Easy access to sophisticated services and specialized personnel if complications develop
- Ability to provide family-centered care for the woman who has a complicated pregnancy

FREESTANDING BIRTH CENTERS

Some communities have birth centers that are separate from, although usually near, hospitals and are similar to outpatient surgical centers. Many birth centers are operated by full-service hospitals and are close enough for easy transfer if the mother, fetus, or newborn develops complications. Certified nurse-midwives often attend the births.

Advantages of freestanding birth centers include the following:

- A homelike setting for the low-risk woman
- Lower costs because the freestanding center does not require expensive departments such as emergency or critical care

Disadvantages include the following:

- A slight but significant delay in emergency care if the mother or child develops life-threatening complications

HOME

Some women give birth at home. Many factors enter into their decision, and most families have carefully weighed the pros and cons of their choice.

Advantages of a home birth include the following:

- Control over persons who will or will not be present for the labor and birth, including children
- No risk of acquiring pathogens from other patients
- A low-technology birth, which is important to some families

Disadvantages vary with the location and may include the following:

- Limited choice of birth attendants (most physicians and nurse-midwives choose not to attend home births; in many communities, only lay midwives are available [whose training, abilities, and licensure status vary widely])
- Significant delay in reaching emergency care if the mother or child develops life-threatening complications
- Possibility of no preestablished relationship with a physician in case an emergency arises that necessitates the woman or newborn to be transferred to a hospital

COMPONENTS OF THE BIRTH PROCESS

Four interrelated components, often called the "four Ps," make up the process of labor and birth: the powers, the passage, the passenger, and the psyche. These factors are discussed in detail in the sections that follow.

Table 6-1   Birth Practices of Selected Cultural Groups

ROLE OF THE WOMAN IN LABOR AND DELIVERY	ROLE OF THE FATHER OR PARTNER IN LABOR AND DELIVERY
American Indian	
Is stoic May have indigenous plants in room May wear special necklaces May commonly use meditation chants Prefers water at room temperature to drink Prefers chicken soup and rice postpartum	Husband avoids eating meat during perinatal phase. Husband may provide support during labor.
Arabic	
Is passive but expressive Views keeping body covered as important May wear protective amulets May have low pain tolerance Values male newborn more than female Expects 20 days of bed rest after birth	Husband is not expected to participate but remains in control. Female family member is preferred as coach. Husband must be present if male health care provider examines woman. Husband may whisper praises in newborn's ear.
African American	
Participates actively Is vocal in labor Wants only sponge bath postpartum Avoids hair washing until lochia ceases	Female attendants are usually preferred.
Cambodian (Khmer)	
Is stoic in labor If walking during labor, must not pause in doorway (thought to delay birth) Does not want head touched without permission Colostrum discarded Will not nurse after delivery or eat vegetables in first week	Individual family preference determines whether father is present during delivery.
Central American (Guatemala, Nicaragua, Salvador)	
Is vocal and active during labor May prefer to wear red (a protective color) If more affluent, prefers bottle feeding Prefers chicken soup, banana, meat, and herbal tea, and showers postpartum Avoids "cold foods"	Husband is expected to be present for support, but female family members participate more.
Chinese	
May be vocal during labor Must not pause in doorway if walking during labor (thought to delay birth) All doors and windows to be unlocked (thought to ease passage of infant) Do not use first name of woman May not shower for 30 days postpartum Covers ears to prevent air from entering body Prefers breastfeeding Needs to be encouraged to ask questions	Husband usually does not play an active role in labor and delivery, but oldest male makes decisions. Woman's mother may participate. Husband may bring long piece of silk material called a *hada* as a sign of greeting and good luck to the child. Husband expects to be called by first and last name.
Cuban	
Is vocal but passive during labor and delivery Uses formal name at introduction Must stay at home 41 days postpartum and be sheltered from stress	Mother of woman preferred as coach. Husband is not usually involved in labor but must be informed first of problems and progress.
Eritrean or Ethiopian	
Is stoic but takes active role Modesty very important; must remain covered Prefers breastfeeding for 2 years Remains in seclusion 40 days postpartum All food and drinks during puerperium must be warm	Traditionally, husbands are not allowed to be present during labor and delivery.

Continued

Table 6-1   **Birth Practices of Selected Cultural Groups—cont'd**

ROLE OF THE WOMAN IN LABOR AND DELIVERY	ROLE OF THE FATHER OR PARTNER IN LABOR AND DELIVERY
Filipino	
Prefers slippery foods (such as eggs) so infant will "slip through birth canal" Prefers midwife support Assumes active role in labor Prefers sponge baths postpartum	Husband is not usually with woman during labor.
Falkland Islands	
Places keys (unlock) and combs (untangle) under pillow of labor bed	Husband is expected to be supportive.
Hindu, Sikh, Muslim, Nepalese, Fijian, Pakistani	
Assumes passive role and follows directions of trained professionals May keep head covered during labor Prenatal care started on day 120 of gestation Should not reveal sex of newborn until after placenta is delivered (to avoid upsetting the mother if the sex is not of her preference) Takes sponge baths postpartum Remains in seclusion 40 days postpartum	Female coach is preferred, although father waits near labor room for consultation. Husband must be present if male attendant examines woman. Ceremony of "A qiqah" involves father shaving head of newborn and whispering praises into ear of newborn. Coach may chant scriptures during birth.
Hmong (Laos, Burma, Thailand)	
Is usually quiet and passive Avoids multiple caregivers Avoids internal examinations Views full genital exposure as unacceptable Prefers squat position Do not remove amulets on wrists or ankles Do not use first name initially Prefers chicken, white rice, and warm fluids postpartum Bottle feeding popular	Husband is usually present and makes all decisions.
Israeli (Orthodox Jewish)	
Prefers nurse-midwife Maintains modesty Must not be intimate with husband until 7 days after lochia stops Males are circumcised on the eighth day Females named on first Saturday after birth	Husband not expected to participate in prenatal classes. Husband may not touch wife during labor, view perineum, or view infant as it is born. Husband may participate from afar with verbal encouragement during labor. Woman's mother participates in birth process.
Japanese	
Modesty is important Will bathe and shower postpartum Infant may be bathed twice each day for a week with loud noise and music to ward off evil spirits Prefers north part of room May cut hair and take special vows Is assertive during labor but may not ask for pain relief	Chanting and throwing rice ward off evil spirits. Modern-day husbands are present and participate during labor and delivery. In modern Japan, husbands are compliant with health education.
Korean	
Is compliant with health care provider Avoids ice water Is an active participant in labor Does not address by first name initially Prefers sponge bath postpartum May breastfeed but needs instruction on pumping and storage of milk May not wish to ambulate early	Husband participates in labor and delivery. Husband prefers not to be told in advance of fetal prognosis. Family makes medical decisions.
Mexican American	
Believes supine position is best for fetus Determines selection of coach Prefers privacy Accepts pain but is active in labor Will not shower postpartum and ambulates only to bathroom Avoids beans postpartum Uses alternative therapies for mother and infant (see Chapter 34)	Husband is in control of decisions but is not present during labor. Female relatives provide support. Husband prefers not to be told in advance of serious fetal prognosis.

Table 6-1   Birth Practices of Selected Cultural Groups—cont'd

ROLE OF THE WOMAN IN LABOR AND DELIVERY	ROLE OF THE FATHER OR PARTNER IN LABOR AND DELIVERY
Puerto Rican	
Is active in labor Prefers hospital care Keeps body covered Does not eat beans, starch, or eggs if breastfeeding Will not wash hair for 40 days postpartum Prefers sponge bath and lotions	Husband assumes supportive role during labor and delivery. If not present during delivery, husband expects to be kept informed.
South American (Brazilian)	
May not participate in coping techniques during delivery Needs to be offered pain relief options Stays at home for 40 days postpartum except for medical appointments	Presence of husband in delivery room is discouraged.
Vietnamese	
Woman expected to "suffer in silence" Offer options for pain relief Prefers upright position for labor and delivery Prefers warm fluids to drink Sponge bathes only for 2 weeks postpartum Newborn is not praised to protect from jealousy	Female family member is preferred. Husband is expected to remain nearby. Sexual intercourse is prohibited during pregnancy and puerperium.
West Indian (Trinidad, Jamaica, Barbados)	
Prefers midwife Maintains passive role and follows instructions Prefers bed rest for 1 week postpartum Do not address by first name initially	Female relative or friend as coach is preferred. Husband is not present in area.

NOTE: Use professional translators whenever possible. Family members may not convey taboo topics accurately.

Data from Lipson JG, Dibble SL: *Culture and nursing care,* ed 2, San Francisco, 2005, University of California, San Francisco, School of Nursing; Murasaki S: *Diary of Lady Murasaki,* New York, 1996, Penguin Books; Bates B, Neuman A, Turner B: Imagery and symbolism in the birth practices of traditional cultures, *Women Health Nurs* (Wiley) 12(1):29-36, 2007; Chalmers B: Childbirth across cultures: research and practice, *Women Health Nurs* (Wiley) 39(4):276-280, 2012; D'Anzo C: *Mosby's pocket guide to cultural health assessment,* ed 4, St Louis, 2008, Mosby.

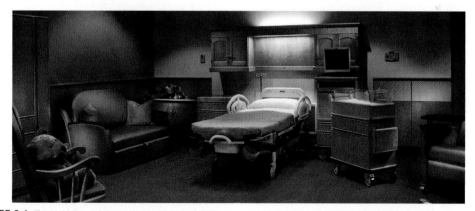

FIGURE 6-1 Typical labor, delivery, and recovery (LDR) room. Homelike furnishings can be quickly adapted to provide essential equipment when woman enters the active phase of labor. (Courtesy Hill-Rom Services, Batesville, Ind.)

Other factors that influence the progress of labor include *preparation,* such as attendance at prenatal classes; *position,* horizontal or vertical; *professional help,* such as knowledgeable nurses in attendance who explain and coach; the *place* or setting, because a lack of privacy and changes in shift personnel can interrupt rapport; *procedures,* such as internal examinations; and *people,* such as the presence of supportive family members (VandeVusse, 1999).

THE POWERS

The powers of labor are forces that cause the cervix to open and that propel the fetus downward through the birth canal. The two powers are the uterine contractions and the mother's pushing efforts.

Uterine Contractions

Uterine contractions are the primary powers of labor during the first of the four stages of labor (from onset until full dilation of the cervix). Uterine contractions are involuntary smooth muscle contractions; the woman cannot consciously cause them to stop or start. However, their intensity and effectiveness are influenced by a number of factors, such as walking, drugs, maternal anxiety, and vaginal examinations.

Effect of Contractions on the Cervix.

Contractions cause the cervix to **efface** (thin) and **dilate** (open) to allow the fetus to descend in the birth canal (Figure 6-2). Before labor begins, the cervix is a tubular structure about 2 to 3.8 cm long. Contractions simultaneously push the fetus downward as they pull the cervix upward (an action similar to pushing a ball out the cuff of a sock). This causes the cervix to become thinner and shorter. Effacement is determined by a vaginal examination and is described as a percentage of the original cervical length. When the cervix is 100% effaced, it feels like a thin, slick membrane over the fetus.

Dilation of the cervix is determined during a vaginal examination. Dilation is described in centimeters, with full dilation being 10 cm (Figure 6-3). Both dilation and effacement are estimated by touch rather than being precisely measured.

Phases of Contractions.

Each contraction has the following three phases (Figure 6-4):
1. *Increment:* The period of increasing strength
2. *Peak, or acme:* The period of greatest strength
3. *Decrement:* The period of decreasing strength

Contractions are also described by their average frequency, duration, intensity, and interval.

Frequency.

Frequency is the elapsed time from the beginning of one contraction until the beginning of the next contraction. Frequency is described in minutes and fractions of minutes, such as "contractions every 4½ minutes." Contractions occurring more often than every 2 minutes may reduce fetal oxygen supply and should be reported.

Duration.

Duration is the elapsed time from the beginning of a contraction until the end of the same contraction. Duration is described as the average number of seconds for which contractions last, such as "duration of 45 to 50 seconds." Persistent contraction durations longer than 90 seconds may reduce fetal oxygen supply and should be reported.

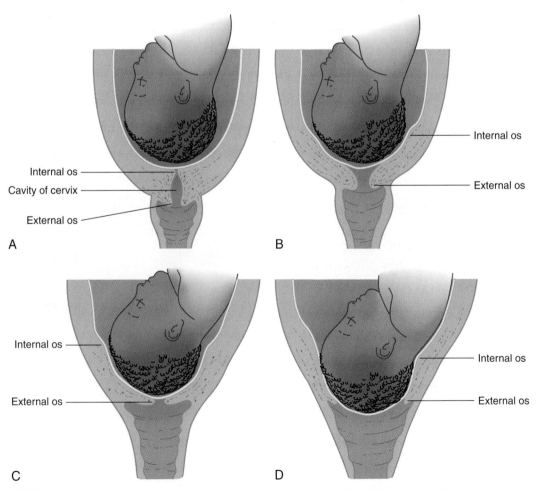

FIGURE 6-2 Cervical effacement and dilation. **A,** No effacement, no dilation. **B,** Early effacement and dilation. **C,** Complete effacement, some dilation. **D,** Complete dilation and effacement. (From Matteson PS: *Women's health during the childbearing years: a community-based approach,* St Louis, 2001, Mosby.)

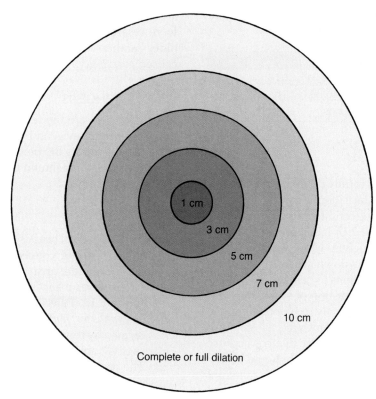

FIGURE 6-3 Cervical dilation in centimeters. Full dilation is 10 cm (1 cm is approximately one finger's width).

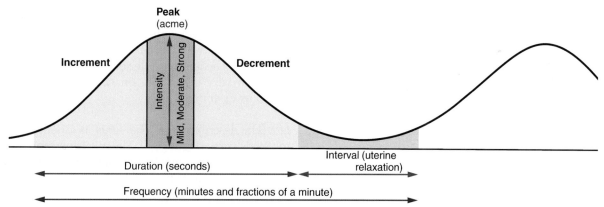

FIGURE 6-4 Contraction cycle. Each contraction can be likened to a bell shape, with an increment, peak (acme), and decrement. The frequency of contractions is the average time from the beginning of one to the beginning of the next. The duration is the average time from the beginning to the end of one contraction. The interval is the period of uterine relaxation between contractions.

Intensity. Intensity is the approximate strength of the contraction. In most cases, intensity is described in words such as "mild," "moderate," or "strong," which are defined as follows:

- *Mild contractions:* Fundus is easily indented with the fingertips; the fundus of the uterus feels similar to the tip of the nose.
- *Moderate contractions:* Fundus can be indented with the fingertips but with more difficulty; the fundus of the uterus feels similar to the chin.

- *Firm contractions:* Fundus cannot be readily indented with the fingertips; the fundus of the uterus feels similar to the forehead.

Interval. The interval is the amount of time the uterus relaxes between contractions. Blood flow from the mother into the placenta gradually decreases during contractions and resumes during each interval. The placenta refills with freshly oxygenated blood for the fetus and removes fetal waste products. Persistent contraction intervals shorter than 60 seconds may reduce fetal oxygen supply.

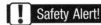
Safety Alert!

Report to the registered nurse any contractions that occur more frequently than every 2 minutes, last longer than 90 seconds, or have intervals shorter than 60 seconds.

Maternal Pushing

When the woman's cervix is fully dilated, she adds voluntary pushing to involuntary uterine contractions. The combined powers of uterine contractions and voluntary maternal pushing in stage 2 of labor propel the fetus downward through the pelvis. Most women feel a strong urge to push or bear down when the cervix is fully dilated and the fetus begins to descend. However, factors such as maternal exhaustion or sometimes epidural analgesia (see Chapter 7) may reduce or eliminate the natural urge to push. Some women feel a premature urge to push before the cervix is fully dilated, because the fetus pushes against the rectum. This should be discouraged, because it may contribute to maternal exhaustion and fetal hypoxia and tearing of maternal soft tissues.

Nursing Tip

Provide emotional support to the laboring woman so she is less anxious and fearful. Excessive anxiety or fear can cause greater pain, inhibit the progress of labor, and reduce blood flow to the placenta and fetus.

THE PASSAGE

The passage consists of the mother's bony pelvis and the soft tissues (cervix, muscles, ligaments, and fascia) of her pelvis and perineum (see Chapter 2 for a review of the structure of the bony pelvis).

Bony Pelvis

The pelvis is divided into the following two major parts: (1) the false pelvis (upper, flaring part); (2) the true pelvis (lower part). The true pelvis, which is directly involved in childbirth, is further divided into the inlet at the top, the midpelvis in the middle, and the outlet near the perineum. It is shaped somewhat like a curved cylinder or a wide, curved funnel. The measurements of the maternal bony pelvis must be adequate to allow the fetal head to pass through, or cephalopelvic disproportion (CPD) will occur, and a cesarean birth may be indicated.

Soft Tissues

In general, women who have had previous vaginal births deliver more quickly than women having their first births, because their soft tissues yield more readily to the forces of contractions and pushing efforts. This advantage is not present if the woman's previous births were cesarean. Soft tissue may not yield as readily in older mothers or after cervical procedures that have caused scarring.

THE PASSENGERS

The passengers are the fetus, the placenta (afterbirth), amniotic membranes, and amniotic fluid. Because the fetus usually enters the pelvis head first (cephalic presentation), the nurse should understand the basic structure of the fetal head.

The Fetus

Fetal Head. The fetal head is composed of several bones separated by strong connective tissue, called **sutures** (Figure 6-5). A wider area, called a **fontanelle,** is formed where the sutures meet. The following two fontanelles are important in obstetrics:

1. The *anterior fontanelle,* a diamond-shaped area formed by the intersection of four sutures (frontal, sagittal, and two coronal)
2. The *posterior fontanelle,* a tiny triangular depression formed by the intersection of three sutures (one sagittal and two lambdoid)

The sutures and fontanelles of the fetal head allow it to change shape as it passes through the pelvis (**molding**). They are important landmarks in determining how the fetus is oriented within the mother's pelvis during birth.

The main transverse diameter of the fetal head is the biparietal diameter, which is measured between the points of the two parietal bones on each side of the head. The anteroposterior diameter of the fetal head can vary depending on how much the head is flexed or extended.

Lie. Lie describes how the fetus is oriented to the mother's spine (Figure 6-6). The most common orientation is the longitudinal lie (greater than 99% of births), in which the fetus is parallel to the mother's spine. The fetus in a transverse lie is at right angles to the mother's spine. The transverse lie may also be called a shoulder presentation. In an oblique lie, the fetus is between a longitudinal lie and a transverse lie.

Attitude. The fetal attitude is normally one of flexion, with the head flexed forward and the arms and the legs flexed. The flexed fetus is compact and ovoid and most efficiently occupies the space in the mother's uterus and pelvis. Extension of the head, the arms, and/or the legs sometimes occurs, and labor may be prolonged.

Presentation. Presentation refers to the fetal part that enters the pelvis first. The cephalic presentation is the most common. Any of the following four variations of cephalic presentations can occur, depending on the extent to which the fetal head is flexed (Figure 6-7):

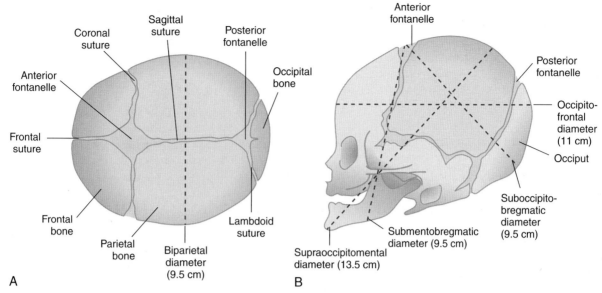

FIGURE 6-5 The fetal skull, showing sutures, fontanelles, and important measurements. **A,** Superior view. Note that the anterior fontanelle has a diamond shape; the posterior fontanelle is triangular. The biparietal diameter is an important fetal skull measurement. **B,** Lateral view. The measurements of the fetal skull are important to determine if cephalopelvic disproportion will be a problem. The mechanisms of labor allow the fetal head to rotate so that the smallest diameter of the head passes through the pelvis as it descends. (From Matteson PS: *Women's health during the childbearing years: a community-based approach,* St Louis, 2001, Mosby.)

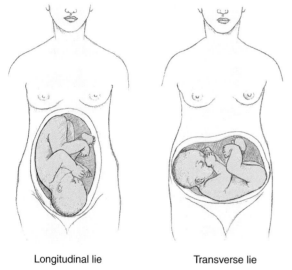

FIGURE 6-6 Lie. In the longitudinal lie, the fetus is parallel to the mother's spine. In the transverse lie, the fetus is at right angles to the mother's spine. The shoulder presents at the cervix.

1. *Vertex presentation:* The fetal head is fully flexed. This is the most favorable cephalic variation, because the smallest possible diameter of the head enters the pelvis. It occurs in about 96% of births.
2. *Military presentation:* The fetal head is neither flexed nor extended.
3. *Brow presentation:* The fetal head is partly extended. The longest diameter of the fetal head is presenting. This presentation is unstable and tends to convert to either a vertex or a face presentation.
4. *Face presentation:* The head is fully extended and the face presents.

The next most common presentation is the breech, which can have the following three variations (see Figure 6-7, *E* to *G*):

1. *Frank breech:* The fetal legs are flexed at the hips and extend toward the shoulders; this is the most common type of breech presentation. The buttocks present at the cervix.
2. *Full or complete breech:* A reversal of the cephalic presentation, with flexion of the head and extremities. Both feet and the buttocks present at the cervix.
3. *Footling breech:* One or both feet are present first at the cervix.

Many women with a fetus in the breech presentation have cesarean births because the head, which is the largest single fetal part, is the last to be born and may not pass through the pelvis easily because flexion of the fetal head cannot occur (see Figure 8-6, p. 190). After the fetal body is born, the head must be delivered quickly so the fetus can breathe; at this point, part of the umbilical cord is outside the mother's body and the remaining part is subject to compression by the fetal head against the bony pelvis.

When the fetus is in a transverse lie, the fetal shoulder enters the pelvis first. A fetus in this orientation must be delivered by cesarean section because it cannot safely pass through the pelvis.

Position. Position refers to how a reference point on the fetal presenting part is oriented within the mother's pelvis. The term *occiput* is used to describe how the head is oriented if the fetus is in a cephalic vertex presentation. The term *sacrum* is used to describe how a fetus in a breech presentation is oriented within the pelvis.

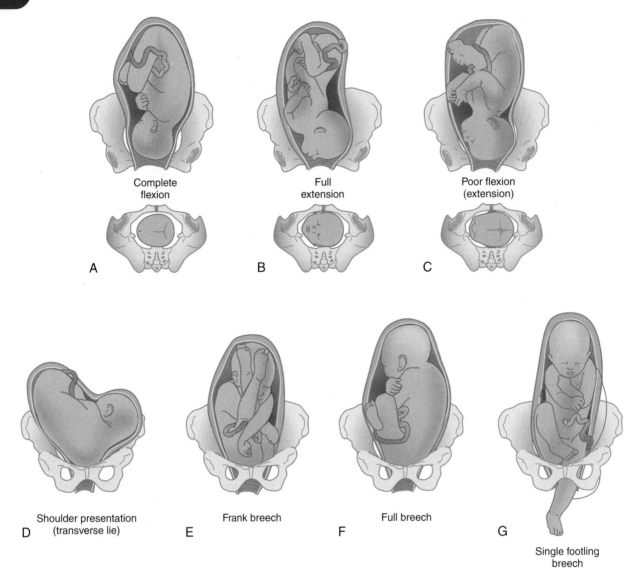

FIGURE 6-7 Fetal presentations. **A,** Cephalic vertex. **B,** Cephalic face. **C,** Cephalic brow. **D,** Shoulder. **E,** Frank breech. **F,** Full or complete breech. **G,** Footling breech (can be single or double). The vertex presentation in which the fetal chin is flexed on the chest is the most common and favorable for a vaginal birth, because it allows the smallest diameter of the head to go through the bony pelvis of the mother. Note how the anterior and posterior fontanelles can be used to determine fetal presentation and position in the pelvis. (From Matteson PS: *Women's health during the childbearing years: a community-based approach,* St Louis, 2001, Mosby.)

The shoulder and back are reference points if the fetus is in a shoulder presentation.

The maternal pelvis is divided into four imaginary quadrants: right and left anterior and right and left posterior. If the fetal occiput is in the left front quadrant of the mother's pelvis, it is described as *left occiput anterior.* If the sacrum of a fetus in a breech presentation is in the mother's right posterior pelvis, it is described as *right sacrum posterior.*

Abbreviations describe the fetal presentation and position within the pelvis (Box 6-1). Three letters are used for most abbreviations:

1. *First letter:* Right or left side of the woman's pelvis. This letter is omitted if the fetal reference point is directly anterior or posterior, such as occiput anterior (OA).

2. *Second letter:* Fetal reference point (occiput for vertex presentations; mentum [chin] for face presentations; and sacrum for breech presentations).

3. *Third letter:* Front or back of the mother's pelvis (anterior or posterior). Transverse (T) denotes a fetal position that is neither anterior nor posterior.

Figure 6-8 shows various fetal presentations and positions.

THE PSYCHE

Childbirth is more than a physical process; it involves the woman's entire being. Women do not recount the births of their children in the same manner that they do surgical procedures. They describe births in emotional terms, such as those they use to describe marriages, anniversaries, religious events, or even deaths.

| Box 6-1 | Classifications of Fetal Presentations and Positions |

CEPHALIC PRESENTATIONS
Vertex Presentations
LOA Left occiput anterior
ROA Right occiput anterior
ROT Right occiput transverse
LOT Left occiput transverse
OA Occiput anterior
OP Occiput posterior
Face Presentations
LMA Left mentum anterior
RMA Right mentum anterior
LMP Left mentum posterior
RMP Right mentum posterior

BREECH PRESENTATIONS
LSA Left sacrum anterior
RSA Right sacrum anterior
LSP Left sacrum posterior
RSP Right sacrum posterior
Abbreviations that designate brow, military, and shoulder presentations are not included here, because they occur infrequently.

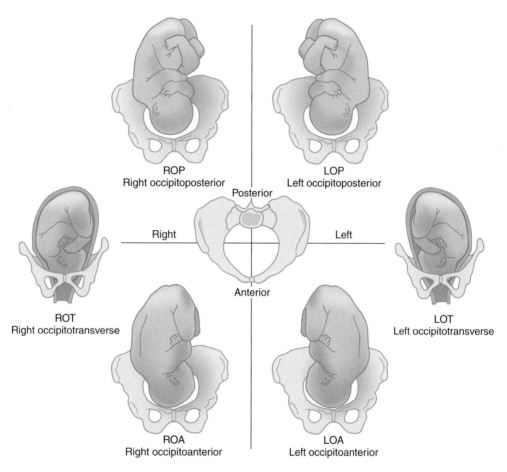

ROP
Right occipitoposterior

LOP
Left occipitoposterior

Posterior

Right

Left

Anterior

ROT
Right occipitotransverse

LOT
Left occipitotransverse

ROA
Right occipitoanterior

LOA
Left occipitoanterior

Lie: Longitudinal or vertical
Presentation: Vertex
Reference point: Occiput
Attitude: Complete flexion

FIGURE 6-8 Fetal position. The right occipitoanterior *(ROA)* or left occipitoanterior *(LOA)* is most favorable for normal labor. When the occiput faces the posterior section of the woman's pelvis, a longer, "back labor" birth process is anticipated. (From Matteson PS: *Women's health during the childbearing years: a community-based approach,* St Louis, 2001, Mosby.)

Families often have great expectations about the *birth experience,* and the nurse can promote a positive childbearing experience by incorporating as many of the family's birth expectations as possible.

A woman's mental state can influence the course of her labor. For example, the woman who is relaxed and optimistic during labor is better able to tolerate discomfort and work with the physiological processes. By contrast, marked anxiety can increase her perception of pain and reduce her tolerance to it. Anxiety and fear also cause the secretion of stress compounds from the adrenal glands. These compounds, called catecholamines, inhibit uterine contractions and divert blood flow from the placenta.

A woman's cultural and individual values influence how she views and copes with childbirth.

NORMAL CHILDBIRTH

The specific event that triggers the onset of labor remains unknown. Many factors probably play a part in initiating labor, which is an interaction of the mother and fetus. These factors include stretching of the uterine muscles, hormonal changes, placental aging, and increased sensitivity to oxytocin. Labor normally begins when the fetus is mature enough to adjust easily to life outside the uterus yet still small enough to fit through the mother's pelvis. This point is usually reached between 38 and 42 weeks after the mother's last menstrual period.

SIGNS OF IMPENDING LABOR

Signs and symptoms that labor is about to start may occur from a few hours to a few weeks before the actual onset of labor.

Braxton Hicks Contractions

Braxton Hicks contractions are irregular contractions that begin during early pregnancy and intensify as full term approaches. They often become regular and somewhat uncomfortable, leading many women to believe that labor has started (see the discussion of true and false labor later in this chapter). Although Braxton Hicks contractions are often called "false" labor, they play a part in preparing the cervix to dilate and in adjusting the fetal position within the uterus.

Increased Vaginal Discharge

Fetal pressure causes an increase in clear and nonirritating vaginal secretions. Irritation or itching with the increased secretions is not normal and should be reported to the physician or certified nurse-midwife (CNM), because these symptoms are characteristic of infection.

Bloody Show

As the time for birth approaches, the cervix undergoes changes in preparation for labor. It softens ("ripens"), effaces, and dilates slightly. When this occurs, the mucous plug that has sealed the uterus during pregnancy is dislodged from the cervix, tearing small capillaries in the process. **Bloody show** is thick mucus mixed with pink or dark brown blood. It may begin a few days before labor, or a woman may not have bloody show until labor is under way. Bloody show may also occur if the woman has had a recent vaginal examination or intercourse.

Rupture of the Membranes

The amniotic sac (bag of waters) sometimes ruptures before labor begins. Infection is more likely if many hours elapse between rupture of the membranes and birth, because the amniotic sac seals the uterine cavity against organisms from the vagina. In addition, the fetal umbilical cord may slip down and become compressed between the mother's pelvis and the fetal presenting part. For these two reasons, women should go to the birth facility when their membranes rupture, even if they have no other signs of labor.

Energy Spurt

Many women have a sudden burst of energy shortly before the onset of labor ("nesting"). The nurse should teach women to conserve their strength, even if they feel unusually energetic.

Weight Loss

Occasionally a woman may notice that she loses 1 to 3 lbs shortly before labor begins, because hormonal changes cause her to excrete extra body water.

MECHANISMS OF LABOR

As the fetus descends into the pelvis, it undergoes several positional changes so that it adapts optimally to the changing pelvic shape and size. Many of these mechanisms, also called cardinal movements, occur simultaneously (Figure 6-9).

Descent

Descent is required for all other mechanisms of labor to occur and for the infant to be born. Descent occurs as each mechanism of labor comes into play. **Station** describes the level of the presenting part (usually the head) in the pelvis. Station is estimated in centimeters from the level of the ischial spines in the mother's pelvis (a 0 [zero] station). Minus stations are above the ischial spines, and plus stations are below the ischial spines (Figure 6-10). As the fetus descends, the minus numbers decrease (e.g., −2, −1) and the plus numbers increase (e.g., +1, +2).

Engagement

Engagement occurs when the presenting part (usually the biparietal diameter of the fetal head) reaches the level of the ischial spines of the mother's pelvis (presenting part is at a 0 station or lower). Engagement often occurs before the onset of labor in a woman who has not previously given birth (a nullipara); if the woman has had previous vaginal births (a multipara), engagement may not occur until well after labor begins.

Flexion

The fetal head should be flexed to pass most easily through the pelvis. As labor progresses, uterine contractions increase the amount of fetal head flexion until the fetal chin is on the chest.

Internal Rotation

When the fetus enters the pelvis head first, the head is usually oriented so the occiput is toward the mother's right or left side. As the fetus is pushed downward by contractions, the curved, cylindrical shape of the pelvis causes the fetal head to turn until the occiput is directly under the symphysis pubis (occiput anterior [OA]).

Extension

As the fetal head passes under the mother's symphysis pubis, it must change from flexion to extension so it can properly negotiate the curve. To do this, the fetal neck

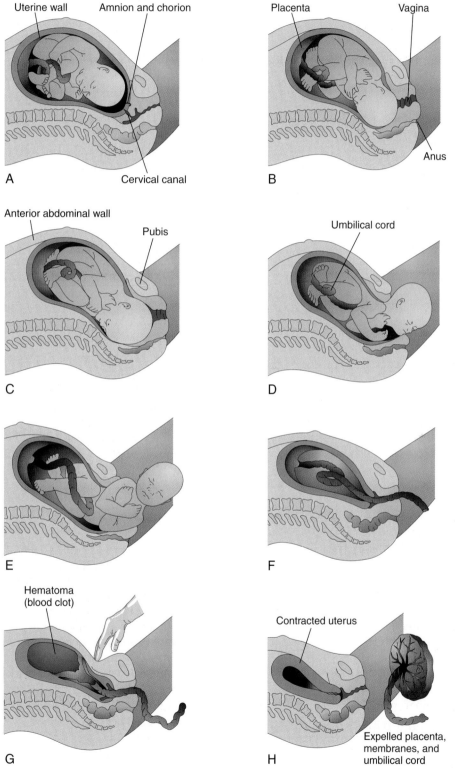

FIGURE 6-9 Mechanisms of labor are also called cardinal movements. The positional changes allow the fetus to fit through the pelvis with the least resistance. **A,** Descent, engagement, and flexion. **B,** Internal rotation. **C,** Beginning extension. **D,** Birth of the head by complete extension. **E,** External rotation, birth of shoulders and body. **F,** Separation of placenta begins. **G,** Complete separation of placenta from uterine wall. **H,** Placenta is expelled and uterus contracts. (From Moore KL, Persaud TVN, Torchia MG: *The developing human: clinically oriented embryology*, ed 9, Philadelphia, 2012, Saunders.)

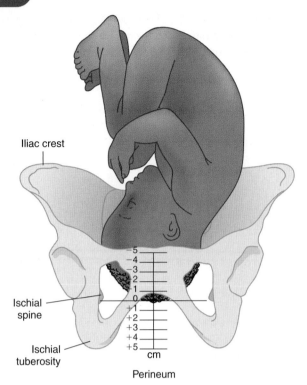

Iliac crest

Ischial spine

Ischial tuberosity

−5
−4
−3
−2
−1
0
+1
+2
+3
+4
+5
cm

Perineum

FIGURE 6-10 Station. The station describes the level of the presenting part in relation to the ischial spines of the mother's pelvis. The "minus" stations are above the ischial spines, and the "plus" stations are below the ischial spines. (From Matteson PS: *Women's health during the childbearing years: a community-based approach*, St Louis, 2001, Mosby.)

stops under the symphysis, which acts as a pivot. The head swings anteriorly as it extends with each maternal push until it is born.

External Rotation
When the head is born in extension, the shoulders are crosswise in the pelvis and the head is somewhat twisted in relation to the shoulders. The head spontaneously turns to one side as it realigns with the shoulders (restitution). The shoulders then rotate within the pelvis until their transverse diameter is aligned with the mother's anteroposterior pelvis. The head turns farther to the side as the shoulders rotate within the pelvis.

Expulsion
The anterior shoulder and then the posterior shoulder are born, quickly followed by the rest of the body.

ADMISSION TO THE HOSPITAL OR BIRTH CENTER

Intrapartum nursing care begins before admission by educating the woman about the appropriate time to come to the facility. Nursing care includes admission assessments and the initiation of necessary procedures. Many women have false labor and are discharged after a short observation period.

WHEN TO GO TO THE HOSPITAL OR BIRTH CENTER

During late pregnancy the woman should be instructed about when to go to the hospital or birth center. There is no *exact* time, but the general guidelines are as follows:

- *Contractions:* The woman should go to the hospital or birth center when the contractions have a pattern of increasing frequency, duration, and intensity. The woman having her first child is usually advised to enter the facility when contractions have been regular (every 5 minutes) for 1 hour. Women having second or later children should go sooner, when regular contractions are 10 minutes apart for a period of 1 hour.
- *Ruptured membranes:* The woman should go to the facility if her membranes rupture or if she thinks they may have ruptured.
- *Bleeding other than bloody show:* Bloody show is a mixture of blood and thick mucus. Active bleeding is free flowing, bright red, and not mixed with thick mucus.
- *Decreased fetal movement:* The woman should be evaluated if the fetus is moving less than usual. Many fetuses become quiet shortly before labor, but decreased fetal activity can also be a sign of fetal compromise or fetal demise (death).
- *Any other concern:* Because these guidelines cannot cover every situation, the woman should contact her health care provider or go to the birth facility for evaluation if she has any other concerns.

ADMISSION DATA COLLECTION

The nurse should observe the appropriate infection control measures when providing care in any clinical area. Water-repellent gowns, eye shields, and gloves are worn in the delivery area, and the newborn infant is handled with gloves until after the first bath. General guidelines for wearing protective clothing in the intrapartal area can be found in Appendix A.

When a woman is admitted, the nurse establishes a therapeutic relationship by welcoming her and her family members. The nurse continues developing the therapeutic relationship during labor by determining the woman's expectations about birth and helping to achieve them. Some women have a written birth plan that they have discussed with their health care provider and the facility personnel. The woman's partner and other family members she wants to be part of her care are included. From the first encounter, the nurse conveys confidence in the woman's ability to cope with labor and give birth to her child.

The three major assessments performed promptly on admission are the following: (1) fetal condition, (2) maternal condition, and (3) impending (nearness to) birth.

Fetal Condition
The fetal heart rate (FHR) is assessed with a fetoscope (stethoscope for listening to fetal heart sounds), a

hand-held Doppler transducer, or an external fetal monitor. When the amniotic membranes are ruptured, the color, amount, and odor of the fluid are assessed, and the FHR is recorded.

Maternal Condition
The temperature, pulse, respirations, and blood pressure are assessed for signs of infection or hypertension.

Impending Birth
The nurse continually observes the woman for behaviors that suggest she is about to give birth, including the following:

- Sitting on one buttock
- Making grunting sounds
- Bearing down with contractions
- Stating "The baby's coming"
- Bulging of the perineum or the fetal presenting part becoming visible at the vaginal opening

If it appears that birth is imminent, the nurse does not leave the woman but summons help or uses the call bell. Gloves should be applied in case the infant is born quickly. Emergency delivery kits (called "precip trays" for "precipitous birth") that contain essential equipment are in all delivery areas. The student should locate this tray early in the clinical experience, because one cannot predict when it will be needed. The nurse's priority is to prevent injury to the mother and infant. The nurse should don gloves and a cover gown and assist with the delivery until help arrives (Skill 6-1).

 Nursing Tip

It is unlikely that a nursing student will be called on to deliver an infant during an unexpected birth, but the process should be reviewed in case this does occur.

Additional Data Collection
If the maternal and fetal conditions are normal, and if birth is not imminent, other data can be gathered in a more leisurely way. Most birth facilities have a pre-printed form to guide admission assessments. Women who have had prenatal care should have a prenatal record on file for retrieval of that information. Examples of the assessment data needed are as follows:

- Basic information should be obtained: the woman's reason for coming to the facility, the name of her health care provider, medical and obstetrical history, allergies, food intake, any recent illness, medication use (including illicit substances), and home environment.
- Woman's plans for birth should be determined.

Assisting with an Emergency Birth

PURPOSE
To prioritize care and to prevent injury to the mother and child

STEPS
1. Obtain an emergency delivery tray ("precip tray").
2. Do not leave the woman if she exhibits any signs of imminent birth, such as grunting, bearing down, perineal bulging, or a statement that the baby is coming. Summon the experienced nurse with the call bell and try to remain calm.
3. Put on gloves and a cover gown. Use of either clean or sterile gloves is acceptable because no invasive procedures will be done. Gloves and a cover gown are used primarily to protect the nurse from exposure to body fluids while supporting the infant during the delivery.
4. Support the infant's head and body as it emerges. Wipe secretions from the infant's face.
5. Feel around the infant's neck for the presence of the umbilical cord (nuchal cord). If the cord is around the infant's neck, it may be long enough to slip over the infant's head or it may be clamped with two clamps and cut.
6. Control delivery of the head to prevent laceration of the perineum, but do not hold the head back.
7. Use a bulb syringe to remove secretions from the mouth and nose; then clamp and cut the cord.
8. Dry the infant quickly and wrap in blankets or place in skin-to-skin contact with the mother to maintain the infant's temperature.
9. Observe the infant's color and respirations. The cry should be vigorous and the color pink (bluish hands and feet are normal).
10. Observe for placental detachment and bleeding. After the placenta detaches, observe for a firm fundus. If the fundus is not firm, massage it. The infant can suckle at the mother's breast to promote the release of oxytocin, which stimulates uterine contraction.
11. Document events as they occurred and include the sex of the infant, the time of birth, and expulsion of the placenta.

- Status of labor should be evaluated. The registered nurse, CNM, or physician does a vaginal examination to determine cervical effacement and dilation as well as fetal presentation, position, and station. Contractions are assessed for frequency, duration, and intensity by palpation and/or with an electronic fetal monitor.
- A woman's general condition should be evaluated by performing a brief physical examination. Any edema, especially of the fingers and face, and any abdominal scars should be further explored. Fundal height is measured (or estimated by an experienced nurse) to determine if it is appropriate for her gestation. Reflexes are checked to identify hyperactivity that may occur with gestational hypertension (GH).

ADMISSION PROCEDURES

Several procedures may be performed when a woman is admitted to a birth facility. Some common procedures are described in the following sections.

PERMISSION AND CONSENT FORMS

The mother signs permission and/or consent forms for her care and the care of her infant during labor, delivery, and the postbirth period. Permission for an emergency cesarean delivery may be included. The health care provider and the nurse must witness all signatures and confirm that proper information was given to the patient.

LABORATORY TESTS

A blood sample for the measurement of hematocrit and a midstream urine specimen for determination of glucose and protein levels are common tests performed on admission. The hematocrit test is often omitted if a woman has had regular prenatal care and a recent evaluation. The woman who did not have prenatal care will have additional tests that may include a complete blood count, urinalysis, a drug screen, tests for sexually transmitted infections, and others as indicated.

INTRAVENOUS INFUSION

An intravenous (IV) line is started to allow for the administration of fluids and drugs. The woman may have a constant fluid infusion, or venous access may be maintained with a saline lock to permit greater patient mobility in early labor.

PERINEAL PREP

Perineal preparation for delivery includes cleansing the perineal area. Removing pubic hair is rarely done, because routine episiotomy is no longer practiced and evidence has shown that it does not prevent infection as it was once believed.

DETERMINING FETAL POSITION AND PRESENTATION

The nurse may assist the health care provider in determining the fetal position and presentation by abdominal

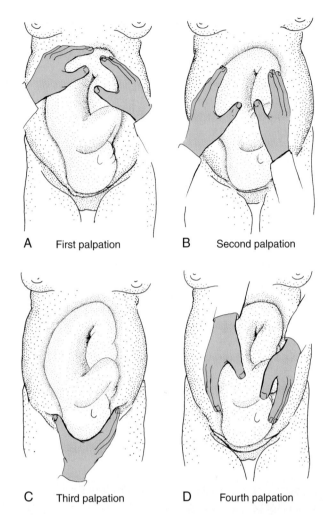

A First palpation

B Second palpation

C Third palpation

D Fourth palpation

FIGURE 6-11 Leopold's maneuver. **A,** Presentation. Hands are placed on either side of the maternal abdomen to palpate the uterine fundus to determine if a round, hard object is felt at the fundus (the fetal head, indicating a breech presentation) or a soft, irregular contour (the fetal buttocks, indicating a vertex presentation). **B,** Position. Hands are placed on either side of the maternal abdomen. Support one side of the abdomen while palpating the other side. Palpating a hard, smooth contour indicates location of the fetal back, whereas feeling soft, irregular objects indicates the small parts or extremities. **C,** Confirm presentation. The suprapubic area is palpated to determine that the vertex or head is presenting. Feeling a hard, round area that does not move may indicate the head is engaged. **D,** Attitude. Attitude of the fetal head is determined by palpating the maternal abdomen with fingers pointing toward the maternal feet. The hand is moved downward toward the symphysis pubis. Feeling a hard, round object on the same side as the fetal back indicates the fetus is in extension. Feeling the hard, round object opposite the fetal back indicates the head is in flexion.

palpations called **Leopold's maneuver** (Figure 6-11). Sometimes performance of this technique at the time of admission shows a previously unidentified multifetal pregnancy. Leopold's maneuver is also helpful in locating the fetal back, which is the best location for hearing the FHR, and thus determining optimal placement of the fetal monitor sensor.

Table 6-2	Comparison of False Labor and True Labor
FALSE LABOR (PRODROMAL LABOR OR PRELABOR)	**TRUE LABOR**
Contractions are irregular or do not increase in frequency, duration, and intensity.	Contractions gradually develop a regular pattern and become more frequent, longer, and more intense.
Walking tends to relieve or decrease contractions.	Contractions become stronger and more effective with walking.
Discomfort is felt in the abdomen and groin.	Discomfort is felt in the lower back and the lower abdomen; often feels like menstrual cramps at first.
Bloody show is usually not present.	Bloody show is often present, especially in women having their first child.
There is no change in effacement or dilation of the cervix.	Progressive effacement and dilation of the cervix occur.

NURSING CARE OF THE WOMAN IN FALSE LABOR

True labor is characterized by changes in the cervix (effacement and dilation), which is the key distinction between true and false labor. Table 6-2 lists other characteristics of true and false labor.

A better term for false labor might be prodromal labor, because these contractions help prepare the woman's body and the fetus for true labor. Many women are observed for a short time (1 to 2 hours) if their initial assessment suggests that they are not in true labor and their membranes are intact. The mother and fetus are assessed during observation as if labor were occurring. Most facilities run an external electronic fetal monitor strip for at least 20 minutes to document fetal well-being. The woman can usually walk about when not being monitored. If she is in true labor, walking often helps to intensify the contractions and bring about cervical effacement and dilation.

After the observation period, the health care provider, who performs another vaginal examination, re-evaluates the woman's labor status. If there is no change in the cervical effacement or dilation, the woman is usually sent home to await true labor. Sometimes, if it is her first child and she lives nearby, the woman in very early labor is sent home because the latent phase of most first labors is quite long (see Table 6-6).

Each woman in false labor (or early latent-phase labor) is evaluated individually. Factors to be considered include the number and the duration of previous labors, distance from the facility, and availability of transportation.

! Safety Alert!

Encourage the woman in false labor to return to the facility when she thinks she should. It is better to have another "trial run" than to wait at home until she is in advanced labor.

If the woman's membranes are ruptured, she is usually admitted even if labor has not begun, because of the risk for infection or a prolapsed umbilical cord (see Chapter 8).

The woman in false labor is often frustrated and needs generous reassurance that her symptoms will eventually change to true labor. No one stays pregnant forever, although it sometimes feels that way to a woman who has had several false alarms and is tired of being pregnant. Guidelines for coming to the facility should be reinforced before she leaves.

NURSING CARE BEFORE BIRTH

After admission to the labor unit, nursing care consists of the following elements:
- Monitoring the fetus
- Monitoring the laboring woman
- Helping the woman cope with labor

MONITORING THE FETUS

Intrapartum care of the fetus includes assessment of FHR patterns and the amniotic fluid. In addition, several observations of the mother's status, such as vital signs and contraction pattern, are closely related to fetal well-being because they influence fetal oxygen supply.

Fetal Heart Rate

The goal of fetal monitoring is to enable early detection of fetal hypoxia, to prevent fetal metabolic acidosis, and to allow prompt interventions that will avoid fetal injury.

The FHR can be assessed by intermittent auscultation, by using a fetoscope or Doppler transducer, or by continuous electronic fetal monitoring. (See Skill 6-2 for the procedure for assessing FHR.) Electronic fetal monitoring is more widely used in the United States, but intermittent auscultation is a valid method of intrapartum fetal assessment when performed according to established intervals and with a 1:1 nurse–patient ratio.

Intermittent Auscultation. Intermittent auscultation allows the mother greater freedom of movement, which is helpful during early labor and is the method used during home births and in most birth centers. However, unlike continuous monitoring, intermittent auscultation does not automatically record the results, so the nurse must provide careful documentation. Intermittent auscultation of the FHR should be performed as noted in Skill 6-2 and Box 6-2. Figure 6-12 shows the approximate locations of the fetal heart sounds according to various presentations and positions of the fetus. **Any FHR outside the normal limits and any slowing of the FHR that persists after the contraction ends is promptly reported to the health care provider.**

Continuous Electronic Fetal Monitoring. Continuous electronic fetal monitoring (EFM) allows the nurse to collect more data about the fetus than intermittent auscultation. FHR and uterine contraction patterns are continuously recorded. Most hospitals use continuous EFM, because the permanent recording becomes part of the mother's chart. Some monitors make use of telemetry (like a cordless telephone) and permit the woman to walk while a transmitter sends the data back to the monitor to be recorded at the nurses' station. In the absence of that capability, intermittent monitoring is a variation that promotes walking during labor. An initial recording of at least 30 minutes is obtained, and then the fetus is remonitored at regular intervals of 30 to 60 minutes (see Skill 6-2).

Determining Fetal Heart Rate

PURPOSE
To assess and document the fetal heart rate (FHR)

STEPS
1. Determine best location for assessing fetal heart rate.
2. Identify where the clearest fetal heart sounds will most likely be found, over the fetal back and usually in the mother's lower abdomen (see Figure 6-12).

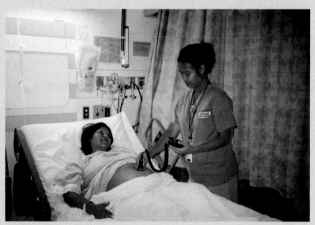

Photo Courtesy Pat Spier, RN-C.

3. Assess fetal heart rate using one of the following methods:

Fetoscope
a. Place the head attachment (if there is one) over your head and the earpieces in your ears.
b. Place the bell in the approximate area of the fetal back and press firmly while listening for the muffled fetal heart sounds. When they are heard, count the rate in 6-second increments for at least 1 minute.
c. Multiply the low and high numbers by 10 to compute the average range of the rate (for example, 130 to 140 beats/min).
d. Assess rate before and after at least one full contraction cycle.

e. Check the mother's pulse rate at the same time if uncertain whether the fetal heart sounds are being heard; the rates and rhythms will be different.

Doppler Transducer
a. Place water-soluble gel on the head of the hand-held transducer.
b. Position the earpieces in your ears, or connect the transducer to a speaker.
c. Turn the switch on and place the transducer head over the approximate area of the fetal back.
d. Count as instructed with fetoscope. If earpieces are used, let the parents hear the fetal heartbeat.

External Fetal Monitor
a. Read the manufacturer's instructions for specific procedures.
b. Connect cable to correct socket on monitor unit.
c. Put water-soluble gel on the transducer and apply as instructed for Doppler transducer.
d. Belts, a wide band of stockinette, or an adhesive ring is used to secure the transducers for external fetal monitoring.
e. The rate is calculated by the monitor and displayed on an electronic panel.
f. The displayed number will change as the machine recalculates the rate.

4. Report the following:
a. Promptly report rates below 110 beats/min or above 160 beats/min for a full-term fetus.
b. Report slowing of the rate that lingers after the end of a contraction.
c. Report a lack of variability in the rate (see Figures 6-13, 6-14, and 6-15).

5. Chart the rate.
The guidelines for a normal FHR at term are as follows:
- Lower limit of 110 beats/min
- Upper limit of 160 beats/min

Box 6-2 When to Auscultate and Document the Fetal Heart Rate

Use these guidelines for charting the fetal heart rate (FHR) when the woman has intermittent auscultation or continuous electronic fetal monitoring.

LOW-RISK WOMEN

Every hour in the latent phase
Every 30 minutes in the active phase
Every 15 minutes in the second stage

HIGH-RISK WOMEN

Every 30 minutes in the latent phase
Every 15 minutes in the active phase
Every 5 minutes in the second stage

ROUTINE AUSCULTATIONS

When the membranes rupture (spontaneously or artificially)
Before and after ambulation
Before and after medication or anesthesia administration or a change in medication
At the time of peak action of analgesic drugs
After a vaginal examination
After the expulsion of enema
After catheterization
If uterine contractions are abnormal or excessive

Modified from ACOG: ACOG guidelines for fetal monitoring: practice bulletin #116, *Obstet Gynecol* 114(1):136-138, 2010.

EFM can be performed with external or internal devices. Internal devices require that the membranes be ruptured and the cervix dilated 1 to 2 cm for device insertion. Internal devices are disposable to reduce transmission of infection. A small spiral electrode applied to the fetal presenting part allows internal FHR monitoring. Two types of devices are used for internal contraction monitoring. One uses a fluid-filled catheter connected to a pressure-sensitive device on the monitor. The other uses a solid catheter with an electronic pressure sensor in its tip.

External fetal heart monitoring is done with a Doppler transducer, which uses sound waves to detect motion of the fetal heart and calculate the rate, just as the hand-held model does. Contractions are sensed externally with a tocotransducer ("toco"), which has a pressure-sensitive button. The toco is positioned over the mother's upper uterus (fundus), about where the nurse would palpate contractions by hand (Skill 6-3).

Evaluating Fetal Heart Rate Patterns. The FHR is recorded on the upper grid of the paper strip and is expressed as beats per minute (beats/min, or bpm); the uterine contraction pattern is recorded on the lower grid. Both grids must be evaluated together for accurate interpretation of FHR patterns. The FHR is evaluated for baseline rate, baseline variability, episodic changes, and periodic changes. Episodic changes are those transient changes in the FHR that are *not* associated with uterine contractions. *Periodic changes* are those transient and brief changes in the FHR that *are* associated with uterine contractions, such as accelerations and decelerations.

- **Baseline fetal heart rate** is the average FHR that occurs for at least 2 minutes during a 10-minute period and are averaged over 30 minutes. It is assessed while there are no uterine contractions. The baseline FHR should be 110 beats/min to 160 beats/min for at least a 2-minute period (ACOG, 2010).
- **Fetal bradycardia** occurs when the FHR is below 110 beats/min for 10 minutes or longer (ACOG, 2010). Causes of fetal bradycardia can be fetal hypoxia, maternal hypoglycemia, maternal hypotension, or prolonged umbilical cord compression. When bradycardia is accompanied by a loss of baseline variability or by late decelerations, immediate intervention is required for a favorable outcome.

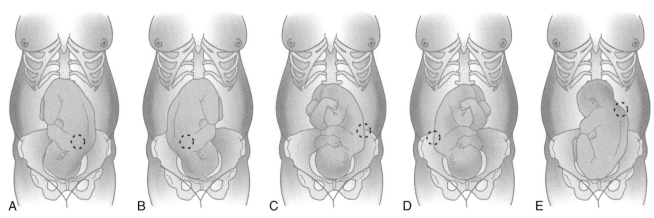

FIGURE 6-12 Determining placement of fetoscope or sensor to assess fetal heart rate (FHR). Approximate the location of the strongest fetal heart sound when the fetus is in various positions and presentations. The fetal heart sounds are heard best in the lower abdomen in a cephalic (vertex) presentation and higher on the abdomen when the fetus is in a breech presentation **(E). A,** LOA; **B,** ROA; **C,** LOP; **D,** ROP; **E,** LSA. (From Matteson PS: *Women's health during the childbearing years: a community-based approach,* St Louis, 2001, Mosby.)

External Electronic Fetal Monitoring

PURPOSE

To monitor the fetal heart rate continuously

STEPS

1. Turn on the fetal monitor device per hospital protocol.
2. Apply and secure the sensors on the mother's abdomen.
   a. Place one sensor over the fundus of the uterus to record uterine contractions.
   b. Place one sensor over the location of the strongest fetal heart sound to record the FHR.

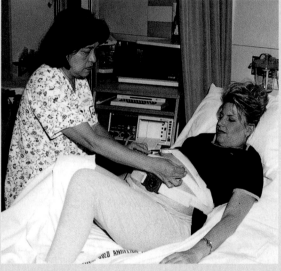

This woman has twins and requires two fetal heart sensors. (Courtesy Loma Linda University Medical Center, Loma Linda, Calif.)

- **Fetal tachycardia** is a baseline FHR greater than 160 beats/min that lasts 2 to 10 minutes or longer (ACOG, 2010). It can be caused by maternal fever or maternal dehydration. When fetal tachycardia occurs along with loss of baseline variability or with late decelerations, immediate intervention is required.
- **Baseline variability** describes fluctuation or constant changes in the baseline fetal heart rate above and below the baseline in a 10-minute window (Figure 6-13). Variability causes a recording of the FHR to have a sawtooth appearance with larger, undulating, wavelike movements. Baseline variability is a reflection of an intact central nervous system and cardiac status of the fetus.
- **Moderate variability**, defined as changes of 6 beats/min to 25 beats/min from the baseline fetal heart

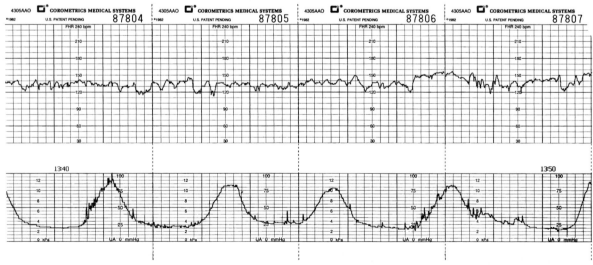

FIGURE 6-13 Recording of the fetal heart rate (FHR) in the upper grid and the uterine contractions in the lower grid. Note the sawtooth appearance of the FHR tracing that is a result of the constant changes in the rate (variability). *Note:* The space between each dark black line on the strip represents 1 minute. The small squares, or the space between each light black line, represents 10 seconds. (Courtesy Corometrics Medical Systems, Wallingford, Conn. Redrawn with permission.)

rate, is desirable, because it indicates good oxygenation of the central nervous system (CNS) and fetal well-being.

- **Marked variability** occurs when there are more than 25 beats of fluctuation over the FHR baseline, and it can indicate cord prolapse or maternal hypotension.
- **Absent variability** is less than 6 beats/min change from baseline for a 10-minute period and is typically caused by uteroplacental insufficiency but can also be caused by maternal hypotension, cord compression, and fetal hypoxia. Nursing interventions for marked or absent variability include positioning the mother on her side, increasing regular IV-fluid flow rate to improve maternal circulation, administering oxygen at 8 to 10 L/min by mask, and notifying the health care provider.
- **Episodic changes** are those changes in the FHR that are *not* associated with uterine contractions. They are brief and quickly return to baseline.
- **Periodic changes** are temporary changes in the baseline rate associated with uterine contractions that quickly return to baseline. Periodic changes include **accelerations** (rate increases) and any of three types of **decelerations** (rate decreases) (Box 6-3).

Accelerations. Accelerations are temporary, abrupt rate increases of at least 15 beats/min above the baseline FHR that last 15 seconds but less than 2 minutes from onset to return to baseline. This pattern suggests a fetus that is well oxygenated and is known as a "reassuring pattern." Accelerations occur with fetal movement and are the basis for interpretation of the non–stress test (NST). An acceleration that lasts 2 to 10 minutes is considered a prolonged acceleration. An acceleration that lasts longer than 10 minutes may be considered a baseline FHR change (Gabbe, 2012).

Early decelerations. Early decelerations are temporary, gradual rate decreases during contractions no more than 40 bpm below baseline; the FHR always returns to the baseline rate by the end of the contraction. The peak of deceleration occurs at the same time as the peak of the contraction. This shows a U-shaped pattern that begins early with the uterine contraction and ends near the end of the uterine contraction. This is caused by compression of the fetal head and is a reassuring sign of fetal well-being.

Variable decelerations. Variable decelerations are abrupt decreases of 15 beats/min below baseline, lasting 15 seconds to 2 minutes. These decreases begin and end abruptly; on the monitor they are V-, W-, or U-shaped (Figure 6-14). They do not always exhibit a consistent pattern in relation to contractions. Variable decelerations suggest that the umbilical cord is being compressed, often because it is around the fetal neck (**nuchal cord**) or because there is inadequate amniotic fluid to cushion the cord. It is not associated with fetal hypoxia but is associated with fetal respiratory acidosis. Variable decelerations are further classified as:

Mild: Deceleration less than 30 seconds and less than 80 bpm below baseline.

Moderate: Deceleration more than 80 bpm below baseline.

Severe: Deceleration more than 70 bpm below baseline for more than 60 seconds.

| Box **6-3** | Reassuring and Nonreassuring Fetal Heart Rate and Uterine Activity Patterns |

REASSURING PATTERNS

Stable fetal heart rate (FHR) with a lower limit of 110 beats/min and an upper limit of 160 beats/min (term fetus)

Moderate variability present

Accelerations: abrupt increase of FHR more than 15 beats/min lasting 30 seconds or less

Uterine contraction frequency greater than every 2 minutes; duration less than 90 seconds; relaxation interval of at least 60 seconds

NONREASSURING PATTERNS

Tachycardia: FHR greater than 160 beats/min for 10 minutes

Bradycardia: FHR rate less than 110 beats/min for 10 minutes

Decreased or absent variability; little fluctuation in rate

Late decelerations: decrease in FHR begins after the contraction starts and persists after the contraction is over

Variable decelerations: if the FHR abruptly falls to less than 60 beats/min, lasting 60 seconds or more, and the return to baseline is prolonged

More than 5 uterine contractions in a 10-minute segment; duration more than 90 seconds, less than 60 seconds relaxation between contractions

---

⚠️ **Safety Alert!**

Report any questionable FHR or contraction pattern to the experienced labor nurse for complete evaluation.

Late decelerations. Late decelerations of the FHR look similar to early decelerations, except that they begin *after* the beginning of the contraction and do not return to the baseline FHR until *after the contraction ends* (Figure 6-15). Late decelerations suggest that the placenta is not delivering enough oxygen to the fetus (**uteroplacental insufficiency**). This is known as a "nonreassuring pattern." Late decelerations under 15 beats/min below baseline are a CNS response to fetal hypoxia. The occurrence of late decelerations greater than 45 beats/min below baseline may be a result of placental aging (postmaturity) or fetal heart depression, and this is an ominous sign. Late decelerations that are accompanied by decreased variability are nonreassuring and require immediate intervention.

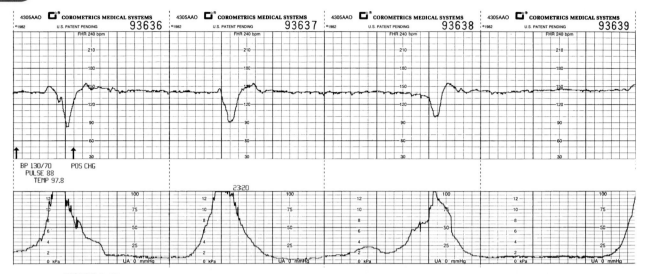

FIGURE 6-14 Variable decelerations, showing their typically abrupt onset and offset. They are caused by umbilical cord compression. The first response to this pattern is to reposition the mother to relieve pressure on the cord. (Courtesy Corometrics Medical Systems, Wallingford, Conn. Redrawn with permission.)

Prolonged decelerations. Prolonged decelerations are abrupt FHR decreases of at least 15 beats/min from baseline that last longer than 2 minutes but less than 10 minutes (ACOG, 2010). The FHR may drop to 90 beats/min during the 2- to 10-minute period. This is caused by cord compression or prolapse, maternal supine hypotension, or regional anesthesia. A prolonged deceleration that lasts longer than 10 minutes may be considered a change in the baseline rate (Gabbe, 2012).

Recurrent decelerations. *Recurrent decelerations* are decelerations that occur in more than 50% of uterine contractions in a 20-minute period.

Intermittent decelerations. *Intermittent decelerations* are decelerations that occur in less than 50% of uterine contractions within a 20-minute period.

Sinusoidal pattern. *Sinusoidal pattern* is a specific FHR pattern that has a smooth, wavelike appearance or undulating pattern that recurs every 3 to 5 minutes and persists for 20 minutes or more. It may be caused by fetal response to medication provided to the mother in labor such as Demerol or Stadol or a fetus who is anemic (Gabbe, 2012).

Nursing Response to Monitor Patterns. The significance of, and therefore the nursing response to, FHR changes depend on the pattern or category identified (Table 6-3). Accelerations and early decelerations are reassuring and thus necessitate no intervention other than continued observation. Repositioning the woman is usually the first response to a pattern of variable decelerations. Changing the mother's position can relieve

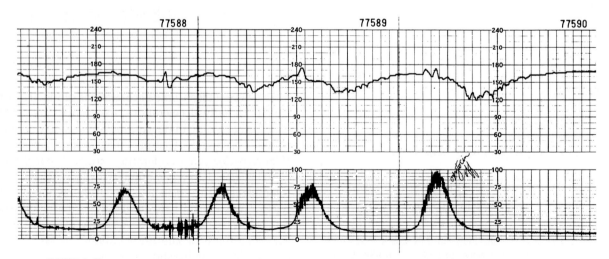

FIGURE 6-15 Late decelerations, showing their pattern of slowing, which persists after the contraction ends. The usual cause is reduced blood flow from the placenta (uteroplacental insufficiency [UPI]). Measures to correct this include repositioning the woman, giving oxygen, increasing nonmedicated intravenous fluid and stopping administration of oxytocin if it is being given, and administering drugs to reduce uterine contractions. (Courtesy Corometrics Medical Systems, Wallingford, Conn. Redrawn with permission.)

Table 6-3	Fetal Heart Rate Categories and Nursing Care	
CATEGORY	**FETAL HEART RATE TRACINGS**	**NURSING RESPONSIBILITIES**
I	Normal baseline rate and variability (no late decelerations)	Provide routine labor care.
II	Variable (other than listed in category I)	Provide close observation and documentation.
III	Abnormal (such as absent baseline variability, recurrent late decelerations, etc.)	Prompt interventions are indicated to have a positive outcome for woman and fetus.

pressure on the umbilical cord and can improve blood flow through it. The woman is turned to her side. Other positions, such as the knee-chest or a slight Trendelenburg (head-down) position may be tried if the side-lying positions do not restore the pattern to a reassuring one. If membranes have ruptured, an **amnioinfusion** technique, in which IV fluid is infused into the amniotic cavity through an intrauterine pressure catheter, may be performed to add a fluid cushion around the cord.

Late decelerations are initially treated by measures to increase maternal oxygenation and blood flow to the placenta. The specific measures depend on the most likely cause of the pattern and may include the following:

- Repositioning to prevent supine hypotension (see Chapter 4)
- Administering oxygen 8 to 10 L/min by face mask to increase the amount in the mother's blood
- Increasing the amount of IV fluid infused to expand the blood volume and make more available for the placenta; this is often needed if regional analgesia or anesthesia causes hypotension
- Stopping oxytocin (Pitocin) infusion because the drug intensifies contractions and reduces placental blood flow
- Preparing to administer tocolytic drugs to decrease uterine contractions

The health care provider is notified of any nonreassuring pattern after initial steps are taken to correct it.

Electronic fetal heart monitoring using "smart technology" is used in the Peri Gen fetal surveillance system that interprets fetal tracings with automatic analysis and documentation in the electronic medical record. It is used to compliment clinical judgment. It can also be used to screen for shoulder dystocia risk (Hamilton, 2012).

Inspection of Amniotic Fluid

The membranes may rupture spontaneously, or the health care provider may rupture them artificially in a procedure called an **amniotomy**. The color, the odor, and the amount of fluid are recorded. The normal color of amniotic fluid is clear, possibly with flecks of white vernix (fetal skin protectant). The amount of amniotic fluid is usually estimated as scant (only a trickle), moderate (about 500 mL), or large (about 1000 mL or more).

Green-stained fluid may indicate the fetus has passed meconium (the first stool) before birth, a situation associated with fetal compromise that can cause respiratory problems at birth. Cloudy or yellow amniotic fluid with an offensive odor may indicate an infection and should be reported immediately.

The FHR should be assessed for at least 1 full minute after the membranes rupture and must be recorded and reported. Marked slowing of the rate or variable decelerations suggests that the fetal umbilical cord may have descended with the fluid gush and is being compressed.

A **nitrazine test** or fern test may be performed if it is not clear whether the mother's membranes have ruptured. Nitrazine paper is a pH paper; alkaline amniotic fluid turns it dark blue-green or dark blue. In the fern test, a sample of amniotic fluid is spread on a microscope slide and allowed to dry. It is then viewed under the microscope; the crystals in the fluid look like tiny fern leaves (Skill 6-4). Commercial high-tech strips are available, such as AmniSure, that involve swabbing vaginal secretions and inserting the swab in a vial to determine the pH of the vaginal fluid.

MONITORING THE WOMAN

Intrapartum care of the woman includes assessing her vital signs, contractions, progress of labor, intake and output, and responses to labor.

Vital Signs

The temperature is checked every 4 hours, or every 2 hours if it is elevated or if the membranes have ruptured (frequency varies among facilities). A temperature of 38° C (100.4° F) or higher should be reported. If the temperature is elevated, the amniotic fluid is assessed for signs of infection. IV antibiotics are usually given to a woman who has a fever because of the risk that the infant will acquire group B streptococcus (GBS) infection. The pulse, blood pressure, and respirations are assessed every hour. Maternal hypotension (particularly if the systolic pressure is below 90 mm Hg) or hypertension (greater than 140/90 mm Hg) can reduce blood flow to the placenta.

Contractions

Contractions can be assessed by palpation and/or by continuous EFM. Some women have sensitive

Testing for the Presence of Amniotic Fluid (Nitrazine Paper Test)

PURPOSE

To determine the presence of amniotic fluid in vaginal secretions

STEPS

1. Place piece of nitrazine paper into fluid from vagina.
2. Read the color on the strip of paper.

   a. A blue-green or deep blue color of the nitrazine paper indicates the fluid is alkaline and most likely amniotic fluid.

   b. A yellow to yellow-green color of the strip paper indicates the fluid is acidic and is most likely urine.

3. Document and report results; offer and provide pericare; remove gloves and wash hands.
4. Document the presence of bloody show, which may alter the accuracy of the results.

---

abdominal skin, especially around the umbilicus. When palpation is used to evaluate contractions, the entire hand is placed lightly on her uterine fundus (Figure 6-16). The nurse should keep the fingers still when palpating contractions. Moving the fingers over the uterus can stimulate contractions and give an inaccurate idea of their true frequency (Skill 6-5 and Table 6-4).

Progress of Labor

The health care provider does a vaginal examination periodically to determine how labor is progressing. The cervix is evaluated for effacement and dilation. The descent of the fetus is determined in relation to the ischial spines (station) (see Figure 6-10). There is no set interval for doing vaginal examinations. The observant nurse watches for physical and behavioral changes associated with progression of labor to reduce the number of vaginal examinations needed. Vaginal examinations are limited to prevent infection, especially if the membranes are ruptured. They are also uncomfortable.

Intake and Output

Women in labor do not usually need strict measurement of intake and output, but the time and approximate amount of each urination are recorded. The woman may not sense a full bladder, so she should be checked every 1 or 2 hours for a bulge above the symphysis pubis. A full bladder is a source of vague discomfort and can impede fetal descent. It often causes discomfort that persists after an epidural block has been initiated.

Policies about oral intake vary among birth facilities. Ice chips are usually allowed to moisten the mouth, unless it is likely that the woman will have a cesarean birth. Many facilities allow Popsicles or hard, sugarless lollipops.

Response to Labor

The nurse assesses the woman's response to labor, including her use of breathing and relaxation techniques, and supports adaptive responses. Nonverbal behaviors that suggest difficulty coping with labor include a tense body posture and thrashing in bed. The health care provider is notified if the woman requests added pain relief, such as epidural analgesia.

⚠ Safety Alert!

Signs that suggest rapid progress of labor are promptly addressed. Bloody show may increase markedly, and the perineum may bulge as the fetal head stretches it. The student nurse or the licensed practical or vocational nurse (LPN/LVN) should summon a registered nurse with the call signal if bloody show or perineal bulging increases or if the woman exhibits behaviors typical of imminent birth (listed earlier in this chapter). Do not leave the woman if birth is imminent! A chart correlating the physiology of the four stages of labor with the related nursing interventions can be used as a guide in planning the care of the woman during labor and delivery (Table 6-5).

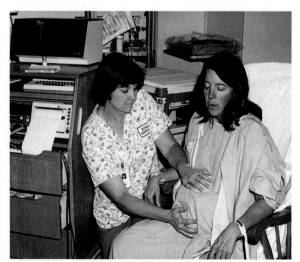

FIGURE 6-16 The nurse helps the mother maintain control and use breathing techniques during active labor. The use of an electronic monitor for fetal heart rate and contractions is *not* a substitute for personal hands-on care during labor. Note that the nurse places the entire hand on the fundus to determine the intensity of the contraction. (Courtesy Loma Linda University Medical Center, Loma Linda, Calif.)

Determining Contractions by Palpation

PURPOSE

To provide intermittent assessment of uterine contractions

STEPS

1. Place the fingertips of one hand lightly on the upper uterus. Keep the fingers relatively still, but move them occasionally so that mild contractions can be felt.
2. Palpate at least three to five contractions for an accurate estimate of their average characteristics.
3. Note the time when each contraction begins and ends.
   a. Calculate the *frequency* by counting the elapsed time from the beginning of one contraction to the beginning of the next.
   b. Calculate the *duration* by determining the number of seconds from the beginning to the end of each contraction.
4. Estimate the *intensity* by trying to indent the uterus at the contraction's peak. If it is easily indented (like the tip of the nose), the contraction is mild; if it is harder to indent (like the chin), it is moderate; if it is nearly impossible to indent (like the forehead), it is firm.
5. Chart the average frequency (in minutes and fractions), duration (in seconds), and intensity.
6. Report contractions more frequent than every 2 minutes or lasting longer than 90 seconds or intervals of relaxation shorter than 60 seconds.

Table 6-4   **Describing Uterine Activity**

UTERINE ACTIVITY	DESCRIPTION
Normal	Five contractions within 10 minutes averaged over a 30-minute period
Tachysystole (increased uterine activity)	More than five contractions within 10 minutes for three consecutive 10-minute periods

Relate the uterine contractions to the occurrence of fetal heart rate (FHR) decelerations or loss of variability and account for frequency, intensity, duration, and relaxation time of the uterine contraction.
Data from Hankins G et al: The 2008 NICHHD workshop report on EFM update of definition, interpretation, and research guidelines, *J Obstet Gynecol* 112(3):661-666, 2008; Gabbe S et al: *Obstetrics: normal and problem pregnancies,* ed 6, St Louis, 2012, Elsevier; ACOG: *Management of intrapartum FHR tracings: practice bulletin #116,* Washington, DC, 2010, American College of Obstetricians and Gynecologists.

HELPING THE WOMAN COPE WITH LABOR

Coping is a dynamic process in which emotions and stress affect and influence each other; coping changes the relationship between the individual and the environment. **Adjustment** is the outcome of coping at a specific point in time. The nurse must understand the physiology of the normal process of labor to recognize abnormalities. The nurse collects, records, and interprets data during labor, such as FHR responses to uterine contractions (see the discussion of electronic fetal monitoring on pp. 131–137), maternal physical responses (e.g., vital signs and duration of contractions), and psychological responses (e.g., anxiety and tension). The nurse also maintains open communication with the health care provider and provides general hygiene and comfort measures for the mother according to the needs presented. In addition to consistent assessment of the fetal and maternal conditions, the nurse helps the woman to cope with labor by comforting, positioning, teaching, and encouraging her (Figure 6-17). Another aspect of intrapartum nursing is care of the woman's partner.

 Nursing Tip

If a laboring woman says her baby is coming, believe her.

Childbirth is a normal and natural process, but today, with modern medicine and technology, few women in the hospital setting give birth without some intervention. These routine interventions include limited oral intake, IV fluids, bed rest, external or internal fetal monitoring, separation of mother and infant immediately after birth, and elective cesarean sections. The Lamaze Institute for normal birth (2007) recommends six basic principles to use as a guide for maternity care whenever possible:

1. Labor should begin on its own.
2. The woman should have freedom of movement.
3. The woman should have a birth support person or doula.
4. No interventions should be performed simply because they are routine.
5. The woman should be in nonsupine positions.
6. The woman should not be separated from the infant.

Table 6-5 Physiologic Changes in Labor and Nursing Interventions

SYSTEM	PHYSIOLOGY	CLINICAL SYMPTOMS	NURSING INTERVENTIONS
Cardiovascular	Uterine contractions release 400 mL of blood into vascular system, causing increase in cardiac output	BP increases by 10 mm Hg; pulse rate slows	Assess BP between contractions Assess level of consciousness
	Ascending vena cava and descending aorta are compressed by weight of uterus	Supine hypotension can occur	Have woman avoid lying on back Encourage left side-lying position
	Holding the breath and forceful pushing increase intrathoracic pressure and reduce venous return and can cause fetal hypoxia	Forceful rather than spontaneous pushing (Valsalva's maneuver) causes redness of face, increase in blood pressure, slowing of pulse rate	Encourage open-glottis pushing and discourage forceful pushing during second stage
	White blood cell (WBC) count increases to 25,000/mm^3	Increase in WBC count is not related to infection	Correct interpretation of laboratory results intrapartum and postpartum is important
	Alterations in the fetal heart rate and rhythm may occur in response to contraction patterns	The normal fetal heart rate is 110-160 beats/min	Monitor the fetal heart rate frequently; time the frequency and duration of contractions
Respiratory	Increased physical activity of labor increases oxygen consumption Anxiety can also increase oxygen consumption	Respiratory rate increases	Encourage relaxation between contractions
	Paced breathing techniques can prevent the development of respiratory alkalosis	Tingling of the hands and feet, dizziness, or numbness may indicate hyperventilation, which can cause respiratory alkalosis	Coach the laboring woman in breathing techniques
Renal (kidneys)	Breakdown in muscle tissue resulting from work of labor can cause proteinuria	Palpate above symphysis pubis to detect full bladder	Encourage voiding every 2 hours; catheterize if bladder is distended and if the woman is unable to void
	Full bladder can be obstructed by full uterus and fetal head	Spontaneous voiding may occur during contractions	Do not confuse spontaneous urination with rupture of bag of waters Nitrazine paper can detect whether fluid discharge is urine or amniotic fluid
Musculoskeletal	Muscle activity increases during labor Increased joint laxity can cause backaches	Observe for diaphoresis, fatigue, increased temperature	Encourage rest between contractions; use comfort measures for diaphoresis and positioning for back and joint pain
Neurological	Euphoria changes to self-centeredness as labor progresses Amnesia during second stage is common, and fatigue and elation occur in third and fourth stages Endorphins produce natural, general sedation, whereas ischemia of perineal tissues by pressure of presenting part causes decrease in perception of perineal pain	Behavior of patient may change during each stage of labor	Provide support and acceptance of behavior; allow sleep whenever possible; provide for safety and privacy

Table 6-5	Physiologic Changes in Labor and Nursing Interventions—cont'd		
SYSTEM	**PHYSIOLOGY**	**CLINICAL SYMPTOMS**	**NURSING INTERVENTIONS**
Gastrointestinal (GI)	Mouth breathing during labor dries the lips and tongue; GI motility is decreased during labor	Dry lips and mouth may be noted Nausea and vomiting of undigested food may occur	Assess for signs of dehydration Use ice chips to moisten lips and/or tongue during active labor Do not allow food or drink during active labor Rectal pressure and urge to defecate may indicate imminent delivery
Endocrine	Estrogen increases and progesterone decreases Metabolism increases during labor; work of labor may decrease glucose levels	Close monitoring of mother with diabetes (including blood glucose levels) during labor is essential	Encourage rest whenever possible between contractions and during fourth stage
Blood	The increased blood volume during pregnancy enables a 500-mL blood loss during delivery without problems unless woman is anemic	Decrease in blood pressure and increase in pulse rate should be reported	Monitor vital signs during labor and delivery
	Increased levels of fibrinogen and other clotting factors during pregnancy prevent hemorrhage during delivery but increase risk for thrombosis	If possible, avoid prolonged use of stirrups to support legs during delivery	
	The increased fetal hemoglobin level enables fetus to carry increased level of oxygen during labor Placental exchange of oxygen and waste occurs between contractions	Contractions that exceed 90 seconds should be reported to the health care provider	Monitor contraction patterns and fetal heart rate closely during labor

BP, Blood pressure.

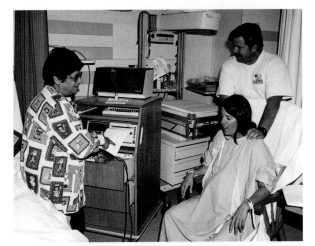

FIGURE 6-17 The nurse explains the external electronic fetal monitor to the woman. The uterine activity sensor is placed on her upper abdomen, over the uterine fundus. The Doppler transducer is placed over her lower abdomen, or wherever the fetal heart rate (FHR) is clearest. The woman and partner are kept informed of progress. (Courtesy Loma Linda University Medical Center, Loma Linda, Calif.)

The nurse should provide continuous labor support in a hands-on, in-person manner rather than rely on monitors viewed from outside the labor room.

Labor Support

The environment of the labor room can be controlled by having the woman listen to familiar music brought from home, which can produce a calming effect. Maintaining an upright position during labor can shorten the first stage (Gabbe, 2012). The recommended positions of comfort for the laboring woman include sitting upright on a rocking chair or birthing ball, which uses the natural force of gravity to promote fetal descent. The "towel-pull" involves the woman pulling on a towel that is secured to the foot of the bed during contractions, which uses the abdominal muscles and aids in expulsion efforts. The lateral Sims position encourages rest and helps prevent pressure on the sacrum.

> **Nursing Tip**
>
> Regular changes of position make the laboring woman more comfortable and promote the normal processes of labor.

Body support can be provided by use of pillows to prevent back strain. This position can also be used to facilitate anterior rotation of the fetus when the woman lies on the side of the fetal spine. The "lunge," in which the mother places her foot on a chair and turns that leg outward, helps the femur press on the ischium to increase pelvic space and facilitates rotation of the fetus that is in occiput posterior (OP) position. The lunge is held for 3 seconds and repeated.

Squatting during a contraction increases the diameter of the pelvis, facilitating fetal rotation and descent (Adams and Bianchi, 2008). In addition to controlling the environment, using nonpharmacological pain relief techniques such as touch, effleurage, massage, back pressure, application of heat or cold, and various relaxation techniques are effective means of labor support. Walking or resting during labor is based on the woman's preference for comfort (Selby, 2012). When IV fluids are administered, 5% dextrose has shown to shorten labor compared to saline (Shrivastava, 2009). Emotional support, encouragement, communication concerning progress, and promoting positive thoughts are also essential.

Teaching

Teaching the laboring woman and her partner is an ongoing task of the intrapartum nurse. Even women who attended prepared childbirth classes often find that the measures they learned are inadequate or need adaptation. Positions or breathing techniques different from those learned in class can be tried. A woman should usually try a change in technique or position for two or three contractions before abandoning it.

Many women are discouraged when their cervix is about 5 cm dilated, because it has taken many hours to reach that point. They think they are only halfway through labor (full dilation is 10 cm); however, a 5-cm dilation signifies that about two thirds of the labor is completed, because the rate of progress increases. Laboring women often need support and reassurance to overcome their discouragement at this point.

The nurse must often help the woman to avoid pushing before her cervix is fully dilated. She can be taught to blow out in short puffs when the urge to push is strong before the cervix is fully dilated. Pushing before full dilation can cause maternal exhaustion and fetal hypoxia, thus slowing progress rather than speeding it.

When the cervix is fully dilated, stage 2 of labor begins, and the nurse teaches or supports effective pushing techniques. If the woman is pushing effectively and the fetus is tolerating labor well, the nurse should not interfere with her efforts. The woman takes a deep breath and exhales at the beginning of a contraction. She then takes another deep breath and pushes with her abdominal muscles while exhaling. Prolonged breath holding while pushing can impair fetal blood circulation (Valsalva's maneuver). The woman should push for about 4 to 6 seconds at a time. If she is in a semisitting position in bed, she should pull back on her knees, with her hands behind her thighs, or use the handholds on the bed.

Providing Encouragement

Encouragement is a powerful tool for intrapartum nursing care, because it helps the woman to summon inner strength and gives her courage to continue. After each vaginal examination, she is told of the progress in cervical change or fetal descent. Liberal praise is given if she successfully uses techniques to cope with labor. Her partner needs encouragement as well, because labor coaching is a demanding job. Some women may use a **doula**, a person whose only job is to support and encourage the woman in the task of giving birth (Figure 6-18).

Laboring down is a term used at the beginning of the second stage of labor when the nurse or doula carefully guides the woman in breathing, pushing, and relaxing through the descent and birth of the infant.

> **⚠ Safety Alert!**
>
> Closed glottis pushing decreases fetal oxygenation and should be avoided (Gabbe, 2012).

The nurse's caring presence cannot be overlooked as a source of support and encouragement for the laboring woman and her partner. Many women feel dependent during labor and are more secure if the nurse is in their room or nearby. Just being present helps, even if no specific care is given, because they see the nurse as the expert.

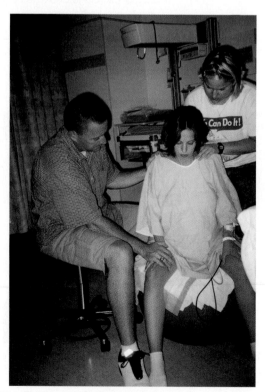

FIGURE 6-18 The doula. The laboring woman sits on a birthing ball as her partner provides encouragement and the doula massages her shoulders. (Courtesy Pat Spier, RN-C.)

Supporting the Partner

Partners, or coaches, vary considerably in the degree of involvement with which they are comfortable. The labor partner is most often the infant's father but may be the woman's mother or friend. Some partners are truly coaches and take a leading role in helping the woman cope with labor (Figure 6-19). Others are willing to assist if they are shown how, but they will not take the initiative. Still other couples are content with the partner's encouragement and support but do not expect him or her to have an active role. The partner should be permitted to provide the type of support comfortable for the couple. The nurse does not take the partner's place but remains available as needed. The partner should be encouraged to take a break and periodically eat a snack or meal. Many partners are reluctant to leave the woman's bedside, but they may faint during the birth if they have not eaten. A chair or stool near the bed allows the partner to sit down as much as possible.

 Patient Teaching

Teaching the Father or Partner What to Expect

The father or partner should be taught the following:
- How labor pains affect the woman's behavior and attitude
- How to adapt responses to the woman's behavior
- What to expect in his or her own emotional responses as the woman becomes introverted or negative
- Effects of epidural analgesia

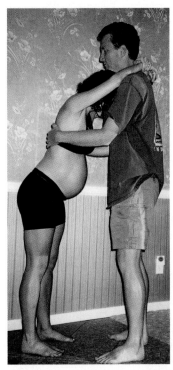

FIGURE 6-19 Standing and walking during early labor and leaning on the partner during contractions use gravity to aid in fetal descent, reduce back pain, and stimulate contractions. Maintaining an upright position can shorten the first stage of labor.

STAGES AND PHASES OF LABOR

Women giving birth display common physical and behavioral characteristics in each of the four stages of labor. Those who receive an epidural analgesic during labor may not exhibit the behaviors and sensations associated with each stage and phase. The nurse must also realize that women are individuals and that each responds to labor in her own way. Table 6-6 summarizes the stages and phases of labor, the related behavioral changes, and the nursing care responsibilities.

 Safety Alert!

If a woman suddenly loses control and becomes irritable, suspect that she has progressed to the transition phase of labor.

VAGINAL BIRTH AFTER CESAREAN

Physicians carefully select women who are appropriate candidates for a **trial of labor after a cesarean section (TOLAC)** and for **vaginal birth after cesarean (VBAC)**. (See p. 181 for more information about cesarean births. The Health Care Provider should discuss the potential risks and benefits of a trial of labor after a cesarean section (TOLAC) and a repeat cesarean section, and documentation of the counseling and plan of care should be included in the medical record.

Nursing care for women who plan to have a VBAC is similar to that for women who have had no cesarean births. The main concern is that the uterine scar will rupture (see p. 182), which can disrupt the placental blood flow and cause hemorrhage. Observation for signs of uterine rupture should be part of the nursing care for all laboring women, regardless of whether they have had a previous cesarean birth.

Women having a VBAC often need more support than other laboring women. They are often anxious about their ability to cope with labor's demands and to deliver vaginally, especially if they have never done so. If their cesarean birth occurred during rather than before labor, they may become anxious when they reach the same point in the current labor. The nurse must provide empathy and support to help the woman cross this psychological barrier. However, the nurse cannot promise the woman that a repeat cesarean birth will not be needed, because one may be required for many reasons. It is essential that an obstetrician and the surgical team be present during all stages of the trial labor after cesarean. Current rates of VBAC have decreased since the year 2000, whereas the rates of cesarean sections have increased (Gabbe, 2012).

NURSING CARE DURING BIRTH

There is no exact time when the woman should be prepared for delivery. In general, the woman having her first child is prepared for delivery when about 3 to

Table 6-6   The Labor Process and the Nurse

CHARACTERISTICS	PATIENT BEHAVIORS	NURSING INTERVENTIONS
First Stage—Dilation and Effacement		
Latent Phase (4-6 Hours)		
Cervix dilation is 1-4 cm.	Cooperative	Establish positive relationships.
Amniotic membranes may be intact.	Alert	Encourage alternating ambulation and rest.
There may be "bloody show."	Talkative	Review breathing and relaxation techniques with
Contractions: q20 minutes decreasing to	Welcomes diversions	coach.
q5 minutes	Urinary frequency	Assess fetal heart rate.
Duration: 15-40 seconds	Thirsty	Time contractions.
Intensity: mild to moderate		Document color of vaginal discharge.
		Assess for distended bladder.
		Provide opportunity to void.
		May provide lollipops for mother to hold and suck on between contractions for carbohydrate and fluid intake.
		Assess vital signs q2 hours.
		Woman may take showers.
		Teach what to expect as labor progresses.
Active Phase (2-6 Hours)		
Cervix dilation is 4-7 cm.	Apprehensive	Help coach implement coping strategies learned in prenatal classes (breathing, relaxation).
Amniotic membranes may rupture.	Anxious	Continue maternal and fetal assessments.
Effacement of cervix occurs.	Introverted	Reassure woman.
Contractions: 2-5 minutes apart	Less social	Praise progress.
Duration: 40-60 seconds	Focused on breathing	Provide back massage.
Intensity: moderate to firm	Perspires	Facilitate position changes (avoid lying flat on back).
	Facial flushing	If taking nothing orally (NPO), moisten mouth.
	Requests pain relief	Maintain communication with health care provider.
	Fears losing control	Monitor intravenous (IV) fluid intake.
	May need epidural analgesia at this time	Watch for bladder distention.
		Encourage voiding.
		Report color, odor, and amount of vaginal discharge; report if meconium is seen.
		Maintain warmth.
		Woman may shower if allowed.
		Provide general comfort measures.
Transition Phase (30 Minutes to 2 Hours)		
Cervix dilation is 7-10 cm; cervix fully effaced.	Irritable	Provide firm coaching of breathing and relaxation techniques, focusing.
Amniotic membranes rupture.	Rejects support person	Support coach.
Contractions: q2-3 minutes	Introverted	Praise and reassure woman.
Duration: 60-90 seconds	Wants to give up	Assess monitor strips of fetal heart rate and contractions.
Intensity: firm	Restless	Assess color of vaginal discharge.
	Tremor of legs	Keep woman informed as to progress with each contraction.
	Fears losing control	Accept negative comments from woman.
	Requests medication	Maintain positive approach.
Second Stage—Expulsion of Fetus (30 Minutes to 2 Hours)		
Cervix dilation is 10 cm.	Bulging perineum	Assist woman to assume position that helps her push.
Contractions: q1½-3 minutes	Mother may pass stool	Assist with open glottis pushing technique and coping strategies.
Duration: 60-80 seconds	Uncontrollable urge to push	Support coach.
Intensity: firm	States "baby is coming"	Maintain communication with health care provider.
Episiotomy may be performed by health care provider.	Exhaustion after each contraction	
Second stage ends with birth of infant.		

Table 6-6   **The Labor Process and the Nurse—cont'd**

CHARACTERISTICS	PATIENT BEHAVIORS	NURSING INTERVENTIONS
Second Stage—Expulsion of Fetus (30 Minutes to 2 Hours)—cont'd		
	Unable to follow directions easily Excitement concerning imminent birth	Monitor contractions and fetal heart rate q5 minutes. Assess perineum and vaginal discharge. Report bulging or crowning. Observe for bladder distention. Prepare sterile supplies for delivery. Prepare infant resuscitation equipment. Provide feedback to woman and partner.
Third Stage—Expulsion of Placenta		
Duration: 5-30 minutes *Contractions:* intermittent *Intensity:* mild to moderate Umbilical cord is cut. Signs of placental separation include the following: • Lengthening of cord • Uterine fundus rises and becomes firm • Fresh blood expelled from vagina Placenta is expelled by Schultze mechanism (shiny fetal side first) or by Duncan's mechanism (dull, rough maternal side first) (see Figure 6-22). Uterus contracts to size of grapefruit. Episiotomy is sutured by health care provider.	Elation Relief Tremors Increased physical energy Curiosity about infant Desire to nurse infant Pain is minimal as placenta is expelled	Observe and document blood loss. Document delivery of placenta. Examine placenta to determine if all of it was expelled (retained placenta causes hemorrhage, because it prevents uterus from contracting). Monitor mother's vital signs q15 minutes. Assess vaginal discharge. Massage uterus until it is firm in midline at or below level of umbilicus. Administer oxytocin to mother as ordered. Obtain cord blood if needed. Note parent–infant interaction. Dry newborn and place in radiant warmer. Attach heart and temperature monitor. Assess and provide immediate newborn care (see p. 150). Perform Apgar evaluation. Apply proper identification to mother, infant, and partner.
Fourth Stage—Recovery		
Uterus remains midline, firmly contracted at or below umbilicus level. Lochia rubra saturates perineal pad (no more than one pad per hour). Cramping may occur. Woman may have shaking chills that may be a thermoregulation response.	A get-acquainted period between woman, partner, and infant Mother breastfeeds infant	Provide proper identification of mother, partner, and newborn. Obtain cord blood if needed. Assess woman's vital signs q15 minutes. Assess maternal voiding. Monitor heart rate and temperature of newborn. Provide warmth to newborn. Assess newborn for anomalies. Assess fundus and massage to maintain firm contraction (a fundus that is displaced to the side indicates a full bladder is pressing against it). Assess lochia (no more than one saturated pad per hour). Change mother's gown and underpads. Encourage breastfeeding. Encourage bonding between parent and infant.

4 cm of the fetal head is visible (**crowning**) at the vaginal opening. The multiparous woman is usually prepared when her cervix is fully dilated but before crowning has occurred. If the woman must be transferred to a delivery room rather than giving birth in a LDR room, she should be moved early enough to avoid a last-minute rush.

If the woman does not have full sensation or movement of the legs because of an epidural anesthetic, padded stirrups may be used, and the woman should be observed closely for excess pressure behind the knees, which can cause thrombophlebitis (blood clot).

A woman can give birth in many different positions. The "traditional" position—semisitting and using foot supports—improves access to her perineum but may not be the most comfortable for her or the best one to expel the infant. She may give birth in a side-lying position, squatting, standing, or in other positions.

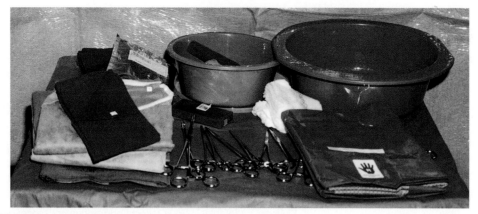

FIGURE 6-20 The table contains the sterile instruments that the health care provider will use for delivery. The table is kept covered with a sterile sheet in the labor, delivery, and recovery (LDR) room until it is ready for use.

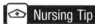
Nursing Tip

Support the woman's partner so that he or she can be the most effective coach possible during labor.

NURSING RESPONSIBILITIES

The registered nurse who cares for the woman during labor usually continues to do so during delivery. Typical delivery responsibilities include the following:

- Preparing the delivery instruments and infant equipment (Figure 6-20)
- Doing the perineal scrub prep (Figure 6-21)
- Administering drugs to the mother or infant
- Providing initial care to the infant, such as suctioning secretions from the airway with a bulb syringe, drying the skin, and placing the infant in a radiant warmer to maintain body heat
- Assessing the infant's Apgar score (Table 6-7)
- Examining the placenta to be sure it is intact and recording if it was expelled via the Schultze or the Duncan mechanism (Figure 6-22)
  - Any abnormalities of the placenta, cord or insertion site should be promptly reported, as they may be correlated with fetal anomalies (Gabbe, 2012).
  - The maternal perineum should be examined for lacerations or bleeding.
- Assessing the infant for obvious abnormalities
- Making a note if the infant has a stool or urinates
- Identifying the mother and infant with like-numbered identification bands (the father or other support person usually receives a band as well; infant footprints and the mother's fingerprints are often obtained)
- Promoting parent–infant bonding and initial breastfeeding by encouraging parents to hold and explore the infant while maintaining the infant's body temperature (observe for eye contact, fingertip or palm touch of the infant, and talking to the infant, all of which are associated with initial bonding; these

observations continue throughout the postpartum period)

Figure 6-23 on pp. 148–149 shows an infant being born in the vertex presentation in a spontaneous vaginal birth.

IMMEDIATE POSTPARTUM PERIOD: THE THIRD AND FOURTH STAGES OF LABOR

The third stage of labor is the expulsion of the placenta. The nurse examines the placenta and monitors the woman's vital signs (see Table 6-6). The fourth stage

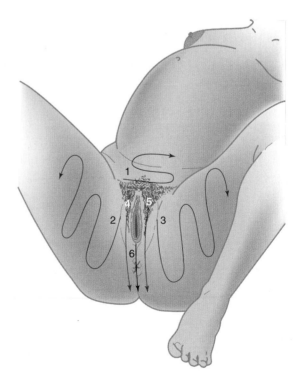

FIGURE 6-21 Perineal scrub preparation is performed just before birth. Numbers and arrows indicate the order and the direction of each stroke. A clean sponge is used for each step. (From Matteson PS: *Women's health during the childbearing years: a community-based approach*, St Louis, 2001, Mosby.)

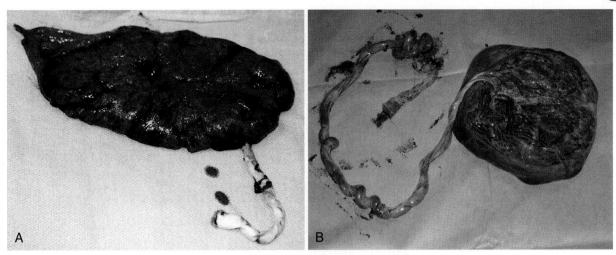

FIGURE 6-22 The placenta after delivery. **A,** Duncan's delivery: The maternal side of the placenta, which is dull and rough, is delivered first. **B,** Schultze delivery: The fetal side of the placenta, which is shiny and smooth, is delivered first. (Courtesy Pat Spier, RN-C.)

of labor is the first 1 to 4 hours after birth of the placenta or until the mother is physiologically stable. Nursing care during the fourth stage of labor includes the following general care:

- Identifying and preventing hemorrhage
- Evaluating and intervening for pain
- Observing bladder function and urine output
- Evaluating recovery from anesthesia
- Providing initial care to the newborn infant
- Promoting bonding and attachment between the infant and family

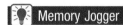 **Memory Jogger**

An easy way to remember placental delivery is **D**uncan: **D**ull; **S**chultze: **S**hiny.

NURSING CARE IMMEDIATELY AFTER BIRTH

CARE OF THE MOTHER

Facility protocols will vary, but a common schedule for assessing the mother during the fourth stage is every 15 minutes for 1 hour, every 30 minutes during the second hour, and hourly until transfer to the postpartum unit. After transfer to the postpartum unit, applicable routine assessments are made every 4 to 8 hours. The following should be included at each assessment during the fourth stage:

- Vital signs (temperature may be taken hourly if normal)
- Skin color
- Location and firmness of the uterine fundus (see Chapter 9)
- Amount and color of lochia (see Chapter 9)
  - Administration of oxytoxin as needed to contract uterus.
- Presence and location of pain

- IV infusion and medications
- Fullness of the bladder or urine output from a catheter
- Condition of the perineum for vaginal birth
- Condition of dressing for cesarean birth or tubal ligation
- Level of sensation and ability to move lower extremities if an epidural or spinal block was used

Observing for Hemorrhage

The uterine fundus is assessed for firmness, height in relation to the umbilicus, and position (midline or deviated to one side). Refer to Chapter 9 for assessment of the fundus. Vaginal bleeding should be dark red (lochia rubra). No more than one pad should be saturated in an hour, and the woman should not pass large clots. A continuous trickle of bright red blood suggests a bleeding laceration. The blood pressure, pulse rate, and respirations are checked to identify a rising pulse rate or falling blood pressure, which suggest shock. An oral temperature is taken and reported if it is 38° C (100.4° F) or higher or if the woman has a higher risk for infection.

Observing for Bladder Distention

The bladder is assessed for distention, which may occur soon after birth. The woman often does not feel the urge to urinate because of the effects of the anesthetic, perineal trauma, and loss of fetal pressure against the bladder. If her bladder is full, the uterus will be higher than expected and often displaced to one side. A full bladder inhibits uterine contraction and can lead to hemorrhage. Catheterization will be needed if the woman cannot urinate.

Promoting Comfort

Many women have a shaking chill after birth yet deny that they are cold. A warm blanket over the woman makes her feel more comfortable until the chill subsides.

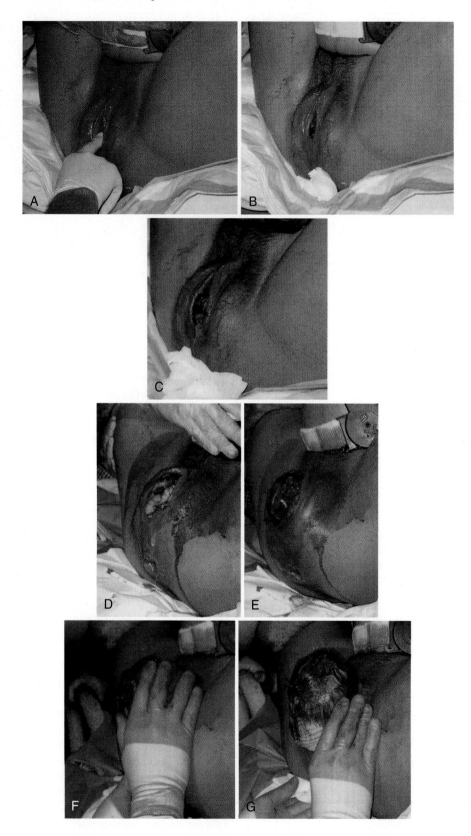

FIGURE 6-23 Vaginal birth of a fetus in vertex presentation. **A,** The health care provider palpates the fontanelle of the fetus to confirm the position of the head. **B,** A portion of the fetal head is visible during a contraction. This is called crowning. **C,** The perineum bulges, and more of the fetal head is visible as the woman bears down. Amniotic fluid drips from the vaginal orifice. **D,** The perineum has been cleansed with an antimicrobial solution as the fetal head begins extension. Head born by extension. Note the distention of the perineum and anus. **E,** The head is about to be delivered by extension. Note the thinning, redness, and distention of the perineal area. An episiotomy may be performed at this stage to enlarge the vaginal opening. Also note the fetal monitor that is in place on the mother's abdomen that allows for continuous monitoring of the fetal heart rate (FHR). **F,** The health care provider supports the perineum as the head emerges. **G,** The health care provider checks for cord around the neck.

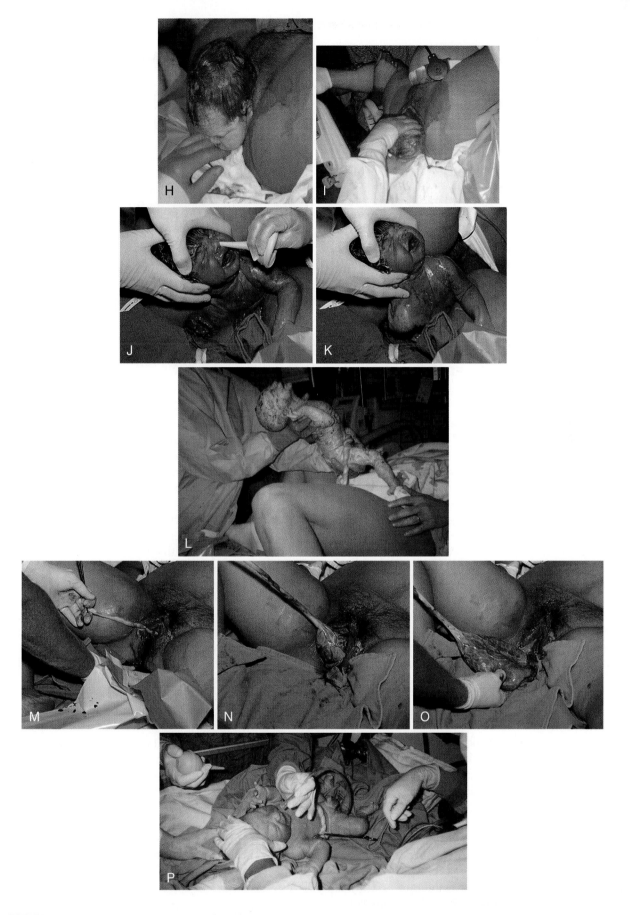

FIGURE 6-23, cont'd H, The perineum is covered as the head is born. **I,** The health care provider exerts gentle pressure on the head to release the anterior shoulder from under the symphysis pubis. **J,** The health care provider uses a bulb syringe to clear the infant's airway. Newborn cries; color is cyanotic. **K,** The posterior shoulder and chest are delivered. **L,** The newborn infant, covered with thick white vernix, is lifted onto the abdomen of the mother, where the cord is cut. **M-O,** Delivery of placenta. **P,** Newborn is placed in the radiant warmer where gentle resuscitative measures, such as bulb syringe suctioning and whiffs of oxygen, are provided. Note that the caregivers are wearing gloves while caring for the unwashed newborn. (**A** to **I** courtesy Pat Spier, RN-C; **J, K, M, N,** and **O** courtesy Michael S. Clement, MD, Mesa, AZ. In Lowdermilk DL, Perry SE, Bobak IM: *Maternity and women's health care,* ed 10, St Louis, 2012, Mosby.)

The warm blanket also maintains the infant's warmth while parents get acquainted.

An ice pack may be placed on the mother's perineum to reduce bruising and edema. A glove can be filled with ice and wrapped in a washcloth. Perineal pads that incorporate a chemical cold pack are often used. These pads do not absorb as much lochia as those without the cold pack, and this must be considered when evaluating the quantity of bleeding. Cold applications are continued for at least 12 hours. A warm pack pad may be used after the first 12 to 24 hours to encourage blood flow to the area.

The infant usually stays with the mother or parents during recovery if there are no complications. The priority care involves promoting respiratory function and maintaining the temperature. (See Chapter 9 for care of the newborn after the fourth stage of labor [phase 2] and Chapter 12 for an in-depth discussion of the normal newborn [phase 3].)

CARE OF THE NEWBORN IMMEDIATELY AFTER DELIVERY

Care of the newborn after delivery is divided into the following "transition phases" that are involved in adapting to extrauterine life:

- *Phase 1:* The immediate care after birth; from birth to 1 hour (usually in delivery room) (discussed in the next section)
- *Phase 2:* From 1 to 3 hours after birth; usually in the transition nursery or postpartum unit (see Chapter 9)
- *Phase 3:* From 2 to 12 hours after birth; usually in the postpartum unit if rooming-in with the mother (see Chapter 12)

Phase 1: Care of the Newborn

Initial care of the newborn includes the following:
- Maintaining thermoregulation
- Maintaining cardiorespiratory function
- Observing for urination and/or passage of meconium
- Identifying the mother, the father or partner, and the newborn
- Performing a brief assessment for major anomalies
- Encouraging bonding and, as the case may be, breastfeeding

The infant will be covered in blood and amniotic fluid at birth. All caregivers should wear gloves when handling the newborn until after the first bath.

Maintaining Thermoregulation. A critical factor in the transition of the newborn is maintaining a **neutral thermal environment** in which heat loss is minimal and oxygen consumption needs are the lowest. *Hypothermia* (low body temperature) can cause hypoglycemia (low blood glucose level), because the infant's body uses glucose to generate heat. *Hypoglycemia* is associated with the development of neurological problems in the

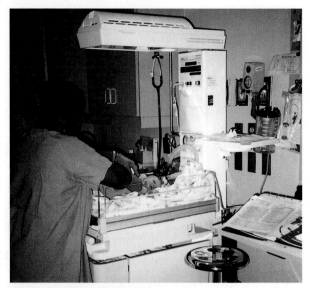

FIGURE 6-24 The nurse applies the sensor and assesses the newborn in the radiant warmer. *Note:* This nurse is wearing purple nitrite (latex-free) gloves when handling the newborn. (Some newborns can be allergic to latex.)

newborn. Hypothermia can also cause **cold stress,** in which the increased metabolic rate required to generate body heat causes increased respiratory rate and oxygen consumption. If the infant cannot supply the increased demand for oxygen, hypoxia will result and cause further problems.

Essential nursing interventions to maintain a neutral thermal environment include the following:
- *Drying the infant* with a towel to prevent heat loss caused by evaporation of amniotic fluid on the skin: the body and head should be gently dried with a warm towel.
- *Placing infant in radiant warmer:* A skin probe can be placed on the right upper abdomen (over the spleen or liver) to act as a thermostat to the radiant warmer so that the proper setting of heat will be supplied (Figure 6-24).
- *Placing a hat on the infant's head* after the head is dried: The head is the largest body surface area in the newborn, and significant heat loss can occur if the moist head is left open to room air.
- *Wrapping the infant* in warm blankets when taken out of the warmer (see Skill 22-1); skin-to-skin (kangaroo) contact between mother and newborn during bonding (see Skill 13-2) or breastfeeding can also prevent heat loss.

An incubator may be necessary if the infant is unable to stabilize body temperature. The first bath is delayed until the infant's temperature is stabilized at 36.5° C to 37° C.

Maintaining Cardiorespiratory Function. Physiological changes in the cardiopulmonary circulation in the newborn are discussed in Chapter 12. Respiratory support immediately after delivery includes the following:

- The face, nose, and mouth are gently wiped to remove mucus and excess amniotic fluid.
- Gentle bulb suctioning of secretions from nose and mouth is performed to clear airways. At birth, the infant may be placed on the mother's abdomen. The health care provider may initiate suctioning before cutting the cord. Further need for suctioning is determined when the infant is placed in the radiant warmer.
- A cord clamp is applied when the infant is stabilized in the radiant warmer (Figure 6-25).

Spontaneous breathing usually begins within a few seconds after birth. The infant's color at birth may be cyanotic (blue) but quickly turns pink (often except for the hands and feet). As the infant cries, the skin color will be pink. **Acrocyanosis** is the bluish color of hands and feet of the newborn that is normal and is caused by sluggish peripheral circulation. Administration of oxygen by facemask may be performed until the infant is crying vigorously.

Some signs of respiratory distress that should be immediately reported include the following:

- Persistent cyanosis (other than the hands and feet)
- Grunting respirations: A noise heard without a stethoscope as the infant exhales
- Flaring of the nostrils
- Retractions: Under the sternum or between the ribs
- Sustained respiratory rate higher than 60 breaths/min
- Sustained heart rate greater than 160 beats/min or less than 110 beats/min

Narcan (naloxone) is kept on hand to reverse narcotic-induced respiratory depression.

Performing Apgar Scoring. Dr. Virginia Apgar devised a system for evaluating the infant's condition and response to resuscitation that was provided at birth (see Table 6-7, p. 152). Five factors are evaluated at 1 minute and 5 minutes after birth and are ranked in order of importance:

1. Heart rate
2. Respiratory effort
3. Muscle tone
4. Reflex response to suction or gentle stimulation on the soles of the feet
5. Skin color

If resuscitative measures are required during the Apgar scoring, a separate chart indicating the interventions and responses are attached to the routine Apgar form (see Table 6-7).

The Apgar score is not a predictor of future intelligence or abilities and disabilities. It was meant to identify only the infant's condition and any response to neonatal resuscitation measures given. Equipment, medications, and personnel must be readily available for resuscitation at any birth, because the need cannot always be anticipated.

Identifying the Infant. Wristbands with preprinted numbers are placed on the mother, the infant, and often the father or other support person in the birthing room as the primary means of identifying the infant. The nurse should check to be sure that all numbers in the set are identical. Other identifying information is completed, such as mother's name, the birth attendant's name, the date and time of birth, the sex of the infant, and usually the mother's hospital identification number. The bands are applied relatively snugly on the infant with only a finger's width of slack, because infants lose weight after birth.

The nurse must check the preprinted wristband numbers to see that they match every time the infant returns to the mother after a separation or the mother goes to the nursery to retrieve her infant. The nurse should either look at the numbers to see that they are identical or have the mother read her own band number while looking at the infant's band.

Footprints of the infant and one or both index fingerprints of the mother are often taken. Many birth facilities take a photograph of the infant in the birthing room or very soon after admission and record birthmarks or unique features. This is primarily for identification of the infant in the event of an abduction and for keepsake purposes.

Observing Urinary Function and Passage of Meconium. Newborns may not urinate for as long as 24 hours after delivery. If the infant voids in the LDR room, it must be documented on the chart. Meconium, the first stool of the newborn, may be passed anytime within 12 to 24 hours. If meconium is passed in the LDR room, it should be documented in the chart. The infant cannot be discharged to the home until documentation is made that the gastrointestinal and genitourinary tracts are functioning. Passing meconium and voiding help determine the status of these systems.

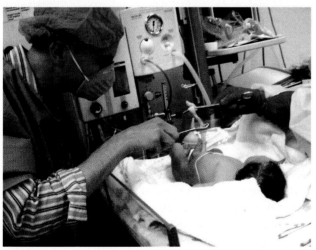

FIGURE 6-25 The nurse assists the father in cutting the umbilical cord to a proper length so the umbilical clamp can be applied.

Table 6-7 Apgar Scoring System

SIGN	0	1	2
Heart rate	Absent	<100 beats/min	≥100 beats/min
Respiratory effort	No spontaneous respirations	Slow; weak cry	Spontaneous, with a strong, lusty cry
Muscle tone	Limp	Minimal flexion of extremities; sluggish movement	Active spontaneous motion; flexed body posture
Reflex irritability	No response to suction or gentle slap on soles	Minimal response (grimace) to stimulation	Prompt response to suction, with cry or active movement with a gentle slap to sole of foot or backrub
Color	Blue or pale	Body pink, extremities blue	Completely pink (light skin) or absence of cyanosis (dark skin)

NOTE: The nurse evaluates each sign in the Apgar and totals the score at 1, 5, 10, and 15 minutes after birth to assess the condition of the infant and to determine what interventions the infant needs. A score of 8 to 10 requires no action other than continued observation and support of the infant's adaptation. A score of 4 to 7 means the infant needs gentle stimulation such as rubbing the back; the possibility of narcotic-induced respiratory depression should also be considered. Scores <3 mean that the infant needs active resuscitation. If resuscitative measures are applied, the following scoring chart is added to the routine Apgar:

MINUTES	1	5	10	15
Oxygen				
PPV/NCPAP				
Endotracheal tube				
Chest compression				
Epinephrine				

NCPAP, nasal continuous positive airway pressure; *PPV*, positive pressure ventilation.

Promoting Maternal–Infant Bonding. Every attempt should be made to facilitate maternal–infant contact. As soon as the infant is dried and warmed, and cardiorespiratory function is stable, the infant should be warmly wrapped and placed in the mother's arms or in skin-to-skin contact with the mother. The infant is alert in the first hour of life, and therefore this is the best time to initiate breastfeeding and bonding. This practice is supported by the awarding of "baby-friendly hospital" designations to those facilities that encourage skin-to-skin contact and breastfeeding immediately after birth in the LDR room (Figure 6-26). Breastfeeding is discussed in Chapter 9. Referral to a nurse who is a lactation specialist may be initiated if the mother needs assistance with breastfeeding.

Eye care. All newborn infants are given specific eye care to prevent **ophthalmia neonatorum**, which is caused by *Neisseria gonorrhoeae*. The American Academy of Pediatrics also recommends protection against *Chlamydia trachomatis*. Therefore, erythromycin eye ointment (administered from single-dose tubes) is placed in each eye (Skill 6-6). Eye care is administered 1 hour after birth (so that the infant and mother can bond in that first hour), but it must be given and documented before the infant leaves the delivery room.

Administering Medications. After the first hour of life the infant begins a sleep pattern with decreased motor activity. This is the best time to place the infant in the warmer for medication administration before leaving the delivery room.

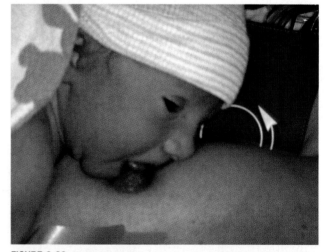

FIGURE 6-26 The naked infant placed on the bare chest of the mother will move toward the breast and breastfeed. Studies show this is beneficial to infant neurodevelopment and behavior and parent–infant bonding. (From Leifer G: *Maternity nursing*, ed 11, St Louis, 2012, Saunders.)

Intramuscular injections: When drawing up medications from a glass ampule, a change of needles is important before injecting the infant, but a change of needles is not necessary if drawing up medication from a vial (Hensel, 2013). The desirable site for an intramuscular injection in an infant is the thickest part of the vastus lateralis muscle in the anteriolateral thigh. Because there are no large vessels in the recommended injection site, aspiration is not necessary (Immunization

Administering Eye Ointment to the Newborn

PURPOSE

To protect against ophthalmia neonatorum and chlamydia infections (all newborns have this prophylactic treatment before leaving the delivery room)

STEPS

1. Apply an antimicrobial ointment to the lower conjunctival sac of the newborn's eyes.

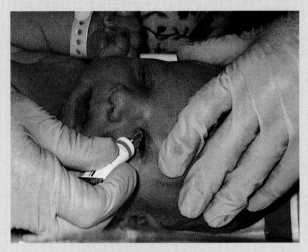

Photo courtesy Pat Spier, RN-C.

Action Coalition, 2010; Crawford, 2012). The medication should be introduced rapidly and the infant held skin to skin, given a sweetened sucrose nipple to suck on, or be breastfed immediately.

Vitamin K (AquaMEPHYTON). Newborns need vitamin K to assist in blood clotting. Vitamin K is naturally produced from intestinal flora, which is absent in the newborn. One single dose of vitamin K is injected into the vastus lateralis muscle (thigh) before the infant leaves the delivery room, usually at age 1 hour (Skill 6-7).

Observing for Major Anomalies. The nurse notes signs of injury or anomalies while performing other assessments and care. The infant's movements and facial expressions during crying are observed for symmetry and equality of movement. The head and face should be assessed for trauma, especially if forceps were used. A small puncture wound is usually apparent on the scalp if an internal spiral electrode was used for fetal monitoring. If the infant was born vaginally in a breech presentation, the buttocks may be bruised.

Many anomalies, such as spina bifida (open lesion over the spine) or a cleft lip (see Chapter 14), are immediately obvious. The fingers and toes should be counted to identify abnormal numbers or webbing. The feet are observed for straightness; if deviated, it should be determined whether they can be returned to the straight position. Length of arms and legs should be checked for equality. Urination or meconium passage is assessed, both of which confirm patency.

A detailed assessment for anomalies and gestational age is completed on admission to the newborn nursery or postpartum unit. See discussion of phases 2 and 3 of newborn care in Chapters 9 and 12.

CORD BLOOD BANKING

Blood from the placenta and umbilical cord has traditionally been treated as a waste product and discarded. Cord blood, like bone marrow, contains regenerative stem cells that can be used for transplant to replace diseased cells or to treat many malignant or genetic diseases in children and adults; these cells are less likely to cause a potentially fatal rejection response. Private cord blood banks have been established in the United States and are accredited by the American Association of Blood Banks.

Families can register and store their infant's cord blood for as long as 15 years for later use. The cost of collection and storage is usually not covered by insurance. Informed consent is essential before collection of cord blood, and privacy of information must be maintained. The cord blood is collected after the healthy infant is delivered and the cord has been clamped and cut. A phlebotomist usually performs collection with appropriate equipment to prevent contamination, and the cord blood bank is notified in advance. The blood must be transported within 48 hours of collection for cryopreservation.

Each unit of cord blood must contain a minimum of 40 mL for use in children and 70 mL for use in adults. In 2004 a bill was introduced in the U.S. Congress to establish a national network of cord blood stem cell banking under the direction of the national Health Resources and Services Administration (HRSA), and in 2008, the

Administering Intramuscular Injections to the Newborn

PURPOSE

To administer an intramuscular injection to the newborn effectively

STEPS

1. Prepare medication for injection.
   a. A 1-mL syringe with a ⅝-inch, 25-gauge needle is often used. A small needle reaches the muscle but potentially prevents striking the bone.
2. Put on gloves to protect against contamination with blood.
3. Locate the correct site. The middle third of the vastus lateralis muscle is the preferred site (see illustration). The middle third of the rectus femoris is an alternate site, but its proximity to major vessels and the sciatic nerve necessitates caution during injection.

4. Cleanse the area with an alcohol wipe.
5. Stabilize leg while grasping tissues (upper thigh) between thumb and fingers to prevent sudden movement by newborn and possible injury. (NOTE: When an injection is administered to the newborn *after* the first bath, the infant should be held in the "hug position" or breastfeeding position and given a sucrose sweetened nipple to suck on (Hensel, 2013).
6. Insert needle at 90-degree angle to the thigh.
7. Do not aspirate and inject rapidly (Hensel 2013).
8. Remove needle quickly and gently massage the site with an alcohol swab. Massage helps medication absorb.
9. Calm, soothe infant; reposition infant. Remove gloves, wash hands, and document in medical record.

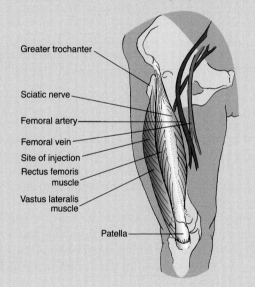

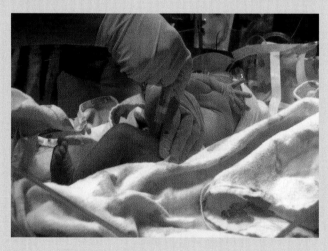

American Congress of Obstetricians and Gynecologists (ACOG) updated the policy recognizing the use of umbilical cord blood as an accepted emerging therapy. It is no longer considered an experimental therapy, as it contains stem cells that make it ideal for use in bone marrow transplants. The data for umbilical cord blood transplantation in children are encouraging, and continued research has demonstrated evidence of success in adults.

EMERGING TECHNOLOGY AND PRACTICES

Fetal blood oximetry was a promising technology but is not endorsed by ACOG and therefore is no longer in use.

STAN Technology is a type of waveform analysis that detects intrapartal changes in fetal ST waveforms

that is indicative of developing fetal metabolic acidosis. It allows for early intervention and possible avoidance of fetal distress and the need for cesarean section (Gabbe, 2012). The technique is being researched by the National Institute of Child Health and Human Development (NICHD) in the United States.

PERICALM-EFM is an FDA-approved computerized "smart technology" interpretation of the real-time FHR patterns that provides automatic analysis of the fetal heart pattern to compliment clinical judgment as well as permanent documentation in the electronic medical record (Saade, 2013).

The use of oral misoprostol solution to replace intravenous oxytoxin to augment labor has been shown to be effective but the safety of outpatient labor induction requires further study (Ho, 2010; Gabbe, 2012).

Unfolding Case Study

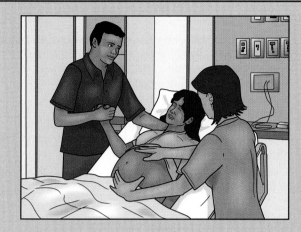

Tess was introduced to the reader in Chapter 4 as a patient in the prenatal clinic and was followed through Chapter 5 where she came to the clinic with specific complaints. The remainder of her pregnancy was without incident.

Tess is admitted to the obstetric unit in her fortieth week of pregnancy, complaining of frequent contractions. She states that a sudden gush of fluid has been expelled into her underwear.

QUESTIONS

1. What is the probable cause of the gush of fluid that she expelled? What is the nursing responsibility when this happens to a woman during pregnancy?
2. What findings would indicate that Tess is close to delivering her infant?
3. The health care provider performs a Leopold's maneuver. What information can be obtained by this procedure?
4. The nurse auscultates the fetal heart. What kind of variations of the FHR are normal, and what findings should immediately be reported to the health care provider?
5. If late decelerations of the fetal heart are noted, what nursing action is indicated?
6. Tess's husband Luis is standing in the corner of the labor room. How can the nurse offer support to Luis during the labor process?

Get Ready for the NCLEX® Examination!

Key Points

- The four components, or "four *P*s," of the birth process are the **p**owers, the **p**assage, the **p**assenger, and the **p**syche. All interrelate during labor either to facilitate or to impede birth.
- True labor and false labor have several differences; however, the conclusive difference is that true labor results in cervical change (effacement and/or dilation).
- The woman should go to the hospital if she is having persistent, regular contractions (every 5 minutes for nulliparas, and every 10 minutes for multiparas); if her membranes rupture; if she has bleeding other than normal bloody show; if fetal movement decreases; or for other concerns not covered by the basic guidelines.
- Three key assessments on admission are fetal condition, maternal condition, and nearness to birth.
- There are four stages of labor, and each stage includes different characteristics. The first stage is the stage of dilation, lasting from labor's onset to full (10 cm) cervical dilation. First-stage labor is subdivided into three phases: latent, active, and transition. Second-stage labor, the stage of expulsion, extends from full cervical dilation until birth of the infant. The third stage, the placental stage, is from the birth of the infant until the placenta is delivered. The fourth stage is the immediate postbirth recovery period and includes the first 1 to 4 hours after placental delivery.
- The main fetal risk during first- and second-stage labor is fetal compromise caused by interruption to the fetal oxygen supply. The main maternal risk during fourth-stage labor is hemorrhage caused by uterine relaxation.
- Nursing care during the first and second stages focuses on observing the fetal and maternal conditions and on assisting the woman to cope with labor.

- Continuous electronic fetal monitoring is most common in hospital births, but intermittent auscultation is a valid method of fetal assessment.
- The normal baseline FHR should be between 110 and 160 beats/min.
- A fetal heart rate tracing demonstrates the relationship between the baseline fetal heart rate and uterine contractions.
- Periodic changes in the FHR are temporary changes from the baseline rate associated with uterine contractions that occur in a pattern over time. The presence of accelerations and moderate variability in the FHR pattern reassures that the fetus is well oxygenated.
- Abnormal FHR patterns must be reported to the health care provider promptly to ensure a favorable outcome.
- Laboring women can assume many positions. Upright positions add gravity to the forces promoting fetal descent. Hands-and-knees or leaning-forward positions promote normal internal rotation of the fetus if "back labor" is a problem (see Chapter 8). Squatting facilitates fetal descent during the second stage. The supine position should be discouraged, because it causes the heavy uterus to compress the mother's main blood vessels, which can reduce fetal oxygen supply.
- The immediate care of the newborn after birth includes maintaining warmth, maintaining cardiorespiratory function, assessing for major anomalies, encouraging parent–infant bonding, and providing proper identification and documentation.

Additional Learning Resources

SG Go to your Study Guide for additional learning activities to help you master this chapter content.

evolve Go to your Evolve website (http://evolve.elsevier.com/Leifer) for the following learning resources:

- Animations
- Answer Guidelines for Critical Thinking Questions
- Answers and Rationales for Review Questions for the NCLEX® Examination
- Glossary with English and Spanish pronunciations
- Interactive Review Questions for the NCLEX® Examination
- Patient Teaching Plans in English and Spanish
- Skills Performance Checklists
- Video clips and more!

 Online Resources
- Coping with labor: www.lamaze.org
- Multilingual facts for prenatal health: www.safemotherhood.org
- Safer childbirth around the world: www.asia-initiative.org

Review Questions for the NCLEX® Examination

1. To determine the frequency of uterine contractions, the nurse should note the time from the:
    1. beginning to end of the same contraction.
    2. end of one contraction to the beginning of the next contraction.
    3. beginning of one contraction to the beginning of the next contraction.
    4. contraction's peak until the contraction begins to relax.

2. Excessive anxiety and fear during labor may result in a(n):
    1. ineffective labor pattern.
    2. abnormal fetal presentation or position.
    3. release of oxytocin from the pituitary gland.
    4. rapid labor and uncontrolled birth.

3. A woman who is pregnant with her first child phones an intrapartum facility and says her "water broke." The nurse should tell her to:
    1. wait until she has contractions every 5 minutes for 1 hour.
    2. take her temperature every 4 hours and come to the facility if it is over 38° C (100.4° F).
    3. come to the facility promptly, but safely.
    4. call an ambulance to bring her to the facility.

4. A laboring woman suddenly begins making grunting sounds and bearing down during a strong contraction. The nurse should initially:
    1. leave the room to find an experienced nurse to assess the woman.
    2. look at her perineum for increased bloody show or perineal bulging.
    3. ask her if she needs pain medication.
    4. tell her that these are common sensations in late labor.

5. A woman in active labor has contractions every 3 minutes lasting 60 seconds, and her uterus relaxes between contractions. The electronic fetal monitor shows the FHR to reach 90 beats/min for periods lasting 20 seconds during a uterine contraction. The appropriate priority nursing action is to:
    1. continue to monitor closely.
    2. administer oxygen by mask at 10 L/min.
    3. notify the health care provider.
    4. prepare for a cesarean section.

Critical Thinking Question

1. A para 0, gravida 1 woman is admitted in active labor. She states she has completed prenatal care and wishes for a natural, unmedicated childbirth. However, she states she now does not feel she can cope with the increasing levels of pain and asks if it is okay if she takes pain medication. What is the best response of the nurse?

Nursing Management of Pain During Labor and Birth

Objectives

1. Define each key term listed.
2. List the common types of classes offered to childbearing families.
3. Describe factors that influence a woman's comfort during labor.
4. Discuss the advantages and limitations of nonpharmacological methods of pain management during labor.
5. Describe the methods of childbirth preparation.
6. Explain nonpharmacological methods of pain management for labor, including the nursing role for each.
7. Discuss the advantages and limitations of pharmacological methods of pain management.
8. Explain each type of pharmacological pain management, including the nursing role for each.

Key Terms

blood patch (p. 169)
Bradley method (p. 161)
cleansing breath (p. 163)
effleurage (ĕf-loo-RĂHZH, p. 162)
endorphins (ĕn-DŌR-fĭnz, p. 160)

focal point (p. 162)
Lamaze method (p. 161)
opioids (Ō-pē-ōydz, p. 165)
pain threshold (p. 159)
pain tolerance (p. 159)

Pregnant women are usually interested in how labor will feel and how they can manage the experience. Preparation for childbirth is important.

EDUCATION FOR CHILDBEARING

Various classes are offered to women during pregnancy by most hospitals and freestanding birth centers to help women adjust to pregnancy, cope with labor, and prepare for life with an infant (Figure 7-1). Women who plan a home birth usually prepare intensely, because they want to avoid medications and other interventions associated with hospital births.

TYPES OF CLASSES AVAILABLE

Classes during pregnancy focus on topics that contribute to good outcomes for the mother and infant (see Health Promotion box). Special classes prepare other family members for the birth and the new infant. Other classes are sometimes available, including:

- Gestational diabetes mellitus classes
- Early pregnancy classes
- Exercise classes for pregnant women
- Infant care classes
- Breastfeeding classes
- Sibling classes
- Grandparent classes
- Adolescent childbirth

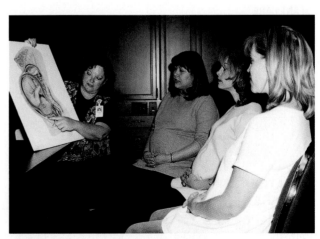

FIGURE 7-1 The nurse teaching this prenatal class discusses the movement of the fetus through the pelvis. (Courtesy Loma Linda University Medical Center, Loma Linda, Calif.)

Health Promotion

Types of Prenatal Classes

CHILDBIRTH PREPARATION
Changes of pregnancy
Fetal development
Prenatal care
Hazardous substances to avoid
Good nutrition for pregnancy
Relieving common pregnancy discomforts
Working during pregnancy and parenthood
Coping with labor and delivery
Care of the infant, such as feeding methods, choosing a
    pediatrician, and selecting clothing and equipment
Early growth and development

EXERCISE
Maintaining the woman's fitness during pregnancy (see Chapter 4)
Postpartum classes for toning and fitness
Positions and environments to avoid

GESTATIONAL DIABETES MELLITUS
Monitoring blood glucose levels
Diet modifications
Need for frequent prenatal visits
Preventing infection and complications

SIBLING
Helping children to prepare realistically for their new brother
    or sister
Helping children to understand that feelings of jealousy and
    anger are normal
Providing tips for parents about helping older children adjust to
    the new baby after birth

GRANDPARENT
Trends in childbirth and parenting styles
Importance of grandparents to a child's development
Reducing conflict between the generations

BREASTFEEDING
Processes of breastfeeding
Feeding techniques
Solving common problems
Some classes with lactation specialists continue after birth

INFANT CARE
Growth, development, and care of the newborn
Needed clothing and equipment
Adolescent classes for birth and parenthood preparation

VAGINAL BIRTH AFTER CESAREAN (VBAC)
What to expect during labor when previous childbirth was by
    cesarean section

VARIATIONS OF BASIC CHILDBIRTH PREPARATION CLASSES

Refresher Classes
Refresher classes consist of one to three sessions to review the material learned during a previous pregnancy. Ways to help siblings adjust to the new baby and a review of infant feeding are often included.

Cesarean Birth Classes
Classes for women who expect a cesarean birth help the woman and her support person to understand the reasons for this method of delivery and anticipate what is likely to occur during and after surgery.

Vaginal Birth after Cesarean Classes
Women in vaginal birth after cesarean (VBAC) classes may need to express unresolved feelings about their previous cesarean birth. Depending on the reason for the cesarean delivery, they may be more anxious about the forthcoming labor.

Adolescent Childbirth Preparation Classes
A pregnant adolescent's needs are different from those of an adult. Adolescents are therefore usually uncomfortable in regular childbirth preparation classes. They are often single mothers and have a more immature perception of birth and child rearing. Some are not old enough to drive or do not have access to a car. They cannot attend classes that target working adults. The content of classes for adolescents is tailored to their special needs. Because acceptance by their peer group is important to adolescents, the girls are a significant source of support for each other. Classes may be held in the school setting. Expectant fathers may be included.

BASIC CONTENT OF ALL CHILDBIRTH PREPARATION CLASSES
Regardless of the specific method taught, most classes are similar in basic content (see the Health Promotion box). Many of the techniques covered can also be used to help the unprepared woman during labor. The woman who learns about the changes produced by pregnancy and childbirth is less likely to respond with fear and tension during labor. Information about cesarean birth is usually included.

Benefits of Exercise
Conditioning exercises such as the pelvic rock, tailor sitting, and shoulder circling prepare the woman's muscles for the demands of birth (see Chapter 4). These exercises also relieve the back discomfort common during late pregnancy.

Pain Control Methods for Labor
The woman and her partner learn a variety of techniques that may be used during labor as needed (Figure 7-2). These are some examples:
- Skin stimulation, such as effleurage (Figure 7-3)
- Diversion and distraction
- Breathing techniques

These techniques are most effective if learned before labor begins. See Box 7-1 for selected nonpharmacological pain-relief techniques.

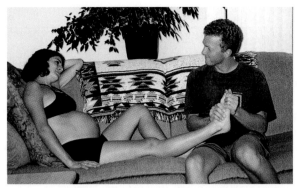

FIGURE 7-2 The partner massages the foot of the pregnant woman. Massage can provide an effective technique for pain relief during labor (see also Chapter 34).

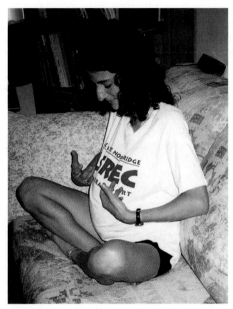

FIGURE 7-3 Effleurage. This woman is practicing effleurage, stroking the abdomen with the fingertips in a circular motion. This technique stimulates large-diameter nerve fibers, thus interfering with pain transmission. Fingertip pressure should be firm enough to prevent creating a tickling sensation.

CHILDBIRTH AND PAIN

Pain is an unpleasant and distressing symptom that is personal and subjective. No one can feel another's pain, but empathic nursing care helps to alleviate pain and helps the woman cope with it.

HOW CHILDBIRTH PAIN DIFFERS FROM OTHER PAIN

Several factors distinguish childbirth pain from other types of pain:
- It is part of a normal birth process.
- The woman has several months to prepare for pain management.
- It is self limiting and rapidly declines after birth.

Pain is usually a symptom of injury or illness, yet pain during labor is an almost universal part of the normal process of birth. Although excessive pain is detrimental to the labor process, pain also can be beneficial.

It may cause a woman to feel vulnerable and seek shelter and help from others. Pain often motivates her to assume different body positions, which can facilitate the normal descent of the fetus. Birth pain lasts for hours, as opposed to days or weeks. Labor ends with the birth of an infant, followed by a rapid and nearly total cessation of pain.

FACTORS THAT INFLUENCE LABOR PAIN

Several factors lead to pain during labor and influence the amount of pain a woman experiences. Other factors influence a woman's response to labor pain and her ability to tolerate it.

Pain Threshold and Pain Tolerance

Two terms are often used interchangeably to describe pain, although they have different meanings. **Pain threshold**, also called pain perception, is the least amount of sensation that a person perceives as painful. Pain threshold is fairly constant, and it varies little under different conditions. **Pain tolerance** is the amount of pain one is willing to endure. Unlike the pain threshold, one's pain tolerance can change under different conditions. A primary nursing responsibility is to modify as many factors as possible so that the woman can tolerate the pain of labor.

Sources of Pain During Labor

The following physical factors contribute to pain during labor:
- Dilation and stretching of the cervix
- Reduced uterine blood supply during contractions (ischemia)
- Pressure of the fetus on pelvic structures
- Stretching of the vagina and perineum

Physical Factors That Modify Pain

Several physical factors influence the amount of pain a woman feels or is willing to tolerate during labor.

Central Nervous System Factors

Gate control theory. The gate control theory explains how pain impulses reach the brain for interpretation. It supports several nonpharmacological methods of pain control. According to this theory, pain is transmitted through small-diameter nerve fibers. However, the stimulation of large-diameter nerve fibers temporarily interferes with the conduction of impulses through small-diameter fibers. Techniques to stimulate large-diameter fibers and "close the gate" to painful impulses include massage, palm and fingertip pressure, and heat and cold applications.

> **Nursing Tip**
>
> Stroking or massage, palm or foot rubbing, pressure, or gripping a cool bed rail stimulate nerve fibers that interfere with the transmission of pain impulses to the brain.

Box 7-1 **Selected Nonpharmacological Pain-Relief Measures**

PROGRESSIVE RELAXATION
The woman contracts and then consciously releases different muscle groups.
Technique helps the woman to distinguish tense muscles from relaxed ones.
The woman can assess and then release muscle tension throughout her body.
Technique is most effective if practiced before labor.

NEUROMUSCULAR DISSOCIATION (DIFFERENTIAL RELAXATION)
The woman contracts one group of muscles strongly and consciously relaxes all others.
The coach checks for unrecognized tension in muscle groups other than the one contracted.
This prepares the woman to relax the rest of her body while the uterus is contracting.
Technique is most effective if practiced before labor.

TOUCH RELAXATION
The woman contracts a muscle group and then relaxes it when her partner strokes or massages it.
The woman learns to respond to touch with relaxation.
Technique is most effective if practiced before labor.

RELAXATION AGAINST PAIN
The woman's partner exerts pressure against a tendon or large muscle of the arm or leg, gradually increasing pressure and then gradually decreasing pressure to simulate the gradual increase, the peak, and the decrease in contraction strength.
The woman consciously relaxes despite this deliberate discomfort.
This gives the woman practice in relaxation against pain.
Technique is most effective if practiced before labor.

EFFLEURAGE
The abdomen or other areas are massaged during contractions (see Figure 7-3).
Massage interferes with transmission of pain impulses, but prolonged continuous use reduces the effectiveness. Therefore the pattern or area massaged should be changed when it becomes less effective.
Massaging in a specific pattern (such as circles or a figure eight) also provides distraction.

OTHER MASSAGE
Massage of the feet, hands, or shoulders often helps relaxation (see Figure 7-2).
Habituation may occur in any type of massage. Change the area massaged if it occurs.

SACRAL PRESSURE
Technique helps to reduce the pain of back labor.
Obtain the woman's input about the best position. Moving the pressure point a fraction of an inch or changing the amount of pressure may significantly improve effectiveness.
Tennis balls in a sock, a warmed plastic container of intravenous solution, or other means may also be used to apply pressure (see Figure 7-4).

THERMAL STIMULATION
Technique is used to stimulate temperature receptors that interfere with pain transmission.
Either heat or cold applications may be beneficial. Examples are cool cloths to the face and ice in a glove to the lower back.

POSITIONING
Any position except the supine position is acceptable if there is no other indication for a specific position.
Upright positions favor fetal descent.
Hands-and-knees positions help to reduce the pain of back labor.
Change positions about every 30 to 60 minutes to relieve pressure and muscle fatigue.

DIVERSION AND DISTRACTION
Technique increases mental concentration on something besides the pain. It may take many forms:
Focal point: Concentrating on a specific object or other point.
Imagery: Creating an imaginary mental picture of a pleasant environment or visualizing the cervix opening and the infant descending.
Music: Serves as a distraction or provides "white noise" to obscure environmental sounds.

HYDROTHERAPY
Water delivered by shower, tub, or whirlpool relieves tired muscles and relaxes the woman.
Nipple stimulation by shower can increase contraction, because it stimulates the pituitary to release oxytocin.

Endorphins. **Endorphins** are natural body substances similar to morphine. Endorphin levels increase during pregnancy and reach a peak during labor. Endorphins may explain why women in labor often need smaller doses of an analgesic or anesthetic than might be expected during a similarly painful experience.

◈ Nursing Tip

Laboring women often tolerate more pain than usual because they have high levels of endorphins and because they are concerned about the infant's well-being.

Maternal Condition
Cervical Readiness. The mother's cervix normally undergoes prelabor changes that facilitate effacement and dilation in labor (see Chapter 6). If her cervix does

not make these changes (ripening), more contractions are needed to cause effacement and dilation.

Pelvis. The size and shape of the pelvis significantly influences how readily the fetus can descend through it. Pelvic abnormalities can result in a longer labor and greater maternal fatigue. In addition, the fetus may remain in an abnormal presentation or position, which interferes with the mechanisms of labor.

Labor Intensity. The woman who has a short, intense labor often experiences more pain than the woman whose birth process is more gradual. Contractions are intense and frequent, and their onset may be sudden. The cervix, vagina, and perineum stretch more abruptly than during a gentler labor. Contractions come so fast that the woman cannot recover from one before another begins. In addition, a rapid labor limits the woman's choices for pharmacological pain control.

Fatigue. Fatigue reduces pain tolerance and a woman's ability to use coping skills. Many women are tired when labor begins, because sleep during late pregnancy is difficult. The active fetus, frequent urination, and shortness of breath when lying down all interrupt sleep.

Fetal Presentation and Position

Various fetal positions and presentations are described in Chapter 6.

The fetal presenting part acts as a wedge to efface and dilate the cervix as each contraction pushes it downward. The fetal head is a smooth, rounded wedge that most effectively causes effacement and dilation of the round cervix. The fetus in an abnormal presentation or position applies uneven pressure to the cervix, resulting in less effective effacement and dilation and thus prolonging the labor and delivery process.

The fetus usually turns during early labor so that the occiput is in the front left or right quadrant of the mother's pelvis (occiput anterior positions) (see Figures 6-7 and 6-8). If the fetal occiput is in a posterior pelvic quadrant, each contraction pushes it against the mother's sacrum, resulting in persistent and poorly relieved back pain (back labor). Labor is often longer with this fetal position.

Interventions of Caregivers

Although they are intended to promote maternal and fetal safety, several common interventions may add to pain during labor. These are some examples:
- Intravenous lines
- Continuous fetal monitoring, especially if it hampers mobility
- Amniotomy (artificial rupture of the membranes)
- Vaginal examinations or other interruptions

Psychosocial Factors That Modify Pain

Several psychosocial variables alter the pain a woman experiences during labor. Many of these variables interrelate with one another and with physical factors.

Culture influences how a woman feels about pregnancy and birth and how she reacts to pain during childbirth. See Table 6-1 for selected traditional cultural practices during labor and delivery.

NONPHARMACOLOGICAL CHILDBIRTH PREPARATION AND PAIN MANAGEMENT

Nonpharmacological pain control methods are important, even if the woman receives medication or an anesthetic. Most pharmacological methods cannot be instituted until labor is well established, because these methods tend to slow the progress of labor. Nonpharmacological methods help the woman to cope with labor before it has advanced far enough for her to be given medication. In addition, most medications for labor do not eliminate pain, and the woman will need nonpharmacological methods to manage the discomfort that remains. Nonpharmacological methods are usually the only realistic option if the woman comes to the hospital in advanced labor.

Advantages

There are several advantages to nonpharmacological methods if pain control is adequate. Poorly relieved pain increases fear and anxiety, thus diverting blood flow from the uterus and impairing the normal labor process. It also reduces the pleasure of this extraordinary experience. Nonpharmacological methods do not harm the mother or fetus. They do not slow labor if they provide adequate pain control. They carry no risk for allergy or adverse drug effects.

Limitations

For best results, nonpharmacological measures should be rehearsed before labor begins. They can be taught to the unprepared woman, preferably during early labor, when she is anxious enough to be interested yet comfortable enough to learn. The nurse may help the woman use several key techniques of nonpharmacological pain control during labor. If the woman and her partner attended childbirth preparation classes, the nurse builds on their knowledge during labor (see Box 7-1).

Childbirth Preparation Methods

Most childbirth preparation classes are based on one of several methods. The basic method is often modified to meet the specific needs of the women who attend.

Dick-Read Method. Grantly Dick-Read was an English physician who introduced the concept of a fear-tension-pain cycle during labor. He believed that fear of childbirth contributed to tension, which resulted in pain. His methods include education and relaxation techniques to interrupt the cycle.

Bradley Method. The **Bradley method** was originally called "husband-coached childbirth" and was the first to include the father as an integral part of labor. It emphasizes slow abdominal breathing and relaxation techniques.

Lamaze Method. The **Lamaze method**, also called the psychoprophylactic method, is the basis of most childbirth preparation classes in the United States. It uses mental techniques that condition the woman to respond to contractions with relaxation rather than tension. Other mental and breathing techniques occupy her mind and limit the brain's ability to interpret labor sensations as painful. The Lamaze breathing technique should be no slower than half of the woman's baseline respiratory rate and no faster than twice the baseline rate.

Nonpharmacological Techniques

Relaxation Techniques. The ability to release tension is a vital part of the expectant mother's "tool kit." Relaxation techniques require concentration, thus occupying the mind while reducing muscle tension. Promoting relaxation is basic to all other methods of pain management and birth preparation, both nonpharmacological and pharmacological. The nurse should adjust the woman's environment and help her with general comfort measures as discussed in Chapter 6. For example, water in a tub or shower helps to refresh her and promotes relaxation. Validating the woman's discomfort and providing support is an essential nursing intervention during all stages of labor.

To reduce anxiety and fear, the woman is oriented to the labor area, any procedures that are done, and what is happening in her body during the normal process of birth. A partnership style of nurse-patient–labor partner is usual in maternity settings.

Looking for signs of muscle tension and teaching her partner to look for these signs help the woman who is not aware of becoming tense. She can change position or guide her partner to massage the area where muscle tension is noted. The laboring woman is guided to release the tension specifically, one muscle group at a time, by saying, for example, "Let your arm relax; let the tension out of your neck...your shoulders..." Specific instructions are repeated until she relaxes each body part.

The woman should change methods at intervals, because constant use of a single technique reduces its effectiveness (habituation).

Skin Stimulation. Several variations of massage are often used during labor. Most can be taught to the woman and partner who did not attend childbirth preparation classes.

Effleurage. Effleurage is a technique that stimulates the large-diameter nerve fibers that inhibit painful stimuli traveling through the small-diameter fibers. The woman strokes her abdomen in a circular movement during contractions (Figure 7-3 and Chapter 34). If fetal monitor belts are on her abdomen, she can massage between them or on her thigh, or she can trace circles or a figure eight on the bed. She can use one hand when she is on her side.

Sacral pressure. Firm pressure against the lower back helps relieve some of the pain of back labor. The woman should tell her partner where to apply the pressure and how much pressure is helpful (Figure 7-4).

Thermal stimulation. Heat can be applied with a warm blanket or a glove filled with warm water. Warmth can also be applied in the form of a shower if there is no contraindication to doing so. Most women appreciate a cool cloth on the face. Two or three moistened washcloths are kept at hand and changed as they become warm.

Positioning. Frequent changing of position relieves muscle fatigue and strain. In addition, position changes can promote the normal mechanisms of labor.

Diversion and Distraction. Several methods may be used to stimulate the woman's brain, thus limiting her ability to perceive sensations as painful. All these methods direct her mind away from the pain.

Focal point. The woman fixes her eyes on a picture, an object, or simply a particular spot in the room. Some women prefer to close their eyes during contractions and focus on an internal **focal point**.

Imagery. The woman learns to create a tranquil mental environment by imagining that she is in a place of relaxation and peace. Preferred mental scenes often involve warmth and sunlight, although some women imagine themselves in a cool environment. During labor, the woman can imagine her cervix opening and allowing the infant to come out, as a flower opens from bud to full bloom. The nurse can help to create a tranquil mental image, even in the unprepared woman (see Chapter 34).

Music. Favorite music or relaxation recordings divert the woman's attention from pain. The sounds of rainfall, wind, or the ocean contribute to relaxation and block disturbing sounds; the woman can also listen to her favorite types of music on an MP3 player or iPod.

Television. Women often enjoy the diversion of television, especially during early labor. The woman may not watch the program, but it provides background noise that reduces intrusive sounds. Some labor rooms have DVD players, and the woman can bring movies to watch during labor or bring an iPad for activities.

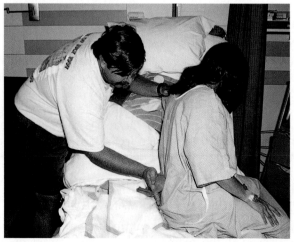

FIGURE 7-4 Sacral pressure. The partner applies firm pressure on the lower back of the woman in labor. Using a tennis ball enhances the effect (see also Chapter 34). (Courtesy Loma Linda University Medical Center, Loma Linda, Calif.)

Breathing. Like other techniques, breathing techniques are most effective if practiced before labor. The woman should not use them until she needs them, generally when she can no longer walk or talk through a contraction. She may become tired if she uses them too early or if she moves to a more advanced technique sooner than she must. If the woman has not had childbirth preparation classes, each technique is taught as she needs it.

Each breathing pattern begins and ends with a **cleansing breath**, which is a deep inspiration and expiration, similar to a deep sigh. The cleansing breaths help the woman to relax and focus on relaxing.

First-stage breathing

Slow-paced breathing. The woman begins with a technique of slow-paced breathing. She starts the pattern with a cleansing breath, then breathes slowly, as during sleep (Figure 7-5, *A*). A cleansing breath ends the contraction. An exact rate is not important, but about six to nine breaths a minute is average. The rate should be at least half her usual rate to ensure adequate fetal oxygenation and prevent hyperventilation.

Modified-paced breathing. This pattern begins and ends with a cleansing breath. During the contraction, the woman breathes more rapidly and shallowly (see Figure 7-5, *B* and *C*). The rate should be no more than twice her usual rate. She may combine slow-paced with modified-paced breathing. In this variation, she begins with a cleansing breath and breathes slowly until the peak of the contraction, when she begins rapid, shallow breathing. As the contraction abates, she resumes slow, deep breathing and ends with a cleansing breath. Hyperventilation is sometimes a problem when the woman is breathing rapidly. She may complain of dizziness, tingling, and numbness around her mouth and may have spasms of her fingers and feet. Box 7-2 lists measures to combat hyperventilation.

Patterned-paced breathing. The technique of patterned-paced breathing is more difficult to teach the unprepared laboring woman, because it requires her to focus on the pattern of her breathing. It begins with a cleansing breath, which is followed by rapid breaths punctuated with an intermittent slight blow (see Figure 7-5, *D*), often called pant-blow, or "hee hoo" breathing. The woman may maintain a constant number of breaths before the blow or may vary the number in a specific pattern, as follows:

- *Constant pattern:* Pant-pant-pant-blow, pant-pant-pant-blow, and so on.
- *Stairstep pattern:* Pant-blow, pant-pant-blow, pant-pant-pant-blow, pant-pant-pant-pant-blow

In another variation, her partner calls out random numbers to indicate the number of pants to take before a blow. If she feels an urge to push before her cervix is fully dilated, the woman is taught to blow in short breaths to avoid bearing down. Blowing out or panting prevents closure of the glottis and the breath-holding urges that often accompany spontaneous pushing. Pushing before full cervical dilation may cause cervical

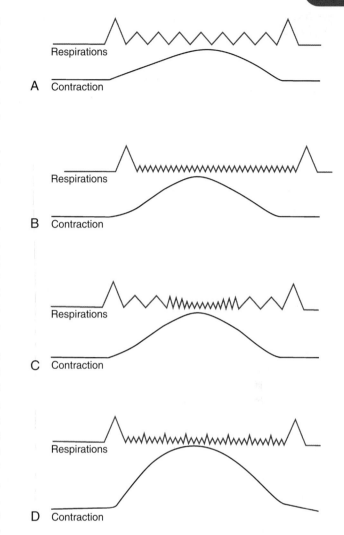

FIGURE 7-5 Breathing patterns. **A,** *Slow-paced breathing.* The pattern starts with a cleansing breath as the contraction begins. The woman breathes slowly, at about half her usual rate, and ends with a second cleansing breath at the end of the contraction. **B,** As labor intensifies, the woman may need to use *modified-paced breathing.* The pattern begins and ends with a cleansing breath. After the opening cleansing breath, the woman breathes rapidly during the contraction, no faster than twice her usual respiratory rate, and makes the closing cleansing breath as the contraction subsides. **C,** In this variation of modified-paced breathing, the woman begins with slow-paced breathing at the beginning of the contraction, switching to faster breathing during its peak. A cleansing breath also begins and ends this pattern. **D,** *Patterned-paced breathing* begins and ends with a cleansing breath. During the contraction the woman emphasizes the exhalation of some breaths. She may use a specific pattern or may randomly emphasize the blow.

edema or lacerations, especially with a woman's first child, because the cervix is not as stretchable as it is after one or more births.

Second-stage breathing. When it is time for the woman to push, the woman takes a cleansing breath, then takes another deep breath and pushes down while exhaling to a count of 10. She blows out, takes a deep breath, and pushes again while exhaling (open glottis pushing).

Box **7-2**	How to Recognize and Correct Hyperventilation

SIGNS AND SYMPTOMS
Dizziness
Tingling of hands and feet
Cramps and muscle spasms of hands
Numbness around nose and mouth
Blurring of vision

CORRECTIVE MEASURES
Breathe slowly, especially in exhalation
Breathe into cupped hands
Place a moist washcloth over the mouth and nose while
   breathing
Hold breath for a few seconds before exhaling

 Nursing Tip

If a woman is successfully using a safe, nonpharmacological pain control technique, do not interfere.

The Nurse's Role in Nonpharmacological Techniques.

When a woman is admitted, the nurse determines whether she had childbirth preparation classes, and the nurse works with what the woman and her partner learned. The nurse helps them to identify signs of tension so the woman can be guided to release it.

If the woman did not have childbirth preparation classes, the nurse teaches simple breathing and relaxation techniques. If the woman is extremely anxious and out of control, she will not be able to comprehend verbal instructions. It may be necessary to make close eye contact with her and to breathe with her through each contraction until she can regain control.

The nurse minimizes environmental irritants as much as possible. The lights should be lowered and the woman kept reasonably dry by regularly changing the underpads on the bed. The temperature should be adjusted; the nurse provides a warm blanket if that offers the most comfort. (See Chapter 6 for other general comfort measures during labor.)

The nurse should be cautious not to overestimate or underestimate the amount of pain a woman is experiencing. The quiet, stoic woman may need analgesia yet be reluctant to ask. A tense body posture or facial grimacing may indicate that she needs additional pain-relief measures.

PHARMACOLOGICAL PAIN MANAGEMENT

Pharmacological pain management methods include analgesics, adjunctive drugs to improve the effectiveness of analgesics or to counteract their side effects, and anesthetics. Analgesics are systemic drugs (affecting the entire body) that reduce pain without loss of consciousness. Anesthetics cause a loss of sensation, especially of pain. Regional anesthetics block sensation from a localized area without causing a loss of consciousness. General anesthetics are systemic drugs that cause a loss of consciousness and sensation of pain. Tables 7-1 and 7-2 summarize intrapartum analgesics, adjunctive drugs, and methods of anesthesia.

Various clinicians administer anesthetics, depending on the type of drug. The physician or the nurse-midwife administers local anesthetics at the time of birth. A specialist in anesthetic administration may provide other anesthetics.

There are two types of anesthesia clinicians:
1. *An anesthesiologist:* a physician who specializes in administering anesthesia
2. *A certified registered nurse anesthetist (CRNA):* a registered nurse who has advanced training in anesthetic administration. State licensing laws and individual facility policies affect which methods of anesthesia each clinician may use.

Physiology of Pregnancy and Its Relationship to Analgesia and Anesthesia

Specific factors in the physiology of pregnancy affect the pregnant woman's response to analgesia and anesthesia:
- The pregnant woman is at a higher risk for hypoxia caused by the pressure of the enlarging uterus on the diaphragm.
- The sluggish gastrointestinal tract of the pregnant woman can result in increased risk for vomiting and aspiration.
- Aortocaval compression (pressure on the abdominal aorta by the heavy uterus when the woman is in supine position) increases the risk of hypotension and the development of shock.
- The effect on the fetus must be considered.

Advantages

Methods that use drugs for reducing pain during birth can help the woman to be a more active participant in birth. They help her relax and work with contractions. Drugs do not usually relieve *all* pain and pressure sensations.

The pain of labor may cause a "stress response" in the mother that results in an increase in autonomic activity, a release of catecholamines, and a decrease in platelet perfusion. This stress response results in fetal acidosis. The pain can also cause maternal hyperventilation and lead to respiratory alkalosis, and then a compensating metabolic acidosis. Metabolic acidosis in the woman results in further fetal acidosis. Therefore appropriate pain relief during labor can play an important role in the positive outcome of pregnancy for mother and infant.

Limitations

Pharmacological methods are effective, but they do have limitations. One important factor to consider is that two persons are medicated—the mother and her fetus. Any drug administered to the mother can affect

Table 7-1   Medications for Labor: Intrapartum Analgesics and Related Drugs

MEDICATION	USE AND EFFECTS
Narcotics	
Meperidine (Demerol)	Given to mothers in labor either intravenously, with a 5-10 minute peak of action, or intramuscularly, with a 50-minute peak of action
	Maternal responses may include hypotension, sedation, nausea and vomiting, and pruritus. If used starting in early labor, it can accumulate in fetal tissues and cause decrease in fetal heart variability and sedation at birth.
	Can cause respiratory depression and sedation in newborn if delivery occurs within 2 hours after the last dose is administered
Fentanyl (Sublimaze)	Rapid onset and short duration of action
	NOTE: fentanyl, sufentanil, and alfentanil are *not* the same drug
	Can cause respiratory depression but less than meperidine can cause
	Often used with epidural analgesia
Combination Opioid Agonist-Antagonist	
Butorphanol (Stadol)	Each have narcotic and narcotic antagonist effect
Nalbuphine (Nubain)	Both drugs reduce pain and are thought to cause less respiratory depression than meperidine
	Should not be used in women who are drug addicts
Opioid Antagonist	
Naloxone (Narcan)	An opioid antagonist that acts within minutes to help resuscitate a newborn who has respiratory depression because of narcotic sedation of the mother during labor; also relieves itching as a maternal side effect of narcotics
	Duration of action is 1-2 hours, so the vital signs of the newborn should continue to be observed
	May cause withdrawal symptoms if administered to a woman who regularly uses illicit drugs (e.g., tremors, perspiration, anxiety, irritability, and seizures)
Ataractics (Analgesic Potentiators)	
Promethazine (Phenergan)	Reduce anxiety and nausea but may reduce analgesic effect of opioids (Gabbe, 2012)
All benzodiazapines	May delay achievement of thermoregulation in newborn (Gabbe, 2012)

NOTE: Consult drug guide for safe doses of drugs.

the fetus, and the effects may be prolonged in the infant after birth. The drug may directly affect the fetus, or it may indirectly affect the fetus because of effects in the mother (such as hypotension).

Several pharmacological methods may slow labor's progress if used early in labor. Some complications during pregnancy limit the pharmacological methods that are safe. For example, a method that requires the infusion of large amounts of intravenous (IV) fluids might overload the woman's circulation if she has heart disease. If she takes other medications (legal or illicit), they may interact adversely with the drugs used to relieve labor pain.

Analgesics and Adjunctive Drugs

Narcotic (Opioid) Analgesics. Systemic **opioids** are the most common means of labor analgesia in the United States. They are used in small doses to avoid causing fetal respiratory depression. Opioids do not provide complete pain relief during labor, but they do help the woman cope with a tolerable level of intermittent labor pains. Drugs used are listed in Table 7-1.

In general, use of narcotic analgesics is avoided if birth is expected within an hour. An attempt is made to time administration so the drug does not reach its peak at the time of birth, or the infant may suffer respiratory depression that may require interventions such as the administration of Naloxone. The nurse must be prepared to support the respiratory efforts of all infants at birth regardless of whether the mother received narcotics during labor.

Narcotic Antagonist. Naloxone (Narcan) is used to reverse respiratory depression, usually in the infant, caused by opioid drugs such as meperidine. It is not effective against respiratory depression from other causes, such as intrauterine hypoxia. It can be given by the IV route, or it may be given through the endotracheal tube during resuscitation. IV naloxone can be administered to the neonate immediately after birth via the umbilical cord vein. The use of naloxone in a woman who is drug dependent can cause withdrawal syndrome in the mother or the neonate.

Adjunctive Drugs. Adjunctive drugs are not pain relievers but are given to relieve nausea and vomiting. All benzodiazepines can disrupt the beat-to-beat variability of the fetal heart rate and delay the newborn infant's ability to regulate temperature (Gabbe, 2012).

Table 7-2 Methods of Anesthesia Administration for Childbirth

ANESTHESIA METHOD	NURSING IMPLICATIONS
Local infiltration: Injection of the perineum with a local anesthetic drug just before vaginal birth; administered by nurse-midwife or physician to site of episiotomy on perineum	Injection may burn until the area becomes numb; adverse effects are rare; check for allergies to -*caine* drugs and for allergies to dental anesthetics.
Pudendal block: Injection of the pudendal nerves with local anesthetic just before vaginal birth; local infiltration of the perineum is also usually done; may be used for some forceps births; administered by nurse-midwife or physician	Similar to local infiltration; warn the woman that the long needle is needed to reach the nerve and is shielded by the needle guide or "trumpet"; observe for hematoma (collection of blood within tissues), which may become evident during the recovery period and is evidenced by excessive perineal or pelvic pain; pelvic infection sometimes occurs but is uncommon.
Epidural block: Injection of local anesthetic drug into the epidural space, which blocks transmission of pain impulses to brain; epidural narcotics are often added to reduce the amount of anesthetic needed and reduce the adverse effects; used for pain relief during labor and vaginal birth, as well as for cesarean birth; administered by physician (obstetrician or anesthesiologist) or by nurse anesthetist when cervix is at least 4 cm dilated	Observe for hypotension and urinary retention; assist the woman to maintain position as needed by anesthesia clinician; initially record blood pressure every 5 minutes after the block is begun and after each reinjection until stable; record fetal heart rates, usually with continuous electronic fetal monitoring; a full bladder may necessitate catheterization if the woman cannot feel the urge to void; ambulate carefully, because sensation will be reduced.
Subarachnoid (spinal) block: Injection of local anesthetic drug under the dura and arachnoid membranes to block transmission of pain impulses to brain; used primarily for cesarean birth; usually administered by anesthesiologist	Observe for hypotension and urinary retention as with epidural block (interventions are the same); suspect postspinal headache (usually during postpartum period) if woman complains of a headache that is worse when she is in an upright position; give oral fluids and analgesics as ordered.
General anesthesia: Uses a combination of intravenous (IV) and inhalational drugs to produce a loss of consciousness; rarely used for vaginal births; used for cesarean births under some conditions: • Woman's refusal of regional block • Contraindication for regional block • Emergency cesarean when there is not time to establish a regional block	Regurgitation, with aspiration of gastric contents, is the primary risk; IV drugs to reduce gastric acidity or speed up stomach emptying may also be provided by the anesthesia clinician; assistant applies cricoid pressure until the woman is intubated to prevent any regurgitated stomach contents from reaching her trachea; anesthesia is light, and woman may move on the operating table; postanesthesia recovery care includes observation of level of consciousness, vital signs, oxygen saturation, plus postcesarean birth care; infant is likely to be born with respiratory depression and require aggressive resuscitation.

Regional Analgesics and Anesthetics

The membranes around the spinal cord are called the meninges. The meninges have three layers:

1. Dura mater
2. Arachnoid mater
3. Pia mater

The *epidural space* is located between the dura mater and the inside bony covering of the brain or spinal cord. The *subdural space* is located between the dura mater and the arachnoid mater, and the *subarachnoid space* is located between the arachnoid mater and the pia mater. Regional anesthesia in obstetrics usually involves the placement of an anesthetic in the epidural or the subarachnoid space (see Figure 7-7).

An *analgesic* blocks pain, whereas an *anesthetic* blocks both pain and motor responses. For example, an epidural block may provide analgesia and allow the woman to ambulate with assistance, but spinal anesthesia prevents ambulation. The role of the nurse in caring for a woman with regional analgesia or anesthesia is to monitor her responses and the status of the fetus. Starting or

managing intermittent dosages of a regional anesthetic is not within the nursing scope of practice for a licensed practical or vocational nurse (LPN/LVN).

Regional anesthetics block sensation in varying degrees, depending on the type of regional block used, the quantity of medication, and the drugs injected. The woman still feels pressure and may feel some pain. The major advantage of regional anesthetics is that they provide satisfactory pain relief, yet they allow the woman to be awake and participate in the birthing process (Table 7-2).

Local and pudendal blocks are administered in the vaginal-perineal area. Epidural and subarachnoid blocks and intrathecal narcotics are given by injecting anesthetic drugs so they bathe the nerves as they emerge from the spinal cord. The spinal cord and nerves are not directly injected.

Local anesthetic agents for childbirth are related to those used for dental work. On admission, the nurse should ask each woman if she is allergic to or has had problems with dental anesthesia. If so, her physician or nurse-midwife should be alerted so she can receive the safest pain-relief measures.

Local Infiltration. Injection of the perineal area for an episiotomy is performed just before birth, when the fetal head is visible. It may also be done after placental expulsion to repair a perineal laceration. There is a short delay between injection of the anesthetic agent and the loss of pain sensation. The physician or nurse-midwife allows the anesthetic to become effective before beginning the episiotomy. There are virtually no risks to this procedure if the woman is not allergic to the drug.

Pudendal Block. The pudendal block is used for vaginal births, although its use has become less common as the popularity of the epidural block has increased. It provides adequate anesthesia for an episiotomy and for most low forceps births. It does not block pain from contractions and, like local infiltration, is given just before birth. There is a delay of a few minutes between injection of the drug and the onset of numbness (paresthesia).

The physician or nurse-midwife injects the pudendal nerves on each side of the mother's pelvis (Figure 7-6). The nerves may be reached through the vagina or by injection directly through her perineum. A long needle (13 to 15 cm [5 to 6 inches]) is needed to reach the pudendal nerves, which are near the mother's ischial spines. If the injection is done through the vagina, a needle guide ("trumpet") is used to protect the mother's tissues. The needle is injected only about 1.3 cm (0.5 inch) into the woman's tissues. The perineum is also infiltrated, because the pudendal block alone does not completely anesthetize the perineum.

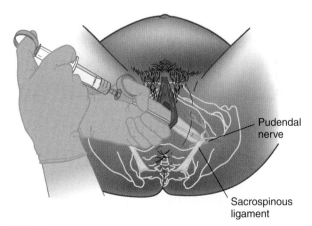

FIGURE 7-6 Pudendal block anesthesia. The two pudendal nerves on each side of the pelvis are injected to numb the vagina and perineum. The illustration shows the technique of inserting the needle beyond the needle guard and passing through the sacrospinous ligament to reach the pudendal nerve. (From Matteson PS: *Women's health during the childbearing years: a community-based approach*, St Louis, 2001, Mosby.)

Adverse effects of pudendal block. The pudendal block includes few adverse effects if the woman is not allergic to the drug. A vaginal hematoma (collection of blood within the tissues) sometimes occurs. An abscess may develop, but this is not common.

Epidural Block. The epidural space is a small space just outside the dura (outermost membrane covering the brain and spinal cord). The woman is in a sitting or side-lying position for the epidural block. Her back is relatively straight, rather than sharply curved forward, to avoid compressing the tiny epidural space, which is about 1 mm (the thickness of a dime).

The physician or nurse anesthetist penetrates the epidural space with a large needle (16- to 18-gauge). A fine catheter is threaded into the epidural space through the bore of the needle (Figure 7-7). A test dose (2 to 3 mL) of local anesthetic agent is injected through the catheter. The woman is not expected to experience effects from the test dose if the catheter is in the right place. Numbness or loss of movement after the small test dose indicates that her dura mater was probably punctured and the drug was injected into the subarachnoid space (as in a subarachnoid block) rather than in the epidural space. Numbness around the mouth, ringing in the ears (tinnitus), visual disturbances, or jitteriness are symptoms that suggest injection into a vein. The test dose is small enough to prevent long-term adverse effects.

If the test dose is normal (no effects), a larger amount of anesthetic agent is injected to begin the block. A few minutes are needed before the onset of the block. If an epidural block is being used for surgery, such as cesarean delivery or tubal ligation, the anesthesiologist or CRNA will test for the level of numbness before surgery begins.

Local anesthetic drugs are usually combined with a small dose of an opioid analgesic such as fentanyl (Sublimaze). The combination of drugs allows quicker and longer-lasting pain relief with less anesthetic agent and minimal loss of movement. An epidural block for labor is more accurately termed *analgesia* (reducing pain) than *anesthesia* (obliterating all sensation).

The woman can sometimes ambulate when a combination-drug epidural is used, because the local anesthetic dose is much lower. She can assume any position with this type of block, although any pregnant woman should avoid the supine position.

To maintain pain relief during labor, the anesthetic drug is constantly infused into the catheter via an infusion pump. Alternatively, intermittently repeated injections of the drug may be given.

Dural puncture. The dura lies just below the tiny epidural space. This membrane is sometimes punctured accidentally ("wet tap") with the epidural needle or the catheter that is inserted through it. If a dural puncture occurs, a relatively large amount of spinal fluid can leak from the hole, which may result in a headache.

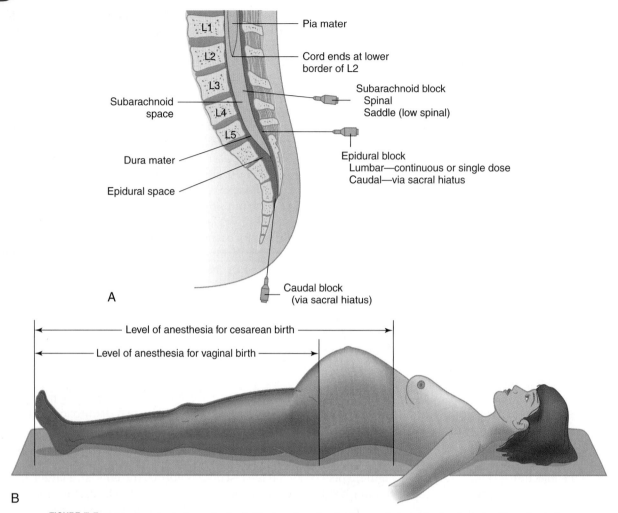

FIGURE 7-7 Epidural and spinal anesthesia. **A,** The insertion sites for the needle in epidural, subarachnoid, and spinal blocks. **B,** Levels of anesthesia for vaginal birth compared with minimum level required for cesarean birth. (From Matteson PS: *Women's health during the childbearing years: a community-based approach,* St Louis, 2001, Mosby.)

Limitations of epidural block. Although it is a popular method of intrapartum pain relief, an epidural block is not used if the woman has any of the following:

- Abnormal blood clotting
- An infection in the area of injection or a systemic infection
- Hypovolemia (inadequate blood volume)

Adverse effects of epidural block. The most common side effects are *maternal hypotension* and *urinary retention*. After initiation of the epidural block, the fetal heart rate and blood pressure should be monitored and documented q5 minutes for 15 minutes and then q30 minutes for 1 hour. To counteract hypotension, which can compromise fetal oxygenation, a large quantity (500 mL to 1000 mL or more) of IV solution, such as Ringer's lactate, is infused rapidly before the block is begun. The large quantity of IV fluids combined with reduced sensation may result in urinary retention. The nurse should palpate the suprapubic area for a full bladder every 2 hours, or more often if a large quantity of IV solution was given. The woman will need catheterization if she is unable to void.

The woman may feel less of an urge to push in the second stage of labor when she has an epidural block, depending on the drugs used for her block. Therefore this stage may be longer if a woman has an epidural block. Maternal and fetal conditions are monitored closely.

! Safety Alert!

Assess the woman for bladder distention regularly if she has received an epidural or subarachnoid block. A full bladder can delay birth and can cause hemorrhage after birth.

Subarachnoid (Spinal) Block. The woman's position for a subarachnoid block is similar to that for the epidural block except that her back is curled around her uterus in a C shape. The dura is punctured with a thin (25- to 27-gauge) spinal needle. A few drops of spinal fluid confirm entry into the subarachnoid space (see Figure 7-7). The local anesthetic drug is then injected. A much smaller quantity of the drug is needed to

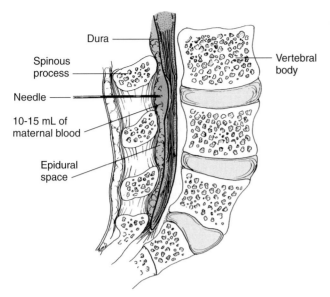

FIGURE 7-8 Epidural blood patch. An epidural blood patch may provide dramatic relief from postspinal headache.

Labels on figure: Dura; Spinous process; Needle; 10-15 mL of maternal blood; Epidural space; Vertebral body

the area of the subarachnoid puncture (Figure 7-8). The blood clots and forms a gelatinous seal that stops spinal fluid leakage. The clot later breaks down and is resorbed by the body.

General Anesthesia

General anesthesia is rarely used for vaginal births or for most cesarean births. Regional blocks are preferred for cesarean births. However, general anesthesia may be necessary in the following circumstances:

- Emergency cesarean birth, when there is not time to establish either an epidural or a subarachnoid block
- Cesarean birth in the woman who refuses or has a contraindication to epidural or subarachnoid block

Combinations of general anesthetic drugs (balanced anesthesia) allow for a quick onset of anesthesia, minimal fetal effects, and prompt maternal wakening after the drug is stopped.

Adverse Effects in the Mother. The major risk of general anesthesia is the same during birth as at any other time: regurgitation with aspiration (breathing in) of the acidic stomach contents. This results in a chemical injury to the lungs, *aspiration pneumonitis,* which can be fatal. Many women begin labor with a full stomach, and their gastric action slows during labor. In addition, the full uterus exerts upward pressure against the stomach. Therefore every pregnant woman is presumed to have a full stomach for purposes of anesthesia.

Adverse Effects in the Neonate. Respiratory depression is the main neonatal risk, because drugs given to the mother may cross the placenta. To reduce this risk, the time from induction of anesthesia to clamping of the umbilical cord is kept as short as possible. The woman is prepped and draped for surgery, and all personnel are scrubbed, gowned, and gloved before anesthesia begins. In addition, the anesthesia is kept as light as possible until the cord is clamped. Aggressive resuscitation of the newborn may be necessary.

The Nurse's Role in Pharmacological Techniques

The nurse's responsibility in pharmacological pain management begins at admission (Nursing Care Plan 7-1). The woman should be questioned closely about allergies to foods, drugs (including dental anesthetics), and latex to identify pain-relief measures that may not be advisable. She should be questioned about her preferences for pain relief. Factors that may have an impact on the choice of pain relief should be noted, such as a history of back surgery, infection in the area where an epidural block would be injected, or blood pressure abnormalities.

The nurse keeps the bed's side rails up if the woman takes pain-relief drugs. Narcotics may cause drowsiness or dizziness. Regional anesthetics reduce sensation and movement to varying degrees, and therefore the woman may have less control over her body. Side rails on the bed may be necessary for safety.

achieve anesthesia using the subarachnoid block than with the epidural block. Anesthesia occurs quickly and is more profound than the epidural block. The woman loses all movement and sensation below the block.

The subarachnoid block is a "one-shot" block, because it does not involve placing a catheter for reinjection of the drug. It is not often used for vaginal births today but remains common for cesarean births. Its limitations are essentially the same as for an epidural block.

Adverse effects of subarachnoid block. Hypotension and urinary retention are the main adverse effects of subarachnoid block, as with the epidural block. They are managed as in the epidural block.

A postspinal headache sometimes occurs, most likely because of spinal fluid loss. The woman may be advised to remain flat for several hours after the block to decrease the chance of postspinal headache. However, there is no absolute evidence that this precaution is effective. Postspinal headache is worse when the woman is upright and often disappears entirely when she lies down. Bed rest, analgesics, and oral and IV fluids help to relieve the headache. A **blood patch**, done by the nurse anesthetist or anesthesiologist, may provide dramatic relief from postspinal headache. The woman's blood (10 mL to 15 mL) is withdrawn from her vein and injected into the epidural space in

> **! Safety Alert!**
>
> To lessen the risk of infection when assisting with spinal anesthesia, the nurse must don a clean face mask, perform hand hygiene, don gloves, and disinfect the injection site per facility protocol (Gabbe, 2012).

★ Nursing Care Plan 7-1   The Woman Needing Pain Management During Labor

PATIENT DATA A woman, para 1, gravida 2, is in active labor and is 4 cm dilated. She is thrashing in bed and is not cooperating with the coaching of her partner.

Selected Nursing Diagnosis: Acute pain related to uterine contractions and descent of fetus in pelvis

Goals	Nursing Interventions	Rationales
The woman will state that her discomfort is manageable during labor using techniques learned in childbirth preparation classes and/or taught by the nurse. The woman will have a relaxed facial and body appearance between contractions.	Continuously determine presence and character of pain during labor: • Statement of pain (assess nature of pain, such as location, intensity, whether intermittent or constant) • Crying, moaning during and/or between contractions • Tense, guarded body posture or thrashing with contractions • "Mask of pain" facial expression	These are common verbal and nonverbal signs of pain; assessment enables the nurse to identify if pain is normal for woman's labor status and to choose the best interventions for pain relief (nonpharmacological and/or pharmacological measures); evaluating verbal and nonverbal communication helps the nurse to evaluate the need for pain relief in women who may not directly communicate their need for pain relief or who do not speak the prevailing language.
	Provide general comfort measures, such as: • Adjust the room temperature and light level for comfort. • Reduce irritants, such as wet underpads. • Provide ice chips, Popsicles, or juices to relieve dry mouth. • Avoid bumping the bed.	These general measures reduce outside irritants that make it harder for the woman to use childbirth preparation techniques and are themselves a source of discomfort. A comfortable environment is conducive to relaxation.
	Encourage the woman to assume positions she finds most comfortable, other than supine.	Position changes promote comfort and help the fetus adapt to the size and shape of woman's pelvis; supine position can result in supine hypotensive syndrome, which reduces placental blood flow and fetal oxygenation.
	Observe for a full bladder every 1 to 2 hours, or more often if the woman receives large amounts of oral or intravenous (IV) fluids.	A full bladder is a source of discomfort and can prolong labor by inhibiting fetal descent; it may cause pain that lingers after epidural analgesia is begun.
	Promote the use of techniques learned in childbirth preparation, including labor partner as appropriate: • Do not stand in front of her focal point. • Offer a back rub or firm sacral pressure; ask her about the best location and amount of pressure; use powder to prevent skin irritation. • Encourage the woman to switch to more complex patterns only when simpler ones are no longer effective. • Breathe along with the woman if she has trouble maintaining patterns; make eye contact.	These are examples of how to assist the woman and her partner in using learned methods most effectively. The use of nonpharmacological pain relief prevents problems associated with pharmacological interventions, and supplements any drug therapy used. Nonpharmacological pain relief measures also provide the woman and her partner with a sense of control and mastery that enhances the perception of birth as a positive experience.
	If the woman has signs of hyperventilation (dizziness, numbness or tingling sensations, spasms of the hands and feet), have her breathe into her cupped hands, a small bag, or a washcloth placed over her mouth and nose.	Hyperventilation often occurs when the woman uses rapid breathing patterns, because she exhales too much carbon dioxide. These measures help her to conserve carbon dioxide and rebreathe it to correct for excess loss.

Nursing Care Plan 7-1   The Woman Needing Pain Management During Labor—cont'd

Goals	Nursing Interventions	Rationales
	Tell the woman and her partner when labor progresses; for example, if she is pushing and her infant's head becomes visible, let her see or feel it.	Labor does not last forever; knowing that her efforts are having the desired results gives her courage to continue and helps her to tolerate pain.

Selected Nursing Diagnosis: Deficient knowledge related to unfamiliar procedures and expected effects of epidural block

Goals	Nursing Interventions	Rationales
After explanations, the woman will state that she understands what will happen during and after epidural block is begun.	Explain what to expect as the epidural block is begun (reinforcing explanations of the anesthesiologist or nurse anesthetist): • An IV line will be started, and she will receive fluids to offset the tendency for blood pressure to fall. • The fetus will be monitored by electronic fetal monitoring. • The nurse anesthetist or anesthesiologist will position her; she should remain still and in this position for insertion of catheter. • A small plastic catheter will be taped to her back to allow constant infusion of medication (or reinjection). • Her blood pressure will be checked every 5 minutes when the block is first begun.	This list reflects a common sequence of events for starting an epidural block. The anesthesia clinician explains the procedure and expected effects; the nurse reinforces explanations as needed, because the woman in pain may not be able to concentrate. Knowledge reduces anxiety and fear of the unknown. If the woman understands that these procedures are a normal part of an epidural block, she is less likely to interpret them as problems.
	If she needs to remain flat briefly to allow the drug to disperse, put a small pillow under her right hip.	Placing a pillow under her hip helps prevent supine hypotensive syndrome.
	Explain that she will feel less pain but will feel pressure; movement and sensation in her legs and feet will vary.	Explanations help the woman to understand that the epidural block is not expected to abolish the pain of labor. Leg movement and sensation are affected to varying degrees. If she understands these possible variations, she is less likely to interpret them as abnormal or as evidence that the block is not working.

Selected Nursing Diagnosis: Risk for injury related to loss of sensation

Goals	Nursing Interventions	Rationales
The woman will not have an injury, such as a muscle strain or fall, while her epidural block is in effect. The fetus will not be born in an uncontrolled delivery.	Check for movement, sensation, and leg strength before ambulating; ambulate cautiously with an assistant. Assist the woman to change positions regularly.	A fall is more likely if the woman does not have sensation and control over her movements. A change of position prevents muscle strain.
	Observe for signs that birth may be near: increase in bloody show, perineal bulging, and/or crowning.	Loss of sensation varies among women having an epidural block. Labor may progress more rapidly than expected. These are signs associated with imminent birth that should be evaluated by the experienced nurse, the nurse-midwife, or the physician.

Critical Thinking Question

1. A woman, para 1, gravida 2, is in active labor. The last examination showed that her cervix was 7 cm dilated and 75% effaced. She states that her contraction pains are almost unbearable, even with the medication she has received. Because getting up and walking helped her earlier, and she needs to go to the bathroom now, she asks the nurse to help her out of bed to walk to the nearby bathroom. What would be the best response of the nurse?

The nurse reinforces the explanations given by the anesthesia clinician regarding procedures and the expected effects of the selected pain-management method. Women often receive these explanations when they are very uncomfortable and do not remember everything they were told. The woman is helped to assume and hold the position for the epidural or subarachnoid block. The nurse tells the anesthesia clinician if the woman has a contraction, because it might prevent her from remaining still. The anesthetic drug is usually injected between contractions.

The woman is observed for hypotension if an epidural or subarachnoid block is administered. Hospital protocols vary, but blood pressure is usually measured every 5 minutes after the block begins (and with each reinjection) until her blood pressure is stable. An automatic blood pressure monitor is often used. Some facilities add a pulse oximeter to monitor oxygen saturation. At the same time, the nurse observes the fetal monitor for signs associated with fetal compromise (see Chapter 6), because maternal hypotension can reduce placental blood flow.

The epidural block is given during labor and may reduce the mother's sensation of rectal pressure. The nurse coaches her about the right time to start and stop pushing with each contraction if needed. The nurse also observes for signs of imminent birth, such as increased bloody show and perineal bulging, because the woman may not be able to feel the sensations distinctly.

Nursing responsibilities related to general anesthesia include assessment and documentation of oral intake and administration of medications to reduce gastric acidity. The woman should be told that all preparations for surgery will be performed *before* she is put to sleep. The nurse should reassure her that she will be asleep before any incision is made. Having a familiar nurse in the operating room full of new people is reassuring to the woman before surgery.

The woman who has received a general anesthetic is usually awake enough to move from the operating table to her bed after surgery. Her respiratory status is observed every 15 minutes for 1 to 2 hours. A pulse oximeter provides constant information about her blood oxygen level. She is given oxygen by face mask or other means until she is fully awake. Her uterine fundus and vaginal bleeding are observed as for any other postpartum woman. Her urine output from the indwelling catheter should be observed for quantity and color at least hourly for 4 hours. The nurse should ambulate the woman cautiously and with assistance to prevent the potential for falling.

Safety Alert!

The following are important admission assessments related to pharmacological pain management: last oral intake (time and type), adverse reactions to drugs (especially dental anesthetics), other medications taken, and any food allergies or latex allergy.

If the woman receives narcotic drugs, the nurse observes her respiratory rate for depression. Because respiratory depression is more likely to occur in the neonate than in the mother, the neonate is closely observed after birth. Narcotic effects in the infant may persist longer than in an adult. The nurse has naloxone on hand in case it is needed to reverse respiratory depression in the mother or neonate.

The nurse observes the woman for late-appearing respiratory depression and excessive sedation if she received epidural narcotics after cesarean birth. This may occur up to 24 hours after administration, depending on the drug given. The woman's vital signs are monitored hourly, and a pulse oximeter may be applied. Facilities often use a scale to assess for sedation so all caregivers use the same criteria for assessment and documentation. Additional analgesics are given cautiously and strictly as ordered. If mild analgesics do not relieve the pain, the health care provider is contacted for additional orders.

Unfolding Case Study

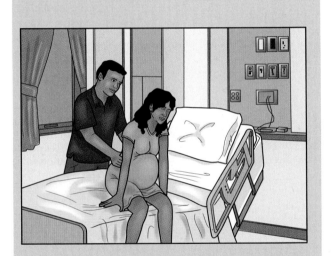

Tess and Luis were introduced to the reader in Chapter 4, and Tess's pregnancy experience has unfolded in each chapter. Refer to earlier chapters for her history and progress.

Tess has been admitted to the labor room in active labor at 40 weeks gestation. She is complaining of very painful contractions. Her husband Luis is at her side.

QUESTIONS

1. What causes Tess's labor pain? What factors influence Tess's labor pain?
2. What are some nonpharmacologic pain-relief measures that the nurse can use to help Tess cope with her pain? With which measures can her husband Luis help?
3. What are some pharmacologic measures for pain relief during labor? What are nursing responsibilities involved in each?
4. What is the effect on the newborn of pharmacologic pain-relief measures used during the labor process?
5. What are the nursing responsibilities in the care of the newborn that relate to Tess having pharmacologic pain relief during labor?

Get Ready for the NCLEX® Examination!

Key Points:

- Pain during childbirth is different from other types of pain, because it is part of a normal process that results in the birth of an infant. The woman has time to prepare for it, and the pain is self limiting.
- A woman's pain threshold is fairly constant. Her pain tolerance varies, and nursing actions can increase her ability to tolerate pain. Irritants can reduce her pain tolerance.
- The pain of labor is caused by cervical dilation and effacement, uterine ischemia, and stretching of the vagina and perineum.
- Poorly relieved pain can be detrimental to the labor process.
- Childbirth preparation classes provide pain-management tools for the woman and her partner to use during labor. Some tools, such as breathing techniques and effleurage, can also be taught to the unprepared woman.
- The nurse should do everything possible to promote relaxation during labor, because it enhances the effectiveness of all other pain-management methods, both nonpharmacological and pharmacological.
- Any drug taken by the expectant mother may cross the placenta and affect the fetus. Effects may persist in the infant much longer than in an adult.
- The use of narcotic antagonist drugs for women who have a drug dependency can cause withdrawal syndrome in the mother or the neonate.
- Observe the mother and infant for respiratory depression if the mother received opioids, including epidural narcotics, during the intrapartum period.
- Regional anesthetics are the most common for birth because they allow the mother to remain awake, including for cesarean birth.
- Closely question the woman about drug allergies when she is admitted. Because drugs used for regional anesthesia are related to those used in dentistry, ask her about reactions to dental anesthetics.
- Observe the mother's blood pressure and the fetal heart rate after epidural or spinal block to identify hypotension or fetal compromise. Urinary retention is also more likely.

Additional Learning Resources

SG Go to your Study Guide for additional learning activities to help you master this chapter content.

evolve Go to your Evolve website (http://evolve.elsevier.com/Leifer) for the following learning resources:
- Animations
- Answer Guidelines for Critical Thinking Questions
- Answers and Rationales for Review Questions for the NCLEX® Examination

- Glossary with English and Spanish pronunciations
- Interactive Review Questions for the NCLEX® Examination
- Patient Teaching Plans in English and Spanish
- Skills Performance Checklists
- Video clips and more!

 Online Resources
- Association of Women's Health, Obstetric and Neonatal Nurses: www.awhonn.org
- Pain relief during birth: www.acog.org/publications/patient_education/bp086.cfm

Review Questions for the NCLEX® Examination

1. Which of the following is most appropriately used for pain relief during labor when the cervix is dilated less than 4 cm?
   1. Stadol (butorphanol) via IM
   2. Demerol (meperidine) via IM
   3. Phenergan (promethazine) via IM
   4. Fentanyl (Sublimaze) via epidural

2. Which technique is likely to be most effective for "back labor"?
   1. Stimulating the abdomen by effleurage
   2. Applying firm pressure in the sacral area
   3. Blowing out in short breaths during each contraction
   4. Rocking from side to side at the peak of each contraction

3. What drug should be immediately available for emergency use when a woman receives narcotics during labor?
   1. Fentanyl (Sublimaze)
   2. Diphenhydramine (Benadryl)
   3. Lidocaine (Xylocaine)
   4. Naloxone (Narcan)

4. Select the **two** most important nursing assessments immediately after a woman receives an epidural block: (Select all that apply.)
   1. Bladder distention
   2. Condition of intravenous site
   3. Respiratory rate
   4. Blood pressure

5. A woman in labor states she wants to have epidural analgesia. When can this method of analgesia best be given?
   1. Anytime during labor
   2. During the transition phase of labor
   3. During the first stage of labor
   4. During the third stage of labor

Objectives

1. Define each key term listed.
2. Discuss each obstetric procedure described in this chapter.
3. Illustrate the nurse's role in each obstetric procedure.
4. Analyze the nurse's role in a cesarean birth.
5. Describe factors that contribute to an abnormal labor.

6. Explain each intrapartum complication discussed in this chapter.
7. Discuss the nurse's role in caring for women with each intrapartum complication.
8. Review the nurse's role in obstetric emergencies.

Key Terms

anaphylactoid syndrome (p. 196)
artificial rupture of membranes (AROM) (p. 176)
augmentation of labor (p. 174)
Bishop score (p. 175)
cephalopelvic disproportion (sĕf-ăh-lō-PĔL-vĭc dĭs-prŏ-PŎR-shŭn, p. 181)
chignon (SHĒN-yŏn, p. 181)
chorioamnionitis (kō-rē-ō-ăm-nē-ō-NĪ-tĭs, p. 192)
dysfunctional labor (p. 183)
dystocia (p. 183)
fibronectin test (fī-brō-NĔK-tĭn tĕst, p. 193)

hydramnios (hī-DRĂM-nē-ŏs, p. 184)
induction of labor (p. 174)
laminaria (lăm-ĭ-NĂ-rē-ăh, p. 176)
macrosomia (măk-rō-SŌM-ē-ă, p. 187)
oligohydramnios (ŏl-ĭ-gō-hī-DRĂM-nē-ŏs, p. 174)
shoulder dystocia (SHŌL-dŭr dĭs-TŌ-sē-ă, p. 189)
spontaneous rupture of membranes (SROM) (p. 176)
tocolytics (tō-kō-LĬT-ĭks, p. 175)
Uterine tachysystole (p. 176)
version (p. 178)

Childbirth is a normal, natural event in the lives of most women and their families. When the many factors that affect the birth process function in harmony, complications are unlikely. However, some women experience complications during childbirth that threaten their well-being or that of the infant.

OBSTETRIC PROCEDURES

Nurses assist with several obstetric procedures during birth; they also care for women after the procedures. Some procedures, such as amniotomy or amnioinfusion, are performed to prevent complications during birth. Other procedures are needed when the woman has a complication that necessitates an intervention to promote a positive outcome for the mother and fetus.

AMNIOINFUSION

An amnioinfusion is the injection of warmed sterile saline or lactated Ringer's solution into the uterus via an intrauterine pressure catheter during labor after the membranes have ruptured. Indications for this procedure include the following:

- **Oligohydramnios** (lower-than-normal amount of amniotic fluid)

- Umbilical cord compression resulting from lack of amniotic fluid
- Goal of reducing recurrent variable decelerations in the fetal heart rate
- Goal of diluting meconium-stained amniotic fluid to prevent meconium aspiration syndrome.

Amnioinfusion replaces the "cushion" for the umbilical cord and relieves the variable decelerations of the fetal heart rate that may occur during contractions when decreased amniotic fluid is present. It can be administered as a one-time bolus for 1 hour or as a continuous infusion. Continuous monitoring of uterine activity and fetal heart rate is essential. The nurse should change the underpads on the bed as needed to maintain patient comfort and should document the color, amount, and any odor of the fluid expelled from the vagina.

INDUCTION OR AUGMENTATION OF LABOR

Induction is the intentional initiation of labor before it begins naturally. **Augmentation** is the stimulation of contractions after they have begun naturally.

Labor involves the complex interaction between fetus and mother. Before labor is induced, it is important that fetal maturity be confirmed by ultrasound;

Table 8-1	Modified Bishop Scoring System			
SCORE	**0**	**1**	**2**	**3**
Dilation of cervix (cm)	0	1-2	3-4	5-6
Consistency of cervix	Firm	Medium	Soft	—
Length of cervix (cm)	>4	2-4	1-2	1-2
Cervical effacement (%)	0-30	40-50	60-70	80
Position of cervix	Posterior	Midline	Anterior	—
Station of presenting part related to ischial spines	−3	−2	−1 or 0	+1 or +2

Modified from Stables D, Rankin J: *Physiology in childbearing: with anatomy and related biosciences*, ed 2, Edinburgh, 2005, Elsevier; Gabbe S et al, editors: *Obstetrics: normal and problem pregnancies*, ed 6, Philadelphia, 2012, Saunders. NOTE: High score is predictive of a successful labor induction, because the cervix has ripened, or softened, in preparation for labor. The American Congress of Obstetricians and Gynecologists (ACOG) recommends a score of 6 or above before induction of labor.

amniotic fluid analysis (lecithin/sphingomyelin [L/S] ratio) (see Chapter 5); presence of increased fetal fibronectin at the cervix and the Bishop score above 6. The **Bishop score** is used to assess the status of the cervix in determining its response to induction (Table 8-1). A score of 6 or more indicates a favorable prognosis for induction. Continuous uterine activity and fetal heart rate monitoring during labor induction is essential.

Indications

Labor is induced if continuing the pregnancy is hazardous for the woman or the fetus. The following are some of the indications for labor induction:

- Gestational hypertension (see Chapter 5)
- Ruptured membranes without spontaneous onset of labor
- Infection within the uterus
- Medical problems in the woman that worsen during pregnancy, such as diabetes, kidney disease, or pulmonary disease
- Fetal problems, such as slowed growth, prolonged pregnancy, or incompatibility between fetal and maternal blood types (see Chapter 5)
- Placental insufficiency
- Fetal death

Convenience for the health care provider or the family is not an indication for inducing labor. However, the woman who has a history of rapid labors and lives a long distance from the birth facility may have her labor induced, because she has a higher risk of giving birth en route if she awaits spontaneous labor.

Contraindications

Labor is *not* induced in the following conditions:

- Placenta previa (see Chapter 5)
- Umbilical cord prolapse (see p. 194)
- Abnormal fetal presentation
- High station of the fetus (head not engaged), which can suggest a preterm fetus or a small maternal pelvis
- Active herpes infection externally or in the birth canal, which the infant can acquire during birth
- Abnormal size or structure of the mother's pelvis
- Previous classic (vertical) cesarean incision (see Figure 8-4, p. 182)

The physician may attempt to induce labor in a preterm pregnancy if continuing the pregnancy is more harmful to the woman or the fetus than the hazards of prematurity would be to the infant.

Pharmacological and Mechanical Methods to Stimulate Contractions

Cervical Ripening. Cervical ripening is the physical softening of the cervix that leads to effacement and dilation. Induction of labor is more effective if the woman's cervix is "ripe" (see Table 8-1). These prelabor cervical changes occur naturally in most women. Methods to hasten the changes, or "ripen" the cervix, ease labor induction, because oxytocic drugs have no effect on the cervix. Oxytoxin used to induce labor without a "ripe cervix" can result in the need for a cesarean section (Gabbe, 2012). Cervical ripening can be achieved by pharmacologic or mechanical means.

The use of prostaglandins to ripen the cervix is contraindicated in women with a history of uterine myomectomy surgery or previous cesarean section because of the risk of uterine rupture.

Prostaglandin E$_2$. Prepidil (Cervidil) vaginal insertion is recommended via a sustained release vaginal insert.

Prostaglandin E$_1$. Cytotec (Misoprostol) was designed for the treatment of peptic ulcer disease, and use as a preinduction medication is considered an "off-label" use approved by ACOG (ACOG, 2011). It can be administered orally (sublingual or buccal) or intravaginally. Prostaglandin E$_1$ is more effective in achieving vaginal delivery within 24 hours, but it is associated with uterine tachysystole and fetal heart abnormalities.

The procedure should be explained to the woman and her family. A fetal heart-rate baseline is recorded. An intravenous (IV) line with saline or heparin sodium (Hep-Lock) may be placed in case uterine tachysystole (hyperstimulation) occurs and IV **tocolytics** (drugs that reduce uterine contractions) are needed. After insertion of the prostaglandin gel, the woman remains on bed rest for 1 to 2 hours and is monitored for uterine contractions. Vital signs and fetal heart rate are also recorded. Oxytocin induction can be started when the insert is removed—usually after 6 to 12 hours. Signs of **uterine tachysystole** (hyperstimulation) include uterine contractions that last longer than 90 seconds and/or more than five contractions in 10 minutes.

The vaginal insert can be removed by pulling on the netted string that protrudes from the vaginal orifice. Some women who receive cervical ripening products begin labor without additional oxytocin stimulation.

Dilating the cervix.

RU486 (Mifepristone). RU486 (Mifepristone) is a steroid receptor agonist that is used for early pregnancy termination.

Stripping the amniotic membranes. Stripping the amniotic membranes involves separation of the chorioamniotic membranes from the wall of the lower uterine segment and cervix by insertion of the examiner's gloved finger through the cervix and beyond the internal cervical os and rotating the finger along the lower uterine segment.

Hydroscopic dilators. Laminaria and Lamicel are mechanical dilators placed in the lower uterine segment that stimulate the release of prostaglandins from the fetal membranes and maternal decidua. They swell inside the cervix, resulting in mechanical cervical dilation.

Transcervical balloon dilators. A 16 Fr catheter with a 30 mL balloon can be inserted through the cervix and inflated. Mechanical pressure by gentle traction against the cervix dilates the cervix.

Extraamniotic saline infusion. An infusion of isotonic saline solution into the extraamniotic space is sometimes used with the balloon dilator. Evidence-based studies do not support the efficacy of this practice (Gabbe, 2012).

AMNIOTOMY

Amniotomy is the **artificial rupture of membranes (AROM)** (amniotic sac) by using a sterile sharp instrument to puncture the amniotic sac and release the amniotic fluid for the purpose of inducing or augmenting labor. It may also be performed to permit internal fetal monitoring (see Chapter 6). A physician or nurse-midwife performs the procedure. The nurse assists the health care provider with the procedure and cares for the woman and fetus afterward. Confirmation of a vertex presentation and the station is essential to prevent umbilical cord prolapse. The amniotomy stimulates prostaglandin secretion, which stimulates labor, but the loss of amniotic fluid may result in umbilical cord compression.

Complications

Three complications associated with amniotomy may also occur if a woman's membranes rupture spontaneously (**spontaneous rupture of membranes [SROM]**).

These complications are prolapse of the umbilical cord, infection, and abruptio placentae.

Prolapse of the Umbilical Cord. Prolapse may occur if the cord slips downward with the gush of amniotic fluid (p. 194).

Infection. Infection may occur because the membranes no longer block vaginal organisms from entering the uterus. Once performed, an amniotomy commits the woman to delivery within a certain time; the physician or nurse-midwife delays amniotomy until he or she is reasonably sure that birth will occur before the risk of infection markedly increases.

Abruptio Placentae. Abruptio placentae (separation of the placenta before birth) is more likely to occur if the uterus is overdistended with amniotic fluid (hydramnios) when the membranes rupture. The uterus becomes smaller with the discharge of amniotic fluid, but the placenta stays the same size and no longer fits its implantation site (see Chapter 5 for more information about abruptio placentae).

Nursing Care

The nursing care after amniotomy is the same as that after spontaneous membrane rupture: observing for complications and promoting the woman's comfort.

⬆ Nursing Tip

Observe for wet underpads and linens after the membranes rupture. Change them as often as needed to keep the woman relatively dry and to reduce the risk for infection or skin breakdown.

Observing for Complications. The fetal heart rate is recorded for at least 1 minute after amniotomy. Rates outside the normal range of 110 to 160 beats/min for a term fetus suggest a prolapsed umbilical cord. A large quantity of fluid increases the risk for prolapsed cord, especially if the fetus is high in the pelvis.

The color, odor, amount, and character of amniotic fluid are recorded. The fluid should be clear, possibly with flecks of vernix (newborn skin coating) and lanugo, and should not have a bad odor. Cloudy, yellow, or malodorous fluid suggests infection. Green fluid means that the fetus passed the first stool (meconium) into the fluid before birth. Meconium-stained amniotic fluid is associated with fetal compromise during labor and infant respiratory distress after birth.

The woman's temperature is taken every 2 to 4 hours after her membranes rupture according to facility policy. A maternal temperature of 38° C (100.4° F) or higher suggests infection. An increase in the fetal heart rate, especially if above 160 beats/min, may precede the woman's temperature increase.

Promoting Comfort. When amniotomy is anticipated, several disposable underpads are placed under the woman's hips to absorb the fluid that continues to leak from the woman's vagina during labor. Disposable underpads are changed often enough to keep her reasonably dry and to reduce the moist, warm environment that favors the growth of microorganisms.

Oxytocin Induction. Initiation or stimulation of contractions with oxytocin (Pitocin) is the most common method of labor induction and augmentation in women with a favorable or "ripe" cervix (Gabbe, 2012). Registered nurses, who have additional training in the induction of labor and electronic fetal monitoring, administer oxytocin. Augmentation of labor with oxytocin follows a similar procedure.

Oxytocin for induction or augmentation of labor is diluted in an IV solution. The oxytocin solution is a secondary (piggyback) infusion that is inserted into the primary (nonmedicated) IV solution line so it can be stopped quickly while an open IV line is maintained. The infusion of oxytocin solution is regulated with an infusion pump. Administration begins at a very low rate and is adjusted upward or downward according to how the fetus responds to labor and to the woman's contractions. The dose is individualized for every woman. When contractions are well established, it is often possible to reduce the rate of oxytocin. Augmentation of labor usually requires less total oxytocin than induction of labor, because the uterus is more sensitive to the drug when labor has already begun.

Continuous electronic monitoring is the usual method to assess and record fetal and maternal responses to oxytocin. Many health care providers prefer internal methods of monitoring when oxytocin is used, because these techniques are more accurate, especially for contraction intensity.

Nonpharmacological Methods to Stimulate Contractions

Walking. Many women benefit from a change in activity if their labor slows. Walking stimulates contractions, eases the pressure of the fetus on the mother's back, and adds gravity to the downward force of contractions. If she does not feel like walking, other upright positions often improve the effectiveness of each contraction. She can sit (in a chair, on the side of the bed, or in the bed), squat, kneel while facing the raised head of the bed for support, or maintain other upright positions.

Nipple Stimulation of Labor. Stimulating the nipples causes the woman's posterior pituitary gland to secrete oxytocin naturally. This improves the quality of contractions that have slowed or weakened, just as IV administration of synthetic oxytocin does. The woman can stimulate her nipples by doing the following:

- Pulling or rolling them, one at a time
- Gently brushing them with a dry washcloth
- Using water in a whirlpool tub or a shower
- Applying suction with a breast pump

If contractions become too strong with these techniques, the woman simply stops stimulation.

Complications of Augmentation of Labor

The most common complications related to overstimulation of contractions are fetal compromise and uterine rupture (see p. 195). Fetal compromise can occur because blood flow to the placenta is reduced if contractions are excessive (tachysystole). Most placental exchange of oxygen, nutrients, and waste products occurs between contractions. This exchange is likely to be impaired if the contractions are too long, too frequent, or too intense.

Water intoxication sometimes occurs because oxytocin inhibits the excretion of urine and promotes fluid retention. Water intoxication is not likely with the small amounts of oxytocin and fluids given intravenously during labor, but it is more likely to occur if large doses of oxytocin and fluids are given intravenously after birth.

Oxytocin is discontinued, or its rate reduced, if signs of fetal compromise or excessive uterine contractions occur. Fetal heart rates outside the normal range of 110 to 160 beats/min, late decelerations, and loss of variability (see Chapter 6) are the most common signs of fetal compromise.

 Safety Alert!

Tachysystole is most often evidenced by contraction frequency greater than every 2 minutes or 5 or more contractions within 10 minutes, durations longer than 90 seconds, or resting intervals shorter than 60 seconds.

The resting tone of the uterus (muscle tension when it is not contracting) is often higher than normal. Internal uterine activity monitoring allows determination of peak uterine pressures and uterine resting tone.

In addition to stopping the oxytocin infusion, the registered nurse chooses one or more of the following measures to correct adverse maternal or fetal reactions:

- Increasing the nonmedicated intravenous solution
- Changing the woman's position, avoiding the supine position
- Giving oxygen by facemask at 8 to 10 L/min

The health care provider is notified after corrective measures are taken. A tocolytic (drug that reduces uterine contractions such as magnesium sulfate or terbutaline) may be ordered if contractions do not quickly decrease after oxytocin is stopped.

In 2007, the Institute of Safe Medical Practices added intravenous oxytocin to a list of high-alert medications. High-alert medications have a higher risk of causing significant adverse reaction when used incorrectly.

The nurse must be aware of signs and symptoms of increased uterine activity and must monitor fetal heart rate every 15 minutes during active labor and every 5 minutes during the transitional phase. Safety interventions for oxytocin-induced uterine contractions or fetal heart rate abnormalities include the following:

- Notifying the health care provider and the registered nurse
- Repositioning the woman to left or right lateral position
- Decreasing the dose of oxytocin to half of the current rate or discontinuing oxytocin
- Preparing an intravenous (IV) bolus of lactated Ringer's
- Administering oxygen at 10 L/min via a nonrebreather facial mask
- Preparing IV terbutaline for administration
- Assessing uterine contractions and fetal heart rate every 5 minutes

Nursing Care

In 2007, the American Academy of Pediatrics (AAP) and the Congress of Obstetricians and Gynecologists (ACOG) recommended that an RN, with 1:1 or 1:2 ratio, care for patients undergoing oxytocin-induced labor. Fetal heart rate must be assessed and recorded every 15 minutes during active labor and every 5 minutes during transition. Baseline maternal vital signs are assessed, and a fetal monitor tracing is performed to identify contraindications to induction or augmentation before the procedure begins.

If abnormalities are noted in either, the nurse stops the oxytocin and begins measures to reduce contractions and increase placental blood flow. The woman's blood pressure, pulse rate, and respirations are measured every 30 to 60 minutes. Her temperature is taken every 2 to 4 hours. Recording her intake and output helps identify potential water intoxication.

✎ Nursing Tip

Women who have oxytocin stimulation of labor may find that their contractions are difficult to manage. Help them to stay focused on breathing and relaxation techniques with each contraction.

VERSION

Version is a method of changing the fetal presentation, usually from breech or oblique to cephalic. There are two methods: external and internal. External version is the more common one. A successful version reduces the likelihood that the woman will need cesarean delivery.

Risks and Contraindications

Few maternal and fetal risks are associated with version, especially external version. Version is not indicated if there is any maternal or fetal reason that vaginal birth should not occur, because that is its goal.

The following are examples of maternal or fetal conditions that are contraindications for version:

- Disproportion between the mother's pelvis and fetal size
- Abnormal uterine or pelvic size or shape
- Abnormal placental placement
- Previous cesarean birth with a vertical uterine incision
- Active herpes virus infection
- Inadequate amniotic fluid
- Poor placental function
- Multifetal gestation
- Malfunctioning placenta

Version may not be attempted in a woman who has a higher risk for uterine rupture, such as several previous cesarean births or high parity. Version is not usually attempted if the fetal presenting part is engaged in the pelvis. The main risk to the fetus is that it will become entangled in the umbilical cord, thus compressing the cord. This is more likely to happen if there is not adequate room to turn the fetus, such as in multifetal gestation (e.g., twins) or when the amount of amniotic fluid is minimal.

Technique

External version is done after 37 weeks of gestation but before the onset of labor. The procedure begins with a non–stress test (NST) or biophysical profile (BPP; see Table 5-1) to determine whether the fetus is in good condition and if there is adequate amniotic fluid to perform the version. The woman receives a tocolytic drug to relax her uterus during the version.

Using ultrasound to guide the procedure, the physician pushes the fetal buttocks upward out of the pelvis while pushing the fetal head downward toward the pelvis in either a clockwise or a counterclockwise turn. The fetus is monitored frequently during the procedure. The tocolytic drug is discontinued after the external version is completed (or the effort abandoned). Rh-negative women receive a dose of Rho (D) immune globulin (RhoGAM) to prevent development of RH positive antibodies if the fetus is RH positive.

Internal version is an emergency procedure. The physician usually performs internal version during a vaginal birth of twins to change the fetal presentation of the second twin.

Nursing Care

Nursing care of the woman having external version includes assisting with the procedure and observing the mother and fetus afterward for 1 to 2 hours. Baseline maternal vital signs and a fetal monitor strip (part of the NST or BPP) are taken before the version. The mother's vital signs and the fetal heart rate are observed to ensure return to normal levels after the version is complete.

Vaginal leaking of amniotic fluid suggests that manipulating the fetus caused a tear in the membranes, and this is reported. Uterine contractions usually decrease or stop shortly after the version. The physician is notified if they do not. The nurse reviews signs of labor with the woman, because version is performed near term, when spontaneous labor is expected.

EPISIOTOMY AND LACERATIONS

Episiotomy is the surgical enlargement of the vaginal opening during birth. Either the physician or a nurse-midwife performs and repairs an episiotomy. A laceration is an uncontrolled tear of the tissues that results in a jagged wound. Lacerations of the perineum and episiotomy incisions are treated similarly.

Perineal lacerations and often episiotomies are described by the amount of tissue involved:

- *First degree:* Involves the superficial vaginal mucosa or perineal skin
- *Second degree:* Involves the vaginal mucosa, perineal skin, and deeper tissues of the perineum
- *Third degree:* Same as second degree, plus involves the anal sphincter
- *Fourth degree:* Extends through the anal sphincter into the rectal mucosa

Women with third- and fourth-degree lacerations may have more discomfort postpartum if they are constipated after birth.

 Nutrition Considerations

Third- or Fourth-Degree Laceration

Pay special attention to a woman's diet and fluids if she had a third- or fourth-degree laceration. A high-fiber diet and adequate fluids help to prevent constipation that might result in a breakdown of the perineal area where the laceration was sutured.

Indications

Fetal indications for an episiotomy are similar to those for forceps or vacuum extraction (see p. 180). Additional maternal indications include the following:

- Better control over where and how much the vaginal opening is enlarged
- An opening with a clean edge rather than the ragged opening of a tear

Episiotomy is no longer routinely performed during vaginal delivery but is used with specific indications when problems occur during the expulsion stage of labor. Perineal massage and stretching exercises before labor are becoming popular techniques to decrease the need for an episiotomy during birth.

Risks

As in other incisions, infection is the primary risk in an episiotomy or laceration. An additional risk is extension of the episiotomy with a laceration into or through the rectal sphincter (third or fourth degree), which can cause prolonged perineal discomfort and stress incontinence.

Technique

The episiotomy is performed with blunt-tipped scissors just before birth. One of the following two directions is chosen (Figure 8-1):

- *Midline (median),* extending directly from the lower vaginal border toward the anus
- *Mediolateral,* extending from the lower vaginal border toward the mother's right or left

A median episiotomy is easier to repair and heals neatly. The mediolateral incision provides more room, but greater scarring during healing may cause painful sexual intercourse. A laceration that extends a median

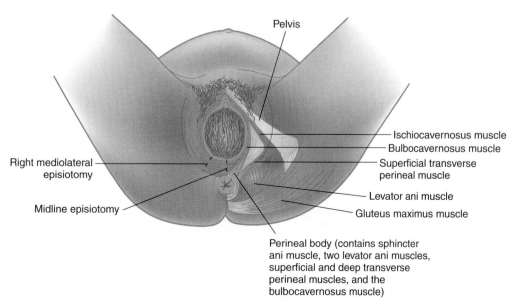

FIGURE 8-1 Episiotomies. The two common types of episiotomies are midline (median) and mediolateral. (From Matteson PS: *Women's health during the childbearing years: a community-based approach,* St Louis, 2001, Mosby.)

episiotomy is more likely to involve the rectal sphincter than one that extends the mediolateral episiotomy.

Nursing Care

Nursing care for an episiotomy or laceration begins during the fourth stage of labor. Cold packs should be applied to the perineum for at least the first 12 hours to reduce pain, bruising, and edema. After 12 to 24 hours of cold applications, warmth in the form of heat packs or sitz baths increases blood circulation, enhancing comfort and healing. Mild oral analgesics are usually sufficient for pain management. See Chapter 9 for postpartum nursing care of the woman with an episiotomy or laceration.

FORCEPS AND VACUUM EXTRACTION BIRTHS

An obstetrician uses obstetric forceps and vacuum extractors to provide traction and rotation to the fetal head when the mother's pushing efforts are insufficient to accomplish a safe delivery. Forceps are instruments with curved blades that fit around the fetal head without unduly compressing it (Figure 8-2). Several different styles are available to assist the birth of the fetal head in a cephalic presentation or the after-coming head in a breech delivery. Forceps may also help the physician extract the fetal head through the incision during cesarean birth.

A vacuum extractor uses suction applied to the fetal head so the physician can assist the mother's expulsive efforts (Figure 8-3). The vacuum extractor is used only with an occiput presentation. One advantage of the vacuum extractor is that it does not take up room in the mother's pelvis, as forceps do. Since 2001, the use of vacuum extractors has increased whereas the use of forceps has decreased during delivery. However, since 2011, the use of cesarean sections has increased whereas both the use of forceps and vacuum extractors has decreased (Gabbe, 2012).

Indications

Forceps or vacuum extraction may be used to end the second stage of labor if it is in the best interest of the mother or fetus. The mother may be exhausted, or

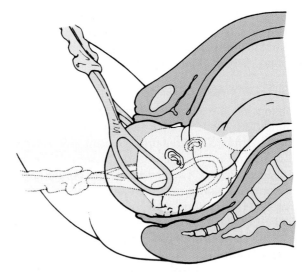

FIGURE 8-2 Use of forceps to assist the birth of the fetal head. After applying the forceps to each side of the fetal head and locking the two blades, the physician pulls, following the pelvic curve.

she may be unable to push effectively. Women with cardiac or pulmonary disorders often have forceps or vacuum extraction births, because prolonged pushing can worsen these conditions. Fetal indications include conditions in which there is evidence of an increased risk to the fetus near the end of labor. The cervix must be fully dilated, the membranes ruptured, the bladder empty, and the fetal head engaged and at +2 station for optimal outcome.

Contraindications

Forceps or vacuum extraction cannot substitute for cesarean birth if the maternal or fetal condition requires a quicker delivery. Delivery by these techniques is not done if they would be more traumatic than cesarean birth, such as when the fetus is high in the pelvis or too large for a vaginal delivery.

Risks

Trauma to maternal or fetal tissues is the main risk when forceps or vacuum extraction is used. The mother may have a laceration or hematoma (collection of blood in the tissues) in her vagina. The infant may have

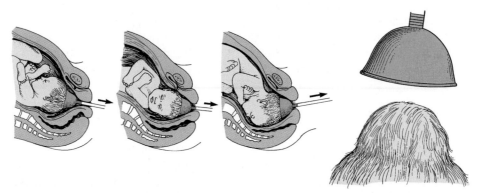

FIGURE 8-3 Use of the vacuum extractor to rotate the fetal head and assist with delivery. The arrows indicate the direction of traction on the vacuum cup. The vacuum cup is positioned on the midline, near the posterior fontanelle. (From Lowdermilk DL, Perry SE, Cashion KL: *Maternity nursing*, ed 8, St Louis, 2013, Mosby.)

bruising, facial or scalp lacerations or abrasions, cephalohematoma (see Chapter 12), or intracranial hemorrhage. The vacuum extractor causes a harmless area of circular edema on the infant's scalp (**chignon**) where it was applied.

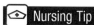 **Nursing Tip**

Many parents are concerned about the marks made by forceps. Reassure them that these marks are temporary and usually resolve without treatment.

Technique

The health care provider catheterizes the woman to prevent trauma to her bladder and to make more room in her pelvis. After the forceps are applied, the physician pulls in line with the pelvic curve. An episiotomy is usually done. After the fetal head is brought under the mother's symphysis pubis, the rest of the birth occurs in the usual way.

Birth assisted with the vacuum extractor follows a similar sequence. The health care provider applies the cup over the posterior fontanelle of the fetal occiput, and suction is created with a machine to hold it there. Traction is applied by pulling on the handle of the extractor cup.

Nursing Care

If the use of forceps or vacuum extraction is anticipated, the nurse places the sterile equipment on the delivery instrument table. After birth, care is similar to that for episiotomy and perineal lacerations. Ice is applied to the perineum to reduce bruising and edema. The physician is notified if the woman has signs of vaginal hematoma, which include severe and poorly relieved pelvic or rectal pain.

The infant's head is examined for lacerations, abrasions, or bruising. Mild facial reddening and molding (alteration in shape) of the head are common and do not necessitate treatment. Cold treatments are not used on neonates, because they would cause hypothermia.

Pressure from forceps may injure the infant's facial nerve. This is evidenced by facial asymmetry (different appearance of right and left sides), which is most obvious when the infant cries. Facial nerve injury usually resolves without treatment. The scalp chignon from the vacuum extractor does not necessitate intervention and resolves quickly.

CESAREAN BIRTH

Cesarean birth is the surgical delivery of the fetus through incisions in the mother's abdomen and uterus. Cesarean section is currently the most common major surgical procedure in the United States. Cesarean birth rates in the United States are 27.6% (National Center for Health Statistics [NCHS], 2008), and the goal of *Healthy People 2020* (U.S. Department of Health and Human Services, 2010) is to reduce cesarean sections to 15%. This is the basis for some of the changes in the management of the second stage of labor, such as the following:

- Position variation (upright or horizontal)
- Epidural analgesia and subarachnoid analgesia that allows ambulation and delivery in squatting position
- Oxytocin (Pitocin) augmentation of labor
- Spontaneous open glottis pushing when fetus is at +1 station
- Use of vacuum-assisted delivery replacing forceps delivery
- Electronic fetal and uterine monitoring

Indications

Several conditions may necessitate cesarean delivery:

- Abnormal labor
- Inability of the fetus to pass through the mother's pelvis (**cephalopelvic disproportion**) (Most breech presentations are delivered by cesarean section)
- Maternal conditions such as gestational hypertension or diabetes mellitus
- Active maternal herpes virus, which may cause serious or fatal infant infection
- Previous surgery on the uterus, including the classic type of cesarean incision
- Fetal compromise, including prolapsed umbilical cord and abnormal presentations
- Placenta previa or abruptio placentae

Contraindications

There are few contraindications to cesarean birth, but it is not usually performed if the fetus is dead or too premature to survive or if the mother has abnormal blood clotting.

Risks

Cesarean birth carries risks to both mother and fetus. Maternal risks are similar to those of other types of surgery and include the following:

- Risks related to anesthesia (see Chapter 7)
- Respiratory complications
- Hemorrhage
- Blood clots
- Injury to the urinary tract
- Delayed intestinal peristalsis (paralytic ileus)
- Infection

Risks to the newborn may include the following:

- Inadvertent preterm birth
- Respiratory problems because of delayed absorption of lung fluid
- Injury, such as laceration or bruising

To help prevent the unintentional birth of a preterm fetus, the physician often performs amniocentesis before a planned cesarean birth to determine if the fetal lungs are mature (see Chapter 5).

Technique

Cesarean birth may occur under planned, unplanned, or emergency conditions. The preparation is similar for each and includes routine preoperative care such as obtaining informed consent. If the woman wears eyeglasses, they should accompany her to the operating room, because she is usually awake to bond with the infant after birth.

Preparations for Cesarean Birth. As with other surgery, several laboratory studies are performed to identify anemia or blood-clotting abnormalities. Complete blood count, coagulation studies, and blood typing and history screening are common, and appropriate consent is obtained. One or more units of blood may be typed and cross-matched if the woman is likely to need a transfusion. The baseline vital signs of the mother and the fetal heart rate are recorded. The woman is placed in a supine position with a wedge under the hip to prevent decreased blood flow to the fetus. A regional anesthetic is administered, and an IV medication to reduce gastric acidity and speed gastric emptying is provided. A prophylactic IV antibiotic may be administered before surgery. Shaving of the skin or hair removal is not necessary.

An indwelling Foley catheter is inserted to keep the bladder empty and to prevent trauma to it. The catheter bag is placed near the head of the operating table so the anesthesiologist can monitor urine output, an important indicator of the woman's circulating blood volume. The circulating nurse scrubs the abdomen with chlorhexidine alcohol by using a circular motion that goes outward from the incisional area. The father or woman's partner may don a hat, mask, and gown and provide support to the mother at the head of the table (see Figure 8-5, *D*).

Types of Incisions. There are two incisions in cesarean birth: a skin incision and a uterine incision. The directions of these incisions are not always the same.

Skin incisions. The skin incision is done in either a vertical or a transverse direction. A vertical incision allows more room if a large fetus is being delivered, and it is usually needed for an obese woman. In an emergency, the vertical incision can be accomplished more quickly. The transverse, or Pfannenstiel, incision is nearly invisible when healed but cannot always be used in obese women or in women with a large fetus.

Uterine incisions. The more important of the two incisions is the one that cuts into the uterus. There are three types of uterine incisions (Figure 8-4): low transverse, low vertical, and classic.

Low transverse incision. A low transverse incision is preferred, because it is not likely to rupture during another birth, causes less blood loss, and is easier to repair. It may not be an option if the fetus is large or if there is a placenta previa in the area where the incision would be made. This type of incision makes VBAC possible for subsequent births.

Low transverse incision

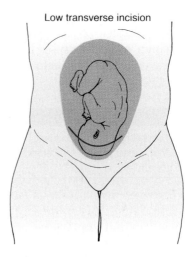

Low vertical incision

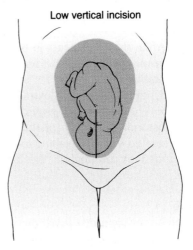

Classic incision

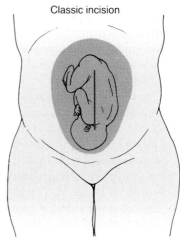

FIGURE 8-4 Three types of uterine incisions for cesarean birth. The low transverse uterine incision is preferred, because it is not likely to rupture during a subsequent birth, allowing vaginal birth after a cesarean birth. The low vertical and classic incisions may occasionally be used. The skin incision and uterine incision do not always match.

Low vertical incision. A low vertical incision produces minimal blood loss and allows delivery of a larger fetus. However, it is more likely to rupture during another birth, although less so than the classic incision.

Classic incision. The classic incision is rarely used, because it involves more blood loss, and of the three types it is the most likely to rupture during another pregnancy. However, it may be the only choice if the fetus is in a transverse lie or if there is scarring or a placenta previa in the lower anterior uterus.

Sequence of Events

After the woman has received a spinal anesthetic and has been scrubbed and draped, the physician makes the skin incision. After making the uterine incision, the physician ruptures the membranes (unless they are already ruptured) with a sharp instrument. The amniotic fluid is suctioned from the operative area, and its amount, color, and odor are noted.

The physician reaches into the uterus to lift out the fetal head or buttocks. Forceps or vacuum extraction may be used to assist birth of the head. The infant's mouth and nose are quickly suctioned to remove secretions, and the cord is clamped. The physician hands the infant to the nurse, who receives the infant into sterile blankets and places the infant into a radiant warmer. A pediatrician is usually available for resuscitation.

After the birth of the infant, the physician scoops out the placenta and examines it for intactness. The uterine cavity is sponged to remove blood clots and other debris. The uterine and skin incisions are then closed and secured in layers with sutures, staples, or dermabond (Figure 8-5).

Nursing Care

The registered nurse assumes most of the preoperative and postoperative care of the woman. This includes obtaining the required laboratory studies, administering medications, performing preoperative teaching, and preparing for surgery. Women who have cesarean births usually need greater emotional support than those having vaginal births. They are usually happy and excited about the newborn, but they may also feel grief, guilt, or anger because the expected course of birth did not occur. These feelings may linger and resurface during another pregnancy. Emotional care of the partner and family is essential; they are included in explanations of the surgery as much as the woman wishes. The partner may be frightened when an emergency cesarean is needed but may not express these feelings because the woman needs so much support. The nurse informs the partner when he or she may enter the operating room, because 30 minutes or longer may be needed to administer a regional anesthetic and for surgical preparations if there is no emergency. The partner dons surgical attire during this time.

The partner may be almost as exhausted as the woman if a cesarean birth is performed after hours of labor. The thoughtful nurse includes the partner and promotes his or her emotional and physical well-being. The mother, neonate, and partner are kept together as much as possible after birth, just as for a vaginal birth. The woman and her partner are encouraged to talk about the cesarean birth so they can integrate the experience. The nurse answers questions about events surrounding the birth. The focus is on the *birth* rather than on the surgical aspects of cesarean delivery.

Nursing assessments after cesarean birth are similar to those after vaginal birth, including assessment of the uterine fundus. Assessments are done every 15 minutes for the first 1 or 2 hours and then every 30 minutes for 1 hour according to hospital policy. Recovery-room assessments after cesarean birth include the following:

- Vital signs to identify hemorrhage or shock; a pulse oximeter is used to better identify depressed respiratory function
- IV site and rate of solution flow
- Fundus for firmness, height, and midline position
- Dressing for drainage
- Lochia for quantity, color, and presence of clots
- Urine output from the indwelling catheter
- Return of sensation to the lower body

The fundus is checked as gently as possible. The woman flexes her knees slightly and takes slow, deep breaths to minimize the discomfort of fundal assessments. While supporting the lower uterus with one hand, the fingers of the other hand are gently "walked" from the side of the uterus toward the midline. Massage is not needed if the fundus is already firm.

> **!** **Safety Alert!**
>
> Although assessing the uterus after cesarean birth causes discomfort, it is important to do so regularly, because the woman may have a relaxed uterus that causes excessive blood loss.

The woman is told to take deep breaths at each assessment and to cough to move secretions from her airways. A small pillow or folded blanket supports her incision when she coughs or moves, which reduces pain. Changing her position every 1 or 2 hours helps expand her lungs and also makes her more comfortable.

Pain relief after cesarean birth may be accomplished by a patient-controlled analgesia (PCA) pump or by intermittent injections of narcotic analgesics. Epidural narcotics provide long-lasting pain relief but are associated with delayed respiratory depression and itching (see Chapter 7), which vary with the drug injected. The woman is changed to oral analgesics after about the first 24 hours. Nursing Care Plan 8-1 on p. 186 details interventions for selected nursing diagnoses that pertain to the woman with an unplanned cesarean birth.

ABNORMAL LABOR

A normal labor evidences a regular progression in cervical effacement, dilation, and descent of the fetus. Abnormal labor, called **dysfunctional labor**, does not progress. **Dystocia** is a term used to describe a difficult labor.

The "four Ps" of labor (see Chapter 6) interact constantly throughout the birth. Abnormalities in the powers, passengers, passage, or psyche may result in a

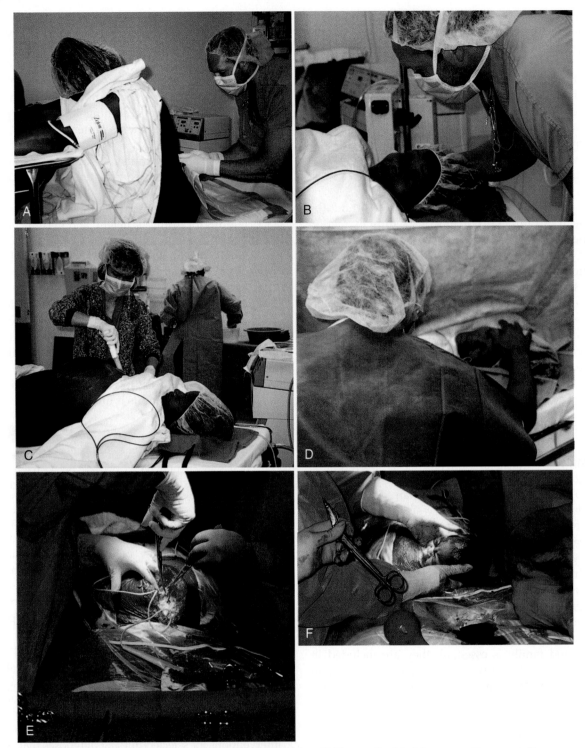

FIGURE 8-5 Cesarean section birth. **A,** Spinal anesthetic is given. **B,** The anesthesiologist reassures the woman. **C,** The nurse preps the abdomen. **D,** The partner encourages the woman. **E,** A vertical incision is made. **F,** The head of the infant is lifted out of the uterus.

dysfunctional labor. In addition, the length of labor may be unusually short or long. Labor abnormalities may necessitate use of forceps or cesarean delivery, and they are more likely to result in injury to the mother or fetus.

It is essential for nurses to understand the normal birth process so that deviations from normal can be recognized and prompt interventions implemented.

Effective support for the woman and her family is part of competent and compassionate care. Risk factors for dysfunctional labor include the following:

- Advanced maternal age
- Obesity
- Overdistention of uterus (**hydramnios** or multifetal pregnancy)

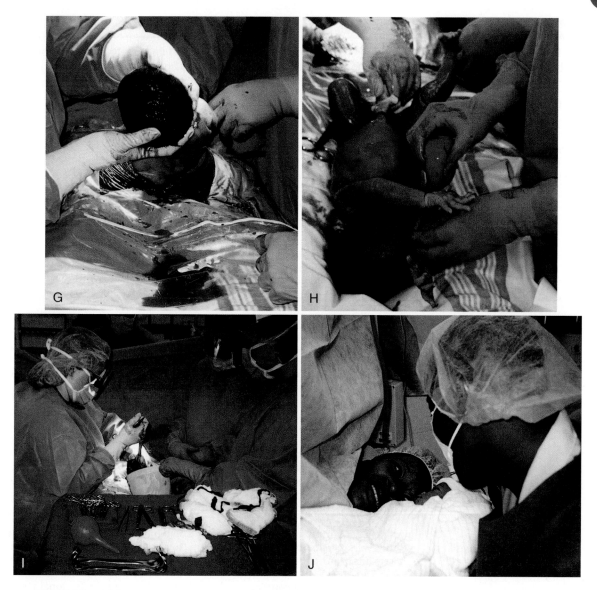

FIGURE 8-5, cont'd   Cesarean section birth. **G,** The body of the infant is lifted out of the uterus. **H,** The infant is placed on the mother's abdomen, and the infant's secretions are suctioned with a bulb syringe. Note the active muscle tone of the newborn. **I,** The placenta is delivered from the uterus. **J,** The parents and the newborn bond. (Courtesy Pat Spier, RN-C.)

- Abnormal presentation
- Cephalopelvic disproportion (CPD)
- Overstimulation of the uterus
- Maternal fatigue, dehydration, fear
- Lack of analgesic assistance

PROBLEMS WITH THE POWERS OF LABOR

Increased Uterine Muscle Tone

Increased uterine muscle tone usually occurs during the latent phase of labor (before 4 cm of cervical dilation) and is characterized by contractions that are frequent, cramplike, and poorly coordinated. These contractions are painful but nonproductive. Even between contractions the uterus is tense, which reduces blood flow to the placenta. Hypertonic labor dysfunction is less common than hypotonic dysfunction. Table 8-2

summarizes the differences between hypertonic and hypotonic labor dysfunction.

Medical Treatment. Medical treatment may include mild sedation to allow the woman to rest. Tocolytic drugs (see p. 193) such as terbutaline (Brethine) may be ordered.

Nursing Care. Women with increased uterine muscle tone are uncomfortable and frustrated. Anxiety about the lack of progress and fatigue impair their ability to tolerate pain. They may lose confidence in their ability to give birth. The nurse should accept the woman's frustration and that of her partner. Both may be exhausted from the near-constant discomfort. Warm

★ Nursing Care Plan 8-1   The Woman with an Unplanned Cesarean Birth

PATIENT DATA A woman, para 0, gravida 1, has been using breathing, relaxation, and imagery techniques during the first stage of labor, and her husband has been helpful and supportive. However, the labor is not progressing, and there are signs of fetal distress. The physician orders that the patient be prepared for an emergency cesarean section.

Selected Nursing Diagnosis: Anxiety related to development of complications

Goals	Nursing Interventions	Rationales
The woman and her partner will express decreased anxiety after explanations about the planned surgery.	Determine stress level and learning needs.	Provides a database to build on to provide information that will decrease anxiety.
	Reinforce all explanations given by physician, expressing them in simpler terms if needed.	Anxiety tends to narrow attention; although physician may have explained the need for surgery, the woman and her partner may not have comprehended everything they were told.
	Encourage the woman to continue using the breathing and relaxation techniques she learned in prepared childbirth classes as long as contractions continue.	Learned pain management techniques increase the woman's sense of control. Control over a situation reduces feelings of helplessness and decreases anxiety.
	Tell the woman what the operating room looks like and who will be present. Explain basic equipment, such as catheter, narrow table, monitors for her heart and blood pressure, anesthesia machine, and large overhead lights. Explain that personnel will wear protective equipment such as masks, eye protection, gowns, gloves, hats, and shoe covers.	Commonplace equipment and attire in an operating room can be intimidating for someone who has not seen them before. Unfamiliarity increases anxiety; preparation reduces anxiety and fear of the unknown.
	Describe the usual postoperative care: assessment of vital signs, fundus, vaginal bleeding, dressing, and catheter. Tell her she will be asked to take deep breaths and change position regularly.	If woman understands common postoperative care, she is more likely to cooperate with it, even if assessments are uncomfortable.
	Encourage her partner to be with her during surgery, and do not separate family afterward, if possible.	Companionship of familiar persons helps to reduce anxiety; keeping new family together promotes attachment to the newborn.
	Stay with the woman. Encourage verbalization and support her coping mechanisms.	The presence of a professional person reduces anxiety.

Selected Nursing Diagnosis: Impaired comfort related to decreased coping ability

Goals	Nursing Interventions	Rationales
The woman will verbalize reduced discomfort or will be able to use effective techniques to decrease perception of pain.	Determine the nature, duration, and location of pain.	Never assume that the pain is related to a contraction. Locating the site of pain helps identify complications that may be occurring (e.g., embolism). Assessing pain and contractions can help identify a prolonged contraction that can cause fetal hypoxia.
	Encourage the woman to continue to use coping mechanisms learned during prenatal classes. Use therapeutic touch to increase comfort.	A feeling of loss of control can increase the perception of pain. Reduction of tension can promote comfort.
	Maintain a calm manner and environment.	A calm manner calms the parents and reduces anxieties and tensions that elevate pain perception.

Critical Thinking Question

1. What are the advantages and disadvantages of a transverse abdominal incision compared to the classic midline incision?

Table 8-2	Differences Between Hypertonic and Hypotonic Labor Dysfunction
HYPERTONIC LABOR	**HYPOTONIC LABOR**
Contractions are poorly coordinated, frequent, and painful	Contractions are weak and ineffective
Uterine resting tone between contractions is tense	Uterine resting tone is not elevated
It is less common than hypotonic labor dysfunction	It is more common than hypertonic labor dysfunction
It is more likely to occur during latent labor, before 4 cm of cervical dilation	It occurs during the active phase, after 4 cm of cervical dilation It is more likely if the uterus is overly distended or if the woman has had many other births
Medical management includes mild sedation and tocolytic drugs	Medical management includes amniotomy, oxytocin augmentation, and adequate hydration
Nursing interventions include acceptance of the woman's discomfort and frustration and the provision of comfort measures	Nonpharmacological stimulation methods include walking, assuming other upright positions, and stimulating the nipples Other nursing interventions include position changes and encouragement

showers or baths may help to promote relaxation. It is important not to equate the amount of pain a woman reports with how much she "should" feel at that point in labor. The nurse provides general comfort measures that promote rest and relaxation.

Decreased Uterine Muscle Tone

A woman who has decreased uterine muscle tone has contractions that are too weak to be effective during active labor. The woman begins labor normally, but contractions diminish (hypotonic labor dysfunction) during the active phase (after 4 cm of cervical dilation), when the pace of labor is expected to accelerate. This is more likely to occur if the uterus is overdistended, such as with twins, a large fetus, or excess amniotic fluid (hydramnios). Uterine overdistention stretches the muscle fibers and thus reduces their ability to contract effectively.

Medical Treatment. The physician usually performs an amniotomy if the membranes are intact. Augmentation of labor with oxytocin or by nipple stimulation increases the strength of contractions. IV or oral fluids may improve the quality of contractions if the woman is dehydrated.

Nursing Care. The woman is reasonably comfortable but frustrated because her labor is not progressing. In addition to providing care related to amniotomy and labor augmentation, the nurse provides emotional support to the woman and her partner. The woman is allowed to express her frustrations. The nurse tells the woman when she is making progress to encourage continuation of her efforts.

Position changes may help to relieve discomfort and enhance progress. Contractions are usually stronger and more effective when the woman assumes an upright position or lies on her side, although they may be less frequent. Walking or nipple stimulation may intensify contractions. Nursing Care Plan 8-2

details interventions for selected nursing diagnoses that pertain to the woman with labor dysfunction.

Ineffective Maternal Pushing

The woman may not push effectively during the second stage of labor because she does not understand which techniques to use or fears tearing her perineal tissues. Epidural or subarachnoid blocks (see Chapter 7) may depress or eliminate the natural urge to push. An exhausted woman may be unable to gather her resources to push appropriately.

Nursing Care. Nursing care focuses on coaching the woman about the most effective techniques for pushing. If she cannot feel her contractions because of a regional block, the nurse tells her when to push as each contraction reaches its peak.

The exhausted woman may benefit from pushing only when she feels a strong urge. The fearful woman may benefit from explanations that sensations of tearing or splitting often accompany fetal descent but that her body is designed to accommodate the fetus. Promoting relaxation, relieving fatigue, changing position, and increasing hydration can help the woman sustain the energy level needed for effective pushing.

PROBLEMS WITH THE FETUS

Fetal Size

A large fetus (**macrosomia**) is generally considered to be one that weighs more than 4000 g (8.8 lb) at birth. The large fetus may not fit through the woman's pelvis. A very large fetus also distends the uterus and can contribute to hypotonic labor dysfunction.

Sometimes a single part of the fetus is too large. For example, the fetus may have hydrocephalus (an abnormal amount of fluid in the brain) (see Chapter 14). In that case the fetal body size and weight may be normal, but the head is too large to fit through the pelvis. These infants are often in abnormal presentations as well.

⭐ Nursing Care Plan 8-2	The Woman with Hypotonic Labor Dysfunction

PATIENT DATA A woman, para 0, gravida 1, is admitted at 7 PM because of premature rupture of the membranes. Contractions remain irregular at 7 AM the next morning. The woman appears anxious and fearful concerning her lack of progress.

Selected Nursing Diagnosis: Risk for infection related to loss of barrier (ruptured membranes)

Goals	Nursing Interventions	Rationales
The woman's temperature will remain under 38° C (100.4° F), and the amniotic fluid will remain clear with a mild odor.	Take the woman's temperature every 2 to 4 hours, or more often if elevated. At the same time, assess the amniotic fluid drainage for color, clarity, and odor.	Elevated temperature is a sign of infection; cloudy, yellow, or foul-smelling fluid suggests infection; and meconium (green) staining suggests fetal compromise but is also seen with prolonged pregnancy.
	Observe fetal heart rates (see Chapter 6).	Fetal tachycardia (rate >160 beats/min) may be the first sign of infection. Poor fetal oxygenation may also occur, especially with abnormal labor.
	Assist the woman to maintain good perineal hygiene (wiping front to back). Keep underpads clean and dry.	Good hygiene reduces the possibility of introducing bacteria into the birth canal.
	Monitor intravenous (IV) line, electrode sites, and incision sites for signs of redness, edema, pain, and drainage.	These are the primary sites where infection can occur.
	After birth, continue to assess the woman's temperature at least every 4 hours. Assess the lochia (postbirth vaginal drainage) for a foul odor or brown color.	The woman may not show these signs of infection until after birth.
	Observe the neonate for a temperature below 36.2° C (97° F) or above 38° C (100.4° F). Observe for poor feeding, lethargy, irritability, or "not looking right."	The neonate may become infected in utero and display these signs of infection after birth. Neonatal sepsis may occur with prolonged rupture of membranes and is a potentially fatal infection.

Selected Nursing Diagnosis: Ineffective coping related to frustration with slow labor and delayed birth

Goals	Nursing Interventions	Rationales
The woman will use breathing and relaxation techniques that she and her partner learned in prepared childbirth class. The woman will verbalize an understanding of what is happening and how she can still participate in the birth process.	If there is no contraindication, encourage the woman to walk or to sit upright in bed or chair. Walking may not be wise if the membranes are ruptured and the fetus is high.	Upright positions enhance fetal descent. Walking strengthens labor contractions; walking when membranes are ruptured and fetal station is high could lead to umbilical cord prolapse.
	Help the woman to use natural methods to stimulate contractions, such as nipple stimulation. Encourage a shower or whirlpool if available and not contraindicated.	Nipple stimulation causes the woman's posterior pituitary gland to secrete natural oxytocin, which strengthens contractions. Water may help the woman relax, which improves labor. All nonpharmacological methods to stimulate labor enhance her sense of control.
	Assist the registered nurse with oxytocin augmentation if it is ordered. Observe contractions for excessive frequency (more frequent than every 2 minutes), duration (>90 seconds), or inadequate rest interval (<60 seconds). Observe fetal heart rate for rates outside the normal range of 110 to 160 beats/min.	The primary risks of oxytocin augmentation or induction of labor relate to overstimulating the uterus. Excessive contractions can reduce fetal oxygen supply. These are signs of potential uterine overstimulation.
	Explain to the woman how each method is expected to help her labor advance. Inform her any time she is making progress, either in improved	If the woman understands the reason for any interventions, she will more likely cooperate with them and feel more in control. Knowing that her efforts are having the desired effect encourages

★ Nursing Care Plan 8-2	The Woman with Hypotonic Labor Dysfunction—cont'd	
Goals	**Nursing Interventions**	**Rationales**
	contractions or with increasing cervical dilation.	her to continue with her learned coping methods.
	Help the woman relax and use the breathing techniques she learned in prepared childbirth class. Praise and support her when she uses them.	Relaxation promotes normal labor. Praise encourages the woman to continue efforts at managing contractions.
	Reposition frequently. Acknowledge the reality of discomfort.	Feeling supported enhances coping.

Critical Thinking Question

1. A woman, para 0, gravida 1, has been admitted with ruptured membranes. Contractions are irregular and ineffective, and progress in dilation and effacement of the cervix is very slow. An oxytocin IV infusion is started after 15 hours. What could happen if the health care provider decided not to augment labor?

Shoulder dystocia may occur, usually when the fetus is large. The fetal head is born, but the shoulders become impacted above the mother's symphysis pubis. A shoulder dystocia is an emergency, because the fetus needs to breathe. The head is out, but the chest cannot expand. The cord is compressed between the fetus and the mother's pelvis. The health care provider may request that the nurse apply firm downward pressure just above the symphysis pubis (suprapubic pressure) to push the shoulders toward the pelvic canal. Squatting or sharp flexion of the thighs against the abdomen may also loosen the shoulders.

Nursing Care. If the woman successfully delivers a large infant, both mother and child should be observed for injuries after birth. The woman may have a large episiotomy or laceration. The large infant is more likely to have a fracture of one or both clavicles (collarbones). The infant's clavicles are felt for crepitus (crackling sensation) or deformity of the bones, and the arms are observed for equal movement (unilateral Moro reflex). The woman is more at risk for uterine atony and postpartum hemorrhage, because after birth her uterus does not contract well to control bleeding at the placental site.

Abnormal Fetal Presentation or Position

Labor is most efficient if the fetus is in a flexed, cephalic presentation and in one of the occiput anterior positions (see Chapter 6). Abnormalities of fetal presentation and position prevent the smallest diameter of the fetal head from passing through the smallest diameter of the pelvis for the effective progress of labor.

Abnormal Presentations. The fetus in an abnormal presentation, such as the breech or face presentation, does not pass easily through the woman's pelvis and interferes with the most efficient mechanisms of labor (see Chapter 6).

In the United States, most fetuses in the breech presentation are born by cesarean delivery. During vaginal birth in this presentation, the trunk and extremities are born before the head. After the fetal body delivers, the umbilical cord can be compressed between the fetal head and the mother's pelvis. The head, which is the single largest part of the fetus, must be quickly delivered to avoid fetal hypoxia. Figure 8-6 illustrates the sequence of delivery for a vaginal breech birth.

Intrapartum nurses must be prepared to assist with a breech birth, because a woman sometimes arrives at the birth facility in advanced labor with her fetus in a breech presentation. External version is sometimes used to avoid the need for cesarean delivery in the case of a breech presentation; however, external version is not always successful, and the fetus sometimes returns to the abnormal presentation.

Abnormal Positions. A common cause of abnormal labor is a fetus that remains in a persistent occiput posterior position (left [LOP] or right [ROP]). The fetal occiput occupies either the left or the right posterior quadrant of the mother's pelvis. In most women the fetal head rotates in a clockwise or counterclockwise direction until the occiput is in one of the anterior quadrants of the pelvis (left [LOA] or right [ROA]).

Labor is likely to be longer when rotation does not occur. Intense and poorly relieved back and leg pain characterize labor when the fetus is in the occiput posterior position. Women with a small or average-sized pelvis may have difficulty delivering infants who remain in an occiput posterior position. The physician may use forceps to rotate the fetal head into an occiput anterior position.

Nursing Care. During labor, the nurse should encourage the woman to assume positions that favor fetal rotation and descent. These positions also reduce some of the back pain. Good positions for back labor include the following:

- Sitting, kneeling, or standing while leaning forward
- Rocking the pelvis back and forth while on hands and knees (Figure 8-7) to encourage rotation

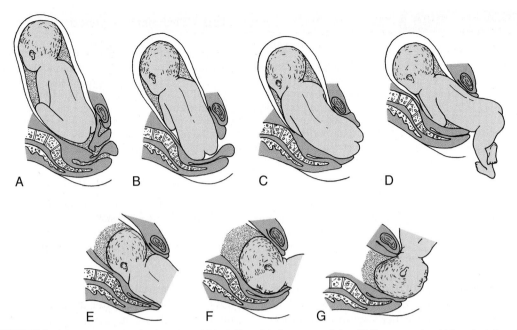

FIGURE 8-6 The mechanism of labor in a breech birth. **A,** Breech before onset of labor. **B,** Engagement and internal rotation of buttocks. **C,** Lateral flexion. **D,** External rotation and restitution of buttocks. **E,** Internal rotation of shoulders and head. **F,** Face rotates to sacrum. Note that there is no flexion of the head so that the smallest diameter of the fetal head is not passing through the pelvis. The umbilical cord is compressed between the fetal head and the bony pelvis. **G,** The head is born as the fetal body is elevated. (From Lowdermilk DL, Perry SE, Cashion KL: *Maternity nursing,* ed 8, St Louis, 2013, Mosby.)

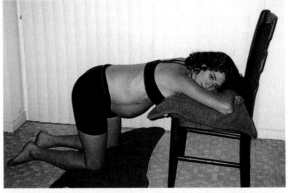

FIGURE 8-7 The hands-and-knees position can help the fetus rotate from an occiput posterior to an occiput anterior position. Gravity causes the fetus to float downward toward the pool of amniotic fluid. This position can be practiced before labor.

- Side-lying (on the left side for an ROP position, on the right side for an LOP position)
- Squatting (for second-stage labor)
- Lunging by placing one foot in a chair with the foot and knee pointed to that side; lunging sideways repeatedly during a contraction for 5 seconds at a time

After birth, the mother and infant are observed for signs of birth trauma. The mother is more likely to have a hematoma of her vaginal wall if the fetus remained in the occiput posterior position for a long time. The infant may have excessive molding (alteration in shape) of the head, caput succedaneum (scalp edema; see Chapter 12), and possibly injury from forceps or the vacuum extractor.

Multifetal Pregnancy

If the woman has more than one fetus, several factors can make dysfunctional labor likely:

- Uterine overdistention contributes to poor contraction quality.
- Abnormal presentation or position of one or more fetuses interferes with labor mechanisms.
- Often one fetus is delivered as cephalic and the second as breech, unless a version is done.

Because of the difficulties inherent in multifetal deliveries, cesarean birth is common. Birth is almost always cesarean if three or more fetuses are involved.

Nursing Care. When the woman has a multifetal pregnancy, each fetus is monitored separately during labor. An upright or side-lying position with the head slightly elevated aids breathing and is usually most comfortable. Labor care is similar to that for single pregnancies, with observations for hypotonic labor.

The nursery and intrapartum staffs prepare equipment and medications for every infant expected. An anesthesiologist and a pediatrician are often present at birth because of the potential for maternal or neonatal problems. One nurse is available for each infant. Another nurse focuses on the mother's needs.

PROBLEMS WITH THE PELVIS AND SOFT TISSUES

Bony Pelvis

Some women have a small or abnormally shaped pelvis that impedes the normal mechanisms of labor. The gynecoid pelvis is the most favorable for vaginal birth. Absolute pelvic measurements are rarely helpful to determine whether a woman's pelvis is adequate for birth. A woman with a "small" pelvis may still deliver vaginally if other factors are favorable. She often delivers vaginally if her fetus is not too large, the head is well flexed, contractions are good, and her soft tissues yield easily to the forces of labor.

In contrast, some women have vaginally delivered several infants much larger than 9 lb (4082 g), yet others cannot deliver one weighing 10 lb (4536 g). Obviously, the pelvis of each was "adequate," or even "large," according to standard measurements. However, the pelvis was not large enough for her largest infant. The ultimate test of a woman's pelvic size is whether her child fits through it at birth. A trial of labor may be indicated, and a cesarean delivery is done if necessary.

Soft Tissue Obstructions

The most common soft tissue obstruction during labor is a full bladder. The woman is encouraged to urinate every 1 or 2 hours. Catheterization may be needed if she cannot urinate, especially if a regional anesthetic or large quantities of IV fluids were given, which fill her bladder quickly yet reduce her sensation to void.

Soft tissue obstructions that are less common include pelvic tumors, such as benign (noncancerous) fibroids. Some women have a cervix that is scarred from previous infections or surgery. The scar tissue may not readily yield to labor's forces to efface and dilate.

PROBLEMS WITH THE PSYCHE

Labor is stressful, but women who have had prenatal care and have adequate social and professional support usually adapt to this stress and can labor and deliver normally. The most common factors that can increase stress and cause dystocia include lack of analgesic control of excessive pain, absence of a support person or coach to assist with nonpharmacological pain-relief measures, immobility and restriction to bed, and a lack of the ability to carry out cultural traditions.

Increased anxiety releases hormones such as epinephrine, cortisol, and adrenocorticotropic hormone that reduce contractility of the smooth muscle of the uterus. The body responds to stress with a "fight-or-flight" reaction that impedes normal labor by the following mechanisms:
- Using glucose the uterus needs for energy
- Diverting blood from the uterus
- Increasing tension of the pelvic muscles, which impedes fetal descent
- Increasing perception of pain, creating greater anxiety and stress and thus worsening the cycle

Nursing Care

Promoting relaxation and helping the woman conserve her resources for the work of childbirth are the principal nursing goals. The nurse uses every opportunity to spare the woman's energy and promote her comfort (see Chapter 7).

ABNORMAL DURATION OF LABOR

Prolonged Labor

Any of the previously discussed factors may be associated with a long or difficult labor (dystocia). The average rate of cervical dilation during the active phase of labor is about 1.2 cm/hr for the woman having her first child and about 1.5 cm/hr if she has had a child previously. Descent is expected to occur at a rate of at least 1.0 cm/hr in a first-time mother and 2.0 cm/hr in a woman who has had a child before (Gee, 2011).

A *Friedman curve* is often used to graph the progress of cervical dilation and fetal descent. The Friedman curve is used as a *guide* to assess and manage the normal progress of labor rather than using a rigid determination of "normal length of labor." Nursing interventions such as encouraging a delay in pushing during the second stage of labor until after full cervical dilation has occurred, alternative positioning of the patient during the first and second stages of labor, and electronic fetal monitoring along with the popular use of epidural anesthesia have had an impact on the length of the first and second stages of labor and on the positive outcome for mother and newborn. Therefore the Friedman curve remains a management guide in assessing cervical dilation in relation to the descent of the fetal head along with other factors and assessments. It may be referred to when determining the need for a cesarean section.

Prolonged labor can result in several problems, including the following:
- Maternal or newborn infection, especially if the membranes have been ruptured for a long time (usually about 24 hours)
- Maternal exhaustion
- Postpartum hemorrhage (see Chapter 10)
- Greater anxiety and fear in an ensuing pregnancy

In addition, mothers who have difficult and long labors are more likely to be anxious and fearful about their next labor.

Nursing Care. Nursing care focuses on helping the woman conserve her strength and encouraging her as she copes with the long labor. The nurse should observe for signs of infection during and after birth in both the mother (see Chapter 10) and the newborn (see Chapter 12).

Precipitate Birth

A precipitate birth is completed in less than 3 hours, and there may be no health care provider present. Labor often begins abruptly and intensifies quickly, rather than having a more subtle onset and gradual progression. Contractions may be frequent and intense, often from the onset. If the woman's tissues do not yield easily to the powerful contractions, she may have uterine rupture, cervical lacerations, or hematoma.

Fetal oxygenation can be compromised by intense contractions, because normally the placenta is resupplied with oxygenated blood between contractions. In precipitate labor, this interval may be very short. Birth injury from rapid passage through the birth canal may become evident in the infant after birth. These injuries can include intracranial hemorrhage or nerve damage.

Nursing Care. Women who experience precipitate birth may have panic responses about the possibility of not getting to the hospital in time or not having their health care provider present. Although they are relieved after birth, they require continued support and reassurance concerning the deviation from their expected experience. After birth, the nurse observes the mother and the infant for signs of injury. Excessive pain or bruising of the woman's vulva is reported. Cold applications limit pain, bruising, and edema. Abnormal findings on the newborn's assessment (see Chapter 12) are reported to the physician.

PREMATURE RUPTURE OF MEMBRANES

Premature rupture of membranes (PROM) is spontaneous rupture of the membranes at term (38 or more weeks of gestation) more than 1 hour before labor contractions begin. A related term, *preterm premature rupture of membranes* (PPROM), is rupture of the membranes before term (before 37 weeks of gestation) with or without uterine contractions. Vaginal or cervical infection may cause prematurely ruptured membranes; it has been associated with nutritional deficiency involving copper and ascorbic acid (Hacker et al, 2010).

Diagnosis is confirmed by testing the fluid with nitrazine paper, which turns blue in the presence of amniotic fluid. A sample of vaginal fluid placed on a slide and sent to the laboratory will show a ferning pattern under the microscope, confirming that it is amniotic fluid (see Chapter 6). Treatment is based on weighing the risks of early delivery of the fetus against the risks of infection in the mother (**chorioamnionitis**, or inflammation of the fetal membranes) and sepsis in the newborn. An ultrasound determines gestational age, and oligohydramnios is confirmed if the amniotic fluid index (AFI) is less than 5 cm. Oligohydramnios in a gestation less than 24 weeks can lead to fetal pulmonary and skeletal defects. If PROM occurs at 36 weeks of gestation or later, labor is induced within 24 hours. Because the cushion of amniotic fluid is lost, the risk for umbilical cord compression is great.

Nursing Care. The nurse should observe, document, and report maternal temperature above 38° C (100.4° F), fetal tachycardia, and tenderness over the uterine area. Antibiotic and steroid therapy may be anticipated, cultures may be ordered, and labor may be induced or a cesarean section may be indicated. Nursing care for the woman who is not having labor induced immediately primarily involves monitoring and teaching the woman. Teaching combines information about infection and preterm labor and includes the following:

- Report a temperature that is above 38° C (100.4° F).
- Avoid sexual intercourse or insertion of anything in the vagina, which can increase the risk for infection.
- Avoid orgasm, which can stimulate contractions.
- Avoid breast stimulation, which can stimulate contractions because of natural oxytocin release.
- Maintain any activity restrictions prescribed.
- Note any uterine contractions, reduced fetal activity, or other signs of infection (see the section on amniotomy).
- Record fetal kick counts daily, and report fewer than 10 kicks in a 12-hour period.

PRETERM LABOR

Preterm labor occurs after 20 and before 37 weeks of gestation. The main risks are the problems of immaturity in the newborn. One goal of *Healthy People 2020* is that 90% of all women will receive prenatal care starting in the first trimester. Preterm delivery is a major cause of perinatal morbidity and mortality, has a major medical and economic impact, and is a factor, for example, in the rising costs of health care. Early prenatal care can prevent premature labor or identify women at risk (Box 8-1).

Early prenatal care allows women to be educated concerning signs of preterm labor so that interventions can occur early. Home uterine activity monitoring can be initiated for women at risk for preterm labor.

Box 8-1   Some Risk Factors for Preterm Labor

- Exposure to diethylstilbestrol (DES)
- Underweight
- Chronic illness such as diabetes or hypertension
- Dehydration
- Preeclampsia
- Previous preterm labor or birth
- Previous pregnancy losses
- Uterine or cervical abnormalities or surgery
- Uterine distention
- Abdominal surgery during pregnancy
- Infection
- Anemia
- Preterm premature rupture of the membranes
- Inadequate prenatal care
- Poor nutrition
- Age less than 18 years or greater than 40 years
- Low education level
- Poverty
- Smoking
- Substance abuse
- Chronic stress
- Multifetal presentation

SIGNS OF IMPENDING PRETERM LABOR

A transvaginal ultrasound showing a shortened cervix at 20 weeks of gestation may be predictive of impending preterm labor. The ultrasound may be advised for high-risk women. The Food and Drug Administration (FDA) has approved a cervical or vaginal fetal **fibronectin test** for clinical use in the United States. Fibronectin is a protein produced by the fetal membranes that can leak into vaginal secretions if uterine activity, infection, or cervical effacement occurs. The presence of increased fibronectin in vaginal secretions between 22 and 24 weeks of gestation is predictive of preterm labor.

Levels of maternal corticotropin-releasing hormone (CRH) increase significantly in the weeks before preterm labor. Stress reduction and improved nutrition are indicated if CRH levels are high. *Diagnosis of preterm labor is based on cervical effacement and dilation of more than 2 cm.*

Maternal symptoms of preterm labor include:
- Contractions that may be either uncomfortable or painless
- Feeling that the fetus is "balling up" frequently
- Menstrual-like cramps
- Constant low backache
- Pelvic pressure or a feeling that the fetus is pushing down
- A change in the vaginal discharge
- Abdominal cramps with or without diarrhea
- Pain or discomfort in the vulva or thighs
- "Just feeling bad" or "coming down with something"

Laboratory tests include glucose level, electrolyte level, urinalysis and culture, and an ultrasound of the fetus to determine maturity, position, and other problems that may exist. Treatment of preterm labor is more aggressive at 28 weeks of gestation than at 34 weeks of gestation. Foot message often given with pedicures are contraindicated in pregnant women at risk for preterm labor.

TOCOLYTIC THERAPY

The goal of tocolytic therapy is to stop uterine contractions and keep the fetus in utero until the lungs are mature enough to adapt to extrauterine life.

Magnesium sulfate is the drug of choice for initiating therapy to stop preterm labor, and it may protect the fetus from developing cerebral palsy. A continuous IV infusion is administered, and therapeutic levels are monitored. The woman should be informed that a warm flush may be perceived during the initiation of therapy. Overdose can affect the cardiorespiratory system, and vital signs are recorded every hour. If the fetus is born during magnesium therapy, drowsiness may be present and resuscitation may be required. The nursery staff should be notified if magnesium sulfate therapy was used within 2 hours before delivery. Calcium gluconate should be on hand to treat adverse effects in the newborn. The FDA recommends limiting the use of magnesium sulfate to fewer than 5 to 7 days, because the fetus can develop low blood calcium and bone problems with prolonged use (FDA, 2013). When magnesium sulfate is used, the nurse should monitor the patient for respiratory rate and lung sounds and signs of fluid overload, urine output, deep tendon reflexes, and bowel sounds, because the intestinal muscles also relax in response to the drug.

β-Adrenergic drugs such as terbutaline (Brethine) are administered subcutaneously to stop uterine contractions. It is an "off-label" use of the drug but is approved by ACOG (Gabbe, 2012). Cardiac side effects such as increased pulse rate and blood pressure can occur, and prolonged parenteral use over 48 hours is not recommended.

Ritodrine (Yutopar) was previously used intravenously to stop preterm labor, but it is no longer approved for use because of the many side effects. Hypotension, cardiac dysrhythmia, and pulmonary edema may occur.

Prostaglandin synthesis inhibitors such as indomethacin are another type of drug that can be used to stop labor contractions. This type of drug causes a reduction in amniotic fluid, which is helpful when polyhydramnios is a problem. However, this drug is not commonly used, because it can stimulate the ductus arteriosus to close prematurely, causing fetal death. Close fetal monitoring is essential.

Calcium channel blockers, such as nifedipine (Procardia), are most commonly used to stop labor contractions. Because the drug causes vasodilation, maternal flushing and hypotension could be side effects, and blood pressure and pulse should be closely monitored. Magnesium sulfate should not be used when nifedipine is used or when intrauterine infection is suspected (Gabbe, 2012).

Antimicrobial therapy is often initiated in women with preterm labor, because studies have shown that subclinical chorioamnionitis is often present.

Contraindications

Tocolytics should not be used in women with preeclampsia, placenta previa, abruptio placentae, chorioamnionitis, or fetal demise. In these cases it would not improve the obstetric outcome to delay birth of the fetus.

Speeding Fetal Lung Maturation. If it appears that preterm birth is inevitable, the physician may give the woman steroid drugs (glucocorticoids) to increase fetal lung maturity if the gestation is between 24 and 34 weeks. Glucocorticoids are often used together with tocolytics. Betamethasone may be administered for this purpose in two intramuscular injections 24 hours apart.

Activity Restrictions. Bed rest was often prescribed for women at risk for preterm birth. However, the benefits of bed rest are not clear, and many adverse maternal effects can occur. Therefore total bed rest is prescribed less frequently than it was in the past. Activity restrictions are often more moderate, such as resting in a semi-Fowler's position or partial bed rest.

Nursing Care. Nurses should be aware of the symptoms of preterm labor, because they may occur in any pregnant woman, with or without risk factors. Symptoms are taught and regularly reinforced for women who have increased risk factors. Nursing care includes positioning the woman on her side for better placental blood flow, assessing vital signs frequently, and notifying the health care provider if tachycardia occurs. Signs of pulmonary edema (chest pains, cough, crackles, or rhonchi) and intake and output should be closely monitored. If the woman is monitored at home, appropriate activities and restrictions are identified, and arrangements for household responsibilities such as childcare should be made with family or with the help of social services. If delivery occurs, monitoring the fetal heart rate is essential, and preparation for admission to the neonatal intensive care unit is initiated. Full emotional support of the parents is offered, because they may be grieving the loss of the normal birth process.

PROLONGED PREGNANCY

A late-term pregnancy lasts between 41 weeks and 41 weeks and 6 days. A post-term pregnancy lasts 42 weeks. The term *postmature* most accurately describes the infant whose characteristics are consistent with a prolonged gestation (see Chapter 13).

RISKS

The greatest risks of prolonged pregnancy are to the fetus. As the placenta ages, it delivers oxygen and nutrients to the fetus less efficiently. The fetus may lose weight, and the skin may begin to peel; these are the typical characteristics of postmaturity. Meconium may be expelled into the amniotic fluid, which can cause severe respiratory problems at birth. Low blood glucose levels are a likely complication after birth.

The fetus with placental insufficiency does not tolerate labor well. Because the fetus has less reserve than needed, the normal interruption in blood flow during contractions may cause excessive stress on the infant. If the placenta continues to function well, the fetus continues growing. This can lead to a large fetus and the problems accompanying macrosomia.

If placental function remains normal, there is little physical risk to the mother other than laboring with a large fetus. Psychologically, however, she often feels that pregnancy will never end. She becomes more anxious about when labor will begin and when her health care provider will "do something."

Medical Treatment

The physician or nurse-midwife will evaluate whether the pregnancy is truly prolonged or if the gestation has been miscalculated. If the woman had early and regular prenatal care, ultrasound examinations have usually clarified her true gestation. Any pregnancy that lasts longer than 40 weeks must be monitored closely with twice weekly non–stress tests (NSTs), amniotic fluid indexes (AFIs), biophysical profiles (BPPs), and daily kick counts (see Chapter 5). Oligohydramnios (decreased amniotic fluid) in a postterm pregnancy is an indication for labor induction (Briscoe et al, 2005). If the woman's pregnancy has definitely reached 41 weeks, 6 days labor is usually induced by oxytocin. Prostaglandin application to ripen the cervix before oxytocin administration increases the probability of successful induction.

Nursing Care

Nursing care involves careful observation of the fetus during labor to identify signs associated with poor placental blood flow, such as late decelerations (see Chapter 6). After birth, the newborn is observed for respiratory difficulties and hypoglycemia.

EMERGENCIES DURING CHILDBIRTH

Several intrapartum conditions can endanger the life or well-being of the woman or her fetus. They necessitate prompt nursing and medical action to reduce the likelihood of damage. Nursing and medical management often overlap in emergencies.

PROLAPSED UMBILICAL CORD

The umbilical cord prolapses if it slips downward in the pelvis after the membranes rupture. In this position, it can be compressed between the fetal head and the woman's pelvis, interrupting blood supply to and from the placenta. It may slip down immediately after the membranes rupture, or the prolapse may occur later. A prolapsed cord (Figure 8-8) can be classified in the following ways:
- *Complete:* The cord is visible at the vaginal opening.
- *Palpated:* The cord cannot be seen but can be felt as a pulsating structure when a vaginal examination is done.
- *Occult:* The prolapse is hidden and cannot be seen or felt; it is suspected based on abnormal fetal heart rates.

! Safety Tip

The risk for prolapsed cord is increased if the membranes rupture before the fetal presenting part is completely engaged in the pelvis. Documenting the fetal heart after the membranes rupture is an essential nursing responsibility.

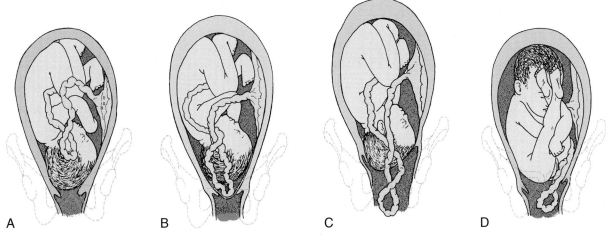

A   B   C   D

FIGURE 8-8 Prolapsed umbilical cord. Note the pressure of the presenting part on the umbilical cord, which will interfere with oxygenation of the fetus. **A,** Occult (hidden) prolapse of cord. The cord will be compressed between the fetal head and the mother's bony pelvis. **B,** Complete prolapsed cord. Note that the membranes are intact. **C,** Cord is presenting in front of the fetal head and may be seen in the vagina. **D,** Frank breech presentation with prolapsed cord. (From Lowdermilk DL, Perry SE, Cashion KL: *Maternity nursing,* ed 8, St Louis, 2013, Mosby.)

Risk Factors

Prolapse of the umbilical cord is more likely if the fetus does not completely fill the space in the pelvis or if fluid pressure is great when the membranes rupture. These conditions are more likely to occur in the following situations:

- The fetus is high in the pelvis when the membranes rupture (presenting part is not engaged).
- The fetus is very small, as in prematurity.
- There are abnormal presentations, such as footling breech or transverse lie.
- Hydramnios (excess amniotic fluid) is present.

Medical Treatment. The experienced physician may push the fetus upward from the vagina. Oxygen and a tocolytic drug such as terbutaline may be administered. The primary focus is to deliver the fetus by the quickest means possible, usually cesarean delivery.

Nursing Care. The main risk of a prolapsed cord is to the fetus. When a prolapsed cord occurs, the first action is to displace the fetus upward to stop compression against the pelvis. Maternal positions such as the knee-chest or Trendelenburg (head down) can accomplish this displacement (Figure 8-9). Placing the mother in a side-lying position with her hips elevated on pillows also reduces cord pressure.

In addition to prompt corrective actions and assisting with emergency procedures, the nurse should remain calm to avoid increasing the woman's anxiety. Prolapsed cord is a sudden development; anxiety and fear are inevitable reactions in the woman and her partner. Calm, quick actions on the part of nurses help the woman and her family to feel that she is in competent hands. After birth, the nurse helps the woman to understand the experience. She may need several explanations of what happened and why.

UTERINE RUPTURE

A tear in the uterine wall occurs if the muscle cannot withstand the pressure inside the organ. There are three variations of uterine rupture:

1. *Complete rupture:* There is a hole through the uterine wall, from the uterine cavity to the abdominal cavity.
2. *Incomplete rupture:* The uterus tears into a nearby structure, such as a ligament, but not all the way into the abdominal cavity.
3. *Dehiscence:* An old uterine scar, usually from a previous cesarean birth, separates.

Risk Factors

Uterine rupture is more likely to occur if the woman has had previous surgery on her uterus, such as a previous cesarean delivery. The low transverse uterine incision (see Figure 8-4) is least likely to rupture. Because the classic uterine incision is prone to rupture, a vaginal birth after this type of incision is not recommended. A woman who has a trial of labor for a vaginal birth after a cesarean section (TOLAC, VBAC) must have a surgical team available to prevent or treat uterine rupture during labor in case a cesarean section is indicated. Surgical intervention must be available within 30 minutes.

Uterine rupture may also occur if tachysystole occurs as a result of labor induction with oxytocin or the woman has sustained blunt abdominal trauma, such as from a motor vehicle accident or from battering.

Characteristics

The woman may have no symptoms, or she may have sudden onset of severe signs and symptoms, such as the following:

- Shock caused by bleeding into the abdomen (vaginal bleeding may be minimal)
- Abdominal pain
- Pain in the chest, between the scapulae (shoulder blades), or with inspiration

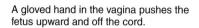

A gloved hand in the vagina pushes the fetus upward and off the cord.

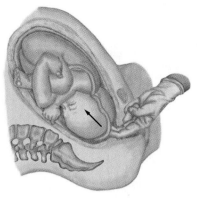

Knee-chest position uses gravity to shift the fetus out of the pelvis. The woman's thighs should be at right angles to the bed and her chest flat on the bed.

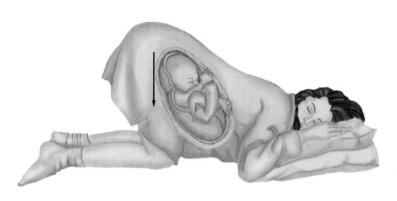

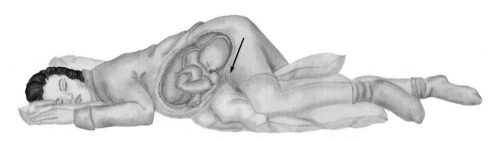

The woman's hips are elevated with two pillows; this is often combined with the Trendelenburg (head down) position.

FIGURE 8-9 Positioning of the mother when the umbilical cord prolapses. These positions can be used to relieve pressure on the prolapsed umbilical cord until delivery can take place. (From Murray SS, McKinney ES: *Foundations of maternal-newborn and women's health nursing*, ed 5, St Louis, 2011, Saunders.)

- Cessation of contractions
- Abnormal or absent fetal heart tones
- Palpation of the fetus outside the uterus because the fetus has pushed through the torn area

Medical Treatment

If the fetus is living when the rupture is detected and/or if blood loss is excessive, the physician performs surgery to deliver the fetus and to stop the bleeding. Hysterectomy (removal of the uterus) is likely to be required for an extensive tear. Smaller tears may be surgically repaired.

Nursing Care

The nurse should be aware of women who are at high risk for uterine rupture, and close monitoring during labor is essential. When uterine rupture occurs, the woman is prepared for immediate cesarean section. Measures to alleviate anxiety in the woman and her partner are necessary as emergency measures are being initiated.

Uterine rupture is sometimes not discovered until after birth. In these cases the woman does not have dramatic symptoms of blood loss. However, she may have continuous bleeding that is brighter red than the normal postbirth bleeding. A rising pulse rate and falling blood pressure reading are signs of hypovolemic shock, which may occur if blood loss is excessive.

AMNIOTIC FLUID EMBOLISM

Amniotic fluid embolism, also known as **anaphylactoid syndrome**, occurs when amniotic fluid, with its particles such as vernix, fetal hair, and sometimes meconium, enters the woman's circulation and obstructs small blood vessels in her lungs. It is more likely to occur during a very strong labor, because the fluid is "pushed" into small blood vessels that rupture as the cervix dilates. Amniotic fluid embolism is characterized by abrupt onset of hypotension, respiratory distress, and coagulation abnormalities triggered by the thromboplastin contained in the amniotic fluid.

Treatment includes providing respiratory support with intubation and mechanical ventilation as necessary, treating shock with electrolytes and volume expanders, and replacing the coagulation factors such as platelets and fibrinogen. Packed red blood cells are sometimes given intravenously.

The woman's intake and output are monitored closely. A pulse oximeter monitors oxygen saturation. The woman may be transferred to the intensive care unit for closer monitoring and nursing care.

Unfolding Case Study

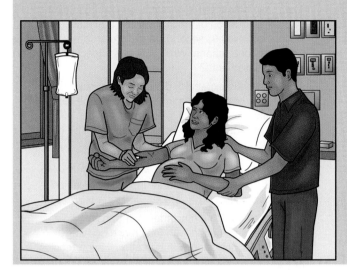

Tess and Luis were introduced to the reader in Chapter 4, and Tess's pregnancy experience has unfolded in each chapter. Refer to earlier chapters for her history and progress.

Tess was admitted to the labor unit and has been in active labor. However, after many hours, her labor contractions stop. The health care provider determines that her Bishop score is 7 and decides to augment her labor.

QUESTIONS

1. What is a Bishop score?
2. What is the difference between induction of labor and augmentation of labor?
3. When is induction or augmentation of labor contraindicated?
4. How can the nurse help Tess stimulate labor contractions using non-pharmacological methods? How can her husband Luis help?
5. What nursing responsibilities are involved during the administration of oxytocin during labor?

Get Ready for the NCLEX® Examination!

Key Points

- An amnioinfusion is the insertion of fluid directly into the uterus to provide a cushion for the umbilical cord after amniotic fluid is lost.
- Induction of labor is the intentional initiation of labor before it occurs naturally.
- Augmentation of labor is the stimulation of contractions after they started naturally.
- A Bishop score above 6 may predict successful labor induction because of a "ripe cervix."
- The nurse observes the character of the amniotic fluid and fetal heart rate when the membranes are ruptured. Fluid should be clear, but it may contain bits of lanugo and have a mild odor; the fetal heart rate should remain near its baseline level and between 110 and 160 beats/min at term.
- The nurse observes the fetal condition and character of contractions if any methods to stimulate labor are used.
- *Dystocia* is a term used to describe a difficult labor, which can be caused by an abnormality of the *power, passenger, passage,* or *psyche* of the woman.
- Nursing measures such as encouraging position changes, aiding relaxation, and reminding the woman to empty her bladder can promote a more normal labor.
- Pharmacologic, nonpharmacologic, or mechanical methods can be used to stimulate labor.
- After version, the nurse observes for leaking amniotic fluid and for a pattern of contractions that may indicate labor has begun. Before discharge, signs of labor are reviewed with the woman so she will know when to return to the birth center.
- Nursing care after episiotomy or perineal lacerations includes comfort measures such as cold applications, analgesics, and wound assessment.

- Nursing care after cesarean birth is similar to that after vaginal birth with the addition of assessing the wound, indwelling catheter patency, and intravenous flow. The woman and her partner may need extra emotional support after cesarean birth.
- Nursing care after births involving instruments (forceps or vacuum extraction) and after abnormal labor and birth include observations for maternal and newborn injuries or infections. Infection is the most common hazard after membranes rupture prematurely, especially if there is a long interval before delivery.
- When oxytocin is given to the woman in labor, the nurse must be aware of signs and symptoms of increased uterine activity and monitor the fetal heart rate every 15 minutes during active labor and every 5 minutes during the transition phase.
- Induction of labor is more effective if cervical ripening is achieved before oxytocin is administered to stimulate contractions.
- Nurses should be aware of the subtle symptoms a woman may experience at the beginning of preterm labor and should encourage her to seek care at the hospital promptly.
- The nurse must be aware of the side effects of tocolytic drugs and monitor the mother and fetus closely.
- Anaphylactoid syndrome occurs when amniotic fluid enters the woman's circulation.
- After any type of emergency, the woman and her family need emotional support, explanations of what happened, and patience with their repeated questions.

Additional Learning Resources

SG Go to your Study Guide for additional learning activities to help you master this chapter content.

evolve Go to your Evolve website (http://evolve.elsevier.com/Leifer) for the following learning resources:
- Animations
- Answer Guidelines for Critical Thinking Questions
- Answers and Rationales for Review Questions for the NCLEX® Examination
- Glossary with English and Spanish pronunciations
- Interactive Review Questions for the NCLEX® Examination
- Patient Teaching Plans in English and Spanish
- Skills Performance Checklists
- Video clips and more!

Online Resources
- *Healthy People 2020:* www.health.gov/healthypeople/document/tableofcontents.htm
- National Center for Health Statistics: www.cdc.gov/nchs/fastats
- Preterm labor: www.merck.com/mmpe/sec18/ch264/ch264k.html

Review Questions for the NCLEX® Examination

1. The nurse notes that a woman's contractions during oxytocin induction of labor are every 2 minutes; the contractions last 95 seconds, and the uterus remains tense between contractions. What action is expected based on these assessments?
   1. No action is expected; the contractions are normal.
   2. The rate of oxytocin administration will be increased slightly.
   3. Pain medication or an epidural block will be offered.
   4. Infusion of oxytocin will be stopped.

2. The nurse can anticipate that which of the following patients may be scheduled for induction of labor? A woman who is:
   1. 38 weeks gestation with fetus in transverse lie.
   2. 40 weeks gestation with fetal macrosomia.
   3. 40 weeks gestation with gestational hypertension.
   4. 40 weeks gestation with a fetal prolapsed cord.

3. A woman has an emergency cesarean delivery after the umbilical cord was found to be prolapsed. She repeatedly asks similar questions about what happened at birth. The nurse's interpretation of the woman's behavior is that she:
   1. cannot accept that she did not have the type of delivery she planned.
   2. is trying to understand her experience and move on with postpartum adaptation.
   3. thinks the staff is not telling her the truth about what happened at birth.
   4. is confused about events because the effects of the general anesthetic are persisting.

4. What nursing intervention during labor can increase space in the woman's pelvis?
   1. Promote adequate fluid intake.
   2. Position her on the left side.
   3. Assist her to take a shower.
   4. Encourage regular urination.

5. A woman is being observed in the hospital because her membranes ruptured at 30 weeks of gestation. While providing morning care, the nursing student notices that the draining fluid has a strong odor. The priority nursing action is to:
   1. caution the woman to remain in bed until her physician visits.
   2. ask the woman if she is having any more contractions than usual.
   3. take the woman's temperature; report it and the fluid odor to the registered nurse.
   4. help to prepare the woman for an immediate cesarean delivery.

Objectives

1. Define each key term listed.
2. Describe how to individualize postpartum and newborn nursing care for different patients.
3. Describe specific cultural beliefs that the nurse may encounter when providing postpartum and newborn care.
4. Describe postpartum changes in maternal systems and the nursing care associated with those changes.
5. Modify nursing assessments and interventions for the woman who has a cesarean birth.
6. Explain the emotional needs of postpartum women and their families.
7. Recognize the needs of a grieving parent.
8. Describe the nursing care of the normal newborn.
9. Identify signs and symptoms that may indicate a complication in the postpartum mother or newborn.
10. Describe nursing interventions to promote optimal infant nutrition.
11. Explain the physiological characteristics of lactation.
12. Compare various maternal and newborn positions used during breastfeeding.
13. Discuss the influences related to the choice of breastfeeding or bottle-feeding the newborn.
14. Identify principles of breast pumping and milk storage.
15. Discuss the dietary needs of the lactating mother.
16. Discuss the principles of weaning the infant from the breast.
17. Illustrate techniques of formula feeding.
18. Plan appropriate discharge teaching for the postpartum woman and her newborn.

Key Terms

afterpains (p. 201)
attachment (p. 220)
bonding (p. 220)
colostrum (kŏ-LŎS-trŭm, p. 223)
diastasis recti (dī-ĂS-tă-sĭs RĔK-tī, p. 208)
episiotomy (p. 204)
foremilk (p. 223)
fundus (p. 200)
galactogogues (gă-LĂK-tō-gŏgz, p. 224)

hindmilk (p. 223)
involution (ĭn-vō-LŪ-shŭn, p. 200)
let-down reflex (p. 223)
lochia (LŌ-kē-ă, p. 202)
postpartum blues (p. 211)
puerperium (pū-ŭr-PĔ-rē-ŭm, p. 199)
rugae (p. 204)
suckling (p. 225)

The postpartum period, or **puerperium**, is the 6 weeks following childbirth. This period is often referred to as the fourth trimester of pregnancy. This chapter addresses the physiological and psychological changes in the mother and her family and the initial care of the newborn.

ADAPTING NURSING CARE FOR SPECIFIC GROUPS AND CULTURES

The nurse must adapt care to a person's circumstances, such as those of the single or adolescent parent, the poor, families who have multiple births, and families from other cultures.

Adolescents, particularly younger ones, need help to learn parenting skills. Their peer group is very important to them, so the nurse must make every effort during both pregnancy and the postpartum period to help them to fit in with their peers. They are often passive in caring for themselves and their infants. They may also be single and poor. Poor, young adolescent mothers often have several children in a short time, which compounds their social problems.

A single woman may have problems making postpartum adaptations if she does not have a strong support system. Often she must return to work very soon, because she is the sole provider for her family.

Poor families may have difficulty meeting their basic needs before a new infant arrives, and a new family member adds to their strain. Women may have inadequate or sporadic prenatal care, which increases their risk for complications that extend into the puerperium and to their child. They may need social service referrals to direct them to public assistance programs or other resources.

Families who add twins (or more) face different challenges. The infants are more likely to need intensive care because of preterm birth, which delays the parents' close contact and ability to provide daily newborn care. It is also difficult for the parents to conceptualize the individuality of each infant, and may be more likely to attach to them as a set, often referring to them as "they." The infants may require care at a distant hospital if their problems are severe. Financial strains mount with each added problem.

CULTURAL INFLUENCES ON POSTPARTUM CARE

The United States has a diverse population. Special cultural practices are often most evident at significant life events such as birth and death. The nurse must adapt care to fit the health beliefs, values, and practices of a specific culture to make the birth a meaningful emotional and social event as well as a physically safe event. See Chapter 6 for specific cultural practices during labor, delivery, and postpartum.

USING TRANSLATORS

The nurse may need an interpreter to understand and provide optimal care to the woman and her family. If possible, when discussing sensitive information the interpreter should not be a family member, who might interpret selectively. The interpreter should not be of a group that is in social or religious conflict with the patient and her family, which is an issue that might arise in many Middle Eastern cultures. It is also important to remember that an affirmative nod from the woman may be a sign of courtesy to the nurse rather than a sign of understanding or agreement. Cultural preferences influence the presence of partners, parents, siblings, and children in the labor and delivery room (Figure 9-1).

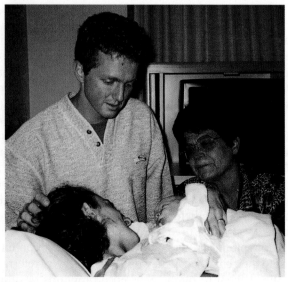

FIGURE 9-1 Mother, husband, and grandmother share relief as they get to see the newborn soon after birth in the delivery room.

DIETARY PRACTICES

Some cultures adhere to the "hot" and "cold" theory of diet after childbirth. Temperature has nothing to do with the foods that are considered hot and those that are considered cold; it is the believed intrinsic property of the food itself that classifies it. For example, "hot" foods include eggs, chicken, and rice. Women may also prefer their drinking water hot rather than cool or cold. Other hot–cold dietary practices include a balance between *yin* foods (e.g., bean sprouts, broccoli, and carrots) and *yang* foods (e.g., broiled meat, chicken, soup, and eggs).

POSTPARTUM CHANGES IN THE MOTHER

Table 9-1 (p. 205) summarizes nursing assessments for the postpartum woman. See Chapter 10 for additional information about postpartum complications.

REPRODUCTIVE SYSTEM

Following the third stage of labor, there is a fall in the blood levels of placental hormones, human placental lactogen, human chorionic gonadotropin, estrogen, and progesterone that help return the body to the prepregnant state. The most dramatic changes after birth occur in the woman's reproductive system. These changes are discussed in the following sections, and the nursing care is discussed for each area as applicable.

Uterus

Involution refers to changes that the reproductive organs, particularly the uterus, undergo after birth to return them to their prepregnancy size and condition. The uterus undergoes a rapid reduction in size and weight after birth. The uterus should return to the prepregnant size by 5 to 6 weeks after delivery. The failure of the uterus to return to the prepregnant state after 6 weeks is called *subinvolution* (see Chapter 10).

Uterine Lining. The uterine lining (called the *endometrium* when not pregnant and the *decidua* during pregnancy) is shed when the placenta detaches. A basal layer of the lining remains to generate new endometrium to prepare for future pregnancies. The placental site is fully healed in 6 to 7 weeks.

Descent of the Uterine Fundus. The uterine **fundus** (the upper portion of the body of the uterus) descends at a predictable rate as the muscle cells contract to control bleeding at the placental insertion site and as the size of each muscle cell decreases. Immediately after the placenta is expelled, the uterine fundus can be felt midline, at or below the level of the umbilicus, as a firm mass (about the size of a grapefruit). After 24 hours the fundus begins to descend about 1 cm (one finger's width) each day. By 10 days postpartum, it should no longer be palpable (see Skill 9-1). A full bladder interferes with uterine contraction, because it pushes the fundus up and causes it to deviate to one side, usually the right side (Figure 9-2).

The Family After Birth

Observing and Massaging the Uterine Fundus

PURPOSE

To prevent excessive postpartum bleeding

STEPS

1. Identify the need for fundal massage. The uterus will be soft and usually higher than the umbilicus. A firm fundus does not need massage.
2. Place the woman in a supine position with the knees slightly flexed. Lower the perineal pad to observe lochia as the fundus is palpated.
3. Place the outer edge of nondominant hand just above the symphysis pubis, and press downward slightly to anchor the lower uterus.
4. Locate and massage the uterine fundus with the flat portion of the fingers of the dominant hand in a firm, circular motion.
5. When the uterus is firm, gently push downward on the fundus, toward the vaginal outlet, to expel blood and clots that have accumulated inside the uterus. *Keep the other hand on the lower uterus to avoid inverting it.*
6. If a full bladder contributes to uterine relaxation, have the mother void. Catheterize her (with a health care provider's order) if she cannot void.
7. Document the consistency and location of the fundus before and after massage.
8. Give any prescribed medications, such as oxytocin, to maintain uterine contraction. Have the mother nurse her infant if she is breastfeeding to stimulate the secretion of natural oxytocin.
9. Report a fundus that does not stay firm.

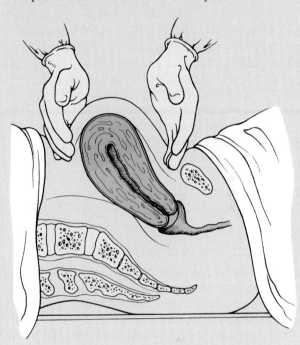

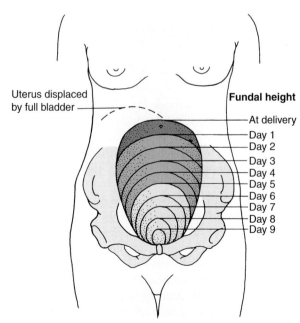

FIGURE 9-2 The height of the uterine fundus changes each day as involution progresses.

Uterus displaced by full bladder

Fundal height

At delivery
Day 1
Day 2
Day 3
Day 4
Day 5
Day 6
Day 7
Day 8
Day 9

 Nursing Tip

If the mother's uterus is soft, massage it (supporting the lower segment), then expel clots so it will remain contracted. If her bladder is also full, massage the uterus until firm, and then address emptying the bladder. Control bleeding first, and then keep it controlled by emptying the bladder.

Afterpains. Intermittent uterine contractions may cause afterpains similar to menstrual cramps. The discomfort is self-limiting and decreases rapidly within 48 hours postpartum. **Afterpains** occur more often in multiparas or in women whose uterus was overly distended. Breast-feeding mothers may have more afterpains, because infant suckling causes their posterior pituitary to release oxytocin, a hormone that contracts the uterus. Mild analgesics may be prescribed. Aspirin is not used postpartum, because it interferes with blood clotting.

Nursing Tip

The nurse should assess the fundus for descent each nursing shift and should teach the mother about the expected changes.

Estimating the Volume of Lochia

PURPOSE

To determine normal progress of the postpartum period

STEPS

1. Assess lochia for quantity, type, and characteristics. A guideline to estimate and chart the amount of flow on the menstrual pad in 1 hour is as follows (see figure):
   a. *Scant:* Less than a 5-cm (2-inch) stain
   b. *Light:* Less than a 10-cm (4-inch) stain
   c. *Moderate:* Less than a 15-cm (6-inch) stain
   d. *Large or heavy:* Larger than a 15-cm stain or one pad saturated within 2 hours
   e. *Excessive:* Saturation of a perineal pad within 15 minutes

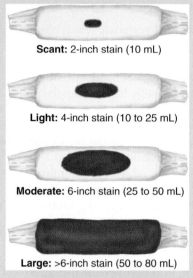

Scant: 2-inch stain (10 mL)

Light: 4-inch stain (10 to 25 mL)

Moderate: 6-inch stain (25 to 50 mL)

Large: >6-inch stain (50 to 80 mL)

(From Murray SS, McKinney ES: *Foundations of maternal-newborn and women's health nursing*, ed 6, St Louis, 2014, Saunders.)

Lochia. Vaginal discharge after delivery, called **lochia**, is composed of endometrial tissue, blood, and lymph. Lochia gradually changes characteristics during the early postpartum period:

- *Lochia rubra* is red, because it is composed mostly of blood; it lasts for about 3 days after birth.
- *Lochia serosa* is pinkish because of its blood and mucus content. It lasts from about the third through the tenth day after birth.
- *Lochia alba* is mostly mucus and is clear and colorless or white. It lasts from the tenth through the twenty-first day after birth.

Lochia has a characteristic fleshy or menstrual odor; it should not have a foul odor. The woman's fundus should be checked for firmness, because an uncontracted uterus allows blood to flow freely from vessels at the placenta insertion site.

Many facilities use perineal pads that contain cold or warm packs. These pads absorb less lochia, and that fact must be considered when estimating the amount (Skill 9-2). If a mother has excessive discharge of lochia, a clean pad should be applied and checked within 15 minutes. The peripads applied during a given time are counted or weighed to help determine the amount of vaginal discharge. One gram of weight equals about a 1-mL volume of blood. The nurse should assess the underpads on the bed to determine if bleeding has overflowed onto the underpad.

The flow of lochia is briefly heavier when the mother ambulates, because lochia pooled in the vagina is discharged when she assumes an upright position. A few small clots may be seen at this time, but large clots should not be present. The quantity of lochia may briefly increase when the mother breastfeeds, because suckling causes uterine contraction. The rate of discharge increases with exercise. Women who had a cesarean birth have less discharge of lochia during the first 24 hours, because the uterine cavity was sponged at delivery. The absence of lochia is not normal and may be associated with blood clots retained within the uterus or with infection.

Nursing Care. The fundus is assessed at routine intervals for firmness, location, and position (see Skill 9-1) in relation to the midline. Women who have a higher risk for postpartum hemorrhage (see Chapter 10) should be assessed more often. While doing initial assessments, the nurse explains the reason they are done and teaches the woman how to assess her fundus. If her uterus stops descending, she should report that to her health care provider.

A poorly contracted (soft or boggy) uterus should be massaged until firm to prevent hemorrhage. Lochia flow may increase briefly as the uterus contracts and expels it. It is essential **not** to push down on an uncontracted uterus to prevent inverting it. If a full bladder contributes to poor uterine contraction, the mother should be assisted to void in the bathroom or on a bedpan if she cannot ambulate. Catheterization may be necessary if she cannot void.

The woman should be taught the expected sequence for lochia changes and the amount she should expect.

The woman should report any of the following abnormal characteristics:

- Foul-smelling lochia, with or without fever
- Lochia rubra that persists beyond the third day
- Unusually heavy flow of lochia
- Lochia that returns to a bright red color after it has progressed to serosa or alba

Medications that may be given to stimulate uterine contraction include the following:

- Oxytocin (Pitocin), often routinely given in an intravenous infusion after birth
- Methylergonovine (Methergine), given intramuscularly or orally

An infant suckling at the breast has a similar effect, because natural oxytocin release stimulates contractions.

Mild analgesics relieve afterpains adequately for most women. The breastfeeding mother should take an analgesic immediately after breastfeeding to minimize sedation and side effects passing to the newborn. Afterpains persisting longer than 48 hours after birth should be reported.

 Nursing Tip

A firm fundus does not need massage.

Cervix

The cervix regains its muscle tone but never closes as tightly as during the prepregnant state. Some edema persists for a few weeks after delivery. A constant trickle of brighter red lochia is associated with bleeding from lacerations of the cervix or vagina, particularly if the fundus remains firm.

Vagina

The vagina undergoes a great deal of stretching during childbirth. The **rugae**, or vaginal folds, disappear, and the walls of the vagina become smooth and spacious. The rugae reappear 3 weeks postpartum. Within 6 weeks, the vagina has regained most of its prepregnancy form, but it never returns to the size it was before pregnancy.

Nursing Care. Couples often are hesitant to ask questions concerning resumption of sexual activity after childbirth, and many resume activity before the 6-week checkup. It is important for the nurse to teach the woman that it is considered safe to resume sexual intercourse when bleeding has stopped and the perineum (episiotomy) has healed. However, the vagina does not lubricate well in the first 6 weeks after childbirth (or longer in the breastfeeding mother). A water-soluble gel such as K-Y or a contraceptive gel can be used for lubrication to make intercourse more comfortable. Instructing the woman to perform the Kegel exercise correctly helps her strengthen muscles involved in urination, bowel function, and vaginal sensations during intercourse.

Perineum

The perineum is often edematous, tender, and bruised. An **episiotomy** (incision to enlarge the vaginal opening) may have been performed, or a perineal laceration may have occurred. Women with hemorrhoids often find that these temporarily worsen because of the pressure exerted during the birth process.

Nursing Care. The perineum should be assessed for normal healing and signs of complications (Skill 9-3). The REEDA acronym helps the nurse remember the five signs to assess.

Assessing the Perineum

PURPOSE

To observe perineal trauma, hemorrhoids, and status of healing

STEPS

1. Provide privacy; explain purpose of procedure.
2. Put on gloves (provide protection from contact of bodily fluids).
3. Ask woman to turn on side and flex upper leg, lower perineal pad, and lift up upper buttock; if necessary, use flashlight to inspect perineum.
4. Observe for edema, bruising, and hematoma.
5. Examine episiotomy or laceration for REEDA (**r**edness, **e**dema, **e**cchymosis, **d**ischarge, **a**pproximation).
6. Observe hemorrhoids for extent of edema (can interfere with bowel elimination).
7. Apply clean peripads, taking care to only touch edges.
8. Reposition woman into position of comfort.
9. Dispose of soiled contents in appropriate waste container, and wash hands.
10. Document care provided in medical record.

Memory Jogger

REEDA is *redness*, *edema*, *ecchymosis*, *discharge*, *approximation*

Redness. Redness without excessive tenderness is probably the normal inflammation associated with healing, but pain with the redness is more likely to indicate infection.

Edema. Mild edema is common, but severe edema interferes with healing.

Ecchymosis (bruising). A few small superficial bruises are common. Larger bruises interfere with normal healing.

Discharge. No discharge from the perineal suture line should be present.

Approximation (intactness of the suture line). The suture line should not be separated. If intact, it is almost impossible to distinguish the laceration or episiotomy from surrounding skin folds.

NOTE: The REEDA acronym is also useful when assessing a cesarean incision for healing.

Comfort and hygienic measures are the focus of nursing care and patient teaching. An ice pack or chemical cold pack is applied for the first 12 to 24 hours to reduce edema and bruising and to numb the perineal area. A disposable rubber glove filled with ice chips and taped shut at the wrist can also be used. The cold pack should be covered with a paper cover or a washcloth to prevent tissue damage. When the ice melts, the cold pack is left off for 10 minutes before applying another for maximum effect. In some cultures, women believe that heat has healing properties and may resist the use of an ice pack.

After 24 hours, heat in the form of a chemical warm pack, a bidet, or a sitz bath increases circulation and promotes healing (Skill 9-4). The sitz bath may circulate either cool or warm water over the perineum to cleanse the area and increase comfort. Sitting in a cool sitz bath and adding ice cubes and remaining in the water for 20 minutes often provides immediate pain relief (Gabbe, 2012).

The woman is taught to do perineal care after each voiding or bowel movement to cleanse the area without trauma. A plastic bottle (peribottle) is filled with warm water, and the water is squirted over the perineum in a front-to-back direction. The perineum is blotted dry. Perineal pads (peripads) should be applied and removed in the same front-to-back direction to prevent fecal contamination of the perineum and vagina (Skill 9-5).

Topical and systemic medications may be used to relieve perineal pain. Topical perineal medications reduce inflammation or numb the perineum. Commonly prescribed medications include the following:

- Hydrocortisone and pramoxine (Epifoam)
- Benzocaine (Americaine or Dermoplast)

In addition to these topical medications, witch hazel pads (Tucks) and sitz baths reduce the discomfort of hemorrhoids.

To reduce pain when sitting, the mother can be taught to squeeze her buttocks together as she lowers herself to a sitting position and then to relax her

Assisting with a Sitz Bath

PURPOSE

To aid healing of perineum through application of moist heat or cold

STEPS

1. Wash hands, explain procedure, and provide privacy.
2. Assess woman's condition; analyze appropriateness of procedure.
3. Place sitz bath on toilet seat; turn flow of water on.
4. Help woman remove pad and sit in flow of water for 20 minutes.
5. When completed, assist woman to pat perineum dry (front to back); apply clean perineal pad.
6. Assist woman in returning to room (then to chair or bed).
7. Wash hands.
8. Record in medical record that sitz bath was taken, condition of woman, and condition of perineum.

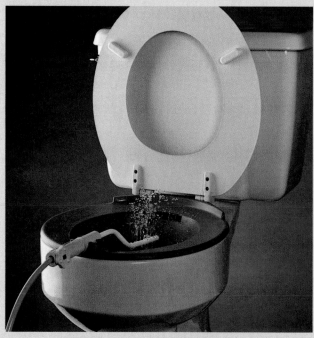

(Courtesy Andermac, Inc., Yuba City, California.)

Table 9-1 Summary of Nursing Assessments Postpartum*

ASSESSMENT	VARIATIONS AND DEVIATIONS	NURSING INTERVENTIONS
Breasts May be soft or engorged	Observe for reddened, tender areas, fissures, and sore nipples	Document and report any alteration; teach breastfeeding principles and assess progress; consult lactation nurse; possible breast massage
Uterus Observe firmness, height of fundus, and location	Check for bladder distention if fundus is not midline; massage a soft, boggy uterus	Document and report any alterations; teach expectations for descent of fundus; teach mother how to massage fundus; discuss "afterpains"
Bladder Observe for bladder distention and urination	Observe for burning or pain on urination	Document and report urine output and abdominal assessment for distended bladder
Bowels Observe for passage of flatus, bowel sounds, and defecation	Report constipation; distended hemorrhoids may be seen	Encourage fluids, ambulation, and fiber in diet; assist with sitz bath for hemorrhoids; possible use of stool softeners
Lochia Observe for character, amount, color, odor, and presence of clots	Observe for large clots and heavy pad saturation; watch for trickle of bright red blood	Document firm, midline fundus; report bleeding and large clots; count peripads saturated in 1 hour; teach the lochial changes to expect
Episiotomy Observe perineum	Observe for vulvar hematoma, perineal bruising; may see hemorrhoids	Document wound assessment in relation to REEDA; teach pericare technique; apply cold packs as indicated; teach how to use sitz bath at home; pad seat area of chair for sitting comfort
Homans' sign Discomfort produced by passive dorsiflexion of the foot is considered a positive Homans' sign indicative of thrombophlebitis	Report if Homans' sign is positive, and assess for other factors that may indicate thrombus formation, such as redness, tenderness, warmth, or increased circumference of the leg	The postpartum value of a positive Homans' sign is limited, because the postpartum woman may have a strained muscle from delivery positioning; clinical symptoms and venous ultrasound are more reliable diagnostic measures (Gabbe, 2012)
Emotions or bonding with newborn Evaluate family interaction, support, and physical contact with newborn	Observe for postpartum depression; observe for "enface contact" with newborn; teach handling and response to newborn needs; assess cultural practices; assess stage of postpartum adaptation	Teach parents about newborn behavior and appearance; teach newborn care; teach self care and *listen* to patient; provide support, nutrition, and periods of rest to prevent fatigue; encourage skin-to-skin contact
Vital signs Bradycardia is common; respirations should be 12-20; vital signs should be stable	Abnormalities may be consistent with comorbidities; deviation in vital signs may also indicate woman is in pain; assess for shock, infection	Record and report tachypnea, elevated temperature, and blood pressure abnormalities; assess for pain, and provide medication as indicated; administer analgesics after breastfeeding to minimize exposure of infant to the medication

REEDA, **R**edness, **e**dema, **e**cchymosis, **d**rainage, **a**pproximation.
*Routine assessments are usually performed every 4 to 6 hours unless risk factors exist.
An acronym that helps remember and organize the postpartum assessment is *BUBBLE-HE:* **B**reast, **U**terus, **B**ladder, **B**owels, **L**ochia, **E**pisiotomy (perineum), **H**omans' sign, **E**motions or bonding.

buttocks. An air ring, or "donut," takes pressure off the perineal area when sitting. The mother should inflate the ring about halfway. (If it is inflated fully, she tends to wobble when she sits on it.) A small egg crate pad is an alternative to the air ring.

Return of Ovulation, Menstruation, and Contraception

The production of placental estrogen and progesterone stops when the placenta is delivered, causing a rise in the production of follicle-stimulating hormone. Menstrual cycles resume in about 5 weeks after delivery if the woman is not breastfeeding or possibly 8 weeks after delivery if the woman is breastfeeding without formula supplementation (Gabbe, 2012). Discussion and teaching concerning contraception should be initiated before discharge, because the mother may not return to her health care provider before 6 weeks postpartum, and she may resume sexual activity before that appointment, which may result in an unplanned pregnancy. Short intervals between pregnancies may result in poor pregnancy outcomes. Natural family planning techniques cannot be effectively used before regular menstrual cycles resume, *but ovulation can occur before menstruation is reestablished, and pregnancy can result.*

Combined oral or transdermal estrogen-progesterone contraceptives can be taken about 2 to 3 weeks after delivery in women who are not

Performing Perineal Care

PURPOSE

To teach the woman the proper technique of perineal care to promote healing and prevent infection

STEPS

1. Wash hands.
2. Explain procedure to woman.
3. Assist the woman to the bathroom.
4. Instruct woman to wash her hands before and after each perineal care.
5. Remove soiled pad from front to back; discard in appropriate waste container.
6. Squeeze peribottle or pour warm water or cleansing solution over perineum without opening labia.
7. Pat dry with clean tissue. Use each tissue one time. Pat from front to back, and then discard tissue.
8. Apply medicated ointments or sprays as directed. Do not apply perineal pad for 1 to 2 minutes (otherwise the medication will be absorbed in the pad).
9. Apply clean perineal pad from front to back, touching only side and outside of pad to lessen risk of infection.
10. Do not flush toilet until woman is standing upright; otherwise, the flushing water can spray the perineum.
11. Always perform perineal care after each voiding, stool, or at least every 4 hours during puerperium.
12. Report clots, increase in lochia flow, or excessive abdominal cramping.

---

breastfeeding, as estrogen does suppress lactation. For breastfeeding women, a low dose progestin-only contraceptive can be started 4 weeks postpartum. Progestin-only contraceptives should be avoided in Hispanic women with gestational diabetes who are breastfeeding, because of the high risk of developing diabetes mellitus type 2 (Gabbe, 2012). Other modes of contraception can be started as soon as lactation is well established.

Breasts

Both nursing and nonnursing mothers experience breast changes after birth. Assessments for both types of mothers are similar, but nursing care differs.

Changes in the Breasts. For the first 2 or 3 days the breasts are full but soft. By the third day the breasts become firm and lumpy as blood flow increases and milk production begins. Breast engorgement may occur in both nursing and nonnursing mothers. The engorged breast is hard, erect, and very uncomfortable. The nipple may be so hard that the infant cannot easily grasp it. The breasts of the nonnursing mother return to their normal size in 1 to 2 weeks.

Nursing Care. At each assessment the nurse checks the woman's breasts for consistency, size, shape, and symmetry. The nipples are inspected for redness and cracking, which makes breastfeeding more painful and offers a port of entry for microorganisms. Flat or inverted nipples make it more difficult for the infant to grasp the nipple and suckle.

Both nursing and nonnursing mothers should wear a bra to support the heavier breasts. The bra should firmly support the nursing mother's breasts but not be so tight that it impedes circulation. Some nonnursing mothers may prefer to wear an elastic binder to suppress lactation.

The nonnursing mother should avoid stimulating her nipples, which stimulates lactation. She should wear a bra at all times to avoid having her clothing brush back and forth over her breasts, and she should stand facing away from the water spray in the shower.

The nipples should be washed with plain water to avoid the drying effects of soap, which can lead to cracking. The nonnursing woman should minimize stimulation when washing her breasts. Breastfeeding is discussed in Chapter 9.

CARDIOVASCULAR SYSTEM

Cardiac Output and Blood Volume

Because of a 50% increase in blood volume during pregnancy, the woman tolerates the following normal blood loss at delivery:

- 500 mL in vaginal birth
- 1000 mL in cesarean birth

Despite the blood loss, there is a temporary increase in blood volume and cardiac output, because blood that was directed to the uterus and the placenta returns to the main circulation. Added fluid also moves from the tissues into the circulation, further increasing her blood volume. The heart pumps more blood with each contraction (increased stroke volume), leading to bradycardia. After the initial postbirth excitement wanes, the pulse rate may be as low as 50 to 60 beats/min for about 48 hours after birth. To reestablish normal fluid balance, the body rids itself of excess fluid in the following two ways:

1. Diuresis (increased excretion of urine), which may reach 3000 mL/day
2. Diaphoresis (profuse perspiration)

Coagulation

Blood clotting factors are higher during pregnancy and for 4 to 6 weeks of the puerperium (Blackburn, 2013), yet the woman's ability to lyse (break down and eliminate) clots is not increased. Therefore she is prone to blood clot formation, especially if there is stasis of blood in the venous system. This situation is more likely to occur if the woman has varicose veins, has had a cesarean birth, or must delay ambulation. Dyspnea (difficult breathing) and tachypnea (rapid breathing) are hallmark signs of a pulmonary embolus and necessitate immediate medical intervention. Women who deliver via cesarean section may receive prophylactic anticoagulant therapy with heparin and/or pneumatic compression devices on the lower extremities to prevent venous congestion and to promote circulation (ACOG, 2011).

Blood Values

The massive fluid shifts just described affect blood values such as hemoglobin and hematocrit, making them difficult to interpret during the early puerperium. Fluid that shifts into the bloodstream dilutes the blood cells, which lowers the hematocrit. As the fluid balance returns to normal, the values are more accurately interpreted, usually by 8 weeks postpartum.

The white blood cell (leukocyte) count may rise as high as 12,000 to 20,000/mm³, a level that would ordinarily suggest infection. The increase is in response to inflammation, pain, and stress, and it protects the mother from infection as her tissues heal. The white blood cell count returns to normal by 12 days postpartum.

Chills

Many mothers experience tremors that resemble shivering or "chills" immediately after birth. These tremors are thought to be related to a sudden release of pressure on the pelvic nerves and a vasomotor response involving epinephrine (adrenaline) during the birth process. Most women will deny feeling cold. These tremors or "chills" stop spontaneously within 20 minutes. The nurse should reassure the woman and cover her with a warm blanket to provide comfort. Chills accompanied by fever after the first 24 hours suggest infection and should be reported.

Orthostatic Hypotension

After childbirth, resistance to blood flow in the vessels of the pelvis drops. As a result, the woman's blood pressure falls when she sits or stands, and she may feel dizzy or lightheaded or may even faint. Guidance and assistance are needed during early ambulation to prevent injury.

Nursing Care. After the fourth stage of labor, vital signs are taken every 4 hours for the first 24 hours. The temperature may rise to 38° C (100.4° F) in the first 24 hours. A higher temperature, or the persistence of a temperature elevation for more than 24 hours, suggests infection. The pulse rate helps to interpret temperature and blood pressure values. Because of the normal postpartum bradycardia, a high pulse rate often indicates infection or hypovolemia.

If diaphoresis bothers the woman, she should be reminded that it is temporary. The nurse should help her shower or take a sponge bath and provide dry clothes and bedding.

The nurse checks for the presence of edema in the lower extremities, hands, and face. Edema in the lower extremities is common, as it is during pregnancy. Edema above the waist is more likely to be associated with pregnancy-induced hypertension, which can continue during the early postpartum period.

The woman's legs should be checked for evidence of thrombosis at each assessment, looking for a reddened, tender area (superficial vein) or edema, pain, and, sometimes, pallor (deep vein). *Homans' sign* (calf pain when the foot is passively dorsiflexed) is of limited value in identifying thrombosis in the postpartum phase (Gabbe, 2012). Early and regular ambulation reduces the venous stasis that promotes blood clots.

The first time the woman gets out of bed, she is at increased risk for a fall because of the physiologic events during delivery that can cause unstable blood pressure and syncope (Lockwood, 2013). Therefore it is a priority nursing responsibility to offer assistance with bedside sitting, toileting, and ambulation following delivery, especially for women who have had epidural analgesia or cesarean births.

 Safety Alert!

All postpartum women, when placed in the postpartum unit following delivery, should be informed of the availability and advisability of asking for assistance the first time they get out of bed to prevent accidental falls.

URINARY SYSTEM

Kidney function returns to normal within a month after birth. A decrease in the tone of the bladder and ureters as a result of pregnancy, combined with intravenous fluids administered during labor, may cause the woman's bladder to fill quickly but empty incompletely during the postpartum period. This can lead to postpartum hemorrhage when the full bladder displaces the uterus, or a possible urinary tract infection because of stasis of the urine in the bladder.

Nursing Care. The nurse should regularly assess the woman's bladder for distention. The bladder may not feel full to the woman, yet the uterus is high and deviated to one side. If she can ambulate, the mother should go to the bathroom and urinate. The first two to three voidings after birth or after catheter removal are measured. Women who receive intravenous infusions or have an indwelling catheter continue to have their urine output measured until the infusion and/or catheter are discontinued. The following measures may help a woman to urinate:

- Provide as much privacy as possible.
- Remain near the woman, but do not rush her by constantly asking her if she has urinated.
- Run water in the sink.
- Have the woman place her hands in warm water.
- Have the woman use the peribottle to squirt warm water over her perineal area to relax the urethral sphincter. Be sure to measure the amount of water in the peribottle when it is filled so the amount used can be deducted from the amount of urine voided.

Some discomfort with early urination is expected because of the edema and trauma in the area. However, continued burning or urgency of urination suggests bladder infection. High fever and chills may occur with kidney infection.

GASTROINTESTINAL SYSTEM

The gastrointestinal system resumes normal activity shortly after birth when progesterone decreases. The mother is usually hungry after the hard work and food deprivation during labor. The nurse should expect to provide food and water to a new mother often!

Constipation may occur during the postpartum period as a result of several factors:

- Medications may slow peristalsis.
- Abdominal muscles are stretched, making it more difficult for the woman to bear down to expel stool. A cesarean incision adds to this difficulty.
- Hemorrhoids or soreness and swelling of the perineum may make the woman fear her first bowel movement.
- Slight dehydration and little food intake during labor make the feces harder.

Nursing Care. The mother is encouraged to drink lots of fluids, add fiber to her diet, and ambulate. A stool softener such as docusate calcium (Surfak) or docusate sodium (Colace) is usually ordered. These measures are generally sufficient to correct the problem. Because constipation is a common problem during pregnancy, measures she has used to relieve it are discussed at that time, and efforts are made to build on the woman's knowledge. A common laxative is bisacodyl (Dulcolax), given orally or as a suppository when a laxative is indicated.

INTEGUMENTARY SYSTEM

Hyperpigmentation of the skin ("mask of pregnancy," or chloasma, and the linea nigra) disappears as hormone levels decrease. Striae ("stretch marks") do not disappear but fade from reddish purple to silver.

MUSCULOSKELETAL SYSTEM

The abdominal wall has been greatly stretched during pregnancy and may now have a "doughy" appearance. Many women are dismayed to discover that they still look pregnant after they give birth. They should be reassured that time and exercise can tighten their lax muscles. Also, some women have **diastasis recti**, in which the longitudinal abdominal muscles that extend from the chest to the symphysis pubis are separated. Abdominal wall weakness may remain for 6 to 8 weeks and contribute to constipation. Hypermobility of the joints that normally occurs during pregnancy usually stabilizes within 6 weeks, but the joints of the feet may remain separated, and the new mother may notice an increase in shoe size. The center of gravity of the body returns to normal when the enlarged uterus returns to its prepregnant size.

A woman can usually begin light exercises as soon as the first day after vaginal birth. Women who have undergone a cesarean birth may wait longer. The woman should consult her health care provider for specific instructions about exercise. Common postpartum exercises include the following:

- *Abdominal tightening.* In the supine or erect position, the woman inhales slowly and then exhales slowly while contracting her abdominal muscles. After a count of 10, she relaxes the muscles. She should begin with 3 repetitions and increase the number to 5, then 10. This may be done 3 times and then 5 times daily, up to 10 times each day.
- *Head lift.* The woman lies flat on her back on her bed with her knees bent and inhales. While exhaling, she lifts her head, chin to chest, and looks at her thighs. She holds this position to a count of three, and then relaxes. This is repeated several times. After the third week (or when the health care provider permits), the head lift may progress to include the head and shoulders. This may be done 5 to 10 times daily.
- *Pelvic tilt.* While lying supine with her knees bent and feet flat, the woman inhales and exhales, flattening her lower back to the bed or exercise surface and contracting her abdominal muscles. She holds the position to a count of three. She begins with 5 repetitions and works up to 10 repetitions daily.

- *Kegel exercises.* Perineal exercises may be resumed immediately after birth to promote circulation and healing. The mother tightens the muscles of the perineal area, as if to stop the flow of urine, and then relaxes them. She should inhale, tighten for a count of 10, exhale, and relax. She may do the exercise five times each hour for the first few days. Then she may increase the number of repetitions. She should not actually stop her urine flow when urinating, however, because this could lead to urine stasis and urinary tract infection.

IMMUNE SYSTEM

Prevention of blood incompatibility and infection are addressed in the postpartum period according to each woman's specific needs.

Rho(D) Immune Globulin

The woman's blood type and Rh factor and antibody status are determined on an early prenatal visit or on admission if she did not have prenatal care. The Rh-negative mother should receive a dose of $Rh_o(D)$ immune globulin **(RhoGAM)** within 72 hours after giving birth to an Rh-positive infant. This prevents sensitization to Rh-positive erythrocytes that may have entered her bloodstream when the infant was born. *RhoGAM is given to the mother, not the infant,* by intramuscular injection into the deltoid muscle. The woman receives an identification card stating that she is Rh negative and has received RhoGAM on that date.

Rubella (German Measles) Immunization

Rubella titers are done early in pregnancy to determine if a woman is immune to rubella. A titer of 1:8 or greater indicates immunity to the rubella virus. The mother who is not immune is given the vaccine in the immediate postpartum period. The vaccine prevents infection with the rubella virus during subsequent pregnancies, which could cause birth defects. A signed informed consent is usually required to administer the rubella vaccine.

The rubella vaccine is given subcutaneously in the upper arm. The woman should not get pregnant for the next month following vaccination. The vaccine should not be administered if the woman is sensitive to neomycin. Women vaccinated during the postpartum period may breastfeed without adverse affects to the newborn (CDC, 2009).

ADAPTATION OF NURSING CARE FOLLOWING CESAREAN BIRTH

The woman who has a cesarean birth has had surgery as well as given birth. Many of her reactions to the surgical birth depend on whether she expected it. The woman who had an unexpected, emergency cesarean often has many questions about what happened to her and why, because there was no time to answer these questions at the time of birth. In addition, her anxiety may have limited her ability to comprehend any explanations given. Occasionally a woman may feel that she failed if she was unable to give birth after laboring. Terms such as *failed induction* and *failure to progress* imply that the woman herself was not competent in some way. Some variations of normal postpartum care are needed for the woman who has experienced a cesarean birth (Nursing Care Plan 9-1).

Uterus

The nurse should check the fundus as on any new mother; it descends at a similar rate. Checking her fundus when a woman has a transverse skin incision is not much different from checking the woman who has had vaginal birth. If she has a vertical skin incision, the nurse should gently "walk" the fingers toward the fundus from the side to her abdominal midline. If the fundus is firm and at its expected level, no massage is necessary.

Lochia

Lochia is checked at routine assessment intervals, which vary with the time since birth. The quantity of lochia immediately after cesarean birth is generally less, because surgical sponges have removed the contents of the uterus.

Dressing

The dressing should be checked for drainage as with any surgical patient. When the dressing is removed, the incision is assessed for signs of infection. The wound should be clean and dry, and the staples should be intact. The REEDA acronym previously described is a good way to remember key items to check as related to an incision: **r**edness, **e**dema, **e**cchymosis, **d**rainage, and **a**pproximation. Staples may be removed and Steri-Strips applied shortly before hospital discharge on the third day. If a woman leaves earlier, the staples may be removed in her health care provider's office.

The woman can shower as soon as she can ambulate reliably. A shower chair reduces the risk for fainting. The dressing or incision can be covered with a plastic wrap and the edges secured with tape. The woman should be told to position herself with her back to the water stream. The dressing is changed after the woman finishes her shower. A similar technique can be used to cover an intravenous infusion site. If the infusion site is in her hand, a glove can cover it.

Urinary Catheter

An indwelling urinary catheter is generally removed within 24 hours of delivery. Urine is observed for blood, which may indicate trauma to the bladder during labor or surgery. The blood should quickly clear from the urine as diuresis occurs. Intake and output are measured until both the intravenous infusion and the catheter are discontinued. The first two to three voidings are measured, and measuring should continue until the

⭐ Nursing Care Plan 9-1   The Woman Having a Cesarean Birth

PATIENT DATA A 32-year-old woman is admitted to the postpartum unit after delivering a healthy 8-lb boy via cesarean section. The woman is lying still in bed and refuses to move, because, she states, she fears postoperative pain.

Selected Nursing Diagnosis: Acute pain related to surgical incision and afterpains

Goals	Nursing Interventions	Rationales
The woman will state that pain relief is adequate with pharmacological and nonpharmacological measures.	Use a 0-to-10 scale to evaluate pain level before and after interventions.	Provides a more objective way for the nurse to evaluate the woman's subjective experience of pain. Evaluates adequacy of pain relief.
	Encourage the woman to change positions regularly (about every 2 hours). Support her body and extremities with pillows as needed.	Reduces discomfort from constant pressure and having body in one position too long. Also helps to mobilize respiratory secretions.
	Teach the woman to use a small pillow pressed to her incision when moving or coughing.	Supports the incision, reducing pain. Increases the likelihood that she will cough adequately, which expels respiratory secretions.
	Provide ordered analgesia: • Patient-controlled anesthesia pump • Intermittent injections • Oral analgesia	Reduces the perception of pain, which facilitates moving, coughing, and ambulating. Reduces anxiety and fatigue.

Selected Nursing Diagnosis: Impaired skin integrity related to abdominal incision

Goals	Nursing Interventions	Rationales
The woman will have no excessive redness or tenderness and no separation or discharge from incision.	Observe dressing for drainage with each assessment.	Red drainage indicates bleeding, which should not increase. Foul-smelling drainage indicates infection.
	When dressing is removed, assess incision using REEDA criteria. Assess amount of tenderness.	Identifies proper healing of incision. A separating suture line, excessive redness or tenderness, or discharge indicates probable infection.
	Determine temperature every 4 hours.	A temperature higher than 38° C (100.4° F) after 24 hours is associated with infection.
The woman will demonstrate knowledge of self-care measures related to her incision by discharge time.	Teach woman self-care measures: • Expected progress of healing and how the incision should look • How to bathe (plastic over incision, if ordered) • What to report (signs of bleeding or infection) • When her staples or sutures should be removed if not done before discharge • Follow-up appointment	Women must assume responsibility for their own care because of short hospital stays. These guidelines give the woman a framework to know what is and is not normal and how to care for herself to prevent infection. Follow-up appointments allow her physician to assess how healing is progressing and to identify complications early.

Critical Thinking Question

1. How will your discharge teaching for a patient who delivered by cesarean section differ from that for a patient who delivered vaginally?

REEDA, **R**edness, **e**dema, **e**cchymosis, **d**rainage, **a**pproximation.

woman urinates at least 150 mL. The nurse should observe and teach the woman to observe for the following signs of urinary tract infection, because use of a catheter increases this risk:

- Fever
- Burning pain on urination
- Urgency of urination

Frequency of urination is difficult to assess in any postpartum woman because of normal postpartum diuresis. However, frequent voidings of small quantities of urine, especially if associated with the described signs and symptoms, suggest a urinary tract infection.

Respiratory Care

Lung sounds should be auscultated each shift for clarity. Diminished breath sounds, crackles, or wheezes indicate that lung secretions are being retained. When she is confined to bed, the woman should take deep breaths and turn from side to side every 2 hours. She should be encouraged to cough to move secretions out of her lungs. To reduce incisional pain from coughing or other movement, the nurse can have the woman hold a small pillow or folded blanket firmly against her incision. An incentive spirometer may be used to give the woman a "target" for deep breaths. The woman should begin ambulating as early as possible to mobilize lung secretions.

Preventing Thrombophlebitis

The woman who has undergone a cesarean birth has a greater risk for thrombophlebitis. She may receive prophylactic heparin anticoagulation therapy and/or pneumatic compression devices applied to her lower extremities to decrease venous congestion and promote circulation until ambulation is established (ACOG, 2011). She should do simple leg exercises, such as alternately flexing and extending her feet or moving her legs from a flexed to an extended position when turning. The nurse should assess for signs of thrombosis as previously described. Early and frequent ambulation also reduces the risk for thrombophlebitis.

Pain Management

Pain control is essential to reduce the woman's distress and facilitate movement that can prevent several complications. The severity, frequency, character, and location of discomfort are assessed. Using a 0-to-10 scale helps to quantify the subjective experience of pain better. Zero would be no pain at all, and 10 would be the worst pain ever. The scale helps the nurse to choose the most appropriate relief methods and provides a method to evaluate the amount of relief the woman receives from the pain interventions.

Some women receive epidural narcotics for long-lasting pain relief. These drugs can cause respiratory depression many hours after they are administered, sometimes up to 24 hours. Therefore hourly respiratory monitoring and a pulse oximeter are usual until the drug's effects have worn off. Naloxone (Narcan) should be readily available to reverse the respiratory depression. If the woman has pain not controlled by the epidural narcotic, the health care provider must be consulted for specific orders.

Many women have a patient-controlled analgesia (PCA) pump to provide them with analgesia. The pump has a syringe with a narcotic analgesic inside. It is programmed to deliver a specific dose of the drug when the woman pushes a button. To prevent overdose, there is a lockout interval during which pushing the button has no effect. As with any narcotic, the drug inside the PCA pump is counted at shift change, and the facility's protocol for record keeping is followed to account for all drug doses received, remaining, or wasted when the PCA drug is discontinued.

Most women change to an oral analgesic on the day after surgery. The woman should be instructed to call for pain medication when she first becomes uncomfortable. Pain is much harder to relieve if it becomes severe.

The breastfeeding mother should be reassured that timing the administration of analgesia immediately after breastfeeding minimizes passage of the drug via breast milk to the infant. It can be explained that adequate pain control helps her to relax so she can breastfeed better and can have the energy to become acquainted with her infant.

EMOTIONAL CARE

The birth of an infant brings about physical changes in the mother but also causes many emotional and relationship changes in all family members.

MOTHERS

The transition to motherhood brings many hormonal changes, changes in body image, and psychological acceptance of the self as a mother figure. Fluctuating hormones in pregnancy and the puerperium have an effect on mood, causing early elation at delivery that can be followed by mild depression with tearfulness, irritability, and fatigue peaking on the fifth day postpartum. Most women recover in a few days. However, the physiological factors that affect mood can interact with minor anxieties and stresses to result in a clinical depression. Rubin (1967) has described three phases of postpartum change that have been a framework for nursing care for 35 years (Table 9-2). More recent studies have shown that women progress through the same three phases, although at a more rapid pace than originally described. The nurse can refer to the three phases when providing postpartum care. The nurse must use the "teaching moments" when the woman enters the take-hold phase, because the woman will be focused on the infant's needs and will be most receptive to teaching.

Postpartum Blues

New mothers often experience conflicting feelings of joy and emotional letdown during the first few weeks after birth, often called the **postpartum blues**, or the baby blues. She may feel let down, but overall she finds pleasure in life. The symptoms are self-limiting. When providing discharge teaching, the nurse should prepare the woman for these feelings and reassure her that they are normal and temporary.

Postpartum Depression

Postpartum depression is a persistent mood of unhappiness and is discussed in Chapter 10. When teaching about the postpartum blues, as described earlier, the nurse should explain that persistent depression is *not* expected and should be reported to her health care provider.

Fatigue

Postpartum assessment typically includes physical assessment and psychological bonding and must also include evaluation for *fatigue*. Today's modern lifestyle often includes the woman working through

Table 9-2	Rubin's Psychological Adaptation of the Puerperium and Related Nursing Interventions
PSYCHOLOGICAL ADAPTATION	**NURSING RESPONSES**
Taking-in Phase	
Mother is passive and willing to let others do things for her. Conversation centers on her birth experience. Has interest in infant but prefers that others care for infant. Has little interest in learning. Focus is on need for food, fluids, and restorative sleep.	Provide opportunity for rest and appropriate nutrition. Provide opportunity to discuss birth experience and vent disappointments or share joys.
Taking-Hold Phase	
Mother begins to initiate action and becomes interested in caring for infant. May be critical about her abilities. Has increased concern about her body functions and assumes self-care needs. Is interested in learning how to care for self and baby.	Provide supportive atmosphere. Identify support system of mother. Use teaching moments. Reinforce self-care and infant caretaking abilities.
Letting-Go Phase	
Mothers and partners work through giving up their previous lifestyle to incorporate new infant. Many mothers must give up their ideal of the birth experience and reconcile it with what really occurred. They give up the fantasy child and accept the real child.	Provide supportive atmosphere. Provide referrals to community agencies as appropriate for assistance needed. Reinforce infant caregiving abilities.

Data from Rubin R: Attainment of the maternal role part 1: processes, *Nurs Res* 16:237-245, 1967.

most of her pregnancy, rooming-in after delivery with responsibility for newborn care, and then returning home after delivery in 48 hours or less to accept complete home responsibilities. Therefore, many women do not have the opportunity to rest and adapt in the postpartum phase. The nurse should assess the level of maternal fatigue and initiate appropriate relief measures such as taking on the care of the newborn for a few hours, or scheduling care that allows for periods of rest. Discussion of the home environment and available support persons should be reviewed before discharge.

FATHERS

New fathers typically display intense interest in their new child (*engrossment*) (Figure 9-3). Their behaviors with their infant parallel those of the new mother. A man's relationship with his own parents, previous experiences with children, and relationship to the mother are important influences on how he will relate to his infant. According to Goodman (2005), new fathers often experience four phases of adjustment to fatherhood characterized by the following:

- Having expectations and personal intentions
- Confronting reality and overcoming frustrations
- Creating one's own personal father role
- Reaping rewards of fatherhood

Adjustment to fatherhood is facilitated by involvement in the infant's care. Fathers should be included when the nurse is sharing instructions about infant care and handling. The nurse must be tactful and supportive of a new father who is trying to assume his new role.

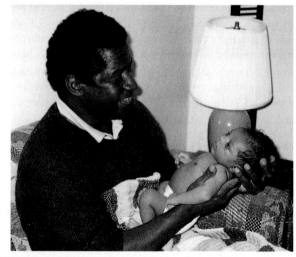

FIGURE 9-3 This father shows intense interest in his new infant (*engrossment*). The father's reaction to the newborn parallels the mother's. Eye-to-eye contact (*en face position*) helps the bonding process. (Courtesy Pat Spier, RN-C.)

SIBLINGS

The influence of a new child's birth on siblings depends on their age and developmental level. Toddlers may respond with regression and anger when the mother's attention turns to the infant. Preschool children typically look at and discuss the newborn but may hesitate to touch actively or hold the infant. Older children often enjoy helping with care of the infant and are very curious about the newcomer.

GRANDPARENTS

The grandparents' involvement with a new child is often dictated by how near they live to the younger family. Grandparents who live a long distance from the family cannot have the close, regular contact that they may desire. Grandparents also differ in what they expect their role to be, and culture sometimes determines their expected role. Some feel that their child-rearing days are in the past, and they want minimal day-to-day involvement in raising the children. Others expect to have regular involvement in the grandchild's life, second only to the parents (Figure 9-4). If parents and grandparents agree on the grandparents' role, little conflict is likely.

GRIEVING PARENTS

The postpartum period is usually a joyful time, but nurses occasionally care for grieving parents. With most of these parents, the nurse should simply listen to them and support them. Therapeutic communication techniques such as open-ended questions or reflection of feelings help the parents express their grief—an early step in resolving it.

It seems strange to talk of grief when a healthy infant is born, but even a healthy child may be much different in size, sex, or appearance from what parents expected. Most parents eventually come to accept their unique infant and his or her characteristics. Their feelings about their child are not right or wrong—feelings simply exist. The nurse should accept and encourage their expressions of grief to allow them to move forward and accept the infant they have.

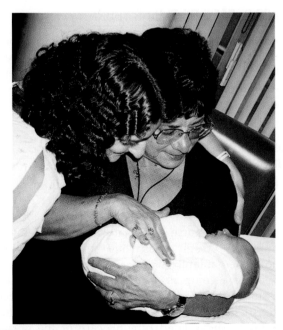

FIGURE 9-4 The daughter's arm around her mother shows how proud she is to introduce her newborn to Grandma. Grandmothers can reinforce cultural customs, help with infant care, and assist with household tasks.

A woman who has experienced the loss of a newborn may experience regret, remorse, and sorrow. This can be one of the most difficult kinds of grief. The woman may question what she could have done differently to prevent the loss. Anniversaries of these events are painful, and feelings often last for many years, if not forever. The birth of a new child may awaken grief that parents thought they had resolved ("We have one child, but we almost had two").

If the condition of a newborn is poor, the parents may wish to have a baptism performed. The minister or priest is notified. In an emergency, the nurse may perform the baptism by pouring water on the infant's forehead while saying, "I baptize you in the name of the Father, and of the Son, and of the Holy Spirit." If there is any doubt as to whether the infant is alive, the baptism is given conditionally: "If you are capable of receiving baptism, I baptize you in the name of the Father, and of the Son, and of the Holy Spirit."

If the infant dies, is stillborn, or has a birth defect, the parents' reactions depend on whether the event was expected. If they have known for some time that the fetus was not living, they may have already begun the grief process and will not display all the typical behaviors. If the death was not expected, the nurse is likely to encounter the following reactions typical of any grieving:

- Shock and disbelief
- Anger (often directed at the physician or staff; rarely at the infant)
- Guilt about what the parents could have done differently
- Sadness and depression
- Gradual resolution of the sadness

The nurse may encounter grieving families at any point in their grieving process and in many settings. When the infant has a birth defect, grieving is often chronic because of the constant reminders of what might have been.

If a newborn dies or is stillborn, nursing units have a protocol to help parents to accept and resolve the event in their minds. The parents should be allowed to progress at their individual pace regarding when or whether they want to see and hold the infant. The parents should be prepared for the infant's appearance. For instance, a stillborn infant may have blue skin, which often is peeling. The nurse should try to keep the infant warm so he or she feels more natural to the parents. If this is not possible, the parents should be prepared for the coolness of the infant's skin and the limp body. The infant should be wrapped in a blanket and the parents should be allowed to unwrap the infant when and if they want to do so. If an anomaly is present, the infant should be wrapped so the most normal part is showing.

The nurse should listen to the parent's responses to determine the level of support needed, to answer questions, and to understand the grief behaviors individual to the family or culture. Providing privacy and planning for an interdisciplinary grief conference before discharge is important in the overall plan of care. Parents should be provided with private time with the infant if possible and given mementos to take home. The support system of the parents (and grandparents) should be examined, and some information concerning the expected grief process, its influence on behavior and the ability to perform activities of daily living, coping mechanisms, and resources for follow-up care should be discussed.

Most nursing units make a memory packet containing items such as a lock of hair, footprints on a hospital birth certificate, the identification band, a photograph, and clothing or blankets. Some type of code, such as a flower or ribbon on the mother's door, alerts personnel from other departments that a grieving family is inside. This reduces the chance that well-intentioned but painful remarks or questions might be made such as, "What did you have, a boy or girl?"

PARENTHOOD

Whether the parents have one or several children, becoming a parent requires learning new roles and making adjustments. Parents having their first child find themselves in a triangular relationship. Many parents say that parenthood, not marriage, made the greatest change in their lives. Adjustments are even greater for women who have professions or who are in the work force, because the changes are more extensive.

The demands of parenthood affect communication between the partners, and there is little doubt that children distract from the relationship at times. It is not unusual for one member to feel left out. The division of responsibility can be a source of conflict, particularly when both parents work. Parents often feel inept, which may cause lower self-esteem, depression, and anger. These feelings can be overwhelming.

Fatigue triggers irritability. Even in the ideal situation, waking up two or three times every night is wearisome for anyone. For the new mother, physiological changes continue to play a part in her emotional lability (instability). Both parents are concerned with increased economic responsibilities. Loss of freedom and a decrease in socialization may give the couple a sense of loneliness.

Ideally, preparing parents for the lifestyle changes that occur with a new child begins before conception. Parenting courses, group discussions, and support from relatives or friends can be explored. Social service agencies, public health nurses, and other professional resources should be suggested as appropriate. Encouraging parents to share their concerns and worries with one another and to keep communication lines open are foremost. Reestablishing a relationship into which the newborn fits with a minimum of disruption can be accomplished when the parents identify their own needs, set priorities, maintain their sense of humor, and relax their standards.

These tools can make the transition to parenthood a rewarding yet sometimes difficult experience—one in which the stable family can grow and become stronger. Parents who find themselves at an impasse should seek early intervention with a professional counselor.

THE FAMILY CARE PLAN

The family care plan is similar to the traditional nursing care plan except that the "patient" is the entire family rather than the woman in the hospital. It is most appropriate to use a family care plan in obstetrics when managing the birth of a child who will have a profound impact on the family processes. Studying the family as the patient, rather than an individual as the patient, can offer insight into community-based care and can help the nurse integrate knowledge of family structure, culture, and composition into a plan of care that will meet some of the goals of *Healthy People 2020* (U.S. Department of Health and Human Services, 2010). The data required in a family care plan are listed in Nursing Care Plan 9-2. The nurse should use information concerning cultural practices (see Chapter 6) and family processes presented in general psychology to recognize the implications of specific nursing diagnoses to the delivery of nursing care to families. The new family should be given telephone numbers or online addresses for follow-up questions, a list of community services available, and a list of available breastfeeding classes and "Mommy and me" programs. Follow-up appointments with the health care provider for both mother and baby should be given to them before they leave the hospital.

PHASE 2: CARE OF THE NEWBORN

This section presents the Phase 2 care of the newborn after transport to the postpartum unit. Care immediately after birth (Phase 1) was discussed in Chapter 6. Newborn assessments and ongoing care (Phase 3) are presented in Chapter 12. Care of the preterm and the postterm infant is presented in Chapter 13.

ADMISSION TO THE POSTPARTUM OR NURSERY UNIT

If the infant has adequate cardiorespiratory and heat-regulating functions, he or she usually remains undisturbed while the parents and infant become acquainted. The nurse can usually assess temperature, heart rate, and respirations while the parents continue to hold their infant. Within an hour, the admitting nurse does a complete physical and gestational age assessment of the infant and gives prophylactic medications. Chapter 12 offers the expected characteristics, deviations, and related nursing care of the normal newborn.

The "intensive care concept" has been introduced to the care of all newborns for the immediate neonatal

✦ Nursing Care Plan 9-2 | The Family Care Plan

PATIENT DATA A woman is admitted to the postpartum unit after delivering a healthy baby girl. The husband, two sons (ages 14 and 10), and the woman's mother are present in the room. The woman tells the nurse she would like to stay in the hospital as long as she can, because she has forgotten everything about baby care.

Selected Nursing Diagnosis: Compromised family coping related to new family member (newborn)

Goals	Nursing Interventions	Rationales
Family members will express satisfaction with adaptation to newborn and confident in their roles.	Determine relationship of family members to one another.	Can help provide a positive experience to prepare the family for new developmental tasks.
	Provide unlimited visiting privileges for family and siblings.	Facilitates the attachment and bonding process.
	Initiate support group concerning breastfeeding and child care.	Verbalization of family culture, roles, and perceived responsibilities enables the appropriate person to be included in instruction concerning breastfeeding and child care.
	Provide anticipatory guidance concerning changes to expect and family adaptation options.	Meeting needs concerning housing, equipment, and community resources available for assisting will help family adapt to changes.
	Discuss sexuality needs and plans for contraception.	Clarification of contraception options acceptable to the cultural group will enhance learning and enable family to make informed decisions.
	Provide written information and suggested books for siblings concerning the new child. Encourage sibling verbalization.	Including the needs of each family member will promote family coping and adaptation.

Critical Thinking Question
1. How does family care differ from the care of an individual patient?

---

period until they have evidenced a normal transition to extrauterine life (Thureen, 2005). The three phases of this transition are as follows:

Phase 1: 0 to 30 minutes (period of reactivity; see Chapter 6)
- Tachycardia, gradually lowering to normal rate
- Irregular respirations
- Rales present on auscultation
- Infant is alert; frequent Moro (startle reaction) reflex, tremors, crying, increased motor activity (because of sudden release from confines of uterus, response to light)
- Hypoactive bowel sounds
- Sucking reflex is present

Phase 2: 30 minutes to 2 hours (decreased responsiveness)
- Decreased motor activity
- Rapid respirations (up to 60 breaths/min)
- Normal heart rate for term newborn
- Audible bowel sounds

Phase 3: 2 to 8 hours (second period of reactivity; see Chapter 12)
- Abrupt, brief changes in color and muscle tone
- Presence of oral mucus (can cause gagging)
- Responsiveness to external stimuli
- Infant stabilizes, begins suck-swallow coordination, and is ready for regular feedings

Supporting Thermoregulation

The temperature of the term newborn is 36° to 36.5° C (96.8° to 97.7° F; skin) or 36.5° to 37° C (97.7° to 98.6° F; axillary). Maintenance of body temperature is very important to the newborn infant, who has less efficient means of generating heat than an older infant. Hypothermia (low body temperature) can cause other problems, such as the following:
- Hypoglycemia (low blood sugar), because the infant uses glucose to generate heat
- Respiratory distress, because the higher metabolic rate consumes more oxygen, sometimes beyond the infant's ability to supply it

Hypoglycemia can be both the cause and the result of hypothermia; therefore the nurse must evaluate both factors. Respiratory distress can also require more glucose for the increased work of breathing, causing hypoglycemia.

Heat is lost by any of the following four means:
- *Evaporation* of liquids from the skin
- *Conduction* caused by direct skin contact with a cold surface
- *Convection* of heat away from the body by drafts
- *Radiation* caused by being near a cold surface, although not in direct contact with it

Conduction, convection, and radiation can also be used to add heat to the body. Newborns lose heat

Table 9-3   Nursing Interventions to Prevent Heat Loss in Newborns

MECHANISM OF HEAT LOSS	SOURCES OF HEAT LOSS	INTERVENTIONS
Evaporation (conversion from liquid to vapor)	Wet skin from amniotic fluid at birth evaporates from skin	Dry infant quickly. Dry and cover head of infant.
Conduction (transfer of heat to a cooler surface)	Cool surface of bed, scale, stethoscope	Prewarm radiant warmer and stethoscope before use. Place scale paper on scale, and place warm blanket on other surfaces.
Convection (loss of heat to the surrounding cooler air)	Drafts from window, air conditioning, oxygen vents	Place crib away from windows and vents.
Radiation (loss of heat to surrounding cold environment)	Cold environment of walls, windows	Place crib away from cold walls. Wrap infant warmly.

quickly after birth, because amniotic fluid evaporates from their body, drafts move heat away, and they may contact cold surfaces (Table 9-3).

The infant remains in a radiant warmer and is monitored until the temperature is stabilized and he or she can be cared for in an open crib, clothed, and wrapped in a blanket. The first bath is delayed until the body temperature is stabilized at 36.5° to 37° C (97.7° to 98.6° F). The temperature should be recorded 30 minutes after the bath and 1 hour after transfer to an open crib. Sponge baths are given to newborns in most hospitals, although research has shown that tub baths can be safely given (AWHONN, 2007).

Observing Bowel and Urinary Function

Newborns may not urinate for as long as 24 hours, and occasionally an infant may not void for 48 hours. If an infant urinates in the birthing or operating room, the staff nurse should be informed and the voiding documented on the delivery record. If a long period elapses before the second voiding, it will have been established that the urinary tract is open. Seventy percent of term newborns pass meconium in the first 12 hours. Meconium should be passed before discharge for assurance of a patent gastrointestinal tract.

Providing for Security

The possibility of abduction must be addressed in any facility that cares for infants and children. In the maternal–newborn setting, security begins with identification bands that the nurse matches every time the infant is reunited with the parent (Figure 9-5).

Identifying the Infant. Wristbands with preprinted numbers are placed on the mother, the infant, and often the father or another support person in the birthing room as the primary means of identifying the infant. The nurse should check to be sure that all numbers in the set are identical (see Figure 9-5). Other identifying information such as mother's name, birth attendant's name, date and time of birth, sex of the infant, and usually the mother's hospital identification number should be completed. The bands are applied relatively snugly

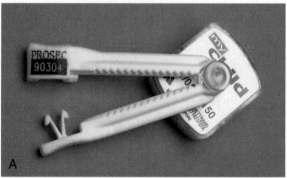

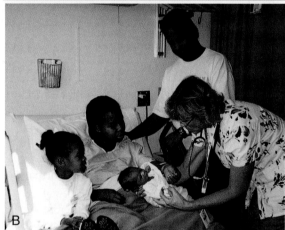

FIGURE 9-5 Identification. **A,** This umbilical clamp can be used as identification (with an identical numbered wristband for the mother) and also as protection from abduction, because it has a lightweight transponder attached to the clamp. When the transponder passes out of the unit, an alarm sounds unless the transponder is neutralized by a coded signal input by the hospital staff. The umbilical clamp is removed before discharge. **B,** The nurse compares the identification bracelet of the newborn with the bracelet on the mother's wrist as the father and sibling look on. (**A** courtesy Prosec Protection Systems, Lakewood, NJ. **B** courtesy Pat Spier, RN-C.)

on the infant with only a finger's width of slack, because infants lose weight after birth.

Each time the infant returns to the mother after a separation, the nurse must check the preprinted band numbers to see that they match. The nurse should either look at the numbers to see that they are identical or have the mother read her own band number while the nurse reads the infant's band. Some identification bands or umbilical clamps have an alarm that alerts the staff if the infant is removed from the hospital unit. These alarm chips are removed at the time of discharge to the home.

> **! Safety Alert!**
>
> Do not check bands by asking, "Is your band number...?" The mother who is sleepy, sedated, or simply distracted may answer affirmatively and receive the wrong infant.

Recognition of Employees. Parents should be able to recognize employees who are authorized to take the infant from the mother's room. Employees wear photo identification badges, and maternal–newborn nurses may have an additional badge. They may wear distinctive uniforms. Some units use a code word that changes on a regular basis. The family is taught very early how to recognize an employee who is allowed to take the infant and to refuse to release their infant to any other person. Security measures should be reinforced when providing care.

Other Security Measures. The mother is taught to keep the infant away from the door to the room. In a semiprivate room the two bassinets are often placed between the mothers. The mother should not leave her infant alone in the room for any reason. If she is alone in her room, she should leave the bathroom door ajar while she toilets or return the infant to the nursery if she showers or naps. These measures also reduce the risk that the infant would aspirate mucus because no one was present for suctioning.

Evaluating Gestational Age

A thorough gestational age assessment is done using a scale such as the Ballard form (see Chapter 13). However, the birthing room nurse does a quick assessment to evaluate whether the infant seems to be of the appropriate gestational age. The infant who seems to be preterm may be admitted to the nursery more rapidly than one who is of the expected term gestation. Characteristics to assess include the following:

- *Skin.* Is the skin thin and somewhat transparent (preterm) or peeling (postterm or possible intrauterine growth restriction [IUGR])?
- *Vernix.* Is this cheesy substance covering most of the skin surface (preterm), is it present only in creases (term), or is it absent (postterm)? Greenish vernix indicates that meconium was passed before birth, which may indicate that the infant is postterm or had poor placental support.
- *Hair.* Is the skin heavily covered with fine lanugo hair (preterm), or is hair only in a few places (term)? Dark-skinned infants often have more lanugo than light-skinned ones.
- *Ears.* When folded toward the lobe, do the ears spring back slowly (preterm) or quickly (term or postterm)? Abundant vernix can stick the ear in

place, so that possibility should be considered if the ear does not quickly return to its erect position.
- *Breast tissue.* Is there no or minimal breast tissue under the nipple (preterm), or is there a palpable mass of tissue 5 mm or more (term)? (A millimeter is about the thickness of a dime.)
- *Genitalia.* For males, is the scrotum smooth and small (preterm) or pendulous and covered with rugae or ridges (term)? For females, are the labia majora and labia minora of nearly equal size (preterm) or do the labia majora cover the labia minora (term)?
- *Sole creases.* Are the sole creases on the anterior third of the foot only (preterm), over the anterior two thirds (term), or over the full foot (term or postterm)? Peeling skin may be obvious on the feet in postterm or IUGR infants.

Observing for Injuries or Anomalies

The nurse notes signs of injury or anomalies while performing other assessments and care. The infant's movements and facial expression during crying are observed for symmetry and equality of movement. The head and face should be assessed for trauma, especially if forceps were used. A small puncture wound is usually apparent on the scalp if an internal spiral electrode was used for fetal monitoring (see Chapter 6). If the infant was born vaginally in a breech presentation, the buttocks may be bruised.

Many anomalies, such as spina bifida (open spine) or a cleft lip, are immediately obvious (see Chapter 14). The fingers and toes should be counted to identify abnormal numbers or webbing. The feet should be observed for straightness or to determine if deviated feet can be returned to the straight position. The length of arms and legs should also be checked for equality. Urination or meconium passage, which confirms patency, must also be noted.

Obtaining Vital Signs

Observation of vital signs begins while parents and infant are bonding. They are measured at 15- to 30-minute intervals at first, then hourly, and every 4 to 8 hours after the infant is stable.

Respiratory Rate. The normal respiratory rate for normal newborn infants is 30 to 60 breaths per minute. For best accuracy, the respiratory and heart rates are assessed before disturbing the infant. The respirations are counted for 1 full minute. Newborn respirations are difficult to count, because they are shallow and irregular. The rate can be auscultated by listening with a stethoscope. Placing a hand lightly over the abdomen or watching the abdomen rise and fall also helps to identify each breath. If the infant is crying, a pacifier or gloved finger to suck may quiet him or her so the respiratory rate can be counted accurately.

Heart Rate. The newborn's heart rate is assessed apically. A small pediatric head is used on the stethoscope if possible to limit extraneous noise. The nurse should count the heartbeat for 1 minute. The normal rate is 110 to 160 beats/min. A consistently low or high heart rate can indicate a pathological condition.

> **Nursing Tip**
>
> In the past, newborns were placed in a prone position to facilitate the drainage of mucus. Because the prone position has been associated with sudden infant death syndrome (SIDS), it is now recommended that newborns be placed on their backs to sleep. Teach all parents this newer information, because they may have been taught previously to keep an infant in a prone position.

Temperature. When the infant is in the radiant warmer, a skin probe on the abdomen records the body temperature. The skin probe should not be placed over bony prominences or areas where brown fat is expected to be found.

An axillary temperature is most commonly used and is safer than a rectal temperature technique, which has a risk of irritating the rectum or perforating the intestinal wall. When taking the axillary temperature, the thermometer is placed in the axilla, keeping it parallel to the chest wall. The infant's arm is folded down firmly against the thermometer for the required time. Tympanic temperatures are less accurate in newborns and are not generally used during the neonatal period.

Blood Pressure. A newborn's blood pressure is measured with an electronic instrument. When blood pressure is assessed on a newborn, all four extremities or one arm and one leg are assessed to identify substantial pressure differences between the upper and lower extremities, which can be a sign of coarctation of the aorta. The normal range of blood pressure is between 65 and 95 mm Hg systolic over 30 to 60 mm Hg diastolic in term infants.

> **Nursing Tip**
>
> When measuring blood pressure in the lower extremity, remember that the artery runs on the posterior aspect of the leg.

Obtaining Weight and Other Measurements

Weight. The infant is weighed in the birthing room or when admitted to the nursery. Disposable paper is put on the scale, and the scale is balanced to zero according to its model. The unclothed infant is then placed on the scale. The nurse's hand should not touch the infant but should be kept just above him or her to prevent falls (see Chapter 12, Figure 12-11). The weight is converted to grams for gestational age assessment. The AAP (2013) recommends the weights of all infants be recorded in kilograms and the kilogram weight reviewed at each shift handoff.

Measurements. Three typical measurements are length, head circumference, and chest circumference. A disposable tape measure is used. To avoid giving a paper cut, the tape should not be pulled out from under the infant. Measurements must also be noted in centimeters for gestational age assessment.

Length. There are several ways to measure the length of the infant. Some facilities have a tape measure applied to the clear wall of a bassinet. The nurse places the infant's head at one end, extends the leg, and notes where the heel ends. Another method is to bring the infant to the bassinet or warmer with the scale paper. The paper is marked at the top of the head, the body and leg are extended, and the paper is marked where the foot is located. Length is measured between the marks. Still another method involves placing the zero end of the tape at the infant's head, extending the body and leg, and stretching the tape to the heel (see Chapter 15, Skill 15-1).

Head circumference. The fullest part of the infant's head is measured just above the eyebrows. Molding of the head may affect the accuracy of the initial measurement (see Chapter 12, Figure 12-5, *A*).

Chest circumference. Chest circumference is measured at the nipple line.

Providing Umbilical Cord Care

The health care provider may leave a long segment of umbilical cord attached. If so, the nurse applies a plastic clamp near the skin and cuts the cord or assists the father to cut the cord just above the clamp. The cord is assessed for the number and type of blood vessels soon after it is cut. The normal umbilical cord has three vessels: two arteries and one vein.

> **Memory Jogger**
>
> The woman's name "**AVA**," for "**A**rtery-**V**ein-**A**rtery," helps the nurse remember the normal number of vessels in the umbilical cord.

A two-vessel cord is associated with other internal anomalies, often of the genitourinary tract. To distinguish the arteries from the vein, the nurse should look at the freshly cut end of the cord. The arteries project slightly from the surface, and the vein looks like a flattened cylinder that does not project from the cut surface.

Umbilical cord care is aimed at preventing infection. Keeping the cord clean and dry shortens the time to cord separation, and only a few hospitals continue to use daily application of triple dye or alcohol to promote drying of the cord. The diaper should be fastened low to allow air circulation to the cord. The cord should become dry and brownish black as it dries. The clamp is removed when the end of the cord is dry and crisp, usually within about 24 hours. The parents are taught to report redness of the area or a moist, foul-smelling umbilical cord. Many parents prefer to give sponge baths for the first week or until the cord stump falls

Providing Umbilical Cord Care

PURPOSE
To assist the cord in drying and falling off

STEPS
1. Identify infant (see Figure 9-5, *B*).
2. Check umbilical clamp placement for tight closure. There should be no bleeding or discharge from the cord.
3. Keep cord dry and exposed to the air.
4. Assess the cord for presence of vessels.
5. When alcohol cord care is ordered, using an alcohol wipe, start from the base of the cord and gently wipe upward and outward. *Note that cord care/observation is completed with every diaper change per facility protocol.*
6. Lift the cord away from the infant's abdomen to facilitate observation or cleansing of all areas.
7. Observe cord and abdominal area for redness, discharge, or foul odor.
8. Diaper infant, and be sure the upper end of diaper is folded down *below* the cord so it does not rub against the cord.
9. Document cord care and observations, solution used to cleanse the area, condition of the cord, teaching of the parents, and the parents' response.

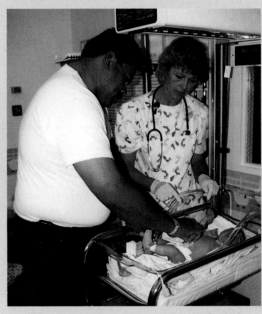

(Courtesy Loma Linda University Hospital Center.)

off, but tub baths are safe (AWHONN, 2007). Baths are given no more often than every other day (Skill 9-6).

Bleeding from the cord during the first few hours usually indicates that the cord clamp has become loose. Because of the newborn's small blood volume, even a small amount of bleeding can be a significant percentage of the blood volume. The clamp should be checked for closure and another applied if needed.

Hypoglycemia
The brain is totally dependent on a steady supply of glucose for its metabolism. Until infants begin regular feedings, they must use the glucose stored in their bodies. A blood glucose level below 45 mg/dL in the term infant indicates hypoglycemia. If the screening test indicates hypoglycemia, a venous blood sample is drawn for a more accurate evaluation. The infant is fed as soon as the sample is obtained to prevent a further drop in blood glucose.

Some infants at risk for low blood glucose after birth include preterm and postterm infants, small for gestational age (SGA) and large for gestational age (LGA) infants, infants of diabetic mothers, and any infant who is stressed because of hypoxia.

These infants undergo a blood glucose evaluation within 1 hour after birth and at intervals until their glucose level is stable. Early feedings or IV glucose may be needed.

Although some infants have a higher risk of developing hypoglycemia, any infant can have a fall in blood glucose levels. Signs of hypoglycemia in the newborn include the following:
- Jitteriness
- Poor muscle tone
- Sweating
- Respiratory difficulty
- Low temperature (which can also cause hypoglycemia)
- Poor suck
- High-pitched cry
- Lethargy
- Seizures

A heel stick is performed when obtaining capillary blood for the glucose-screening test. The heel stick should avoid the center of the heel where bone, nerves, and blood vessels are near the surface (Figure 9-6).

Screening Tests
Several tests are undertaken to screen for abnormalities that are known to cause physical or mental disability. The mandatory tests vary according to the state. Most of the disorders are associated with therapy that can

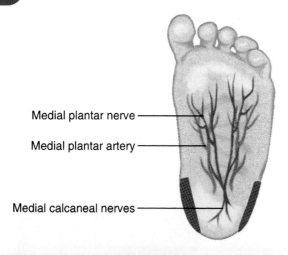

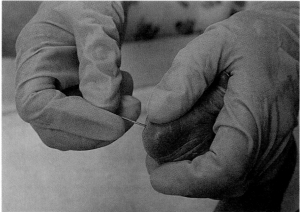

Medial plantar nerve

Medial plantar artery

Medial calcaneal nerves

FIGURE 9-6 Heel stick. The shaded areas at the sides of the heel are used for heel sticks in newborns to avoid nerves, blood vessels, and bony areas. Warming the heel before puncture will promote better blood flow.

prevent many, if not all, of the disabilities that would result if the disorder were left untreated. A test for phenylketonuria (PKU) is mandatory in all states. If the infant has this disorder, a special formula begun in the first 2 months of life can reduce disability and prevent severe mental retardation in most cases. The PKU test is done on the day of discharge for better accuracy, and it is repeated during early clinic visits. Other tests may include those for hypothyroidism, galactosemia, sickle cell disease, thalassemia, maple syrup urine disease, and homocysteinuria. The Centers for Disease Control and Prevention (CDC) highly recommend routine screening for all newborns for cystic fibrosis (CF) by measuring immunoreactive trypsinogen levels, which are elevated in infants with CF. A Masimo pulse oximeter is capable of noninvasively monitoring oxygen saturation, hemoglobin, and respiratory distress. In 2013, New York State became the first state to mandate pulse oximetry testing for congenital heart disease for all newborns, and currently 9 states screen newborns by oximetry for early detection of heart abnormalities. As research is published and distributed, more states will require this noninvasive test for congenital heart disease for all newborns.

Skin Care

Initial skin care after the infant's condition is stable involves washing off the blood and amniotic fluid that may be present on the infant's skin. To preserve skin integrity, vigorous removal of all remnants of vernix is not advised. There should be little vernix present on the skin of the term infant. Until the infant's first sponge bath and shampoo, the nurse must wear gloves while handling the infant. Care of the skin of the newborn is discussed in Chapter 12.

Promoting Bonding and Attachment

Bonding and attachment are terms often used interchangeably, although they differ slightly. **Bonding** refers to a strong emotional tie that forms soon after birth between the parents and the newborn. **Attachment** is an affectionate tie that occurs through time as infant and caregivers interact. It is important for nurses to promote these processes to help parents claim the infant as their own. Bonding actually begins during pregnancy as the fetus moves and shows individual characteristics on sonogram.

Both partners should view, hold, and—most important—*touch* the infant as soon as possible after birth. They must do this to reconcile the fantasy child of pregnancy with the real child they now have. Many parents are not surprised to know the sex of their infant at birth if the sonogram showed it earlier. However, some do not want to know the infant's sex before birth, and some are surprised when the predicted sex differs from the actual one. Most parents count all fingers and toes.

To prevent infant hypothermia, the unclothed infant is kept near the mother's skin, and both are covered with a warm blanket (skin-to-skin contact). Parents soon identify individual characteristics, such as a nose that looks like Grandpa's, long fingers like the father's, or a cry just like an older sibling. All of these parental behaviors help to identify the infant as a separate individual (Figure 9-7).

For some, parental feelings do not come naturally. Difficulty in bonding, rejection, or indifference in one or both parents should be recorded, and a referral to social services should be considered. Mothers who have little social support may have difficulty forming attachments with their newborns.

Nursing Tip

Observe the interaction between parents and infant to evaluate the attachment process.

Nursing Care to Promote Bonding and Attachment. The nurse observes parenting behaviors, such as the amount of affection and interest shown to the infant. The amount of physical contact, stimulation, eye-to-eye contact (*en face position;* see Figure 9-3), and time spent interacting with the infant are significant. Adults tend to talk with infants in high-pitched voices. The extent to which the parents encourage involvement of

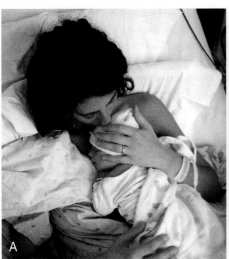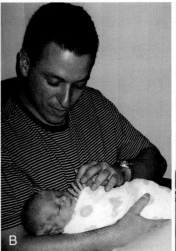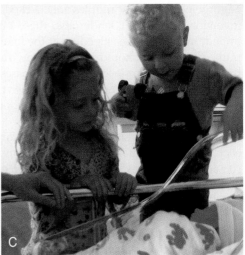

FIGURE 9-7 **A,** Mother–infant bonding is obvious in this picture of a mother and her newborn infant. **B,** An uncle bonds with the newborn as he examines features and fingers. **C,** Siblings get their first introduction to their newborn brother.

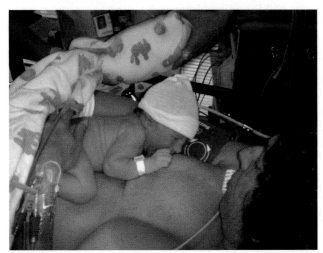

FIGURE 9-8 Placing the naked infant on the bare chest of the mother, covered by a blanket, encourages both breastfeeding and bonding.

siblings and grandparents with the newborn should be noted. This information provides a basis for nursing interventions that may encourage bonding and foster positive family relationships (Figure 9-8).

Parents must learn what their infant's communication cues mean. Soon after birth, most parents begin to recognize when an infant is signaling discomfort from hunger as opposed to discomfort from other causes, such as a wet diaper or boredom. In addition, the parents should quickly be able to distinguish their infant's cry from the cries of other infants. Although this process is just beginning when the mother and infant leave the birth facility, the nurse should note its early signs.

The nurse should observe for parent–infant interactions that dictate a need for additional interventions. Some of these include indifference to the infant's signals of hunger or discomfort, failure to identify their infant's communication, avoidance of eye contact with the infant, or discussing the infant in negative terms. However, the family's culture should also be considered.

Nursing interventions to facilitate parent–infant attachment vary. Calling the infant by name, holding the infant en face, providing skin-to-skin contact, and talking in gentle, high-pitched tones help the nurse to model appropriate behavior for the parent. Role modeling is especially important to adolescent mothers who may feel self-conscious when interacting with their child. Expected infant behaviors should be discussed and unique characteristics pointed out to enhance the bonding process. This is especially important if the parents' "fantasy" child differs from the "real" child in sex, physical attributes, or health.

Providing and Teaching Routine Care

A newborn infant stays in the mother's room most of the time unless either mother or infant has a problem that necessitates separation. Routine assessments and care provide an opportunity for the nurse to teach the parents normal newborn characteristics, signs of problems that should be reported, and how to provide care for the infant. Involving the parents in care of their infant helps them to learn most successfully. First-time parents may be sensitive to critical remarks, and therefore the nurse should praise their efforts while tactfully giving suggestions for needed improvement.

Feeding and elimination patterns are assessed by discussing them with the mother as well as observing at diaper changes. The mother should be asked how many wet and soiled diapers the infant has had since the last assessment. Voidings are usually totaled for the shift. Stools are also tallied and are described. Meconium stools are expected during the birth facility stay, although they may change to transitional stools before discharge.

If the infant is breastfed, the nurse should discuss with the mother how well the infant is nursing, the frequency and duration of the nursing sessions, and any difficulty she is having. Her breasts are checked for engorgement, and her nipples are checked for flatness, inversion, trauma, or tenderness; these problems can impede successful breastfeeding. If the infant is fed formula, the mother should be asked how many ounces the infant has taken since the previous assessment. This is also a good time to remind the mother that bacteria multiply rapidly in formula, so she should discard any leftovers.

The infant's skin should be observed for jaundice at each assessment. Infants have a large number of erythrocytes, because they live in a low-oxygen environment in utero. Excess erythrocytes are broken down after birth, which releases bilirubin into the bloodstream. High levels of bilirubin cause yellow skin color, starting at the head and progressing downward on the body. Extremely high levels of bilirubin can cause kernicterus (see Chapter 14).

The infant needs only a shirt and diaper for clothing. A light receiving blanket is used to swaddle the infant, and another receiving blanket is placed over the child. A cap is used, because the infant's head is the largest body surface area and can be a source of significant heat loss.

Teaching is an important part of mother–infant care. Parent teaching of infant care includes the following:

- Maintenance of an open airway by positioning and use of the bulb syringe
- Temperature maintenance and assessment after discharge
- Expected increase in the number of voidings
- Changes in the stools
- Feeding
- Signs of illness to report
- Follow-up appointments for well-baby care

The first feeding should be observed carefully, because anomalies that cause choking could be present.

BREASTFEEDING

Nutrition is especially important in the first few months of life, because the brain grows rapidly. Energy use is high because of the newborn's rapid growth. More in-depth discussions of the nutritional needs of the infant are found in Chapters 15 and 16. The mother may choose to nurse her infant or bottle-feed. The nurse should support the mother in either decision.

ADVANTAGES AND DISADVANTAGES

Breastfeeding has many advantages for the newborn:

- Breast milk contains the full range of nutrients that the infant needs and in the right proportions. No commercial formula has the exact nutritional composition of breast milk.
- Breast milk is easily digested by the infant's maturing digestive system.
- Breast milk does not cause infant allergies.

- Breastfeeding provides natural immunity, because the mother transfers antibodies through the milk. Colostrum is particularly high in antibodies.
- Breast milk promotes elimination of meconium. Breastfed infants are rarely constipated.
- Suckling at the breast promotes mouth development.
- Breastfeeding is convenient and economical.
- Breastfeeding eliminates the risks of a contaminated water supply or improper dilution.
- Infant suckling promotes a return of the uterus to its prepregnant state.
- Breastfeeding may play a significant role in improving brain development of the infant.
- Breast milk production uses maternal fat stores, which facilitates maternal weight loss.
- Breastfeeding enhances a close mother–child relationship.
- Breastfeeding may decrease the occurrence of childhood respiratory disorders.

There are some contraindications to breastfeeding (Gabbe, 2012).

- There is a potential for most maternal medications to enter breast milk. Use of antimetabolites, antineoplastic drugs, or chloramphenicol is an absolute contraindication to breastfeeding.
- True galactosemia is a contraindication to breastfeeding.
- Women who have untreated active tuberculosis, infection with human immunodeficiency virus (HIV), or active herpes zoster infection of the breast should not breastfeed. Cancer may become worse with the hormonal changes of lactation.

Infectious Diseases and Breastfeeding

The only infections that are absolute contraindications to breastfeeding are HIV and the human T cell lymphotrophic viruses (HTLV 1 and 2), all of which can be transmitted to the infant via breast milk. Maternal hepatitis A infection is *not* a contraindication to breastfeeding, because the infant can receive immunoglobulin and hepatitis A vaccine therapy. Infants of hepatitis B virus–positive (HBV) mothers should receive HBV vaccine therapy before discharge and can breastfeed. In mothers who are infected with the hepatitis C virus, breastfeeding is contraindicated in the presence of liver failure. In mothers infected with the herpes simplex virus or the varicella zoster virus, breastfeeding is contraindicated when lesions on the breast are present.

Mothers who have active pulmonary tuberculosis (TB) must be isolated from their newborn infants, but infants can be fed breast milk that is pumped, because the breast milk does not contain the tubercle bacilli. Certain drugs decrease the breast milk volume, such as levodopa, barbiturates, antihistamines, pyridoxine, estrogens, androgens, and bromocriptine, and whenever possible these drugs should be avoided.

PHYSIOLOGY OF LACTATION

Hormonal Stimulation

To better support the nursing mother, the nurse must understand how breast milk production occurs and how the milk changes with time. The following two hormones have a major role in the production and expulsion of breast milk:

- *Prolactin* from the anterior pituitary gland causes the production of breast milk.
- *Oxytocin* from the posterior pituitary gland causes the milk to be delivered from the alveoli (milk-producing sacs) through the duct system to the nipple (*milk ejection,* or **let-down reflex**). The mother usually feels a tingling in her breasts and sometimes abdominal cramping as her uterus contracts (Figure 9-9).

During pregnancy, the glandular tissue of the breasts grows under the influence of several hormones. The woman also secretes high levels of prolactin, which is the hormone that causes milk production. However, other hormones from the placenta inhibit the breasts' response to prolactin. The influence of prolactin is unopposed after birth and after the expulsion of the placenta, and milk production begins. If milk is not removed from the breast, prolactin secretion abates, and the breasts return to their prepregnant state.

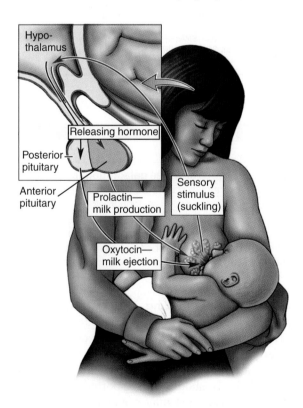

FIGURE 9-9 Lactation reflex arc. The infant suckling on the breast stimulates nerve fibers in the areola of the nipple that travel to the hypothalamus. The hypothalamus stimulates the anterior pituitary to secrete prolactin; this stimulates milk production and stimulates the posterior pituitary to release oxytocin, which causes a "let-down" reflex, contracting the lobules in the breast and squeezing milk out into the nipple and to the infant. (From Herlihy B: *The human body in health and illness,* ed 5, St Louis, 2014, Saunders.)

Infant suckling at the breast stimulates the release of oxytocin so that milk is delivered to the nipple, where it is ingested by the newborn. Prolactin secretion increases as milk is removed from the breasts, thus stimulating further milk production. Therefore feedings that are infrequent or too short can reduce the amount of milk produced. The opposite is also true, which explains why a mother can produce enough milk for twins.

Very little milk is stored between feedings. Most is manufactured as the infant nurses. The composition of milk changes slightly from the beginning of a feeding until the end of that feeding, as follows:

- **Foremilk** is the first milk the infant obtains. It is more watery and quenches the infant's thirst.
- **Hindmilk** is the later milk that has a higher fat content. It helps satisfy the infant's hunger. Feedings that are too short do not allow the infant to obtain the hunger-satisfying hindmilk.

>  **Nursing Tip**
>
> Anticipatory guidance concerning possible problems associated with breastfeeding helps the mother to see these challenges as common occurrences and not as complications.

Phases of Milk Production

Milk production changes after birth in the following three phases:

1. Colostrum
2. Transitional milk
3. Mature milk

Late in pregnancy and for the first few days after birth, **colostrum** is secreted by the breasts. This yellowish fluid is rich in protective antibodies. It provides protein, vitamins A and E, and essential minerals, but it is lower in calories than milk. It has a laxative effect, which aids in eliminating meconium.

Approximately 7 to 10 days after birth, the *transitional milk* emerges as the breasts gradually shift from production of colostrum to production of mature milk. Transitional milk has fewer immunoglobulins and proteins but has increased lactose (milk sugar), fat, and calorie content.

Mature milk is secreted by 14 days after birth. Mature human breast milk has a bluish color, which leads women to think that it is not "rich" enough to nourish the infant. The nurse should explain that the apparent "thinness" of the milk is normal and that the milk contains 20 kcal/oz and all the nutrients the infant needs.

ASSISTING THE MOTHER TO BREASTFEED

Infants are more likely to be breastfed and to breastfeed longer if they had skin-to-skin contact and initiated breastfeeding in the delivery room (Gabbe, 2012). The first nursing session includes the following advantages:

- Promotes mother–infant bonding
- Maintains infant temperature
- Infant suckling stimulates oxytocin release to contract the mother's uterus and control bleeding

Table 9-4   Teaching the New Mother How to Breastfeed

INSTRUCTION	RATIONALE
Wash hands before feeding; wash nipples with warm water and no soap.	Prevents infection of the newborn and breast; use of plain water prevents nipple cracking and irritation.
Position self (sitting or side-lying).	Alternating positions facilitates breast emptying and reduces nipple trauma.
Sit comfortably in chair or raised bed with back and arm support; hold infant with cradle hold or football hold, supported by pillows.	Pillow support of mother's back and arm and the infant's body in any position reduces fatigue; infant is more likely to remain in correct position for nursing.
Side-lying with pillow beneath head, arm above head; support infant in side-lying position.	Side-lying position reduces fatigue and pressure on abdominal incision.
Turn body of infant to face mother's breast.	Prevents pulling on nipple or poor position of mouth on nipple.
Stroke infant's cheek with nipple.	Elicits rooting reflex to cause infant to turn toward nipple and open mouth wide.
Infant's mouth should cover entire areola.	Compresses ducts and lessens tension on nipples; suction is more even.
Avoid strict time limits for nursing; nurse at least 10 minutes before changing to other breast, or longer if infant is nursing vigorously.	Let-down reflex may take 5 minutes; a too-short feeding will yield infant foremilk only, not the hunger-satisfying hindmilk. Strict time limits do not prevent sore nipples.
Use a safety pin on the bra as a reminder about which breast to start with at the next feeding.	Alternating breasts increases milk production.
Lift infant or breast slightly if breast tissue blocks nose.	Provides a small breathing space.
Break suction by placing finger in corner of infant's mouth or indenting breast tissue.	Removing infant in this way prevents nipple trauma.
Nurse infant after birth and every 2-3 hours thereafter.	Early, regular, and frequent nursing reduces breast engorgement. Breast milk is quickly digested. Early suckling stimulates oxytocin from mother's pituitary to contract her uterus and control bleeding.
Burp infant halfway through feeding and following feeding.	Rids stomach of air bubbles and reduces regurgitation.

The newborn should be put to breast within the first hours when the alert state allows for suckling and bonding. Breastfeeding should not be delayed beyond 6 hours after delivery. If the mother is too tired or uncomfortable to nurse at this time, or if the infant seems disinterested, she should be reassured that she can still breastfeed successfully. Table 9-4 reviews techniques the nurse can teach a new mother who wants to breastfeed.

The focus of the nurse in the early hours of breastfeeding should be to help the mother position the infant correctly and to help the infant obtain an open, gaping mouth in preparation for suckling. Frequent reassurance and praise of the mother's efforts are essential.

 Communication

Cross-Cultural Communication

To verify that a woman (or family) understands what the nurse has told her, have the woman repeat the teaching in her own words. An affirmative nod may indicate courtesy, not understanding, when the primary languages and the cultures of the nurse and family are different.

 Cultural Considerations

Galactogogues

Mothers from many cultures use **galactogogues** (breast-milk stimulators), and nurses should be aware of these practices. Beer, brewer's yeast, rice, gruel, fenugreek tea, and sesame tea are commonly used postpartum. Garlic eaten by the mother to prevent newborn illness will flavor her breast milk but will not harm the newborn. Cultural practices should be respected.

Positions for Breastfeeding

Any of several positions may be used for breastfeeding. The mother may sit in bed or in a chair and hold the infant in a cradle hold, with the head in her antecubital area (Figure 9-10, *A*). To prevent arm fatigue, the infant's body should be supported with pillows or folded blankets. She may prefer the football hold (see Figure 9-10, *B*), supporting the infant's head with her hand while the infant's body rests on pillows alongside her hip. The football hold is good for mothers who have a cesarean incision. The mother may prefer to lie on her side with the infant's body parallel to hers (see Figure 9-10, *C*). Pillows or folded

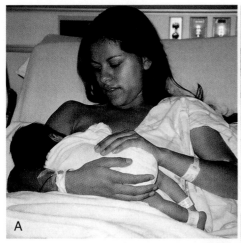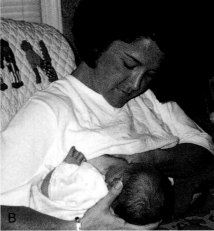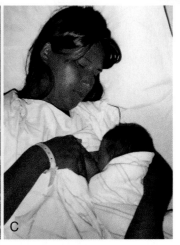

FIGURE 9-10 Positions for nursing. **A,** Cradle hold. **B,** Football hold. The mother supports the infant's head with her hand while the infant's body rests on pillows alongside her hip. The mother has control of the infant's head and can see the position of the infant's mouth on the breast. The football hold avoids pressure on a cesarean incision and is comfortable for mothers with large breasts. **C,** Side-lying position. (**A** and **C** courtesy Pat Spier, RN-C; **B** from Perry SE, Lowdermilk DL, Hockenberry MJ, Wilson D: *Maternal child nursing care*, ed 4, St Louis, 2010, Mosby.)

blankets can be used to support the infant in the proper position. Mothers often use the side-lying position when feeding the infant during the night. The side-lying position is also good for mothers who have had a cesarean birth.

Regardless of the position selected for breastfeeding, the infant's body should be in "chest-to-chest" position with the mother, with the head and neck in alignment. If the infant's chest faces the ceiling of the room, then the infant will have to turn his or her head away from midline to grasp the breast nipple. This position makes swallowing difficult for the infant. The infant should be at the level of the breast nipple to allow easy flow of milk. Holding the infant above the level of the nipple works against gravity flow; holding the infant below the level of the nipple exerts a pressure on the nipple that can cause soreness and bruising. The nipple should be centered to the nose of the infant with the nipple aimed to the roof of the infant's mouth so that the lower jaw latches on first. When the infant's mouth is wide open before latch-on, a more effective latch-on will occur as the mother moves her arm to bring the infant closer to the breast (Box 9-1).

Box 9-1   Essential Techniques in Breastfeeding

- Proper body alignment of infant
- Infant's mouth is wide open for areola grasp
- Proper hand position of mother on breast
- Infant's mouth moves in rhythmic motion to compress areola
- Audible swallow is heard
- Mother in relaxed, supported position
- Room is warm and private
- Infant ends feeding relaxed and appears satiated
- Mother has soft, nonengorged breasts at end of feeding

Breastfeeding Techniques

The mother is taught to wash her hands before each breastfeeding session. She should wash her breasts gently with plain water. Manually expressing a few drops of colostrum will make the nipple more erect in preparation for breastfeeding. Breastfeeding should begin with the opposite breast from the one that began the previous feeding session.

Position of the Mother's Hands. The mother should hold her breast in a C position, with the thumb above the nipple and the fingers below it. The thumb and fingers should be well back from the nipple, and the nipple should not tip upward. She can also use the scissors hold to grasp the breast between her index and middle fingers, but her fingers are more likely to slip downward over the nipple. Most infants do not need to have the breast indented for breathing room. The mother can lift the infant's hips higher if her breasts are very large or if the infant buries the nose in her breast.

Latch-on. The mother is taught to allow the infant to become alert and hungry but not frantic. To elicit latch-on, the mother should hold her breast so the nipple brushes against the infant's lower lip. A hungry infant usually opens the mouth wide with this stimulation. As soon as the infant's mouth opens wide, the mother should bring the infant close to her breast so that her areola is well into the mouth. The infant's lips should flare outward. The infant's tongue position can be checked to be sure it is under the nipple by gently pulling down on the lower lip (Figure 9-11).

Suckling Patterns. **Suckling** is the term that specifically relates to giving or taking nourishment at the breast. Infants have different suckling patterns when they breastfeed. Some suck several times before swallowing,

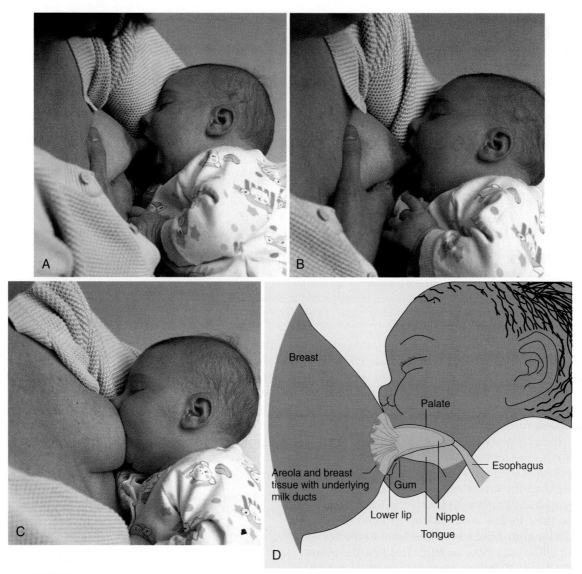

FIGURE 9-11   A, The newborn responds to touch on the lips and opens the mouth wide. **B,** After the mouth is open, quickly pull the newborn close to enable latch-on. **C,** The baby should have as much areola in his or her mouth as possible, not just the nipple. **D,** Correct attachment (latch-on) at breast. (From Perry SE, Hockenberry MJ, Lowdermilk DL, Wilson D: *Maternal child nursing care*, ed 5, St Louis, 2014, Mosby.)

and others swallow with each suck. After 4 days, the infant generally swallows with every suck at the beginning of breastfeeding, taking in approximately 0.14 mL of fluid, and has about two sucks per swallow near the end of the feeding, taking in 0.01 mL with each suck. A soft "ka" or "ah" sound indicates that the infant is swallowing colostrum or milk (nutritive sucking). Noisy sucking or smacking sounds or dimpling of the cheeks usually indicates improper mouth position. "Fluttering" sucking motions indicate nonnutritive suckling.

Removing the Infant from the Breast. When the infant must be repositioned or changed to the other breast, the mother should break the suction and remove the infant quickly. She can break the suction by inserting a finger in the corner of the infant's mouth or by indenting her breast near the mouth (Figure 9-12). Pulling the infant away from the breast can cause sore nipples.

Evaluating Intake of the Infant

Often the mother must be reassured that she is providing adequate milk for her infant, because she cannot see the milk consumed as she can with bottle feeding. Signs that breastfeeding is successful include the following:

- Breast feels firm before feedings and softer after.
- "Let-down" reflex occurs—a tingling sensation with milk dripping from breasts when a feeding is due.
- Infant nurses at the breast for 10 to 15 minutes per breast 8 to 10 times a day.
- An audible swallow is heard as the infant sucks.
- Infant demands feeding and appears relaxed after feeding.
- Infant has six to eight wet diapers per day.
- Infant passes stools several times a day.

By 14 days of age, the breastfed infant should regain his birth weight (Gabbe, 2012).

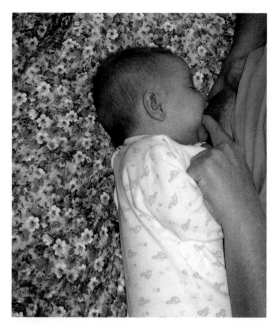

FIGURE 9-12 Breaking suction. The mother should always first break the suction before removing the infant from the breast. She can break the suction by inserting a finger in the corner of the infant's mouth.

Preventing Problems

Teaching can help new mothers prevent many problems with breastfeeding. Pain, anxiety, and insecurity can inhibit the "let-down-reflex" and are the most common reasons for breastfeeding problems. If the mother can avoid problems, she is less likely to become discouraged and stop nursing early. Lactation consultants are available in many birth settings to help with breastfeeding problems. Local chapters of La Leche League may be available to the mother for ongoing support after discharge. Most birth centers have "warm lines" to help with breastfeeding or other problems that occur in mothers and infants after birth.

Frequency and Duration of Feedings. Breastfed infants usually nurse every 2 to 3 hours during the early weeks, because their stomach capacity is small and because breast milk is easily digested. Some infants cluster several feedings at frequent intervals and then wait a longer time before nursing again. It is best to maintain flexibility during the early weeks. However, if the infant has not nursed for 3 hours, the mother should gently waken the infant and try to breastfeed.

If feedings are too short, the infant's hunger will not be satisfied, because the calorie density of the foremilk is lower. It may take as long as 5 minutes for the woman's let-down reflex to occur. The infant will soon be hungry again if he or she does not receive the richer hindmilk. This can frustrate the mother, because her infant wants to "eat all the time." Engorgement will occur if milk is not removed from the breasts, and milk production will decrease or stop. Mothers should be taught how to recognize signs of early hunger in their infants. Crying is usually a late sign of hunger (Box 9-2).

Box **9-2** Recognizing Hunger in Newborns
• Hand-to-mouth movements • Mouth and tongue movements • Sucking motions • Rooting movements • Clenched fists • Kicking of legs • Crying (a late sign of hunger; may result in shut-down and poor feeding if needs are not met)

The infant should nurse at least 15 minutes on the first breast, or longer if still nursing vigorously. The mother should then remove the infant from the first breast and have the infant nurse at the second breast until he or she is satisfied. The total duration of early feedings should be at least 15 minutes per breast. The mother should not switch back and forth between breasts several times during a feeding session.

Infants who breastfeed usually do not swallow much air. To burp the infant, the mother can hold the infant in a sitting position in her lap and pat or rub the back to assist (Figure 9-13). Alternately, the infant can be placed against the mother's shoulder for burping. A soft cloth protects the adult's clothing from any "spit-ups."

The mother should begin the next nursing session using the breast that was not used first in the previous session. A safety pin attached to her bra helps her to remember which breast to use first the next time.

The Baby-Friendly Hospital. A baby-friendly hospital initiative was launched in 1991 by UNICEF and the World Health Association (WHO) with a goal of

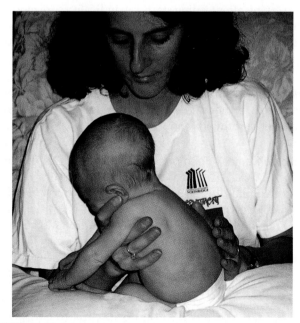

FIGURE 9-13 The mother can burp the infant by holding the infant in a sitting position on her lap, supporting the chin and chest, and gently patting or rubbing the back. In this position the mother can see the infant's face in case of spit-ups.

supporting and promoting breastfeeding. A baby-friendly hospital is defined as a facility that meets specific criteria and has been recognized by external assessment (Moore, 2012). To be recognized as a baby-friendly hospital, the following criteria must be met:

1. The hospital must have a written breastfeeding policy and must teach related skills to staff.
2. Parents are educated concerning values and techniques of breastfeeding.
3. Breastfeeding is initiated in the delivery room or is maintained if mother and infant are separated.
4. The infant is fed only breast milk, and feeding on demand is encouraged.
5. Mother and infant room-in 24 hours a day. No pacifiers or artificial nipples are used.
6. Formula samples are not distributed at discharge, and referral to support groups is offered.

The Sleepy Infant. Some newborns are sleepy and need to be awakened for feedings until a routine of feeding on demand is established. To bring the infant to an alert state in preparation for feeding, the infant should be unwrapped, the diaper can be changed, the mother should hold the infant upright and talk softly to him or her, or she may provide a gentle massage of the back, palms, or soles of the feet. When the infant is awake, feeding will be more successful.

The Fussy Infant. Some infants awaken from sleep crying lustily, eliminating the opportunity to observe for early cues of hunger (see Box 9-2). These infants must be calmed before successful feeding can be attempted. The infant is wrapped snugly (swaddled) and held close. The mother should talk calmly to the infant. When the infant calms, feeding can begin. Stiffening and crying after feeding starts can indicate a sore mouth from thrush, gas, cramps, or some illness that requires a health care provider's intervention. Collaboration with a lactation consultant is advisable.

Flat or Inverted Nipples. To help the nipples become erect for feedings, the mother can gently roll them between her thumb and forefinger.

Supplemental Feedings and Nipple Confusion. Supplemental feedings of formula or water should not be offered to the healthy newborn who is breastfeeding. Successful breastfeeding is based on supply and demand. The hungry infant will nurse and stimulate maternal milk production to meet physiological needs. A form of "imprinting" may occur if a newborn is given a bottle of formula and finds it easy to obtain fluid from the nipple with minimal effort and specific movements of the tongue. When the infant is then placed at the breast, considerably more effort is needed to obtain the breast milk, and a different movement of the tongue is required for success. As a result, the hungry infant may become fretful and irritable, which causes the mother to lose confidence and decide the infant prefers the formula and artificial nipple. This is often called "nipple confusion." When lactation is firmly established, usually after the neonatal period, the use of a pacifier to meet nonnutritive sucking needs will not cause nipple confusion.

⚠ Safety Alert!

If a pacifier is used to provide extra sucking, teach parents to use a one-piece type to prevent choking. They should use a clip to secure the pacifier to the infant's clothing and should not place it on a string around the infant's neck, which can cause strangulation.

Breast Engorgement. Early, regular, and frequent nursing helps to prevent breast engorgement. If engorgement does occur, and the breast and areola are very tense and distended, the mother can pump her breasts to get the milk flow started and soften the areola. She may use a breast pump or manual expression of milk. Cold applications between feedings and heat just before feedings may help to reduce discomfort and engorgement.

Manual massage of all segments of the breasts helps to soften them and express milk downward in the duct system. The mother cups her hands around the breast near the chest wall and firmly slides her fingers forward toward the nipple. She rotates her hands to massage all areas of the breast.

Nipple Trauma. Cracks, blisters, redness, and bleeding may occur. Correct positioning of the infant is the best preventive measure. Feeding formula at this time can worsen the trauma and pain, because it is likely to cause engorgement because less milk is removed. Warm water compresses applied to the breasts offer some relief. Rubbing a small amount of breast milk into the nipples may aid healing. Ointments are not effective; if used, they should be removed before nursing.

Hygiene. The mother should not use soap on her breasts. She should wear a supportive and not excessively tight bra 24 hours a day.

SPECIAL BREASTFEEDING SITUATIONS
Multiple Births

The mother's body adjusts the milk supply to the greater demand of multiple infants. Twins can be fed one at a time or simultaneously. The mother may want to use the crisscross hold when nursing simultaneously. She will need help to position two infants at the breasts in a cradle hold in each arm. She positions the first infant in a cradle hold, then her helper positions the second infant at the other breast in the crook of her arm. Their bodies cross over each other. The infant's and the mother's arm are supported with pillows.

Premature Birth

Breastfeeding is especially good for a preterm infant because of its immunological advantages (see Chapter 13 for more information on the preterm infant). If the infant cannot nurse, the mother can pump her breasts and freeze the milk for gavage (tube) feedings. When nursing the preterm or small infant, the mother may prefer the cross-cradle hold. She holds the infant's head with the hand opposite the breast that she will use to nurse. She uses the same arm to support the infant's body. The hand on the same side as the nursing breast is used to guide the breast toward the infant's mouth.

Breast Surgery

Previous breast surgery for breast augmentation or reduction may influence successful breastfeeding if the incision was around the areola of the breast, as nerves or lactiferous ducts may be damaged. A silicone breast implant does not negatively influence breastfeeding (Gabbe, 2012). A lactation specialist should be consulted.

Delayed Feedings

When breastfeeding must be temporarily delayed, the mother should be taught how to pump her milk to resume full breastfeeding (Figure 9-14). Portable breast pumps enable the mother to return to work and continue pumping and storing the breast milk to be available later for the infant.

STORING AND FREEZING BREAST MILK

Breast milk should be used within 1 hour of pumping to avoid the potential for bacterial contamination. Various commercial containers are available for the storage of breast milk, each with advantages and disadvantages. The container size should hold about as much milk as the infant will consume at one feeding.

Milk may be safely stored in glass or hard plastic. Leukocytes may stick to the glass, but they are not destroyed. Several types of plastic bottles are available in stores. Clear hard plastic bottles are made of polycarbonate, and, although little research is available, they are considered safe for storing and freezing milk. Dull or cloudy hard plastic bottles are polystyrene or milky white polypropylene. Polystyrene bottles are not designed for frozen milk storage. Polymers become unstable when heating after freezing. When used for freezing, polypropylene bottles alter the lysozyme, lactoferrin, and vitamin C content of breast milk. Polyethylene containers are usually clear plastic bags that may be at risk for puncture and invasion by microorganisms; some brands contain a special nylon between the polyethylene layers to reduce the puncture risk. The loss of lysozyme and fat is significant, and some valuable antibodies that adhere to polyethylene are lost to the infant. Any plastic material used for infants should be labeled as bisphenol A (BPA)–free.

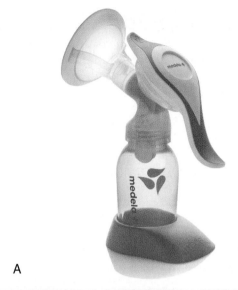

A

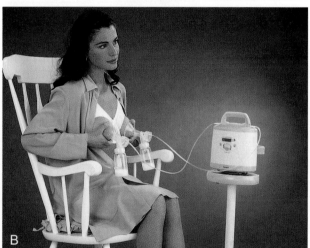

B

FIGURE 9-14 Breast pumps. Breast pumps can be manual **(A)**, battery-operated or electric **(B),** and pump directly into a bottle or freezer bag. One or both breasts can be pumped, and suction pressure is adjustable. Most hospitals and breastfeeding clinics help new mothers establish breastfeeding and breast pumping schedules to fit their individual needs. (Courtesy of Medela, Inc., McKenry, IL. Copyright © Medela, Inc., used with permission.)

Milk can be thawed in the refrigerator for 24 hours (best to preserve immunoglobulins) or by holding the container under running lukewarm water or placing it in a container of lukewarm water, rotating (not shaking) the bottle often. Microwaving is not advised, because it destroys some immune factors and lysozyme contained in the milk and can cause hot spots to develop because of uneven heating.

Milk can be stored in a tightly capped container in the back of the refrigerator (4° C [39° F]) up to 5 to 8 days without significant changes occurring or in the freezer section of the refrigerator for 2 weeks; or in a deep freezer (−4° C [−18° F]) for up to 6 months. Freezing can destroy some antimicrobial factors in the breast milk. See Table 9-5 for details regarding breast milk storage.

Containers should hold a portion appropriate for one feeding, should be labeled with the date, and should not be refrozen after thawing.

Table 9-5	Storing Breast Milk	
FRESHLY EXPRESSED MILK	**TEMPERATURE**	**STORAGE LIMIT**
Room temperature	66° to 72° F 19° to 22° C	6 to 8 hours
Insulated cooler with blue ice packs	5° to 39° F −15° to 4° C	24 hours
Refrigerated milk	39° F or 4° C	5 to 8 days
Refrigerated thawed milk	32° to 39° F 0° to 4° C	24 hours
Freezer inside refrigerator	0° F or −15° C	2 weeks
Separate freezer unit	0° F or −15° C	3 to 6 months
Separate deep freeze	−4° F or −20° C	6 to 12 months

Data from USDHHS Office of Women's Health: *Guide to breastfeeding* (2012). Available at: www.Womenshealth.gov/publications/our-publications/breastfeeding-guide. Accessed May 2013; Lawrence R, Lawrence R: *Breastfeeding: a guide for the medical profession,* ed 7, Philadelphia, 2011, Mosby; Riordan J: *Breastfeeding and human lactation,* ed 4, Sudbury, Mass., 2011, Jones & Bartlett.
NOTE: Use a tight cap when storing. Nipples allow entrance of organisms. Do not save milk left in a used bottle for future feeding. Do not add fresh milk to frozen milk. Place freshly expressed milk in the freezer within 24 hours. Store milk in the back of refrigerator/freezer. Label and date container of milk.

MATERNAL NUTRITION

To maintain her own nutrient stores while providing for the infant, the mother needs 500 additional calories each day beyond what her nonpregnant diet provided (see Figure 4-7). She should choose foods from each of the following groups in the MyPlate food guide:

- Meat, fish, poultry, eggs, beans, and nuts
- Milk and other dairy products
- Vegetables
- Fruits
- Breads, cereals, and grains

Women who are lactating need a 20% to 30% increase of vitamins and minerals, double the prepregnancy needs of folic acid, and a 40% to 50% increase of calcium and phosphorus. These increases are easily attainable by adding the following foods:

2 cups of milk
2 ounces of meat or peanut butter
A slice of whole wheat bread
A citrus fruit
A salad with $^1/_2$ cup of dark green or yellow vegetables

About a liter of uncaffeinated fluid is needed each day to replace the fluid lost to breastfeeding.

Women with lactose intolerance may use substitutes such as tofu, soy milk, and canned salmon with bones as a substitute for milk products. The health care provider usually recommends that the nursing mother continue taking prenatal vitamins during lactation, although routine supplementation has been shown as unnecessary for the well-nourished mother.

Some foods eaten by the mother may change the taste of the milk or cause the infant to have gas. Foods that often cause problems are chocolate, cabbage, beans, and broccoli. If the mother suspects that a particular food is causing fussiness or gas in the infant, she can eliminate it from her diet for a few days to determine whether the infant has fewer problems. These problems do not indicate an allergy to breast milk but only an irritation with some food by-product contained in the milk.

Many medications taken by the mother are secreted in breast milk but in varying concentrations depending on the drug. In general, timing the drug dose so that it passes its peak of action before the infant's nursing sessions begin can reduce the amount delivered to the infant.

WEANING

Gradual weaning is preferred to abrupt weaning, which can cause engorgement, can lead to mastitis, and can be upsetting to the infant. There is not a particular "best" time to wean. Even a short period of breastfeeding provides the infant with many immunological and digestive advantages. As the infant matures, he or she will gradually become less interested in the breast, especially when solid foods are added to the diet around 6 months.

The nurse can teach mothers the following tips when they want to wean their infants:

- Eliminate one feeding at a time. Wait several days and eliminate another one. The young infant will need formula from a bottle; the older infant may be weaned from the breast to a cup.
- Omit daytime feedings first, starting with the one in which the infant is least interested.
- Eliminate the infant's favorite feeding last. This will often be the early morning or bedtime feeding.
- Expect the infant to need "comfort nursing" if he or she is tired, ill, or uncomfortable.

If the mother must wean abruptly for some reason, breast engorgement is likely to occur. A supportive bra, ice packs, analgesics, or cabbage leaves applied to the breasts may relieve discomfort. Breast pumping is not advised, because the breast must remain full enough to decrease the milk supply cycle.

FORMULA FEEDING

Women choose to formula feed for many reasons. Some are embarrassed by breastfeeding or may have little social support. Others are uncomfortable when they cannot see the amount of milk the infant takes at each feeding. Women who have many other commitments and cannot maintain the flexibility needed when lactation is established may find that formula feeding is the only realistic choice. A few women must take medications or may have other illnesses that make breastfeeding unwise. When a woman who has been fully informed about the advantages of breastfeeding for both the mother and the infant chooses to formula feed, regardless of the reason for choosing to formula feed, the nurse should fully support the mother and reassure her that her infant can receive good nutrition and emotional closeness.

TYPES OF INFANT FORMULAS

Before the first formula feeding, most hospitals have a policy of offering water to the newborn to assure patency of the gastrointestinal tract. If the infant sucks, swallows, and retains the water, formula is then offered. If the infant has an anomaly such as esophageal atresia (tracheoesophageal fistula) (see Chapter 28), aspiration can occur. Aspiration of water involves less risk than aspiration of formula.

Most formulas are modifications of cow's milk. Similac Advance and Enfamil Premium are examples of cow's milk–based formulas. Infants who do not tolerate cow's milk formulas or who come from a family with many allergies may be prescribed soy or protein hydrolysate formulas, such as Nutramigen. Soy formulas include ProSobee and Isomil. Other formulas are available to meet special needs, such as those of the preterm infant or the infant with PKU. Common formulas are available in three forms:

1. Ready-to-feed, either in cans or in glass bottles
2. Concentrated liquid
3. Powdered

Specific types of infant formulas are discussed in Chapter 16.

PREPARATION

The parent should wash the hands before preparing formula and feeding the infant. Bottles and nipples can be washed in hot, soapy water, using a nipple brush, and rinsed well. Bottles can be washed in a dishwasher, but nipples should be washed by hand to slow their deterioration. Bottles of formula can be prepared one at a time, or a 24-hour supply can be prepared. Formula should be refrigerated promptly and kept refrigerated until ready to use.

Ready-to-feed formulas require no dilution. Diluting them with water reduces the amount of nutrients the infant receives and can be dangerous. Ready-to-feed formula for home use comes in bottles and cans. The

mother should wash the can's lid and open it with a freshly washed can opener. She then pours the approximate amount the infant will take at a feeding into a bottle and caps the bottle.

 Safety Alert!

Overdilution or underdilution of concentrated liquid or powdered formulas can result in serious illness.

Concentrated liquid formula also comes in a can. After washing the can and opening it, the mother pours recommended proportions of concentrated liquid formula and tap water into the bottles and caps them. The usual proportions are one part concentrated liquid formula plus one part tap water. Water for formula dilution does not need to be boiled unless its safety is questionable.

Powdered formula is a popular choice for nursing mothers who want to feed their infant an occasional bottle of formula. It is also less expensive than ready-to-feed liquid formulas. The parent measures the amount of tap water into the bottle and adds the number of scoops recommended for that quantity. Sterilization is not required unless the quality of the water is in doubt.

Bottled cow's milk and evaporated milk are nutritionally inadequate for use as infant formula and stress the kidneys of the newborn and young infant.

FEEDING THE INFANT

Formula is digested more slowly than breast milk, and most formula-fed infants initially feed about every 3 to 4 hours (Skill 9-7). Like the breastfeeding mother, the formula-feeding mother should be encouraged to avoid rigid scheduling.

Many mothers prefer to warm the formula somewhat, but this is not necessary. Placing the bottle in a container of hot water takes the chill off the milk. Microwave heating of infant formula is *not* recommended, because heating is uneven and may result in hot spots that can cause mouth burns in the infant.

The nurse should caution parents not to prop the bottle, even when the infant is older. Propping the bottle may cause the infant to aspirate formula and is associated with dental caries (cavities) and ear infections.

Fathers or partners are encouraged to assist with feedings. When teaching new parents about infant care, the father or other support person should be involved to aid his or her involvement and attachment to the infant as well as to enhance support for the mother. Tips concerning safe bottle feeding of the infant can be found in Chapter 16.

DISCHARGE PLANNING

Discharge planning begins on admission or even earlier, when parents attend childbirth classes. Because

Bottle Feeding the Infant

PURPOSE

To provide necessary nutrients for growth and development

STEPS

1. Wash hands.
2. Identify infant.
3. Verify formula prescribed and expiration date on the bottle.
4. Change diaper and provide cord care (see Skill 9-6).
5. Wash and sanitize hands.
6. Select an appropriate nipple. Crosscut nipple offers rapid feedings; single-hole nipple offers regular milk flow; preemie nipple offers softer nipple that requires less sucking effort from the infant.
7. Open bottle (you should hear a "pop" to indicate bottle was previously unopened); place selected nipple on the bottle and tighten securely. Use room-temperature formula.
8. Hold infant in "cradle position" with infant's head slightly elevated above the body (see figure).
9. Touch infant's lips with nipple and gently insert nipple along infant's tongue. Hold bottle so nipple is *always* full of formula.
10. Feed infant slowly. Stop to "burp or bubble" infant after feeding 1 to 1.5 oz (30 to 45 mL) and at end of feeding.
11. If formula runs out of the side of the mouth during infant feeding, the nipple holes may be too large. The nipple should be discarded and replaced with a different one.
12. To burp the infant, sit the infant on your lap with his or her body leaning slightly forward. Support

the head and gently pat the middle or upper back (see Figure 9-13).
13. Place the infant in the crib on his or her side or back after feeding.
14. Leftover formula should be discarded, because microorganisms from the infant's mouth grow rapidly in warm formulas.
15. Document the amount taken; type of formula; any regurgitation; sucking strength; and parent teaching that was provided.

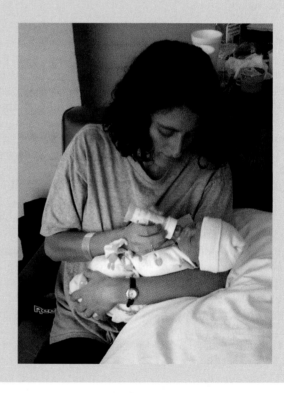

mothers and infants are discharged quickly after birth, self-care and infant care teaching must often begin before the mother is psychologically ready to learn. Some birth facilities use *clinical pathways* (also called care maps, care paths, or multidisciplinary action plans [MAPs]) to ensure that important care and teaching are not overlooked (see Chapter 12). These plans guide the nurse to identify areas of special need that necessitate referral as well as a means to keep up with the many facets of routine care needed after birth. The nurse must take every opportunity to teach during the short stay in the birth facility. Ample written materials for both new mother

and infant care should be provided to refresh the memory of parents who may be tired and uncomfortable when teaching occurs.

POSTPARTUM SELF-CARE

The nurse teaches the new mother how best to care for herself to reduce her risk for complications. The health care provider may prescribe more specific instructions for some patients.

Follow-Up Appointments

Most health care providers want to see postpartum women 2 weeks and 6 weeks after birth. The nurse should emphasize the importance of these follow-up appointments that verify that involution is proceeding normally and identify any complications as soon as possible. Signs of problems the woman should report have been discussed in previous sections, and danger signs are discussed later in the chapter.

At the 2-week appointment, the healing of the mother's perineum or cesarean incision is assessed. At the 6-week appointment, the mother's general health and recuperation from birth are assessed. The health care provider does a vaginal examination to check the uterus to ensure that involution is complete. Any incision is assessed for healing. The breasts are carefully examined for any signs of problems. Occasionally a complete blood count is done, and vitamins or iron supplements, or both, are ordered if anemia is present.

The woman has the opportunity to discuss any physical or psychological problems she may be having. The health care provider and the nurse usually inquire about how she is adapting to motherhood. Is she getting enough rest? How is breastfeeding progressing? Does she have help at home? How is the partner adapting to this new role?

Hygiene

A daily shower is refreshing and cleanses the skin of perspiration that may be more profuse in the first days after birth. Perineal care should be continued until the flow of lochia stops. Douches and tampons should not be used for sanitary protection until after the 6-week checkup.

Sexual Intercourse

Coitus should be avoided until the episiotomy is fully healed and the lochia flow has stopped. Having sexual relations earlier can lead to infection, trauma, and/or another pregnancy. A water-soluble lubricant can make intercourse more comfortable for the woman.

Ovulation, and therefore pregnancy, can occur before the 6-week checkup. The health care provider usually discusses contraception with the woman, but the nurse must often clarify or reinforce any explanations. It is important to emphasize that breastfeeding is *not* a reliable contraceptive.

Diet and Exercise

A well-balanced diet and moderate exercise promote healing and recovery from birth. Because constipation may be a problem, the mother is taught about high-fiber foods (e.g., whole-grain breads, and fruits and vegetables with the skins). Breastfeeding mothers should not try to lose weight while nursing. The formula-feeding mother should delay a strict reducing diet until released by her health care provider to do so. Moderate exercise can aid in the return of the uterus to its prepregnancy

state and promote a feeling of well-being. Most health care providers recommend that new mothers continue any prescribed prenatal vitamins until after the 6-week checkup.

Danger Signs

By teaching the mother about changes to expect as she returns to the prepregnant state, the nurse gives her a framework to recognize when something is not progressing normally. Hemorrhage, infection, and thrombosis are the most common complications. The mother should report the following:

- Fever higher than 38° C (100.4° F)
- Persistent lochia rubra or lochia that has a foul odor
- Bright red bleeding, particularly if the lochia has changed to serosa or alba
- Prolonged afterpains, pelvic or abdominal pain, or a constant backache
- Signs of a urinary tract infection
- Pain, redness, or tenderness of the calf
- Localized breast tenderness or redness
- Discharge, pain, redness, or separation of any suture line (cesarean, perineal laceration, or episiotomy)
- Prolonged and pervasive feelings of depression or being let down; generally not enjoying life

NEWBORN DISCHARGE CARE

Discharge planning for the infant begins at birth. Because of short stays after birth, the nurse must teach the parents how to care for their newborn at every opportunity. Discharge teaching will then be more of a summary than an attempt to crowd all teaching into a short time.

Most newborns are checked by a health care professional at birth and before discharge. The infant is assessed at this early check for jaundice, feeding adequacy, urine and stool output, and behavior. If the newborn is discharged before 72 hours of age, the American Academy of Pediatrics (AAP) recommends that a follow-up visit be scheduled within 2 days of discharge to assess the infant for jaundice, because the bilirubin level usually peaks between 3 and 5 days of age.

Infants are usually seen again at 6 to 8 weeks after birth to begin well-baby care. When providing discharge teaching, the nurse should emphasize the value of these visits. It should be explained that immunizations can be administered to prevent many illnesses. The health care provider assesses the infant for growth and development, nutrition, and any problems the parents or infant are having. Teaching parents about the infant's upcoming needs (anticipatory guidance) helps them to plan ahead to prevent injuries and to promote healthy growth and development.

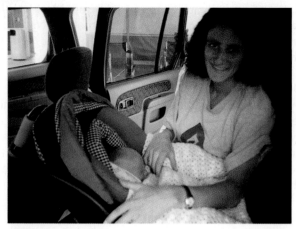

FIGURE 9-15 A new mother prepares to leave the birth facility. The infant is placed in a car seat that will be rear-facing and secured by the car's seat belt for the ride home.

The nurse should teach parents the importance of infant car safety seats and their correct use (Figure 9-15). The newborn should be placed in semireclining position in the car seat in the car's back seat (never in the front), facing the rear until 2 years of age (AAP, 2011). The seat's harness is snugly fastened, and the seat is secured to the automobile seat with the seat belt. Parents should consult their car's instruction manual for specific instructions on securing safety seats. The U.S. Department of Transportation has a toll-free vehicle safety hotline to help parents solve problems when using car safety seats: 800-424-9393.

Nursing Tip

If siblings are waiting when mother and baby return from the hospital, it is helpful if the father arrives carrying the infant. This leaves the mother's arms free for hugs before turning attention to the new child.

The nurse must emphasize to the parent that even in a low-impact accident, the infant will probably be thrown from his or her arms—or even from the car safety seat if the infant is improperly restrained—and will become a "missile" within the car or will even be ejected from it. Death is a likely result. Air bags can prevent serious injuries to older children and adults in motor vehicle accidents. However, the air bag thrusts an infant toward the rear, causing a whiplike motion that can seriously injure the neck or head.

New parents should be given written instructions, because they are often overwhelmed at the volume of information provided in such a short time. They should be reassured that the birth facility staff is available 24 hours a day to help them to care for their infant and to refresh their memories if they forget what they have been told (see Discharge Planning and Parent Teaching in Chapter 12).

Nursing Tip

Advise parents to limit the newborn's exposure to crowds during the early weeks of life, because infants have difficulty forming antibodies against infection until about 2 months of age.

Unfolding Case Study

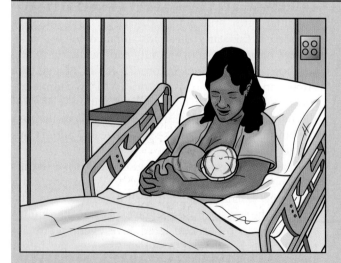

Tess and Luis were introduced to the reader in Chapter 4, and Tess's pregnancy experience has unfolded in each chapter. Refer to earlier chapters for her history.

Tess has delivered twins! Baby A, a girl named Sofia, has been admitted to the NICU and will be discussed in Chapter 14. Husband Luis follows Sofia to the NICU with his cell phone, taking pictures of the unexpected event. Baby B, a boy named Marco, is admitted to the postpartum unit with his mother Tess. Tess is tired but very talkative about her delivery experience, which included an episiotomy. She complains of having afterpains that seem to be worse during breastfeeding. She is also worried that she is having vaginal bleeding, because she thought her menstrual period would not return so quickly.

QUESTIONS

1. Explain (according to Rubin's theory of psychological changes during the puerperium) why Tess is so talkative after delivery and state how these stages influence when parent teaching would be most effective.
2. What are afterpains and why do they often worsen during breastfeeding?
3. Explain how the nurse can evaluate Tess's vaginal bleeding after childbirth and state what the nurse will teach Tess about what she can expect in the next few days and weeks concerning her vaginal discharge.
4. How will the nurse assess the perineum after Tess's episiotomy and what nursing care can be implemented?
5. Explain "phase 2" care of Baby Marco after he arrives in the postpartum unit with Tess.

Get Ready for the NCLEX® Examination!

Key Points

- It is essential to consider all patients individually to better incorporate their culture and special needs into the plan of care.
- From its level at the umbilicus, the uterus should descend about one finger's width per day after birth. It should no longer be palpable at 10 days postpartum.
- A slow pulse is common in the early postpartum period. A maternal pulse rate that would be high normal at other times may indicate hemorrhage or infection in the postpartum patient.
- A full bladder interferes with uterine contraction, which can lead to hemorrhage.
- Measures to prevent constipation should be emphasized at each assessment: fluid intake, a high-fiber diet, and activity.
- RhoGAM is given within 72 hours to the Rh-negative mother who delivers an Rh-positive infant.
- The postpartum check should include the status of fundus, lochia, breasts, perineum, bowel and bladder elimination, vital signs, Homans' sign, pain, and evidence of parent–infant attachment.
- Neonatal screening tests such as the phenylketonuria (PKU) test identify disorders that can be treated to reduce or prevent disability.
- The nurse must always keep the possibility of infant abductions in mind when providing care.
- The facility's specific protocol for security should be maintained during care. Most persons will not be offended by precautions but will be grateful for the protection.
- Bonding and attachment require contact between parents and infant. The nurse should promote this contact whenever possible.
- More breast milk removed means more milk produced. Early, regular, and frequent nursing promotes milk production and lessens engorgement.
- Duration of nursing on the first breast should be at least 15 minutes to stimulate milk production.
- The nursing mother needs 500 extra calories each day plus enough fluid to replace liquid lost via breastfeeding (about 1 liter).
- Weaning from the breast should be gradual, starting with the feeding the infant is least interested in and ending with the one in which he or she has the most interest.
- Commercially prepared formulas are available in ready-to-feed, concentrated liquid or in powdered form. Dilution, if required, must be followed exactly according to instructions.
- Discharge planning should take place with every instance of mother or newborn nursing care as the nurse teaches the mother normal findings, significance, and what to report. Written materials should be provided to augment all teaching.

Additional Learning Resources

SG Go to your Study Guide for additional learning activities to help you master this chapter content.

evolve Go to your Evolve website (http://evolve.elsevier.com/Leifer) for the following learning resources:
- Animations
- Answer Guidelines for Critical Thinking Questions
- Answers and Rationales for Review Questions for the NCLEX® Examination
- Glossary with English and Spanish pronunciations
- Interactive Review Questions for the NCLEX® Examination
- Patient Teaching Plans in English and Spanish
- Skills Performance Checklists
- Video clips and more!

 Online Resources
- Breastfeeding Support Consultants Center for Lactation Education: www.bsccenter.org
- Car safety seats: Information for families: www.aap.org/family/Carseatguide.htm
- International Lactation Consultant Association: www.ilca.org
- La Leche League International: www.lalecheleague.org

Review Questions for the NCLEX® Examination

1. Which assessments are expected 24 hours after birth? (Select all that apply.)
   1. Scant amount of lochia alba on the perineal pad.
   2. Fundus firm and in the midline of the abdomen.
   3. Breasts distended and hard with flat nipples.
   4. Bradycardia.

2. Nursing the infant promotes uterine involution, because it:
   1. uses maternal fat stores accumulated during pregnancy.
   2. stimulates additional secretion of colostrum.
   3. causes the pituitary to secrete oxytocin to contract the uterus.
   4. promotes maternal formation of antibodies.

3. The best way to maintain the newborn's temperature immediately after birth is to:
   1. dry the infant thoroughly, including the hair.
   2. give the infant a bath using warm water.
   3. feed 1 to 2 oz of warmed formula.
   4. limit the length of time that parents hold the infant.

4. Eight hours postpartum the woman states she prefers the nurse to take care of the infant. The woman talks in detail about her birthing experience on the phone and to anyone who enters her room. She complains of being hungry, thirsty, and sleepy

and is unable to focus on the infant care teaching offered to her. The nurse would interpret this behavior as:

1. inability to bond with the infant.
2. development of postpartum psychosis.
3. inability to assume the parenting role.
4. the normal taking-in phase of the puerperium.

5. Which of the following is a nursing intervention that does not require the written order of the health care provider? (Select all that apply.)

1. Administer an analgesic for pain.
2. Teach the patient how to perform perineal care.
3. Apply topical anesthetic for perineal suture pain.
4. Turn patient q2h.

Nursing Care of Women with Complications After Birth

Objectives

1. Define each key term listed.
2. Describe signs and symptoms for each postpartum complication.
3. Identify factors that increase a woman's risk for developing each complication.
4. Explain nursing measures that reduce a woman's risk for developing specific postpartum complications.
5. Describe the medical and nursing management of postpartum complications.
6. Explain general and specific nursing care for each complication.
7. Compare and contrast mood disorders in the postpartum period.

Key Terms

atony (ĂT-ŏ-nē, p. 240)
curettage (KYŪ-rĕ-tăhzh, p. 242)
endometritis (ĕn-dō-mē-TRĪ-tĭs, p. 244)
hematoma (hē-mă-TŌ-mă, p. 241)
hypovolemic shock (hī-pō-vō-LĒ-mĭk shŏk, p. 238)
involution (ĭn-vō-LŪ-shŭn, p. 242)

mania (MĀ-nē-ă, p. 247)
mastitis (măs-TĪ-tĭs, p. 246)
mood (p. 246)
psychosis (sī-KŌ-sĭs, p. 246)
puerperal sepsis (pū-ĔR-pŭr-ăl SĔP-sĭs, p. 243)
subinvolution (sŭb-ĭn-vō-LŪ-shŭn, p. 242)

Most women who give birth recover from pregnancy and childbirth uneventfully. However, some experience complications after birth that slow their recoveries and may interfere with their ability to assume their new role. A woman can have any medical problem after a birth, but most complications related to childbirth fall into one of six categories:

1. Shock
2. Hemorrhage
3. Thromboembolic disorders
4. Puerperal infections
5. Subinvolution of the uterus
6. Mood disorders

SHOCK

Shock is defined as a condition in which the cardiovascular system fails to provide essential oxygen and nutrients to the cells. Postpartum shock related to childbearing includes the following:

- *Cardiogenic shock:* Caused by pulmonary embolism, anemia, hypertension, or cardiac disorders
- *Hypovolemic shock:* Caused by postpartum hemorrhage or blood clotting disorders
- *Anaphylactic shock:* Caused by allergic responses to drugs administered
- *Septic shock:* Caused by puerperal infection

The inherent danger of obstetric shock is that body compensation can mask the signs until the condition becomes life threatening. The vigilance of the nurse can enable detection of early signs and then prompt intervention.

HEMORRHAGE

Postpartum hemorrhage complicates 1 in 100 deliveries (Gabbe, 2012) and is traditionally defined as blood loss greater than 500 mL after vaginal birth or 1000 mL after cesarean birth, resulting in signs or symptoms of hypovolemia. Because the average-sized woman has 1 to 2 L of added blood volume from pregnancy, she can tolerate up to these amounts of blood loss better than would otherwise be expected.

Most cases of hemorrhage occur immediately after birth, but some are delayed up to several weeks. *Early postpartum hemorrhage* occurs within 24 hours of birth. *Late postpartum hemorrhage* occurs after 24 hours and within 6 weeks after birth.

The major risk of hemorrhage is *hypovolemic (low-volume) shock,* which interrupts blood flow to body cells. This prevents normal oxygenation, nutrient delivery, and waste removal at the cellular level. Although a less dramatic problem, anemia is likely to occur after hemorrhage.

HYPOVOLEMIC SHOCK

Hypovolemic shock occurs when the volume of blood is depleted and cannot fill the circulatory system. The woman can die if blood loss does not stop and if the blood volume is not corrected.

Body's Response to Hypovolemia

The body initially responds to a reduction in blood volume with increased heart and respiratory rates. These reactions increase the oxygen content of each erythrocyte (red blood cell) and faster circulation of the remaining blood. **Tachycardia (rapid heart rate) is usually the first sign of inadequate blood volume (hypovolemia).** The first blood pressure change is a narrow pulse pressure (a falling systolic pressure and a rising diastolic pressure). The blood pressure continues falling and eventually cannot be detected.

Blood flow to nonessential organs gradually stops to make more blood available for vital organs, specifically the heart and brain. This change causes the woman's skin and mucous membranes to become pale, cold, and clammy (moist). As blood loss continues, flow to the brain decreases, resulting in mental changes, such as anxiety, confusion, restlessness, and lethargy. As blood flow to the kidneys decreases, they respond by conserving fluid. Urine output decreases and eventually stops.

 Safety Alert!

Because postpartum women often have a slow pulse rate, the caregiver should suspect hypovolemic shock or infection if the pulse rate is greater than 100 beats/min.

Medical Management

Medical management of hypovolemic shock resulting from hemorrhage may include any of the following actions:

- Stopping the blood loss
- Giving intravenous (IV) fluids to maintain the circulating volume and to replace fluids
- Giving blood transfusions to replace lost erythrocytes
- Giving oxygen to increase the saturation of remaining blood cells; a pulse oximeter is used to assess oxygen saturation of the blood
- Placing an indwelling (Foley) catheter to assess urine output, which reflects kidney function

Nursing Care. Routine postpartum care involves assessing vital signs every 15 minutes until stable so that the signs of postpartum hemorrhage are identified as early as possible. The woman should be observed closely for early signs of shock, such as tachycardia, pallor, cold and clammy hands, and decreased urine output. Decreased blood pressure may be a late sign of hypovolemic shock. Routine frequent assessment

of lochia in the fourth stage of labor helps identify early postpartum hemorrhage. When the amount and character of lochia are normal and the uterus is firm, but signs of hypovolemia are still evident, the cause may be a large hematoma. Excessive bright red bleeding despite a firm fundus may indicate a cervical or vaginal laceration. The occurrence of petechiae, bleeding from venipuncture sites, or oliguria may indicate a blood clotting problem. In the first hours postpartum, the perineal pad should be weighed to determine the output amount, with 1 g equaling 1 mL (see Chapter 9). Intake and output should be recorded and IV therapy monitored. Oxygen saturation levels are also monitored in early postpartum hemorrhage.

 Safety Alert!

Saturation of a peripad within 15 minutes to 1 hour after delivery must be promptly reported.

Careful explanations to the mother and family are essential, and providing emotional support and maintaining the integrity of the woman's support system are key nursing roles. Even if the mother is separated from her infant, information concerning the infant's condition should be readily accessible. Rooming-in should be established as soon as the woman's condition permits.

Intensive care may be required to allow invasive hemodynamic monitoring of the woman's circulatory status. Nursing Care Plan 10-1 specifies interventions for the woman at high risk for altered tissue perfusion related to hemorrhage.

ANEMIA

Anemia occurs after hemorrhage because of the erythrocytes that are lost. Anemia resulting from blood loss occurs suddenly, and the woman might be dizzy or light-headed and is likely to faint as a result. These symptoms are more likely to occur if she changes position quickly, particularly from a lying to an upright position. Until her hemoglobin and hematocrit levels return to near normal, she will probably be exhausted and have difficulty meeting her needs and those of her infant.

Iron supplements are prescribed to provide adequate amounts of this mineral for manufacture of more erythrocytes. Many health care providers have the woman continue taking the remainder of her prenatal vitamins, which usually provide enough iron to correct mild anemia.

EARLY POSTPARTUM HEMORRHAGE

Early postpartum hemorrhage results from one of the following three causes:

1. Uterine atony (the most common cause)
2. Lacerations (tears) of the reproductive tract
3. Hematomas in the reproductive tract

Nursing Care Plan 10-1   The Woman with Postpartum Hemorrhage

PATIENT DATA A woman is admitted to the postpartum unit. She appears anxious and frightened, and her lochia has saturated three perineal pads in the last hour.

Selected Nursing Diagnosis: Ineffective tissue perfusion related to excessive blood loss secondary to uterine atony or birth injury

Goals	Nursing Interventions	Rationales
The woman's blood pressure and pulse rate will be within 10% of her values when she was admitted.	Identify whether woman has added risk factors for postpartum hemorrhage. Observe the following: • Fundus for height, firmness, and position • Lochia for color, quantity, and clots; count pads and degree of saturation (weigh pads for greater accuracy); check blood pressure, pulse rate, and respiratory rate per hospital protocol	Women who have risk factors should be assessed more often than those who do not. The fundus must be firm to compress bleeding vessels at the placenta site. Bladder distention interferes with uterine contraction and causes the fundus to be high and displaced to one side. A rising pulse rate is often the first sign of inadequate blood volume. A rising pulse rate and falling blood pressure reading also occur. Most blood lost after birth is visible rather than concealed. Observing lochia provides an estimate of actual blood loss.
	Observe for less obvious signs of bleeding: • Constant trickle of brighter red blood with a firm fundus • Severe, poorly relieved pain, especially if accompanied by changes in the vital signs or shock signs and symptoms	Most postpartum hemorrhage is caused by uterine atony, which often produces dramatic blood loss. However, blood loss from a laceration or hematoma can be significant, even though it is less obvious.
The woman will not have signs or symptoms of hypovolemic shock.	Observe for other signs and symptoms of hypovolemic shock. If signs of hemorrhage are noted, take appropriate actions according to the probable cause for hemorrhage: • *Uterine atony:* Massage uterus until firm—do not overmassage; expel blood from uterine cavity when uterus is firm; have breastfeeding woman nurse infant; notify registered nurse and/or health care provider for orders and medication if uterus does not become firm and stay firm. • *Lacerations:* Notify registered nurse and/or health care provider to examine woman. • *Hematomas on the vulva:* Place cold pack on the area.	Excessive blood loss can result in hypovolemic shock. Hemorrhage can cause death of a new mother if not promptly corrected. Most minor episodes of uterine atony are easily corrected with fundal massage and infant suckling. If the uterus does not remain firm, the health care provider examines the woman to identify and correct cause of bleeding. Oxytocin (Pitocin) infusions are often ordered to contract the uterus. Other drugs, such as methylergonovine (Methergine) or prostaglandin, may be needed. Excessive massage of uterus can tire it, possibly resulting in inability to contract. Trauma such as laceration or hematoma may necessitate repair by health care provider. Small hematomas on the vulva can be limited by cold applications, because these applications reduce blood flow to area; cold also numbs area and makes woman more comfortable.

Selected Nursing Diagnosis: Fear, related to powerlessness

Goals	Nursing Interventions	Rationales
Woman will be able to cope with the unexpected complication. Anxiety will be at a manageable level.	Identify woman's reaction to unexpected complication and correct misconceptions and exaggerations of fact or myth. Be calm and reassuring when in contact with the woman. Encourage woman to verbalize her fears and perceptions. Stay with the woman and her partner.	Supplying factual information reduces fear. Identifying reaction establishes basis for intervention. Anxiety can be transferred by voice or body language. This helps establish a basis for patient teaching and identification of fears. Having a professional person present promotes a feeling of security.

Critical Thinking Question

1. A woman is admitted to the postpartum unit after delivery of an infant weighing 9-lb, 12-oz. She voids 600 mL. The fundus is difficult to locate, and lochia is heavy. What are the priority nursing actions?

Table 10-1 Types of Early Postpartum Hemorrhage

UTERINE ATONY	LACERATIONS	HEMATOMA
Characteristics		
Soft, high uterine fundus that is difficult to feel through woman's abdominal wall	Continuous trickle of blood that is brighter than normal lochia	If visible, appears as blue or purplish mass on vulva
Heavy lochia, often with large clots or sometimes a persistent moderate flow	Fundus that is usually firm	Severe and poorly relieved pain and/or pressure in vulva, pelvis, or rectum
Bladder distention that causes uterus to be high and usually displaces it to one side	Onset of hypovolemic shock that may be gradual and easily overlooked	Large amount of blood lost into tissues, which causes signs and symptoms of hypovolemic shock
Possible signs of hypovolemic shock		Lochia that is normal in amount and color
Contributing Factors		
Bladder distention	Rapid labor	Prolonged or rapid labor
Abnormal or prolonged labor	Use of instruments such as forceps or vacuum extractor during birth	Large infant
Overdistended uterus		Use of forceps or vacuum extractor
Multiparity (five or more births)		
Use of oxytocin during labor		
Medications that relax uterus		
Operative birth		
Low placental implantation		

Table 10-1 summarizes the types of early postpartum hemorrhage.

Uterine Atony

Atony describes a lack of normal muscle tone. The postpartum uterus is a large, hollow organ with three layers of muscle. The middle layer includes interlacing "figure-eight" fibers. The uterine blood supply passes through this network of muscle fibers to supply the placenta.

After the placenta detaches, the uterus normally contracts and the muscle fibers compress bleeding vessels. If the uterus is atonic, however, these muscle fibers are flaccid and do not compress the vessels. Uterine atony allows the blood vessels at the placenta site to bleed freely and usually massively. Uterine overdistention, retained placental fragments, prolonged labor, or the use of drugs during labor that relax the uterus may cause atony.

Normal Postpartum Changes. After a full-term birth, the uterus should easily be felt through the abdominal wall as a firm mass about the size of a grapefruit. After the placenta is expelled, the fundus of the uterus is at the umbilicus level and then begins descending at a rate of about 1 finger's width (1 cm) each day.

Lochia rubra should be dark red. The amount of lochia during the first few hours should be no more than one saturated perineal pad per hour. A few small clots may appear in the drainage, but large clots are not normal.

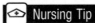 Nursing Tip

Perineal pads containing cold packs absorb less than regular perineal pads.

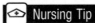 Nursing Tip

To determine blood loss most accurately, weigh perineal pads before and after applying them: 1 g in weight equals about 1 mL in volume of blood lost.

Characteristics of Uterine Atony. When uterine atony occurs, the woman's uterus is difficult to feel and, when found, it feels boggy (soft). The fundal height is high, often above the umbilicus. If the bladder is full, the uterus is higher and pushed to one side rather than located in the midline of the abdomen (Figure 10-1). The uterus may or may not be soft if the bladder is full. A full bladder interferes with the ability of the uterus to contract and, if not corrected, eventually leads to uterine atony.

Lochia is increased and may contain large clots. The bleeding may be dramatic but may also simply be slightly above normal for a long time. Some lochia will be retained in the relaxed uterus, because the cavity is enlarged. Thus the true amount of blood loss may not be immediately apparent. Collection of blood within the uterus further interferes with contraction and worsens uterine atony and postpartum hemorrhage. A woman who has risk factors for postpartum hemorrhage (see Table 10-1) should have more frequent postpartum assessments of the uterus, lochia, and vital signs.

Medical Management and Nursing Care. Care of the woman with uterine atony combines nursing and medical measures. When the uterus is boggy, it should be massaged until firm (see Chapter 9), but it should not be overly massaged. Because the uterus is a muscle, excessive stimulation to contract it will tire it and can

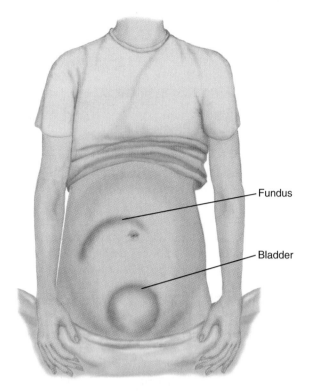

FIGURE 10-1 A distended bladder pushes the uterus upward and usually to one side of the abdomen. The fundus may be boggy or firm. If not emptied, a distended bladder can result in uterine atony and hemorrhage, because it interferes with normal contraction of the uterus. (From McKinney ES, James SR, Murray SS, et al: *Maternal-child nursing*, ed 4, St. Louis, 2013, Saunders.)

— Fundus

— Bladder

actually worsen uterine atony. If the uterus is firmly contracted, it should be left alone.

Bladder distention is an easily corrected cause of uterine atony. The nurse should catheterize the woman if she cannot urinate on the toilet or in a bedpan. Pressing toward the vagina should expel any clots or blood pooled in the vagina *after the uterus is firm.* Most health care providers include an order for catheterization to prevent delaying this corrective measure. First the uterus is massaged to firmness, and then the bladder is emptied to keep the uterus firm.

The infant suckling at the breast stimulates the woman's posterior pituitary gland to secrete oxytocin, which causes uterine contraction. A dilute oxytocin (Pitocin) IV infusion is the most common drug ordered to control uterine atony. Other drugs to increase uterine tone include methylergonovine (Methergine) or prostaglandins such as Hemabate or Cytotec. Methylergonovine increases blood pressure and should not be given to a woman with hypertension. Excessive bleeding may also be managed by providing a uterine tamponade (packing), using an intrauterine balloon, selective arterial embolization, or surgical ligation of the artery. Intravenous calcium gluconate may be used to counteract a tocolytic drug that may have been administered to relax the uterus during labor.

The health care provider may examine the woman in the delivery or operating room to determine the source of her bleeding and to correct it. Rarely, a hysterectomy is needed to remove the bleeding uterus that does not respond to any other measures. The woman should have nothing by mouth (NPO) until her bleeding is controlled.

> **! Safety Alert!**
>
> The woman who develops a hemorrhagic complication should be kept on NPO status until the health care provider evaluates her condition, because she may need general anesthesia for correction of the problem.

Lacerations of the Reproductive Tract

Lacerations of the perineum, vagina, cervix, or area around the urethra (periurethral lacerations) can cause postpartum bleeding. The vascular beds are engorged during pregnancy, and bleeding can be profuse. Trauma is more likely to occur if the woman has a rapid labor or if forceps or a vacuum extractor is used. Blood lost in lacerations is usually a brighter red than lochia and flows in a continuous trickle. Typically, the uterus is firm.

Treatment. The health care provider should be notified if the woman has signs of a laceration—(bleeding with a firmly contracted uterus). The injury is usually sutured in the delivery or operating room.

Nursing Care. Signs and symptoms of a bleeding laceration should be reported. A continuous trickle of blood can result in as much or more blood loss than the dramatic bleeding associated with uterine atony. The woman should be kept on NPO status until further orders are received, because she may need a general anesthetic for repair of the laceration. Genital trauma can cause long-term effects such as cystocele, prolapsed uterus, or urinary incontinence (see Chapter 11).

Hematomas of the Reproductive Tract

A **hematoma** is a collection of blood within the tissues. Hematomas resulting from birth trauma are usually on the vulva or inside the vagina. They may be easily seen as a bulging bluish or purplish mass. Hematomas deep within the vagina are not visible from the outside.

Discomfort after childbirth is normally minimal and easily relieved with mild analgesics. The woman with a hematoma usually has severe, unrelenting pain that analgesics do not relieve. Depending on the amount of blood in the tissues, she also may describe pressure in the vulva, pelvis, or rectum. She may be unable to urinate because of the pressure.

The woman does not have unusual amounts of lochia, but she may develop signs of concealed blood loss if the hematoma is large. Her pulse and respiratory rates rise, and her blood pressure falls. She may develop other signs of hypovolemic shock if blood loss into the tissues is substantial.

See Table 10-1 for risk factors for the development of a hematoma.

Treatment. Small hematomas usually resolve without treatment. Larger ones may require incision and drainage of the clots. The bleeding vessel is ligated or the area packed with a hemostatic material to stop the bleeding.

Nursing Care. An ice pack to the perineum is sufficient for most small perineal hematomas and requires no physician prescription. The nurse should observe and report for the classic symptom: excessive, poorly relieved pain. Signs of concealed blood loss accompanied by maternal complaints of severe pain, perineal or vaginal pressure, or the inability to void should be reported. The woman is kept NPO until the health care provider examines her and prescribes treatment.

LATE POSTPARTUM HEMORRHAGE

Late postpartum hemorrhage (bleeding that occurs 24 hours to 6 weeks after childbirth) usually occurs after discharge from the hospital and usually results from the following:

- Retention of placental fragments
- Subinvolution of the uterus

Placental fragments are more likely to be retained if the placenta does not separate cleanly from its implantation site after birth or if there is disruption of the placental scab. Clots form around these retained fragments and slough several days later, sometimes carrying the retained fragments with them. Retention of placental fragments is more likely to occur if the placenta is manually removed (removed by hand rather than being pushed away from the uterine wall spontaneously as the uterus contracts). These placental fragments are also more likely to exist if the placenta grows more deeply into the uterine muscle than is normal.

Treatment. Treatment consists of the administration of drugs such as oxytocin, methylergonovine, or prostaglandins such as carboprost to contract the uterus. Firm uterine contraction often expels the retained fragments and no other treatment is needed. Ultrasonography may be used to identify remaining fragments. If bleeding continues, **curettage** (scraping or vacuuming the inner surface of the uterus) is performed to remove small blood clots and placental fragments. This procedure is known as dilation and curettage (D&C) or dilation and evacuation (D&E). Antibiotics are prescribed if infection is suspected.

Nursing Care. The nurse should teach each postpartum woman what to expect about changes in the lochia (see Chapter 9). The woman should be instructed to report the following signs of late postpartum hemorrhage to her health care provider:

- Persistent bright red bleeding
- Return of red bleeding after it has changed to pinkish or white

If a late postpartum hemorrhage occurs, the nurse assists in implementing pharmacological and surgical treatment.

SUBINVOLUTION OF THE UTERUS

Involution is the return of the uterus to its nonpregnant condition after birth. The muscles of the uterus contract and constrict the blood vessels at the placental site, stopping the bleeding. Normally the uterus descends at the rate of 1 cm (one finger's width) per day and is no longer palpable by 12 days postpartum. The placental site heals by 6 weeks postpartum. **Subinvolution** is a slower-than-expected return of the uterus to its nonpregnant condition. Infection and retained fragments of the placenta are the most common causes. Typical signs of subinvolution include the following:

- Fundal height greater than expected for the amount of time since birth
- Persistence of lochia rubra or a slowed progression through the three phases
- Pelvic pain, heaviness, fatigue

Treatment. Medical treatment is selected to correct the cause of the subinvolution. It may include the following:

- Methylergonovine (Methergine) to maintain firm uterine contraction
- Antibiotics for infection
- Dilation of the cervix and curettage to remove fragments of the placenta from the uterine wall

Nursing Care. The mother will almost always have been discharged when subinvolution of the uterus occurs. All new mothers should be taught about the normal changes to expect so they can recognize a departure from the normal pattern. Women should report fever, persistent pain, persistent red lochia (or return of bleeding after it has changed), or foul-smelling vaginal discharge. The woman should be taught how to palpate the fundus and what normal changes to expect.

The woman may be admitted to the hospital on the gynecology unit. Nursing care involves assisting with medical therapy and providing analgesics and other comfort measures. Specific nursing care depends on whether the subinvolution results from infection or another cause.

THROMBOEMBOLIC DISORDERS

A *venous thrombosis* is a blood clot within a vein and occurs in 1 in 1500 pregnancies (Gabbe, 2012). The size of the clot can increase as circulating blood passes over it and deposits more platelets, fibrin, and cells. It often causes an inflammation of the vessel wall. The pregnant woman is at increased risk for venous thrombosis because of the venous stasis that can occur from compression of the blood vessels by the heavy uterus or by pressure behind the knees when the legs are placed in stirrup leg supports for episiotomy repair. Blood vessel injury during cesarean section can also cause a thrombus. The levels of fibrinogen and other clotting factors normally increase during pregnancy, whereas levels of clot-dissolving factors (such as plasminogen activator and antithrombin III) are normally decreased, resulting in a state of hypercoagulability (increased susceptibility to develop blood clots). If the woman has varicose veins or remains on bed rest, her state of hypercoagulability places her at increased risk for thrombus formation.

Preventative measures include use of pneumatic compression devices on the lower extremities or prophylactic heparin for women undergoing cesarean sections or who are on prolonged bed rest (Gabbe, 2012).

There are three types of thromboembolic disorders:

1. *Superficial venous thrombosis (SVT)* involves the saphenous vein of the lower leg and is characterized by a painful, hard, reddened, warm vein that is easily seen.
2. *Deep venous thrombosis (DVT)* can involve veins from the feet to the femoral area and is characterized by pain, calf tenderness, leg edema, color changes, pain when walking, and sometimes a positive Homans' sign (pain when the foot is dorsiflexed), although the Homans' sign is not always reliable during the postpartum period, as it is not specific to blood clots postpartum. An increase in leg circumference greater than 2 cm accompanied by redness, tenderness, and edema should be promptly reported. Diagnosis is confirmed via ultrasound with or without a Doppler (Gabbe, 2012).
3. *Pulmonary embolism (PE)* occurs when the pulmonary artery is obstructed by a blood clot that breaks off (*embolizes*) and lodges in the lungs. It may have dramatic signs and symptoms, such as sudden chest pain, cough, dyspnea (difficulty breathing), decreased level of consciousness, and signs of heart failure. A small pulmonary embolism may have nonspecific signs and symptoms, such as shortness of breath, palpitations, hemoptysis (bloody sputum), faintness, and low-grade fever.

Treatment. Superficial venous thrombosis is treated with administration of analgesics, local application of heat, and elevation of the legs to promote venous drainage. Deep venous thrombosis is treated similarly, with the addition of subcutaneous or IV anticoagulation drugs such as heparin. Low molecular weight heparin (LMWH) such as Lovenox may be used, because it is long acting and requires less frequent doses and less frequent lab testing. Anticoagulant therapy, with drugs such as warfarin (Coumadin) or heparin, may be started 6 to 12 hours after birth if needed, and continued for 6 weeks after birth to minimize the risk of embolism. Antibiotics are prescribed if infection is a factor. The woman with a pulmonary embolism is usually transferred to the intensive care unit.

> **⚠ Medication Safety Alert!**
>
> The antidote for a warfarin overdose is vitamin K.

Nursing Care. The woman should be observed before and after birth for signs and symptoms that suggest venous thrombosis. Dyspnea, coughing, and chest pain suggest pulmonary embolism (PE) and must be reported immediately.

Prevention of thrombi is most important. Pregnant women should not cross their legs, because this impedes venous blood flow. When the legs are elevated, there should not be sharp flexion at the groin or pressure in the popliteal space behind the knee, which would restrict venous flow. Measures to promote venous flow should be continued during and after birth, because levels of clotting factors remain high for several weeks.

Early ambulation or range-of-motion exercises are valuable aids to preventing thrombus formation in the postpartum woman. Antiembolic stockings may be used if varicose veins are present. The nurse should teach the woman how to put on the stockings properly, because rolling or kinking of the stocking can further impede blood flow. If stirrups are used during birth or episiotomy repair, they should be padded to prevent pressure at the popliteal angle.

The woman who will be undergoing anticoagulant therapy at home should be taught how to give herself the drug and about signs of excess anticoagulation (prolonged bleeding from minor injuries, bleeding gums, nosebleeds, unexplained bruising). She should use a soft toothbrush and avoid minor trauma that can cause prolonged bleeding or a large hematoma. Home nursing visits are often prescribed to obtain blood for laboratory clotting studies and to help the woman cope with therapy.

INFECTION

PUERPERAL SEPSIS

Puerperal sepsis is infection or septicemia after childbirth. Tissue trauma during labor, the open wound of the placental insertion site, surgical incisions, cracks in the nipples of the breasts, and the increased pH of the vagina after birth are all risk factors for the postpartum woman. About 7% of women develop a fever of 38° C (100.4° F) or higher after the first postpartum day. Fever after cesarean section occurs in about 14% of patients (Hacker et al, 2010). The fever is most often caused by **endometritis**, an inflammation of the inner lining of the uterus. Blockage of the lochial flow because of retained placenta or clots increases susceptibility to infection. The danger of postpartum infection is that a localized infection of the perineum, vagina, or cervix can ascend the reproductive tract and spread to the uterus, fallopian tubes, and peritoneum, causing peritonitis, which is a life-threatening condition. Table 10-2 lists characteristics, medical treatment, and nursing care for these infections. Regardless of their location or the causative organism, postpartum infections have several common features.

Manifestations. Puerperal (postpartum) fever is defined as a temperature of 38° C (100.4° F) or higher after the first 24 hours and for at least 2 days during the first 10 days after birth. Slight temperature elevations with no other signs of infection often occur during the first 24 hours because of dehydration. The nurse should look for other signs of infection if the woman's temperature is elevated, regardless of the time since delivery. A pulse rate that is higher than expected and an elevated temperature often occur when the woman has an infection. Other signs and symptoms of infection may be localized (in a small area of the body) or systemic (throughout the body).

White blood cells (leukocytes) are normally elevated during the early postpartum period to about 20,000 to 30,000 cells/mm^3, which limits the usefulness of the blood count to identify infection. Leukocyte counts in the upper limits are more likely to be associated with infection than lower counts.

> **! Safety Alert!**
>
> Proper hand hygiene is the primary method to prevent the spread of infectious organisms. Gloves should be worn when in contact with any blood or body fluid or any other potentially infectious materials.

Table 10-2 Postpartum Infections

WOUND INFECTIONS	ENDOMETRITIS (UTERUS)	URINARY TRACT INFECTIONS	MASTITIS (BREAST)
Characteristics			
Signs of inflammation (redness, edema, heat, pain) Separation of suture line Purulent drainage	Tender, enlarged uterus Prolonged, severe cramping Foul-smelling lochia Fever and other systemic signs of infection Signs of uterine subinvolution	Cystitis (bladder) Low-grade fever Burning, urgency, and frequency of urination Pyelonephritis (kidneys) High fever with pattern of spikes Chills Pain in costovertebral angle or flank Nausea and vomiting	Reddened, tender, hot area of breast Edema and feeling of heaviness in breast Purulent drainage (may occur if an abscess forms)
Medical Management			
Culture and sensitivity of wound exudate Antibiotics	Culture and sensitivity test of uterine cavity Antibiotics by intravenous (IV) route initially	Clean-catch or catheterized urine specimen for culture and sensitivity testing Antibiotics (initially by IV route for pyelonephritis)	Antibiotics (usually oral, although may be IV initially if woman has abscess) Incision and drainage of abscess
Nursing Care			
Use aseptic or sterile technique for all wound care as indicated Teach proper perineal hygiene to reduce fecal contamination Use sitz baths for perineal wound infections	Teach woman usual progression of lochia, because infection often occurs after discharge Use Fowler's position to facilitate drainage of infected lochia Administer analgesics Observe for absent bowel sounds, abdominal distention, and nausea or vomiting, which suggest spread of infection	Teach perineal hygiene Encourage fluid intake of 3 L/day Teach which foods increase acidity of urine, such as apricots, cranberry juice, plums, and prunes	Teach effective breastfeeding techniques Encourage moist heat applications with warm pack Use warm shower before nursing to start milk flow Massage affected area to reduce congestion and start milk flow Encourage regular and frequent nursing or pumping to keep breasts empty

Treatment. The goals of medical treatment are to limit the spread of infection, to prevent it from reaching the blood and other organs, and to eliminate the infection. A culture and sensitivity sample from the suspected site of infection is taken to determine the antibiotics that will be most effective. A culture and sensitivity test typically requires 2 or 3 days to complete. In the meantime, antibiotics that are effective against typical organisms that cause the infection are provided to limit the spread of infection to nearby structures.

Nursing Care. Nursing care objectives focus on preventing infection and, if an infection occurs, on facilitating medical treatment. To achieve these goals, the nurse should do the following:

- Use and teach hygienic measures to reduce the number of organisms that can cause infection (e.g., hand washing, perineal care).
- Promote adequate rest and nutrition for healing.
- Observe for signs of infection.

- Teach signs of infection that the woman should report after discharge.
- Teach the woman to take all of the antibiotics prescribed rather than stopping them after her symptoms are eliminated.
- Teach the woman how to apply perineal pads (front to back).

Women should be taught to wash their hands before and after performing self-care that may involve contact with secretions. The nurse should explore ways to help the woman get enough rest. Nursing Care Plan 10-2 details interventions for the woman at high risk for infection.

Ultimately, a woman's own body must overcome infection and heal any wound. Nutrition is an essential component of her body defenses. The nurse, and sometimes a dietitian, teaches her about foods that are high in protein (meats, cheese, milk, legumes) and vitamin C (citrus fruits and juices, strawberries, cantaloupe), because these nutrients are especially important for healing. Foods high in iron to correct anemia include

---

✳ Nursing Care Plan 10-2 | The Woman with Risk for Postpartum Infection

PATIENT DATA A woman is admitted to the postpartum unit after delivering a baby boy via cesarean section. Her husband is at her bedside, and she is resting in bed.

Selected Nursing Diagnosis: Risk for infection related to loss of skin integrity (cesarean incision) and increased risk factors (blood loss, invasive procedures)

Goals	Nursing Interventions	Rationales
The woman will not have signs of infection as evidenced by an oral temperature less than 38° C (100.4° F) and by normal progression of lochia that does not have a foul odor.	Perform proper hand hygiene when providing care. Teach woman personal hygiene measures, such as hand washing, perineal care, and regular changes of perineal pads.	Limits the transfer of infectious organisms between patients and from one area of the body to another. Regular pad changes also reduce the amount of time organisms have to multiply in this warm, dark, and moist environment.
	Determine vital signs every 4 hours or more frequently if signs of infection are present.	An elevated temperature and rising pulse rate are signs of infection. If they occur, woman should be assessed for other signs and symptoms of infection.
	Observe lochia for amount, color, and odor when assessing vital signs.	Infection is evidenced by foul-smelling lochia that may increase or decrease in amount; it is sometimes brown.
	Observe the wound each shift for redness, edema, ecchymosis, discharge, and approximation (REEDA).	Signs of inflammation characterize a wound infection. The suture line may separate if there is infection in the area.
	Maintain medical and surgical asepsis when in contact with the woman.	Reduces the potential for infection for the woman at risk because of postpartum complications.
The woman will not self-contaminate.	Teach woman wound care protocols and general hygiene.	Decreases the spread of infection by self-contamination.
	Promote fluid and nutritional intake. Record intake and output.	Adequate nutrition is essential for healing. Decreased output can indicate kidney shutdown.

Critical Thinking Question

1. The nurse is caring for a woman who had an emergency cesarean delivery and is 1 day postpartum. She is sleepy and asks the nurse to care for the infant. Her temperature at 8 AM was 38° C (100.4° F) and at 10 AM was 38.3° C (101.0° F). What nursing intervention(s) are appropriate?

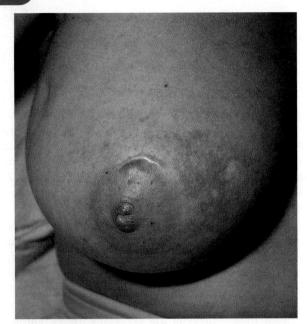

FIGURE 10-2 Mastitis typically occurs several weeks after birth in the woman who is breastfeeding. Bacteria usually enter the breast through small cracks in the nipples. Breast engorgement and milk stasis increase the risk for mastitis. (From Swartz MH: *Textbook of physical diagnosis: history and examination*, ed 6, Philadelphia, 2009, Saunders.)

meats, enriched cereals and breads, and dark green, leafy vegetables.

MASTITIS AND BREASTFEEDING

Mastitis is an infection of the breast. It usually occurs about 2 or 3 weeks after giving birth (Figure 10-2). Mastitis occurs when organisms from the skin or the infant's mouth enter small cracks in the nipples or areolae. These cracks may be microscopic. Breast engorgement and inadequate emptying of milk are associated with mastitis. Mastitis often involves only one breast.

Signs and symptoms of mastitis include the following:
* Redness and heat in the breast
* Tenderness
* Edema and a heaviness in the breast
* Purulent drainage (may or may not be present)

The woman usually has fever, chills, and other systemic signs and symptoms. If not treated, the infected area becomes encapsulated (walled off) and an abscess forms. The infection is usually outside the ducts of the breast, and the milk is not contaminated.

Treatment. Antibiotics and the continued removal of milk from the breast are the primary treatments for mastitis. Mild analgesics make the woman more comfortable. The woman may need an incision and drainage of the infected area and intravenous antibiotics if an abscess forms. The mother can usually continue to breastfeed. If she should stop nursing for any reason, she should pump her breasts. She should not wean her infant when she has mastitis, because weaning leads to engorgement and stasis of milk, which worsens the mastitis.

Nursing Care. The nursing mother should be taught proper breastfeeding techniques to reduce the risk for mastitis (see Chapter 9). Nursing care for mastitis centers on relieving pain and on maintaining lactation. Heat promotes blood flow to the area, comfort, and complete emptying of the breast. Moist heat can be applied with chemical packs. Placing a warm wet cloth in a plastic bag and applying it to the breasts can create an inexpensive warm pack. A warm shower provides warmth and cleanliness and stimulates the flow of milk if done just before nursing.

Patient Teaching

Mastitis

* Wash hands thoroughly before breastfeeding.
* Maintain breast cleanliness with frequent breast pad changes.
* Expose nipple(s) to air when possible.
* Ensure correct newborn latch-on and removal from breast.
* Encourage the newborn to empty the breast, because milk provides a medium for bacterial growth.
* Frequently breastfeed to encourage milk flow.
* If an area of the breast is distended or tender, breastfeed from the uninfected side *first* at each feeding (to initiate let-down reflex in the affected breast).
* Massage distended area as the newborn nurses.
* Report redness and fever to health care provider.
* Apply ice packs or moist heat to relieve discomfort.

Both breasts should be emptied regularly to reduce milk stasis, which increases the risk for abscess formation. If the affected breast is too painful for the mother to breastfeed, she can use a breast pump to empty it. She can massage the area of inflammation to improve milk flow and reduce stasis. Nursing first on the unaffected side starts the milk flow in both breasts and can improve emptying with less pain. Other nursing measures include the following:
* Encouraging fluid intake
* Advising the woman to wear a good support bra to support the breasts and to limit movement of the painful breast; the bra should not be too tight or it will cause milk stasis
* Supporting the woman emotionally and reassuring her that she can continue to breastfeed

MOOD DISORDERS

A **mood** is a pervasive and sustained emotion that can color one's view of life. "Postpartum blues" or "baby blues" are common after birth. The woman has periods when she feels let down, but overall she finds pleasure in life and in her new role as mother. Her roller-coaster emotions are usually self-limiting as she adapts to the changes in her life. A **psychosis** involves serious impairment of one's perception of reality. Postpartum depression and postpartum psychosis are disorders that are more serious than "postpartum blues."

POSTPARTUM DEPRESSION

Postpartum depression is a nonpsychotic depressive illness that is usually manifested within 2 to 4 weeks after delivery and affects 10% to 20% of postpartum women in the United States. The onset of depression during this time may interfere with the mother's ability to respond to her infant's cues and interferes with the developing maternal–infant bonding. Formal postpartum screening for depression is not standard practice in the United States, which places the responsibility on the nurse to detect and refer problems to prevent progression to chronic depression. The nurse can promote the behaviors that improve mental health. Risk factors for postpartum depression include inadequate social support, poor relationship with partner, life and childcare stress, low self-esteem, and unplanned pregnancy. Those having close contact with the woman notice the depression. Signs and symptoms may include the following:

- Lack of enjoyment in life
- Disinterest in others; loss of normal give-and-take in relationships
- Intense feelings of inadequacy, unworthiness, guilt, inability to cope
- Loss of mental concentration; inability to make decisions
- Disturbed sleep or appetite
- Constant fatigue and feelings of ill health

Postpartum depression strains the coping mechanisms of the entire family at a time when all are adapting to the birth of a child. As a result of the strained relationships, communication is often impaired, and the depressed woman may withdraw further, which distances her even further from her support system. The woman usually remains in touch with reality.

> **Nursing Tip**
>
> If a postpartum woman seems depressed, the nurse should not assume that she has the common "baby blues" or that she will "snap out of it." Explore her feelings to determine if they are persistent and pervasive.

Treatment. Treatment of postpartum depression includes psychotherapy and increased social support and may include antidepressant medications. However, many breastfeeding mothers are reluctant to take medications. Prompt referral to a multidisciplinary health care team can improve the long-term outcome for mother, infant, and family. Light therapy (phototherapy) and exercise are complementary and alternative (CAM) treatment strategies that may help in the management of postpartum depression (see Chapter 34 for other types of CAM therapy). The influence of hormones on mood changes before, during, and after menstruation supports the theory that fluctuating hormone levels postpartum may also have an effect on the woman's mood. Falling estrogen levels affect the dopamine levels in the brain, which are thought to be responsible for emotion and thought. Therefore hormonal skin patches are sometimes used in the treatment of postpartum depression. Referral for follow-up with a case manager, and counseling that includes the woman's partner and family, are essential treatment plans.

Nursing Care. The nurse is more likely to encounter the woman with postpartum depression in the health care provider's office or an outpatient clinic. The nurse may help the mother by being a sympathetic listener. Women may be reluctant to express dissatisfaction with their new role, especially if they have waited a long time for a child.

The nurse should elicit the new mother's feelings about motherhood and her infant. She must observe for complaints of sleeplessness or chronic fatigue. The mother's expressions of feelings should be pursued to help her express them better. The nurse must help the mother see that there is hope for her problem yet not minimize her feelings by saying things such as, "You'll get over it."

Isolation can be both a cause and a result of depression. The new mother should be helped to identify sources of emotional support among her family and friends. Many of her friends may have stopped including her in activities, because she has withdrawn from them. She may not have the emotional energy to reach out to them again.

The woman who is physically depleted often has exaggerated feelings of disappointment and depression. The nurse should determine whether the mother is getting enough exercise, sleep, and proper nutrition to improve her physical health and sense of well-being. The mother should be helped to identify ways to meet her own needs and be reassured that she is not being selfish.

A new mother may feel guilty because she is not happy all the time. The nurse can explain that these feelings are not right or wrong—feelings simply exist. She should be referred to support groups if these are available. Discussing her feelings with others who have similar difficulties can help her realize that she is not alone.

POSTPARTUM PSYCHOSIS

Women experiencing a postpartum psychosis have an impaired sense of reality. Psychosis is much less common than postpartum depression. A woman may have any psychiatric disorder, but two are most often encountered:

1. *Bipolar disorder:* A disorder characterized by episodes of **mania** (hyperactivity, excitability, euphoria, and a feeling of being invulnerable) and depression
2. *Major depression:* A disorder characterized by deep feelings of worthlessness and guilt, serious sleep and appetite disturbances, and sometimes delusions about the infant being dead

Postpartum psychosis can be fatal for both mother and infant. The mother may endanger herself and her infant during manic episodes, because she uses poor judgment and has a sense of being invulnerable. Suicide and infanticide are possible, especially during depressive episodes.

If the woman has resources, such as private health insurance or a health maintenance organization (HMO), case managers, home visits, and outpatient psychiatric counseling may be available. In some cases, social workers within the community may refer the woman for counseling. In other cases, an inpatient psychiatric treatment center is the appropriate environment for treatment. Virtually all psychotropic medications prescribed for psychoses pass through the breast milk and will affect the newborn infant. Therefore breastfeeding is typically contraindicated when psychotropic medications are prescribed for the mother.

THE HOMELESS MOTHER AND NEWBORN

Homelessness is defined as a lack of a permanent home and is not limited to women who must live on the street. Some women live in single-room hotels, and others stay with friends or extended family. Homeless women often have difficulty accessing care, receive care from different health care providers at different sites, and have incomplete medical records. Follow-up is difficult. Before discharging a mother with her newborn infant, it is essential to determine that she has a place to go and has a way of accessing help for herself or her newborn. The nurse can be a key link in facilitating referrals to outreach programs, support services, counseling, shelters, and follow-up medical care.

Unfolding Case Study

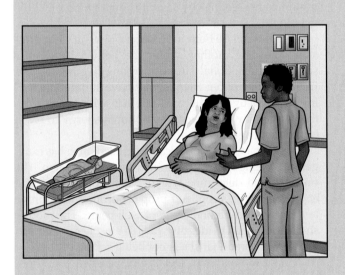

Tess and Luis were introduced to the reader in Chapter 4, and Tess's pregnancy experience has unfolded in each chapter. Tess has delivered twins and has transferred to the postpartum unit with one twin infant, while her husband, Luis, stays with the other twin infant in the NICU.

Tess has been resting in the postpartum unit for 4 hours with the infant at her bedside. She states that she is worried that her lochia is heavy and still red, and she believes she may be bleeding too heavily. She has not ambulated at all, because she says she is too tired.

QUESTIONS

1. What factors during delivery may contribute to postpartum hemorrhage for Tess?
2. What assessments would the nurse make to determine if her lochia is excessive?
3. Since Tess has not yet ambulated to the bathroom, what safety precautions need to be initiated for Tess?
4. What safety precautions need to be initiated for the baby?
5. What teaching would the nurse offer?

Get Ready for the NCLEX® Examination!

Key Points

- The nurse must be aware of women who are at higher risk for postpartum hemorrhage and assess them more often.
- A constant small trickle of blood can result in significant blood loss, as can a larger one-time hemorrhage.
- Pain that is persistent and more severe than expected is characteristic of a hematoma in the reproductive tract.
- It is essential to identify and limit a local infection before it spreads to the blood or other organs.
- The nurse should teach new mothers about normal postpartum changes and indications of problems that should be reported.

- Early ambulation can prevent thrombosis formation.
- Types of obstetric shock include *cardiogenic* (from anemia or cardiac disorders), *hypovolemic* (from hemorrhage), *anaphylactic* (from a drug response), and *septic* (caused by puerperal infection).
- Careful listening and observation can help the nurse identify a new mother who is suffering from postpartum depression.
- Postpartum psychoses are serious disorders that are potentially life threatening to the woman and others, including her infant.

Additional Learning Resources

SG Go to your Study Guide for additional learning activities to help you master this chapter content.

evolve Go to your Evolve website (http://evolve.elsevier.com/Leifer) for the following learning resources:

- Animations
- Answer Guidelines for Critical Thinking Questions
- Answers and Rationales for Review Questions for the NCLEX® Examination
- Glossary with English and Spanish pronunciations
- Interactive Review Questions for the NCLEX® Examination
- Patient Teaching Plans in English and Spanish
- Skills Performance Checklists
- Video clips and more!

 Online Resources

- Association of Women's Health, Obstetric, and Neonatal Nurses: www.awhonn.org
- Behavioral health care: www.naphs.org
- Child passenger safety: www.saferoads.org/issues/fs-child.htm

Review Questions for the NCLEX® Examination

1. The earliest finding in postpartum hypovolemic shock is usually:
   1. low blood pressure.
   2. rapid pulse rate.
   3. pale skin color.
   4. soft uterus.

2. A bleeding laceration is typically manifested by:
   1. a soft uterus that is difficult to locate.
   2. low pulse rate and blood pressure.
   3. bright red bleeding and a firm uterus.
   4. profuse dark red bleeding and large clots.

3. During the postpartum period the white blood cell (leukocyte) count is normally:
   1. higher than normal.
   2. lower than normal.
   3. unchanged.
   4. unimportant.

4. A postpartum mother who is breastfeeding has developed mastitis. She states that she does not think it is good for her infant to drink milk from her infected breast. The best response from the nurse would be to:
   1. instruct her to nurse the infant from only the unaffected breast until the infection clears up.
   2. suggest that she discontinue breastfeeding and start the infant on formula.
   3. encourage breastfeeding the infant to prevent engorgement.
   4. apply a tight breast binder to the infected breast until the infection subsides.

5. A woman has delivered her newborn several hours previously, and her uterus remains soft and boggy. Which of the following medications should the nurse anticipate that the health care provider would prescribe to increase uterine tone and firm the uterus? (Select all that apply.)
   1. Methergine (Methylergonovine)
   2. Carboprost (Hemabate)
   3. Magnesium sulfate
   4. Pitocin (Oxytoxin)

Objectives

1. Define each key term listed.
2. Explain aspects of preventive health care for women.
3. Describe each menstrual disorder and its care.
4. Explain each gynecological infection in terms of cause, transmission, treatment, and care.
5. Describe the various methods of birth control, including indications, side effects and contraindications of each.
6. Describe how to use natural family family-planning methods for contraception or infertility management.
7. Describe possible causes and treatment of infertility.
8. Explain the changes that occur during the perimenopausal period and after menopause.
9. Explain the medical and nursing care of women who are nearing or have completed menopause.
10. Discuss the medical and nursing care of women with pelvic floor dysfunction or problems related to benign growths in the reproductive tract.
11. Describe the nursing care and treatment of a woman with leiomyoma.

Key Terms

amenorrhea   (ă-měn-ŏ-RĒ-ă, p. 253)
climacteric   (klī-MĂK-ŭr-ĭk, p. 274)
coitus interruptus   (KŌ-ĭ-tŭs ĭn-tŭr-RŬP-tŭs, p. 268)
dysmenorrhea   (dĭs-měn-ō-RĒ-ă, p. 254)
dyspareunia   (dĭs-pă-RŪ-nē-ă, p. 254)
endometriosis   (ĕn-dō-mē-trē-Ō-sĭs, p. 254)
leiomyomas   (lī-ō-mī-Ō-măz, p. 278)
menopause   (MĚN-ō-păwz, p. 274)
menorrhagia   (měn-ō-RĀ-zhă, p. 253)

metrorrhagia   (mě-trō-RĀ-zhă, p. 253)
mittelschmerz   (MĬT-ěl-shmārts, p. 253)
myomas   (mī-Ō-măz, p. 272)
osteoporosis   (ŏs-tē-ō-pă-RŌ-sĭs, p. 274)
polycystic ovary syndrome   (p. 278)
retrograde ejaculation   (p. 270)
spermicides   (p. 264)
spinnbarkeit   (SPĬN-băhr-kīt, p. 261)
stress incontinence   (p. 277)

Today women from all ethnic backgrounds choose to be active participants in their health care and therefore need information about their bodies, health promotion, self-care techniques, and choices concerning treatment options. Culturally competent communication is the key to empowering the woman to feel confident about her ability to care for herself and her family. In some cultures, women ask when they have questions; in other cultures, women wait to be told what to do. To be an effective teacher about health behaviors, the nurse must understand the cultural practices, past experiences, and individual goals of the patient. The nurse offers support, knowledge, and caring behaviors that help the woman cope with screening tests or problems.

GOALS OF *HEALTHY PEOPLE 2020*

Some *Healthy People 2020* (U.S. Department of Health and Human Services [USDHHS], 2010) goals and strategies related to women's health include the following:

- Increasing the number of women over the age of 40 who have mammograms according to

established guidelines to help curb the rise in breast cancer
- Increasing the number of women over the age of 21 who have Papanicolaou (Pap) tests according to established guidelines to reduce the number of deaths from cervical cancer
- Reducing the occurrence of vertebral/hip fractures in older women with osteoporosis
- Reducing the occurrence of sexually transmitted infections (STIs [formerly known as sexually transmitted diseases—STDs]) and pelvic inflammatory disease (PID)

Achievement of these goals requires preventive care, screening, and increased accessibility to health care.

PREVENTIVE HEALTH CARE FOR WOMEN

The goal of preventive health care, or health maintenance, is the prevention or early identification of disease. The value of preventive health care is that some disabling conditions can be prevented or their severity lessened by specific measures, such as altering the diet or detecting the disorder early and at a more treatable stage. Preventive care for women may include disorders with the characteristics that follow:

- Exclusive to women, such as cervical cancer
- Dominant in women, such as breast cancer or osteoporosis
- Prevalent in the general population, such as hypertension or colorectal cancers

This chapter focuses on those disorders that are exclusive to or dominant in women. Much of preventive health care involves screening tests. These tests are not diagnostic but can identify whether additional testing is needed. Examples of screening tests that are common in women's health care include mammography to identify breast cancer and Pap tests for cervical cancer.

 Nursing Tip

Encouraging women to practice preventive health care can help prevent some disorders or identify them early, when they are the most treatable.

BREAST CARE

Three approaches are needed for early detection of breast cancer:

1. Monthly breast self-examination
2. Annual professional breast examination
3. Mammography as appropriate

The nurse's role is to educate women about the benefit of all three examinations and techniques of self-examination. The reader should consult a medical-surgical text for additional information about the diagnosis and treatment of breast cancer.

 Nursing Tip

Preventive care for breast health involves self-examination, professional examinations, and mammography at the appropriate ages.

Breast Self-Examination

All women after age 20 years should perform breast self-examination (BSE) at about the same time each month. The best time for BSE is 1 week after the beginning of the menstrual period. If she is not menstruating, the woman may choose any day that is easy for her to remember, such as the first day of each month. Skill 11-1 describes how to teach a woman to perform BSE.

The chief value of BSE is that a woman learns how her own breasts feel. This is particularly valuable if she has fibrocystic breast changes, in which there are often many lumps that may change with hormonal fluctuations. The woman, who knows her own breasts, is more likely to notice when something is different about them.

Professional Breast Examination

BSE is a supplement to, rather than a substitute for, regular professional examinations. Although the woman who does regular BSE knows what is usual for her own breasts, professionals have the training and experience to identify suspicious breast masses. Breast examination is part of every annual gynecological examination and is done more frequently for women who have a high risk for breast cancer. It is recommended at yearly intervals for all women older than 20 years. The professional examination is similar to that for BSE.

Mammography

Mammography uses very low-dose x-rays to visualize the breast tissue. Mammography can detect breast tumors very early—long before the woman or a professional can feel them. The breast is compressed firmly between two plates, which is briefly uncomfortable. Scheduling the mammogram after a menstrual period reduces the discomfort, because the breasts are less tender at that time. The American Cancer Society currently recommends an annual mammogram for all women age 40 years or older. Women at higher risk for breast cancer may begin mammography earlier.

VULVAR SELF-EXAMINATION

Women over 18 years of age (or younger, if sexually active) should perform a monthly examination of the external genitalia to identify lesions or masses that may indicate infection or malignancy. The woman should use a hand mirror in a good light to inspect systematically and to palpate her vulva and mons pubis for any new growths of any type, any painful or inflamed areas, ulcers, sores, or changes in skin color. She should report any abnormalities to her health care provider.

PELVIC EXAMINATION

The pelvic examination should be scheduled between menstrual periods, and the woman should not douche or have sexual intercourse for at least 48 hours before the examination to avoid altering the Pap test. The purpose of the pelvic examination is to identify conditions such as tumors, abnormal discharge, infections, or unusual pain.

The health care provider first checks the external genitalia to identify signs or problems similar to those noted in vulvar self-examination. Next, a speculum is inserted to visualize the woman's cervix and vagina for inflammation, discharge, or lesions. The speculum is warmed and lubricated with warm water only. A Pap test is obtained to screen for changes in the vaginal and cervical tissues that may be precancerous. The current guidelines for routine Pap test are on p. 253 (ACOG, 2012).

How to Perform Breast Self-Examination

PURPOSE

To learn to know how the breasts feel and detect any changes

NOTE: Perform breast self-examination monthly. If you are menstruating, do the examination 1 week after the beginning of your period, because your breasts are less tender at this time. If you are not menstruating, choose any day that you can easily remember, such as the first day of each month. Examine your breasts three ways: before a mirror, lying down, and in the shower.

STEPS

Before a Mirror

1. Inspect your breasts in four steps:
   a. With arms at your sides
   b. With arms over your head
   c. With your hands on your hips, pressing them firmly to flex your chest muscles
   d. Bending forward.
2. At each step, note any change in the shape or appearance of your breasts.
3. Note skin or nipple changes such as dimpling of the skin.
4. Squeeze each nipple gently to identify any discharge.

3. Use a systematic pattern to check the entire breast:
   a. One pattern is to feel the tissue in a circular pattern, spiraling inward toward the nipple.
   b. Another method is to use an up-and-down pattern. Use the same systematic pattern to examine the underarm area, because breast tissue is also present here.
4. Repeat for the other breast.

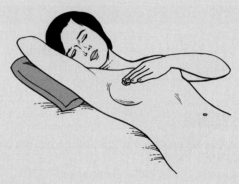

In the Shower

1. Raise your arm.
2. Use your soapy fingers to feel the breast tissue in the same systematic pattern described under "Lying Down."

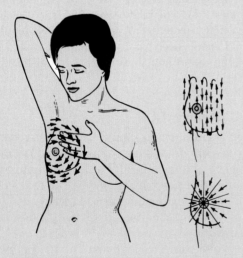

Lying Down

1. Place a small pillow under your right shoulder and put your right hand under your head while you examine your right breast with your left hand.
2. Use the sensitive pads of your fingers to press gently into the breast tissue.

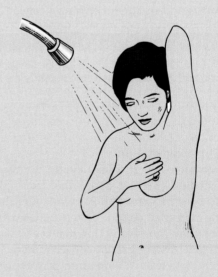

For Additional Information:

Contact the American Cancer Society at 1-800-ACS-2345, or visit the website at www.cancer.org.

(Figures from Lowdermilk DL, Perry SE: *Maternity and women's health care*, ed 8, St Louis, 2004, Mosby.)

- Start at 21 years or older regardless of sexual activity
- Every 3 years for women age 21 to 29
- Every 5 years for women age 30 to 65
- No screening necessary for women over the age of 65 with negative screening for past 10 years

A Pap test and HPV coscreening are often completed together. Women with a history of exposure to diethylstilbestrol (DES) in utero or having positive or atypical findings in previous tests may be scheduled for more frequent checkups.

After the Pap test is obtained, the health care provider will perform an internal, or bimanual, examination to evaluate the internal organs. The index and middle fingers of one hand are inserted into the vagina, and the other hand is placed on the abdomen to permit palpation of the cervix, uterus, and ovaries between the fingers. After the internal examination, a single lubricated finger is inserted into the rectum to identify hemorrhoids or other lesions. A test for fecal occult blood may be performed at this time (see a medical-surgical text for details).

MENSTRUAL DISORDERS

Menstrual cycle disorders can cause distress for many women. The nursing role in each depends on the disorder's cause and treatment. Common nursing roles involve explaining any recommended treatments (e.g., medications) and caring for the woman, including emotional support, before and after procedures.

AMENORRHEA

Amenorrhea is the absence of menstruation. It is normal before menarche, during pregnancy, and after menopause. Amenorrhea that is not normal may fall into one of two categories:

1. *Primary:* Failure to menstruate by age 16 years; failure to menstruate by age 14 years if she has not developed any secondary sex characteristics
2. *Secondary:* Cessation of menstruation for at least three cycles or 6 months in a woman who previously had an established pattern of menstruation

Treatment of amenorrhea begins with a thorough history, physical examination, and laboratory examinations to identify the cause. Pregnancy testing is completed for any sexually active woman.

The specific treatment depends on the cause that is identified. For example, women who are very thin or who have a low percentage of body fat may experience amenorrhea, because fat is necessary for estrogen production. This group of women may include athletes but may also include patients who have eating disorders such as anorexia or bulimia. Therapy for the eating disorder may result in the resumption of normal periods. Other treatments are aimed at correcting the cause, which may be an endocrine imbalance.

ABNORMAL UTERINE BLEEDING

Abnormal uterine bleeding is defined as being (1) too frequent, (2) too long in duration, or (3) excessive in amount. **Metrorrhagia** (intermenstrual bleeding) is uterine bleeding that is usually normal in amount but occurs at irregular intervals. **Menorrhagia** refers to menstrual bleeding that is excessive in amount. The average woman loses about 35 mL of blood during normal menstruation. Blood loss greater than 80 mL/month is considered excessive and often results in anemia. Heavy menstrual bleeding is manifested by soaking through a menstrual pad/tampon within 1 hour, for several hours; passing clots the size of a quarter; and a gushing sensation often leaking through protection (Holland-Hall, 2012).

Common causes for any type of abnormal bleeding include the following:

- Bleeding disorders
- Pregnancy complications, such as an unidentified pregnancy that is ending in spontaneous abortion
- Lesions of the vagina, cervix, or uterus (benign or malignant)
- Breakthrough bleeding (BTB) that may occur in the woman taking oral contraceptives
- Endocrine disorders such as hypothyroidism
- Failure to ovulate or respond appropriately to hormones secreted with ovulation (dysfunctional uterine bleeding)

Treatment of abnormal uterine bleeding depends on the identified cause. Pregnancy complications and benign or malignant lesions are treated appropriately. BTB may be relieved by a change in the oral contraceptive used. Abnormal hormone secretion is treated with the appropriate medications. Antifibrolytic agents can be used for heavy menstrual bleeding but risks for thrombus formation must be evaluated. Surgical dilation and evacuation (D&E [formerly known as dilation and curettage, or D&C]) may serve to remove intrauterine growths or aid in diagnosis. Hysterectomy may be performed for some disorders if the woman does not desire additional children. A technique called laser ablation can permanently remove the abnormally bleeding uterine lining without a hysterectomy. Menorrhagia can be treated with mefenamic acid (a nonsteroidal antiinflammatory drug, or NSAID) or tranexamic acid (an antifibrinolytic) if hormone therapy is contraindicated (Bond, 2013).

MENSTRUAL CYCLE PAIN

Mittelschmerz

Mittelschmerz ("middle pain") is pain that many women experience around ovulation, near the middle of their menstrual cycle. Mild analgesics are usually sufficient to relieve this discomfort. The nurse can teach the woman that this discomfort, although annoying, is harmless.

Dysmenorrhea

Dysmenorrhea, painful menses or "cramps," affects many women. It occurs soon after the onset of menses and is spasmodic in nature. Discomfort is in the lower abdomen and may radiate to the lower back or down the legs. Some women also have diarrhea, nausea, and vomiting. It is most common in young women who have not been pregnant (nulliparas).

There are two types of dysmenorrhea: *primary*, in which there is no evidence of pelvic abnormality, and *secondary*, in which a pathological condition is identifiable.

Primary dysmenorrhea is a leading cause of short-term recurrent school absenteeism in adolescent girls in the United States. Characteristics include the following:

- Onset occurs shortly after menarche with heavy menstrual flow.
- Pain begins no more than a few hours before menstruation starts and lasts no more than 72 hours.
- Pelvic examination results are normal.

Secondary dysmenorrhea most commonly results from endometriosis, the use of an intrauterine device (IUD) to prevent pregnancy, pelvic inflammatory disease, uterine polyps, or ovarian cysts. Treatment involves identifying and treating the cause.

Vasopressins and prostaglandins from the endometrium (uterine lining) play an important role in dysmenorrhea. Some women produce excessive amounts of prostaglandins from the endometrium, and these substances are potent stimulants of painful uterine contractions. Three treatments may provide relief:

1. Prostaglandin-inhibitor drugs, such as ibuprofen (Motrin, Advil) or naproxen (Naprosyn, Anaprox) (Prostaglandin inhibitors are most effective if taken before the onset of menstruation and cramps.)
2. Heat application to the lower abdomen or back
3. Oral contraceptives, which reduce the amount of endometrium built up each month and therefore reduce prostaglandin secretion.

ENDOMETRIOSIS

Endometriosis is the presence of tissue that resembles endometrium outside the uterus. This tissue responds to hormonal stimulation just as the uterine lining does. The lesions may cause pain, pressure, and inflammation to adjacent organs as they build up and slough during menstrual cycles.

Endometriosis causes pain in many women that is either sharp or dull. It is more constant than the spasmodic pain of dysmenorrhea. **Dyspareunia** (painful sexual intercourse) may be present. Endometriosis appears to cause infertility in some women.

Treatment of endometriosis may be either medical or surgical. Medications such as danazol and agonists of gonadotropin-releasing hormone (GnRH) may be administered via nasal spray to reduce the buildup of tissue by inducing an artificial menopause. The woman may have hot flashes and vaginal dryness, similar to symptoms occurring at natural menopause. She is also at increased risk for other problems that occur after menopause, such as osteoporosis and serum lipid changes. Surgical treatment includes the following:

- Hysterectomy with removal of the ovaries and all lesions if the woman does not desire another pregnancy
- Laser ablation (destruction) of the lesions if she wants to maintain fertility

PREMENSTRUAL DISORDERS

Premenstrual syndrome (PMS), and the more serious premenstrual dysphoric disorder (PMDD), are associated with abnormal serotonin response to normal changes in the estrogen levels during the menstrual cycle. The following symptom criteria (which are used to diagnose PMDD) occur between ovulation and the onset of menstruation, begin to improve between the menstruation and ovulation phase, and are not present in the week after the menstrual period. Five or more of the following symptoms usually occur regularly:

- Depressed mood
- Anxiety, tension, feeling "on edge"
- Increased sensitivity to rejection
- Irritability
- Decreased interest in usual activities
- Difficulty in concentrating
- Lethargy
- Change in appetite—food cravings
- Change in sleep habits
- Feeling overwhelmed
- Physical symptoms such as breast tenderness, bloating, weight gain, headaches

Diagnosis is often based on an established pattern throughout more than 3 months. Treatment includes a diet rich in complex carbohydrates and fiber (to lengthen effects of the carbohydrate meal), stress management, and exercise. Medical management includes oral contraceptives (low-estrogen, progestin-dominant), diuretics during the luteal phase of the menstrual cycle (between ovulation and onset of menstruation), and NSAIDs.

Patient education concerning maintenance of a monthly calendar of symptoms, stress management, and dietary guidance are important concepts for the nurse to teach. Reduction of caffeine, simple sugars, and salty foods, regular exercise, and prevention of hypoglycemia are important lifestyle changes. Although eating chocolate has been shown to elevate depressed moods, excessive consumption should be avoided. Serotonin reuptake inhibitors (SRIs) such as fluoxetine (Sarafem) or sertraline (Zoloft, or short-acting antianxiety drugs such as alprazolam [Xanax]) may be initiated 2 weeks before menses and discontinued when menses begins. Remission usually occurs during the follicular stage with no signs and symptoms the week after menses.

THE NORMAL VAGINA

At birth, the infant's vaginal epithelium is controlled by estrogen from the mother and is rich in glycogen, with a low pH of 3.7 to 6.3. When the maternal estrogen effect decreases, the vaginal epithelium atrophies, contains little glycogen, and the pH rises to 7. Estrogen influence returns at puberty, and glycogen increases. The interaction of glycogen and estrogen in the vaginal epithelium results in the growth of lactobacilli, which produce a bacteriostatic action. The pH falls to 3.5 to 4.5. The types of bacteria found in the vagina vary with the pH of the vagina. Factors that change the normal flora of the vagina and predispose to vaginal infection include the following:

- *Antibiotics:* Encourage yeast overgrowth
- *Douching:* Changes pH
- *Sexual intercourse:* Raises pH to 7 or higher for 8 hours after coitus
- *Uncontrolled diabetes mellitus:* Increases glucose that promotes organism growth

The normally acidic pH for the vagina is the first line of defense against vaginal infections. Normal vaginal secretions are made up of creamy white epithelial cells and mucus from the cervix, Skene glands, and Bartholin glands. The secretions prevent dryness and infection. Immediately after menstruation the mucus is thin, but as ovulation approaches, the estrogen level increases; at ovulation, the mucus is clear and slippery and can be stretched without breaking (spinnbarkeit) (see Figure 11-2). After ovulation the mucus is cloudy and sticky. At menopause, lowered estrogen causes vaginal dryness, and the pH may change, predisposing the woman to vaginal discomfort and infections. Other factors that can alter the pH of the vagina temporarily include the following:

- Deodorant soap
- Perfumed toilet tissue
- Douching
- Spermicides
- Tampons
- Hot tubs and swimming pools
- Tight clothing made of synthetic fabrics

🏃 Health Promotion

Preventing Vaginal Infections

By promoting vaginal health, nurses can enhance the quality of life for the women they counsel. The promotion of vaginal health includes wearing cotton underwear, avoiding tight-fitting nylon or spandex pants, wiping front to back after toileting, and frequent hand washing. A healthy lifestyle, with a high-fiber, low-fat diet and exercise, strengthens the immune system and can prevent many infections. Douching increases the risk for vaginal infections. Women should not douche or use internal feminine hygiene products without first consulting their health care provider.

GYNECOLOGICAL INFECTIONS

Vaginal infections are the most common reason for women to seek health care. Nurses play a key role in educating women concerning vaginal health and the prevention of sexually transmitted infections. Identifying high-risk behaviors and providing nonjudgmental, sensitive counseling and education should be part of every physical checkup. Safe sex practices, a reduction in the number of partners, and avoiding the exchange of body fluids are part of primary prevention of STIs. Community-based education in schools and churches is also important in primary prevention.

There are three classes of gynecological infections:
1. Toxic shock syndrome
2. Sexually transmitted infections
3. Pelvic inflammatory disease

TOXIC SHOCK SYNDROME

Toxic shock syndrome (TSS) is a rare and potentially fatal disorder. It is caused by strains of *Staphylococcus aureus* that produce toxins that can cause shock, coagulation defects, and tissue damage if they enter the bloodstream. TSS is associated with the trapping of bacteria within the reproductive tract for a prolonged time. Factors that increase the risk of TSS include the use of high-absorbency tampons for prolonged periods of time and the use of a diaphragm or cervical cap for contraception. Signs and symptoms of TSS include the following:

- Sudden spiking fever
- Flulike symptoms
- Hypotension
- Generalized rash that resembles sunburn
- Skin peeling from the palms and soles 1 to 2 weeks after the illness

The incidence of TSS has decreased, but nurses continue to play a role in prevention. The nurse's role is primarily one of education. The following teaching points should be included:

Tampon use:
- Wash hands before and after inserting a tampon.
- Change tampons at least every 4 hours.
- Do not use superabsorbent tampons.
- Use pads rather than tampons when sleeping, because tampons will likely remain in the vagina longer than 4 hours.

Diaphragm or cervical cap use:
- Wash hands before and after inserting the diaphragm or cervical cap.
- Do not use a diaphragm or cervical cap during the menstrual period.
- Remove the diaphragm or cervical cap at the time recommended by the health care provider.

Treatment is supported and includes vasopressor drugs, antimicrobial medication, and fluid replacement.

! **Safety Alert!**

To prevent toxic shock syndrome, the woman should be taught to wash her hands well when using tampons or a diaphragm. The diaphragm should not be used during menstruation. Tampons should be changed every 4 hours and not used during sleep, which usually lasts longer than 4 hours.

SEXUALLY TRANSMITTED INFECTIONS

STIs are those that can be spread by sexual contact, although several of these infections have other modes of transmission as well. It is important that all sexual contacts of the infected person, even those persons who are asymptomatic, be completely treated to eradicate the infection. Table 11-1 provides specific information about STIs that the nurse may encounter. Certain STIs must be reported to the health department.

Nursing care related to STIs primarily focuses on patient education to prevent the spread of these infections, including the following:

- Teaching signs and symptoms that should be reported to the health care provider
- Explaining diagnostic tests
- Teaching measures to prevent the spread of infection, such as the use of condoms
- Explaining treatment measures
- Emphasizing the importance of completing treatment and follow-up and of treating all partners to eliminate the spread of infection

The incidence of STIs has increased during the past few decades. Teaching STI prevention to women across the life span is important, because some viral STIs remain in the body for life and can include long-term complications.

Human papillomavirus (HPV) is the most common viral STI, with more than 100 variations. HPV types 16 and 18 are associated with serious cervical cancer, and women who are immunocompromised are at the greatest risk. The use of condoms may not protect the woman if the male's lesion is on the scrotum or inguinal folds. It may take 3 to 6 months after infection to develop visible warts. Treatment includes cryotherapy, laser vaporization, electrodiathermy, and electrofulguration with a loop electrode excision procedure. Topical agents are used, such as podofilox (Condylox), imiquimod (Aldara), and bichloroacetic acid (BCA). Lidocaine cream may be used 20 minutes before painful treatments. 5-Fluorouracil (5-FU) is no longer used for this condition because of serious side effects. The CDC recommends a 3-dose series of vaccinations for all males and females between the ages of 11 and 26 to prevent the most common strains of HPV.

Herpes simplex virus II (HSV II) is another example of a viral STI that is recurrent and incurable. HSV infection during pregnancy can have serious consequences for the newborn.

Hepatitis B can be sexually transmitted if sexual practices include anal–oral sexual contact, digital rectal sexual intercourse, or multiple sex partners. Symptoms are nonspecific and include malaise, anorexia, nausea, and fatigue. Liver failure can develop. Hepatitis B vaccine can prevent the disease, and immunoglobulin can be administered if known exposure has occurred.

Chlamydia trachomatis is the most common bacterial STI in the United States (Centers for Disease Control and Prevention [CDC], 2008). Treatment tends to be delayed, because infection is often asymptomatic.

Gonorrhea (GC) is the second most common reportable infectious disease in the United States and a major cause of *pelvic inflammatory disease (PID)*. The occurrence of gonorrhea in 2007 declined except for an increase of 1.8% in the black population. Casual sex in the 15- to 19-year-old age group and sex associated with drug use are the highest-risk practices for GC infection (CDC, 2008). Several nucleic acid amplification tests are now available to detect chlamydia, GC, and trichomoniasis with a simple noninvasive urine sample, with results available in a few hours. Fluoroquinolones are no longer recommended for treatment of GC infections (CDC, 2008).

The rate of *syphilis* reached an all-time low in 2000. However, since 2006 the rate has been increasing. Between 2006 and 2007, a 15.2% increase in the diagnosis of syphilis has been noted (CDC, 2008). Untreated syphilis is a risk factor in the spread of *human immunodeficiency virus (HIV)* infection and also leads to central nervous system (CNS), musculoskeletal, and heart complications. Most newborns of mothers infected with syphilis will have congenital syphilis or will die. An external chancre is a characteristic first sign that resolves within 6 weeks without treatment; however, the disease spreads internally. A rash also occurs and resolves, and then the latent period of syphilis occurs and progresses to tertiary syphilis. Aortic aneurysms, dementia, and death can occur.

The number of women infected with HIV worldwide is staggering. Patient education plays a key role in prevention, quality of life, and compassionate and knowledgeable referral. Early diagnosis, access to care, medications, and safe sex practices are improving outcomes and decreasing occurrence. Universal HIV screening at pregnancy is a goal of the National Academy of Sciences Institute of Medicine, because many women in the early stages do not realize they are infected. Education for prevention is essential. Nurses may be less likely to consider the older age group at risk and may miss opportunities for early detection and education for prevention. Sexual contact and intravenous (IV) drug use are the most common risk behaviors for HIV infection.

Prevention of disease is the key role of the nurse. The nurse must develop strategies, use initiatives, and contact adolescents in the community setting, schools, and

Text continued on p. 260

Table 11-1   Sexually Transmitted Infections

INFECTION (CAUSATIVE ORGANISM)	SIGNS AND SYMPTOMS	DIAGNOSIS	PREGNANCY, FETAL, AND NEONATAL EFFECTS	TREATMENT	COMMENTS
Candidiasis (yeast) (*Candida albicans*)	Itching and burning on urination, inflammation of vulva and vagina, "cottage cheese" appearance to discharge	Signs and symptoms; identification of the spores of the causative fungus	Can infect newborn at birth	Miconazole nitrate (Monistat), clotrimazole (Gyne-Lotrimin), nystatin (Mycostatin), fluconazole (Diflucan)	Medications are available over the counter (OTC), but the woman should seek medical attention to diagnose her first infection or if she has persistent or recurrent infections.
Trichomoniasis (*Trichomonas vaginalis*)	Thin, foul-smelling, greenish yellow vaginal discharge, vulvar itching, edema, redness	Identification of the organism under microscope in a wet-mount preparation and rapid antibody test; DNA and PCR testing can be performed now for this organism so that providers are able to prescribe more definitive therapy	Does not cross placenta Can cause postpartum infection	Metronidazole (Flagyl) contraindicated during first trimester; clotrimazole (Gyne-Lotrimin) for symptom relief during first trimester	Organism thrives in an alkaline environment. Most infections are thought to be transmitted by sexual contact.
Bacterial vaginosis (*Gardnerella vaginalis*)	Thin, grayish white discharge that has a fishy odor	Microscopic evidence of clue cells (epithelial cells with bacteria clinging to their surface) and rapid detection tests	Associated with preterm delivery	Bacteria is normal inhabitant of vagina but overgrows Treatment aims to restore normal balance of vaginal bacterial flora Metronidazole (Flagyl) may relieve symptoms	Avoid alcohol during treatment with metronidazole and for 24 hours afterward. Flagyl cannot be used during first trimester of pregnancy.

Continued

Table 11-1   Sexually Transmitted Infections—cont'd

INFECTION (CAUSATIVE ORGANISM)	SIGNS AND SYMPTOMS	DIAGNOSIS	PREGNANCY, FETAL, AND NEONATAL EFFECTS	TREATMENT	COMMENTS
Chlamydia (*Chlamydia trachomatis*)	Yellowish discharge and painful urination Often asymptomatic in women, which delays treatment	Culture, rapid detection tests; DNA probe using urine specimen is noninvasive nucleic acid amplification test (NAAT)	Transmitted via birth canal Causes conjunctivitis and pneumonia in newborn	Azithromycin, doxycycline, erythromycin in pregnancy All newborns have prophylactic eye care	Untreated infection can ascend into fallopian tubes, causing scarring. Infertility or ectopic pregnancy may result. Can spread to neonate's eyes by contact with infected vaginal secretions.
Gonorrhea (*Neisseria gonorrhoeae*)	Purulent discharge, painful urination, dyspareunia	Culture of organism, NAAT	Transmitted to newborn's eyes during birth, causing blindness (ophthalmia neonatorum)	Antibiotics All newborns have prophylactic eye care	Can result in pelvic inflammatory disease with tubal scarring.
Syphilis (*Treponema pallidum*)	Three stages: *Primary:* painless chancre on the genitalia, anus, or lips *Secondary:* 2 months after primary syphilis; enlargement of spleen and liver, headache, anorexia, generalized skin rash, wartlike growths on the vulva *Tertiary:* may occur many years after secondary syphilis and cause heart, blood vessel, nervous system damage	*Primary:* examining material scraped from the chancre with darkfield microscopy to identify the spirochete organism; serological tests are not positive at this early stage *Secondary or tertiary:* serological test (Venereal Disease Research Laboratory [VDRL] [less specific], and rapid plasma reagin (RPR) and fluorescent treponemal antibody absorption [FTA-ABS] [more specific])	Transmitted across placenta Causes congenital syphilis, stillbirth, spontaneous abortion	Penicillin; doxycycline, tetracycline, or erythromycin if allergic Tetracycline is not recommended during pregnancy; desensitization of the woman is recommended	Primary and secondary stages are the most contagious. Spread is through sexual contact, by inoculation (sharing needles), or through the placenta from an infected mother.

Condition	Signs and symptoms	Diagnosis	Effects on pregnancy/neonate	Treatment	Comments
Herpes genitalis (herpes simplex virus [HSV], types I and II) 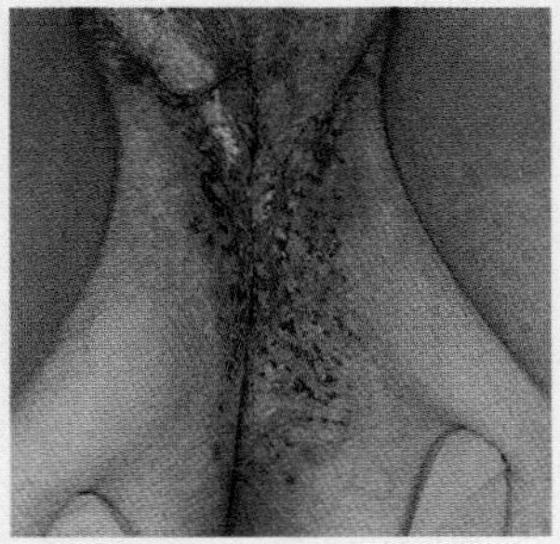	Clusters of painful vesicles (blisters) on the vulva, perineum, and anal areas. Vesicles rupture in 1 to 7 days and heal in 12 days	By signs and symptoms; confirmed by viral culture antibody or DNA-based rapid test	Can cause spontaneous abortion, stillbirth. Active genital infection necessitates cesarean delivery. Causes neonatal central nervous system problems	No cure exists; acyclovir (Zovirax) or valacyclovir (Valtrex) reduces symptoms. Treated with hygiene, sitz baths during pregnancy	HSV II usually causes genital lesions. The first episode is usually the most uncomfortable. The virus "hides" in the nerve cells and can reemerge in later outbreaks that are as contagious as the first.
Condylomata acuminata (human papillomavirus [HPV]) 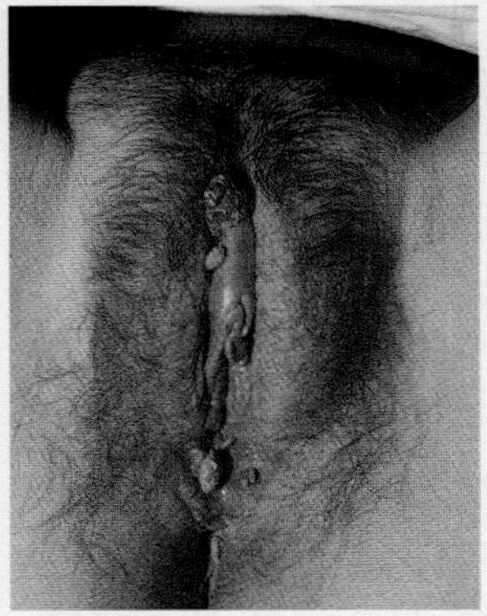	Dry, wartlike growths on vagina, labia, cervix, and perineum	By typical appearance and location	Growth may obstruct birth canal. Infant may have laryngeal papillomas. **The CDC recommends vaccination of all males and females between 11-21 years of age.**	Removal with cryotherapy (cold), electrocautery, laser, or podophyllin applications are alternatives	Also known as venereal or genital warts; associated with higher rates of cervical cancer. Women should have routine HPV and Papanicolaou (Pap) tests.
Acquired immunodeficiency syndrome (AIDS) (human immunodeficiency virus [HIV])	Initially, no symptoms; later symptoms include weight loss, night sweats, fever and chills, fatigue, enlarged lymph nodes, skin rashes, diarrhea. Late symptoms include immune suppression, opportunistic infections, and malignancies	Serology tests: positive enzyme-linked immunosorbent assay (ELISA), followed by positive Western blot test	Prevent breaks in skin of mother and fetus during birth process. Transmitted antepartum to newborn. Drug therapy advised. Infant should be bottle fed	No cure available yet; zidovudine (AZT, Retrovir) and didanosine (Videx) may slow progression. Lamivudine and nelfinavir are administered during pregnancy	Transmitted through contact with nonintact skin or mucous membranes with infectious secretions, exposure to blood, and transmission from mother to fetus. Standard precautions reduce risk for caregivers. Condom use reduces risk for sexual transmission.

(Unnumbered figure 1 from Grimes DE, Grimes RM: *AIDS and HIV infection*, St Louis, 1994; unnumbered figures 2 and 3 from Jarvis C: *Physical examination and health assessment*, ed 3, Philadelphia. 2000, Saunders; unnumbered figure 4 from Callen JP, Greer KE, Paller AS, Swinyer LJ: *Color atlas of dermatology*, ed 2, Philadelphia, 2000, Saunders.)

churches. Teaching all age groups healthy behaviors such as abstinence, safe sex practices, and discussion of STI prevention is essential. Improving access to care and early detection are also important. The CDC offers various free programs that are available through the Internet that can be used by nurses and teachers in the community to teach STI prevention.

PELVIC INFLAMMATORY DISEASE

Pelvic inflammatory disease (PID) is an infection of the upper reproductive tract. Asymptomatic STIs are a common cause of PID. The cervix, uterine cavity, fallopian tubes, and pelvic cavity are often involved. Infertility may be the result.

The woman's symptoms vary according to the area affected. Fever, chronic pelvic pain, abnormal vaginal discharge, nausea and anorexia, and irregular vaginal bleeding are common. When examined, the abdomen and pelvic organs are often very tender. Laboratory tests identify common general signs of infection, such as elevated leukocytes and an elevated sedimentation rate. Cultures of the cervical canal are done to identify the infecting organism, which most commonly are *S. gonorrhoeae* or *C. trachomatis*. Urinalysis is usually done to identify infection of the urinary tract. The pelvic inflammation can result in scarring of the fallopian tubes that can cause blockage and infertility or ectopic pregnancy.

Treatment includes antibiotics and patient education to prevent reinfection. Treatment may be administered on an inpatient or outpatient basis depending on the severity of the infection. Antibiotics are begun promptly to treat the infection. A change in antibiotic(s) is made if culture and sensitivity testing indicates that another antibiotic would be more effective.

Douching results in changes in the vaginal flora and predisposes the woman to the development of PID, bacterial vaginosis, and ectopic pregnancies. However, many women practice regular douching in the belief that it is cleansing. The nurse can play an important role in educating the woman to prevent PID.

FAMILY PLANNING

CONTRACEPTION

Contraception (birth control) may be part of the nurse's responsibility in family-planning clinics, in physician or nurse-midwife practices, or on the postpartum or gynecology units of an acute care hospital. In addition, family members and friends may turn to the nurse as a resource person who can answer their questions about contraception. The nurse can play a part in helping couples choose and correctly use contraceptive methods that enable them to have children who are both wanted and well timed. The nurse's role in family planning includes the following:

- Answering general questions about contraceptive methods
- Explaining different methods that are available, including accurate information about their advantages and disadvantages
- Teaching the correct use of the method or methods of contraception that the patient chooses

A couple's choice of contraception often changes as needs change. Factors that influence the choice of a contraceptive include the following:

- Age
- Health status, including risk for STI
- Religion
- Culture
- Impact of an unplanned pregnancy on the woman or family
- Desire for children in the future
- Frequency of intercourse
- Convenience and degree of spontaneity that is important to the couple
- Expense
- Degree of comfort the partners have with touching their bodies
- Number of sexual partners

Contraception does not always prevent pregnancy. An important consideration for patients is how likely the method is to fail. A contraceptive technique may fail because the method is ineffective, or the user is using the method inappropriately. The following two *Healthy People 2020* (USDHHS, 2010) goals are relevant to the provision of family-planning services:

- Reduce the percentage of unintended pregnancies to no more than 30%.
- Reduce the percentage of women who have an unintended pregnancy despite the use of a contraceptive method to no more than 7%.

NATURAL FAMILY PLANNING

Natural family planning, also called fertility awareness, involves learning to identify the signs and symptoms associated with ovulation. The couple either abstains from intercourse or uses a barrier method during the period that is presumed to be fertile. The ovum is viable up to 24 hours after ovulation, and sperm are viable for 48 to 72 hours in the fallopian tube, although most die within 24 hours.

Natural family planning methods are acceptable to most religions. They require no administration of systemic hormones or insertion of devices. They are not only reversible but also can actually be used to increase the odds of achieving pregnancy when the couple desires a child.

Natural family planning requires extensive assessment and charting of all the changes in the menstrual cycle. The woman must be highly motivated to track the many factors that identify ovulation. Both partners must be willing to abstain from intercourse for much of the woman's cycle if the method is used to prevent

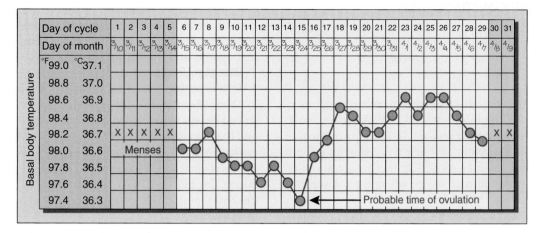

FIGURE 11-1 Basal body temperature chart. By taking and recording her temperature, the woman can determine the probable time of ovulation.

pregnancy. They must also be willing to accept the relatively high failure rate of 20%. Most women use a combination of the following four methods for predicting when they are fertile to increase the predictive value over that of each method on its own.

Basal Body Temperature

The basal body temperature (BBT) is taken on awakening and before any activity (Figure 11-1). This technique is based on the fact that the basal temperature rises very slightly at ovulation (about 0.2° C [0.4° F]) and remains higher in the last half of the cycle. Unfortunately, BBT is better at identifying that ovulation has *already* occurred rather than predicting when it is *about* to occur. The most important time point to identify in attempting conception or contraception is *the day before* ovulation, rather than the day of ovulation (Fehring, 2008).

A *basal thermometer* is calibrated in tenths of a degree or uses an electronic digital format to detect these tiny changes. The woman charts each day's temperature to identify her temperature pattern. A rise in the BBT for the last 14 days of the cycle means that ovulation has probably occurred. Some electronic models have a memory to retain each day's temperature, and they display the pattern on a small screen.

Many factors can interfere with the accuracy of the BBT in predicting ovulation. Poor sleep, illness, jet lag, sleeping late, alcohol intake the evening before, or sleeping under an electric blanket or on a heated waterbed can make the BBT unreliable.

Cervical Mucus

The cervical mucus method of predicting ovulation is also called the *Billings method*. The character and amount of cervical mucus changes during the menstrual cycle, because estrogen and progesterone influence the mucus-secreting glands of the cervix. Immediately after menstruation, the cervical mucus is sticky, thick, and white. As ovulation nears, the mucus increases and becomes thin, slippery, and clear to aid

the passage of sperm into the cervix. The slippery mucus can be stretched 6 cm or more and has the consistency of egg white (Figure 11-2). The stretching characteristic of the mucus is called **spinnbarkeit**. After ovulation the mucus again becomes thicker. Factors that interfere with the accuracy of cervical mucus assessment include the use of antihistamines, vaginal infections, contraceptive foams or jellies, sexual arousal, and recent coitus. The noticeable changes in vaginal mucus before ovulation can aid in natural family planning and fertility awareness (Speroff, 2011).

Calendar, or Rhythm, Method

The woman charts her menstrual cycles on a calendar for several months. If the cycles are regular, she may be able to predict ovulation. The rhythm method is based on the fact that ovulation usually occurs about 14 days *before* the subsequent menstrual period. This would be about halfway through a 28-day cycle, but would be on day 16 of a 30-day cycle.

Marquette Method

The Marquette method of natural family planning incorporates the use of an electronic hormonal fertility monitor that tracks the changing levels of a urinary metabolite of estrogen and luteinizing hormone (LH). The method can be used in combination with other traditional methods such as BBT and cervical mucus to identify a 6-day fertile window that can be used to plan or help prevent pregnancy (Fehring, 2008).

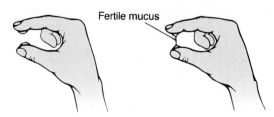

FIGURE 11-2 Spinnbarkeit. The woman tests the capacity of her cervical mucus to stretch. This helps to determine the time of ovulation.

TEMPORARY CONTRACEPTION

Reversible contraception is defined as the temporary prevention of fertility.

Abstinence

Abstinence is 100% effective in preventing pregnancy and STIs, including infection with HIV; however, most couples believe that their sexual relationship adds to the quality of life. Therefore abstinence is rarely an option the couple will consider. Most religious groups support abstinence among unmarried people and adolescents.

Hormonal Contraceptives

Hormonal contraceptives include one or more of the following contraceptive effects:

- Prevent ovulation
- Make the cervical mucus thick and resistant to sperm penetration
- Make the uterine endometrium less hospitable if a fertilized ovum does arrive
- Hormonal contraceptives do not protect either partner from STIs, including HIV infection.

Oral Contraceptives ("The Pill"). Oral contraceptives (OCs) are a popular, highly effective, and reversible method of birth control (Figure 11-3). They contain either combined hormones (estrogen and progestin) or progestin alone ("minipill"). Progestin-only contraceptives should be avoided for postpartum Hispanic women with gestational diabetes who are breastfeeding because of an increased risk of later development of type 2 diabetes (Gabbe, 2012). Combined hormones can be taken about 3 weeks after delivery, although progestin-only pills have a positive effect on lactation (Gabbe, 2012).

Oral contraceptives require a prescription. The woman's history is obtained, and she will have a physical examination, including breast and pelvic examinations and a Pap test. She should have a yearly physical examination, Pap test, breast examination, and blood pressure check. See Treatment Options on p. 274 regarding the use of oral contraceptives for treating menopause and menstrual irregularities.

Dosage regimens

Monthly contraception. Combination OCs are available in 21- or 28-pill packs. If the woman has a 21-pill pack, she takes one pill each day at the same time for 21 days, and then stops for 7 days. The woman who has a 28-day pack takes a pill each day; the last seven pills of the pack are inert (inactive) but help her maintain the habit of taking the pill each day. Menstruation occurs during the 7-day period when either no pills or inert pills are ingested.

Some pills are multiphasic in that their estrogen and progestin content changes during the cycle to mimic natural hormonal activity. If the woman takes multiphasic pills, it is very important that she take each pill in order. Taking the pills at the same time each day is important, regardless of the type of OC, to maintain a stable blood level of the hormones.

It is most important that the medication-free interval not be extended beyond 7 days. Taking the first pill of the cycle on time is most critical in preventing accidental pregnancies.

Extended-dose contraception. Extended-dose contraception is also known as *induced amenorrhea*. Research has shown that there are no specific health benefits to monthly menstruation (Fontenot, 2008). Ethinyl-estradiol and norethindrone (Loestrin 24 Fe) contains 24 days of active hormone and 4 days of ferrous fumarate tablets instead of placebo pills. Ethinyl-estradiol and levonorgestrel 30/150 (Seasonale) is an extended-cycle oral contraceptive. The woman takes the active hormone for 84 days and then the hormone-free placebo for 7 days, resulting in a menstrual period once every 3 months. There has been no noted evidence of adverse effects with the extended-dose regimen, and its failure rate is 0.9% compared to 1.3% with conventional (monthly) administration (Fontenot and Harris, 2008). Levonorgestrel and ethinyl-estradiol 90/20 (Lybrel), a continuous low-dose OC, was approved by the U.S. Food and Drug Administration (FDA) in 2007 and extends the menstrual cycle to once a year. There are no planned withdrawal bleeds, but some women report spotting or breakthrough bleeding about 3 days/month when they start the regime (Speroff, 2011).

Benefits. OCs have a failure rate of 9% for combined pills and 9% for minipills. They reduce the risk for ovarian and endometrial cancer. Their effect on the risk for breast and cervical cancer risks is not yet definitively established. Women tend to have less cramping and lighter periods (and therefore less anemia) when taking OCs. OCs may improve premenstrual symptoms for some women. In some formulations, iron and folic acid supplementation has been added to the OC pill.

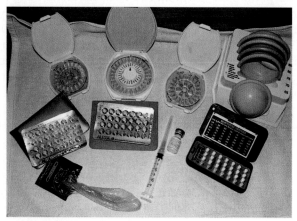

FIGURE 11-3 Contraceptives. This photo shows common types of contraceptives: condoms, diaphragms, oral contraceptives, transdermal patch, and parenteral contraceptives.

Side effects and contraindications. Common side effects of OCs include nausea, headache, breast tenderness, weight gain, and spotting between periods or amenorrhea. These effects generally decrease within a few months and are seen less frequently with low-dose OCs.

Women with the following disorders should not take OCs or should take them with caution:

- Thromboembolic disorders (blood clots)
- Cerebrovascular accident or heart disease
- Estrogen-dependent cancer or breast cancer
- A smoking pattern of more than 15 cigarettes a day for women older than 35 years (the pill is safe for women older than 35 years if they do not smoke)
- Impaired liver function
- A confirmed or possible pregnancy
- Undiagnosed vaginal bleeding

> **⚠ Safety Alert!**
>
> Smoking increases the chance of experiencing complications related to oral contraceptives, particularly in women older than 35 years.

The first episode of menstrual bleeding after an abortion is usually preceded by ovulation, and therefore contraception should begin immediately to prevent pregnancy. However, after a term delivery there is a high risk of thromboembolism; therefore, the contraceptive is usually started 3 to 4 weeks postpartum.

The use of combination OCs also may decrease breast milk production, and OC use is therefore contraindicated in the breastfeeding woman until lactation is well established. Women, who breastfeed at least 10 times per day, usually do not ovulate for 10 weeks postpartum, but breastfeeding is *not* a reliable method of contraception. Progestin-only OCs (minipill) may be used until menstruation returns in women who breastfeed regularly.

Extended-dose oral contraceptives have been used successfully to minimize the bloating, fluid retention, and symptoms of PMDD usually associated with oral contraceptives. Serum potassium levels should be monitored for women who take this medication with other medications known to increase serum potassium levels.

> **💡 Memory Jogger**
>
> The acronym *ACHES* can help a woman recall the warning signs to report when taking OCs:
> - **A**bdominal pain (severe)
> - **C**hest pain, dyspnea, bloody sputum
> - **H**eadache (severe), weakness, or numbness of the extremities
> - **E**ye problems (blurring, double vision, vision loss)
> - **S**evere leg pain or swelling, speech disturbance

Some medications decrease the effectiveness of OCs, including the following:

- Some antibiotics, such as ampicillin and tetracycline
- Anticonvulsants
- Rifampin, barbiturates

Nursing care. The woman needs thorough teaching if the pill is to be a satisfactory contraceptive for her. Teaching should be done in her own language and should be supplemented by generous written materials if she can read. Teaching points should include the following:

- How to take the specific drug
- What to do if a dose is missed or if she decides to stop using it and does not want to become pregnant
- Common side effects and signs and symptoms that should be promptly reported
- Backup contraceptive methods, such as barrier methods (discussed later in this chapter)
- Supplemental barrier methods of contraception to use, in addition to OCs, that also reduce the risk of STIs (including HIV infection)

> **🔲 Nursing Tip**
>
> The more birth control pills a woman misses, the greater her risk that pregnancy will occur.

Hormone Implants. Etonogestrel implant (Implanon), approved by the FDA in 2006, is a single-rod system that involves the placement of one implant under the skin of the upper, nondominant arm, which provides contraception for 3 years and does not affect bone mineral density (Fontenot, 2008). Implanon can be used during lactation, and when it is discontinued, the woman will have a rapid return to fertility. Intradermal implants can be removed in the outpatient clinic with the use of a local anesthetic. The typical failure rate is 0.05%

Medroxyprogesterone acetate (Depo-SubQ Provera 104). Medroxyprogesterone acetate (Depo-SubQ Provera 104) is an injectable form of slow-release progestin. Its contraceptive action is similar to that of the minipill and hormone implant. It provides 3 months of highly effective contraception; therefore, it must be administered every 3 months. Fertility returns about 1 year after stopping the medication (Hacker, 2011).

The injection is given subcutaneously within 5 days of the menstrual period. If administered later than 5 days after the menstrual period, the woman should use another form of contraception as well, because ovulation may have already occurred. The breastfeeding woman usually starts hormone injections 6 weeks after birth, and the nonlactating woman may start 5 days after delivery. Depo-SubQ Provera 104 may result in decreased bone density and is not recommended for long-term use by teens; however, the decreased bone density is reversible (Fontenot, 2008).

Side effects and contraindications. The side effects and contraindications of hormone injections are similar to those of OCs and hormone implants. Menstrual irregularities, breakthrough bleeding, and amenorrhea are common complaints and are often the reason that women stop taking the drug. There is no STI protection with this method. The typical failure rate is 6%.

Nursing care. The woman should be taught about the side effects and problems to report. It should be emphasized that she must return for continued injections if she wants to maintain a constant hormone level, thus preventing pregnancy. A backup contraceptive method should be taught for use if she decides to stop the injections or is delayed in returning for subsequent injections. Women with seizure disorders can use this method of contraception without fear of interaction with their antiseizure medication. Women with coagulation problems or with sickle cell anemia benefit from this type of contraception, which suppresses ovulation and reduces blood loss (Fontenot, 2008).

Intrauterine Devices. An intrauterine device (IUD) is a reversible method of birth control that requires a prescription and a health care provider to insert it. They are effective (98% or greater) and reversible, and no specific actions are required related to intercourse. The ParaGard is a small, T-shaped, copper-containing plastic device that is effective for 10 years. Other devices, such as Mirena, carry a sleeve on one segment that contains a reservoir of progestin or levonorgestrel that is diffused into the uterus each day. The action is local in the uterine cavity, and blood levels do not increase. The levonorgestrel type of IUD (LNG-IUS) must be replaced every 5 years. The LNG-IUS is also used to control menorrhagia. The main mechanism of contraceptive action of a copper IUD is the production of a hostile environment for the sperm that impedes sperm transport and viability in the cervical mucus and within the uterus. On removal of the IUD, fertility rapidly returns. The IUD does not protect against STIs.

Side effects and contraindications. Cramping and bleeding are likely to occur with insertion. Insertion should not be attempted during menses. Increased menstruation and dysmenorrhea may occur, and these are common reasons that a woman decides to have the IUD removed. The woman who has heavier periods may need iron supplementation.

Nursing care. The woman is taught about side effects and how to take iron supplements if they are prescribed. The woman will need to feel for the fine plastic strings (tail) that protrude from the vagina and are connected to the IUD to verify that it is in place. She should check the tail weekly for the first 4 weeks after insertion, then monthly. The woman is taught to report if she cannot feel the tail that protrudes into the vagina, or if it is longer or shorter than previously. The nurse can teach her the signs of infection (fever, pain, change in vaginal discharge) and the signs of ectopic pregnancy (see Chapter 5) that should be reported promptly.

! Safety Alert!

Only women who have no current pelvic infection and who are in a relationship that is monogamous for both partners should use an intrauterine device.

Transdermal Patch. Ortho-Evra is a transdermal adhesive patch containing hormones (norelgestromin/ethinyl-estradiol) that is applied to the skin once a week for 3 weeks, followed by a 1-week patch-free interval to allow for menstruation to occur. The patch provides safe and effective contraception similar to oral contraceptives for women weighing less than 198 pounds. Studies concerning the effects on the health of the woman and the development of nonestrogen patches are ongoing (Ortho-McNeil-Janssen, 2009; Skopp, 2009). The FDA warns that counterfeit contraceptive patches, which may provide little or no protection against pregnancy, have been sold on foreign websites.

Vaginal Ring. A flexible, one-size vaginal ring (Nuva-Ring) that releases estrogen and progestin locally instead of systemically has been approved for contraceptive use in the United States. The ring is worn in the vagina for 3 weeks and is removed for 1 week to allow for withdrawal bleeding (Hacker, 2011). The typical use failure rate is 9%.

Barrier Methods

Barrier methods work by blocking the entrance of semen into the woman's cervix. **Spermicides** (sperm-killing chemicals) play a part in some of these methods. They help the woman avoid the use of systemic hormones. Some barrier methods offer some protection against STIs by providing a barrier to contact.

Some barrier methods must be applied just before intercourse (condoms, spermicidal foams, and suppositories), whereas others can be inserted several hours earlier (diaphragm, cervical cap). Spermicidal foams and suppositories are messy and may drip from the vagina. These methods are not suitable for people who are uncomfortable with touching their bodies. They are often used as a backup method for contraception.

Barrier methods are inexpensive per use. The diaphragm and cervical cap require a fitting and prescription, which adds to their initial cost. Other barrier methods are over-the-counter purchases. These methods are often chosen as backup methods or when the woman is lactating, or if she cannot tolerate OCs or an IUD.

Diaphragm and Cervical Cap. Diaphragms and cervical caps are rubber domes that fit over the cervix and are used with spermicides to kill sperm that pass the mechanical barrier (Skill 11-2). A health care provider fits the diaphragm and cervical cap. The woman must learn how to insert and remove the diaphragm or cervical cap and to verify proper placement. User misplacement, especially of the small cervical cap, is a common reason for unintended pregnancy. The typical failure rate is 12%.

How to Use a Diaphragm

PURPOSE

To learn to use a diaphragm for contraception

NOTE: A diaphragm can be inserted up to 4 hours before intercourse. Insertion and removal skills increase with practice.

STEPS

1. Apply spermicidal cream or gel inside at center and around the rim of the diaphragm. This aids the insertion and offers a more complete seal.

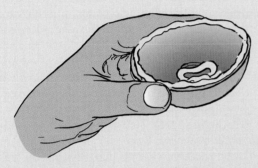

2. Hold diaphragm between your thumb and finger and compress diaphragm. Use fingers of other hand to spread the labia (lips of the vagina).
3. Begin to insert diaphragm into vagina with spermicide toward the cervix. Squatting or placing one foot on a chair makes insertion (and removal) easier.
4. Insert diaphragm into vagina. Direct it inward and downward behind and below the cervix.

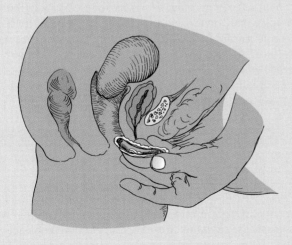

5. Tuck the front of the rim of diaphragm behind the pubic bone.

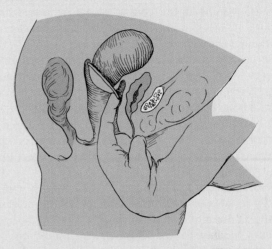

6. Feel your cervix through the center of the diaphragm.
7. Leave diaphragm in place at least 6 hours after intercourse.
8. To remove diaphragm, assume squatting position and bear down. Hook a finger over the top rim to break suction, and pull diaphragm down and out.

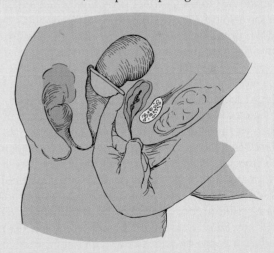

9. Wash diaphragm with mild soap and dry well after each use.
10. Dust diaphragm with cornstarch. Scented talc or baby powder can weaken the rubber.
11. Inspect it occasionally for small holes by holding it up to light.

Before insertion, the woman should check either device for weak spots or pinholes by holding it up to the light. Spermicidal jelly or cream is applied to the ring and the center of the diaphragm before inserting it and positioning it over the cervix. It may be inserted several hours before intercourse, and it should remain in place for at least 6 hours after intercourse, but not more than 24 hours to prevent pressure on local tissue. More spermicidal jelly or cream must be inserted into the vagina if the couple repeats coitus within 6 hours. The diaphragm must be refitted after each birth or after a weight change of 10 pounds or more. The cap must be refitted yearly and after birth, abortion, or surgery.

The *FemCAP* is a latex-free cap that fits over the cervix and must be fitted, prescribed, and initially inserted by a health care provider. Spermicide can be added to the dome of the cap. *Lea's shield*, a silicone reusable shield, is used with a spermicide and has been FDA approved since 2002.

Side effects and contraindications. Women who have an allergy to latex or spermicides are not good candidates for the diaphragm or cervical cap. Pressure on the bladder may increase the risk of urinary tract infection.

Nursing care. The health care provider who fits the device will provide much of the teaching on insertion, verification of placement, and removal. The nurse often reinforces the teaching, especially about the use and reapplication of spermicide for repeat intercourse. The nurse should teach the woman about signs of uterine infection (pain, foul-smelling drainage, or fever) and of sensitivity to the product (irritation or itching). The woman also should be taught to report signs and symptoms of urinary tract infection: fever, pain, or burning with urination, urgency, or urinary frequency.

Male Condom. Male condoms are sheaths of thin latex, polyurethane, or natural membrane ("skins") worn on the penis during intercourse. Condoms collect semen before, during, and after ejaculation. They come in various styles, such as ribbed, lubricated, and colored, and with or without spermicide. They are single-use, low-cost items that are widely available from vending machines, drugstores, and family-planning clinics. Latex condoms provide some protection from STIs, including HIV. Natural membrane condoms do not prevent the passage of viruses, including HIV. See Skill 11-3 for the correct use of the condom.

To prevent condom breakage, water-soluble lubricants should be used if the condom or vagina is dry. Unlike other, oil-based lubricants, water-soluble lubricants do not damage the latex or cause breakage. The penis should be withdrawn from the vagina immediately if the man feels that the condom is breaking or is becoming dislodged. The condom is removed and a new one is applied. Condoms are not reused, because even a pinhole can lead to pregnancy or permit the entry of viruses, including HIV. The condom package should be checked for expiration date.

The nurse should educate patients to prevent common condom mistakes, including the following:
- Allowing the penis to lose erection while still in the vagina
- Opening the condom package with the teeth or a sharp object, which can tear the condom
- Unrolling the condom before applying it to the penis
- Using out-of-date condoms (condoms with spermicide last for 2 years; others last for 5 years)
- Using baby oil, cold cream, vegetable oil, or petroleum jelly to lubricate the condom
- Reusing the condom
- Storing condoms in the wallet (heat destroys spermicide)
- Not leaving space between the tip of the penis and the condom to provide a reservoir for ejaculate

Side effects and contraindications. Side effects of and contraindications to condom use are rare. Either of the partners may be allergic to latex, in which case a polyurethane condom can often be used successfully. The failure rate for condoms is 18%.

Female Condom. Female condoms are essentially used for the same purpose as male condoms—to prevent pregnancy and to protect the woman from HIV and other STIs (Figure 11-4). Two styles of female condoms are currently available:
1. Two flexible rings, one that fits into the vagina and one that remains outside, connected by a polyurethane sheath
2. A bikini-panty style that has a pouch that fits inside the vagina and can be inserted up to 8 hours before intercourse.

In 2005, a latex-free nitrile condom was introduced with a soft sponge rather than a firm ring to hold it in place (Kaplan, 2008a).

Female condoms are prelubricated, single-use items that are available over the counter. They allow the woman control over her exposure to infections without having to rely on the cooperation of her partner. Its failure rate in pregnancy prevention is 5%. Many women find it unattractive.

Side effects and contraindications. There are few problems with the use of the female condom. The typical failure rate is 21%.

 Nursing Tip

Adolescents must be educated about contraception, reproductive health, and the dangers of unprotected sex.

Spermicides. Spermicidal foam, cream, jelly, film, and suppository capsules are over-the-counter contraceptives. They are inserted into the vagina before intercourse to neutralize vaginal secretions, destroy sperm, and block entrance to the uterus. Each product has specific directions for use. Vaginal films and suppositories must melt before they are effective, which takes about 15 minutes. Most spermicides are effective

How to Use the Male Condom

PURPOSE

To learn to use a condom for contraception

STEPS

1. Use a new condom each time you have intercourse.
2. Check the expiration date on packages, because condoms deteriorate over time.
3. Apply the condom before you have any contact with the woman's vagina, because there are sperm in the secretions before you ejaculate.
4. Squeeze the air from the tip when placing the condom over the end of your penis. Leave a half-inch of space at the tip to allow sperm to collect and to prevent breakage.

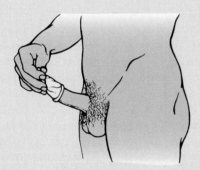

5. Hold the tip while you unroll the condom over the erect penis.

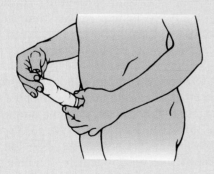

6. Do not use petroleum jelly, grease, or oil as lubricants because they can cause the condom to burst. Instead, use a water-soluble lubricant such as K-Y Jelly.
7. Hold on to the condom at the base of the penis to prevent spillage as you withdraw from the vagina.

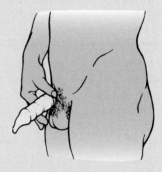

8. Remove the condom carefully to be sure that no semen spills from it.
9. Place the condom in the trash or in some safe disposal.

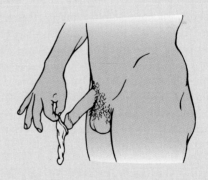

for no more than 1 hour. Reapplication is needed for repeated coitus. The woman should not douche for at least 6 to 8 hours after intercourse.

Adolescents often choose this type of contraception, because it is inexpensive and easy to obtain. Teenagers should be taught that products labeled "for personal hygiene use" do not have contraceptive action. Spermicides have an actual failure rate of 21%. The use of a condom with the spermicide increases the contraceptive effectiveness.

Side effects and contraindications. Spermicides can cause local irritation in the vagina or on the penis. The irritation can cause tiny cracks that provide portals of entry for infection, including HIV.

EMERGENCY CONTRACEPTION

The "morning after" pill is a method of preventing pregnancy after unprotected sexual intercourse. It can be used if contraceptives fail (such as a condom that tears), in cases of rape, or in other situations as needed.

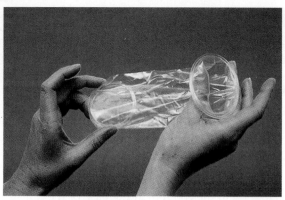

FIGURE 11-4 Female condom. (From Grimes DE, Grimes RM: *AIDS and HIV infection*, St Louis, 1994, Mosby.)

The one-step emergency contraception Plan B contains the progestin levonorgestrel in a one-dose pill "morning after" regime that is available in pharmacies without a prescription. It is most effective if used within 72 hours of unprotected intercourse, but may be effective if used within 120 hours after unprotected sexual intercourse. The one-step emergency contraceptive plan may not be effective in women weighing over 165 pounds.

Legislation was passed in 2013 to remove age restrictions to over-the-counter access of levonorgestrel-containing emergency contraceptives Plan B and Plan B One-Step. The AAP, ACOG, and Planned Parenthood organizations were in favor of this legislation. Emergency contraceptives using medicines containing estrogen were not as well tolerated, and estrogen is known to increase cardiovascular risk; therefore, the Plan B progestin-only package is in use today (Hatcher, 2011).

An emergency contraceptive, uliprisal acetate (Ella), has been approved by the FDA and requires a prescription. It prevents pregnancy by prolonging ovulation and can be taken within 5 days of unprotected sex. The woman should be referred for counseling and follow-up care after use of the emergency contraceptive. Information can be obtained by accessing www.not-2-late.com.

UNRELIABLE CONTRACEPTIVE METHODS

Withdrawal
Withdrawal, or **coitus interruptus**, is withdrawal of the penis before ejaculation. It demands more self-control than most men can achieve. Preejaculatory secretions often contain sperm that can fertilize an ovum.

Douching
Douching after intercourse is not a form of birth control and may actually transport sperm farther into the birth canal.

Breastfeeding
Breastfeeding inhibits ovulation in many women as long as the infant receives at least 10 feedings in 24 hours, because the prolactin secreted to stimulate milk production also inhibits ovulation. If the woman supplements with formula, or when the infant begins taking solids, milk intake (and thus prolactin secretion) falls. Ovulation is then likely, and pregnancy can occur. Remember that ovulation precedes menstruation—pregnancy can occur before the first menstrual period after birth.

 Nursing Tip

A woman can become pregnant while breastfeeding.

PERMANENT CONTRACEPTION

Sterilization
Sterilization is a permanent method of birth control that is almost 100% effective in preventing pregnancy. Although the procedures may be reversed in some cases, reversal is expensive and not always successful. Therefore patients should think carefully about this decision and should consider it permanent.

Advantages. The advantages of sterilization relate to the fact that the person can consider the risk of pregnancy to be near zero. Minimal anxiety about becoming pregnant may help the individual to enjoy the sexual relationship more.

Disadvantages. A major disadvantage of sterilization is the same as its primary advantage: permanence. Divorce, marriage, death of a child, or a change in attitude toward having children may make the person regret his or her decision. The procedures require surgery, and, although the risks are small, they are the same as for other surgical procedures: hemorrhage, infection, injury to other organs, and anesthesia complications.

Male Sterilization. Male sterilization, or *vasectomy*, is performed by making a cut in each side of the scrotum and cutting each vas deferens, the tube through which the sperm travel (Figure 11-5, *A*). Because sperm are already present in the system distal to the area of ligation, sterility is not immediate. Another method of birth control must be implemented until all sperm have left the system, usually about 1 to 3 months. The man should return to his physician for analysis of his semen to verify that it no longer contains sperm. Many men need information about the anatomy and physiology of their sex organs. They need reassurance that they will still have erections and ejaculations and that intercourse will remain pleasurable.

The surgery takes about 20 minutes and is performed on an outpatient basis with a local anesthetic. There is some pain, bruising, and swelling after the surgery. Rest, a mild analgesic, and the application of an

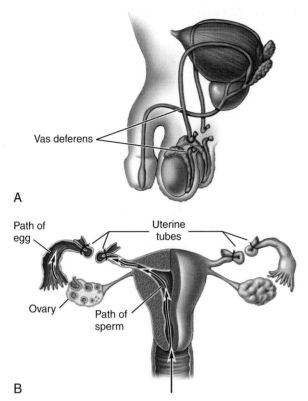

A

B

FIGURE 11-5 Surgical methods of birth control. **A,** Vasectomy, the cutting and ligation (tying off) of the vas deferens. **B,** Tubal ligation, the ligation of the fallopian tubes. (From Herlihy B: *The human body in health and illness*, ed 5, St Louis, 2014, Saunders.)

ice pack are comfort measures. As in other surgeries, the man should report the following:

- Bleeding or substantial bruising
- Separation of the suture line, drainage, or increasing pain

Female Sterilization

Tubal ligation. Tubal ligation involves blocking or ligating the fallopian tubes. This can be accomplished by using electrocautery or clips. Tubal ligation is easy to perform during the immediate postpartum period, because the fundus, to which the tubes are attached, is large and near the surface. Three methods may be used:

1. A *minilaparotomy*, nicknamed "Band-Aid surgery," uses an incision near the umbilicus in the immediate postpartum period or just above the symphysis pubis at other times. The surgeon makes a tiny incision, brings each tube through it, and ligates and cuts the tube.
2. *Laparoscopic surgery* is similar, but the tubes are identified and ligated through a lighted tube called a laparoscope (Figure 11-5, *B*).
3. The traditional approach is performed during other abdominal surgery, usually a cesarean birth.

The discomfort after the minilaparotomy or laparoscopy is usually easily relieved with oral analgesia. Some

women experience nausea from the anesthesia. Even though this is not considered major surgery, the woman requires 1 or 2 days to recuperate. She should report signs of bleeding or infection, as with the male vasectomy.

Hysteroscopic sterilization. A hysteroscope can be placed through the vagina into the cervix. Saline distends the uterus and an Essure microinsert is placed into the fallopian tubes. A benign inflammation occurs that results in permanent closure of the fallopian tubes within 3 months. This type of procedure helps the woman avoid hospitalization, anesthesia, and abdominal scarring. Contraceptives must be used for 3 months until tubal fibrosis occurs. A hysterosalpingogram can confirm closure of the tubes (Hatcher, 2011).

> **Nursing Tip**
>
> When discussing sexual issues with a couple, the nurse should use the word partner until the couple indicates a preference for an alternative term.

INFERTILITY

Infertility is the inability to conceive when desired. The strict definition of infertility is that a couple who has regular, unprotected sexual intercourse for 1 year cannot conceive. Infertility is primary if conception has never occurred and secondary when there have been one or more pregnancies before the infertility. The definition is usually expanded to couples that conceive but repeatedly lose a pregnancy.

More couples are seeking help for infertility for many reasons, including the following:

- Couples are delaying childbearing until their mid- to late 30s, when a natural decline in fertility occurs.
- New treatments may cause couples to reconsider their acceptance of childlessness and initiate or resume infertility therapy.

SOCIAL AND PSYCHOLOGICAL IMPLICATIONS

The role of parent is one that most people expect to assume at some time in their lives. Because parenting is such an expected and common part of society, infertility has implications that go far beyond the physical.

Assumption of Fertility

Most couples assume they are fertile and work hard to prevent pregnancy as they pursue educational or career goals. When they do decide to have a child, couples expect to conceive in a few months at the most. They enjoy being with parents and expectant parents and often begin making preparations for living space and supplies that an infant will need. As months pass and the woman's period comes each month, the couple becomes less certain that they will become parents themselves. Once-joyful occasions, such as baby showers, become melancholy or anxiety-provoking events. The potential grandparents may think their children are waiting too long to start a family or may even believe they are selfish, if they do not realize that the younger couple is trying to conceive.

Psychological Reactions

Shock. Shock is often a couple's first reaction to infertility. Their reactions vary based on how easily the infertility is alleviated and based on their personalities, their self-images, and their relationship.

Guilt. The partner who has the identified problem may feel guilty, believing that he or she is depriving the other one of children. Either partner may regret past choices that now affect fertility, such as sexual practices that resulted in infections that scarred the fallopian tubes.

> **Nursing Tip**
>
> Avoid using the word *fault* when discussing the situation with the member of the infertile couple who has the identified problem. Although a problem may be identified in only one person, many unknown factors affect fertility.

Isolation. Infertile couples often feel different from those who have no problem conceiving. They may isolate themselves from these people to avoid emotional pain. In doing so, they may also isolate themselves from sources of support.

Depression. Infertility challenges one's sense of control and self-image. The couple may experience a roller coaster of hope alternating with despair as the woman has her period each month. They may become judgmental and angry with others.

Stress on the Relationship. Either or both partners may feel unlovable, because their self-esteem has been shaken. A man often finds it difficult to perform sexually "on demand" for semen specimens or at specific times each month. Their sexual relationship may take on a clinical air rather than one of love and support.

Cultural and Religious Considerations

In many cultures, fertility (or the lack thereof) is considered strictly a female problem. It may be closely linked to the woman's social status. The stigma of infertility can lead to divorce and rejection from family and society. To choose treatment for infertility may go against the couple's societal norms, particularly if the male must be treated to achieve pregnancy in the woman.

Religious norms influence what tests and treatments a couple is willing to pursue. Surrogate parenting, in vitro fertilization, or other techniques may not be acceptable in terms of the couple's personal or religious beliefs. Conflict can arise if a potentially successful therapy is acceptable to one member of the couple but not to the other.

FACTORS AFFECTING INFERTILITY

Many factors that cause infertility are unknown. Some couples may have a problem that makes it unlikely that they would conceive; yet they have several children. Others have no identified problem but still cannot conceive.

Male Factors

Abnormal Sperm. To produce a pregnancy, the man must deposit a sufficient number of normal sperm near the cervix, and the sperm must be protected from the acidic vaginal secretions until they enter the cervix. The sperm must be able to swim purposefully to the waiting ovum. A man may have a sperm count that is too low to achieve fertilization. He may have a sufficient number of sperm, but too many of these are weak or abnormally formed. Sperm are continuously formed, and many factors can affect their formation. Some factors that can interfere with normal sperm formation and function include the following:

- High scrotal temperature from hot tubs, saunas, or fever
- Abnormal hormone stimulation
- Infections
- Anatomic abnormalities such as a varicocele (enlarged veins in the testicles)
- Medications, illicit drugs, excessive alcohol intake
- Exposure to toxins

Abnormal Erections. Anything that impairs nervous system function or blood flow to the penis can interfere with erections. Some drugs, notably antihypertensives, reduce or shorten the duration of erections.

Abnormal Ejaculation. Some drugs and nervous system disorders may cause **retrograde ejaculation**, in which semen is released into the bladder rather than from the penis. *Hypospadias* (urethral opening on the underside of the penis rather than the tip) causes semen to be deposited closer to the vaginal outlet rather than near the cervix.

Abnormal Seminal Fluid. Seminal fluid carries the sperm into the vagina, but only sperm enter the cervix to fertilize the ovum. Semen coagulates immediately after ejaculation, and then liquefies within 30 minutes to allow sperm to swim toward the cervix. Sperm will be trapped or will not survive if the seminal fluid remains thick or if its composition does not protect the sperm from the vaginal secretions.

Female Factors

A woman's fertility depends on regular production of normal ova, having an open path from the ovary to the uterus, and having a uterine endometrium that supports the pregnancy.

Disorders of Ovulation. Normal ovulation depends on a balanced and precisely timed interaction between the hypothalamus, the pituitary, and the ovary (see Chapter 2). If the hypothalamus and/or pituitary do not properly stimulate the ovary, ovulation will not occur. Conversely, the ovary may not respond despite normal hormonal stimulation. Chemotherapeutic drugs for cancer, excessive alcohol intake, and smoking can interfere with ovulation. Sometimes ovulation does not occur because the woman is entering the climacteric (menopause) early.

Abnormal Fallopian Tubes. Infections such as chlamydia and gonorrhea can cause scarring and adhesions of the fallopian tubes that result in blockage of the tubes. Adhesions may also occur because of endometriosis, pelvic surgery, appendicitis, peritonitis, or ovarian cysts. If the tubal obstruction allows the smaller sperm to pass but is too narrow for the resulting fertilized ovum, ectopic tubal pregnancy may occur (see Chapter 5). The same conditions may cause abnormal transport of the ovum through the tube.

Abnormal Uterus, Cervix, or Ovaries. Congenital abnormalities of the reproductive tract or uterine **myomas** (benign uterine muscle tumors) may interfere with normal implantation of the ovum, or they may result in repeated spontaneous abortion or early preterm labor. Women with polycystic ovaries experience abnormalities of ovulation and menstruation that accompany the hormonal dysfunction associated with this disorder.

Hormone Abnormalities. In addition to interfering with ovulation, abnormal hormone stimulation can interfere with proper development of the uterine lining, resulting in an inability to conceive or in repeated spontaneous abortions. Abnormalities in the amount or timing of any hormone necessary for endometrial buildup, ovum development and release, or support of the conceptus can result in infertility.

Other Factors That May Influence Fertility

Coital Frequency. Intercourse more than three times per week is best for conception. The window of opportunity to conceive opens 2 days before ovulation and closes 1 day after ovulation.

Age. Women over 35 years of age have a somewhat decreased (but not absent) chance of conceiving.

Cigarette Smoking. Cigarette smoking of more than 15 cigarettes per day suppresses the function of the immune system, leading to an early loss of reproductive function. Nicotine has an effect on tubal motility, resulting in an increased risk of ectopic pregnancies.

Exercise, Diet, and Weight. Excessive exercise and weight loss may be linked to decreased fertility. A low-calorie vegetarian diet is associated with a short luteal phase, and excessive weight loss may influence the release of gonadotropins. Ovarian dysfunction is common in obese women, especially those who gain weight rapidly. However, extra weight is thought to be a cofactor of infertility rather than a direct cause.

Emotional Factors. Emotional factors do not cause infertility, but many infertile couples experience stress and anxiety and require emotional understanding. A strong support system is helpful in the decision to start or stop fertility treatments.

Medical Problems. Pelvic adhesions can obstruct the fallopian tube and cause infertility. Adhesions can result from abdominal and/or pelvic surgery, Crohn's disease, ulcerative colitis, or celiac disease. PID and STIs are also associated with infertility.

Drugs and Chemicals. Pollutants in the environment and medications or chemicals ingested may influence fertility. Chemotherapeutic agents used in the treatment of cancer are related to infertility. Research is ongoing concerning the protective effect of suppressing ovarian function or storing ova during chemotherapeutic treatments. Recreational drugs such as marijuana and cocaine pose an increased risk for infertility. Cocaine use in men has been shown to affect the motility of sperm and contribute to infertility of the couple. Antihistamines can decrease vaginal lubrication, antihypertensives can decrease erectile ability, barbiturates can inhibit the release of gonadotropin, and NSAIDs can block egg release. The use of cimetidine, monoamine oxidase (MAO)-inhibitor antidepressants, and lithium are also thought to alter male reproduction. Reprotox is a center that maintains a database of reproductive effects of industrial chemicals. This database can be found at www.reprotox.org/Default.aspx and requires membership to access.

EVALUATION OF INFERTILITY

Both members of a couple are evaluated for infertility. The evaluation begins with a thorough history and physical examination to identify evidence of other conditions that may also be affecting their fertility. Testing proceeds from the simple to the complex; however, it may be accelerated in the older woman because of her natural decline in fertility with age.

Male Testing

A semen analysis is the first male test performed. Semen is best collected by masturbation; if this is not an option, semen can be collected in a condom that does not contain spermicide. Endocrine tests identify the presence of hormonal stimulation that is necessary for sperm formation. Ultrasonography can identify anatomical abnormalities. Testicular biopsy is an invasive procedure to obtain a sample of testicular tissue for analysis.

Female Testing

The methods for predicting ovulation discussed in the section on natural family planning can also be used to evaluate infertility. Ultrasonography is used to assess the structure of reproductive organs, to identify the maturation and release of the ovum, and to ensure proper timing for other tests, such as the postcoital test. Ultrasonography is also used to identify multifetal pregnancies. The postcoital test is performed 6 to 12 hours after intercourse to evaluate the action of sperm within the woman's cervical mucus at the time of ovulation. Endocrine tests evaluate the hormone stimulation of ovulation and the buildup of the uterine lining to prepare for pregnancy. More invasive tests are sometimes required. The hysterosalpingogram is an x-ray study using contrast medium to evaluate the structure of the reproductive organs. An endometrial biopsy is done to obtain a sample of uterine lining to assess its response to hormones. Hysteroscopy and laparoscopy use an endoscope (instrument that allows visual inspection of internal organs) to examine the uterine interior and the pelvic organs.

THERAPY FOR INFERTILITY

The specific therapy depends on what cause, if any, was identified by testing.

Medications

Medications may be given to the man to improve semen quality or to the woman to induce ovulation, to prepare the uterine endometrium for pregnancy, or to support the pregnancy after it is established. Several drugs are provided in combination with another drug to mimic natural function. Medications are continued for six to nine cycles for optimum outcome. Some of the drugs that may be prescribed include the following:

- *Bromocriptine (Parlodel):* Corrects excess prolactin secretion by the pituitary, which stimulates ovulation and supports pregnancy
- *Clomiphene (Clomid):* Induces ovulation; may be used with human chorionic gonadotropin (hCG)
- *Gonadotropin-releasing hormone (GnRH, Lutrepulse):* Stimulates production of other hormones that, in turn, stimulate ovulation in the female and production of testosterone and sperm in the male
- *Leuprolide (Lupron):* Reduces endometriosis
- *Menotropin (e.g., Pergonal):* Stimulates ovulation and sperm production
- *Nafarelin (Synarel):* Reduces endometriosis; stimulates ovulation and spermatogenesis
- *Progesterone:* Promotes implantation of the fertilized ovum
- *Sildenafil (Viagra):* Increases erectile function

- *hCG (Pregnyl):* Stimulates ovulation and sperm production

Medications administered to induce ovulation also increase the risk of multifetal gestations. Although most of these multiple gestations are twins, higher multiples present a much higher risk for maternal, fetal, and neonatal complications. The parents of high multiples may need to make a decision about which, if any, of their fetuses to abort so that the others have a better chance of achieving maturity. This situation presents a difficult ethical situation for both parents and professionals.

Surgical Procedures

Surgery may be used to correct anatomical abnormalities such as varicocele, adhesions, or tubal obstruction.

Therapeutic Insemination

Once called "artificial insemination," therapeutic insemination may use the male partner's sperm or sperm from an anonymous donor. A woman who wants to bear a child biologically on her own also may use therapeutic insemination. If sperm are placed directly in the uterus, they are washed and concentrated to improve their chances of fertilizing an ovum. Donors are screened for genetic defects, infections, and high-risk behaviors. Donor sperm is held frozen for 6 months to reduce the risk of transmitting a disease that was not apparent at the initial screening. Reputable centers limit the number of times a man may donate his sperm to reduce the chance of inadvertent consanguinity (blood relationship) between his offspring when they grow up.

Surrogate Parenting

A surrogate mother may donate the use of her uterus only, with the sperm and ovum coming from the infertile couple who have a problem carrying a pregnancy. Or, she may be inseminated with the male partner's sperm, thus supplying both her genetic and her gestational components. Surrogate mothering cannot be anonymous, and the birth mother inevitably forms bonds with the fetus during the months of pregnancy.

Bypassing Obstacles to Conception. Reproductive technology provides new hope to couples who may have once considered their infertility to be irreversible; however, some of the techniques are not covered by insurance.

Various techniques place intact sperm and ova together to allow fertilization. Each begins with ovulation induction by medications to obtain several ova and thus improve the likelihood of a successful pregnancy (Table 11-2). In general, gamete intrafallopian transfer (GIFT) and tubal embryo transfer (TET) have a higher pregnancy rate than in vitro fertilization (IVF). These techniques can result in multifetal pregnancy. Rarely do all the ova placed in the uterus implant successfully.

Table 11-2	Summary of Assisted Reproductive Therapies (ARTs)
THERAPY	**DESCRIPTION**
Therapeutic insemination	Donor sperm are placed in the uterus or fallopian tube; sperm may be the partner's or a donor's.
In vitro fertilization (IVF)	After inducing ovulation, ova are recovered by laparoscopy or transvaginal aspiration under sonography; they are then fertilized with sperm from the partner or a donor in the laboratory and 2 days later are transferred to the uterus.
Gamete intrafallopian transfer (GIFT)	Oocytes are retrieved into a catheter that contains prepared sperm; up to two ova are injected into each fallopian tube, where fertilization occurs. The woman must have at least one open tube.
Tubal embryo transfer (TET), also called zygote intrafallopian transfer (ZIFT)	Ova are fertilized as in IVF but are transferred to the fallopian tube as soon as fertilization occurs. The resulting embryos enter the uterus normally for implantation.
Donor oocyte	Multiple ova are retrieved from a woman. They are fertilized and placed in the prepared uterus of the infertile woman.
Surrogate mother	A woman allows her ova to be inseminated by the partner or another donor. She then carries the fetus and agrees to relinquish the infant after birth.
Gestational surrogate	The infertile couple undergoes IVF, but the resulting embryos are placed in the prepared uterus of a woman who has agreed to carry the fetus for them. The woman does not donate any of her genetic components.
Intracytoplasmic sperm injection (ICSI)	Sperm are inserted directly into ova via microsurgery.

Outcomes of Infertility Therapy

Three outcomes are possible after infertility therapy:
1. Achievement of a "take-home" infant
2. Unsuccessful therapy resulting in a decision about adoption
3. Pregnancy loss after treatment

Becoming pregnant changes the couple's anxiety but does not eliminate it. Because of past disappointments, they may be reluctant to invest emotionally in the pregnancy. They may delay preparations for birth, because they expect to be disappointed again or fear that something will go wrong. Even when their infant is born, they may have unrealistic expectations of themselves as parents after all the difficulties in achieving pregnancy.

Couples who decide to pursue adoption must consider their preferences and the realities of the adoption "market." Most couples prefer to adopt an infant of the same race, but that child may not be available. Some couples fear that they will have a biological child after adoption and wonder if they can love the two children equally.

When a pregnancy is lost after treatment, the couple may feel optimism mixed with sadness. On one hand, they proved that they could conceive. On the other hand, the conception did not result in the live birth of an infant.

Legal and Ethical Factors in Assisted Reproduction

Noncoital reproduction brings with it many legal and ethical issues. In most cases, assisted reproductive techniques (ARTs) are used to assist infertile couples. However, a couple can also use these techniques to avoid known genetic anomalies carried by one partner. Donors and surrogates involve third parties, and their emotional bonds and legal rights must be considered. Homosexual couples or single persons can parent a child through surrogacy, and a changed family structure evolves.

Interpreting and protecting parental rights are legal challenges. It is now possible for a child to have five parents: a sperm donor, an egg donor, a gestational surrogate, and the parents who will rear the child. The right to bear a child is protected by the United States Constitution; the government cannot usually interfere. The nontraditional family is therefore entitled to constitutional protection.

Cloning one's lost child is now a possibility. The fate of a frozen embryo when the parents divorced has been challenged in court. The sale of frozen embryos has a growing impact on our legal system. Federally funded research on fetal tissue can affect future research and development. State laws can also prevent funding of private research. The problems of insurance coverage and access to care are also highly debated issues.

Nursing Care Related to Infertility Treatment

Much of the nursing role involves supporting the couple as they undergo diagnosis and make decisions concerning treatment. The nurse must use tactful therapeutic communication to help each member of the couple discuss his or her feelings. Partners are encouraged to accept their feelings. The normality of feelings that seem out of place (such as ambivalence about a pregnancy after working so hard to achieve it) is reinforced. The couple is helped to identify ways to communicate with each other and to discuss available options that empower them with control.

The couple's sense of control should be increased as much as possible. Their positive coping skills are reinforced, and more constructive alternatives to poor coping are explored. They may benefit from relaxation techniques, support groups, and other stress-management methods. Support groups can also reduce their sense of isolation. The couple should be helped to explore their options at each decision point. Only the person(s) involved can make the decision, but the nurse can help them to explore their feelings.

MENOPAUSE

The definition of **menopause** according to the World Health Organization (WHO) is the cessation of menstrual periods for a 12-month period because of changes in estrogen production. The **climacteric** (change of life) is also known as the perimenopausal period, which extends for 2 to 8 years before menstruation ceases. The last menstrual period occurs between approximately 45 to 50 years of age. In the 2- to 8-year period before this time, the ova slowly degenerate and menstrual cycles are often anovulatory and irregular. Estrogen production by the ovaries decreases. Pregnancy can occur during the climacteric, and the woman should be encouraged to continue any birth control that she has used in the past. Decreasing estrogen in the woman increases her risk for osteoporosis, arteriosclerosis, and increases in cholesterol levels in the blood. Menopause may be induced at any age by surgery, pelvic irradiation, or extreme stress.

PHYSICAL CHANGES

The decrease in estrogen specifically causes the following:
- Changes in the menstrual cycle
- Vasomotor instability (hot flashes)
- Decreased moisture and elasticity of vagina that can cause dyspareunia (painful intercourse)

Other symptoms such as mood swings and irritability are also experienced. Hot flashes are a well-known phenomenon. The woman suddenly feels a burning or hot sensation of her skin followed by perspiration. Hot flashes often occur during the night, and some women have several sleep interruptions because of them. They are more likely to occur when menopause is artificial, such as through oophorectomy (removal of the ovaries), rather than when it occurs naturally. The woman may also notice chills, palpitations, dizziness, and tingling of the skin as part of the vasomotor instability.

The reproductive organs are estrogen dependent, leading to changes as the estrogen level declines. The uterus shrinks, and the ovaries atrophy. The sacral ligaments relax, and pelvic muscles weaken, which can result in pelvic floor dysfunction. The cervix becomes pale and shrinks. The vagina becomes shorter, narrower, and less elastic. There is less lubrication. Some women notice a change in *libido* (sexual desire) at this time. Coitus may be uncomfortable because of vaginal dryness. Urinary incontinence may be a problem, because the muscles controlling urine flow atrophy. The breasts atrophy.

Loss of estrogen secretion also means an end to its protective effect on the woman's cardiovascular and skeletal systems. Estrogen increases the amount of high-density lipoproteins, which carry cholesterol from body cells to the liver for excretion. The incidence of heart disease rises after menopause, because low-density lipoproteins, which carry cholesterol into body cells (including blood vessels), increase.

Estrogen assists the deposition of calcium in the bones to strengthen them. Loss of bone mass accelerates as estrogen levels fall, resulting in **osteoporosis**. Osteoporosis is a leading cause of vertebral, hip, and other fractures in postmenopausal women, because the bones become very fragile. Both males and females lose bone mass as they age. Females, who have a lower bone mass to begin with because they are smaller, lose more in proportion to the total amount as they age. In addition, women generally live longer than men, so the loss continues longer. Therefore, problems such as hip fractures related to age affect many more women than men. The bones may be so fragile that a fracture occurs and causes a fall, rather than the fracture being the result of a fall.

PSYCHOLOGICAL AND CULTURAL VARIATIONS

Women from different cultures experience menopause differently. How the society views aging, the role of the female, and femininity itself have a bearing. In countries in which age is revered, menopause is practically a "nonevent." In the United States, with its emphasis on youth, sex appeal, and physical beauty, menopause can threaten the woman's feelings of health and self-worth. A positive aspect of menopause is that it is a time of liberation from monthly periods, cramps, and the fear of unwanted pregnancy. It can be the beginning of a satisfying postreproductive life.

TREATMENT OPTIONS

Culture, finances, and access to health care are factors that must be considered. Partnership-building communication with the health care team can help the woman cope with lifestyle changes that may be necessary to maintain health. The nurse can help educate the woman to understand the changes that are occurring and develop coping mechanisms to promote comfort in handling minor discomforts. Vaginal dryness can be relieved by the use of lubricants, Kegel exercises can counter genital atrophy, and maintaining good hydration and techniques to prevent urinary tract infections can promote general well-being. Exercise, an increase in the dietary intake of calcium and magnesium, and a high-fiber, low-fat diet rich in antioxidants are essential.

In the past, hormone replacement therapy (HRT) was advocated for most women as a treatment for menopausal symptoms that interfered with activities of daily living and for its protective effect on the cardiovascular and skeletal systems. However, in 2002 a large study (Women's Health Initiative [WHI]) was stopped, because evidence indicated the women experienced increased occurrence of heart attack or stroke, breast cancer, and thrombophlebitis. The risks of HRT were thought to outweigh the benefits. The U.S. Preventive Services Task Force (USPSTF), the American Congress of Obstetricians and Gynecologists (ACOG), the American Heart Association, the North American Menopause Society, and the Canadian Task Force on preventive health care all recommend against the use of hormone replacement therapy for the prevention of chronic diseases in postmenopausal women.

Today, HRT decisions are based on the individual patient, with the benefits and risks clearly identified. Nurses should counsel their patients who are taking HRT to have regular follow-up care and to report any signs of complications, such as headache, vision changes, signs of thrombophlebitis, or cardiac symptoms (Hacker, 2010).

Contraindications for HRT include estrogen-dependent breast cancer, endometrial cancer, thromboembolic disease, a history of malignant melanoma, chronic liver disease, severe hypertriglyceridemia, gallbladder disease, and seizure disorders. Although women who are *BRCA-1* gene carriers have a 60% to 80% chance of developing breast cancer, prophylactic surgery before menopause lowers the risk of developing cancer. Annual breast examinations and regular self-breast assessments are advised for women undergoing HRT.

Complementary and Alternative Therapies

The use of over-the-counter complementary therapy during menopause has become very popular. Some examples include the following:

- Yam root contains natural progesterone in the form of diosgenin but does not provide a proven progesterone effect; it is available in oral and topical forms.
- Ginseng may help relieve menopausal symptoms such as hot flashes and headaches.
- Soy products contain phytoestrogens and are thought to reduce problems such as hot flashes and to help convert vitamin D into calcitonin.
- Vitamin E is thought to stabilize estrogen levels.
- Black cohosh, marketed as Remifemin, is thought to reduce luteinizing hormone.
- Calcium and vitamin D supplements are recommended for women who cannot spend at least 30 minutes a day in the sun.

Homeopathy, acupuncture, and relaxation techniques can also be helpful. See Chapter 34 for more information concerning complementary and alternative

medicine (CAM) therapies. Excessive caffeine intake and alcohol ingestion may increase calcium excretion, and smoking further decreases estrogen utilization; thus they should be avoided. See Chapter 34 for detailed discussion of complementary and alternative therapies used in maternal–child care.

Therapy for Osteoporosis

Osteoporosis occurs when the loss of calcium from the bones is faster than its deposition in the bones. Signs of osteoporosis include a loss of height, the development of a "dowager's hump" (a dorsal kyphosis and cervical lordosis), curvature of the upper spine, and increased susceptibility to hip and spinal fractures. Calcium intake from food sources such as dairy products, dark green leafy vegetables, soybeans, and wheat bread and/or calcium and vitamin D supplements can prevent complications of osteoporosis. A daily intake of 1200 mg calcium is needed for the menopausal woman and 600 to 800 mg of vitamin D per day is needed to absorb calcium from the gastrointestinal tract (ACOG, 2010). Weight-bearing exercises such as walking, hiking, stair climbing, and dancing are advisable to strengthen the musculoskeletal system. High-impact exercises should be avoided. To assess risk for osteoporosis, bone mineral density (BMD) testing is recommended for postmenopausal women older than 65 years. Alendronate (Fosamax) may be prescribed to prevent potential fractures. Esophageal and gastric irritation are common side effects of alendronate, and the woman should be instructed to drink 8 ounces of plain water and to sit upright for 30 minutes after taking the drug and before eating a meal. Parathyroid hormones and calcitonin show promise to reduce the risk of fractures and possibly to increase bone formation. Denosumab (Prolia) may be prescribed to reduce bone loss.

NURSING CARE OF THE MENOPAUSAL WOMAN

Nursing Care Plan 11-1 offers further nursing interventions in addition to those discussed here. The woman's knowledge of the changes surrounding menopause is assessed. If she is near the age for the climacteric to begin, any symptoms are identified. Treatments or tests that the woman will have, such as bone density studies, are clarified. The nurse must determine the woman's understanding of the risks and benefits of HRT when helping her to decide about the therapy, with written information provided to reinforce verbal teaching.

The woman is taught the signs and symptoms that she should report, such as vaginal bleeding that recurs after the cessation of menstrual periods. She should also report signs of vaginal irritation or signs of urinary tract infection, because these are more common with atrophy of vaginal tissues.

The woman is also taught how to take prescribed medications properly. For example, the nurse must teach the woman that calcium is best absorbed if she also takes vitamin D. Taking foods or other medications

Nursing Care Plan 11-1   **The Woman Experiencing Perimenopausal Symptoms**

PATIENT DATA A 49-year-old woman tells the nurse that she is experiencing a lot of discomfort relating to her beginning menopause. She states she is having hot flashes and does not enjoy having sex anymore, among other "embarrassing" symptoms.

Selected Nursing Diagnosis: Impaired comfort related to vasomotor symptoms (hot flashes)

Goals	Nursing Interventions	Rationales
The woman will verbalize measures to increase her comfort during vasomotor symptoms.	Suggest that she wear layered cotton clothes.	This allows the woman to take off or put on clothes during hot flashes or chills; cotton allows easier passage of air than synthetic fabric.
	Advise her to avoid caffeine (coffee, tea, colas, chocolate).	Hot flashes often occur at night; caffeine is a stimulant and will contribute to insomnia and perspiration.
	Explain that stress exacerbates the condition; explore activities that she finds relaxing.	Stress affects virtually every system of the body, including the endocrine and cardiovascular systems, worsening the hot flashes.
	Suggest she discuss hormone replacement therapy (HRT) with her physician.	HRT is effective at relieving vasomotor symptoms, but the individual patient must evaluate its benefits and risks.
	Vitamin E, ginseng, and other herbs may reduce vasomotor symptoms.	Some women should not take or choose not to take HRT, and these measures provide an alternative.

Selected Nursing Diagnosis: Ineffective sexuality patterns related to painful intercourse

Goals	Nursing Interventions	Rationales
The woman will state measures to reduce vaginal dryness. The woman will express no discomfort with coitus.	Teach the woman to use water-soluble lubricant before intercourse.	Thinning of vaginal walls and drying of secretions can lead to discomfort during intercourse unless additional lubrication is used; oil-based lubricants can promote bacterial growth.
	Teach that products such as Replens and Lubrin are available without a prescription to provide relief for vaginal dryness for several days.	These products lubricate the vagina for a longer time, reducing tissue trauma.
	If estrogen vaginal cream is prescribed, teach that it should be inserted at bedtime.	Topical applications of estrogen reduce vaginal atrophy; applying at bedtime reduces loss and increases absorption.

Selected Nursing Diagnosis: Stress urinary incontinence and infection related to genital atrophy

Goals	Nursing Interventions	Rationales
The woman will restate measures to promote urinary tract health.	Teach Kegel exercises: Contract muscles as if to stop urine flow. Repeat 10 times. Do the cycle of 10 Kegel exercises five times each day. Do not actually stop urine flow while urinating.	Kegel exercises increase muscle tone around the urinary meatus and the vagina. Repeatedly stopping the stream of urine could cause retention that could lead to infection.
	Drink at least eight glasses of water each day. Caffeine-containing drinks should not be included in the target amount of fluid.	Adequate intake of liquid dilutes urine and promotes regular emptying, both of which discourage bacterial growth. Caffeine acts as a diuretic, which reverses some of the benefits of the fluid ingested.
	Urinate regularly; do not allow the bladder to become overly distended.	Prevents the stasis of urine that promotes the growth of bacteria.
	Wipe from front to back after toileting.	Prevents bringing anal organisms to the urinary meatus or vagina, where they could cause infection.

Critical Thinking Question

1. A woman, age 49 years, requests help in controlling her anxiety level. She reports hot flashes, night sweats, sleep pattern disturbances, and mood swings. She is afraid her husband will leave her, and she wants medication to "calm her down." Based on her age and history, what is the best response of the nurse?

before allowing at least 30 minutes (preferably 1 hour) for alendronate to be absorbed will negate the benefit of that dose. Lying down after taking alendronate can cause severe esophageal irritation.

The woman should be informed of medication-related side effects to report. She should contact her health care provider if she has headaches, visual disturbances, signs of thrombophlebitis, heaviness in her legs, chest pain, or breast lumps, because these symptoms may indicate adverse side effects associated with HRT. Basic education concerning the use of CAM therapies and their side effects (see Chapter 34) and interactions should be included in the teaching plan.

The woman should be taught about the value of weight-bearing exercise in slowing bone loss. She must be helped to identify suitable exercises that she enjoys and cautioned about the high-impact ones that she should avoid. Because even minor falls can result in disabling fractures in women who have osteoporosis, the nurse should teach the woman ways to make her environment safer. Safety needs may be as simple as making sure there are adequate lights with handy switches and that loose cords and obstructions are secured outside of walking paths. Nonskid bath and shower floors and convenient grab bars reduce the risk of falls when bathing.

The nurse should identify the woman's perception of her menopausal status with consideration of cultural factors, sexuality concerns, access to care, and use of self-medication. Teaching the woman about available support groups in the community and the physiology of menopause can increase compliance with preventive health measures.

PELVIC FLOOR DYSFUNCTION

Pelvic floor dysfunction occurs when the muscles, ligaments, and fascia that support the pelvic organs are damaged or weakened. The dysfunction may occur as a result of childbirth injury but often does not become obvious until the perimenopausal period. There are two classifications of pelvic floor dysfunction that often occur together:

1. Vaginal wall prolapse, which includes cystocele and rectocele
2. Uterine prolapse

VAGINAL WALL PROLAPSE

The vaginal wall may prolapse in either the anterior or posterior wall or in both walls.

Cystocele

A *cystocele* occurs when the anterior vaginal wall becomes too weak to support the bladder that contains urine. Stress incontinence may result and cause the woman to lose urine when there is a sudden increase in intraabdominal pressure, such as when laughing, coughing, or sneezing.

Rectocele

A *rectocele* occurs when the posterior vaginal wall becomes weakened. When the woman strains to defecate, feces are pushed against the weakened wall rather than being directed toward the rectal sphincter for elimination. The woman may use digital pressure against her posterior vaginal wall to facilitate defecation.

UTERINE PROLAPSE

A *uterine prolapse* occurs when the ligaments that support the uterus and vagina are weakened. The uterus sags downward in the vagina. It is more likely to occur in the woman who has had several vaginal births or the woman who has given birth to large infants. Symptoms of uterine prolapse include pelvic fullness, a dragging sensation, pelvic pressure, fatigue, and a low backache. In addition, the woman will often have symptoms characteristic of vaginal wall prolapse.

MANAGEMENT OF PELVIC FLOOR DYSFUNCTION

Medical management of pelvic floor dysfunction depends on several factors, such as age, physical condition, sexual activity, and extent of the problem. Surgical correction provides the most definitive relief. The vaginal wall(s) may be repaired, and a vaginal hysterectomy is often performed for uterine prolapse. The two surgeries are often combined. If the woman cannot undergo surgery, a *pessary* (a device to support the pelvic structures) may be inserted into her vagina. Contraindications to the use of a pessary include pelvic infections, PID, and latex allergy. Careful hygiene and follow-up care are essential when a pessary is inserted to prevent complications such as ulcerations or infections.

NURSING CARE OF THE WOMAN WITH PELVIC FLOOR DYSFUNCTION

Kegel exercises can help to strengthen the pubococcygeal muscle, a major support for the urethra, vagina, and rectum. The woman performs these exercises by contracting her pelvic muscles as if to stop the flow of urine. She should not actually do the exercise while urinating. She should repeat the contraction 10 times and perform this cycle five times daily. The woman should continue Kegel exercises for the rest of her life to maintain pelvic muscle tone.

To reduce some of the low back and pelvic discomforts associated with pelvic relaxation, the woman can be taught to lie down with her feet elevated. Assuming the knee-chest position for a few minutes may also help. Measures to prevent constipation, such as adequate fluid and fiber intake, reduce hard feces that would put further pressure on a rectocele.

URINARY INCONTINENCE

Urinary incontinence is an uncontrollable leakage of urine from the bladder. **Stress incontinence** is leakage caused by a sudden increase in intraabdominal pressure (as occurs when sneezing or coughing). *Urge incontinence* is the inability to control the urge to urinate because of an overactive bladder. Urinary incontinence in women is often related to genital trauma during childbirth and is most common in multiparous women. It can be worsened by drugs such as antidepressants, diuretics, caffeine, anticholinergics, alcohol, beta-blockers, and angiotensin-converting enzyme (ACE) inhibitors.

TREATMENT AND NURSING CARE

The nurse can teach the woman how to do Kegel exercises, which can be enhanced by the use of vaginal weights to strengthen the pelvic floor muscles. Electrical muscle stimulation (TENS) may also be prescribed. Medications used for an overactive bladder include oxybutynin (Ditropan XL), tolterodine (Detrol), imipramine (Tofranil), dicyclomine (Bentyl), and hyoscyamine (Cystospaz).

Surgical procedures for stress incontinence include injection of collagen into periurethral tissue. Extracorporeal magnetic innervation is a noninvasive stimulation of muscles that has shown promise in both stress incontinence and overactive bladder. Intraurethral occlusive plugs, which are valved catheters that act as an artificial urinary sphincter control, are rapidly replacing absorbent pads and surgical intervention.

OTHER FEMALE REPRODUCTIVE TRACT DISORDERS

A woman may have other reproductive tract disorders during her life. An overview of some common benign disorders is presented in the following sections. A medical-surgical text should be consulted for more information about these and for information about malignant female reproductive tract disorders.

UTERINE FIBROIDS

Uterine fibroids are also known as **leiomyomas**, myomas, and myofibromas. Uterine fibroids are benign growths of uterine muscle cells and are a very common gynecological condition. They grow under the influence of estrogen, and they are thus most prominent during the childbearing years and often atrophy after menopause. Nulliparity and obesity are risk factors, whereas oral contraceptives reduce the risk of forming fibroids. Many women have no problems with fibroids, but they sometimes cause irregular bleeding, pressure on the bladder, pelvic pressure, dysmenorrhea, and menorrhagia with blood loss exceeding 200 mL/month.

Treatment

Uterine fibroids that are asymptomatic are observed and periodically reevaluated. If the woman is symptomatic, there are surgical and nonsurgical options. Surgical interventions include hysteroscopic myomectomy, where the fibroid is removed with a hysteroscope rather than a surgical incision, but this is not an option for large or multiple lesions. A hysterectomy (removal of the entire uterus) can be performed if the woman is past her childbearing years or does not desire additional children. Medical treatment before surgery improves outcome. A laparoscopic myomectomy, the surgical removal of fibroids, preserves fertility. Myolysis is the laser or electrosurgical destruction of fibroids, and it also preserves fertility.

Uterine fibroid embolization is a nonsurgical technique of treating uterine fibroids that involves fewer physiological effects than drug therapy, fewer psychological effects than surgery, and a faster recovery time. The nurse should help the woman understand her options in relation to her childbearing goals. Some women feel sexual functioning is related to having a uterus, and the nurse can help clarify misconceptions and reduce anxieties. The preoperative and postoperative care is similar to that for any abdominal surgery (a medical-surgical text should be consulted).

OVARIAN CYSTS

A follicular ovarian cyst may develop if the follicle fails to rupture and release its ovum during the menstrual cycle. This type of cyst usually regresses with the next menstrual cycle. A lutein cyst may occur when the corpus luteum that develops after ovulation fails to regress. The lutein cyst is more likely to cause pain. An ovarian cyst that ruptures or becomes twisted and infarcted as its blood supply is cut off can cause pelvic pain and tenderness.

Diagnosis is by transvaginal ultrasound examination. A laparoscopy may aid in diagnosing and differentiating the ovarian cyst pain from that caused by endometriosis. Laparotomy may be required to remove the cyst.

Polycystic Ovary Syndrome

Polycystic ovary syndrome (PCOS) is an endocrine disorder that involves hormonal imbalance and ovarian cysts. Common symptoms include obesity, infertility, amenorrhea, and excessive hair growth. If untreated, PCOS can lead to the development of diabetes mellitus type 2, increased blood lipids, and heart disease. A poor body self-image and infertility are major problems involved with this condition. Treatment includes dietary management and weight loss to prevent development of diabetes mellitus and other problems related to obesity. Medications such as metformin combined with clomophine have been used with success as well as hormonal therapy, laparoscopic ovarian diathermy (to cauterize testosterone-producing tissue of the ovary), and treatments to increase fertility (McFarland, 2012). CAM therapy such as acupuncture and Chinese herbal medicine has also shown promise in increasing efficacy of assisted reproductive techniques. Psychological support is valuable in treating this condition (McFarland, 2012).

CULTURAL ASPECTS OF PAIN CONTROL

Pain is considered the fifth vital sign for nurses to assess on a regular basis. Culture and ethnicity may have an impact on the accuracy of pain assessment. Asian women may understand a vertical pain score, because they read downward rather than left to right (see Chapter 21 for pain rating scales). Descriptive words for pain can imply intensity, such as "aches" versus "hurt." In general, any pain score above 5 on a scale of 0 to 10 can interfere with activities of daily living and requires nursing intervention.

Ethnicity can affect drug metabolism so that a dose that is effective for one ethnic group may not be the same in others. Drug research often uses white males as subjects.

Diet can affect drug absorption. For example, griseofulvin requires fat in the diet for adequate absorption. Malnutrition can interfere with the absorption and excretion of medications. Smoking is known to have an impact on the metabolism of some drugs.

CAM therapy can affect the action of prescribed drugs. For example, ginseng alters metabolism and therefore affects the absorption and elimination of drugs (see Chapter 34 for details of CAM therapy). Patients should be asked what type of self-care they use for chronic pain. Many patients report using CAM therapy in addition to prescribed drugs. Some women suffer in silence with pain that is not relieved by prescribed medication, believing nothing more can be done. These women need guidance, counseling and referral to available pain clinics. Members of some cultural groups will not report embarrassing side effects, such as diarrhea, and they may stop taking the medication because of these side effects. Careful, sensitive questioning by the nurse is essential, because this information may not be volunteered.

Understanding pain, its symptoms, and its causes as well as the influence of culture, ethnicity, diet, and CAM therapy on pain relief is essential if nurses are to provide comprehensive care to their patients.

Unfolding Case Study

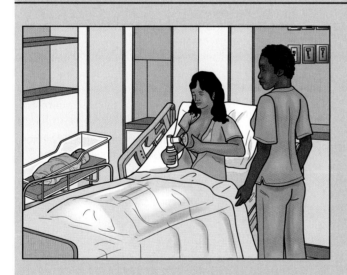

Tess and Luis were introduced to the reader in Chapter 4, and Tess's pregnancy experience has unfolded in each chapter. Tess has given birth to twins unexpectedly. Refer to earlier chapters for additional history.

Both Tess and Luis are interested in finding a plan for contraception so she will not become pregnant again until they are ready. Tess is breastfeeding her babies and asks if breastfeeding will protect her from becoming pregnant.

QUESTIONS
1. What can the nurse tell Tess about the contraceptive protection offered by breastfeeding her babies?
2. What options for temporary birth control are available for Tess?
3. How soon can Tess begin hormonal contraception after delivery of her twins?
4. What can the nurse teach Tess about possible side effects of contraceptives that she should report to her health care provider?

Get Ready for the NCLEX® Examination!

Key Points

- Preventive care is cost-effective, because health problems can be caught early and treated.
- Teaching a woman that breast self-examination can reduce her risk of death from breast cancer.
- Several self-help measures can relieve some symptoms of premenstrual syndrome.
- Prevention of toxic shock syndrome involves not allowing microorganisms the time to grow in the woman's reproductive tract.
- Sexually transmitted infections (STIs) must be adequately treated in all sexual contacts to stop the transmission and to prevent resistance to antibiotics.

- Contraception is an individual choice. The nurse must avoid incorporating personal preferences when educating patients about contraceptive methods.
- Contraceptive choices include temporary contraception, such as barrier methods or hormones, or permanent contraception, such as hysteroscopic sterilization or vasectomy.
- Emergency contraception, Plan B, is a progestin-only medication taken within 72 hours of unprotected sexual intercourse and is available without a prescription.
- Fertility awareness methods can be used both to prevent pregnancy and to increase the chance of achieving it.
- Except for abstinence, condoms (male and female) offer the best protection from STIs, including HIV.

- Nursing care of infertile couples includes helping them to evaluate their options at different phases during evaluation and treatment.
- Common menopausal symptoms, such as hot flashes and vaginal dryness, stem from the cessation of ovulation and the decrease in hormonal activity, particularly that of estrogen and progesterone.
- Prevention of disabling osteoporosis begins with adequate calcium and vitamin D intake during youth to achieve maximum bone mass. Reducing risk for osteoporosis after menopause is best accomplished by adequate calcium and vitamin D intake combined with exercise.
- Alternative therapies for hormone replacement are available for women who cannot take estrogen (see Chapter 34).
- Pain is considered a fifth vital sign and should be assessed with cultural sensitivity.

Additional Learning Resources

SG Go to your Study Guide for additional learning activities to help you master this chapter content.

e**volve** Go to your Evolve website (http://evolve.elsevier.com/Leifer) for the following learning resources:
- Animations
- Answer Guidelines for Critical Thinking Questions
- Answers and Rationales for Review Questions for the NCLEX® Examination
- Glossary with English and Spanish pronunciations
- Interactive Review Questions for the NCLEX® Examination
- Patient Teaching Plans in English and Spanish
- Skills Performance Checklists
- Video clips and more!

Online Resources
- American Congress of Obstetricians and Gynecologists (ACOG): www.ACOG.org
- Managing contraception: www.managingcontraception.com
- Marquette Method: www.marquette.edu/efficacy.php; http://nursing.slu.edu/ncfe/index.html
- Menopause: www.menopause.org/psht08.pdf
- National Osteoporosis Foundation: www.nof.org
- National Women's Health Information Center: www.4women.gov
- Planned Parenthood: www.plannedparenthood.org

- Prevention and early detection of cervical cancer: www.cancer.org/docroot/CRI/content/CRI_2_6x_cervical_cancer_prevention_and_early_detection_8.asp?sitearea=PED
- Reproductive toxicology database: www.reprotox.org

Review Questions for the NCLEX® Examination

1. Choose the correct teaching for breast self-examination (BSE):
   1. Monthly BSE eliminates the need for a professional examination until after age 40 years.
   2. BSE should be done 1 week after the beginning of each menstrual period.
   3. Dry fingers make it easier to feel very small lumps that are just under the skin.
   4. Use the palm of the hand to palpate the breast.

2. Factors that change the normal flora of the vagina and predispose to vaginal infection include (Select all that apply.):
   1. use of antibiotics.
   2. douching.
   3. sexual intercourse.
   4. daily baths.

3. What is a reliable temporary (reversible) birth control method?
   1. Douching
   2. Breastfeeding
   3. Transdermal patch
   4. Vasectomy

4. To relieve or reduce symptoms of premenstrual dysphoric disorder, what should the nurse recommend that the woman do?
   1. Avoid simple sugars and caffeine consumption.
   2. Use oral contraceptive medication.
   3. Avoid physical exercise.
   4. Limit water intake to 1000 mL/day.

5. The nurse should teach the woman who is experiencing menopause that (Select all that apply.):
   1. calcium is best absorbed when vitamin D intake is adequate.
   2. weight bearing exercise is important.
   3. lying down and resting after each meal is important.
   4. an increased intake of vitamin C will enhance calcium absorption.

Objectives

1. Define each key term listed.
2. Briefly describe three normal reflexes of the newborn, including the approximate age of their disappearance.
3. Demonstrate the details of the physical assessment of the newborn.
4. State four methods of maintaining the body temperature of a newborn.
5. Define the following skin manifestations in the newborn: lanugo, vernix caseosa, mongolian spots, milia, acrocyanosis, and desquamation.
6. State the cause and describe the appearance of physiological jaundice in the newborn.
7. State the methods of preventing infection in newborns.
8. Interpret discharge teaching for the mother and her newborn.

Key Terms

acrocyanosis (ăk-rō-sī-ă-NŌ-sĭs, p. 294)
caput succedaneum (KĂP-ŭt sŭk-sĕ-DĀ-nē-ŭm, p. 283)
cephalohematoma (sĕf-ă-lō-hē-mă-TŌ-mă, p. 283)
circumcision (sŭr-kŭm-SĬZH-ŭn, p. 292)
dancing reflex (p. 283)
Epstein's pearls (p. 294)
fontanelles (fŏn-tă-NĔLZ, p. 283)
head lag (p. 282)
icterus neonatorum (ĬK-tŭr-ŭs nē-ō-nā-TŌR-ŭm, p. 294)
lanugo (lă-NŪ-gō, p. 294)

meconium (mĕ-KŌ-nē-ŭm, p. 299)
milia (MĬL-ē-ă, p. 294)
molding (p. 283)
Mongolian spots (p. 294)
Moro reflex (p. 282)
rooting reflex (p. 282)
scarf sign (p. 291)
tissue turgor (p. 294)
tonic neck reflex (p. 283)
vernix caseosa (VŪR-nĭks kā-sē-Ō-să, p. 294)

The arrival of the newborn, or *neonate,* begins a highly vulnerable period during which many psychological and physiological adjustments to life outside the uterus must be made. The fetus, that remains in the uterus until maturity has reached a major goal. The infant's genetic background, the health of the recent uterine environment, a safe delivery, and the care during the first month of life further contribute to this adjustment.

The *infant mortality rate* is the ratio of the number of deaths of infants younger than age 1 year during any given year to the number of live births occurring in the same year. The rate is usually expressed as the number of deaths per 1000 live births. The infant death rate is highest in the first month and is referred to as the *neonatal mortality rate.* The first 24 hours of life are the most dangerous. The infant mortality rate is considered to be one of the best means of determining the health of a country. To obtain accurate figures, all births and deaths must be registered. In the United States, law requires this registration. Each birth certificate is permanently filed with the state bureau of vital statistics.

Morbidity (*morbidus,* "sick") refers to the state of being diseased or sick. Morbidity rates show the incidence of disease in a specific population during a certain time frame. *Perinatology* is the study and support of the fetus and neonate. The term *perinatal mortality* designates fetal and neonatal deaths related to prenatal conditions and delivery circumstances. See Chapter 1 for details concerning statistics in the United States.

Low-birth-weight newborns and limited access to health care are major causes of infant morbidity. Reducing infant morbidity rates can reduce the resulting incidence of disability, which can have an impact on the growth and development of children. The nurse can play a vital role in educating new parents about health care and the developmental needs of their newborn.

ADJUSTMENT TO EXTRAUTERINE LIFE

When a child is born, an orderly, continuous adaptation from fetal life to extrauterine life takes place. All the body systems undergo some change. Respirations are stimulated by chilling and by chemical changes within the blood. Sensory and physical stimuli also appear to play a role in respiratory function. The first breath opens the alveoli. The infant then enters the world of air exchange, at which time an independent existence begins. This process also initiates cardiopulmonary interdependence. The newborn's ability to metabolize food is hampered by the immaturity of the digestive system, particularly because of deficiencies in enzymes from the pancreas and liver. The kidneys are structurally developed, but their ability to concentrate urine and maintain fluid balance is limited because of a decreased rate of glomerular flow and limited renal tubular reabsorption. Most neurological functions are primitive (see the discussion of the individual body systems in this chapter).

PHASE 3: CARE OF THE NEWBORN

Phase 3 care of the newborn covers the physical characteristics and nursing assessment of the normal term newborn, by body system. Refer to Chapter 6 for care of the newborn immediately after birth (Phase 1) and Chapter 9 for care of the newborn on admission to the nursery or postpartum unit (Phase 2).

When observing the newborn, the nurse identifies expected normal findings as well as *variations* of normal and *deviations from* normal, which must be reported to the health care provider.

NERVOUS SYSTEM: REFLEXES

The nervous system directs most of the body's activity. Newborns can move their arms and legs vigorously but cannot control them. When the infant is lifted from the bed, the head will fall back, because the newborn cannot maintain neutral position of the head. This is called a **head lag** (Figure 12-1). The reflexes that full-term infants are born with, such as blinking, sneezing, gagging, sucking, and grasping (Figure 12-2), help to keep them alive. They can cry, swallow, and lift their heads slightly when lying on their abdomen.

If the crib is jarred, infants draw their legs up and the arms fan out and then come toward midline in an embrace position. This is normal and is called the **Moro reflex** (Figure 12-3). Its absence may indicate abnormalities of the nervous system. The **rooting reflex** causes the infant's head to turn in the direction of anything that

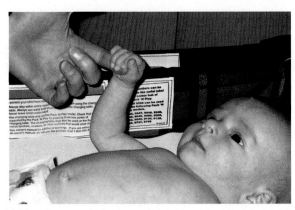

FIGURE 12-2 Grasp reflex. Touching the hands near the base of the fingers causes a reflex flexion of the hands. This grasp reflex is replaced after age 3 months by a voluntary grasp.

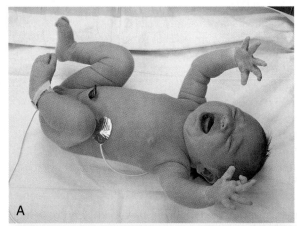

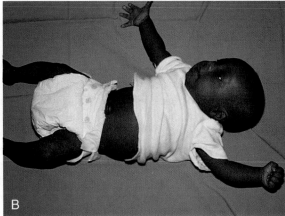

FIGURE 12-3 A, Moro reflex. Sudden jarring causes extension and abduction (an embracing motion) of the extremities and spreading of the fingers, with the index finger and the thumb forming a C shape. A unilateral (one-sided) Moro reflex may indicate a fractured clavicle. Absence of the Moro reflex may indicate a pathological condition of the central nervous system. **B,** Abnormal Moro reflex. Note the clenched fist of one hand that does not follow a symmetrical embracing motion. This infant requires follow-up care. (**A** from Murray SS, McKinney ES, Gorrie TM: *Foundations of maternal-newborn nursing,* ed 3, Philadelphia, 2002, Saunders. **B** from Zitelli BJ, Davis HW: *Zitelli and Davis' atlas of pediatric physical diagnosis,* ed 6, St. Louis, 2012, Saunders.)

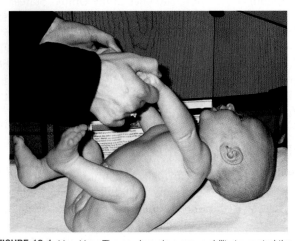

FIGURE 12-1 Head lag. The newborn has some ability to control the head in some positions. When placed on the abdomen, the newborn may be able to raise the chin from the bed briefly. However, head lag and hyperextension normally occur when the newborn is raised from the bed in a supine position. Significant head lag after age 6 months indicates a need for follow-up care.

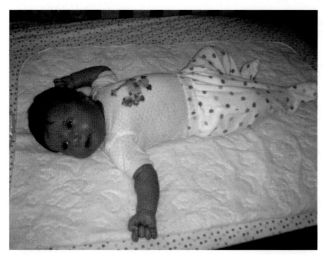

FIGURE 12-4 Spontaneous tonic neck reflex. The infant turns the head to one side, and the arm and leg are extended on that side. The opposite arm and leg flex. Often called the "fencing" reflex, it disappears by age 5 to 7 months as the central nervous system matures.

touches the cheek, in anticipation of food. The nurse uses this when helping a mother to breastfeed her infant. A breast touching the cheek causes the infant to turn toward it to find the nipple (see Chapter 9).

The **tonic neck reflex** is a postural reflex that is sometimes assumed by sleeping infants. The head is turned to one side, the arm and leg are extended on the same side, and the opposite arm and leg are flexed in a "fencing" position. This reflex disappears by the seventh month of life (Figure 12-4). Prancing movements of the legs, seen when an infant is held upright on the examining table, are termed the **dancing reflex**. Table 12-1 lists the ages at which the neurological signs of infancy appear and disappear.

Head

The brain grows rapidly before birth, and therefore the newborn's head is large in comparison with the rest of the body. The normal limits of head circumference range from 32 to 36 cm (12.5 to 14.1 inches) (Skill 12-1). The head may be out of shape from **molding** (the conforming of the fetal head to the size and shape of the birth canal) (Figure 12-5, *A*). There may also be swelling of the soft tissues of the scalp, which is termed **caput succedaneum**. It gradually subsides without treatment. Occasionally, a **cephalohematoma** (*cephal*, "head," *hemato*, "blood," and *toma*, "tumor") protrudes from beneath the scalp (see Figure 12-5, *B* and *C*). This condition is caused by a collection of blood beneath the periosteum of the cranial bone. It may be seen on one or both sides of the head but does not cross the suture line. This condition usually recedes within a few weeks without treatment.

The **fontanelles** are unossified spaces or soft spots on the cranium of a young infant. They protect the head during delivery by permitting the process of molding and allow for further brain growth during the next

1½ years. The anterior fontanelle is diamond shaped and is located at the junction of the two parietal and two frontal bones. It usually closes by age 12 to 18 months. The posterior fontanelle is triangular and is located between the occipital and parietal bones. It is smaller than the anterior fontanelle and is usually ossified by the end of the second month. A tough membrane covers these areas, and there is little chance of their being injured during ordinary care. The features of the newborn's face are small. The mouth and lips are well developed, because they are necessary to obtain food. The newborn can both taste and smell. In fact, the newborn can recognize the scent of the mother's milk on the breast pad.

Eyes

The healthy newborn can see and can fixate on points of contrast. The newborn shows a preference for observing a human face and follows moving objects. *Visual stimulation* is thus an important ingredient in newborn care. Toys that make sounds and have contrasting colors attract the newborn.

Most newborns appear cross-eyed, because their eye muscle coordination is not fully developed. At first, the eyes appear to be blue or gray; the permanent coloring becomes fixed between ages 6 and 12 months. The eyelids are closed most of the time. Tears do not appear until approximately age 1 to 3 months because of the immaturity of the lacrimal gland ducts.

A small conjunctival hemorrhage may be seen in the eye, or mild conjunctivitis may be seen as a result of a response to eye medication instilled at birth, but these conditions are considered *variations* rather than *deviations* from normal, usually require no specific follow-up, and will resolve spontaneously.

Ears

The ears are well developed but small at birth. The ears are assessed for placement, because low-set ears may indicate a congenital abnormality in another part of the body. An imaginary line drawn from the outer canthus of the eye should be even with the upper tip of the pinna of the ear (Figure 12-6). An "ear tag" is a small skin tag or pit on the outside of the ear that is sometimes seen as a variation in newborns, and, although its presence should be documented on the physical assessment record, it is rarely of medical significance. The hearing ability of the newborn is well developed at birth, but the sick or premature newborn may not respond to sounds that are heard. The presence of amniotic fluid in the ear canal can diminish hearing, but normal drainage and sneezing that occur shortly after birth help clear the ear canal.

The newborn will react to a sudden sound with an increase in pulse rate and respirations or a display of the startle reflex. Increased responses to vocal stimulation, particularly higher-pitched female voices, have been documented. The ability to discriminate between

Table 12-1 **Ages of Appearance and Disappearance of Neurological Signs Unique to Infancy**

RESPONSE	HOW TO ELICIT	AGE AT TIME OF APPEARANCE	AGE AT TIME OF DISAPPEARANCE
Reflexes of Position and Movement			
Moro reflex	A loud noise, bumping the surface of crib, or suddenly lowering the head while holding will cause the infant to symmetrically extend and abduct the arms and then adduct in an embracelike motion (see Figure 12-3)	Birth	3-6 months
Tonic neck reflex	Turn infant's head to one side, and the arm and leg will extend on that side with a flexion of the opposite arm and leg (see Figure 12-4) (This is a postural reflex that is assumed by sleeping infants)	Birth	5-7 months (unsustained)*
Palmar grasp reflex	Place object in the hand of the newborn, and the newborn will grasp it tightly (plantar reflex involves curling of the toes when pressure is applied to the sole of the foot)	Birth	4 months
Babinski reflex	Stroke the side of the foot: the big toe will dorsiflex, and the toes will flare out	Birth	Variable, but before the infant begins walking†
Responses to Sound			
Blinking response	The infant will blink on hearing a loud noise	Birth	NA
Turning response	The infant will turn its head toward the source of the noise	Birth	NA
Reflexes of Vision‡			
Eye opening	Holding the newborn infant upright, under the arms, and tipping the infant forward will induce eye opening	Birth	3 months
Blinking to threat	Bringing an object close to the eye at a fast pace will induce blinking	6-7 months	NA
Horizontal following	Moving an object side to side within the infant's visual field will elicit this response	4-6 weeks	NA
Vertical following	Moving a colorful object up and down within the visual field of the infant will induce this response	2-3 months	NA
Food Reflexes			
Rooting response	Infant's head turns in the direction of anything that touches the cheek in anticipation of food	Birth	3-4 months
Sucking response	Infant will suck on a finger or nipple placed in the mouth	Birth	7-12 months
Other Signs			
Stepping reflex	Hold infant upright above a table: the infant will lift the foot up on contact with the firm surface of the table	Birth	4-5 months

NA, Not applicable.
*The infant can break arm and leg posturing after a few minutes, despite continued neck stimulus.
†Usually of no diagnostic significance until after age 2 years.
‡Holding the newborn infant upright under the arms will induce eye opening.
NOTE: Absence of these reflexes or prolonged appearance may indicate a neurological problem and requires further follow-up.

the mother's voice and the voices of others may occur as early as age 3 days. Hearing is important to the development of normal speech. The nurse observes and records how the newborn reacts to sound, such as a rattle or the voice of the caretaker. The infant will respond to voices by decreasing motor activity and sucking activity and turning the head toward the sound.

One type of test used to measure infant hearing is the ALGO hearing screening test, which analyzes hearing by sending a series of soft clicks into the sleeping infant's ear (Figure 12-7). The infant's brain responds with a specific brain wave that is referred to as an auditory brainstem response (ABR). A computer compares the response to normal responses, and a pass/fail score is recorded. Another type of test is the otoacoustic emissions test (OAE) that measures sounds from the cochlea in response to sound stimulation. Newborn hearing screening programs have become part of the protocol of care in hospital nurseries across the United States.

Taking Head and Chest Measurements

PURPOSE

To determine baseline measurements of the head and the chest

STEPS

1. The circumference of the head is measured from the top of the eyebrow to the widest part of the occiput.

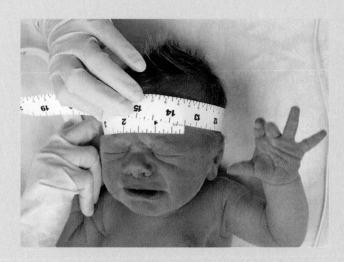

2. To obtain the size of the fontanelle, measure the widest point of the width and the widest point of the length, add the measurements together, and divide by 2.

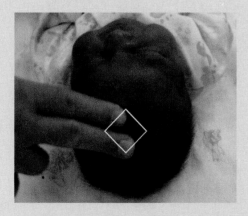

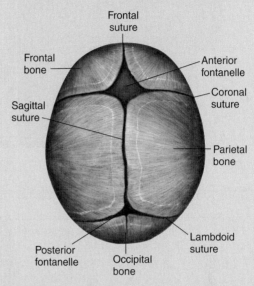

3. The normal anterior fontanelle in a newborn measures between 3.6 and 6 cm. The fontanelles should appear flat with the contour of the skull. A bulging fontanelle may indicate increased intracranial pressure. A depressed fontanelle may indicate dehydration and should be reported to the health care provider.

4. When measuring the chest circumference, the measuring tape is placed at the nipple line.

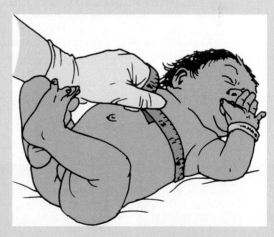

5. Lift the infant to remove the paper tape in order to prevent paper cuts to the infant's skin.

6. Document findings and report any abnormal measurements.

   NOTE: The head circumference should be equal to and no more than 2 cm greater than the chest circumference until age 2. See normal growth charts to compare findings and to determine need for follow-up referral.

(Unnumbered figures 1-3: from Hockenberry MJ, Wilson D: *Wong's essentials of pediatric nursing,* ed 8, St Louis, 2009, Mosby; unnumbered figure 4: from Leifer G: *Maternity nursing,* ed 11, St Louis, 2012, Saunders.)

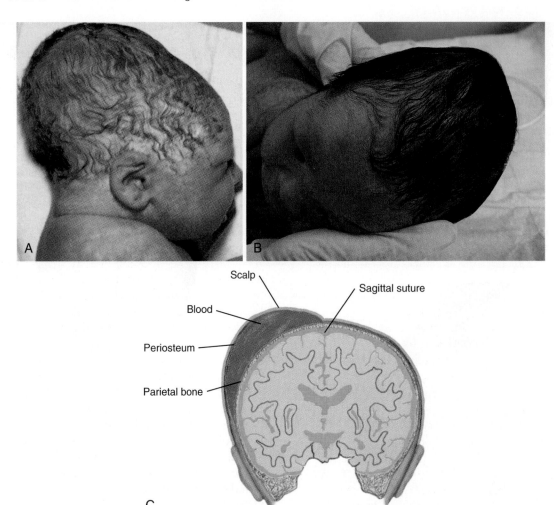

FIGURE 12-5 **A,** Molding of the head occurs as a result of the parietal bones overriding each other as the head passes through the birth canal. Often a collection of fluid under the scalp caused by edema of the presenting part (caput succedaneum) causes the head to appear longer than normal and soft to the touch. This condition disappears without treatment within a few weeks. **B,** Cephalohematoma appears as a lump on one side of the head. **C,** With a cephalohematoma, the blood collects between the surface of the cranial bone and the periosteal membrane. The swelling does not cross the suture lines. (**A** from Beischer NA, Mackey EV, Colditz PB: *Obstetrics and the newborn,* ed 3, Philadelphia, 1997, Saunders. **B** from McKinney, ES, James SR, Murray SS, Ashwill JW: *Maternal-child nursing,* ed 4, Philadelphia, 2013, Saunders.)

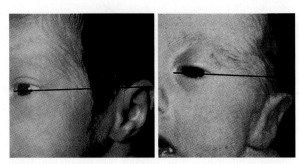

FIGURE 12-6 Ear position. The ears are assessed for placement because low-set ears may indicate a congenital abnormality. An imaginary line drawn from the outer canthus of the eye should be even with the upper tip of the pinna of the ear. (From Thureen PJ, Deacon J, O'Neill P, Hernandez JA: *Assessment and care of the well newborn,* ed 2, Philadelphia, 2005, Saunders.)

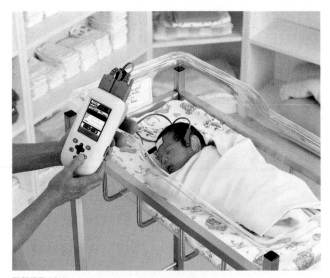

FIGURE 12-7 ALGO hearing screener shows how the test is accomplished. Immediate pass/fail results indicate whether the infant needs further audiological testing.

The ears and nose need no special attention except for cleansing with a soft cloth during the bath. Occasionally they may be *externally* cleansed with a cotton ball moistened slightly with water. The bony canal of the external ear is not well developed, and the tympanic membrane is vulnerable to injury. The nurse should *not* insert applicators. They may cause serious injury to the tympanic membrane if inserted too far into the ear canal or if the infant moves suddenly.

Sensory Overload. *Sensory overload* can occur if there is too much stimulation. This detrimental overload can occur in the hospital environment, where lights are bright and voices carry. The nurse can help to modify this situation by responding quickly to alarms and by speaking quietly when working near the infant.

Sleep

The neonate sleeps approximately 15 to 20 hours a day. There is a gradual change in the quantity and quality of sleep as the newborn matures. At birth the newborn passes through the phases of sleep–wake states as part of the adjustment to life outside of the uterus:

- *First reactive phase:* During the first 30 minutes of life the newborn is alert, and this is the best time to initiate bonding between the parent and newborn.
- *Sleep phase:* During the next few hours of life the infant gradually becomes sleepier and less responsive.
- *Second reactive phase:* After a deep sleep the infant again becomes responsive and alert.
- *Stability phase:* After age 24 hours the sleep–wake pattern becomes more stabilized. The pattern of sleep gradually develops into one in which the newborn is awake during the day and asleep during the night.

The environment plays a large role in the infant's sleep behavior. The nurse can help the parent to understand that normal conversational tones can quiet a newborn, whereas high noise levels can cause increased crying. Wrapping an infant snugly can maintain temperature and promote sleep, as can gentle horizontal rocking. An infant held upright on the shoulder and rocked in a vertical fashion is likely to maintain an alert state. Newborns exhibit a specific pattern of reactivity that can influence the response to stimuli and bonding, as follows:

- *Quiet sleep:* Infant sleeps and does not move.
- *Rapid eye movement (REM) sleep:* Respirations are more irregular during REM sleep. Eye movements are evident beneath the eyelid, and limb and mouth movement may be seen.
- *Active alert:* The infant displays diffuse motor activity.
- *Quiet alert:* The infant is awake, relaxed, and quiet. In this state the infant is most responsive to testing and to bonding efforts.

- *Crying:* The infant's cry is accompanied by vigorous motor activity of extremities.
- *Transitional:* The infant is moving between one of the previously described states. The infant may be quiet and relaxed but not very responsive to the environment.

> **⚠ Safety Alert!**
>
> Even the youngest of infants can roll off a changing table or bed when left unattended.

Pain

In the past it was believed that newborns did not experience pain because of immaturity of the nerve pathways to the brain. It is now thought that fibers that conduct pain stimuli to the spinal cord are in place early in fetal life. These are called *nociceptors* (*noci,* "pain," and *ceptus,* "to receive"). The newborn also produces catecholamines and cortisol in response to stress. Heart rate and respiratory rates change. Blood pressure increases, and blood glucose levels rise. Newborns should be medicated for pain when discomfort is anticipated.

The nurse is responsible for understanding the physiological and behavioral responses to pain and providing appropriate pain relief measures. Untreated pain in early infancy can have long-term effects, because the pain pathways and structures required for long-term memory are well developed by 24 weeks of gestation. Unrelieved pain can also cause exhaustion and irritability and can slow the healing process. Some infants may be too weak to demonstrate a visible response to pain, and so behavioral responses and physiological changes must both be monitored. There are several pain assessment tools available for preterm and term infants. Pain assessment tools appropriate for the older child are discussed in Chapter 21. Examples of pain assessment tools for infants include the following:

- *COMFORT scale:* A 7-point scale that includes alertness, calmness, muscle tone, movement, facial tension, and respiratory response, and two physiologic items (heart rate and mean arterial blood pressure). Each item is scored from 1 to 5, with a high cumulative score indicating increased distress.
- *CRIES:* This 10-point scale (with each component scored from 0 to 2) includes facial expression, cry, movement of the arms and legs, consolability, and oxygen saturation in its scoring. Letters of the acronym are defined as follows: **C** = **c**ry, **R** = **r**equires oxygen, **I** = **i**ncreased vital signs, **E** = **e**xpression on face, **S** = **s**leeplessness.
- *FLACC:* This pain tool measures the pain of infants. The parameters include **f**ace, **l**egs, **a**ctivity, **c**ry, and **c**onsolability. Each parameter is scored from 0 to 2, with a higher cumulative score indicating increased distress.

- *PIPP:* The **P**remature **I**nfant **P**ain **P**rofile is based on scales similar to the CRIES scale. This rates eye squeeze, nasal labial furrow, heart rate, oxygen saturation, and the brow furrow on a 0-to-3 scale, with 21 indicating the worst level of pain.
- *NIPS:* The **N**eonatal **I**nfant **P**ain **S**cale is based on scales similar to the CRIES scale. This scale rates facial expression, arm movement, cry, leg movement, respiration, and arousal on a 0-to-2 scale with a score of 7 indicating the worst level of pain.
- *NPASS:* The **N**eonatal **P**ain, **A**gitation, and **S**edation **S**cale considers the previous criteria in addition to behavior and is considered to be a very reliable and valid assessment tool, even for premature infants on ventilators. Scores are given for crying or irritability, behavioral state, facial expression, tone of extremities, vital signs, and oxygen saturation. Scores in each category range from −2 for sedated infants to +2 for agitated infants. A normal response indicating no pain or sedation is scored as 0 (zero).

The pain assessment findings should be documented and appropriate nursing interventions implemented.

Adequate pain relief in newborns who undergo painful procedures (e.g., circumcision) can reduce postoperative morbidity. Evaluation of pain in the neonate can be based on changes in vital signs and behavior of the infant and decreased oxygen saturation rates (Figure 12-8). Swaddling with the hand near the mouth, cuddling, rocking, nonnutritive sucking, and a quiet environment are noninvasive methods of pain relief for newborn infants. Oral sucrose is an effective pain reliever for minor procedures (Harrison et al, 2010). Morphine, fentanyl, and topical anesthetics can be used safely for severe pain. The nurse must be aware of safe dosage ranges and must observe infants closely for side effects or signs of withdrawal when the medication is gradually decreased and then discontinued.

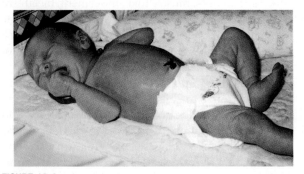

FIGURE 12-8 Pain in the newborn. Note furrowed brow, clenched fist, irritability or cry, chin quiver, increased muscle tone and activity, tightly closed eyes, facial grimace, raised cheeks, deepened nasolabial fold, and open mouth. Diaphoresis; rapid, shallow respirations; and increased heart rate and blood pressure also can be observed in the neonate experiencing pain. Pain relief for the neonate during any medical procedure is very important.

Conditioned Responses

A conditioned response or reflex is one that is learned over time. It is an unconscious response to an external stimulus. An example is the hungry infant who stops crying merely at the sound of the caregiver's footsteps, even though food is not yet available. Emotions are particularly subject to this type of conditioning. As an infant matures, the mere sight of an object that once caused pain can precipitate fear.

Neonatal Behavioral Assessment Scale

The Neonatal Behavioral Assessment Scale, developed by T.B. Brazelton (1973), has increased the understanding of the newborn's capabilities. Among other areas of assessment, this scale measures the inherent neurological capacities of the newborn and responses to selected stimuli. Areas tested include alertness, response to visual and auditory stimuli, motor coordination, level of excitement, and organizational process in response to stress.

RESPIRATORY SYSTEM

The unborn fetus is completely dependent on the mother for all vital functions. The fetus needs oxygen and nourishment to grow. These nutrients are supplied through the bloodstream of the pregnant woman by way of the placenta and the umbilical cord. The fetus is relieved of the waste products of metabolism by the same route. The lungs are not inflated and are almost completely inactive. The circulatory system is adapted only to life within the uterus. Little blood flows through the pulmonary artery because of natural openings within the heart and vessels that close at birth or shortly thereafter.

When the umbilical cord is clamped and cut, the lungs take on the function of breathing oxygen and removing carbon dioxide. The first breath helps to expand the collapsed lungs, although full expansion does not occur for several days. The health care provider assists the first respiration by removing mucus from the passages to the lungs. The infant's cry should be strong and healthy. The most critical period for the newborn is the first hour of life, when the drastic change from life within the uterus to life outside the uterus takes place.

Mucus may be seen draining from the nose or mouth, and can be wiped away. Gently clearing mucus with a bulb syringe may be indicated (Skill 12-2). When this procedure is done orally, the tip is inserted into the side of the mouth to avoid stimulating the gag reflex. Parents are taught how to use the bulb syringe and are instructed to keep one next to the newborn during the early weeks of life.

The nurse can assist newborns to maintain a patent airway by positioning them on their back or side and dressing them in clothing that maintains warmth while allowing expansion of the lungs. The nurse should

Bulb Suctioning

PURPOSE

To clear the airway of mucus

STEPS

1. Compress the ball of the bulb syringe.
2. Insert the narrow portion of the bulb syringe into the side of the infant's mouth to avoid stimulating the gag reflex. Suction the mouth first to prevent inhalation and aspiration of mucus during a gasp reflex, which is stimulated by nasal suctioning.
3. Release the pressure on the ball of the bulb syringe and listen for the sound of mucus being suctioned.
4. Remove the bulb syringe and empty the contents into a receptacle by compressing the bulb.
5. Compress the bulb syringe and insert into one nostril; then release pressure on the bulb to suction the mucus out.
6. Remove the bulb syringe and empty it into a receptacle. Repeat for the other nostril.

7. The nurse should demonstrate to parents the technique of suctioning with a bulb syringe and review cleaning and storage of the bulb syringe.

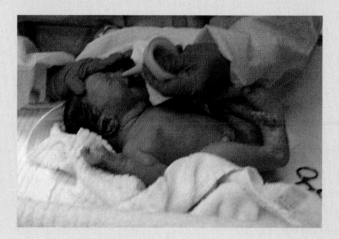

record vital signs and should suction mucus as needed, first from the mouth and throat and then from the nose.

Apgar Score

The Apgar score is a standardized method of evaluating the newborn's condition immediately after delivery. Five objective signs are measured: heart rate, respiration, muscle tone, reflexes, and color. The score is obtained 1 minute after birth and again after 5 minutes (see Chapter 6, Table 6-7). On admission of the newborn to the nursery, the Apgar score is reviewed to determine any particular difficulties encountered during the birth process. The health care provider's orders are noted. The nurse must observe the newborn *very closely*. Respiratory distress may be evidenced by the rate and character of respirations, color (cyanosis), and general behavior (see Chapter 13). Sternal retractions are reported immediately.

CIRCULATORY SYSTEM

The mother's blood carried essential oxygen to the placenta, which sent it to each cell of the fetus while in the uterus. The health care provider cuts off this supply by severing the umbilical cord. Thereafter the newborn depends on his or her own systemic circulation and pulmonary circulation (see Figure 3-7).

The newborn has approximately 300 mL of circulatory blood volume. The circulation of blood in the fetus differs from that in the newborn in that most fetal blood bypasses the lungs (see Chapter 3). Some of the blood goes from the right atrium to the left atrium of the heart through an opening (the foramen ovale) in the septum. Some passes from the pulmonary artery to the thoracic aorta by way of the ductus arteriosus. These normal openings close soon after birth. If they fail to close, the infant may be cyanotic, because part of the blood continues to bypass the lungs and does not pick up oxygen.

Murmurs are sounds heard when auscultating the heart and are caused by blood leaking through openings that have not yet closed. Murmurs may be functional (innocent) or organic (caused by improper heart formation). Functional murmurs result from blood passing through normal valves. Organic murmurs are caused by blood passing through abnormal openings. The majority of heart murmurs are not serious, but they should be checked periodically to rule out other pathological conditions.

Providing Warmth

The newborn has an unstable heat-regulating system. Body temperature falls immediately after birth, but within a few hours it climbs slowly to a range of 36.6° to 37.2° C (97.8° to 98.9° F), aided by the metabolism of brown adipose tissue (brown fat) and that process is called *nonshivering thermogenesis*. The temperature of the room and the number of blankets covering the infant influence the body temperature of the newborn. The temperature of the nursery, or of the mother's room in the case of rooming-in, is kept at 21° to 24° C (69° to 75° F). The humidity should be between 45% and 55%. The air in the room must be fresh, but there should be no drafts.

The newborn's hands and feet are not used as guides to determine warmth, because the infant's extremities are cooler than the rest of the body. *Acrocyanosis* (*acro*, "extremity," and *cyanosis*, "blue color") is also evident because of sluggish peripheral circulation. The newborn cannot adapt to changes in temperature. The nurse wraps the infant in a blanket whenever the infant leaves the nursery, and the head, which is the largest body surface area, is covered (Skill 12-3). The infant's heat perception is poor, so the nurse must be careful when applying any form of external heat.

Because the sweat glands do not function effectively during the neonatal period, the newborn infant is at risk for developing an elevated temperature if overdressed or if placed in an overheated environment. A red skin rash may develop in response to overheating. A quivering or shivering-like tremor of the chin may be noticed in the newborn but it is evidence of an immature neurological system and not an indication of response to a cold environment. Maintaining body temperature in the newborn is summarized in Figure 12-9. See also Table 9-3.

Obtaining Temperature, Pulse Rate, and Respirations

Some birth facilities recommend that the initial temperature of the newborn be taken by rectum to determine that the rectum is patent. When the temperature is taken rectally, the nurse must be gentle to avoid injuring the rectal mucosa. Daily routine temperatures are taken by axilla. To obtain the axillary temperature, the thermometer is held firmly in the center of the newborn's axilla. During this time, the arm is held against the infant's side. Digital thermometers are read when the indicator sounds.

The newborn's pulse rate and respirations are counted before the temperature is taken because the infant is apt to cry when disturbed. Figure 12-10 illustrates the apical pulse rate being obtained from a newborn infant. The newborn's pulse is irregular and rapid and varies from 110 to 160 beats/min. Blood pressure is low and may vary with the size of the cuff used. The average blood pressure at birth is 80/46 mm Hg. The respirations are approximately 30 to 60 breaths/min. The nurse always reports the following changes:

- Temperature elevated above 37.7° C (99.8° F) or below 36.2° C (97.1° F)
- Pulse rate greater than 160 beats/min or less than 110 beats/min
- Respirations greater than 60 breaths/min or less than 30 breaths/min
- Noisy respirations
- Nasal flaring or chest retraction

MUSCULOSKELETAL SYSTEM

The bones of the newborn are soft, because they are composed mostly of cartilage, in which there is only a small amount of calcium. The skeleton is flexible, and the joints are elastic to accommodate the passage

---

Swaddling the Newborn

PURPOSE

To provide warmth and a sense of security to the newborn

STEPS

1. Place a small blanket flat on the bed in the shape of a diamond, with the top corner folded down slightly.
2. Place the newborn with the shoulders at the upper edge of the blanket. The arm may be placed at the infant's side or positioned so the hand is near the mouth. Wrap the right corner of the blanket around the newborn and tuck it under the left side of the infant. Fold the left corner of the blanket over the newborn and tuck it under the right side of the infant.
3. Pull the bottom of the blanket up to the infant's chest and secure each corner around the newborn and under its back (snugly, not tightly).

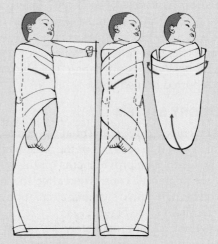

(From Leifer G: *Principles and techniques in pediatric nursing*, ed 4, Philadelphia, 1982, Saunders.)

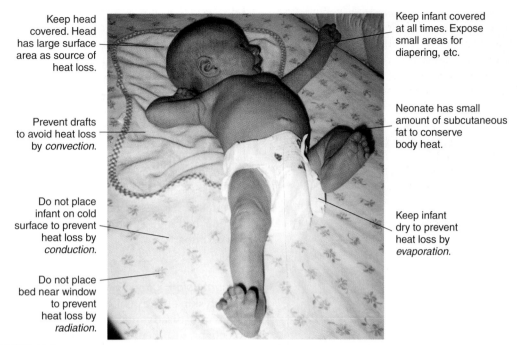

Keep head covered. Head has large surface area as source of heat loss.

Prevent drafts to avoid heat loss by *convection*.

Do not place infant on cold surface to prevent heat loss by *conduction*.

Do not place bed near window to prevent heat loss by *radiation*.

Keep infant covered at all times. Expose small areas for diapering, etc.

Neonate has small amount of subcutaneous fat to conserve body heat.

Keep infant dry to prevent heat loss by *evaporation*.

FIGURE 12-9 Maintaining body temperature of the newborn. Chilling causes "cold stress"—an increased metabolism and oxygen consumption in the neonate—because the infant cannot shiver, as the adult can, to raise body temperature.

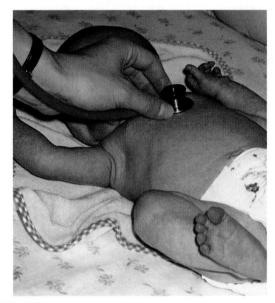

FIGURE 12-10 Assessing an apical pulse. The most accurate method of assessing the heart rate in the neonate is by determining the apical pulse rate.

through the birth canal. Because the bones of the infant are easily molded by pressure, the infant's position must be changed frequently. If the infant lies constantly in one position, the bones of the head can become flattened.

The movements of the newborn are random and uncoordinated. Most newborns appear cross-eyed because their eye muscle coordination is not fully developed. The newborn lacks the muscular control to hold the head steady. The development of muscular control proceeds from head to foot and from the center of the body to the periphery (see the discussion of cephalocaudal and proximodistal control in Chapter 15). Therefore the infant holds the head up before sitting erect. In fact, the head and neck muscles are the first ones to come under control. The newborn's legs are small and short and may appear bowed. There should be no limitation of movement. Fingers clenched in a fist should be separated and observed.

An examination of the newborn for gestational maturity includes checking for the **scarf sign** (see Figure 13-3, *D*). This refers to the full-term infant's resistance to attempts to bring one elbow farther than the midline of the chest. No resistance is observed in the preterm infant.

The infant needs freedom of movement. The infant stretches, sucks, and makes faces and vigorously moves the entire body when crying. Tremors of the lips and extremities during crying are normal. Constant tremors during sleep may be pathological. These are often accompanied by eye movements, are not related to particular stimuli, and should be reported to the health care provider. The morning bath provides excellent opportunities for the newborn to exercise and the nurse to inspect and assess the infant's condition. When handled, the infant should not feel limp. General body proportions are observed in the following section. Bathing is also an excellent form of stimulation for the newborn.

Length and Weight

The length of the average newborn is 46 to 56 cm (19 to 21.5 inches). The weight varies from 2722 to 4082 g (6 to 9 lb). In general, girls weigh a little less than boys. African American, Asian American, and Native American infants may be somewhat smaller. In the first 3 to 4 days

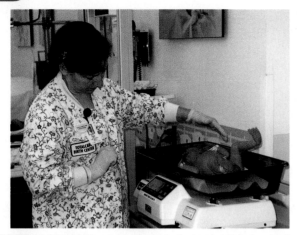

FIGURE 12-11 Weighing the infant. Note the barrier placed under the infant and the nurse's hand held above the infant for safety and protection. The scale used may be a balance scale or digital scale that locks in and displays the weight in kilograms. Some scales enable conversion of kilograms to pounds when the parents request to know the birth weight in pounds. Gloves should be worn when handling a nude infant. (Courtesy Pat Spier, RN-C.)

after birth, the infant loses about 5% to 10% of the birth weight. This loss may be as high as 15% for preterm infants. This may result from withdrawal from maternal hormones, fluid shifts, and the loss of feces and urine. Mothers should be prepared for this and reassured that the weight will normalize after 3 or 4 days and that the infant will regain his or her birth weight by 10 days of age. Newborns are weighed at the same time each day, when morning care is given. (Instructions for measuring and weighing the infant are provided in Figure 12-11 and Chapter 15.)

The weight of the baby *in kilograms* should be recorded on the medical record and reviewed at each hand-off report (AAP, 2013).

GENITOURINARY SYSTEM

The kidneys function at birth but are not fully developed. The glomeruli are small. Renal blood flow is only about one third that of the adult. The ability to handle a water load is reduced, as is the excretion of drugs. The renal tubules are short and have a limited capacity for reabsorbing important substances such as glucose, amino acids, phosphate, and bicarbonate. There is a decrease in the ability to concentrate urine and to cope with fluid imbalances. It is important to note the first voiding of the newborn. This may occur in the delivery room or may not occur for several hours. If voiding does not occur within the first 24 hours, the health care provider is notified. The nurse must keep an accurate record of the frequency of urination. Anuria, changes in color, and any unusual findings are brought to the attention of the health care provider. The newborn should have about six wet diapers per day.

Male Genitalia

The genitalia of the male are developed at birth, although their maturation varies. The testes of the male descend into the scrotum before birth. Occasionally, they remain in the abdomen or the inguinal canal. This condition is called cryptorchidism, or undescended testes, and is described in Chapter 29. With proper surgical treatment, the prognosis is good. The location of the urethral opening should be at the tip of the penis in newborn boys. A white cheesy substance called smegma is found under the foreskin and is thought to be bacteriostatic. The school-age child can be taught to retract the foreskin gently about once a week during routine bathing. Full retraction may not be possible before puberty.

Circumcision. **Circumcision** is the surgical removal of the foreskin on the penis. Circumcision has both advantages and disadvantages. The disadvantages include infection and hemorrhage. Infants with congenital anomalies of the penis, such as *hypospadias* (the opening of the urethra is on the undersurface of the penis), should not be circumcised because the skin may be needed for surgery. The benefits of circumcision include possible prevention of cancer, fewer urinary tract infections, and fewer occurrences of sexually transmitted disease later in life.

A discussion of the pros and cons of this procedure is included as part of prenatal and postpartum education. In 2012 the American Academy of Pediatrics (AAP) position on circumcision stated, "Existing scientific evidence demonstrates potential benefits outweigh the risks for circumcision and further research is needed. Regardless of whether the male is circumcised, at an appropriate age he is taught daily hygiene of the genitalia. This includes special attention to skin folds, retraction and replacement of the foreskin, cleansing of the penis, and examination for lumps or swelling of the penis or the scrotum.

The infant should be physiologically stabilized before circumcision. The newborn is restrained on a circumcision board (Figure 12-12, *A*). The *Gomco clamp* and the *Plastibell clamp* are two devices commonly used for performing circumcisions. If the Gomco clamp is used, a thin layer of petroleum jelly (Vaseline) or petroleum jelly–impregnated gauze may be applied to the end of the penis to protect it from moisture and from sticking to the diaper. The area is observed for bleeding, infection, and irritation. Voidings are recorded.

When a Plastibell clamp is used, the foreskin is tied over a fitted plastic ring and the excess prepuce cut away. The rim usually drops off 5 to 8 days after circumcision. Parents are instructed not to remove it prematurely. No special dressing is required, and the infant is bathed and diapered as usual. A dark brown or black ring encircling the plastic rim is natural.

Families of the Muslim faith also favor circumcision, and it is considered a rite of passage for many African tribes.

The nurse's role in circumcision includes assessing parental knowledge, checking to see that the surgical consent has been signed, and preparing the newborn. The infant is not fed for 1 to 2 hours before the procedure to prevent possible vomiting and aspiration. A bulb syringe is kept handy in case suctioning is required. A light blanket is placed under the infant on the "circ" board, and the diaper is removed. A heat lamp is positioned to prevent cold stress, or the infant may be placed in a radiant warmer. The physician may administer a local anesthetic to minimize pain during the procedure and to prevent irritability and sleep disturbances after it. Additional comfort measures include holding and soothing the infant and using a pacifier or a small amount of sucrose solution. If bleeding occurs, gentle pressure is applied to the site with a sterile gauze pad and the physician is notified. The amount and characteristics of the urinary stream are recorded, because edema could cause an obstruction. Parents should be provided with written instructions concerning the care of the circumcised or uncircumcised penis.

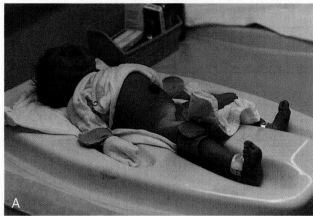
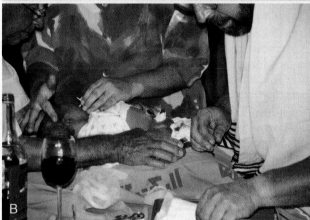

FIGURE 12-12 Circumcision. **A,** A circumcision board is used to restrain the newborn during circumcision in the hospital, which is usually done by the obstetrician without the family present. A eutectic mixture of local anesthetics (EMLA) is a local skin anesthetic that may be used before the procedure. A sucrose-sweetened pacifier is a helpful pain relief measure during this procedure. **B,** A ritual circumcision. In the Jewish faith, a circumcision is called a *bris milah* and is performed at home on the eighth day of life. It is performed by a specially trained individual called a *mohel* (seen in this picture wearing a *tollis*, or religious scarf). The person who restrains the newborn during the procedure is known as the *sandek* (pictured on the left); this honor is often bestowed on an elder in the family. The presence of a minimum of 10 adults is customary, but not required, for the ceremony. A few drops of the wine in the foreground are fed to the newborn by a nipple for pain relief during the procedure. The naming ceremony is often combined with the circumcision ceremony. Understanding and respecting the rituals and traditions of others is an integral part of cultural competence. Written instructions concerning the care of the circumcised penis should be given to the parents in a language they understand. (**A** from Hockenberry MJ, Wilson D, Winkelstein M, Klein ME: *Wong's nursing care of infants and children,* ed 7, St Louis, 2003, Mosby.)

Patient Teaching
Home Care of the Penis

CARE OF THE CIRCUMCISED PENIS
Keep area clean; change diaper.
Wash area with warm water; avoid alcohol-containing wipes.
Do not remove yellow crust from penis.
Apply diaper loosely to prevent pressure.
Report redness and bleeding or drainage.
Observe for at least six wet diapers per day.

CARE OF THE UNCIRCUMCISED PENIS
Avoid forcefully pulling back the foreskin over the glans (retraction).
Wash penis with water. White lumps (smegma) are normal.
At toddler age, gentle retraction after bathing prevents moisture collection; be sure to replace foreskin after retraction.
At school age, the child can be taught to gently retract foreskin for cleansing; this should be done once a week during bathing.
Retraction of the foreskin should never be forced.

This disappears when the rim drops off. Parents are instructed to consult their physician if there are any questions, if there is increased swelling, or if the ring has not fallen off within 8 days; parents should contact their physician immediately if the ring has slipped onto the shaft of the penis. The Jewish religious custom of circumcision, comparable to baptism in the Christian faith, is performed on the eighth day after birth if the newborn's condition permits. The infant usually receives his Hebrew name at that time (see Figure 12-12, *B*).

Female Genitalia
The female genitalia may be slightly swollen. A thin, white or blood-tinged mucus, (pseudomenstruation) may be discharged from the vagina. This discharge is caused by hormonal withdrawal from the mother at birth. The nurse cleanses the vulva **from the urethra to the anus,** using a clean cotton ball or different sections of a washcloth for each stroke to prevent fecal matter from infecting the urinary tract. The importance of this is stressed to parents.

INTEGUMENTARY SYSTEM

Skin

Tissue turgor refers to the hydration or dehydration of the skin. To test tissue turgor (elasticity), the nurse gently grasps and releases the skin (Figure 12-13). It should spring back to place immediately in the well-hydrated infant. When the skin remains distorted ("tented"), tissue turgor is considered poor.

The skin of newborn Caucasian infants is red to dark pink. The skin of African American infants is reddish brown. Infants of Latin descent may appear to have an olive or yellowish tint. The body is usually covered with fine hair called **lanugo**, which tends to disappear during the first week of life. This is more evident in premature infants. **Vernix caseosa**, a cheeselike substance that covers the skin of the newborn, is made of cells and glandular secretions; it is thought to protect the skin from irritation and the effects of a watery environment in utero (Figure 12-14). White pinpoint "pimples" caused by the obstruction of sebaceous glands may be seen on the nose and chin. These are called **milia** and

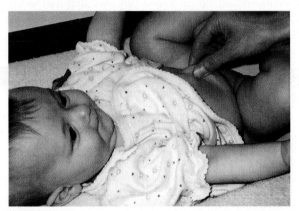

FIGURE 12-13 Testing tissue turgor. The term turgor refers to the elasticity of the skin, which is affected by the extent of hydration. The nurse tests skin turgor by gently grasping the skin. When the skin is released, it should instantly spring back into place; if it does not, tissue turgor is considered poor.

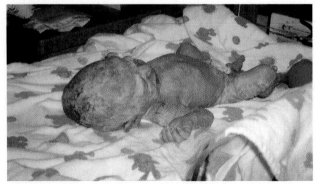

FIGURE 12-14 Vernix is the thick, white, cheesy substance covering the skin of the newborn. Preterm newborns are heavily covered in vernix, whereas postterm newborns have little vernix protection on their skin. Note the heavy covering of vernix on this newborn.

disappear within a few weeks. Lesions on the midline of the hard palate of the milia type are called **Epstein's pearls** and are caused by a collection of epithelial cells. Stork bites (telangiectatic nevi) are flat, red areas seen on the nape of the neck and on the eyelids. They result from the dilation of small vessels. See Table 12-3 for other skin manifestations seen in the newborn.

Mongolian spots, which are bluish discolorations of the skin, are common in infants of African American, Native American, and Mediterranean descent. They are usually found over the sacral and gluteal areas (see Table 12-3). They disappear spontaneously during the early years of life. Mongolian spots can be differentiated from a hematoma resulting from abuse, because the hematoma will change color each day, but the Mongolian spot remains the same color and hue for years.

Acrocyanosis, or peripheral blueness of the hands and feet, is normal and results from poor peripheral circulation. The hands or feet should not be used to determine general body warmth in the newborn. Central body areas are not cyanotic in normal newborns. Pallor is not normal and should be reported because it may indicate neonatal anemia or another more serious condition.

Desquamation, or peeling of the skin, occurs during the early weeks of life. Skin in areas such as the nose, knees, elbows, and toes may break down because of friction from rubbing against the sheets. The involved area is kept dry, and the infant's position is changed frequently. The buttocks need special attention. A wet diaper should be changed immediately to prevent chafing. The buttocks are washed and dried well.

Physiological jaundice, also called **icterus neonatorum**, is characterized by a yellow tinge of the skin. It is caused by the rapid destruction of excess red blood cells, which the infant does not need now because he or she is in an atmosphere that contains more oxygen than was available during prenatal life. Plasma levels of bilirubin increase from a normal 1 mg/dL to an average of 5 to 6 mg/dL between the second and fourth days (Table 12-2). Physiological jaundice becomes evident between the second and the third days of life and lasts for about 1 week. This is a normal process and is not harmful to the infant. However, genetic and ethnic factors may affect its severity, resulting in pathological hyperbilirubinemia. Evidence of jaundice is reported and charted, and the newborn is evaluated frequently to ensure safety (Skill 12-4).

Table **12-2** Changing Laboratory Values			
	NEWBORN	**7 DAYS**	**3 MONTHS**
Hemoglobin (Hgb) (g/dL)	18.5	17	11.3
Hematocrit (Hct)	56	44	35
White blood cell count (WBC)/mm³	18,000	12,000	10,800
Bilirubin (mg/dL)	6	12	1

Assessing for Jaundice

PURPOSE

To determine if a blood test for bilirubin level is indicated

STEPS

1. Observe skin in a well-lit room.
2. Press skin over the nose or sternum with the thumb until the skin blanches (lightens).
3. Observe the level of jaundice. (NOTE: There is a cephalocaudal progression of jaundice in term infants. As the bilirubin level increases, the jaundice progresses from the head toward the feet (Kliegman, 2011).
4. Jaundice seen below the sternum or present in the arms, lower abdomen, or feet may indicate that a serum bilirubin test is required (Kliegman, 2011).

Two commonly used methods to assess jaundice are the following:

1. *Icterometer:* The icterometer is a plastic strip with increasingly deeper yellow stripes representing levels of jaundice. The strip is placed against the infant's nose until the skin blanches. The underlying skin tone is matched to the corresponding shade of yellow.
2. *Transcutaneous bilirubin measurement (TcB):* Transcutaneous measurement of jaundice is noninvasive. The U.S. Food and Drug Administration (FDA) has approved the Colormate III bilirubinometer as a screening device to determine whether a more accurate blood test or follow-up is indicated. The machine is unaffected by the level of melanin in the skin (Maisels et al, 2004). Jaundice is discussed further in Chapter 13.

Table 12-3 discusses nursing interventions for common skin manifestations of the newborn infant.

> **Safety Alert!**
>
> Jaundice that appears in the first day of life is not normal and should be recorded and reported.

The Interactive Bath

Initial skin care after the newborn is stable involves washing blood, amniotic fluid, and excessive vernix from the skin. Until the infant's first bath and shampoo, the nurse wears gloves when handling the newborn (Skill 12-5). The bath provides an opportunity for teaching as well as assessment of the infant and infant–parent interaction. The nurse should emphasize certain basic principles of care such as hand hygiene, cleansing the tub, organizing supplies to be within easy reach, safe water temperature, and techniques for holding the wet infant securely.

Principles of eye and ear care are reviewed. Cotton swabs should not be inserted into the ear or the nose. Alkaline soaps, oils, and lotions are not advised as they can alter the normal pH of the newborn's skin, making it vulnerable to bacterial infection. Powders should be avoided because of the high risk of aspiration of small particles. Some health care providers advise giving sponge baths until the cord falls off and heals (about 1 to 2 weeks), but tub baths are acceptable. The infant need only be bathed 2 or 3 times a week using plain warm water during the neonatal period. Daily bathing with soap and water is no longer recommended (Association of Women's Health, Obstetric and Neonatal Nurses [AWHONN], 2007). The bath is an excellent time to provide basic hygiene and to observe the naked newborn for behavior, muscle activity, and general well-being.

The temperature of the bath water should be approximately 37.8° C (100° F) in a warm room environment at 24° to 27° C (75° to 80° F). Special care should be taken to keep the infant covered to prevent chilling. Parents should be taught to start bathing the face and then proceed in a cephalocaudal (head-to-toe) direction, turning the surface of the washcloth as the bath progresses. The eyes should be cleansed with a moist cotton ball from the inner canthus to the outer canthus, using a clean cotton ball for each eye. The genitalia should be cleansed with a front-to-back motion to prevent urinary tract infection.

The nurse may wrap the infant in a towel and use a football hold to shampoo the hair. The shampooing is administered last because the large surface area of the head predisposes the infant to heat loss. Observing the cues and responses of the infant to the warmth of the water and the touch of the washcloth, drying, and dressing are discussed with the parent in relation to opportunities to promote parent–infant bonding during the bath experience. The general principles of the infant bath should be explained to parents to foster good techniques at home. Cord care is discussed in Chapter 9 (see Skill 9-6).

> 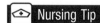 **Nursing Tip**
>
> The infant bath provides not only cleaning but an opportunity to assess and bond.

Table 12-3	Common Skin Manifestations of the Newborn	
	APPEARANCE	**INTERVENTION**
Acrocyanosis 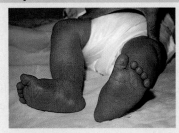	Cyanosis of the hands and feet in the first week of life is caused by a combination of a high hemoglobin level and vasomotor instability.	Parent education concerning this normal phenomenon is helpful.
Cutis Marmorata 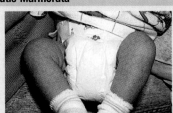	Lacelike red or blue pattern on the skin surface of a newborn's body	Normal vasomotor response to low environmental temperature. Wrap infant warmly. Intense or persistent appearance should be reported.
Desquamation 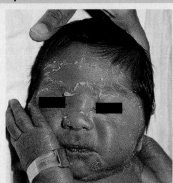	Peeling of the skin at birth may indicate postmaturity. Early removal of vernix can be followed by desquamation in term newborns.	Instruct parents to avoid harsh soaps. Some hospitals do not vigorously remove vernix from the skin of newborns.
Epstein's Pearls 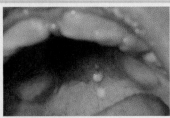	Pearly white pinpoint papules in midline of upper palate	Distinguish from a thrush lesion (see Chapter 28).
Erythema Toxicum 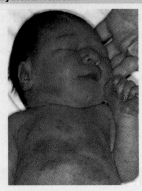	Splotchy erythema with firm yellow-white papules that have a red base	Can occur at age 2 days; no intervention is required because erythema will spontaneously clear.

Continued

Table 12-3 Common Skin Manifestations of the Newborn—cont'd

	APPEARANCE	INTERVENTION
Forceps Marks		
	Bruised area on skin in the shape of forceps or pattern of vacuum extractor	Bruising and swelling fade within a few days and do not necessitate intervention other than parental support and teaching.
Harlequin Color Change		
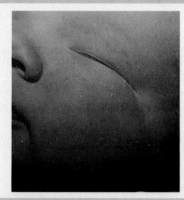	Imbalance of autonomic vascular regulatory mechanism; deep red color over half of body; pallor on the longitudinal half of body; usually occurs with preterm infants who are placed on their sides	Phenomenon disappears with muscular activity. Changing position of infant is helpful. Condition is temporary and does not usually indicate a problem.
Milia		
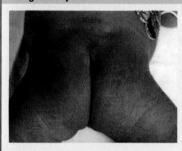	Pearly white pinpoint papules on face and nose of newborn	No treatment. Will spontaneously disappear. Educate parents not to attempt to "squeeze out" the white material because infection can occur.
Mongolian Spots		
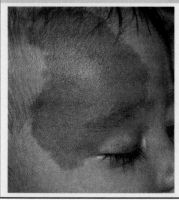	Dark blue or slate grey discolorations most commonly found in lumbosacral area; intensity and hue of color remain until fading occurs	Caused by melanin deposits in dark-skinned persons and will gradually disappear in a few years. Nurse must distinguish these lesions from hematoma of child abuse.
Nevi		
	Known as *stork bites;* pink, easily blanched patches that can appear on eyelids, nose, lips, and nape of neck (see Chapter 30)	Marks gradually fade and are of no clinical significance.
Port-Wine Stain		
	Known as *nevus flammeus;* a collection of capillaries in the skin. It is a flat, red-purple lesion that does not blanch on pressure.	This is a permanent skin marking that darkens with age and can become elevated and vulnerable to injury. If a large area of face or neck is involved, laser surgery may be indicated to preserve the child's self-image. Can be associated with genetic disorders.

(Unnumbered figures 1, 2, 3, 6: from Eichenfield LF, Friden IJ, Esterly NB: *Textbook of neonatal dermatology,* Philadelphia, 2001, Saunders; unnumbered figures 4 and 7: from Zitelli BJ et al: *Atlas of pediatric physical diagnosis,* ed 6, St Louis, 2012, Mosby; unnumbered figure 5: from Swartz MH: *Textbook of physical diagnosis,* ed 5, Philadelphia, 2006, Saunders; unnumbered figure 8: from Murray SS, McKinney ES: *Foundations of maternal-newborn and women's health nursing,* ed 6, St Louis, 2014, Saunders; unnumbered figure 9: from Swartz MH: *Textbook of physical diagnosis,* ed 7, Philadelphia, 2014, Saunders.)

Bathing the Newborn

PURPOSE

To cleanse the skin and interact with the newborn

A sponge bath may be given until the umbilical cord site and circumcision site are healed; however, tub baths can be given before the cord falls off without risk of infection (Association of Women's Health, Obstetric and Neonatal Nurses [AWHONN], 2007).

- Give bath between feedings at most convenient time for baby and family.
- Complete baths are not necessary more than two or three times a week because specific areas are washed after diaper changes and when milk is spit up.
- After the bath, the baby will likely want to sleep.
- A bath should not be given immediately after feeding, because excessive handling may cause regurgitation.
- Carefully wash and dry each area to prevent heat loss.
- Keep the baby warm by exposing only the area you are washing.

STEPS

Sponge Bath

1. Test bath water. (It should be approximately 37.2° to 38° C [99° to 100.4° F]). A bath thermometer should be used; many have preset temperature alerts.
2. Proceed from the cleanest to the most soiled area of the body: from eyes and face to the trunk and extremities and finally to the diaper area. Shampooing the hair is always done last to prevent excessive heat loss from the head.
   a. Wash the baby's face with clear water. Use a separate clean area of the washcloth (or use cotton ball) to wipe each eyelid. Use a clean area to wash outer ear (do not put anything inside ear or nose).
   b. Wash behind ears, where milk that is spit up may accumulate.
   c. If necessary, clean nose with a clean corner of the washcloth.
   d. Put hand under the baby's shoulders and lift slightly. This allows the creases of the neck to be washed.
   e. Wash the vulva of a female newborn by wiping from front to back to prevent contamination of the vagina or urethra by rectal content. In the male newborn, do not force back the foreskin of the uncircumcised penis. Clean the penis and scrotal area gently. It is important to clean under the scrotum and the folds of the scrotum.
   f. The easiest way to wash the hair is to hold the baby (wrapped in a towel to prevent chilling) in one arm using the football hold over the basin of water. Soap hair and rinse by pouring water from a container over the head. Then dry hair to prevent chilling.

Tub Bath

1. Use a plastic tub or a clean sink for the bath.
2. Place a small blanket or pad at the bottom of the tub for comfort and to prevent slipping.
3. Place approximately 3 to 4 inches of warm water in the tub. The water temperature should be 36.6° to 37.2° C (98° to 99° F).
4. Using a clean, dampened washcloth, wash eyes and face with plain water.
5. Place the baby in the tub. The baby may seem frightened and cry when first put in the water. Holding the baby securely and talking with a soft voice will often help baby adjust to the bath, which is a new experience.
6. Be sure all soap is rinsed off the baby before removing him or her from the tub.
7. Remove newborn from the tub and immediately wrap in a dry towel.
8. With the baby wrapped in a towel and held in a football hold, gently shampoo the hair; rinse thoroughly with warm water and dry with a clean towel.

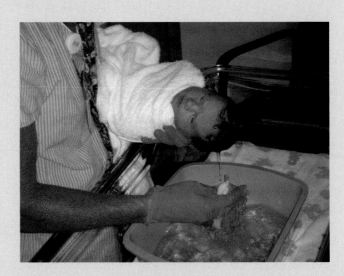

GASTROINTESTINAL SYSTEM

Stools

The intestinal tract functions as an outlet for amniotic fluid as early as the fifth month of fetal life. The normal functions of the gastrointestinal tract begin after birth. Food is digested and absorbed into the blood, and waste products are eliminated. **Meconium**, the first stool, is a mixture of amniotic fluid and secretions of the intestinal glands. It is dark greenish black, thick, and sticky (tarry) and is passed 8 to 24 hours after birth. The stools gradually change during the first week. They become loose and are greenish yellow with mucus. These are called *transitional stools* (Figure 12-15).

The stools of a breastfed infant are bright yellow, soft, and pasty. There may be three to six stools a day. The number of stools decreases with age. The bowel movements of a bottle-fed infant are more solid than those of the breastfed infant. They vary from yellow to brown and are generally fewer in number. There may be one to four a day at first, but this gradually decreases to one or two a day. The stools are darker when an infant is receiving oral iron supplements, and they are green when an infant is under the phototherapy lamp. Small, puttylike stools or diarrhea and bloody stools are abnormal. When there is a question, the nurse saves the stool specimen for the physician to observe. The nurse keeps an accurate

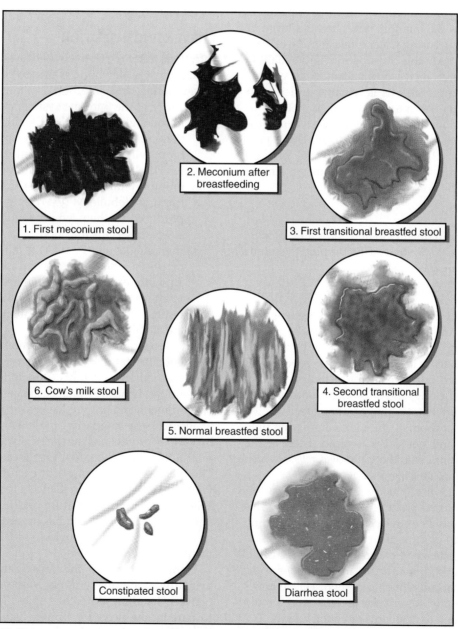

FIGURE 12-15 The normal infant stool cycle. The first meconium is dark, black, and tarry. It gradually changes to a greenish yellow transitional stool. The breastfed infant's "milk" stool is golden yellow, whereas the bottle-fed infant has a pale yellow stool. A green, watery stool is indicative of diarrhea and should be reported to the health care provider. (Redrawn from Clinical Education Aid #3. Courtesy Ross Laboratories, Columbus, Ohio, 1978.)

record of the number and characteristics of stools that each newborn passes daily.

Constipation

Constipation refers to the passage of hard dry stools. Newborns differ in regularity. Some pass a soft stool every other day. This is not constipation. The nurse explains to parents that straining in the newborn period results from undeveloped abdominal musculature. This is normal, and no treatment is required. In the first month of life, a breastfed infant will pass at least four stools a day. After the second month of life, the infant will increase stool volume and decrease stool frequency. Even if 5 to 6 days pass without a stool, it is not considered constipation if the stool passed is large in volume and soft or pasty in character. Constipation is sometimes seen as the infant matures and if a formula change is made. Increasing water intake may be all that is necessary to remedy this constipation. If the infant is eating solid foods, an increased intake of fruits, vegetables, and whole-grain cereals is usually sufficient to help the situation. The nurse encourages mothers to telephone their health care provider's office when questions arise and to ask to speak to the nurse. This is particularly emphasized for new mothers, who may be afraid of appearing "ignorant." Very often a simple solution can relieve hours of anxiety.

Hiccoughs

Hiccoughs appear frequently in newborns and are normal. Most disappear spontaneously. Burping the infant and offering warm water may help.

Digestion

Breastfeeding and formula feeding are discussed in Chapters 9 and 16. Breastfed infants may be put to the breast in the first hour after delivery for psychological benefits and to help stimulate milk production. Bottle feedings are begun in about 5 hours. Crying, restlessness, fist sucking, and an evident rooting reflex give evidence to an infant's hunger. The capacity of the infant's stomach is about 90 mL (3 oz). Emptying time is 2 to 3 hours, and peristalsis is rapid. Feeding the newborn often stimulates the *gastrocolic reflex*, which results in the infant passing a stool.

The immature cardiac sphincter of the stomach causes the young infant to be prone to regurgitation. For this reason parents should be educated to avoid overfeeding their infant and to position the infant on the right side after feeding. Deficiency of pancreatic enzymes such as lipase limits fat absorption. Breast milk contains some lipase enzyme that aids infant digestion. Whole cow's milk does not contain this enzyme and therefore should not be fed undiluted to newborns or young infants.

The salivary glands do not secrete saliva until the infant is age 2 to 3 months. Drooling in the newborn is considered a sign of pathological disturbance and should be reported. The liver is immature, especially in its ability to conjugate bilirubin, regulate blood glucose, and coagulate blood.

Vitamins

Infants need extra vitamins C and D. Breast milk contains sufficient vitamin C if the mother's diet is rich in citrus fruits and certain vegetables. Vitamin D may be added to commercial milk (labeled "vitamin D milk") that the mother consumes. Commercial concentrated vitamin preparations may also be prescribed. The fluid is drawn up in the dropper to the prescribed amount (0.3 or 0.6 mL) and is placed directly in the infant's mouth. This is done at approximately the same time each morning to prevent forgetting the vitamins.

PREVENTING INFECTION

Infections that are relatively harmless to an adult may be fatal to the newborn. The newborn's response to inflammation and infection is slow because of the immaturity of the immune system, as follows:

- Immunoglobulin G (IgG) is an immunoglobulin that crosses the placenta and provides the newborn with passive immunity to infections to which the mother was immune. This type of immunity rarely lasts longer than 3 months.
- Immunoglobulin M (IgM) is an immunoglobulin produced by the newborn, and an elevated level suggests serious infection.
- Immunoglobulin A (IgA) is an immunoglobulin produced after the neonatal period (about age 1 month) that is contained in breast milk and provides some resistance to respiratory and gastrointestinal infections. Before 1 month of age, infants are at risk for such infections.

An open wound (such as the umbilical cord) can be a portal of entry for infection. Measures to prevent infections in the newborn nursery include using standard precautions, hand washing, cleansing and replacement of equipment, and proper disposal of soiled diapers and linens. Nursery standards are developed and enforced by various professional agencies, such as the AAP, hospital accreditation boards, and local health agencies. The infection control nurse in each hospital also provides education and surveillance. Provisions governing space, control of temperature and humidity, lighting, and safety from fire and other hazards are also considered. Each newborn has an individual crib, bath equipment, and linen supply.

Hand washing is the most reliable precaution available. The nursery nurse washes his or her hands between handling different babies. The nurse stresses to parents the need for proper hand washing in the home. In many hospitals, nursery personnel wear clean scrub gowns while in the nursery for the purpose of infection control and/or security. Health care providers, technicians, and other nonnursery personnel wear cover gowns when entering the nursery and when handling infants.

Health examination of personnel before employment minimizes the spread of infection by unhealthy persons. The nurse who has signs of a cold, earache, skin infection, or intestinal upset should not work in the nursery or care for ill children. Visitors are instructed not to come to the hospital or be around hospital patients if they are not feeling well.

> ### ! Safety Alert!
> The nurse must adhere to standard precautions while working in the delivery room and/or nursery. These guidelines are of particular importance during the initial care of the newborn when exposure to secretions, blood, and amniotic fluid is high.

DISCHARGE PLANNING AND PARENT TEACHING

Discharge teaching ideally begins with the admission of the woman to the hospital or birthing center. Many hospitals have flow sheets that are helpful in ensuring that all topics have been addressed and that patients understand what has been explained to them. Areas of teaching include the following:

- Basic care of the infant, including bathing, cord care, circumcision care, feeding, and elimination
- Safety measures including position for sleep
- Immunizations
- Support groups, such as La Leche League
- Return appointments for well-baby care
- Telephone number of nursery (note 24-hour availability)
- Proper use of car safety seats (see Figure 9-15)
- Signs and symptoms of problems and who to contact; for example, temperature greater than 38° C (100.4° F) by axilla, refusal of two feedings in a row, two green watery stools, frequent or forceful vomiting, lack of voiding or stooling

The nurse should guide the parents in assessing, bathing, and feeding the newborn so that questions can be answered early and parents can demonstrate understanding of skills and behaviors. Clinical Pathway 12-1 specifies nursing interventions for assisting the mother, the parents, or other caregivers in caring for the infant before and after discharge from the hospital.

Home Care
Feeding. Feeding the newborn is discussed in Chapter 9.

Furnishings. It helps if the newborn has a separate room or a separate area within a room. Simple, durable, easy-to-clean furnishings are necessary. A crib

with a firm mattress is a suitable place for the infant to sleep. Crib slats should adhere to safety standards. Mattress covers are usually waterproof. Fitted sheets are convenient, and blankets of lightweight cotton are warm and easy to launder. For safety reasons, a pillow should not be placed in the crib of the newborn.

> ### ! Safety Alert!
> Instruct parents about the danger of suffocation if the infant sleeps in the same bed with the parents.

Pictures should be attached securely to the wall with wall tape. The growing child may swallow thumbtacks. A chest of drawers for clothing, an adult chair (preferably a rocker), and a flat-topped table for changing clothes are necessary. A plastic basin may be used for the first few months to bathe the infant. A tray containing frequently used articles saves time and energy. These items might include a digital thermometer, hairbrush and comb, baby wipes, and baby lotion. A separate linen hamper for the infant's clothes and a closed receptacle for soiled diapers are also necessary.

Clothing. Clothing must be soft, washable, of the proper size, and easy to put on and take off. Parents are instructed to launder new clothing and sheets before using them to prevent skin irritation. Use of nightgowns with drawstring necks is avoided because they may lead to strangulation. Buttons must be sewn on tightly. Snaps or Velcro fasteners are safer. If the mother does not have a clothes dryer, she needs a clothes rack to dry the infant's garments during inclement weather.

Disposable diapers are most commonly used in hospitals and homes. They have an outer waterproof layer. Diapers made of gauze, knitted cotton, or bird's-eye or cotton flannel are available in contoured shapes or prefolded styles. However, they take longer to dry when laundered at home and are more costly. Diaper liners are specially treated tissues placed within the cloth diaper. When diapers are soiled, the liner and stool are rinsed into the toilet. The diapers are soaked in cold water, washed with a mild laundry soap, rinsed thoroughly, and dried by a clothes dryer or outdoors in the sun. Diapers that have been improperly washed and rinsed may aggravate rashes. If a rash is present, the buttocks are kept exposed to the air as often as possible. Diapers are changed as soon as they are wet. If a rash becomes increasingly worse, the health care provider is consulted.

The quantity of items that the mother needs is determined by her washing facilities and the climate of the area in which she lives. Figure 12-16 shows how the diaper is folded so that the edge is below the

Clinical Pathway 12-1

Documentation Codes

Initial = Meets standard

★ = Exception on pathways identified

C = Chronic problems

N/A = Not applicable

Patient/Family Problems

1. Thermoregulation
2. Nutrition
3. Parent-infant attachment
4. Potential alteration in newborn metabolism
5. Risk for infection
6. Infant safety
7. _____
8. _____

CLINICAL PATHWAY	DATE AND TIME	EXPECTED PATIENT/FAMILY OUTCOMES	MULTIDISCIPLINARY ASSESSMENT	TESTS	CONSULT	TREATMENTS	MEDICATIONS	NUTRITION	EDUCATION AND DISCHARGE PLANNING
Immediate Newborn Care		Apgar score >7 at 5 min [4]	Apgar score 1 and 5 min	Hypoglycemia protocol when indicated		Clamp cord	Neonatal eye prophylaxis and AquaMEPHYTON	Determine if bottle feeding or breastfeeding	Initiate safety and security measures with parent(s)/family
		Maintains axillary temp of 36.5°–37.2° C while in radiant warmer or in double blankets [1]	Transitional newborn assessment q 30 min			Dry newborn	HBIG if indicated	Assist with initial breastfeeding	Teach breastfeeding mother proper latch
		Physiological parameters WNL [4]	Suck reflex			Radiant warmer or double blanket while being held until temp stable			
		Demonstrates proper latch response when breastfeeding [2]				ID bands			
Newborn Admission		Maintains axillary temp of 36.5°–37.2° C while in radiant warmer or in double blankets [1]	Weight	Hypoglycemia protocol when indicated		Cord care		Initial feeding:	
		Physiological parameters WNL [4]	V/S q 30 min × 4			Admission bath			
		Tolerates initial feeding [2]	Multisystem admission assessment						
		Mother's blood type O/Rh negative	Suck reflex						
Day of Birth		NDE	NDE	NDE	NDE	NDE	NDE	NDE	NDE
		Maintains axillary temp of 36.5°–37.2° C independent of external heat source [1]	Temp, apical pulse, neuro, cardiac, resp, GI, GU, integumentary q shift	Hypoglycemia protocol when indicated	Social service consult if indicated	Cord care		Breast/bottle feed on demand (breast: q 2-3 hr; bottle: q 3-4 hr)	Reinforce safety and security measures with parent(s)/family
		Parent(s)/family verbalize understanding of safety and security measures [6]	Parent/infant attachment			Circumcision care when indicated			Observe and reinforce proper latch and instruct breastfeeding mother/family in alternative positioning
		Physiological parameters WNL [4]	Positioning and LATCH score of breastfed newborn						Give and review new pamphlets:
		Parent(s)/family and infant demonstrate attachment behaviors [3]	Frequency and amount of bottle feeding						• Message to mothers
		Feeding [2]							• Newborn screening
		LATCH score is 7 or greater for breastfed newborn [2]							• Car seat
		No jaundice [4]							• Health insurance for newborns
		Infant seen by physician within 12 hours [6]							• Preparing formula
									• Breastfeeding: A Guide for Success

Continued

Clinical Pathway 12-1

CLINICAL PATHWAY	DATE AND TIME	EXPECTED PATIENT/FAMILY OUTCOMES	MULTIDISCIPLINARY ASSESSMENT	TESTS	CONSULT	TREATMENTS	MEDICATIONS	NUTRITION	EDUCATION AND DISCHARGE PLANNING
Day 1		NDE ☐ Maintains axillary temp of 36.5°-37.2° C independent of external heat source [1] ☐ Parent(s)/family and newborn demonstrate attachment behaviors [3] ☐ Physiological parameters WNL [4] ☐ Feeding [2] LATCH score 7 or greater for breastfed newborn [2] ☐ No jaundice [4] ☐ No signs of infection [5]	NDE ☐ Temp, apical pulse, cardiac, resp, neuro, GI, GU, integumentary q 8 hr ☐ N/A N/A Weight ☐ Parent(s)/family and infant attachment behaviors ☐ LATCH score of breastfed newborn ☐ Frequency and amount of bottle feeding	NDE ☐	NDE ☐ Referral made to lactation consultant for LATCH score <7 ☐	NDE ☐ N/A N/A Cord care Circumcision care when indicated ☐	NDE ☐	NDE ☐ Breast/bottle feed on demand (breast: q 2-3 hr; bottle: q 3-4 hr)	NDE ☐ Observe return demonstration: • Breastfeeding mother's use of alternative positioning • Infant's suck, swallow ☐ Observe parent (s) providing appropriate newborn care; reinforce ☐
Day 2		NDE ☐ Maintains axillary temp of 36.5°-37.2° C independent of external heat source [1] ☐ Parent(s)/family and newborn demonstrate attachment behaviors [3] ☐ Physiological parameters WNL [4] ☐ Feeding [2] LATCH score 7 or greater for breastfed newborn [2] ☐ No jaundice [4] ☐ No signs of infection [5]	NDE ☐ Temp, apical pulse, cardiac, resp, neuro, GI, GU, integumentary q 8 hr ☐ N/A N/A Weight ☐ Parent(s)/family and infant attachment behaviors ☐ LATCH score of breastfed newborn ☐ Frequency and amount of bottle feeding	NDE ☐	NDE ☐ Referral made to lactation consultant for LATCH score <7 ☐	NDE ☐ N/A N/A Cord care Circumcision care when indicated ☐	NDE ☐	NDE ☐ Breast/bottle feed on demand (breast: q 2-3 hr; bottle: q 3-4 hr)	NDE ☐ Observe return demonstration: • Breastfeeding mother's use of alternative positioning • Infant's suck, swallow ☐ Observe parent (s) providing appropriate newborn care; reinforce ☐

Continued

303

Clinical Pathway 12-1

CLINICAL PATHWAY	DATE AND TIME	EXPECTED PATIENT/FAMILY OUTCOMES	MULTIDISCIPLINARY ASSESSMENT	TESTS	CONSULT	TREATMENTS	MEDICATIONS	NUTRITION	EDUCATION AND DISCHARGE PLANNING
Discharge		☐ Maintains axillary temp of 36.5°–37.2° C independent of external heat source [1] ☐ Parent(s)/family and newborn demonstrate attachment behaviors and appropriate care of newborn [3] ☐ Physiological parameters WNL [4] ☐ Circumcision without bleeding [5] ☐ Voided at least × 1 [4] ☐ Stooled at least × 1 [4] ☐ Feeding [2] ☐ LATCH score 7 or greater for breastfed newborn [2] ☐ Parent(s)/family verbalize newborn discharge instructions [6] ☐ No jaundice [4] ☐ Physician aware of Coombs results ☐ Discharge Day 2 ☐ No signs of infection	☐ Temp, apical pulse, cardiac, resp, neuro, GI, GU, integumentary q 8 hr ☐ Weight ☐ Parent(s)/family and infant attachment behaviors ☐ LATCH score of breastfed newborn ☐ Frequency and amount of bottle feeding	☐ Newborn screening tests before discharge ____	☐ Referral made to lactation consultant for LATCH score <7 ☐ ____	☐ Cord care ☐ Circumcision care when indicated ☐ Cord clamp removed before discharge	☐ Hepatitis B vaccine per order ____ ☐	☐ NPO for circumcision when indicated ☐ Breast/bottle feed on demand (breast: q 2-3 hr; bottle: q 3-4 hr)	☐ Review discharge instructions with parent(s)/family ☐ Discuss plan for follow-up care ☐ Discharge to mother's care
Name		**Initials**		**Name**		**Initials**		**Name**	**Initials**

An example of a clinical pathway for a newborn from birth to discharge on the second day. This is used by all caregivers to plan and document care. (Courtesy Women's and Children's Services of the York Health System, York, PA. Modified with permission.)

NOTE: Each patient requires an individual assessment and treatment plan. This clinical pathway is a recommendation for the average patient that requires modification when necessary by the professional staff.

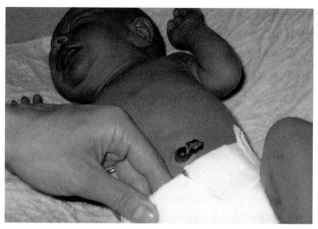

FIGURE 12-16 Note that the diaper is folded so that it does not touch the umbilical cord stump. The umbilical cord stump is kept dry and it usually falls off between 8 and 10 days after delivery.

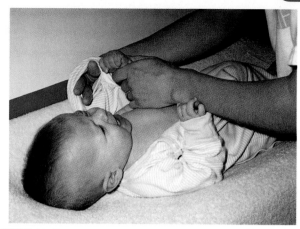

FIGURE 12-17 Dressing the newborn. The simplest technique of dressing the newborn is to place the hand through the sleeve, grasp the infant's hand, and gently pull it through the sleeve.

umbilical cord stump to keep the cord clean and dry. Figure 12-17 illustrates the simplest way to dress the newborn.

The social service department may be of help in ensuring that the home environment is satisfactory and that any special needs of the infant or parent are met. The home health nurse is a key member of the interdisciplinary health care team who can help with after-discharge needs of the family.

Unfolding Case Study

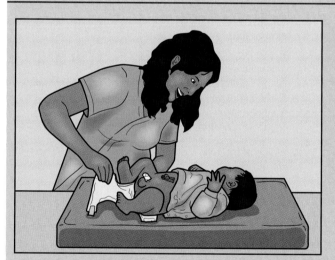

Tess and her husband Luis were introduced to the reader in Chapter 4, and each chapter has followed Tess through her labor and delivery. She has delivered twins and their daughter, Sofia, was admitted to the NICU accompanied by Luis. (Sofia will be discussed in Chapter 14.) After 1 hour in the delivery room, their son Marco is admitted to the postpartum unit with Tess.

Baby Marco's weight is 3.19 kg and he has had one black-green tarry stool and one void since delivery. The cord clamp is in place and the umbilical cord stump is clean and dry. He is circumcised at 12 hours of age and returned to the postpartum

room with his mother Tess. Tess says she is unsure how to care for the surgical site at home.

QUESTIONS
1. What are the general principles of care of the newly circumcised penis that the nurse can explain to the mother?
2. What can the nurse tell Tess about the normal changes in the appearance of her infant's stool that she will see in the next week when she is at home?
3. What will the nurse tell Tess about the care of the umbilical cord when she is at home? How should Tess modify the diapering technique while the umbilical cord stump is still in place?
4. Baby Marco's weight is documented in kilograms. Tess is only interested in how many pounds her infant weighs. Why is it necessary to record the weight in kilograms instead of just pounds and ounces?
5. Tess is worried that she will not have enough breast milk for the twins. How can she tell if the infants are receiving enough breast milk when they are discharged at home?
6. Tess states that Marco must be cold because she sees his chin quiver and his hands are a bit blue so she wants to delay bathing the baby. What can the nurse teach Tess about her baby's quivering chin, his blue hands, and how often baths should be given to newborn infants?

Get Ready for the NCLEX® Examination!

Key Points

- Assessment of the newborn includes gestational age, weight and length measurements, reflexes, system assessment, and bonding with parents.
- Heat loss occurs in the newborn via conduction, convection, evaporation, and radiation.
- The newborn is born with certain reflexes. Three of these are the Moro reflex, the rooting reflex, and the tonic neck reflex.
- The Apgar score is a standardized method of evaluating the newborn's condition at 1 and 5 minutes after delivery. Five objective signs are measured: heart rate, respirations, muscle tone, reflexes, and color.
- The most critical period for the newborn is the first hour of life, when the drastic change from life within the uterus to life outside it takes place.
- Physiological jaundice becomes evident after the second and third days of life and lasts for about 1 week.
- The newborn has an unstable heat-regulating system and must be kept warm.
- Although the kidneys function at birth, they are not fully developed. Likewise, the immune system is not fully activated.
- Vernix caseosa is a cheeselike substance that covers the skin of the newborn at birth.
- Meconium, the first stool of the newborn, is a mixture of amniotic fluid and secretions of the intestinal glands. These stools change in color from tarry greenish black, to greenish yellow (transitional stools), to yellow gold (milk stools).
- Proper hand washing is essential for preventing infection in newborn infants.
- Nursery standards are developed and enforced by various professional agencies.
- The hydration status of newborns can be evaluated by determining the number and consistency of stools, frequency of voiding, appearance of sunken fontanelles, and status of tissue turgor.
- The normal newborn infant will lose about 10% of the birth weight in the first few days of life but will return to the birth weight by the age of 10 days.
- The fontanelles are spaces between the skull bones of the newborn that allow for molding and provide space for the brain to grow. They are known as "soft spots" on the infant's head.
- Caput succedaneum is edema of the infant's scalp that occurs during the birth process.
- Cephalohematoma is a collection of blood under the periosteum of a cranial bone. The swelling does not cross the suture lines of the skull bones.
- The goal of the infant bath is to cleanse the skin and to assess the newborn.
- Discharge teaching begins before birth and continues to discharge date. It includes infant care, follow-up visits, evaluation of support systems, and the use of car safety seats.

Additional Learning Resources

SG Go to your Study Guide for additional learning activities to help you master this chapter content.

 Go to your Evolve website (http://evolve.elsevier.com/Leifer) for the following learning resources:

- Animations
- Answer Guidelines for Critical Thinking Questions
- Answers and Rationales for Review Questions for the NCLEX® Examination
- Glossary with English and Spanish pronunciations
- Interactive Review Questions for the NCLEX® Examination
- Patient Teaching Plans in English and Spanish
- Skills Performance Checklists
- Video clips and more!

Online Resources
- Circumcision: www.cirp.org; www.circinfo.com/prepandcare/ccc.html
- Growth and development: www.cdc.gov/growthcharts
- Newborn care: www.parenthood.com
- Tips for parents: www.healthvideo.com/childrens-health

Review Questions for the NCLEX® Examination

1. The mother of a newborn reports to the nurse that her infant has had a black tarry stool. The nurse would tell the mother that:

   1. this is most likely caused by blood the infant may have swallowed during the birth process.
   2. the health care provider will be promptly notified.
   3. the infant will be given nothing by mouth (remain NPO) until a stool culture is taken.
   4. this is a normal stool in newborn infants.

2. Which of the following observations of the newborn infant should be promptly reported to the health care provider? (Select all that apply.)

   1. A respiratory rate of 24/min.
   2. Temperature of 98.4° F
   3. Pulse rate of 88/min.
   4. Nasal flaring.

3. Infections in the newborn require prompt intervention because:

   1. they spread more quickly.
   2. infections that are relatively harmless to an adult can be fatal to the newborn.
   3. the portals of entry and exit are more numerous.
   4. the newborn has no defenses against infection.

4. The mother states that her newborn has white pinpoint "pimples" on his nose and chin and she plans to squeeze them to make them disappear. The best response of the nurse would be:

1. "Be sure to wipe the area with an alcohol sponge to avoid infection."
2. "Ask your health care provider to prescribe an antibiotic ointment for the pimples."
3. "These pimples are called 'Epstein's pearls' and are a normal occurrence."
4. "These pimples are called 'milia' and will disappear on their own in a week or two."

5. Which observation of the newborn should be reported to the health care provider as soon as possible?

1. A swelling beneath the scalp on one side of the head
2. A respiratory rate of 55 breaths/min
3. A unilateral Moro reflex
4. Cyanosis of the hands and feet

Critical Thinking Question

1. A new mother brings her 5-day-old infant to the clinic and states she wants to stop breastfeeding and start formula because her infant weighs less now than he did at birth. She states that her breasts are small anyway, so she probably is not providing enough milk to help him gain weight. What is the best response of the nurse?

Preterm and Postterm Newborns

Objectives

1. Define each key term listed.
2. Differentiate between the preterm and the low-birth-weight newborn.
3. List three causes of preterm birth.
4. Describe selected problems and needs of preterm newborns and the nursing goals associated with each problem.
5. Describe the symptoms of cold stress and methods of maintaining thermoregulation.
6. Contrast the techniques for feeding preterm and full-term newborns.
7. Discuss two ways to help facilitate maternal–infant bonding for a preterm newborn.
8. Describe the family reaction to preterm infants and nursing interventions.
9. List three characteristics of the postterm infant.

Key Terms

apnea (ĂP-nē-ă, p. 312)
Ballard scoring system (p. 309)
bradycardia (brād-ē-KĂHR-dē-ă, p. 312)
bronchopulmonary dysplasia (brŏn-kō-PŬL-mŏ-nār-ē dĭs-PLĀ-zhă, p. 312)
cold stress (p. 314)
early term infant (p. 309)
full term infant (p. 309)
gestational age (p. 309)
hyperbilirubinemia (hī-pŭr-bĭl-ē-rū-bĭ-NĒ-mē-ă, p. 316)
hypocalcemia (hī-pō-kăl-SĒ-mē-ă, p. 314)
hypoglycemia (hī-pō-glī-SĒ-mē-ă, p. 314)
hypoxia (p. 312)
icterus (ĬK-tŭr-ŭs, p. 316)
kangaroo care (p. 317)

lanugo (lă-NŪ-gō, p. 321)
late term infant (p. 309)
necrotizing enterocolitis (NEC) (NĔK-rō-tīz-ĭng ĕn-tĕr-ō-kō-LĪ-tĭs, p. 315)
neutral thermal environment (p. 316)
postterm infant (p. 309)
preterm infant (p. 309)
previability (p. 309)
pulse oximetry (p. 313)
respiratory distress syndrome (RDS) (p. 310)
retinopathy of prematurity (ROP) (p. 315)
sepsis (SĔP-sĭs, p. 313)
surfactant (sŭr-FĂK-tănt, p. 311)
thermoregulation (p. 316)
total parenteral nutrition (TPN) (TŌT-ăl pă-RĔN-tŭr-ăl nū-TRĬ-shŭn, p. 318)

THE PRETERM NEWBORN

The preterm (also known as premature) newborn is the most common admission to the intensive care nursery. With increased specialization and sophisticated monitoring techniques, many infants who in the past would have died are now surviving. The nurse's role continues to be increasingly complex, with greater emphasis placed on subtle clinical observations and technology. In acquainting the student with the preterm infant, one goal of this chapter is to encourage an appreciation of the preterm infant's struggle for survival and the intense responsibility placed on those entrusted with his or her care. The words *preterm* and *premature* are used synonymously, although the former is now considered more accurate. Any newborn whose life or quality of existence is threatened is considered to be in a high-risk category and requires close supervision

by professionals in a special neonatal intensive care unit (NICU). Preterm newborns constitute a majority of these patients. Preterm birth is responsible for more deaths during the first year of life than any other single factor. Preterm infants also have a higher percentage of birth defects. Prematurity and low birth weight are often concomitant, and both factors are associated with increased neonatal morbidity and mortality. The less an infant weighs at birth, the greater the risks to life during delivery and immediately thereafter.

In the past, a newborn was classified solely by birth weight. The emphasis is now on gestational age and level of maturation. Figure 13-1 shows two different term infants of the same gestational age. One newborn would be classified as small for gestational age (SGA), which may be the result of intrauterine growth restriction (IUGR) because of its weight and size. Term infants

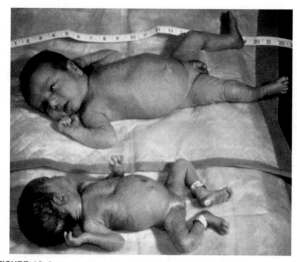

FIGURE 13-1 Two different term infants of the same gestational age. These infants are discordant twins. The variation in size and weight resulted from a malformation of the placenta. (From Zitelli BL, Davis HW: *Zitelli and Davis' atlas of pediatric physical diagnosis*, ed 6, St Louis, 2012, Saunders.)

over 4000 g (8.8 lb) may be classified as large for gestational age (LGA). Current data also indicate that intrauterine growth rates are not the same for all infants and that individual factors must be considered. **Gestational age** refers to the actual time, from conception to birth, that the fetus remains in the uterus. For the **preterm infant** this is less than 37 weeks. An **early term infant** is born between 37 weeks and 38 weeks, 6 days. The **full term infant** is one born between 39 and 40 weeks, 6 days, and the **late term infant** is one born between 41 weeks and 41 weeks, 6 days. The **postterm infant** is born beyond 42 weeks, and all of these newly defined categories are also considered a high-risk newborn regardless of birth weight. The ACOG redefined "term pregnancy" and "term infant" in 2013 to emphasize that every week in utero up to 39 weeks is important for optimal fetal development. One standardized method used to estimate gestational age within 1 to 2 weeks is the **Ballard scoring system**, which is based on the infant's external characteristics and neurological development (Figures 13-2 and 13-3). The Ballard score, the estimated gestational age based on the mother's last normal menstrual period, and ultrasound evaluations all are methods used to evaluate the gestational age of the newborn infant.

Level of maturation refers to how well developed the infant is at birth and the ability of the organs to function outside the uterus. The physician can determine much about the maturity of the newborn by careful physical examination, observation of behavior, and family history. An infant who is born at 34 weeks of gestation, weighs 1588 g (3.5 lb) at birth, has not been damaged by multifactorial birth defects, and has had a good placenta may be healthier than a full-term, "small-for-date" infant whose placenta was insufficient for any of a number of reasons. Such an infant is also probably in better condition than the heavy but immature infant

of a diabetic mother. Each infant has different and distinct needs.

CAUSES

The predisposing causes of preterm birth are numerous; in many instances the cause is unknown. Prematurity may be caused by multiple births, illness of the mother (e.g., malnutrition, heart disease, diabetes mellitus, or infectious conditions), or the hazards of pregnancy itself, such as gestational hypertension, placental abnormalities that may result in premature rupture of the membranes, placenta previa (in which the placenta lies over the cervix instead of higher in the uterus), and premature separation of the placenta. Studies also indicate the relationships between prematurity and poverty, smoking, alcohol consumption, and abuse of cocaine and other drugs.

Adequate prenatal care to prevent preterm birth is extremely important. Some preterm infants are born into families with numerous other problems. The parents may not be prepared to handle the additional financial and emotional strain imposed by a preterm infant. After delivery, early parental interaction with the infant is recognized as essential to the bonding (attachment) process. The presence of parents in special care nurseries is commonplace. Multidisciplinary care (including parent aides and other types of home support and assistance) is vital, particularly because current studies indicate a correlation between high-risk births and child abuse and neglect.

PHYSICAL CHARACTERISTICS

Preterm birth deprives the newborn of the complete benefits of intrauterine life. The infant the nurse sees in the incubator may resemble a fetus of 7 months of gestation. The skin is transparent and loose. Superficial veins may be seen beneath the abdomen and scalp. There is a lack of subcutaneous fat, and fine hair (lanugo) covers the forehead, shoulders, and arms. The cheeselike vernix caseosa is abundant. The extremities appear short. The soles of the feet have few creases, and the abdomen protrudes. The nails are short. The genitalia are small. In girls the labia majora may be open (see Figure 13-3).

RELATED PROBLEMS
Inadequate Respiratory Function
Important structural changes occur in the fetal lungs during the second half of the pregnancy. The alveoli, or air sacs, enlarge, which brings them closer to the capillaries in the lungs. The failure of this phenomenon to occur leads to many deaths attributed to **previability** (*pre*, "before," *vita*, "life," and *able* "capable of"). In addition, the muscles that move the chest are not fully developed; the abdomen is distended, creating pressure on the diaphragm; the stimulation of the respiratory center in the brain is immature; and the gag and cough reflexes are weak because of immature nerve supply. Oxygen may be required and can be administered via

MATURATIONAL ASSESSMENT OF GESTATIONAL AGE (New Ballard Score)

NEUROMUSCULAR MATURITY

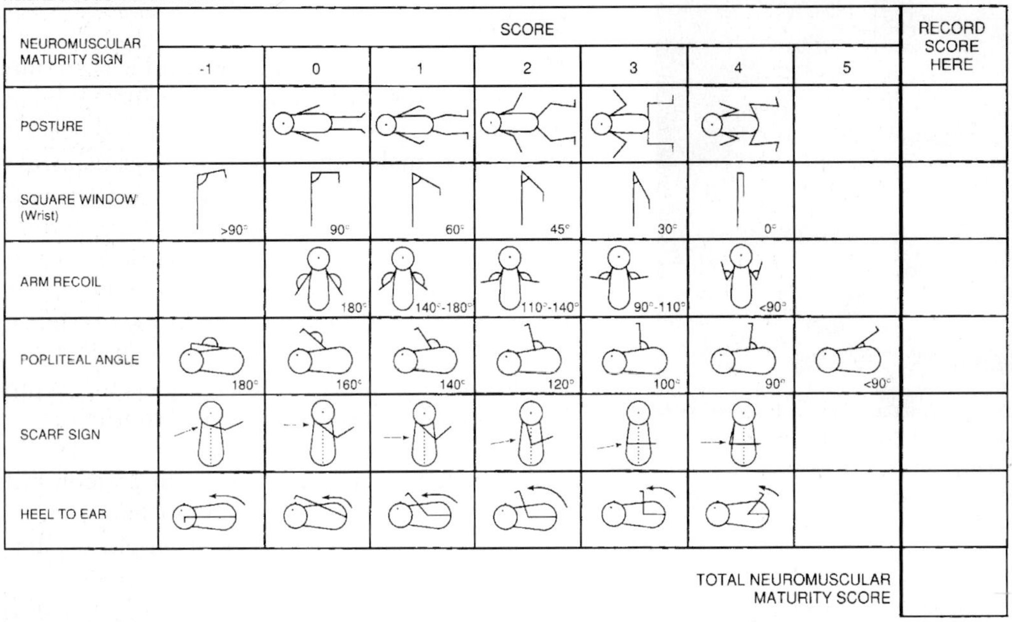

NEUROMUSCULAR MATURITY SIGN	SCORE							RECORD SCORE HERE
	-1	0	1	2	3	4	5	
POSTURE								
SQUARE WINDOW (Wrist)	>90°	90°	60°	45°	30°	0°		
ARM RECOIL		180°	140°-180°	110°-140°	90°-110°	<90°		
POPLITEAL ANGLE	180°	160°	140°	120°	100°	90°	<90°	
SCARF SIGN								
HEEL TO EAR								

A

TOTAL NEUROMUSCULAR MATURITY SCORE

PHYSICAL MATURITY

PHYSICAL MATURITY SIGN	SCORE							RECORD SCORE HERE
	-1	0	1	2	3	4	5	
SKIN	sticky friable transparent	gelatinous red translucent	smooth pink visible veins	superficial peeling &/or rash, few veins	cracking pale areas rare veins	parchment deep cracking no vessels	leathery cracked wrinkled	
LANUGO	none	sparse	abundant	thinning	bald areas	mostly bald		
PLANTAR SURFACE	heel-toe 40-50 mm:-1 <40 mm:-2	>50 mm no crease	faint red marks	anterior transverse crease only	creases ant. 2/3	creases over entire sole		
BREAST	imperceptible	barely perceptible	flat areola no bud	stippled areola 1-2 mm bud	raised areola 3-4 mm bud	full areola 5-10 mm bud		
EYE/EAR	lids fused loosely: -1 tightly: -2	lids open pinna flat stays folded	sl. curved pinna; soft; slow recoil	well-curved pinna; soft but ready recoil	formed & firm instant recoil	thick cartilage ear stiff		
GENITALS (Male)	scrotum flat, smooth	scrotum empty faint rugae	testes in upper canal rare rugae	testes descending few rugae	testes down good rugae	testes pendulous deep rugae		
GENITALS (Female)	clitoris prominent & labia flat	prominent clitoris & small labia minora	prominent clitoris & enlarging minora	majora & minora equally prominent	majora large minora small	majora cover clitoris & minora		

B

TOTAL PHYSICAL MATURITY SCORE

SCORE

Neuromuscular _____

Physical _____

Total _____

MATURITY RATING

score	weeks
-10	20
-5	22
0	24
5	26
10	28
15	30
20	32
25	34
30	36
35	38
40	40
45	42
50	44

GESTATIONAL AGE (weeks)

By dates _____

By ultrasound _____

By exam _____

C

FIGURE 13-2 The new Ballard scale estimates gestational age based on the neonate's neuromuscular maturity **(A)** and physical maturity **(B)**. A newborn will score 45 for a 42-week gestation, or only 20 for a 32-week gestation **(C)**. An accurate assessment of the newborn's maturity can aid in the development of an individualized plan of care for that newborn infant. (From Ballard JL, Khoury J, Wedig K, et al: New Ballard score expanded to include extremely premature infants, *J Pediatr* 119:417-423, 1991.)

nasal catheter, incubator, or oxygen hood (Figure 13-4). The oxygen must be warmed and humidified to prevent drying of the mucous membranes. Mechanical ventilation may be required. Oxygen saturation levels should be monitored. The infant is usually admitted to the NICU.

Respiratory Distress Syndrome. **Respiratory distress syndrome (RDS)**, also called hyaline membrane disease, is also known as respiratory distress syndrome type 1 (RDS type 2 is discussed in Chapter 14). RDS type 1 is a result of lung immaturity, which leads to decreased gas exchange. An estimated 30% of all neonatal deaths

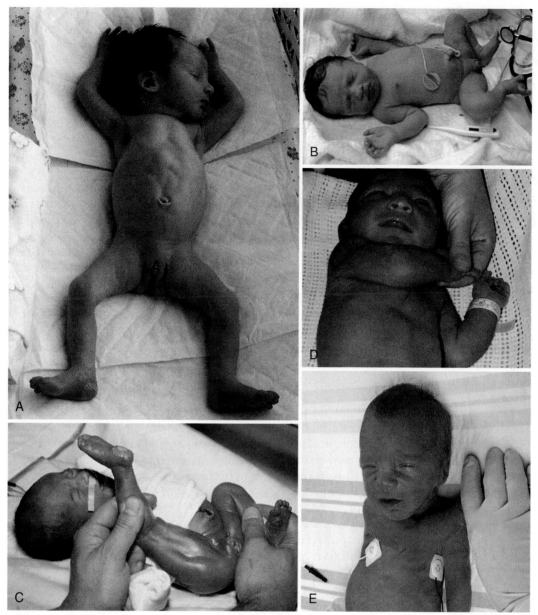

FIGURE 13-3 A, The preterm newborn. This infant evidences the extended posture of the arms and legs characteristic of the preterm infant. The skin is thin and transparent, and the labia are open and gaping. (See Ballard scale, Figure 13-2.) **B,** The full-term newborn. Compare the completely flexed arms and legs evidencing good muscle tone in this full-term newborn. The flexed position of the newborn limits the loss of body heat, as less skin surface is exposed to the air. **C,** Popliteal angle. This heel-to-ear maneuver demonstrates the easy extension of the leg consistent with a 30-week gestation. A full-term infant would show muscle resistance to this maneuver. (See Ballard scale, Figure 13-2.) **D,** When the arm of the full-term infant is pulled across the chest, the elbow goes only as far as the chin in the midline. This is called the *scarf sign.* **E,** When the arm is pulled across the chest of the preterm infant, it can be pulled into a straight line, with the elbow passing the chin at the midline (abnormal scarf sign). (**C** and **D** from Zitelli BL, Davis HW: *Zitelli and Davis' atlas of pediatric physical diagnosis,* ed 6, St Louis, 2012, Saunders. **E** from Murray SS, McKinney ES: *Foundations of maternal-newborn and women's health nursing,* ed 6, St Louis, 2014, Saunders.)

result from RDS or its complications (Kliegman, 2011). In this disease, there is a deficient synthesis or release of **surfactant**, a chemical in the lungs. Surfactant is high in lecithin, a fatty protein necessary for the absorption of oxygen by the lungs. Testing for the lecithin/sphingomyelin (L/S) ratio provides information about the amount of surfactant in amniotic fluid.

Manifestations. In general, the symptoms of respiratory distress are apparent after delivery, but they may not manifest for several hours (Figure 13-5). Respirations increase to 60 breaths/min or more. Rapid respirations (tachypnea) are accompanied by gruntlike sounds, nasal flaring, cyanosis, and intercostal and sternal retractions. Edema, lassitude, and apnea occur as

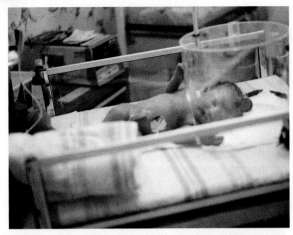

FIGURE 13-4 Oxygen administration via an oxygen hood. Oxygen is administered to this infant by means of a plastic hood. The infant is accessible for treatments without interrupting the oxygen supply.

the condition becomes more severe. Mechanical ventilation may be necessary. The treatment of these infants is ideally carried out in the NICU.

Treatment. Surfactant begins to appear in the fetal alveoli at approximately 24 weeks of gestation and is at a level to enable the infant to breathe adequately at birth by 34 weeks of gestation. If insufficient amounts of surfactant are detected through amniocentesis, it is possible to increase its production by giving the mother injections of corticosteroids such as betamethasone. Administration 1 or 2 days before delivery may reduce the chances of RDS. In preterm newborns, surfactant can be administered via endotracheal (ET) tube at birth or when symptoms of RDS occur, with improvement of lung function seen within 72 hours. Surfactant production is altered during episodes of cold stress or hypoxia and when there is poor tissue perfusion, and such conditions are often present in the preterm infant in the first days of life.

Vital signs are monitored closely, arterial blood gases are analyzed, and the infant is placed in a warm incubator with gentle and minimal handling to conserve energy. The concept of *cluster care* involves combining and coordinating the handling required for assessment and treatments so as to provide adequate blocks of time for uninterrupted rest. Intravenous fluids are prescribed, and the nurse observes for signs of overhydration or dehydration. Oxygen therapy may be given via hood (see Figure 13-4) or ventilator in concentrations necessary to maintain adequate tissue perfusion. Oxygen toxicity is a high risk for infants receiving prolonged treatment with high concentrations of oxygen. **Bronchopulmonary dysplasia** is the toxic response of the lung to oxygen therapy. Atelectasis, edema, and thickening of the membranes of the lung interfere with ventilation. This often results in prolonged dependence on supplemental oxygen and ventilators and has long-term complications.

Apnea. **Apnea** is defined as the cessation of breathing for 20 seconds or longer. It is not uncommon in the preterm newborn and is believed to be related to immaturity of the nervous system. An apneic episode may be accompanied by **bradycardia** (heart rate of fewer than 100 beats/min) and cyanosis. Apnea monitors alert nurses to this complication. Gentle rubbing of the infant's feet, ankles, and back may stimulate breathing after this occurrence. When these measures fail, suctioning of the nose and mouth and raising of the infant's head to a semi-Fowler's position usually facilitates breathing. If breathing does not begin, an Ambu bag is used.

Neonatal Hypoxia. Neonatal **hypoxia** is inadequate oxygenation at the cellular level in a newborn infant. A deficiency of oxygen in the arterial blood is known

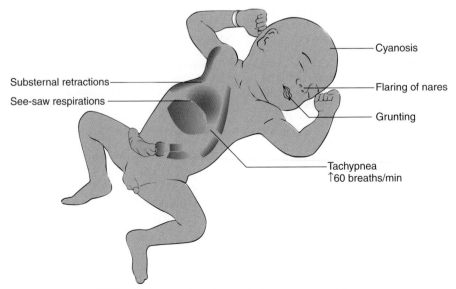

Substernal retractions

See-saw respirations

Cyanosis

Flaring of nares

Grunting

Tachypnea
↑60 breaths/min

FIGURE 13-5 Signs of respiratory distress in a preterm infant.

as hypoxemia. The degree of hypoxemia present can be detected by a noninvasive pulse oximetry reading. **Pulse oximetry** is defined as the measure of oxygen on the hemoglobin in the circulating blood divided by the oxygen capacity of the hemoglobin. A pulse oximeter saturation level of 92% or higher is normal (see Skill 13-1). There must be at least 5 g/dL of desaturated hemoglobin (unoxygenated blood) to produce clinical cyanosis. Therefore the severely anemic infant may have severe hypoxia yet not manifest clinical cyanosis. If the hemoglobin present is an abnormal fetal hemoglobin, hypoxia can be present even when the pulse oximeter shows a normal reading, because fetal hemoglobin does not readily release oxygen to the tissues and end organs (Rohan and Golombek, 2009).

Advances in Pulse Oximetry Technology. The new Masimo-Pronto-7 is a pulse oximeter that can noninvasively measure the transcutaneous hemoglobin level as well as provide an accurate oxygen saturation level. The FDA has cleared the device to screen newborns for congenital heart disease. The bedside pulse oximeter, Radical-7, can display simultaneous oxygen saturation, and total hemoglobin simultaneously. The device can also be set to display the respiratory rate and carboxyhemoglobin and methemoglobin levels with additional sensors (Schuman, 2012).

Sepsis. **Sepsis** is a generalized infection of the bloodstream. Preterm newborns are at risk for developing this complication because of the immaturity of many body systems. The liver of the preterm infant is

Applying a Pulse Oximeter

PURPOSE

To determine oxygen saturation of the blood

STEPS

1. Prepare the infant and explain procedure to the family.
2. Turn on oximeter.
3. Set alarm switch to minimum acceptable oxygen saturation (Sao_2) of approximately 92%-95%.
4. Apply the oximeter sensor to the toe or the side of the foot (see illustration).

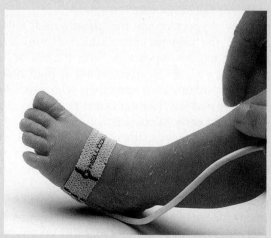

5. The probe must be flush with the skin and be secured firmly with the wing tapes.
6. The sensors, a light-emitting diode and photo detector, must be lined up opposite each other to obtain an accurate reading. Use the circles on the external surface of the lead to align the sensors. A red light passes from one sensor on the toe or foot through the vascular bed and registers on the sensor on the opposite side.
7. Check the monitor reading for level of oxygen saturation.
8. Compare the heart rate reading on the monitor with the infant's heart rate. Matching heart rates indicate the saturation level reading is accurate. If heart rates do not match, reapply or adjust sensors.
9. Document time that oximetry is initiated, heart rate and oxygen saturation readings, and location of sensor on the infant's body. Any oxygen administered and method of administration should also be recorded.

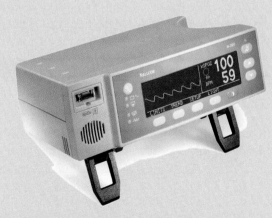

(Figures copyright © 2014 Covidien. All rights reserved. Used with permission of Covidien.)

immature and forms antibodies poorly. Body enzymes are inefficient because of the abbreviated stay in the uterus. There is little or no immunity received from the mother, and stores of nutrients, vitamins, and iron are insufficient. There may be no local signs of infection, which also hinders diagnosis. Some signs of sepsis include a low temperature, lethargy or irritability, poor feeding, and respiratory distress. Maternal infection and complications during labor can also predispose the preterm infant to sepsis.

Treatment involves administration of intravenous antimicrobials, maintenance of warmth and nutrition, and close monitoring of vital signs, including blood pressure. Keeping nursing care as organized as possible will help conserve energy. An incubator separates the infant from other infants in the unit and facilitates close observation. Maintenance of strict Standard Precautions is essential (see Appendix A).

Poor Control of Body Temperature

Keeping the preterm infant warm is a nursing challenge. Heat loss in the preterm infant results from the following factors:

- The preterm infant has a lack of brown fat, which is the body's insulation.
- There is excessive heat loss by radiation from a surface area that is large in proportion to body weight. The large surface area of the head predisposes the infant to heat loss.
- The heat-regulating center of the brain is immature.
- The sweat glands are not functioning to capacity.
- The preterm infant is inactive, has muscles that are weak and are less resistant to cold, and cannot shiver.
- The posture of the preterm infant's extremities is one of leg extension. This increases the surface area exposed to the environment and increases heat loss.
- Metabolism is high, and the preterm infant is prone to low blood glucose levels (hypoglycemia).

These and other factors make the preterm newborn vulnerable to **cold stress**, which increases the need for oxygen and glucose. Early detection can prevent complications.

Nursing Tip

Signs and symptoms of cold stress include the following:
- Decreased skin temperature
- Increased respiratory rate with periods of apnea
- Bradycardia
- Mottling of skin
- Lethargy

Nursing Care. The infant's skin temperature will decrease before the core temperature falls. Therefore a skin probe is used to monitor the temperature of preterm infants. The skin probe is placed in the right upper quadrant of the abdomen. Care should be taken to ensure that the probe is not directly over a bony prominence, in the line of cool oxygen input, or under a diaper.

The infant is placed under a radiant warmer or in an incubator to maintain a warm environment. The temperature of the incubator is adjusted so that the infant's body temperature is at an optimal level (36.2° to 37° C [97.1° to 98.6° F]).

Hypoglycemia and Hypocalcemia

Hypoglycemia (*hypo*, "less than," and *glycemia*, "sugar in the blood") is common among preterm infants. They have not remained in the uterus long enough to acquire sufficient stores of glycogen and fat. This condition is aggravated by the need for increased glycogen in the brain, the heart, and other tissues as a result of asphyxia, sepsis, RDS, unstable body temperature, and similar conditions. Any condition that increases energy requirements places more stress on these already deficient stores. Plasma glucose levels lower than 40 mg/dL indicate hypoglycemia in a term infant, and in a preterm infant, lower than 30 mg/dL.

The brain needs a steady supply of glucose, and hypoglycemia must be anticipated and treated promptly. Any condition that increases metabolism increases glucose needs. Preterm infants may be too weak to suck and swallow formula and often require gavage or parenteral feedings to supply their 120- to 150-kcal/kg/day needs. Nursing responsibilities include frequent glucose monitoring and nasogastric or parenteral feedings.

Hypocalcemia (*hypo*, "below," and *calcemia*, "calcium in the blood") is also seen in preterm and sick newborns. Calcium is transported across the placenta throughout pregnancy, but in greater amounts during the third trimester. Early birth can result in infants with lower serum calcium levels.

In **early** hypocalcemia the parathyroid fails to respond to the preterm infant's low calcium levels. Infants stressed by hypoxia or birth trauma or who are receiving sodium bicarbonate are at high risk for this problem. Infants born to mothers who are diabetic or who have had low vitamin D intake are also at risk for developing early hypocalcemia.

Late hypocalcemia usually occurs about age 1 week in newborn or preterm infants who are fed cow's milk. Cow's milk increases serum phosphate levels, which cause calcium levels to fall.

Administering intravenous calcium gluconate is the treatment for hypocalcemia. During intravenous therapy, the nurse should monitor the infant for bradycardia. Adding calcium lactate powder to the formula also lowers phosphate levels. (Calcium lactate tablets are insoluble in milk and must not be used.) When calcium lactate powder is slowly discontinued from the formula, the nurse should again monitor the infant for signs of neonatal tetany.

Nursing Tip

Signs of hypoglycemia in the preterm infant include the following:
- Tremors
- Weak cry
- Lethargy
- Convulsions
- Plasma glucose level lower than 40 mg/dL (term) or 30 mg/dL (preterm)

⚠ **Safety Alert!**

When an infant is given intravenous calcium gluconate, the nurse should monitor the heart rate closely and report bradycardia if it occurs.

Increased Tendency to Bleed

Preterm infants are more prone to bleeding than full-term infants because their blood is deficient in prothrombin, a factor of the clotting mechanism. Fragile capillaries of the head are particularly susceptible to injury during delivery, causing intracranial hemorrhage. Ultrasonography is helpful in detecting this problem. The nurse should monitor the neurological status of the infant and report bulging fontanelles, lethargy, poor feeding, and seizures. The bed should be in a slight Fowler's position, and unnecessary stimulation that can cause increased intracerebral pressure should be avoided.

Retinopathy of Prematurity

Retinopathy of prematurity (ROP) is a disorder of the developing retina in premature infants that can lead to blindness. The condition was formerly termed *retrolental fibroplasia,* but the term *ROP* is currently used because it is more precise. It is the leading cause of blindness in newborns weighing less than 1500 g (3.3 lb). Premature infants are at risk, because their immature retinas are incompletely vascularized at birth. After birth, often accompanied by high levels of oxygen required for the infant's survival, the retina completes an abnormal vascularization process that causes fibrous tissue to form behind the lens of each eye resulting in blindness and retinal detachment (Gabbe, 2012). Full-term infants who have fully developed vascular systems in the retina at birth are not affected (AAP, 2013). In 2013, the AAP revised standards that had been set in 2006 to include routine retinal exams by certified ophthalmologists in the NICU for infants with birth weight between 1500 g and 2000 g or gestational age less than 30 weeks. Examination at 4 weeks of age and at proper intervals for follow-up can result in early detection and prompt treatment. Retinal ablative therapy using laser photocoagulation of the fibrous tissue, or intravitreal injection of bevacizumab, has been used with success in preventing blindness (AAP, 2013). Follow-up for other eye problems such as strabismus, refractive errors, or cataracts should be provided within 4 to 6 months after discharge from the NICU. The nurse must teach the parents concerning the importance of follow-up care.

Prevention of preterm births and the problems that beset preterm infants are the key to preventing ROP. Careful monitoring of oxygen saturation in high-risk infants with a pulse oximeter continues to be a priority in the nursery (Skill 13-1). It is the level of oxygen in the blood, rather than the amount of oxygen received, that is of importance in oxygen therapy. There is no "safe level" of oxygen. Infants must be provided with the level of oxygen required to sustain life and prevent neurological damage. Maintaining a sufficient level of vitamin E and avoiding excessively high concentrations of oxygen may help to prevent this condition.

Poor Nutrition

The stomach capacity of the preterm infant is small. The sphincter muscles at both ends of the stomach are immature, which contributes to regurgitation and vomiting, particularly after overfeeding. Sucking and swallowing reflexes are immature. The infant's ability to absorb fats is poor (this includes fat-soluble vitamins). The inadequate store of nutrients in the preterm infant and the need for glucose and nutrients to promote growth and prevent brain damage contribute to the nutritional problems of the preterm infant. Parenteral or gavage feedings are usually required until the infant is strong enough to tolerate oral feedings without compromising cardiorespiratory status.

Necrotizing Enterocolitis

Necrotizing enterocolitis (NEC) is an acute inflammation of the bowel that leads to bowel *necrosis.* Preterm newborns are particularly susceptible to NEC. Factors implicated include a diminished blood supply to the lining of the bowel wall because of hypoxia or sepsis that causes a decrease in protective mucus and results in bacterial invasion of the delicate tissues. A source for bacterial growth occurs when the infant is fed a milk formula or hypertonic gavage feeding.

Signs of NEC include abdominal distention, bloody stools, diarrhea, and bilious vomitus. Specific nursing responsibilities include observing vital signs, maintaining infection control techniques, and carefully resuming oral fluids as ordered. Measuring the abdomen and listening for bowel sounds are also important measures. Treatment includes antimicrobials and the use of parenteral nutrition to rest the bowels. Surgical removal of the necrosed bowel may be indicated.

Immature Kidneys

Improper elimination of body wastes contributes to electrolyte imbalance and disturbed acid-base relationships. Dehydration occurs easily. Tolerance to salt is limited, and susceptibility to edema is increased.

The nurse should document the intake and output for all preterm infants. The nurse should weigh the dry diaper and subtract its weight from the infant's wet diaper to determine the urine output. The urine output should be between 1 and 3 mL/kg/hr. The infant should be observed closely for signs of dehydration or overhydration. The nurse should document the status of the fontanelles, tissue turgor, weight, and urine output.

Jaundice

The liver of the newborn is immature, which contributes to a condition called **icterus** or jaundice. Jaundice causes the skin and the whites of the eyes to assume a yellow-orange cast. The liver is unable to clear the blood of bile pigments that result from the normal postnatal destruction of red blood cells. The amount of bile pigment in the blood serum is expressed as milligrams of bilirubin per deciliter (mg/dL). The higher the blood bilirubin level is, the deeper the jaundice, and the greater the risk for neurological damage. An increase of more than 5 mg/dL in 24 hours or a bilirubin level greater than 12.9 mg/dL requires careful investigation (Kliegman, 2011). Physiological jaundice is normal and is discussed in Chapter 12. Pathological jaundice is more serious, occurs within 24 hours of birth, and is secondary to an abnormal condition such as ABO-Rh incompatibility (see Chapter 13). In preterm infants the normal rise in bilirubin levels (icterus neonatorum) is slower than in full-term infants and lasts longer, which predisposes the infant to **hyperbilirubinemia** (*hyper*, "excessive," *bilirubin*, "bile," and *emia*, "blood"), or excessive bilirubin levels in the blood.

There is more evidence of jaundice in infants who are breastfed. Breast milk jaundice begins to be seen about the fourth day, when the mother's milk supply develops. The newborn usually does well but is carefully monitored to rule out problems. In early-onset jaundice of the breastfed infant, inadequate infant suckling at the breast causes jaundice and necessitates an increase in breastfeeding. Glucose water feedings should *not* be offered to the infant, because this practice may decrease milk intake and can serve to further increase bilirubin levels. In late-onset jaundice of the breastfed infant, the breast milk itself may inhibit conjugation of bilirubin, and therefore formula may be substituted for 24 to 48 hours to reduce bilirubin levels. The total serum bilirubin level typically peaks 3 to 5 days after birth. The early discharge of a newborn

necessitates follow-up visits within 2 days to check total serum bilirubin and to prevent the development of kernicterus (Kliegman, 2011).

The goals of treatment for hyperbilirubinemia are to prevent kernicterus (a serious neurological complication that can cause brain damage, which is also known as bilirubin encephalopathy) and to avoid the continued increase of bilirubin levels in the blood. The nursing care for hyperbilirubinemia consists of observing the infant's skin, sclera, and mucous membranes for jaundice. (Blanching the skin over bony prominences enhances the evaluation for jaundice.) Observing and reporting the progression of jaundice from the face to the abdomen and feet is important, because the progression may indicate increasing bilirubin blood levels. Treatment includes monitoring and reporting bilirubin laboratory values and documenting the response of the infant to phototherapy See Chapter 12 and Skill 12-4 for assessing jaundice.

SPECIAL NEEDS

The physician appraises the physical status of the preterm newborn at delivery. The immediate needs are to clear the infant's airway and to provide warmth. The infant is given care for the umbilical cord and care for the eyes and is then properly identified. The infant is placed naked in an incubator and taken to the nursery. The nurse in charge receives a report on the general condition of the newborn, the type of delivery, and any complications that have occurred. Many hospitals transfer their preterm infants to special medical centers geared to care for them. The transport team is briefed by the neonatologist and is dispatched to the referring hospital. A life-support infant-transport incubator that can be carried by ambulance (and sometimes helicopter) is used. Box 13-1 lists some nursing goals for care of the preterm newborn.

Thermoregulation (Warmth)

Thermoregulation (*thermo*, "heat," and *regulation*, "maintenance of") involves maintaining a stable body temperature and preventing hypothermia (low temperature) and hyperthermia (high temperature). A stable body temperature is essential to the survival and management of preterm infants.

Incubator. The preterm newborn is placed in an incubator designed to provide a **neutral thermal environment** wherein temperature, air, radiating surface

---

Box 13-1	Nursing Goals for the Preterm Newborn

The nursing goals in caring for the preterm newborn include the following:
- Improve respiration
- Maintain body heat (keep the "preemie" warm)
- Conserve energy

- Prevent infection
- Provide proper nutrition and hydration
- Give good skin care
- Observe the infant carefully and record observations
- Support and encourage the parents

temperatures, and humidity are controlled to maintain the infant's temperature within a normal range with minimal oxygen consumption required. The incubator also provides isolation and protection from infection. The top of the incubator is transparent to enable personnel to view the newborn clearly at all times. Different models include alarms to indicate overheating or a lack of circulating air, facilities for positioning, and a scale to weigh the infant without removal from the warm environment. Nurses must understand how to use the incubators available in the nurseries to which they are assigned (Figure 13-6). They should request assistance if needed.

The temperature of the incubator is adjusted to a level that will maintain an optimal body temperature in the infant. Smaller infants may require higher incubator temperatures. The nurse records the temperature of the infant and the incubator every 2 hours. The infant's temperature is monitored with a heat-sensitive probe that is taped to the abdomen. Axillary temperatures may also be taken. A relative humidity of 60% or higher is desirable. Overheating should be avoided because it increases the infant's oxygen and caloric requirements.

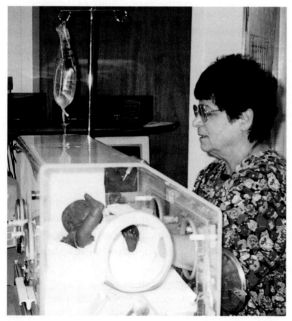

FIGURE 13-6 The incubator. The infant is dressed only in a diaper. Portholes facilitate routine infant care without disturbing the atmospheric conditions in the incubator. The infant can be assessed through Plexiglas windows. Levers under the mattress can place the bed in the Fowler's or the Trendelenburg position. Openings at the head and foot of the incubator can be used to remove soiled linen using the principles of aseptic technique. The door of the incubator can be lowered to form a platform that makes the infant accessible for special treatments or tests. The nurse must make sure the door is *locked* in the closed position when the incubator is in use. To promote circadian rhythms, a blanket may be placed over the top of the incubator to shield the infant from environmental lights.

Radiant Heat. Radiant heat cribs that supply overhead heat have the advantage of providing easier access to the patient while maintaining a neutral thermal environment. Nursing Care Plan 13-1 lists nursing interventions for selected nursing diagnoses pertinent to care of the preterm newborn.

Kangaroo Care. **Kangaroo care** is a method of care for preterm infants that uses skin-to-skin contact. This method of holding the infant is similar to the way a kangaroo keeps its offspring warm in its pouch (Skill 13-2). The practice began in 1979 in Bogota, Colombia, in response to a shortage of incubators and staff and is currently a popular practice in the United States. The infant, wearing only a diaper and a small cap, rests on the mother or father's naked chest. The skin provides warmth and calms the child, and the contact promotes bonding. Kangaroo care has shown to be superior to holding a blanket wrapped infant in enhancing the stabilization of infants as well as promoting later development (Neu, 2013). Skin-to-skin contact is an important practice in hospitals that are designated as "baby friendly."

Nutrition

Feeding of the preterm newborn varies with gestational age and health status. The ability to coordinate breathing, sucking, and swallowing does not develop before 34 weeks of gestation. Therefore a very preterm infant may require gavage feedings (via a tube placed through the nose or mouth into the stomach). Infants weighing more than 1500 g (3.3 lb) may be able to bottle feed if a small, soft nipple with a large hole is used to minimize the energy and effort required for sucking. Human milk is ideal, because the fat is absorbed readily. Breast milk may be manually expressed by the mother and placed in a bottle for her preterm infant. If the infant is gavage fed, the tube is replaced every 3 to 7 days. Intravenous fluids may be provided to meet fluid, calorie, and electrolyte needs in small, weak preterm infants. Often the infants are fed while still in the incubator. Early initiation of feedings reduces the risk of hypoglycemia, hyperbilirubinemia, and dehydration.

The nurse should observe and record bowel sounds and the passage of meconium, which indicate intestinal readiness for oral feedings. When the infant is gavage fed, the contents of the stomach should be aspirated before the feeding is started. If only mucus or air is aspirated, the feeding can be given as planned. If a residual of liquid contents is aspirated, the physician should be notified before proceeding to feed the infant. Infants older than 28 weeks of gestation usually have the digestive enzymes required for the digestion of breast milk. Formulas designed for the term infant are not well tolerated by preterm infants because they are a burden to their kidneys and can cause central nervous system problems. Formulas designed for preterm infants are not well tolerated by infants older than 34 weeks of

★ Nursing Care Plan 13-1 | The Preterm Newborn

PATIENT DATA A newborn infant of 30 weeks gestation is admitted to the neonatal intensive care unit (NICU). The infant is placed in a prewarmed incubator, and cardiorespiratory sensors are applied.

Selected Nursing Diagnosis: Hypothermia related to decreased subcutaneous tissue and immature body temperature control

Goals	Nursing Interventions	Rationales
Infant's temperature will remain at 36.5° to 37° C (97.6° to 98.6° F).	Monitor temperature with skin probe or by axillary method.	These methods provide the best indication of the infant's core temperature and are less invasive.
	Adjust incubator or radiant warmer to maintain skin temperature.	A neutral thermal environment permits the infant to maintain a normal core temperature with minimum oxygen consumption and caloric expenditure.
	Observe for signs of cold stress, such as decreased temperature, pallor, and lethargy.	Preterm infants have little or no muscular activity; they remain in an extended posture because of lack of muscle tone; they cannot shiver.
	Use discretion in bathing.	The temperature of a wet infant drops quickly as a result of evaporation.
	Avoid cold surfaces.	Conductive heat loss occurs when an infant is weighed on a cold scale; prewarm surfaces or use a receiving blanket for protection.

Selected Nursing Diagnosis: Risk for impaired skin integrity, related to immature skin, poor nutrition, and immobility

Goals	Nursing Interventions	Rationales
Skin will remain intact.	Change position regularly.	This prevents pressure sores and aids respiration and circulation.
	Be gentle when removing dressings, tape, and electrodes.	The preterm infant's skin is fragile and bruises easily; use as little tape as possible.
	Cleanse skin with clear water or approved cleansers.	Avoid hexachlorophene cleaners because of their toxic effect; all products must be carefully assessed before use, because permeability of the preterm infant's skin fosters absorption of ingredients.
	Observe skin for signs of infection while recognizing that there may be no local inflammatory response, but only vague signs and symptoms.	Heel pricks and other invasive procedures are often necessary; the preterm infant's immune system is immature, and healing becomes difficult.

Critical Thinking Question

1. A mother comes to visit her preterm son in the NICU. She states she wants to see her infant, but she is afraid to touch anything and fears she will hurt her fragile newborn. What is the nurse's best response?

---

gestation or term infants because hypercalcemia may develop. Supplemental vitamins are usually prescribed for the preterm infant. If the infant is too premature or too ill to tolerate oral feedings, **total parenteral nutrition (TPN)**—the intravenous infusion of lipids and nutrients—may be prescribed to meet the infant's nutritional and growth needs. Gavage and gastrostomy tube feedings are discussed in Chapter 22.

Close Observation

The physician examines the preterm newborn and writes specific orders for treatment and nursing care. When the physician leaves the nursery, the nurse is responsible for reporting any significant changes in the infant's condition. The experienced nurse in the preterm nursery observes and charts care and treatment in great detail. Table 13-1 lists the *general* observations to guide care of the preterm newborn. Sudden changes are reported immediately.

Positioning and Nursing Care

The preterm newborn is positioned on the side or prone, with the head of the mattress slightly elevated unless contraindicated. In this position the abdominal contents do not press against the diaphragm and impede breathing.

Positioning the preterm infant should be compatible with the drainage of secretions and the prevention of aspiration. Propping the infant on the side or placing the infant prone can decrease respiratory effort, improve oxygenation, promote a more organized sleep pattern, and lessen physical activity that burns up energy needed for growth and development. An enclosed space, or *nesting,* can provide a calming, supportive environment that promotes body flexion for the preterm infant (Figure 13-7). Infants should be gradually weaned from the prone position when the physical condition becomes stable, and they should be placed in the supine position well before discharge from the

Kangaroo Care

PURPOSE

To maintain skin-to-skin contact to promote warmth and bonding

STEPS

1. Explain the rationale and principles of care to the parents.
2. Provide comfortable chair and privacy.
3. Have parent wear a gown that opens in the front, leaving the chest bare.
4. Remove newborn's clothes except for diaper.
5. Place newborn in vertical position between the breasts of the bare chest of the parent.
6. Place a blanket over the newborn.
7. Monitor the temperature of the newborn throughout this form of care.
8. Document the procedure, the infant's vital signs, and responses.

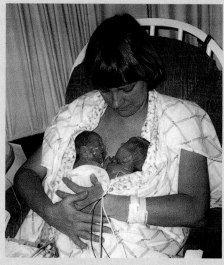

The mother provides kangaroo care for her preterm infants. Skin-to-skin contact is provided, with warmth maintained by the outer covering.

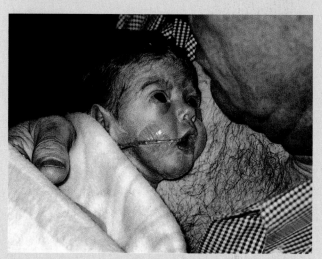

The father can also provide effective kangaroo care. The infant shows a positive response to this contact. (Courtesy Loma Linda University Medical Center, Loma Linda, CA.)

Table 13-1 Nursing Observations in Care of the Preterm Infant

OBSERVATION	SIGNS TO REPORT
General activity	Increase or decrease in movements, lethargy, twitching, frequency and quality of cry, hyperactivity
Fontanelles	Sunken, flat, or bulging
Eyes	Discharge
Respirations	Regularity, apnea, sternal retractions, labored breathing
Pulse	Rate and regularity
Abdomen	Distention
Cord	Discharge; odor
Feeding	Sucking ability, vomiting or regurgitation, degree of satisfaction
Voiding	Initial, frequency
Stools	Frequency, color, consistency
Mucous membranes	Dryness of lips and mouth, signs of thrush
Color	Paleness, cyanosis, jaundice
Skin	Rashes, irritations, pustules, edema

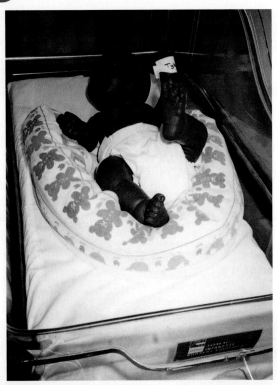

FIGURE 13-7 Infant nesting. An enclosed space bounded by small blanket rolls encircling the preterm infant provides a calming, supportive environment.

NICU (McMullen, 2013). It is important to teach the parent about the importance of the "back-to-sleep" concept to prevent SIDS. The infant should not be left in one position for long periods, because it is uncomfortable and may harm the lungs. Changing the position also prevents breakdown from pressure on the infant's delicate skin. If such a breakdown should occur, the area is exposed to the air, and a suitable ointment is applied as prescribed by the health care provider. Alkaline-based soap, alcohol, and medicated wipes should not be used on the preterm infant's thin and sensitive skin. Hydrocolloid adhesives or using gauze or cotton under adhesive tape is advisable. Daily cleansing of eyes, mouth, and diaper area, and baths two or three times weekly with the application of emollients such as Eucerin or Aquaphor, promote skin integrity (Association of Women's Health, Obstetric, and Neonatal Nurses [AWHONN], 2007) (see Chapter 12 for a more extended discussion of the skin of the newborn).

Every effort should be made to maintain a quiet environment and organize nursing care so that overstimulation of the preterm infant is avoided. Blankets can be placed over the top of the incubator to reduce external stimulation and to establish a normal *circadian rhythm* (night–day sleep pattern), and eye patches can be placed over the infant's eyes to protect against the bright procedure lights. Observing physical and behavioral responses of the preterm infant enables a developmentally appropriate care plan to be developed. The preterm infant should be awakened slowly and gently for procedures or nursing care and should be moved gently, maintaining flexion of the limbs close to the infant's body.

Some studies have shown that cobedding of twins (placing them together in one incubator) may improve their growth and development, but further research is needed to determine the risks related to transmission of infection.

PROGNOSIS

In the absence of severe birth defects and complications, the growth rate of the preterm newborn nears that of the term infant by about the second year. Very low–birth weight infants may not catch up, especially if there has been chronic illness, insufficient nutritional intake, or inadequate care taking (Kliegman, 2011). Additional studies are needed to determine the effects of these factors at various age levels. Parents must be prepared for relatives' comments on the infant's small size and slower development. In general, growth and development of the preterm infant are based on current age minus the number of weeks before term that the infant was born; for example, if born at 36 weeks of gestation, a 1-month-old infant would be at a newborn's achievement level. This calculation ensures that no one has unrealistic expectations for the infant.

FAMILY REACTION

The nurse should assist the parents to cope with their responses to having a small, preterm infant. Parents need guidance throughout the infant's hospitalization to help to prepare them for this new experience. They may be disheartened by the unattractive appearance of the preterm newborn. They may believe that they are to blame for the infant's condition. They may fear that the infant will die but may be unable to express their feelings. They need time to look at and touch the infant and begin to see the child as uniquely their own (Figure 13-8). This touch and immediate human contact are vital for the infant as well. The mother is usually concerned with her ability to care for such a small and helpless creature. When she feels ready, she may assist the nurse in diapering, bathing, feeding, and other activities. Other aspects of infant care are also stressed during this time.

Nursing care of the preterm infant includes measures to provide short periods of stimulation during the alert phase of activity. The parents can be taught to provide stimulation by using a black-and-white mobile, stroking gently, talking to the infant, rocking, or providing range-of-motion activity or kangaroo care. A pacifier may be used during gavage feeding to provide nonnutritive sucking. Care should be taken not to overly stimulate or tire the infant. There should be minimal stimulation during feeding to enable the infant to concentrate energy on the sucking and swallowing

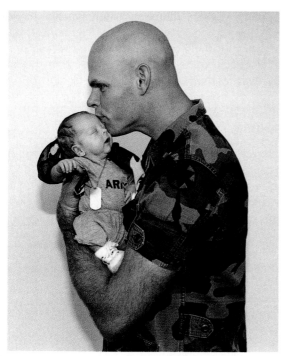

FIGURE 13-8 This father holds his preterm infant in a moment of bonding.

process. Stimulation and interaction with parents should be provided between feedings.

The nurse should collaborate with pediatricians, social workers, nutritionists, psychologists, and staff from other disciplines to plan and coordinate follow-up care of the preterm infant after discharge. Often a mother is discharged without her infant. This is difficult for the entire family and makes attachment and bonding more complicated. The nurse encourages the family to keep in touch by telephone and by visits. Parents can help siblings to accept the infant by addressing the child by name, sharing news of progress, taking pictures of the infant, and encouraging communication by means of drawings and cards. Listening to what siblings are saying provides information for discussion.

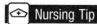 **Nursing Tip**

Encourage parents to talk about their feelings and fears concerning the preterm infant. Answer questions about home care.

THE POSTTERM NEWBORN

The newborn is considered *postterm* if the pregnancy goes beyond 42 weeks. *Postmaturity* refers to the infant showing characteristics of the postmature syndrome. Identification of infants who are not tolerating the extra time in the uterus is the major goal of treatment. Death of the postterm infant is uncommon today because of early detection and intervention. The cause of postmaturity is not yet clear; however, it is known that the placenta does not function adequately as it ages, which could result in fetal distress. The mortality rate of late infants is higher than that of newborns delivered at term. Morbidity rates are also higher. After the infant survives delivery, the risks are fewer.

The late birth is a psychological strain on the mother, the father, and other members of the family, who are eagerly awaiting the arrival of the child. The nurse encourages parents to verbalize their feelings and concerns about the delay. Very large newborns, such as those of diabetic mothers, are not necessarily postmature but are larger than normal because of rapid, abnormal growth before delivery.

The following problems are associated with postmaturity:

- Asphyxia caused by chronic hypoxia while in the uterus because of a deteriorated placenta
- Meconium aspiration: hypoxia and distress may cause relaxation of the anal sphincter, and meconium can be aspirated into the fetal lungs
- Poor nutritional status; depleted glycogen reserves cause hypoglycemia
- Increase in red blood cell production (polycythemia) because of intrauterine hypoxia
- Difficult delivery because of increased size of the infant
- Birth defects
- Seizures as a result of the hypoxic state

PHYSICAL CHARACTERISTICS

The postterm infant is long and thin and looks as though weight has been lost. The skin is loose, especially about the thighs and buttocks. There is little **lanugo** (downy hair) or vernix caseosa. The loss of the cheeselike vernix caseosa leaves the skin dry; it cracks, peels, and is almost like parchment in texture. The nails are long and may be stained with meconium. The infant has a thick head of hair and looks alert.

Nursing Care

Labor induction or cesarean deliveries are commonly performed if testing determines that the pregnancy is past 42 weeks or if there are signs of fetal distress or maternal risk. Many postterm infants suffer few adverse effects from the delay, but they still require careful observation in the nursery. Nursing care involves observing for respiratory distress (usually because of aspiration of meconium-stained amniotic fluid), hypoglycemia (caused by depleted glycogen stores), and hyperbilirubinemia (as a result of polycythemia). The infant may be placed in an incubator, because fat stores have been used in utero for nourishment, and the infant is vulnerable to cold stress.

TRANSPORTING THE HIGH-RISK NEWBORN

Transportation of the high-risk newborn to a regional neonatal center requires the organization and expertise of a special team. A nurse and sometimes a physician accompany the infant unless specialists in emergency medical transport are part of the transport team. Stabilization of the infant before discharge is important. Baseline data, such as vital signs and blood work (blood gases and glucose levels), are obtained. The infant is weighed if this is not contraindicated. Copies of all records are made, including the infant's record, the mother's prenatal history and delivery, and pertinent admission data. A transport incubator is provided for warmth, and the batteries are kept fully charged.

The nurse is responsible for placing an identification band on the infant before transport and for verifying the identification name and number with the mother's identification band. The mother should be reassured that the identification will stay with the infant. The parents should be given the name and location of the receiving hospital and the name and telephone number of a physician to contact for follow-up information and visits.

Parents are shown the newborn before departure. If the mother is unable to hold the infant because of the baby's condition, the incubator is wheeled to her bedside for her observation. A picture is taken and given to the parents. On occasion, a mother is unable to see her infant because of her own unstable condition. Such situations require special empathy from nursing personnel. After the infant has safely reached its destination, the parents are contacted by telephone. It is also thoughtful for the receiving hospital personnel to provide feedback to the transport team so that they may enjoy hearing the results of their efforts.

DISCHARGE OF THE HIGH-RISK (PRETERM BIRTH) NEWBORN

Discharge planning begins at birth. The parents will need to demonstrate and practice routine and/or specialized care. Visits by the nurse to assess home care and to provide additional support are valuable. Continued medical supervision is important. The nurse stresses the importance of well-baby examinations, immunizations, and prevention of infection. Good prenatal care for subsequent pregnancies is emphasized (especially after a preterm birth, because the mother is at high risk for future preterm births).

Parents are often anxious about taking their high-risk newborn home. The nurse must familiarize the parent with the newborn's care. The newborn's behavioral patterns are discussed, and realistic expectations concerning the preterm infant's catch-up development are reviewed. Communication is maintained with "warm-lines" and "hot-lines" provided to parents, and the social services department may be of help in ensuring that the home environment is satisfactory and that special needs can be met. Support group referrals are given to parents, and newborn CPR techniques are reviewed.

Unfolding Case Study

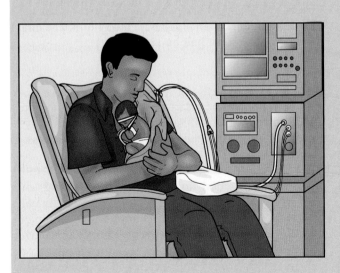

Tess and her husband Luis were introduced to the reader in Chapter 4, and each chapter has followed Tess through her labor and delivery. She has delivered twins unexpectedly. Baby Marco is in the postpartum unit with Tess. Baby Sofia showed signs of respiratory distress and was transported to the NICU accompanied by Tess's husband Luis.

Sofia was admitted to the NICU and has been diagnosed with respiratory distress and inadequate thermoregulation. She has been placed in an incubator.

QUESTIONS

1. What are the signs of respiratory distress in the newborn?
2. What are the nursing responsibilities involved in applying a pulse oximeter and monitoring Sofia's oxygen saturation?
3. The health care provider suggests kangaroo care for baby Sofia. What is kangaroo care? Can Sofia's father give kangaroo care to Sofia? What guidance and teaching will the nurse offer Sofia's father?
4. While in the NICU, Sofia's vital signs will be monitored. What are the normal vital signs of a newborn infant?

Get Ready for the NCLEX® Examination!

Key Points

- Every week in utero up to 39 weeks gestation is important for optimal fetal development.
- Early identification of the high-risk fetus facilitates treatment and nursing care.
- Studies indicate that there is a relationship between prematurity and poverty, smoking, alcohol consumption, narcotics use, and lack of prenatal care.
- Preterm infants have poor muscle tone and less subcutaneous fat but more vernix and lanugo than full-term infants.
- The preterm infant is observed for jaundice, low oxygen saturation levels, and unstable vital signs. The intake and output of all preterm infants is monitored.
- The care of preterm infants is organized and "clustered" to minimize handling and stimulation.
- Blanket rolls are used to provide an enclosed space for preterm infants.
- Nurses support parents and encourage participation in care.
- Respiratory distress syndrome has a high mortality rate, and it may precipitate long-term effects.
- Hypoxia is lack of oxygen on the cellular level, and hypoxemia is decreased oxygen in the circulating blood.
- Problems associated with prematurity include asphyxia, meconium aspiration, hypoglycemia, hypocalcemia, hemorrhage from fragile vessels, poor resistance to infection, and inadequate nutrition.
- Hypoglycemia is defined as glucose level lower than 40 mg/dL in the term infant or lower than 30 mg/dL in the preterm infant.
- Heat or thermoregulation is essential for the preterm newborn's survival. Cold stress is to be avoided.
- Nursing goals in caring for the preterm newborn are improving respirations, maintaining body heat, conserving the infant's energy, preventing infection, providing nutrition and hydration, providing good skin care, and supporting and encouraging the parents.
- Kangaroo care promotes stabilization of the infant as well as enhancing later development.
- Retinopathy of prematurity is a disorder of the developing retina that can lead to blindness in the preterm infant.
- The postterm newborn is born after 42 weeks of gestation and shows certain characteristics that place the infant at risk, such as hypoxia, poor nutritional stores, and polycythemia.
- The postterm newborn has little lanugo and vernix, and the skin is dry and peeling.

Additional Learning Resources

SG Go to your Study Guide for additional learning activities to help you master this chapter content.

evolve Go to your Evolve website (http://evolve.elsevier.com/Leifer) for the following learning resources:

- Animations
- Answer Guidelines for Critical Thinking Questions
- Answers and Rationales for Review Questions for the NCLEX® Examination
- Glossary with English and Spanish pronunciations
- Interactive Review Questions for the NCLEX® Examination
- Patient Teaching Plans in English and Spanish
- Skills Performance Checklists
- Video clips and more!

 Online Resources
- March of Dimes Annual Report: www.marchofdimes.com/797.asp
- Premature birth: www.mayoclinic.com/health/premature-birth/DS00137
- Premature birth complications: www.americanpregnancy.org/labornbirth/complicationspremature.htm

Review Questions for the NCLEX® Examination

1. Hypocalcemia is a common problem in preterm infants. When IV calcium gluconate is given to the newborn, what would a priority nursing intervention be?
   1. Monitor infant for bradycardia.
   2. Monitor infant for passage of stool.
   3. Prepare to give sodium bicarbonate.
   4. Monitor infant for bleeding.

2. Some preterm infants are fed by gavage because of:
   1. poor digestion.
   2. overdeveloped gag and cough reflexes.
   3. refusal of formula.
   4. weak sucking and swallowing reflexes.

3. A characteristic sign of necrotizing enterocolitis (NEC) in the newborn is:
   1. bloody diarrhea.
   2. necrosis of the abdomen.
   3. projectile vomiting.
   4. high fever.

4. Which of the following observations of a preterm neonate would indicate presence of respiratory distress? (Select all that apply.)
   1. Substernal retractions
   2. Respiratory rate of 70/min
   3. Grunting
   4. Lethargy

5. An infant is born at 43 weeks gestation. The nurse should monitor the infant for common problems such as (select all that apply):
   1. respiratory distress caused by possible meconium aspiration.
   2. increased weight gain resulting from increased glucose availability.
   3. hypoglycemia resulting from decreased glucose reserves.
   4. presence of increased amounts of lanugo.

The Newborn with a Perinatal Injury or Congenital Malformation

Objectives

1. Define each key term listed.
2. List and define the more common disorders of the newborn.
3. Describe the classifications of birth defects.
4. Outline the nursing care for the newborn with hydrocephalus.
5. Discuss the prevention of neural tube anomalies.
6. Outline the preoperative and postoperative nursing care of a newborn with spina bifida cystica.
7. Differentiate between cleft lip and cleft palate.
8. Discuss the early signs of developmental hip dysplasia.
9. Discuss the dietary needs of a newborn with phenylketonuria.
10. Discuss the care of the newborn with Down syndrome.
11. Outline the causes and treatment of hemolytic disease of the newborn (erythroblastosis fetalis).
12. Devise a plan of care for a newborn receiving phototherapy.
13. Describe home phototherapy.
14. Describe the symptoms of increased intracranial pressure.
15. Discuss the assessment and nursing care of a newborn with macrosomia.

Key Terms

birth defects (p. 324)
cheiloplasty (KĪ-lō-plăs-tē, p. 331)
cleft lip (p. 330)
cleft palate (p. 331)
clubfoot (p. 332)
congenital malformations (p. 325)
erythroblastosis fetalis (ĕ-rĭth-rō-blăs-TŌ-sĭs fĕ-TĂL-ĭs, p. 340)
habilitation (p. 329)
hydrocephalus (hī-drō-SĔF-ă-lăs, p. 325)
hyperbilirubinemia (hī-pŭr-bĭl-ē-rū-bĭ-NĒ-mē-ă, p. 342)
kernicterus (p. 342)
macrosomia (măk-rō-SŌ-mē-ă, p. 347)
meconium aspiration syndrome (MAS) (p. 346)

meningocele (mă-NĬNG-gō-sēl, p. 328)
meningomyelocele (mă-nĭng-gō-MĪ-ĕ-lō-sēl, p. 328)
myelodysplasia (mī-ă-lō-dĭs-PLĂ-zhă, p. 328)
neonatal abstinence syndrome (p. 346)
Ortolani's sign (p. 334)
Pavlik harness (p. 334)
phototherapy (p. 342)
RhoGAM (p. 341)
shunt (p. 326)
spica cast (p. 335)
spina bifida (SPĪ-nă BĬF-ĭ-dă, p. 328)
transient tachypnea of the newborn (TTN) (p. 346)
transillumination (p. 325)

Birth defects, abnormalities that are apparent at birth, occur in 3% to 4% of all live births. The rate is even higher if the defects that become evident later in life are counted. An abnormality of structure, function, or metabolism may result in a physical or mental disability, may shorten life, or may be fatal. Box 14-1 shows the system of classification of birth defects. Because these disorders include so many conditions, it is necessary to limit the number discussed in this chapter and to place others in relevant areas of the text (see the Index for specific conditions). Fetal alcohol syndrome and environmental influences on fetal growth are discussed in Chapter 5. Congenital heart disease is discussed in Chapter 26.

Defects present at birth often involve the skeletal system; limbs may be missing, malformed, or duplicated. Some abnormalities (e.g., congenital hip dysplasia) are more subtle, and the nurse must be alert to detect them. *Inborn errors of metabolism* include a number of inherited diseases that affect body chemistry. There may be an absence or a deficiency of a substance necessary for cell metabolism. The deficient substance is usually an enzyme. Almost any organ of the body may be damaged. Examples of inborn errors of metabolism include cystic fibrosis and phenylketonuria (PKU). In *disorders of the blood*, there is a reduced or missing blood component or an inability of a component to function adequately. Sickle cell disease, thalassemia, and hemophilia fall into this category. *Chromosomal abnormalities* number in the thousands. Most involve some type of mental retardation, and others are incompatible with life. The newborn with Turner's syndrome or Klinefelter's syndrome may have impaired physical growth and sexual development. *Perinatal injuries* have

Classification of Birth Defects

MALFORMATIONS PRESENT AT BIRTH
Structural Defects
Hydrocephalus,* spina bifida,* congenital heart malformations, cleft lip and palate,* clubfoot,* developmental hip dysplasia,* tracheoesophageal fistula, hypospadias, and others
Metabolic Defects (Body Chemistry)
Cystic fibrosis, phenylketonuria,* Tay-Sachs disease, family hypercholesterolemia (high cholesterol that often causes early heart attack), and others

BLOOD DISORDERS
Sickle cell disease, hemophilia, thalassemia, defects of white blood cells and immune defense, and others (see Chapter 27)

CHROMOSOMAL ABNORMALITIES
Down syndrome,* Klinefelter's syndrome, Turner's syndrome, trisomies 13 and 18, and many others; most involve some combination of mental retardation and physical malformations that range from mild to fatal

PERINATAL INJURY
Infections, drugs, maternal disorders, abnormalities unique to pregnancy (e.g., Rh disease,* difficult labor or delivery, premature birth)

*Topics discussed in this chapter. More detailed discussions of other conditions can be found in other chapters within this text.

many causes and are seen in various forms, the most common of which is premature birth.

As the March of Dimes Birth Defect Foundation (2006) points out, "Few birth defects can be attributed to a single cause. The majority are thought to result from an interplay between environment and heredity, depending on inherited susceptibility, stage of pregnancy, and degree of environmental hazard." Newborns with birth defects may need to remain in the neonatal unit for an extended period of time for intensive care and treatment.

MALFORMATIONS PRESENT AT BIRTH

The following sections discuss some **congenital malformations**, or those defects present at birth, according to body systems.

NERVOUS SYSTEM
Neural Tube Defects
Neural tube defects are most often caused by failure of neural tube closure at either the cranial (top) or the caudal (lower) end of the spinal cord. These defects often result in hydrocephalus and spina bifida.

Hydrocephalus
Pathophysiology. **Hydrocephalus** (*hydro,* "water," and *cephalo,* "head") in the newborn is a condition characterized by an increase of cerebrospinal fluid (CSF) within the ventricles of the brain, which causes pressure changes in the brain and an increase in head size. It results from an imbalance between the production

and absorption of CSF or improper formation of the ventricles. Hydrocephalus may be congenital or acquired. It is most commonly acquired by an obstruction, such as a tumor, or as a sequela of infections (encephalitis or meningitis) or perinatal hemorrhage. The symptoms depend on the site of obstruction and the age at which it develops.

Hydrocephalus is classified as noncommunicating (obstructive) or communicating. *Noncommunicating hydrocephalus* results from the obstruction of CSF flow from the ventricles of the brain to the subarachnoid space. *Communicating hydrocephalus* results when CSF is not obstructed in the ventricles but is inadequately reabsorbed in the subarachnoid space (Figure 14-1).

Manifestations. The signs and symptoms of hydrocephalus depend on the time of onset and the severity of the imbalance. The classic sign is an increase in head size. If hydrocephalus occurs in utero, the enlarged head will necessitate a cesarean section delivery. At birth, the head enlarges rapidly and the fontanelles bulge. The cranial sutures separate to accommodate the enlarging mass. The scalp is shiny, and the veins are dilated. In advanced cases the pupils of the eyes may appear to be looking downward and the sclera may be seen above the pupils, much like the look of a setting sun (Figure 14-2). A foreshortened occiput suggests pathology of the fourth ventricle, with the brain stem protruding through the cervical canal. This is called the Arnold-Chiari malformation (Kliegman et al, 2011). When the enlarged head involves a prominent occiput, the condition usually involves an atresia of the foramen of Lushka and the foramen of Magendie and is known as the Dandy-Walker syndrome. The infant is helpless and lethargic. The body becomes thin, and the muscle tone of the extremities is often poor. The cry is shrill and high pitched. Irritability, vomiting, and anorexia are present, and convulsions may occur.

When hydrocephalus occurs in the older child, the head cannot enlarge because the cranial sutures are fused; therefore headache is the predominant symptom, with cognitive slowing, personality changes, spasticity, and other neurological signs.

Diagnosis. **Transillumination** (*trans,* "across," and *illuminare,* "to enlighten")—the inspection of a cavity or organ by passing a light through its walls—is a simple diagnostic procedure useful in visualizing fluid. A flashlight with a sponge-rubber collar is held tightly against the infant's head in a dark room. The examiner observes for areas of increased luminosity. A small ring of light is normal, but a large halo effect is not. The child's head is measured daily. Echoencephalography, computed tomography (CT) scanning, and magnetic resonance imaging (MRI) are used to visualize the enlarged ventricles and to identify the area of

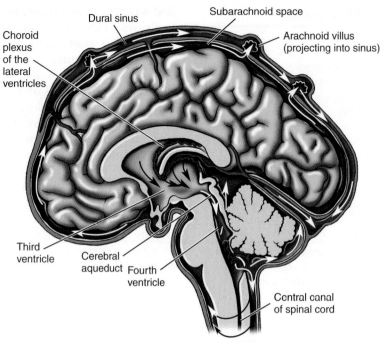

FIGURE 14-1 Cerebrospinal fluid circulation. Cerebrospinal fluid (CSF) is formed in the choroid plexus. The total volume of CSF is approximately 50 mL in the infant and 150 mL in the adult. It flows from the lateral ventricles through the foramen of Monro to the third ventricle. From the third ventricle, the CSF fluid flows through the aqueduct of Sylvius to the fourth ventricle, and then through the foramen of Luschka and the foramen of Magendie into the cisterns at the base of the brain. Flow continues to the spinal canal. The CSF is then absorbed by the arachnoid villi (which are also known as pacchionian bodies). Communicating or nonobstructive hydrocephalus occurs when the arachnoid villi are malformed or malfunction. Noncommunicating or obstructive hydrocephalus results when the tiny aqueduct of Sylvius is obstructed within the ventricles. When hydrocephalus occurs, excessive CSF causes the ventricles to enlarge and press the brain tissue against the bony skull. (From Herlihy B, Maebius NK: *The human body in health and illness,* ed 4, Philadelphia, 2011, Saunders.)

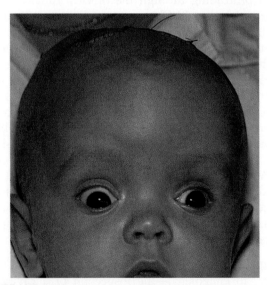

FIGURE 14-2 Marked hydrocephalus with "setting sun" sign of the eyes. Note the characteristic large head, distended scalp veins, and full fontanelle. (Courtesy Dr. Albert Biglan, Children's Hospital of Pittsburgh. In Zitelli BL, Davis HW: *Zitelli and Davis' atlas of pediatric physical diagnosis,* ed 6, St Louis, 2012, Saunders.)

obstruction. A ventricular tap or puncture may be performed using a sterile technique to determine pressure and to drain CSF. The equipment needed is the same as that for a lumbar puncture. A specimen is labeled and sent to the laboratory for analysis.

Treatment. The use of acetazolamide and furosemide reduces the production of CSF and may provide some relief, but most often surgery is indicated (Kliegman et al, 2011). The surgeon attempts to bypass, or **shunt**, the point of obstruction. The CSF may thus be carried to another area of the body, where it is absorbed and finally excreted. This is accomplished by inserting special tubing, which is replaced at intervals as the child grows. The procedure, known as a ventriculoperitoneal shunt (Figure 14-3), allows the excess fluid to drain into the peritoneal cavity where it is absorbed.

The prognosis for the child with hydrocephalus has improved with modern drugs and surgical techniques. If the brain is not seriously damaged before the operation, mental function may be preserved. Motor development is sometimes slower if the child cannot lift the head, normally because of its increased weight. Complications of shunts are usually mechanical (kinking or plugging of tubing) or infectious. The shunt acts as a focal spot for infection and may need to be removed if infection persists.

Preoperative Nursing Care. Most often, surgical correction can be accomplished in utero via fetal surgery or shortly after birth to prevent brain damage caused by increased intracranial pressure. The immediate preoperative care is routine, involving assessment of vital signs and skin preparation and emotional support

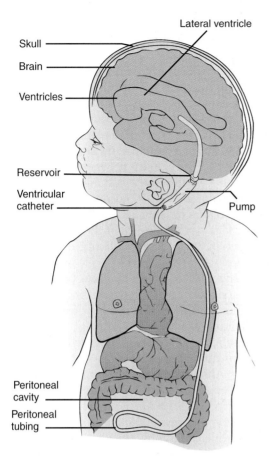

Skull
Brain
Ventricles
Lateral ventricle
Reservoir
Ventricular catheter
Pump
Peritoneal cavity
Peritoneal tubing

FIGURE 14-3 Shunting procedure for hydrocephalus, in which a catheter drains the ventricular system into the peritoneal cavity. Note the pump behind the ear, which can be depressed intermittently to clear obstructions.

of the parents. However, when the infant does not have access to corrective surgery, the general nursing care of an infant with hydrocephalus who has not undergone surgery presents several challenges. As the child grows, the child may be barely able to raise the head. Mental development is delayed. Lack of appetite, a tendency to vomit easily, and poor resistance to infections complicate the management of these infants.

The position of the infant must be changed frequently to prevent hypostatic pneumonia and pressure sores. Hypostatic pneumonia occurs when the circulation of the blood in the lungs is poor and the infant remains in one position too long. It is particularly prevalent in infants who are poorly nourished or weak or who have a debilitating disease. When the nurse turns an infant who has hydrocephalus, the head must always be supported. To turn the infant in bed, the weight of the head is borne in the palm of one hand, and the head and body are rotated together to prevent a strain on the neck. When the infant is lifted from the crib, the head must be supported by the nurse's arm and chest.

The tissues of the head, ears, and bony prominences tend to break down. A pad of lamb's wool or sponge rubber placed under the head may help to prevent these

lesions. If the skin becomes broken, it is given immediate attention to prevent infection. The infant must be kept dry, especially around the creases of the neck where perspiration may collect.

In most cases the nurse may hold the infant for feedings. The nurse sits with the arm supported because the infant's head is heavy. A calm, unhurried manner is necessary. The room should be as quiet as possible. After the feeding, the infant is placed in a side-lying position. The infant is not disturbed once settled, because vomiting occurs easily. The nurse must organize daily care so that it does not interfere with meals.

Observations to be recorded and reported include the type and amounts of food taken, any vomiting, the condition of the skin, motor abilities, restlessness, irritability, and changes in vital signs. Fontanelles are inspected for size and signs of bulging. Head circumference is measured around the occipitofrontal area and is recorded on the chart.

Symptoms of increased pressure within the head are an increase in blood pressure and a decrease in pulse rate and respirations. Signs of a cold or other infection are immediately reported to the nurse in charge and are recorded.

Postoperative Nursing Care. In addition to routine postoperative care and observations, the nurse observes the patient for signs of increased intracranial pressure (ICP) and of infection at the operative site or along the shunt line. As with any postoperative care, pain control management is essential.

Bacterial infection is a life-threatening complication that sometimes necessitates shunt removal. Signs of infection include an increase in vital signs, poor feeding, vomiting, pupil dilation, decreased levels of consciousness, and seizures. The operative area is observed for signs of inflammation. An internal flushing device may be used to ensure patency of the shunt tube when increased ICP is suspected. The surgeon may order the pump to be routinely depressed a certain number of times each day to facilitate drainage. This is accomplished by compressing the antechamber or reservoir that is under the skin behind the ear (see Figure 14-3).

Positioning of the infant depends on several factors and may vary with the infant's progress. If the fontanelles are sunken, the infant is kept flat because too rapid a reduction of fluid may lead to seizures or cortical bleeding. If the fontanelles are bulging, the infant is usually placed in the semi-Fowler's position to promote drainage of the ventricles through the shunt. The infant is always positioned in a way that prevents pressure on the operative site. The surgeon leaves orders for the patient's position and activity. Assessment of skin remains a priority. Head and chest measurements are recorded. In patients with peritoneal shunts, the abdomen is measured or observed to detect malabsorption of fluid.

The infant should be observed for signs of increased ICP. The development of a high-pitched cry, unequal pupil size or response to light, bulging fontanelles, irritability or lethargy, poor feeding, or abnormal vital signs should be reported and recorded. (Evidence of increased ICP in the older child may be manifested by a change in personality, a change in level of consciousness, and complaints of headaches that are unrelieved by over-the-counter medications.) The need for pain control should be assessed and medications given as needed. Intake and output are carefully recorded, and the infant is observed closely for signs of fluid overload. The infant is usually fed after active bowel sounds are heard. The surgical suture lines should be kept clean and dry and the infant's diaper kept well below the abdominal suture line to prevent contamination.

Parent education, support, and guidance are essential. Parents are taught signs that indicate shunt malfunction, how and when to "pump" the shunt by pressing against the valve behind the ear, and the need for multidisciplinary follow-up care. Signs of tube malfunction in the *older* child involve signs of increasing ICP such as headache, lethargy, and changes in level of consciousness. Community resources, such as the National Hydrocephalus Foundation and information concerning special car seats for children with special needs, should be made known to the parents. There is approximately an 80% survival rate for infants treated early, and approximately one third of the cases result in normal physical and neurological functioning. Other survivors may have varying degrees of developmental disabilities.

Spina Bifida

Spina bifida, also known as **myelodysplasia**, refers to a group of central nervous system disorders characterized by malformation of the spinal cord.

Pathophysiology. **Spina bifida** (divided spine) is a congenital embryonic neural tube defect in which there is an imperfect closure of the spinal vertebrae. There are two forms: occulta (hidden) and cystica (sac or cyst) (Figure 14-4).

Spina bifida occulta is a relatively minor variation of the disorder in which the opening is small and there is no associated protrusion of structures. It often goes undetected and occurs most commonly at the L5 and S1 levels. There may be a tuft of hair (Figure 14-5), dimple, lipoma, or discoloration at the site. In general, treatment is not necessary unless neuromuscular symptoms appear. These symptoms consist of progressive disturbances of gait, such as footdrop, or disturbances of bowel and bladder sphincter function.

Spina bifida cystica consists of the development of a cystic mass in the midline of the opening in the spine. Meningocele and meningomyelocele are two types of spina bifida cystica. A **meningocele** (*meningo*, "membrane," and *cele*, "tumor") contains portions of the membranes and CSF. The size varies from that of a walnut to that of a newborn's head.

More serious is a protrusion of the membranes and spinal cord through this opening, which is a **meningomyelocele**. Although it resembles a meningocele, there may be associated paralysis of the legs and poor control of bowel and bladder functions. Hydrocephalus is a common complication. Prenatal detection is possible through ultrasonography and testing for increased alpha-fetoprotein (AFP) in the amniotic fluid of the mother (see Chapter 5).

Prevention. The specific cause of meningomyelocele is unknown. The use of drugs during early pregnancy and poor nutrition may contribute to the development of a neural tube defect. The American Academy of Pediatrics (AAP) recommends that all women of childbearing age take a daily multivitamin that contains 0.4 mg of folic acid and continue the intake of folic acid until the twelfth week of pregnancy, when basic neural tube development is completed. Studies have shown that the intake of folic acid before

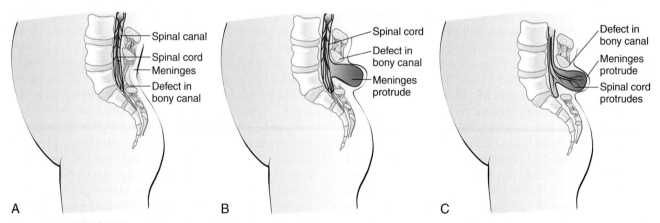

FIGURE 14-4 Types of spina bifida. **A,** Spina bifida occulta. There is a defect in the bony canal. The meninges and spinal cord are normal. **B,** Spina bifida cystica meningocele. The spinal cord is normal, but there is a defect in the bony canal. The meninges protrude through this defect. **C,** Spina bifida cystica meningomyelocele. There is a defect in the bony canal. The meninges protrude, and the spinal cord protrudes through the defect.

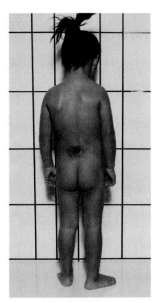

FIGURE 14-5 A child with a hairy patch in the lumbosacral region indicating the site of a spina bifida occulta. (Courtesy Dr. A.E. Chudley, Section of Genetics and Metabolism, Department of Pediatrics and Child Health, Children's Hospital and University of Manitoba, Winnipeg, Manitoba, Canada. From Moore KL, Persaud TVN, Torchia MG: *The developing human: clinically oriented embryology*, ed 9, Philadelphia, 2013, Saunders.)

conception dramatically decreases the occurrence of neural tube defects such as spina bifida.

> 🔲 **Nursing Tip**
>
> The intake of a daily multivitamin containing 0.4 mg of folic acid before conception can reduce the risk of neural tube defects such as spina bifida. A higher dose of folic acid may be prescribed if the mother has a previous history of giving birth to a child with a neural tube defect.

Treatment. The treatment for spina bifida is surgical closure. The prognosis for patients with these conditions depends on the extent of involvement. When a patient with meningocele has no weakness of the legs or sphincter involvement, surgical correction is performed with excellent results. Surgery is also indicated for a patient with meningomyelocele for cosmetic purposes and to help prevent infection. A multidisciplinary approach is necessary, because, depending on the extent of the defect, the child may have difficulties associated with hydrocephalus, orthopedic problems, and problems relating to urinary and bowel function.

Habilitation is necessary after the operation because the legs remain paralyzed and the patient is incontinent of urine and feces. **Habilitation**, rather than *rehabilitation*, is the term used to describe this treatment, because the patient is disabled from birth and therefore is learning rather than relearning. The aim of habilitation is to minimize the child's disability and put to constructive use the unaffected parts of the body. Every effort is made to help the child develop a healthy personality so that he or she may experience a happy and productive life.

Eventually the child can be taught to use a wheelchair and possibly to walk with braces, crutches, or other walking devices. The implantation of an artificial urinary sphincter in early childhood can help some children to become continent and prevent the complications associated with constant urinary dribble. Medications such as oxybutynin chloride (Ditropan) are available to increase bladder storage. Children can also be "bowel trained" with the use of suppositories that promote timed bowel movements, helping the child avoid the social rejection that can be caused by bowel incontinence.

Nursing Care. The main objectives of nursing care include prevention of infection of or injury to the sac, correct positioning to prevent pressure on the sac and development of contractures, good skin care (particularly if the infant is incontinent of urine and feces), adequate nutrition, accurate observations and charting, education of the parents, continued medical supervision, and habilitation.

Immediate care of the sac is essentially the same regardless of whether the cord is involved. On delivery, the newborn is placed in an incubator. Moist, sterile dressings of saline or an antibiotic solution may be ordered to prevent drying of the sac. Some method of protecting the mass is necessary if surgery is to be delayed. Protection from injury and maintenance of a sterile environment for the open lesion are essential.

Along with routine observations made for every newborn, other pertinent nursing observations must be made and recorded:

- The size and area of the sac are checked for any tears or leakage.
- The extremities are observed for deformities and movement. (There may be spasticity or paralysis of the limbs, or they may be normal depending on the type and location of the cyst.)
- The head circumference is measured to determine the possibility of associated hydrocephalus.
- Fontanelles are observed to provide baseline data.
- The lack of anal sphincter control and dribbling of urine are significant in the differential diagnosis (Figure 14-6). In general, the higher the defect on the spine, the greater the neurological deficit.

Positioning of the infant is important. The goal is to prevent pressure on the sac and to prevent postural deformities. When positioning infants with multiple deformities, the nurse must try to guard against aggravating existing problems. The infant is usually placed prone with a pad between the legs to maintain abduction and to counteract hip subluxation. A small roll is placed under the ankles to maintain foot position. Some infants may be supported in a side-lying posture to provide periods of relief. The disadvantage of this position is that it reduces movement of the arms and flexes the hips. The physical therapy staff may provide a helpful consultation. Surgery is generally done early.

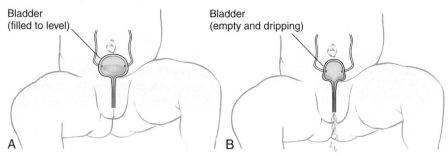

FIGURE 14-6 Incontinence in the newborn. **A,** Normally when the bladder fills to a certain level, a sensor stimulates contraction of the bladder, and expulsion of a volume of urine into the diaper occurs. A normal newborn has about six wet diapers a day. **B,** A newborn is considered incontinent when the sensor does not function and the bladder does not fill to its capacity before emptying. There is a constant dribble of urine into the diaper. The diaper is always wet.

Postoperative nursing care involves neurological assessment and prevention of infection. The status of the fontanelles and any signs of increased ICP, such as irritability or vomiting, are significant. Sometimes a shunt is performed shortly after closure of the spine, if hydrocephalus is present. Complications that can be life threatening include meningitis, pneumonia, and urinary tract infection.

Urological monitoring is essential, because many of these infants have urinary incontinence (see Figure 14-6). Medication to prevent urinary tract infection is routinely given. The Credé method of bladder emptying (applying pressure above the symphysis pubis) may be used for infants. Older children may be taught intermittent, clean self-catheterization. This technique can be performed by parents and learned by children.

Skin care is a challenge. Constant dribbling of feces and urine irritates the perineal area and can infect the sac or the incision. Meticulous cleanliness is necessary. The bedding must be dry and free of wrinkles. Frequent cleansing, application of a prescribed ointment or lotion, and light massage help to maintain skin integrity. If range of motion exercises are ordered, they are performed gently.

Feeding is facilitated by early closure of the defect. In delayed cases, gavage may be used. These patients need cuddling and sensory stimulation. An infant who cannot be held can be soothed by touch. The nurse talks to the infant and, when possible, provides face-to-face (en face) communication. Mobiles are placed appropriately. Periodically moving the incubator or crib provides diversity of view. Soft music is also soothing.

Many infants with spina bifida develop a latex allergy. A latex-free environment should be adopted whenever possible. Parents should be informed that latex products such as balloons, "koosh" balls, tennis balls, and adhesive strips can cause allergic reactions that may include rashes and wheezing. The parents should be informed about food sensitivities that are common to children with latex allergies. Foods to avoid include bananas, avocados, and kiwi. Other commonly used items to avoid include latex-based pacifiers, feeding nipples, and water toys. The child should wear a

medical identification tag indicating the latex allergy. In some cases, antihistamines and steroids may be prescribed before and after surgery. Nurses should wear nitrile gloves instead of latex gloves while caring for these patients.

Special consideration must be given to the establishment of parent–infant relationships. This problem is complicated if the infant is transferred to a large medical center. Understanding and support are given to the parents, who may be overwhelmed. It is not unusual for them to be repulsed by the cyst. Most experience a sense of loss for what was to have been their "perfect baby." The astute nurse may recognize steps of the grieving process. Information and education about this disorder can be obtained from the Spina Bifida Association of America.

GASTROINTESTINAL SYSTEM

Cleft Lip

Pathophysiology. A **cleft lip** is characterized by a fissure or opening in the upper lip (Figure 14-7). It is a result of the failure of the maxillary and median nasal processes

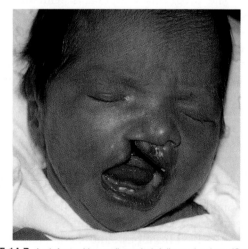

FIGURE 14-7 An infant with a unilateral cleft lip and palate. (Courtesy Dr. A.E. Chudley, Section of Genetics and Metabolism, Department of Pediatrics and Child Health, Children's Hospital and University of Manitoba, Winnipeg, Manitoba, Canada. From Moore KL, Persaud TVN, Torchia MG: *The developing human: clinically oriented embryology,* ed 9, Philadelphia, 2013, Saunders.)

to unite during embryonic development, usually between the seventh and eighth weeks of gestation. In many cases it seems to be caused by hereditary predisposition, but occasionally it can be caused by environmental influences during the stage of oral development. This disorder appears more frequently in boys than in girls and may occur on one or both sides of the lip. The extent of the defect may vary from slight to severe. Sometimes it is accompanied by a *cleft palate*—a fissure in the midline of the roof of the mouth. Cleft lip and cleft palate are common congenital anomalies and occur in about 1 in 750 births. Transculturally, they occur more often in Asian Americans and Native Americans and less commonly in African Americans (Kliegman, 2011).

Treatment and Nursing Care. The initial treatment for cleft lip is a surgical repair known as **cheiloplasty**. The cleft lip is repaired before age 6 months when weight gain is established and the infant is free of infection (Cassell, 2009). Surgery not only improves the infant's sucking ability but also greatly improves appearance. Indirectly, this influences bonding and the amount of affection the infant receives, because some parents refrain from cuddling an infant who is obviously disfigured.

A complete physical examination is done and routine blood tests are ordered before surgery. Photographs may also be taken. Any signs of oral, respiratory, or systemic infection are reported to the registered nurse. The physician may order elbow restraints to prevent the infant from scratching the lip and to acquaint the infant with them because they may be necessary postoperatively. A syringe with a rubber tip, a long nipple with a large hole attached to a squeeze bottle, or a medicine dropper can be used to feed the infant formula or breast milk before and after surgery, because sucking motions must be avoided to keep from applying tension on the suture line.

Postoperative Nursing Care. Postoperative nursing goals for the infant undergoing a cheiloplasty include the following:

- Preventing the infant from sucking and crying, which could cause tension on the suture line.
- Careful positioning (never on the abdomen) to prevent injury to the operative site.
- Preventing infection and scarring by gentle cleansing of the suture line to prevent crusts from forming.
- Preventing injury to the operative site by using elbow restraints. A Logan bow (a device used to immobilize the upper lip) may be applied for a short time postoperatively.
- Providing for the infant's emotional needs by cuddling and other forms of affection. This is of particular importance because the infant cannot obtain the usual satisfactions from sucking.
- Providing appropriate pain relief and sedation, which may be required for active infants.

Feeding. The infant receives feedings by dropper until the wound is completely healed (1 to 2 weeks). The infant is usually fed breast milk or formula as soon as clear liquids are tolerated postoperatively. Care should be taken to avoid touching the suture line when inserting the medicine dropper. Sucking is prevented as much as possible until the suture line is healed. Placing a small amount of breast milk or formula into the infant's mouth and allowing time for swallowing will prevent aspiration. Offering small amounts of sterile water will cleanse the mouth after feeding. Formula or drainage is gently cleaned from the suture line with saline solution, and an ointment may be applied to the skin as prescribed. Holding the infant during feedings, burping frequently, and placing the infant in an infant seat after feeding or on the right side propped with a rolled blanket will aid in a positive outcome for this infant. The mother who has fed her infant preoperatively and has been allowed to assist with feedings during hospitalization will feel more confident after discharge. The immediate improvement as a result of surgery is encouraging to the parents, particularly if the child must have further surgery for cleft palate repair.

Cleft Palate

Pathophysiology. A **cleft palate** is a failure of the hard palate to fuse at the midline during the seventh to twelfth weeks of gestation. This separation forms a passageway between the nasopharynx and the nose, which not only complicates feeding but also easily leads to infections of the respiratory tract and middle ear that can result in hearing loss. It is generally responsible for speech difficulties that occur in later life. The cleft may not be readily apparent at birth, and for this reason careful examination of the oral cavity and upper palate at birth is essential. Feeding is a problem because the cleft prevents negative pressure from being formed within the mouth, which is necessary for successful sucking.

Treatment. The goals of therapy are union of the cleft, improved feeding, improved speech, improved dental development, and the nurturing of a positive self-image. Some surgeons prefer to operate between 1 year and 18 months of age, if at all possible, so that speech patterns are minimally affected and tooth buds are protected (Cassell, 2009). If surgery has been deferred, a dental speech appliance may be used to facilitate communication. This appliance must be changed periodically as the child grows.

Treatment of the child with a cleft lip and palate requires multidisciplinary teamwork with a surgeon, pediatrician, pediatric dentist, orthodontist, nurse, psychologist, speech therapist, and social worker. The public health nurse should be responsible for coordinating parental counseling and referral as needed. The emotional problems that sometimes occur with this condition require more extensive attention than does the repair itself. A child born with a facial deformity encounters many problems. Feedings are difficult and are not relaxed in the initial period. As the child grows, irregular tooth eruptions, drooling, delayed speech, and the need for intermittent hospitalization and frequent clinic appointments can be frustrating. High-resolution ultrasound can detect cleft palate by 13 weeks of gestation, and therefore its correction (without scarring) by fetal surgery appears promising for the near future.

> **!** **Safety Alert!**
>
> Suctioning the mouth should be avoided in infants who have a cleft palate repair.

Psychosocial Adjustment of the Family. A mother's first reaction to a disfigured newborn is one of shock, hurt, disappointment, and guilt. Some parents regard the deformity as a result of their inadequacies. They may desire to hide the child from relatives and friends. The developing child senses the parents' feelings and acquires either a positive or a negative self-image. The patient and family need understanding, a concrete basis for hope, and practical advice. Family stress often occurs because of the multiple surgeries that may be required throughout childhood.

Follow-Up Care and Home Care. In large cities, special cleft palate clinics are available in which several specialists can work together in convenient consultation. The parents are instructed about the resources available in the state in which they live. The American Cleft Palate–Craniofacial Association, the Cleft Palate Foundation, the March of Dimes Birth Defect Foundation, and state programs for children with special needs are examples of community referrals that should be offered to parents.

Postoperative Treatment and Nursing Care

Nutrition. Fluids are taken by a cup, although a gravity feeder may be desirable in some cases. The method varies with the plastic surgeon. The diet is progressive, at first consisting of clear fluids and then full fluids. By the time of discharge, a soft diet can generally be taken. Hot foods and liquids are avoided to prevent injury to the operative site. The patient must not suck on a straw. When feeding with a spoon, the nurse should place the spoon into the side of the mouth. The spoon must not touch the roof of the mouth. The nurse teaches parents to keep objects such as the child's thumb, tongue blades, toast, cookies, forks, and pacifiers out of the mouth. Elbow restraints are used to prevent the child from placing his or her fingers or objects in the mouth. The diet is advanced only on consultation with the physician.

Oral hygiene. The mouth is kept clean at all times. Feedings are followed by a little water. The physician may prescribe a mild antiseptic mouthwash.

Speech. It is helpful to speak slowly and distinctly to the child. The child is encouraged to pronounce words correctly. Children who have undergone extensive repairs or have associated deafness need the help of a speech therapist. The speech therapist evaluates the child and assists the parents in specific activities that facilitate speech development.

Diversion. Crying is to be prevented as much as possible. Play should be quiet, particularly in the immediate postoperative period. The nurse reads, draws, or colors with the child.

Complications. Ear infections and dental decay may accompany cleft palate. Parents are instructed to take the child to the health care provider at the first sign of earache. Regular visits to the dentist are scheduled. Throughout the long-term care, a stable goal in the care of this infant is to promote optimal growth and development and to establish positive self-esteem.

MUSCULOSKELETAL SYSTEM

Clubfoot

Pathophysiology. **Clubfoot**, one of the most common deformities of the skeletal system, is a congenital anomaly characterized by a foot that has been twisted inward or outward. The incidence is about 1 in 1000 live births. Many mild forms are caused by improper position in the uterus, and these clear up with manipulative exercises. In contrast, true clubfoot does not respond to simple exercise. Several types are recognized. Talipes (*talus*, "heel," and *pes*, "foot") equinovarus (*equinus*, "extension," and *varus*, "bent inward") is seen in 95% of patients. The feet are turned inward, and the child walks on the toes and the outer borders of the feet. It generally involves both feet (Figure 14-8).

Treatment and Nursing Care. The treatment of clubfoot is started as early as possible, or the bones and muscles will continue to develop abnormally. Conservative treatment that consists of splinting or casting to hold the foot in the right position is performed during infancy. Passive stretching exercises may also be recommended. If these methods are not effective by

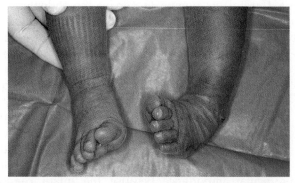

FIGURE 14-8 Clubfoot. A child with a clubfoot showing a flexed ankle, turned heel, and adducted forefoot. (From Bowden VR, Dickey SB, Greenberg SC: *Children and their families: the continuum of care*, Philadelphia, 1998, Saunders.)

age 3 months, surgery may be indicated. The infant with a clubfoot is under medical supervision for a long time. Parents must be instructed in developmental behaviors of the infant as well as the clinical aspects of care. Ongoing support is paramount.

Cast care. Casts are made of plaster or synthetic materials such as fiberglass or polyurethane. The plaster cast consists of crinoline that has powdered plaster in its meshwork. It is placed in warm water before being applied over cotton wadding or a stockinette. The wet plaster of Paris hardens as it dries. This type of cast dries from the inside out and takes 24 to 48 hours to dry.

If the patient returns to the unit before the cast is dry, the cast must be left uncovered and protected from pressures that could cause a depression in it. If the physician orders that the leg and foot be elevated on pillows to prevent swelling, the nurse who assists must use the palms of the hands, not the fingers, to lift the cast. Indentations made in a wet cast by fingers can press on the underlying skin and cause damage. This precaution is also explained to parents. Lighter synthetic casts dry in less than 30 minutes, are lighter in weight and water resistant if a water-resistant stockinette is applied. Often a mixture of fiberglass and plaster of Paris materials are used for a cast to provide strength and decrease weight of the cast.

The toes are left exposed for observation. The nurse checks them for capillary refill and signs of poor circulation, pallor, cyanosis, swelling, coldness, numbness, pain, or burning. If circulation is impaired, the physician may split the cast to relieve the pressure, or the cast may need to be removed and reapplied. The nurse also reports irritation of the skin around the edges of the cast and lack of movement of the toes. Adhesive petals may be placed around the edges of the cast to prevent skin irritation.

As the infant grows, the cast may need to be removed and reapplied. Because an infant grows rapidly, parents should be taught how to check for circulation impairments, which could be caused by a tight cast.

If surgery on tendons and bones has been performed, the nurse also observes the cast for evidence of bleeding. If a discolored area appears on the cast, it is circled and the time is recorded. Further bleeding can then be estimated. If bleeding is noted, the patient's vital signs are also checked and compared with preoperative readings. After surgery the cast is changed approximately every 3 weeks to bring the foot gradually into position. When the cast is removed for the final time, exercise and use of special shoes may be indicated.

Emotional support. The nurse is an important figure in the care of the long-term patient with clubfoot. Nurses review the normal growth and development of children in the patient's age range to anticipate problems and to educate caretakers in parenting.

Children in a cast may be slow in developing certain motor abilities. Education concerning the therapy and referral for follow-up care is an important nursing responsibility. The financial burdens of hospitalization, surgery, special shoes, and continued medical supervision may pose a serious problem. If the nurse suspects that the parents need financial help, a social service referral is made.

Nursing Tip

In the long-term care of orthopedic patients, educating the parents about orthopedic devices, cast care, exercise, hygiene, and treatment goals is necessary. The nurse explains the importance of frequent clinic visits, reinforces physicians' information, and clarifies directions as necessary.

Developmental Hip Dysplasia

Pathophysiology. **Developmental hip dysplasia,** formerly known as congenital hip dysplasia, is a common orthopedic deformity. The incidence is about 1 in 1000 births. The term *hip dysplasia* is a broad description applied to various degrees of deformity: subluxation or dislocation, either partial or complete. The head of the femur is partly or completely displaced as a result of a shallow hip socket (acetabulum). Hereditary and environmental factors appear to be causal factors. Hip malformation, joint laxity, breech position, and maternal hormones may all contribute. Developmental hip dysplasia is seven times more common in girls than in boys. Newborn infants seldom have complete dislocation. However, the child beginning to walk exerts pressure on the hip, which can cause complete dislocation. Therefore early detection and treatment are of particular importance.

There is a high risk for developmental hip dysplasia in cultures in which the newborn is wrapped snugly with the hips in adduction and extension. There is a lower risk for developmental hip dysplasia in cultures in which the infant is carried straddled on the mother's waist with the infant's hips flexed and widely abducted.

Manifestations. A dislocation of the hip is commonly discovered at the periodic health examination of the infant during the first or second month of life. One of the most reliable signs is a limited abduction of the leg on the affected side. When the infant is placed on the back with knees and hips flexed, the physician can press the thigh of the normal hip backward until it almost touches the examining table. This can be accomplished only partially on the affected side. The knee on the side of the dislocation is lower, and the skin folds of the thigh are deeper and often asymmetrical (Figure 14-9). When the infant is in a prone position, one buttock appears higher than the other.

A physician performs a *Barlow's test* to detect an unstable hip in the newborn. The physician adducts and extends the hips while stabilizing the pelvis and may "feel" the dislocation occur as the femur leaves the acetabulum.

In infants aged 1 to 2 months with developmental dislocation of the hip, the physician can actually feel

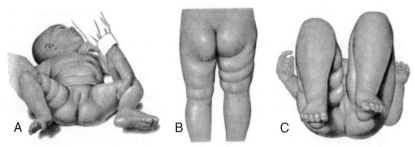

FIGURE 14-9   Early signs of dislocation of the right hip. **A,** Limitation of abduction. **B,** Asymmetry of skin folds. **C,** Shortening of femur. (From Ross Laboratories: *Clinical education aid no. 15,* Columbus, Ohio, 1986, Author. Reproduced with permission of Ross Laboratories.)

and hear the femoral head slip back into the acetabulum under gentle pressure. This is called **Ortolani's sign** or Ortolani's click and is also considered diagnostic of the disorder. The child who is walking and has had no treatment displays a characteristic limp. Bilateral (*bi,* "two," and *latus,* "side") dislocation may occur; however, unilateral (*uni,* "one," and *latus,* "side") dislocation is more common. Radiographic studies confirm the diagnosis.

Treatment. Treatment begins immediately on detection of the dislocation. The hips are maintained in constant flexion and abduction for 4 to 8 weeks to keep the head of the femur within the hip socket. This constant pressure enlarges and deepens the acetabulum; thus, it can correct the dislocation.

A triple-thick diaper may be used in the newborn to maintain a "froglike" abduction of the legs until a Pavlik harness can be fitted properly (Kliegman, 2011). In infants more than 2 months of age, soft tissue contractures prevent stabilization of the hip, and longer-term immobilization with a **Pavlik harness** may be required (Figure 14-10). Traction may be necessary if the dislocation is severe or is not detected until the child begins to walk. This pulls the head of the

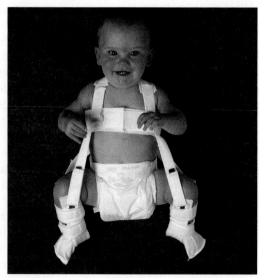

FIGURE 14-10   The Pavlik harness is used with infants aged 1 to 6 months to maintain hips in a position of flexion and abduction. (Wheaton Pavlik Harness. Courtesy Wheaton Brace Co.)

femur down to the correct position opposite the acetabulum and helps to overcome muscle spasm. Casting in a froglike position is then done. This type of cast, known as a body *spica cast,* is shown in Figure 14-11. The spica cast may be made from fiberglass or a mixture of fiberglass and plaster of Paris. (See Chapter 24 for care of the orthopedic patient.)

The length of time spent in a cast varies according to the patient's progress and growth and the condition of the cast; however, it is usually several months. During this time the cast may be changed about every 6 weeks. Surgery may be required in infants more than 18 months of age who do not respond to treatment. In such cases, open reduction of the dislocation or repair of the shelf of the hipbone is performed. After surgery a cast may be applied to keep the femur in the correct position.

Nursing care. The nursery nurse carefully observes each infant during the bath to detect signs of a hip dysplasia:

- When the infant is prone, the nurse observes the buttocks for variation in size.
- The legs of the infant should be equal in length.
- The infant should be kicking both legs, not just one leg.
- The depth and number of skin folds of the infant's upper thighs should be symmetrical.
- In the well-baby clinic the nurse notes the posture and gait of older children and records observations.

Infants who progress well with the Pavlik harness or Frejka splint (or a similar brace) remain at home with regular visits to the physician. The parents need assurance that the infant may be held and may sit in a chair. They should be encouraged to ask questions of the clinic nurse and physician.

The child who is admitted to the hospital with a diagnosis of developmental hip dysplasia is given as much personal attention as possible. The first admission sets the pattern for future hospitalization; therefore, the child must make a satisfactory adjustment. The nurse becomes familiar with the child's habits and plan of care. Every effort is made to provide a homelike environment for children who are hospitalized for many weeks.

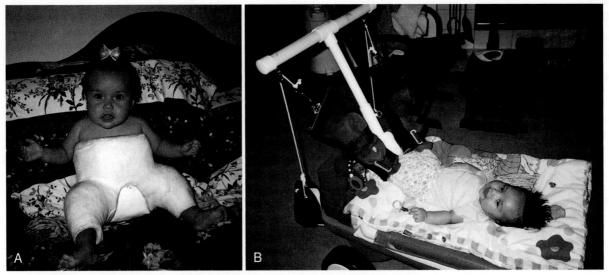

FIGURE 14-11 **A,** Infant in a spica body cast. This cast maintains the legs in a froglike position and is used to treat developmental hip dysplasia. Note that the infant is able to move her toes freely. A diaper tucked inside prevents the cast from becoming soiled with urine or feces. **B,** Traction is sometimes necessary before surgery or casting. Home care enables the child to be in familiar surroundings that will nurture growth and development.

The spica cast. The body **spica cast** encircles the waist and extends to the ankles or toes. Neurovascular assessment, discussed in Chapter 24, should be reviewed at this point. Nursing Care Plan 14-1 provides selected nursing diagnoses and interventions for the patient with a spica cast.

Firm, plastic-covered pillows are required. These are placed beneath the curvatures of the cast for support. Older children may benefit from an overhead bar and trapeze. The room should be adequately ventilated. A fracture pan should be available at the bedside for toileting as developmentally appropriate.

The head of the patient's bed is slightly elevated so that urine or feces drain away from the body of the cast. One should not use pillows to elevate the head or shoulders of a child in a body cast, because this thrusts the patient's chest against the cast and causes discomfort or respiratory difficulty. The child who is not toilet trained may be placed on a Bradford frame to facilitate nursing care. Frequent changes of position are important; immobilized patients must be turned often. Infants may be held in the nurse's lap after the cast has dried. A ride on a wagon or gurney to the playroom or around the hospital provides changes of position and scenery.

The supporting bar between the legs should not be used as a lever when turning the child (Skill 14-1). All body curvatures are supported with pillows or sheet rolls. Whenever possible, the older child should be on his or her abdomen during mealtime to facilitate swallowing and self-feeding. When placing a child in a body cast on a fracture pan, the upper back and legs are supported with pillows so that body alignment is maintained.

Itching is a problem for the patient in a body cast. If at all possible, a strip of gauze is placed beneath the cast before it is applied; this gauze extends through the opened area required for toilet needs. It is gently moved back and forth to relieve itching. When the strip becomes soiled, a clean one is tied to one end of the soiled gauze and pulled through the cast; this soiled portion is then removed. Other methods to relieve itch that might cause injury to the skin beneath the cast are discouraged, because any break in the skin under a cast is difficult to heal.

Toys small enough to be "hidden" inside the cast should not be given to the child. Toys that can be used when the child is in a prone position are best.

The child with this long-term disability requires help in meeting his or her everyday needs. This child is growing and developing rapidly, and therefore frequent adjustments in home and clinic care are necessary. Dressing and clothing are a problem. The child cannot fit into regular furniture or much of the play equipment enjoyed by other children. Transportation is difficult. A special wagon built up with pillows may be used (see Figure 14-11). The child should be included in everyday family and play activities to encourage normal growth and development. A referral for home health care should be made on discharge.

METABOLIC DEFECTS

The infant with an inborn error of metabolism has a genetic defect that may not be apparent before birth. As the infant adjusts to the birth process and begins to ingest nourishment, symptoms can rapidly emerge that quickly become life threatening. Symptoms such as lethargy, poor feeding, hypotonia, a unique odor to the body or urine, tachypnea, and vomiting must be reported by the nurse in the newborn nursery to prevent long-term or life-threatening sequelae. The nurse must also be prepared to offer psychological support

Nursing Care Plan 14-1   The Infant or Child with a Spica Cast

PATIENT DATA An infant returns from the cast room after having a spica cast applied. The infant is scheduled for discharge after the cast is dry.

Selected Nursing Diagnosis: Ineffective tissue perfusion because of cast constriction

Goals	Nursing Interventions	Rationales
Tissues and circulation will appear adequate as evidenced by pink, warm skin, good capillary refill, and lack of numbness or swelling.	Observe exposed extremities and skin distal to the cast every 30 minutes for the first few hours of a new cast and every 1 to 4 hours thereafter; watch for signs of pallor, cyanosis, swelling, coldness, numbness, pain, or burning.	Circulation can be impaired, leading to ischemia. Peripheral nerves, in contrast to muscles, do not degenerate with disuse, but loss of *innervation* can take place if nerves are damaged by pressure or if the blood supply is disrupted.
Parents will understand signs of inadequate circulation and explain importance of seeking immediate assistance if these signs appear.	Circle any drainage on cast with date and time; monitor and record findings.	An increase in size of circle indicates further bleeding or possibly a draining infection.
	Observe nonverbal communication for signs of pain; ask older child if pain is experienced.	Unrelieved pain, especially after a few days, may indicate *compartment syndrome*; compartment syndrome appears in a group of muscles and fascia where an increase in pressure within this closed space may disrupt circulation within the space.
	Educate parents and patient, if old enough, in all of above.	Education reduces stress for parents and patient.
	Provide written instructions.	Written instructions provide reinforcement and help to ensure the success of other interventions.

Selected Nursing Diagnosis: Risk for injury, related to awkwardness and weight of cast

Goals	Nursing Interventions	Rationales
Patient will remain safe and as independent as possible.	Inform older child when turning as to how and when you are going to proceed (e.g., "ready, set, go").	Involving child in procedure, as age appropriate, gives him or her a sense of control; procedure will go more smoothly.
	Leave articles and toys within reach.	Child will not need to strain or move awkwardly to reach articles; patient will feel greater control if articles can be obtained independently.
	Some car seats are adapted to accommodate a small child in a spica cast.	These children need protection in a car.

Critical Thinking Question

1. A mother brings her 2-year-old child to the clinic complaining that the spica cast has a strong, unpleasant odor. The child has a temperature of 37.8° C (100° F). He appears to be in no acute distress and is playing with a small toy car in one hand and has a half-eaten cracker in the other hand. What nursing intervention is indicated?

Technique for Turning the Child in a Body Cast

PURPOSE

To change position of child for comfort and prevention of pressure areas on skin

STEPS

Two people, one on each side of the bed, are needed to turn a child in a body cast, as follows:

1. Move the child to the edge of the bed as far as possible so that the nurse who will receive the child is farther away from him or her.

2. The nurse nearer to the child places one hand under the head and back and one hand under the leg part of the cast and turns the child to the midway point on the side.

3. The nurse farther away then accepts the support of the child and cast as turning is completed.

and to help parents deal with the impact of having an infant with a genetic problem.

PHENYLKETONURIA

Pathophysiology. **Classic phenylketonuria** (PKU) is a genetic disorder caused by the faulty metabolism of phenylalanine, an amino acid that is essential to life and is found in all protein foods. This inborn error of metabolism, which is transmitted by an autosomal recessive gene, is termed classic PKU and is associated with blood phenylalanine levels above 20 mg/dL. The hepatic enzyme phenylalanine hydrolase, which is normally needed to convert phenylalanine into tyrosine, is missing. When the infant is fed breast milk or formula, phenylalanine begins to accumulate in the blood. It can increase to as high as 20 times the normal amount. Its by-product, phenylpyruvic acid, appears in the urine within the first weeks of life.

Classic PKU results in severe retardation that is evidenced in infancy. Early detection and treatment are paramount. By the time the urine test is positive, brain damage has already occurred. The infant appears normal at birth but begins to show delayed development at about 4 to 6 months of age. The child may show evidence of failure to thrive, have eczema or other skin conditions, have a peculiar musty odor, or have personality disorders. About one third of the children have seizures. PKU occurs mainly in blonde and blue-eyed children; these features result from a lack of tyrosine, a necessary component of the pigment melanin. Less severe forms of the disorder are now recognized. They are designated as "atypical PKU" and "mild hyperphenylalaninemia."

Diagnosis. The *Guthrie blood test* is widely used and is currently considered the most reliable test for PKU. Blood is obtained from a simple heel stick. A few drops of capillary blood are placed on filter paper and mailed to the laboratory for screening. It is recommended that the blood be obtained after 48 to 72 hours of life, preferably after the ingestion of proteins, to reduce the possibility of false-negative results. Many states require that the test be done on all newborns before they leave the nursery, but because of early discharge the test may be repeated within 2 weeks. The infant can be tested at home by a public health nurse or at the clinic or physician's office. Confirmation of the diagnosis requires quantitative elevations of phenylalanine compound in the blood (Kliegman, 2011). Screening programs for pregnant women have also been advocated to detect elevated phenylalanine levels that could have an effect on the newborn.

Treatment and Nursing Care. Treatment of PKU consists of close dietary management and frequent evaluation of blood phenylalanine levels. Because phenylalanine is found in all natural protein foods, a food that provides enough protein for growth and tissue repair, but little phenylalanine, must be substituted.

The most commonly used formulas are Lofenalac or Phenex-1 for infants, Phenyl-Free for children, and Phenex-2 for adolescents. The goals of the diet are to provide enough essential proteins to support growth and development while maintaining phenylalanine blood levels between 2 and 10 mg/dL. A phenylalanine level below 2 mg/dL may result in growth retardation, whereas levels above 10 mg/dL can result in significant brain damage.

There is a low phenylalanine content in breast milk, and infants can be partially breastfed and supplemented with Lofenalac while phenylalanine blood levels are monitored. Solid foods that are low in phenylalanine are added at the same age that solid foods are added for infants without PKU. Phenyl-Free is introduced between ages 3 and 8 years. Cookbooks and family recipes provide ideas for variety. Eventually the child learns to assume full management of the diet.

A dietitian may be consulted concerning parental guidance and support in maintaining the dietary regimen, especially for the school-age child and adolescent. Many foods that contain a high level of phenylalanine are clearly labeled and provide easier choices for parents at the supermarket. A single 12-oz can of diet cola containing NutraSweet or Equal (aspartame) will not significantly raise blood levels of phenylalanine, but the intake of most meat, dairy products, and diet drinks must be restricted. An exchange list for food selection can aid the child in participating in and monitoring his or her progress. Flavoring the milk substitute with a fruit-flavored powder or chocolate flavoring can increase the child's compliance. Sapropterin dihydrochloride (Kuvan), is the first drug on the market to treat this inherited disorder and is designed to break down excess phenylalaline in the blood (Keil, 2013). The tablets are dissolved in juice and administered by mouth. Genetic counseling is important for the affected child for future family planning. Women of childbearing age who have PKU must follow a low-phenylalanine diet before conception to prevent brain damage of the fetus during development. Phenylalanine levels greater than 6 mg/dL in pregnant women can affect development of the embryo.

⚠ Safety Alert!

Children with PKU must avoid the sweetener aspartame (NutraSweet or Equal) because it is converted to phenylalanine in the body.

MAPLE SYRUP URINE DISEASE

Pathophysiology. **Maple syrup urine disease** is caused by a defect in the metabolism of branched-chain amino acids. It causes marked serum elevations of leucine, isoleucine, and valine. This results in acidosis, cerebral degeneration, and death within 2 weeks if left untreated.

Manifestations. The infant with maple syrup urine disease appears healthy at birth but soon develops feeding difficulties, loss of the Moro reflex, hypotonia, irregular respirations, and convulsions. The infant's urine, sweat, and cerumen (earwax) have a characteristic sweet or maple syrup odor. This is caused by ketoacidosis, a process similar to that which may occur in diabetic children, and causes a fruity odor of the breath. However, the condition does not resolve with the correction of blood glucose levels. The urine contains high levels of leucine, isoleucine, and valine. Diagnosis is confirmed by blood and urine tests.

Treatment and Nursing Care. Early detection in the newborn period is extremely important. The nursery nurse should report any newborn whose urine has a sweet aroma. Initial treatment consists of removing these amino acids and their metabolites from the tissues of the body. This is accomplished by hydration and peritoneal dialysis to decrease serum levels. The patient is placed on a lifelong diet that is low in the amino acids leucine, isoleucine, and valine. Several formulas specifically for this disease are available. Exacerbations are most often related to the degree to which the leucine level is abnormal. These exacerbations are frequently related to infection and can be life threatening. The nurse must frequently assess the patient and instruct parents about the need to prevent infections.

GALACTOSEMIA

Pathophysiology. In **galactosemia** the body is unable to use the carbohydrates galactose and lactose. In the healthy person, the liver converts galactose to glucose. In the patient with galactosemia, an enzyme is defective or missing and therefore there is a disturbance in a normally occurring chemical reaction. The result is an increase in the amount of galactose in the blood (galactosemia) and in the urine (galactosuria). This can cause cirrhosis of the liver, cataracts, and mental retardation if left untreated. Because galactose is present in milk sugar, early diagnosis is necessary so that a milk substitute can be used.

Manifestations. The symptoms of galactosemia begin abruptly and worsen gradually. Early signs consist of lethargy, vomiting, hypotonia, diarrhea, and failure to thrive. These commence as the newborn begins breastfeeding or ingesting formula. Jaundice may be present. Diagnosis is made by observing galactosuria, galactosemia, and evidence of decreased enzyme activity in the red blood cells. Screening tests are available.

Treatment and Nursing Care. Milk and lactose-containing products are eliminated from the diet of the patient with galactosemia. The nursing mother must discontinue breastfeeding. Lactose-free formulas and those with a soy-protein base are often substituted.

The nurse must realize the frustration and anxiety that this diagnosis creates. Parents experience periods of feeling overwhelmed and inadequate. They can also become totally absorbed in the dietary program. A rare disease creates feelings of isolation and uncertainty. Because surveillance is ongoing, some of the emotional characteristics of the family with a child who has a chronic disease are pertinent.

CHROMOSOMAL ABNORMALITIES

DOWN SYNDROME

Pathophysiology. Down syndrome is one of the most common chromosomal abnormalities. Its incidence is approximately 1 in 1000 live births worldwide (WHO, 2012). It is the most common cause of genetic intellectual disability, and children born with this birth defect may also have some physical abnormalities. In the past, children with this condition were called "mongoloid" because of the Oriental ("Mongolian") appearance of their faces, but this term is now considered inappropriate.

There are three phenotypes (genetic make-ups) of Down syndrome: trisomy 21, mosaicism, and translocation of a chromosome. The most common type, trisomy 21 syndrome, accounts for 95% of patients. In this instance there are three number 21 chromosomes rather than the normal two. This is a result of *nondisjunction*, the failure of a chromosome to follow the normal separation process into daughter cells. The earlier in the embryo's development this occurs, the greater the number of cells affected. When nondisjunction occurs late in development, both normal and abnormal cells are present in the newborn. This condition is *mosaicism*, and patients tend to be less severely affected in physical appearance and intelligence. The third condition is *translocation*. In translocation, a piece of chromosome in pair 21 breaks away and attaches itself to another chromosome. Scientists at the University of Massachusetts have developed a type of "chromosome therapy" for Down syndrome that involves prenatal injection of a chromosome called Xist that inactivates the extra chromosome that causes the problem. However, ethical problems arise that may inhibit the refining of this technique, because other cells in the fetus may be genetically altered as well (Lockwood, 2013).

Screening for Down syndrome is offered during the first trimester of pregnancy and includes an ultrasound assessment of the thickness of the fetal nuchal fold (called nuchal translucency) and absence of the nasal bone. This early screening allows parents to discuss options of terminating or continuing the pregnancy with preparation for the outcome. A second trimester "quad test" involves testing of the blood for levels of AFP, unconjugated estriol (UE), inhibin-A (a placental hormone), and human chorionic gonadotropin (hCG) (see Chapter 5). A low AFP or a high hCG and inhibin-A with a low UE may indicate a high risk for

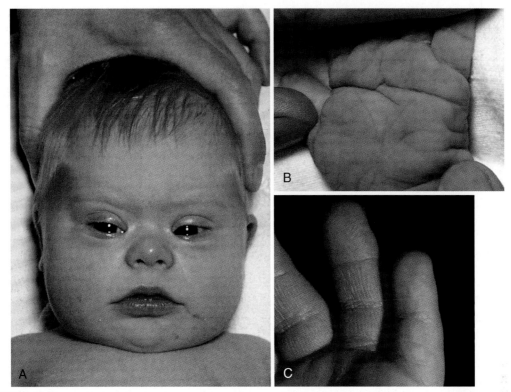

FIGURE 14-12 Down syndrome. **A,** The typical facial appearance of an infant with Down syndrome shows the upward slant of the canthal folds of the eyes, protruding tongue, and short, thick neck. **B,** The straight simian crease in the palm of the hand is a typical finding in children with Down syndrome. **C,** The short fifth finger is a typical finding in children with Down syndrome. The tip of the fifth finger does not extend to the distal joint of the adjoining finger. (From Zitelli BL, Davis HW: *Zitelli and Davis' atlas of pediatric physical diagnosis,* ed 6, St Louis, 2012, Saunders.)

Down syndrome in the developing fetus. A test of pregnancy-associated plasma protein A (PAPP-A) may also indicate a risk for Down syndrome. Positive tests in the first or second trimester may indicate the need for amniocentesis to confirm the diagnosis.

Manifestations. Down syndrome can be diagnosed by the clinical manifestations, but a chromosomal analysis will confirm the specific type. The signs of Down syndrome, which are apparent at birth, are close-set and upward-slanting eyes, small head, round face, flat nose, protruding tongue that interferes with sucking, and mouth breathing (Figure 14-12, *A*). There is a deep straight line across the palm, which is called the *simian crease* (Figure 14-12, *B*). The hands of the infant are short and thick, and the little finger is curved (Figure 14-12, *C*). There is also a wide space between the first and the second toes. The undeveloped muscles and loose joints enable the child to assume unusual positions. Physical growth and development may be slower than normal (Tables 14-1 and 14-2). The child is limited intellectually. Some children have been found to have intelligence quotients (IQs) in the borderline to low-average range. Congenital heart deformities are also associated with this condition.

Children with Down syndrome are very lovable. They may be restless and somewhat more difficult to train than the normal youngster. Their resistance to

Table 14-1 Time of Occurrence of Developmental Milestones in Normal Children and Those with Down Syndrome (in Months)

MILESTONE	CHILDREN WITH DOWN SYNDROME		NORMAL CHILDREN	
	AVERAGE	RANGE	AVERAGE	RANGE
Sitting	2	1.5-4	1	0.5-3
Rolling over	8	4-22	5	2-10
Sitting alone	10	6-28	7	5-9
Crawling	12	7-21	8	6-11
Creeping	15	9-27	10	7-13
Standing	20	11-42	11	8-16
Walking	24	12-65	13	8-18
Talking, words	16	9-31	10	6-14
Talking, sentences	28	18-96	21	14-32

From Carey W, Feldman H, Coleman W, Crocker A, Elias E: *Developmental-behavioral pediatrics,* ed 5, Philadelphia, 2009, Saunders.

infection is poor, and they are prone to respiratory and ear infections as well as speech and hearing problems. The life span of children with Down syndrome has increased with the widespread use of antibiotics. The incidence of acute leukemia is higher in these children than in the normal population, and Alzheimer's

| Table 14-2 | Time of Occurrence of Self-Help Skills in Normal Children and Those with Down Syndrome (in Months) |

MILESTONE	CHILDREN WITH DOWN SYNDROME		NORMAL CHILDREN	
	AVERAGE	RANGE	AVERAGE	RANGE
Eating				
Finger feeding	12	8-28	8	6-16
Using spoon and fork	20	12-40	13	8-20
Toilet Training				
Bladder	48	20-95	32	18-60
Bowel	42	28-90	29	16-48
Dressing				
Undressing	40	29-72	32	22-42
Putting on clothes	58	38-98	47	34-58

From Carey W, Feldman H, Coleman W, Crocker A, Elias E: *Developmental-behavioral pediatrics*, ed 5, Philadelphia, 2009, Saunders.

disease is common to those who reach middle adult life (Jackson et al, 2009).

The limp, flaccid posture of the infant is caused by hypotonicity of the muscles; it makes positioning and holding more difficult and contributes to heat loss from the exposed surface areas. The infant should be warmly wrapped to prevent chilling. The hypotonicity of muscles also causes respiratory problems and excess mucus accumulation. Bulb suctioning may be necessary before feedings. In addition, the hypotonicity of muscles contributes to the development of constipation, which can be controlled by dietary intervention.

Nursing Care

Counseling parents. The counseling of families of Down syndrome children is ongoing. Maternity nurses must be aware of their own feelings before they can effectively support parents. They, too, will feel saddened at the birth of an imperfect child. They may identify with the parents. It is appropriate to express one's feelings of initial helplessness, and it may encourage the parents to verbalize their concerns. The nurse must listen and provide honest, tactful, and compassionate support.

Empathy from the nurse is particularly important. Involving parents in the care and planning for the infant from the start facilitates bonding. The need for the staff's warm concern cannot be overestimated. Pampering the infant by putting a little curl in the hair, for example, shows that others care.

Counseling siblings. Siblings of the patient must be informed and included in discussions about the newborn. Even very young children are aware of parental distress, and the situations the children imagine can be more frightening than the reality. Early and open communications will prevent isolation and misconceptions and promote an easier transition period. The effects on siblings have been identified and not all effects are negative. Some siblings state a deeper understanding of others who are different and are more appreciative of what they have (Hyunkyung, 2013). Social support from friends and parent–child relationships, which may be influenced by family demands, should be recognized and resources in the community identified (Hyunkyung, 2013). The nurse should connect the family with a Down syndrome support group in their area if there is one. Other parents with a Down syndrome child are an important resource. The National Association for Down Syndrome is one organization that provides education and support to families. (See Chapter 23 for further discussion of nursing care of the cognitively impaired child.)

PERINATAL INJURIES

HEMOLYTIC DISEASE OF THE NEWBORN: ERYTHROBLASTOSIS FETALIS

Pathophysiology

Erythroblastosis fetalis (*erythro*, "red," *blast*, "a formative cell," and *osis*, "disease condition") is a disorder that becomes apparent during fetal life or soon after birth. It is one of many congenital hemolytic diseases found in the newborn. It is caused when an Rh-negative mother and an Rh-positive father produce an Rh-positive fetus. Although fetal and maternal blood does not mix during pregnancy, small leaks may allow fetal blood to enter the maternal circulation and sensitize the mother. The mother's body responds by producing antibodies that cross the placenta and destroy the blood cells of the fetus, causing anemia and possible heart failure (see Chapter 5). The terms *isoimmunization* and *sensitization* refer to this process (Box 14-2). The incidence of erythroblastosis fetalis has greatly decreased as a result of the protective administration of an Rh immune

| Box 14-2 | Terms Helpful in Understanding Rh Sensitization |

Antigen (*anti*, "against," and *gen*, "to produce"): A substance that induces the formation of antibodies; the antigen-antibody reaction is the basis of immunity

Coombs' test: **Indirectly** measures Rh-positive antibodies in the mother's blood; directly measures antibody-coated Rh-positive red blood cells in the **infant's** blood

Erythroblastosis fetalis: The severe form of this disease produces anemia in the **fetus** as a result of the incompatibility between the red blood cells of the mother and those of the fetus

Rh$_o$(D) immune globulin (RhoGAM): Immunoglobulin given to an Rh-negative mother after delivery of an Rh-positive fetus to prevent the maternal Rh immune response

Sensitization (isoimmunization): The phenomenon in which an Rh-negative mother develops antibodies against an Rh-positive fetus

Box **14-3**	ABO Incompatibility

Hemolytic disease with symptoms similar to those of erythroblastosis can occur with ABO incompatibility. A mother who has an O blood type and who gives birth to an infant with an A or B blood group constitutes the most commonly seen ABO incompatibility. Treatment and nursing care are the same as for erythroblastosis.

globulin (RhoGAM) to women at risk (see following discussion of prevention). Incompatibility of ABO factors is now more common and generally less severe than Rh incompatibility (Box 14-3).

The process of maternal sensitization is depicted in Figure 14-13. The mother accumulates antibodies with each pregnancy; therefore the chance that complications may occur increases with each gestation. If large numbers of antibodies are present, the infant may be severely anemic. In the gravest form, *hydrops fetalis*, the progressive hemolysis causes anemia, heart failure, fetal *hypoxia,* and *anasarca* (generalized edema). This is rare today because of early detection methods.

Diagnosis and Prevention. An extensive maternal health history is obtained. Of particular interest are previous Rh sensitizations, an ectopic pregnancy, abortion, blood transfusions, or children who developed jaundice or anemia during the neonatal period. The mother's blood titer is carefully monitored. An *indirect Coombs'* test on the mother's blood will indicate previous exposure to Rh-positive antigens.

Diagnosis of the disease in the prenatal period is confirmed by amniocentesis and monitoring of bilirubin levels in the amniotic fluid. Information gained from these tests helps to determine the necessity of early interventions such as induction of labor or intrauterine fetal transfusions that allow the fetus to remain in utero until the lungs mature. Repeated transfusions may be required (Kliegman et al, 2011). Fetal Rh$_o$(D) status can be determined noninvasively via free DNA in maternal plasma, and this new technique can be used in other areas of genetic testing (Moise, 2005a).

Prevention of erythroblastosis by the use of Rh$_o$(D) immune globulin (**RhoGAM**) is now routine. An intramuscular injection is given to the mother within 72 hours of delivery of an Rh-positive infant. RhoGAM may also be given to the pregnant woman at 28 weeks of gestation. It is also administered, when appropriate, after a spontaneous or therapeutic abortion, after amniocentesis, and to women who have bleeding during pregnancy, because fetal blood may leak into the mother's circulation at these times.

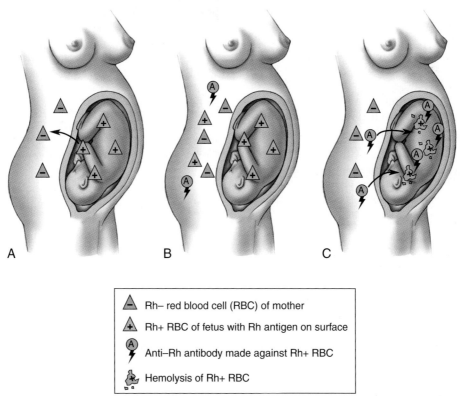

A   B   C

△ Rh− red blood cell (RBC) of mother

△ Rh+ RBC of fetus with Rh antigen on surface

Ⓐ Anti–Rh antibody made against Rh+ RBC

Hemolysis of Rh+ RBC

FIGURE 14-13 Maternal sensitization producing erythroblastosis in the newborn. **A,** During the first pregnancy, the mother is sensitized to the Rh-positive antigen from the fetus. **B,** The mother produces Rh antibodies to the Rh antigen to which she was exposed. **C,** During a second pregnancy, these Rh antibodies cross the placenta to the fetus and destroy the fetal Rh-positive blood cells. (From Herlihy B, Maebius NK: *The human body in health and illness,* ed 4, Philadelphia, 2011, Saunders.)

Nursing Tip

RhoGAM is administered to Rh-negative mothers by the intramuscular route after a normal delivery, after an ectopic pregnancy, or after an abortion to prevent the development of Rh-positive antibodies. RhoGAM has no effect on existing Rh-positive antibodies.

Manifestations. At the time of delivery, a sample of the infant's cord blood is sent to the laboratory. The *direct Coombs' test* detects damaging antibodies. The symptoms of erythroblastosis fetalis vary with the intensity of the disease. Anemia and jaundice are present. The anemia is caused by hemolysis of large numbers of erythrocytes. This *pathological jaundice* differs from *physiological jaundice* in that it becomes evident within 24 hours after delivery. The liver is unable to handle the massive hemolysis, and bilirubin levels rise rapidly, causing **hyperbilirubinemia** (*hyper*, "excess," *bilis*, "bile," *rubor*, "red," and *emia*, "blood"). Early jaundice is immediately reported to the physician. Techniques of assessing for jaundice are discussed in Chapter 12.

Enlargement of the liver and spleen and extensive edema may develop. The circulating blood usually contains an excess of immature nucleated red blood cells (erythroblasts) caused by the infant's attempts to compensate for the destruction of cells. The oxygen-carrying power of the blood is diminished, as is the blood volume, and therefore shock or heart failure may result. Jaundice (with symptoms such as irritability, lethargy, poor feeding, and high-pitched shrill cry), muscle weakness progressing to opisthotonos positioning (arched back), and seizures are indications of bilirubin toxicity that could lead to kernicterus. **Kernicterus** (accumulation of bilirubin in the brain tissues) may cause serious brain damage and permanent disability.

Safety Alert!

Jaundice that occurs on the first day of life is always pathological and necessitates prompt intervention.

Treatment and Nursing Care. Treatment includes prompt identification, laboratory tests, drug therapy, phototherapy, and exchange transfusion if indicated. **Phototherapy** may be used to reduce serum bilirubin levels. It may be used alone or in conjunction with an exchange transfusion. The newborn is placed in an incubator under a bank of fluorescent lights (Figure 14-14, *A*). The eyes are protected from the lights (Figure 14-14, *B*); the infant is turned frequently and hydration is monitored closely as the infant often develops loose stools. Intensive phototherapy may involve standard light sources above an incubator and an appropriately sized fiberoptic pad placed under the infant to increase the exposed body surface

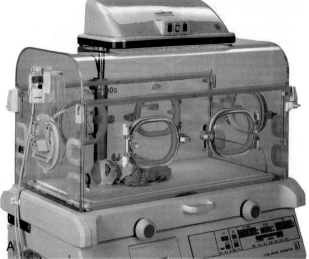

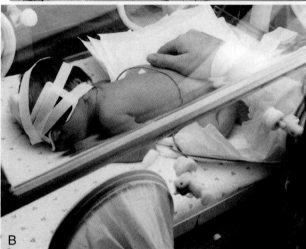

FIGURE 14-14 Phototherapy. **A,** The neoBLUE provides a high-intensity, narrow band of blue light that helps break down excess bilirubin. A flip of a switch allows change from conventional to intense phototherapy treatment. *Note:* In the clinical setting, the infant would be diapered only, not fully clothed. **B,** When an infant receives phototherapy in an incubator, the eyes are protected from the fluorescent lights. The infant is turned frequently so that all skin surfaces are exposed to the lights. (**A** courtesy Natus Medical Inc., San Carlos, Calif.)

area. Phototherapy is usually discontinued when the bilirubin level steadily declines to 14 mg/dL.

Phototherapy is contraindicated in infants with a history of congenital porphyria (a metabolic disorder involving sensitivity to light) or the use of photosensitizing drugs. Although phototherapy may prevent an increase in the level of bilirubin, it has no effect on the underlying cause of jaundice. The nursing care of the infant receiving phototherapy is presented in Nursing Care Plan 14-2. If phototherapy fails to keep the total serum bilirubin at acceptable levels to prevent kernicterus, an exchange transfusion may be indicated.

During an exchange transfusion, a plastic catheter is inserted into the umbilical vein of the newborn, small

✦ Nursing Care Plan 14-2   The Infant Receiving Phototherapy

PATIENT DATA A newborn, 12 hours of age, is diagnosed with hyperbilirubinemia and is placed in an incubator for phototherapy.

Selected Nursing Diagnosis: Risk for injury to eyes and gonads related to phototherapy

Goals	Nursing Interventions	Rationales
Infant does not have eye drainage or irritation.	Apply eye patches over infant's closed eyes before placing infant under lights.	Closing eyes prevents corneal abrasion and protects retina from damage by high-intensity light.
	Remove patches at least once per shift to assess eyes for conjunctivitis.	Facilitates early detection of inflammation and jaundice (sclera may yellow).
	Remove patches to allow eye contact during feeding.	Provides for visual stimulation and bonding.
Genitals are protected.	Cover ovaries or testes with diaper.	Protects gonads from damage by heat.

Selected Nursing Diagnosis: Impaired skin integrity related to immature structure and function, immobility

Goals	Nursing Interventions	Rationales
Skin will remain intact as evidenced by absence of skin rash, excoriation, or redness.	Observe for maculopapular rash.	Rashes and burns have been known to occur as a result of phototherapy.
	Cleanse rectal area gently, because stools are often green and liquid.	Frequent stools may cause breakdown of skin; loose stools are a result of increased bilirubin excretion.
	Reposition at least every 2 hours.	Repositioning provides exposure of all skin areas.
	Observe for jaundice or bronzing. (NOTE: Serum bilirubin level may be high even though infant may not appear jaundiced under lights.)	Jaundice may be initial sign of hyperbilirubinemia. Bronze baby syndrome appears in preterm infants who do not excrete the photooxidation products adequately.
	Observe for pressure areas.	Early intervention prevents skin breakdown.

Selected Nursing Diagnosis: Risk for deficient fluid volume, related to increased water loss through skin and loose stools

Goals	Nursing Interventions	Rationales
Infant will not become dehydrated as evidenced by good skin turgor, normal fontanelles, and moist tongue and mucous membranes.	Monitor intravenous fluids.	Intravenous (IV) fluids are sometimes used to prevent dehydration or in anticipation of exchange transfusion.
	Check skin turgor.	Helps to determine extent of dehydration.
	Observe for depressed fontanelle.	Sign of dehydration.
	Anticipate the need for additional water between feedings.	Adequate hydration facilitates elimination and excretion of bilirubin.
Weight maintenance and urine output will be satisfactory.	Measure weights daily unless contraindicated.	Assess progress; helps to determine extent of dehydration.

Selected Nursing Diagnosis: Risk for hyperthermia or hypothermia

Goals	Nursing Interventions	Rationales
Infant will not become overheated or chilled; temperature will be maintained between 36.3° and 37.4° C (97.4° and 99.4° F).	Monitor infant's temperature.	Hyperthermia and hypothermia are common complications of phototherapy.
	Adjust incubator to maintain neutral thermal environment.	Avoid overheating incubator or warming unit.

Selected Nursing Diagnosis: Risk for injury (neurological), related to nature of hyperbilirubinemia

Goals	Nursing Interventions	Rationales
Infant will show no signs of neurological involvement (e.g., lethargy, twitching).	Anticipate measurement of daily bilirubin blood levels.	Phototherapy success determined by frequently measuring serum bilirubin levels.
	Turn off phototherapy lights when blood is being drawn to prevent false readings.	Promotes accuracy of blood test.
	Observe parameters for neurological deficit (e.g., twitching, lethargy).	Kernicterus (brain damage) is rare but is evidenced by neurological sequelae such as hypotonia, diminished reflexes, twitching, and lethargy.

Continued

⭐ **Nursing Care Plan 14-2** | **The Infant Receiving Phototherapy—cont'd**

Selected Nursing Diagnosis: Imbalanced nutrition: less than body requirements

Goals	Nursing Interventions	Rationales
Infant will receive adequate nutrients as evidenced by stabilization of weight and laboratory reports.	Provide feedings as ordered.	Early feedings within 4 to 6 hours after delivery tend to decrease high bilirubin levels and provide nourishment.
	Assist mother to reestablish breastfeeding if temporarily halted.	Encourages mother, helps her feel more in control, promotes bonding; opinions of physicians vary regarding discontinuance of breastfeeding, because the cause of breast milk jaundice is not known.

Selected Nursing Diagnosis: Parental anxiety related to deficient knowledge crisis of having an infant with jaundice

Goals	Nursing Interventions	Rationales
Parents express fears concerning infant's welfare.	Explain procedures and treatment. Provide reassurance. Provide follow-up care.	Information decreases parental stress. Parents are in need of support persons. Follow-up care is reassuring to parents and medical personnel that family is progressing nicely without complications.

Critical Thinking Question

1. The mother of an infant receiving phototherapy states she has other children and always fed them every 4 hours. She states she does not want her infant to become "fat" and therefore does not want to feed more often. What is the appropriate response of the nurse?

---

amounts of blood (10 to 20 mL) are withdrawn, and equal amounts of Rh-negative blood are injected. The amount of donor blood used is about twice the infant blood volume to a limit of 500 mL. In this way, healthy cells are added to the infant's blood, and antibodies are removed. Additional small transfusions may be necessary later. After a second exchange transfusion, approximately 85% of the infant's blood will have been replaced. Antibiotics may be given to prevent infection.

Nursing Tip

An infant born with cardiac failure and edema as a result of hemolytic disease is a candidate for immediate exchange transfusion with fresh whole blood.

The nurse is usually responsible for the following: observing the newborn's color and reporting any evidence of jaundice during the first and second days; stressing to mothers the importance of good prenatal care for subsequent pregnancies; helping to interpret the treatment to parents by giving reassurance as needed; and observing and assisting the physician with the exchange transfusion. A classification of drug called metalloporphyrins, (SnMP), is under study for approval by the U.S. Food and Drug Administration (FDA). This drug, given by intramuscular injection, is designed to treat hyperbilirubinemia, eliminating the need for exchange transfusions and perhaps even phototherapy. At present, the drug is reserved for use in extremely low-birth-weight infants who may

experience neurological complications during phototherapy (Kliegman, 2011).

Nursing Tip

Tips on assessing jaundice:
- The skin and the whites of the eyes assume a yellow-orange cast.
- Blanching the skin over the bony prominences enhances the evaluation of jaundice.

Home Phototherapy. Home phototherapy programs are being used for newborns with mild to moderate physiological (normal) jaundice. These programs are advocated because bilirubin levels generally begin to increase on the third day after birth, when the mother and newborn are discharged. An increase in bilirubin levels may necessitate the newborn's return to the hospital and the possible separation of mother and infant. Home therapy is less costly. A referral for home care is made by the infant's pediatrician on the basis of the newborn's health, bilirubin levels (generally between 10 and 14 mg/dL), evidence of jaundice, and suitability of the family for complying with the home program.

A phototherapy blanket in a bassinet (Figure 14-15) or a fiberoptic pad (Figure 14-16) can be used. These allow for holding the infant and decrease the risk of eye damage. Written instructions are given to the parents. Parents keep a daily record of their infant's temperature, weight, intake and output, stools, and feedings (see Nursing Care Plan 14-2). Phototherapy tips are listed in Box 14-4.

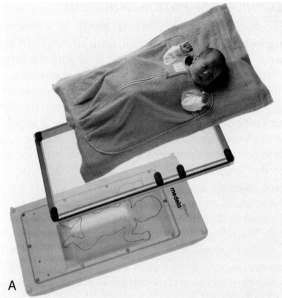

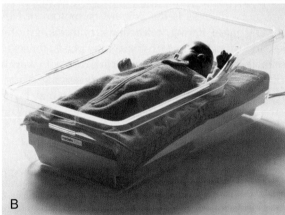

FIGURE 14-15 Phototherapy Bilibed. **A,** The infant is diapered and placed in the therapy blanket, which fits on a light-permeable infant support. This plastic support is placed over the irradiation unit, which fits into the standard bassinet instead of the mattress. **B,** The infant in the Bilibed can room-in with the mother and requires no eye-patch protection. The therapeutic light focuses directly on the infant's skin through the underside of the phototherapy blanket. (Photos courtesy Medela.)

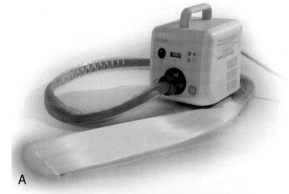

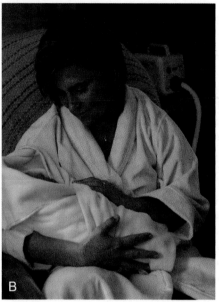

FIGURE 14-16 Biliblanket Plus High Output Phototherapy System. **A,** A pad of woven fibers is used to transport light from a light source to the infant. This fiberoptic pad is wrapped directly on the infant's skin to bathe the skin in light. **B,** The infant can then be diapered, clothed, held, and nursed during treatment at home. (Photos courtesy Medela.)

INTRACRANIAL HEMORRHAGE

Pathophysiology. **Intracranial hemorrhage,** the most common type of birth injury, may result from trauma or anoxia. It occurs more often in the preterm infant, whose blood vessels are fragile. Blood vessels within the skull are broken, and bleeding into the brain occurs. When the diagnosis is made, the specific location of the hemorrhage may be noted (i.e., subdural, subarachnoid, or intraventricular). This injury may also occur during precipitate delivery or prolonged labor or when the newborn's head is large in comparison with the mother's pelvis.

Manifestations. The signs of intracranial hemorrhage may occur suddenly or gradually. Some signs or all signs may be present depending on the severity of

---

Box **14-4** **Phototherapy Tips**

IF THE INFANT IS IN AN INCUBATOR:
- Cover the infant's eyes while under lights.
- Place a small diaper over the gonad area.
- Turn the infant frequently to expose all skin surfaces.
- The infant does not need to be dressed or wrapped because incubator environment will prevent chilling.
- Distinguish loose, greenish stools caused by photo degradation products from true diarrhea.

IF THE INFANT IS WRAPPED IN A BILIBLANKET:
- Put the light source on a flat, nonabsorbent surface and not on a carpet or crib mattress.
- Use a 3-pronged plug for safety, and set the intensity knob on the light box to the highest setting.
- Do not put anything on top of the light source box or the fiberoptic cable.
- Expose as much of the infant's skin as possible to the Bililight pad while keeping a diaper in place.
- Be sure there is a clean disposable cover between the light-emitting side of the pad and the infant's skin.

the hemorrhage, and can include poor muscle tone, lethargy, poor sucking reflex, respiratory distress, cyanosis, twitching, forceful vomiting, a high-pitched shrill cry, and convulsions. Opisthotonos posturing may be observed (see Figure 23-8). The fontanelle may be tense and under pressure rather than soft and compressible. The pupil of one eye is likely to be small (constricted) and the other large (dilated).

If the symptoms are mild, most patients have a good chance of complete recovery. Death results if there is a massive hemorrhage. The infant who survives an extensive hemorrhage may suffer residual effects such as mental retardation or cerebral palsy. The diagnosis is established by the history of the delivery, CT scan, MRI, evidence of an increase in ICP, and the symptoms and course of the disease.

Treatment and Nursing Care. The newborn is placed in an incubator, which allows proper temperature control, ease in administering oxygen, and continuous observation (see Chapter 13). The infant is handled gently and as little as possible. The head is elevated. The physician may prescribe vitamin K to control bleeding and phenobarbital if twitching or convulsions are apparent. Prophylactic antibiotics and vitamins may be used. The infant is fed carefully because the sucking reflex may be affected. The infant vomits easily. The nurse observes the infant for signs of increased ICP (see Chapter 23) and convulsions and assists the physician with procedures such as lumbar punctures and aspiration of subdural hemorrhage. Performing neurochecks, monitoring vital signs and head circumference, and palpating fontanelles are essential.

If a convulsion occurs, observation of its character aids the physician in diagnosing the exact location of the bleeding. The following are of particular importance: Were the arms, legs, or face involved? Was the right or left side of the body involved? Was the convulsion mild or severe? How long did it last? What was the condition of the infant before and after the seizure? The nurse records observations and notifies the team leader or health care provider.

TRANSIENT TACHYPNEA OF THE NEWBORN

Transient tachypnea of the newborn (TTN) usually occurs after a cesarean section birth or an uneventful vaginal delivery of a term infant. It is characterized by tachypnea (rapid respirations) and may also include chest retractions, grunting, and mild cyanosis. The condition is often referred to as *respiratory distress syndrome, type II* (type I is discussed in Chapter 13). The distinctive feature of this condition is that it typically resolves suddenly after 3 days. TTN is thought to be caused by slow absorption of the fluid in the lungs after birth. Treatment is supportive, providing warmth, energy conservation, and supplemental oxygen.

MECONIUM ASPIRATION SYNDROME

Meconium aspiration syndrome (MAS) is a group of symptoms that occur when the fetus or newborn aspirates meconium-stained amniotic fluid into the lungs.

In utero, the fetus often expels some meconium into the amniotic fluid during the prolonged labor process, especially if there is cord compression or another condition that temporarily interrupts fetal circulation. If asphyxia and acidosis occur in utero, the fetus may make gasping movements that draw meconium-stained amniotic fluid into the lungs. This condition can also occur when the infant takes its first breath before the nose and mouth are suctioned and meconium-stained amniotic fluid that is present in the upper airway passages is drawn into the lungs. Meconium aspiration can be prevented by giving the mother amnioinfusion (see Chapter 8) when fetal distress occurs because of loss of amniotic fluid and also by suctioning the nose and mouth of the infant as soon as the head is delivered, before the infant takes its first breath. Respiratory distress is the primary symptom of MAS, including nasal flaring, retractions, cyanosis, grunting, rales, and rhonchi. The tachypnea may persist for several weeks. Treatment includes supportive care with warmth, supplemental oxygen, and energy-conserving plans of care. Intubation and mechanical ventilation may be necessary, and the infant is transferred to the neonatal intensive care unit (NICU).

NEONATAL ABSTINENCE SYNDROME

Neonatal abstinence syndrome occurs when the fetus has prenatal exposure to drugs such as opiates, amphetamines, tranquilizers, or multiple illicit drugs while in utero. Because these drugs cross the placenta, the infant born to an addicted mother is physiologically dependent on the drugs and suffers withdrawal symptoms after birth and possible long-term developmental and neurological deficits. Body tremors and hyperirritability are the principal signs of this condition in the newborn. Wakefulness, diarrhea, poor feeding, sneezing, and yawning may also be present. Treatment includes providing a quiet environment with swaddling (see Skill 12-3), reduction of external stimuli, and close observation for seizures. Continued treatment of the mother with methadone during breastfeeding is supported by the American Academy of Pediatrics (Gabbe, 2012). *Fetal alcohol syndrome* (FAS) and parent teaching are discussed in Chapter 5.

INFANT OF A DIABETIC MOTHER

Diabetes in the mother presents various problems for the newborn. These are determined by the severity and duration of the disease in the mother, the degree of control of her condition, and the gestational age of the infant. Diabetes in pregnancy is discussed in Chapter 5. When diabetes of the mother is under good control from conception and throughout pregnancy, the adverse effects on the newborn infant are minimal.

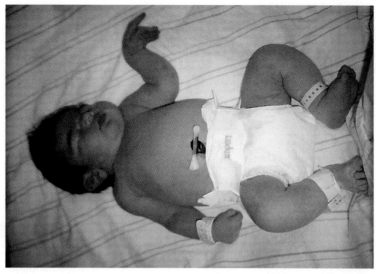

FIGURE 14-17 Macrosomia. A newborn with macrosomia caused by maternal diabetes mellitus during pregnancy. This infant weighed 5.5 kg (11 lb) at birth. Macrosomic infants often have respiratory disorders and other problems. (Courtesy Pat Spier, RN-C.)

Many newborn infants of diabetic mothers have serious complications. When the mother is hyperglycemic, large amounts of glucose are transferred to the fetus. This makes the fetus hyperglycemic. In response, the fetal pancreas (islet cells) produces large amounts of fetal insulin. Hyperinsulinism, along with excess production of protein and fatty acids, often results in a newborn infant who weighs more than 4082 g (9 lb). Such an infant is designated "large for gestational age" (LGA), and this condition is termed **macrosomia** (*macro,* "large," and *soma,* "body"). This infant is prone to injuries at birth because of his or her size (Figure 14-17).

After delivery the infant often has low blood glucose levels because of the abrupt loss of maternal glucose and hypertrophy of the pancreatic islet cells, which results in a temporary overproduction of insulin. The infant has a characteristic cushingoid appearance because of increased subcutaneous fat. The face is round and appears puffy, and the infant appears lethargic. The size of these newborn infants makes them appear healthy, but this is deceptive because they often have developmental deficits and may suffer complications of respiratory distress syndrome (RDS) or congenital anomalies. In contrast, some infants born to a mother with severe diabetes may be small for gestational age (SGA) because of poor placental perfusion. These infants suffer from hypoglycemia, hypocalcemia, and hyperbilirubinemia.

The nursing care of the infant of a diabetic mother includes close monitoring of vital signs, early feeding, and frequent assessment of blood glucose levels for the first 2 days of life. Hypoglycemia in the first days of life is defined as a blood glucose level that falls below 40 mg/dL. It can result in rapid and permanent brain damage. The infant should be closely watched for signs of irritability, tremors, and respiratory distress.

Unfolding Case Study

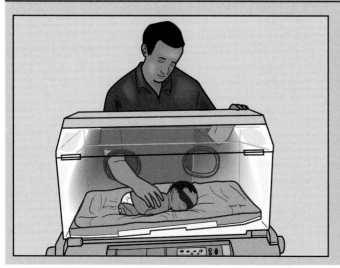

Tess and her husband Luis were introduced to the reader in Chapter 4 and were followed through each chapter as her labor progressed and she delivered twins. After 1 hour in the delivery room, baby Marco was taken to the postpartum unit with his mother Tess but baby Sofia evidenced respiratory distress and was transported to the NICU accompanied by her father.

Sofia's respiratory distress has resolved but increasing jaundice is now noted and the bilirubin level is reported to be 16. She has been diagnosed with hyperbilirubinemia possibly caused by erythroblastosis fetalis. Sofia is diapered and placed in an incubator under phototherapy lights.

QUESTIONS

1. What factors lead to hyperbilirubinemia caused by erythroblastosis fetalis?

Continued

Unfolding Case Study—cont'd

2. What are the signs of bilirubin toxicity that leads to kernicterus that the nurse should watch for and document?
3. What are the safety measures involved in the nursing care of Sofia while she is in the incubator?
4. If an exchange transfusion is needed, the nurse is responsible to check the label on the blood container to be infused. Tess is Rh-negative and baby Sofia is Rh-positive. Which type of blood will Sofia be given? Why?

5. What are the priorities of nursing care for Sofia? Can she be fed breast milk?
6. When Sofia is removed from the incubator and discharged home, what follow-up care is required?
7. Based on Sofia's diagnosis, what treatment should Sofia's mother have before discharge?

Get Ready for the NCLEX® Examination!

Key Points

- The nurse manages communication between parents and the multidisciplinary health care team to meet the needs of the newborn with congenital problems and of their families.
- Measuring head size is important in infants with hydrocephalus.
- Spina bifida is a congenital embryonic neural tube defect in which there is an imperfect closure of the spinal vertebrae.
- Folic acid supplementation during the early weeks of pregnancy can prevent neural tube anomalies.
- Postoperative nursing care of the infant with a cleft lip includes preventing the infant from sucking and crying, which could impair healing of the suture line.
- Newborns feel pain, and adequate pain control after invasive procedures and surgery is essential.
- The body spica cast encircles the waist and extends to the ankles or toes. It is used to treat developmental hip dysplasia.
- A positive Barlow's test and Ortolani's sign are indicative of developmental hip dysplasia.
- Newborn infants are routinely screened for phenylketonuria.
- Lofenalac is a formula used for infants with phenylketonuria.
- RhoGAM is given to an Rh-negative mother after delivering an Rh-positive fetus to prevent maternal Rh sensitization.
- Hyperbilirubinemia results from rapid destruction of red blood cells.
- Jaundice that occurs in the first 24 hours of life is considered pathological.
- Distinguishing pathological jaundice from physiological jaundice can facilitate early intervention and prevent serious complications.
- Macrosomia is a condition in which the infant is large for gestational age (LGA) and usually occurs in infants of diabetic mothers.
- In intracranial hemorrhage, blood vessels within the skull are broken and there is bleeding into the brain.

Additional Learning Resources

SG Go to your Study Guide for additional learning activities to help you master this chapter content.

evolve Go to your Evolve website (http://evolve.elsevier.com/Leifer) for the following learning resources:
- Animations
- Answer Guidelines for Critical Thinking Questions
- Answers and Rationales for Review Questions for the NCLEX® Examination
- Glossary with English and Spanish pronunciations
- Interactive Review Questions for the NCLEX® Examination
- Patient Teaching Plans in English and Spanish
- Skills Performance Checklists
- Video clips and more!

 Online Resources
- Centers for Disease Control and Prevention: www.cdc.gov
- Cleft Palate Foundation: www.cleftline.org
- March of Dimes: www.marchofdimes.com
- National Association for Down Syndrome: www.nads.org
- Spina Bifida Association of America: www.spinabifidaassociation.org

Review Questions for the NCLEX® Examination

1. The postop nursing care of an infant who has had a cheiloplasty includes (select all that apply):
   1. Feed formula using a soft nipple.
   2. Apply elbow restraints.
   3. Provide pain relief measures.
   4. Position infant on its abdomen.

2. Characteristic signs of developmental hip dysplasia that the nurse should observe and report include (select all that apply):
   1. inability to move legs.
   2. unequal skin folds in the upper thigh.
   3. straight simian crease.
   4. limited ability to abduct legs.

3. The postoperative care for a newborn who has had a ventriculoperitoneal shunt includes observing for increased intracranial pressure, which is manifested by (select all that apply):
   1. a high pitched cry.
   2. bulging fontanelles.
   3. a personality change.
   4. unequal eye pupil size.

4. A Pavlik harness is often used to correct:
   1. clubfoot.
   2. juvenile arthritis.
   3. developmental hip dysplasia.
   4. fractured femur.

5. When bathing an infant, the nurse observes the hips for dislocation. What observation may indicate developmental hip dysplasia?
   1. Toes turned inward
   2. Limitation of abduction of legs
   3. Asymmetry of epicanthal folds
   4. Shortening of patella

Objectives

1. Define each key term listed.
2. Discuss the nursing implications of growth and development.
3. Explain the differences between growth, development, and maturation.
4. Recognize and read a growth chart for children.
5. List five factors that influence growth and development.
6. Discuss the importance of family-centered care in pediatrics.
7. Recognize the influence of the family and cultural practices on growth, development, nutrition, and health care.
8. Describe three developmental theories and their impact on planning the nursing care of children.
9. Discuss the nutritional needs of growing children.
10. Differentiate between permanent and deciduous teeth, and list the times of their eruption.
11. Understand the characteristics of play at various age levels.
12. Describe the relationship of play to physical, cognitive, and emotional development.
13. Understand the role of computers and computer games in play at various ages.
14. Define therapeutic play.
15. Understand the use of play as an assessment tool.

Key Terms

adolescent (p. 352)
cephalocaudal (sĕf-ă-lō-KĂW-dăl, p. 353)
cognition (kŏg-NĬ-shŭn, p. 367)
community (p. 360)
competitive play (p. 384)
cooperative play (p. 384)
deciduous (dĕ-SĬD-ū-ŭs, p. 380)
dysfunctional family (p. 359)
Erikson's stages (p. 368)
extended family (p. 359)
fluorosis (flū-RŌ-sĭs, p. 382)
growth (p. 352)
height (p. 353)
infant (p. 352)
Kohlberg (p. 367)

length (p. 353)
Maslow (p. 360)
maturation (p. 352)
metabolic rate (p. 353)
neonate (p. 352)
nuclear family (p. 359)
nursing caries (p. 382)
parallel play (p. 384)
personality (p. 360)
Piaget (pē-ă-ZHĀ, p. 367)
preschool (p. 352)
proximodistal (prŏk-sĭ-mō-DĬS-tăl, p. 353)
school-age (p. 352)
therapeutic play (p. 384)
toddler (p. 352)

GROWTH AND DEVELOPMENT

The main difference between caring for the adult and caring for the child is that the latter is in a continuous process of growth and development. This process is orderly and proceeds from the simple to the more complex (Box 15-1). Although the process is orderly, it is not steadily paced. Plateaus often follow growth spurts. One of the most noticeable growth spurts is at the time of puberty. The rate of growth varies with the individual child. Each infant has an individual timetable that revolves around established norms. Siblings within a family vary in growth rate. Growth is measurable and can be observed and studied. This is done by comparing height, weight, increase in vocabulary, physical skills, and other parameters. There are variations in growth within the systems and the subsystems. Not all parts mature at the same time. Skeletal growth approximates whole-body growth, whereas the brain, lymph, and reproductive tissues follow distinct and individual sequences.

Box 15-1	Emerging Patterns of Behavior from Age 1 to 5 Years

12 MONTHS

Motor: Walks with one hand held; rises independently; takes several steps

Adaptive: Picks up pellet with pincer action of thumb and forefinger; releases object to another person on request

Language: Says "mama," "dada," and a few similar words

Social: Plays simple ball game; makes postural adjustment to dressing

15 MONTHS

Motor: Walks alone; crawls up stairs

Adaptive: Makes tower of three cubes; makes a line with crayons; inserts pellet in bottle

Language: Jargon; follows simple commands; may name a familiar object (ball)

Social: Indicates some desires or needs by pointing; hugs caregivers

18 MONTHS

Motor: Runs stiffly; sits on small chair; walks up stairs with one hand held; explores drawers and wastebaskets

Adaptive: Makes tower of four cubes; imitates vertical stroke; imitates scribbling; dumps pellet from bottle

Language: 10 words (average); names pictures; identifies one or more parts of body

Social: Feeds self; seeks help when in trouble; may complain when wet or soiled; kisses caregivers with pucker

2 YEARS

Motor: Runs well; walks up and down stairs, one step at a time; opens doors; climbs on furniture; jumps

Adaptive: Tower of seven cubes (six at 21 months); circular scribbling; imitates horizontal stroke; folds paper once imitatively

Language: Puts three words together (subject, verb, object)

Social: Handles spoon well; often tells immediate experiences; helps to undress; listens to stories with pictures; plays in parallel with other children

2½ YEARS

Motor: Goes up stairs alternating feet

Adaptive: Tower of nine cubes; makes vertical and horizontal strokes but generally will not join them to make a cross; imitates circular stroke, forming a closed figure

Language: Refers to self by pronoun "I"; knows full name

Social: Helps put things away; pretends in play

3 YEARS

Motor: Rides tricycle; stands momentarily on one foot

Adaptive: Tower of 10 cubes; imitates construction of "bridge" of three cubes; copies a circle; imitates a cross

Language: Knows age and sex; counts three objects correctly; repeats three numbers or a sentence of six syllables

Social: Plays simple games (cooperative play is highly imaginative); helps in dressing (unbuttons clothing and puts on shoes); washes hands

4 YEARS

Motor: Hops on one foot; throws ball overhand; uses scissors to cut out pictures; climbs well

Adaptive: Copies bridge from model; imitates construction of "gate" of five cubes; copies cross and square; draws a man with two to four parts besides head; identifies longer of two lines

Language: Counts four pennies accurately; tells a story

Social: Plays with several children with the beginning of social interaction and role playing; goes to toilet alone

5 YEARS

Motor: Skips

Adaptive: Draws triangle from copy; identifies heavier of two weights

Language: Names four colors; repeats sentence of 10 syllables; counts 10 pennies correctly

Social: Dresses and undresses; asks questions about meaning of words; domestic role playing

NOTE: After 5 years, the Stanford-Binet, the Wechsler-Bellevue, and other scales offer the most precise estimates of developmental level. To have the greatest value only an experienced and qualified person should administer them.

Modified from Kliegman R, Stanton B, St Geme III J, Schor N, Behrman R: *Nelson's textbook of pediatrics,* ed 19, Philadelphia, 2011, Saunders. Data are derived from those of Gesell (as revised by Knobloch), Shirley, Provence, Wolf, Bailey, and others.

THE IMPACT OF GROWTH AND DEVELOPMENT ON NURSING CARE

Pediatrics is a subspecialty of medical-surgical nursing. Adult acute care units in a hospital may contain a separate neurology unit, a separate cardiac unit, a separate medical unit, and a separate surgical unit. On the pediatric acute care unit in the general hospital, all medical-surgical specialties are usually housed on one unit—for patients ranging from newborn to adolescent. The developmental needs of the child have an impact on his or her response to illness and on the approach the nurse must take in developing a plan of care. Choosing the right words to explain to a child what will happen is essential. For example, if the nurse states that the child will be "put to sleep" before the operation, will the child relate that to a pet at home being "put to sleep" and never heard from again? The fractured jaw of an 8-month-old after a motor vehicle accident may affect his developmental process more seriously than the same injury in a 4-year-old, because the 8-month-old is in the oral phase of development.

Because the child differs from the adult both anatomically and physiologically, differences in response to therapy as well as in manifestations of illness can be anticipated. The nurse must understand the normal to recognize deviations within any age group and to plan care that takes these developmental differences into consideration (Box 15-2).

Nursing Tip

The developmental level of the child and family values should govern the nursing approach, with choices and active participation offered when appropriate.

Box 15-2	The Nursing Process Applied to Growth and Development

DATA COLLECTION

Obtain height and weight and plot a standard growth chart.
Record developmental milestones achieved as they relate to age.
Observe infant; interview parents.

ANALYSIS AND NURSING DIAGNOSIS

Determine appropriate nursing diagnoses related to parenting, coping skills, and unmet developmental needs.

OUTCOMES IDENTIFICATION AND PLANNING

Offer guidance and teaching to family, school personnel, and child to meet child's developmental needs. For example, the toddler and preschooler may have specific needs related to safety or the use of age-appropriate toys.

IMPLEMENTATION

Interventions that foster growth and development in the hospital setting can include encouraging age-appropriate self-care. In the home, the school-age child with diabetes may be taught to participate in performing blood glucose tests and administering insulin.
Anticipatory guidance may be given to parents so they understand changes in behavior, eating habits, and play of the growing child.

EVALUATION

Ongoing evaluation of growth and development of the child and follow-up of teaching and guidance offered at previous clinic/home visits are essential.

An understanding of growth and development, including its predictable nature and individual variation, has value in the nursing process. Such knowledge is the basis of the nurse's anticipatory guidance of parents. For example, the nurse who knows when the infant is likely to crawl can, at the appropriate age, expand teaching on safety precautions. The nurse also incorporates these precautions into nursing care plans in the hospital. Age-appropriate care cannot be administered without an understanding of growth and development.

While explaining various aspects of child care to families, the nurse stresses the importance of individual differences. Parents tend to compare their children's development and behavior with those of other children and with information in popular magazine articles. This may relieve their anxiety or cause them to impose impossible expectations and standards. In addition, many parents had poor role models who influenced their own experiences as children. The nurse can recognize lack of knowledge about parenting, and suitable interventions can be implemented.

The nurse who understands that each child is born with an individual temperament and "style of behavior" can help frustrated parents cope with a newborn who has difficulty settling into the new environment. Specific parameters can be used to determine whether an infant is merely on an individual timetable or whether the infant varies from normal.

The nurse must also recognize when to intervene to prevent disease and/or accidents. For example, a brief visit with a caregiver may show that the child's immunizations are not up to date. A review with a teenage mother of the characteristics of a 2-year-old may prevent the ingestion of poisons. Complications of the newborn can be avoided by advising the expectant mother to avoid alcohol and cigarettes. Other threats to health may likewise be anticipated. Knowing that specific diseases are prevalent in certain age groups, the nurse maintains a high level of suspicion when interacting with these patients. This approach, based on developmental knowledge, experience, and effective communication, helps to ensure a higher level of family care. Finally, the nurse must understand how to provide nursing care to children of various ages to enhance their physical, mental, emotional, and spiritual development according to their specific needs and comprehension.

Nursing Tip

Arnold Gesell, founder of the Clinic for Child Development at Yale University, was the first to study children scientifically over time. He coined the term *child development.*

TERMINOLOGY

The following stages of growth and development are referred to throughout this text:

- *Fetus:* Ninth gestational week to birth
- *Neonate:* Birth to 4 weeks
- *Infant:* 4 weeks to 1 year
- *Toddler:* 1 to 3 years
- *Preschool:* 3 to 6 years
- *School-age:* 6 to 12 years
- *Adolescent:* 12 to 18 years

Growth refers to an increase in physical size and is measured in inches and pounds. *Development* refers to a progressive increase in the function of the body. These two terms are inseparable. **Maturation** (*maturus,* "ripe") refers to the total way in which a person grows and develops, as dictated by inheritance (Box 15-3). Although maturation is independent of environment, its timing may be affected by environment.

Box 15-3	Key Terms in Child Development

Development: A progressive increase in the function of the body (e.g., infant's increasing ability to digest solids)
Growth: An increase in physical size, measured in feet or meters and pounds or kilograms
Maturation: The total way that a person grows and develops, as dictated by inheritance

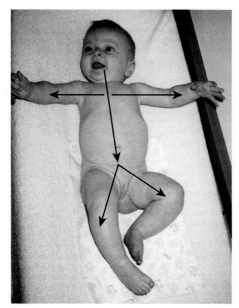

FIGURE 15-1 The development of muscular control proceeds from head to foot (cephalocaudally) and from the center of the body to its periphery (proximodistally).

DIRECTIONAL PATTERNS

Directional patterns are fundamental to all humans. **Cephalocaudal** development proceeds from head to toe. The infant is able to raise the head before being able to sit, and he or she gains control of the trunk before walking. The second pattern is **proximodistal**, or from midline to the periphery. Development proceeds from the center of the body to the periphery (Figure 15-1). These patterns occur bilaterally. Development also proceeds from the general to the specific. The infant grasps with the hands before pinching with the fingers.

SOME DEVELOPMENTAL DIFFERENCES BETWEEN CHILDREN AND ADULTS

Height

Height refers to standing measurement, whereas **length** refers to measurement while the infant is in a recumbent position. At birth the newborn has an average length of about 50 cm (20 inches). Linear growth is caused mainly by skeletal growth. Growth fluctuates until maturity is reached. Infancy and puberty are both rapid growth periods. Height is generally a family trait, although there are exceptions. Good nutrition and general good health are instrumental in promoting linear growth. Height is measured during each well-child visit (Skill 15-1). The length of the infant usually increases about 2.5 cm (1 inch) per month for the first 6 months. By age 1 year, the birth length increases by 50% (mostly in the trunk area).

Weight

Weight is another good index of health. However, the weight of a newborn infant does not always imply gestational maturity (see Chapter 13 and Figure 13-1). The average full-term newborn weighs 2.72 to 4.08 kg (6 to 9 lb), with an average of 3.4 kg (7.5 lb). Approximately 5% to 10% of the birth weight is lost by age 3 or 4 days as the result of the passage of stools and a limited fluid intake. The infant usually regains his or her birth weight by age 10 to 12 days. **Birth weight usually doubles by age 5 to 6 months and triples by age 1 year.** After the first year, weight gain levels off to approximately 1.81 to 2.72 kg (4 to 6 lb) per year, until the pubertal growth spurt begins.

Weight is determined at each office visit. A marked increase or decrease necessitates further investigation. The body weight of a newborn is composed of a higher percentage of water than in the adult. This extracellular fluid falls from 40% in the newborn to 20% in the adult. The high proportion of extracellular fluid in the infant can cause a more rapid loss of total body fluid, and therefore every infant must be closely monitored for dehydration. (See technique of weighing infants in Chapter 12 and Figure 12-11.)

Body Proportions

Body proportions of the child differ greatly from those of the adult (Figure 15-2). The head is the fastest-growing portion of the body during fetal life. During infancy the trunk grows rapidly, whereas during childhood, growth of the legs becomes the predominant feature. At adolescence, characteristic male and female proportions develop as childhood fat disappears. Alterations in proportions in the size of head, trunk, and extremities are characteristic of certain disturbances. Routine measurements of head and chest circumference are important indices of health.

Metabolic Rate

The **metabolic rate** (energy use and oxygen consumption) is higher in children than in adults. Infants require more calories, minerals, vitamins, and fluid in proportion to weight and height than adults. Higher metabolic rates are accompanied by an increased production of heat and waste products. The body surface area (BSA) of young children is far greater in relation to body weight than that of adults. The young child loses relatively more fluid from the pulmonary and integumentary systems.

Respirations

The respirations of infants are irregular and abdominal. Small airways can become easily blocked with mucus. The short, straight eustachian tube connects with the ear and predisposes the infant to middle ear infections. The chest wall is thin, and the muscles are immature, and therefore pressure on the chest can interfere with respiratory efforts.

Cardiovascular System

In neonates, the muscle mass of the right and left ventricles of the heart is almost equal. An increased need for cardiac output is often met by an increase in heart rate. Newborns have high oxygen consumption and require a high cardiac output in the first few months of life. The presence of fetal (immature) hemoglobin in the first months of life also contributes to the need for a high cardiac output. The disappearance of fetal hemoglobin along with the loss of maternal iron stores contributes to the development of physiological anemia in infants after 3 or 4 months of age.

Assessing the Length and Height of Infants and Children

PURPOSE

To determine height in order to calculate body surface area (BSA) measurement and to determine status on growth chart

STEPS

Infants from Birth Until 2 Years

1. Measure infants from birth until age 2 years in the recumbent position.
2. Exert *mild* pressure on the knee to straighten the leg for crown–heel measurement. Use a tape measure or measuring mat (the leg should *not* be "pulled" to straighten by exerting pressure on the ankle.)
3. Plot the measurement on an established growth chart.
4. Document findings and report any abnormalities.
   Infants from birth to age 2 years are measured in the recumbent position. Exerting mild pressure on the knee will straighten the leg for crown–heel measurement with tape measure or measuring mat. The leg should not be "pulled" to straighten by exerting pressure on the ankle.

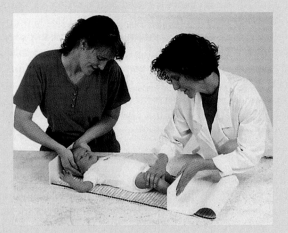

Children from 2 to 18 Years

1. Measure children ages 2 to 18 years in the standing position. The body should be in alignment, with the head erect and the child looking straight ahead and shoulders, buttocks, and heels touching the wall. The child should not be wearing shoes and should stand on a paper barrier.

2. Plot the measurement on an established growth chart.
3. Document findings and report any abnormalities.
   Children from 2 to 18 years are measured in the standing position. The body should be in alignment with the child looking straight ahead and shoulders, buttocks and heels touching the wall. The child should not be wearing shoes and should stand on a paper barrier. The height should be measured accurately and recorded.

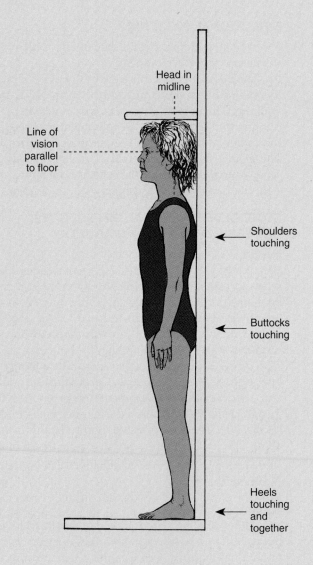

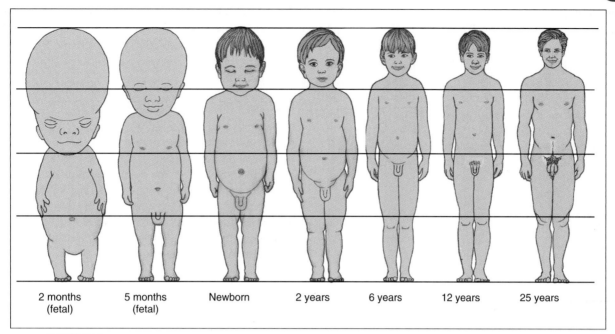

FIGURE 15-2   Changes in body proportions. Approximate changes in body proportions from fetal life through adulthood are shown. These changes in body proportions affect calculations of body surface area that are used to determine the percentages of body burns in burn injuries. (See the "rule of nines" in Chapter 30, Figure 30-15.) (From McKinney ES, Ashwill JW, Murray SS, James SR, Gorrie TM, Droske SC: *Maternal-child nursing,* 4 ed, Philadelphia, 2013, Saunders.)

Immunity

For the first 3 months of life, the newborn is protected from illnesses to which the mother was exposed. The infant gradually produces his or her own immunoglobulin until adult levels are reached by puberty. Therefore the infant and child must be protected from health care–associated infections in the hospital and from unnecessary exposure to pathogens. Immunizations against common childhood communicable diseases are discussed in Chapter 32.

Kidney Function

Kidney function is not mature until the end of the second year of life. Therefore drugs that are eliminated via the kidney can accumulate in the body to dangerous levels before age 2 years. Immature kidney function also predisposes the infant to dehydration. Nursing responsibilities for children less than 2 years of age include monitoring for dehydration and observing closely for toxic effects of drug therapy.

Nervous System

Maturation of the brain is evidenced by increased coordination, skills, and behaviors in the first years of life. Purposeful controlled movement such as voluntarily grasping an object within view, replaces primitive reflexes such as the involuntary grasp reflex. Head circumference increases 1.5 cm (0.6 inch) per month to an approximate total of 43 cm (17 inches) at age 6 months. During the second 6 months of life, head circumference increases 0.5 cm (0.2 inch) per month to an approximate total of 46 cm (18 inches) at 1 year of age.

The age-appropriate toy is correlated with nervous system maturation. When selecting play activities, the nurse should consider the diagnosis and the child's developmental level and abilities to be sure the toy is safe.

Sleep Patterns

Sleep patterns vary with age. The neonate sleeps 8 to 9 hours per night and naps an equal amount of time during the day. The 2-year-old may sleep 10 hours during the night and have only one short daytime nap. The 7-year-old usually requires 11 to 13 hours of sleep and rarely has a daytime nap. These patterns may be altered by cultural practices. For example, Israeli *kibbutzim* often have *all* family members nap after work or school, before dinner.

Bone Growth

Bone growth provides one of the best indicators of biological age. Bone age can be determined by x-ray studies. In the fetus, bones begin as connective tissue, which later is converted to cartilage. Cartilage is converted to bone through ossification. The rate of bone growth and the age of maturity vary within individuals, but the progression remains the same. Growth of the long bones continues until *epiphyseal* fusion occurs. Bone is constantly synthesized and resorbed. In children, bone synthesis is greater than bone destruction. Calcium reserves are stored in the ends of the long bones. Vitamin A, vitamin D, sunlight, and fluorine are necessary for the growth and development of skeletal and soft tissue.

CRITICAL PERIODS

There appear to be certain periods when environmental events or stimuli have their maximum impact on the child's development. The embryo, for example, can be adversely affected during times of rapid cell division. Certain viruses, drugs, and other agents are known to cause congenital anomalies during the first 3 months after conception. It is believed that issues such as developing a sense of trust during the first year of life and learning readiness are also subject to these periods of particular sensitivity.

INTEGRATION OF SKILLS

As the child learns new skills, they are combined with those previously mastered. The child who is learning to walk may sit, pull the body up to a table by grasping it, balance, and take a cautious step. Tomorrow the child may take three steps! Children connect and perfect each skill in preparation for learning a more complex one.

GROWTH STANDARDS

Growth is measured in dimensions such as height, weight, volume, and thickness of tissues. Measurement alone, without any standard of comparison, limits the interpretation of the data. A number of standards have been developed to make it possible to compare (1) the measurement of a child to others of the same age and sex (and, ideally, race), and (2) the child's present measurements with the former rate of growth and pattern of progress. These standards, available as *growth charts*, are among the tools that have been used to assess the child's overall development (Figure 15-3).

Length refers to horizontal measurement; it is used before a child can stand, usually from birth to 2 years. Height is measured with the child standing, usually between 2 and 18 years. Some pointers in reading and interpreting growth charts are as follows:

- Children who are in good health tend to follow a consistent pattern of growth.
- At any age, there are wide individual differences in measured values.
- Percentile charts are customarily divided into either seven or eight percentile levels designated by lines. In general, these lines are labeled 95th, 90th, 75th, 50th, 25th, 10th, and 5th; or 97th, 95th, 90th, 75th, 50th, 25th, 10th, and 3rd.
- A solid black line designates the median (middle) or 50th percentile. Percentile levels show the extent to which a child's measurements deviate from the 50th percentile or middle measurement. A child whose weight is at the 75th percentile line is *one percentile above* the median. A child whose height is at the 25th percentile is *one percentile below* the median.
- A difference of two or more percentile levels between height and weight may suggest an underweight or overweight condition and prompts further investigation.
- Deviations of two or more percentile levels from an established growth pattern necessitate further evaluation.

DEVELOPMENTAL SCREENING

Developmental screening is a vital component of child health assessment. One widely used tool is the Denver II, a revision of the Denver Developmental Screening test. This tool assesses the developmental status of children during the first 6 years of life in four categories: personal-social, fine motor-adaptive, language, and gross motor. It is *not* an intelligence test. Its purpose is to identify children who are unable to perform at a level comparable to their age-mates. A low score merely indicates a need for further evaluation. Both professionals and paraprofessionals can use this test. Proper administration and interpretation will aid in developing an individualized plan of care for the child.

> **Nursing Tip**
>
> "Catch-up" growth refers to the process by which a child who has been sick or malnourished and whose growth has slowed or stopped experiences a period of more rapid growth after recovery as the body attempts to compensate.

INFLUENCING FACTORS

Growth and development are influenced by many factors, such as heredity, nationality, race, ordinal position in the family, gender and environment. These factors are closely related and dependent on one another in their effect on growth and development. They make each person unique. If a child is ill, physically or emotionally, the developmental processes may be delayed.

Hereditary Traits

Characteristics derived from our ancestors are determined at the time of conception by countless genes within each chromosome. Each gene is made of a chemical substance called deoxyribonucleic acid (DNA), which plays an important part in determining inherited characteristics. Examples of inherited traits are eye color, hair color, and physical resemblances within families.

Nationality and Race

Many physical differences among people of various nationalities and races, who were formerly distinguished with ease, have become less apparent in our age of common environment and customs. For instance, a person of Japanese origin might be thought of as being of short stature. However, Japanese children living in the United States are comparable in height to other children in this country. Nevertheless, ethnic differences extend into many areas including speech, food

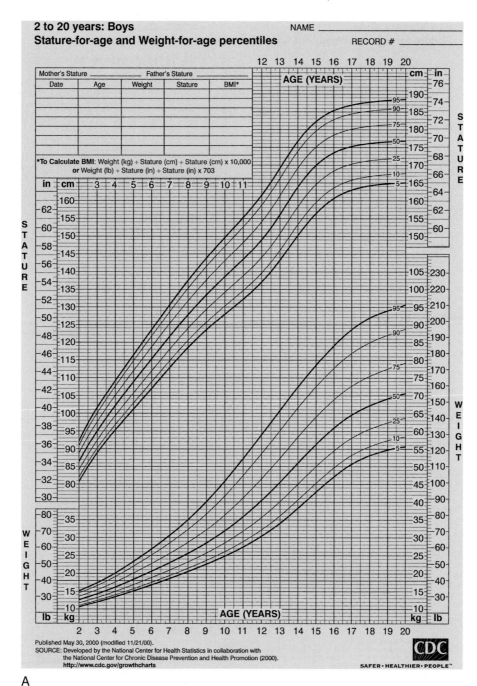

2 to 20 years: Boys
Stature-for-age and Weight-for-age percentiles

Published May 30, 2000 (modified 11/21/00).
SOURCE: Developed by the National Center for Health Statistics in collaboration with
the National Center for Chronic Disease Prevention and Health Promotion (2000).
http://www.cdc.gov/growthcharts

A

FIGURE 15-3 Sample of a complete growth chart, United States. Note the percentiles for height and weight. *BMI*, Body mass index. (Developed by the National Center for Health Statistics in collaboration with the National Center for Chronic Disease Prevention and Health Promotion [2000].)

(Continued)

preferences, family structure, religious orientation, and code of conduct. The nurse should ascertain cultural beliefs and practices when collecting data for nursing assessment (see Table 15-2).

Ordinal Position in the Family
Whether the child is the youngest, the middle, or the oldest in the family has some bearing on growth and development. The youngest and middle children learn from their older sisters and brothers. However, motor development of the youngest may be prolonged if the

others in the family baby the child. The only child or the oldest child may excel in language development because his or her conversations are mainly with adults. These children are often the objects of greater parental expectations.

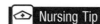

Nursing Tip

Acceptance of the child's value system and cultural beliefs will assist in positive nurse–child interactions.

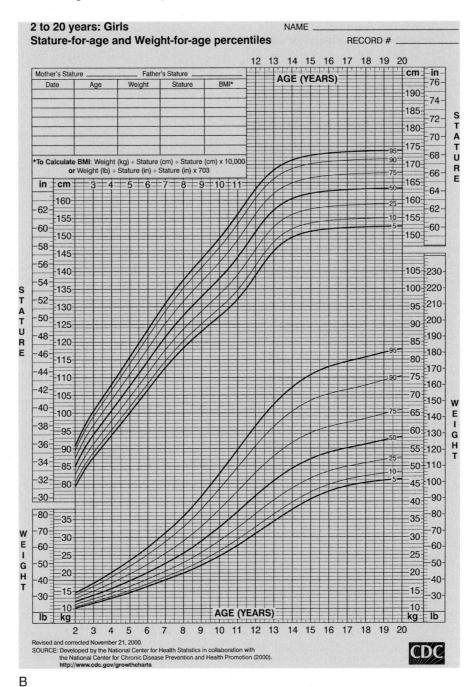

2 to 20 years: Girls
Stature-for-age and Weight-for-age percentiles

NAME _____
RECORD # _____

*To Calculate BMI: Weight (kg) ÷ Stature (cm) ÷ Stature (cm) x 10,000
or Weight (lb) ÷ Stature (in) ÷ Stature (in) x 703

Revised and corrected November 21, 2000.
SOURCE: Developed by the National Center for Health Statistics in collaboration with
the National Center for Chronic Disease Prevention and Health Promotion (2000).
http://www.cdc.gov/growthcharts

B

FIGURE 15-3, cont'd Sample of a complete growth chart, United States.

Gender

The male infant often weighs more and is slightly longer than the female. He grows and develops at a slightly different rate. Parents and relatives may treat boys differently from girls by providing "gender-appropriate" toys and play and by having different expectations of them. Current trends promote unisex activities in play and career development.

Environment

The prenatal environment influences the physical condition of the newborn. The health of the mother at the time of conception and the amount and quality of her diet during pregnancy are important for proper fetal development. Infections or diseases may lead to malformations of the fetus. A healthy and strong newborn can easily adapt to its surroundings.

The home greatly influences the infant's physical and emotional growth and development. If an added member financially strains a family, and the parents are unable to provide nourishing foods and suitable housing, the infant is directly affected. An uneducated mother may not know how to cook foods properly to preserve their nutritional value. Immunizations and other medical attention may be neglected. The infant senses tension within the family and is affected by it.

In contrast, energies can be directed toward positive development when the surroundings are secure and stable and the infant feels secure, wanted, and loved. Most environments are neither completely positive nor completely negative but fall somewhere between the two extremes. Intelligence plays an important role in social and mental development. It is believed that potential intelligence is inherited but is greatly affected by the environment.

 Nursing Tip

"Different" does not mean "inferior."

The Family

The *family* has been defined in many different ways and fulfills many different purposes. Generally, a family is defined as two or more person's living and interacting together. Traditionally, the **nuclear family**, or biological family, has been the basic unit of structure in American society (mother, father, siblings). Today many nuclear families do not share the same household because of single parenthood, divorce, and remarriage. Kinship lines have become blurred, and fundamental changes from what was once perceived as standard are occurring in the family. The **extended family** refers to three generations: grandparents, parents, and children. Because of an increasing life span, however, there are a greater number of living grandparents and great-grandparents, and the proportion of them living in the family home may increase. Table 15-1 lists the various types of families and gives a description of each.

The *interactions* of family unit members are by far the most influential aspect of family life in the growth and development of the child. The nurse must understand the interaction of the family unit to be able to effect a positive change that may be necessary to prevent or treat childhood illnesses. Some families have solid support systems and use available community resources to maintain health. Other families may lack support systems and require closer follow-up care and encouragement by the health team. Parenting is a learned behavior, often modeled by past experience and modified by the acceptance of specific roles and responsibilities. A family that does not provide for the optimum physical, psychological, and emotional health of the children is called a **dysfunctional family**. A dysfunctional family does not necessarily imply that its members are not loving and caring. A dysfunctional family does not know how to be successful in its efforts and interactions and requires intervention.

Historically, in middle-class families the father was the breadwinner and the mother managed the home and raised the children. This model has shifted. Because of changing economic conditions, both parents' earnings may be necessary to maintain the family's standard of living. In dual-career families, both the father and the mother are often absent for most of the day because of long commutes or the demands of the working environment. Both parents may share child care and domestic chores. The parents may need to transfer to different locations to maintain their careers. This decreases extended family support and makes it necessary for children to change schools frequently.

Divorce, separation, death, and pregnancy outside marriage create many one-parent families. The percentage of children living in single-parent families has more than doubled since the 1970s. Most single-wage families have an economic disadvantage, but families with women as the sole wage earner often have considerably lower incomes than those in which men are sole wage earners. The problem of providing good, affordable child care is a serious one for both dual-career families and single parents. Relatives and the noncustodial parent may assist in raising the child. Many single parents remarry, creating the *blended* family. The addition may be merely a stepfather or stepmother, or two families may unite. These family units must make many adjustments. To succeed, parents and children have to learn problem-solving techniques, communication skills, and flexibility.

Table **15-1**	Variations of Family Living
TYPE OF FAMILY*	**DESCRIPTION**
Nuclear	Traditional—husband, wife, children (natural or adopted)
Extended	Grandparents, parents, children, relatives
Single-parent	Women or men establish separate households through individual preference, divorce, death, illegitimacy, or desertion
Foster-parent	Parents who care for children requiring parenting because of a dysfunctional family, no family, or individual problems
Alternative	Communal family
Dual-career	Both parents work outside the home because of desire or need
Blended	Remarriage of persons with children
Polygamous	More than one spouse
Homosexual	Two persons of the same sex adopt children or have children from a previous marriage
Cohabitation	Heterosexual or homosexual couples live together but remain unmarried

*Not all family types may be legally sanctioned. A family is two or more persons who live and interact together.

A *family APGAR,* first described by Smilkstein and colleagues (1984), is a tool that can be used as a guide to assess family functioning. This assessment is valuable in determining the approach to home care needs:

- *Adaptation:* How the family helps and shares resources
- *Partnership:* Lines of communication and partnership in the family
- *Growth:* How responsibilities for growth and development of child are shared
- *Affection:* Overt and covert emotional interactions among family members
- *Resolve:* How time, money, and space are allocated to prevent and solve problems

Questions concerning each of these areas should be posed and evaluated. The goal in family assessment is to enable the nurse to develop interventions that aid the family to achieve a healthier adaptation to the child's health needs or problems.

Nursing Tip

An infant who is hypersensitive to noise or touch needs the parent to understand the need for quiet surroundings. A chronically depressed parent may interpret fussiness or lack of smiling as rejection. Therefore an assessment of parent–child interaction is essential in the home, clinic, or hospital setting.

Nursing Tip

Special care may be required to assist in the growth and development of infants who are blind or whose parents are chronically depressed.

The Family as Part of a Community. The term **community** is defined in many ways, but here it is used to refer to the immediate geographical area in which the family lives and interacts (e.g., "I come from the South Side"). Families are greatly influenced by the communities in which they reside. Nurses must understand the culture of the community in which they work or to which the patient will return (Table 15-2). Assessment of the community is particularly important in creating discharge plans for families from various cultures. Their lives may be broadened or restricted depending on the facilities within the community. A few factors to consider are housing, access to public transportation, city services, safety, and health care delivery systems. The nurse has immediate access to the patient and therefore becomes an important liaison between various agencies that address specific needs.

The Homeless Family. The homeless family with children is a modern-day problem that has an impact on the growth, development, and health of the child. Support systems and financial resources are often lacking, and the school nurse or emergency department nurse may be the first to identify the status of this family. Community referrals to provide shelter, food, education, and financial aid are primary needs that must be met before health teaching can be effective.

It is imperative that nurses take advantage of the strengths of the family while attending to its weaknesses. Nurses are in an excellent position to help the health profession move toward truly contemporary models of family-centered care. The nuclear family of the past is no longer dominant. Pediatric nursing research and care must reflect this phenomenon.

PERSONALITY DEVELOPMENT

Most people tend to equate personality with social attractiveness: "She has a lot of personality, and he has no personality"; or "*There's* an example of personality plus." The term "personality" is more broadly defined by psychologists. One definition states that **personality** is a "unique organization of characteristics that determine the individual's typical or recurrent pattern of behavior." No two persons are exactly alike. An individual's personality is the result of interaction between biological and environmental heritages.

Although no one group of theories can explain all human behavior, each can make a useful contribution to it. Many experts have devoted their lives to understanding why children and families behave as they do. Some experts, called *systems theorists,* believe that everyone in the family or system is affected by each of its members. This theory focuses on the interrelatedness of the various persons as opposed to an analysis of an individual in the group. Nurses using systems theory focus on caring for the child by caring for the whole family. They see the family as protector, educator, resource, and health provider for the child. In turn, they see the child's health as having an impact on each member of the family as a whole.

Many experts see human development through a composite lens of various theories. The hierarchy of needs developed by Abraham **Maslow** is depicted in Figure 15-4, and the developmental theories of

Text continued on p. 367

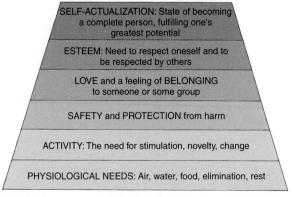

FIGURE 15-4 Maslow's hierarchy of basic needs. The needs at the bottom of the pyramid must be met before one can fulfill needs at the next higher level.

Table 15-2 **Cultural Influences on the Family**

CULTURAL GROUP	FAMILY AND KINSHIP STRUCTURE	COMMUNICATION	HEALTH BELIEFS AND PRACTICES	FAMILY AND CHILD CARE PRACTICES
Hispanic				
Mexican American	Family is an extensive network composed of nuclear and extended family members. Father is provider and decision maker; mother is family caregiver. Decisions are made by father after discussion with older or extended family members. Divorce is uncommon. Out-of-wedlock relationships are common. Children are the center of family life.	Eye contact may be considered rude. Looking at or admiring an infant without touching the child can bring about *mal ojo* (evil eye).	Health represents an equilibrium between hot and cold, wet and dry. An imbalance in these forces causes disease. Cold remedies are used to treat hot diseases, and hot remedies are used to treat cold diseases. Balance and harmony are accomplished through avoiding some foods and consuming others. Seek *curandero,* a folk healer, for treatment remedies and spiritual healing ceremonies. May combine advice from *curandero* with the antibiotics or other therapies from a physician. Resort to prayer or home remedies *(remedias caseras)* before seeking help from folk practitioner or health care provider. Often delay seeking medical attention and obtaining screening examinations and immunizations. Higher incidence of jobs with no health insurance. Mother is unlikely to sign consent for child's health care without discussion with the father.	Delay breastfeeding until milk comes in. Believe that stress and anger make milk bad, and infant can become ill. Neutralize infant bowel when weaning from breast to bottle by feeding only anise tea for 24 hours. More likely to have children without prenatal or postnatal care. *Mal ojo,* or "evil eye," is an illness that affects children and occurs when someone with special powers looks at or admires a child but does not touch or hold the child. A *curandero* can treat the child through massage and prayer. Wearing special amulets or charms can protect child from the evil eye. The practice of binding the umbilicus of the newborn is done to prevent bad air from entering the infant. Parent–child relationship is warm and nurturing. Parents are often quite permissive in respect to their child's behavior.
Puerto Rican	Extended and patriarchal family.	Bilingual—Spanish and English.	Avoid iron supplements because they are considered "hot" medications. Classify foods and medications as hot, cold, and cool.	Children are viewed as a gift from God. Children are taught to obey and respect their parents. Male–female roles are taught.

Continued

Table 15-2   Cultural Influences on the Family—cont'd

CULTURAL GROUP	FAMILY AND KINSHIP STRUCTURE	COMMUNICATION	HEALTH BELIEFS AND PRACTICES	FAMILY AND CHILD CARE PRACTICES
Hispanic, cont'd				
Cuban	Family ties are strong, and this continues as children grow into adulthood. Several generations live together.	Bilingual—Spanish and English.	Health promotion is important. Believe in the biomedical model, although supernatural forces (evil eye) are thought to cause some illnesses that can be cured by ethnic treatments or magic spells. Amulets on a bracelet or necklace may be worn to ward off the evil eye. Diet is high in fat, cholesterol, sugar, and fried foods.	Mother is the primary child caregiver. Plump infants and young children are idealized. School system assumes much of the childrearing responsibilities. Fathers make the family decisions.
Haitian				
	Extended family is important as the support system. Matriarchal society with male as figurehead.	Rely on native language.	Believe that God's will must prevail. Rely on folk foods and treatments for illness management. Believe in hot–cold theory. Avoid eggplant, okra, tomatoes, black pepper, cold drinks, milk, rice, bananas, and fish during pregnancy. White foods are believed to cause increased vaginal discharge in pregnancy.	Usually breastfeed and believe strong emotions affect quality of milk. Folk medicine is the first line of treatment.
African American				
	Family is of great importance. Many are headed by mother in absence of a father. In two-parent families, egalitarian structure is most prominent. It is not uncommon to have extended family living together and older members assisting with child care.	English	Wife or mother is the source of advice on medical ailments and when to seek medical treatment. Many believe that illness comes from germs. Others believe that illness can result from natural causes (e.g., exposure to wind, rain) or unnatural causes (witchcraft, voodoo, punishment for sin).	Begin cereal consumption in infancy at early age. This culture is least likely to breastfeed. Religious orientation is strong (Baptist predominant). Use belly band or binder to protect newborn's umbilicus from dirt, injury, or hernias.

Table 15-2 Cultural Influences on the Family—cont'd

CULTURAL GROUP	FAMILY AND KINSHIP STRUCTURE	COMMUNICATION	HEALTH BELIEFS AND PRACTICES	FAMILY AND CHILD CARE PRACTICES
African American, cont'd				
			Poverty and lack of health insurance lead to inadequate health care. Many rely on folk remedies passed from one generation to next before seeking care from physician. "Granny" or "old lady" is woman in community with knowledge of herbs to treat common illnesses. Spiritualist is someone with a special gift from God to heal certain diseases. Prayer is commonly used in response to illness. A diet high in fat and sodium is considered an indication of well-being. Many individuals have lactose intolerance; therefore milk may be inadequate in the diets of pregnant women and children.	Strict parenting practices are encouraged and are meant to develop effective coping abilities in children to prepare them for the racial discrimination they are likely to encounter in society. There is a high respect for authority figures, a strong work ethic, and an emphasis on achievement. Expression of emotions by males and females is encouraged. Children are expected to use their time wisely, assume responsibilities at an early age, and participate in decision making. Physical forms of discipline are often used.
Asian				
Vietnamese	Patriarchal in structure. Extended families are predominant. Primogeniture (first son inherits family's worth).	Avoid confrontations with health care professionals, perhaps answering questions with what they believe the other person wants to hear. May consider health practitioners to be loud and boisterous. Do not touch children on the head. The head is considered sacred because it is where one's consciousness lies. Eye contact may be considered rude.	Forces of *yang* (light, heat, or dryness) and *yin* (darkness, cold, and wetness) influence the balance and harmony of a person's state of health. Seek a shaman (a physician-priest) for treatment remedies and spiritual healing ceremonies. Evil spirits enter the body through open orifices such as ears, nose, and mouth, causing infection. If the opening is covered, the bad spirits cannot enter and the illness is cured.	Breastfeeding may be delayed for 3 days because the colostrum is considered "dirty." Breastfeeding is low among immigrant Southeast Asians. Boys are breastfed longer than girls. Delay the introduction of solid foods up to 18 months. Diet may consist of breast milk and rice water; the diet is low in calcium and iron.

Continued

Table 15-2	Cultural Influences on the Family—cont'd			
CULTURAL GROUP	**FAMILY AND KINSHIP STRUCTURE**	**COMMUNICATION**	**HEALTH BELIEFS AND PRACTICES**	**FAMILY AND CHILD CARE PRACTICES**
Asian, cont'd				
		Beckoning with one's hand or finger is the gesture used with dogs and is considered insulting when used with people.	Health represents an equilibrium between hot and cold, wet and dry. An imbalance in these forces causes disease.	Excessive consumption of cow's milk (up to eight bottles a day) in the second year of life is common, as is the continual use of the bottle instead of the cup into the third year of life. Avoid praising an infant for fear that a spirit may overhear the praise and be tempted to steal the infant. Parents have an approach to childrearing that is more controlling, achievement oriented, and more encouraging of independence than that of parents in many other cultures. Balance and harmony are valued.
Chinese	Needs of the family come before the needs of the individual. Children repay their parents' love and care by providing for them in their old age. Extended family important, with older adults respected and cared for in the homes of the adult children. Interracial marriages are frowned upon.	Silence does not necessarily indicate the end of a conversation; it may mean the speaker wishes the listener to consider the content before the speaker continues.	Forces of *yang* (light, heat, or dryness) and *yin* (darkness, cold, and wetness) influence the balance and harmony of person's state of health. Health is a state of physical and spiritual harmony with nature. Prevention is key to healthy living. Traditional Chinese medicine is sought before Western medical services. Use acupuncture, herbal medicines, massage, cupping, skin scraping, and moxibustion as therapies to restore *yin* and *yang*. Avoid eating soy sauce during pregnancy because it is believed to darken the infant's skin; shellfish is believed to cause allergies in the infant, and iron supplements are believed to harden bones and lead to difficult delivery.	Primary responsibility for child care belongs to mother. Grandparents may be asked to assist in child care. Cultural healing practices can cause visible bruising or injury to child's skin. It is important for children to exhibit self-control. Children are socialized not to challenge authority. Pregnancy means woman has "happiness in her body." Many children are breastfed until they are 4 to 5 years of age. Jade is often worn in the form of a charm to keep the child safe. Believe physical illness is caused by an imbalance of *yin* and *yang* in body.

Table 15-2 Cultural Influences on the Family—cont'd

CULTURAL GROUP	FAMILY AND KINSHIP STRUCTURE	COMMUNICATION	HEALTH BELIEFS AND PRACTICES	FAMILY AND CHILD CARE PRACTICES
Asian, cont'd				
Japanese	Value social group harmony above individual needs and autonomy. Family structure is extended and patriarchal. Women are traditionally passive.	Silence does not necessarily indicate the end of a conversation; it may mean the speaker wishes the listener to consider the content before the speaker continues. Handshakes are acceptable; a pat on the back is not acceptable. Direct eye contact considered lacking in respect.	When in pain, patients stoically withstand it. Women labor in silence. After delivery, long periods of rest and recuperation are encouraged. Use natural herbs—kampo—medicine. Use both Western and traditional Oriental healing methods.	Mother has primary responsibility for childrearing and ensuring the child's success in school. Mother may sleep with her child. Colostrum is not fed to infants. Only half of all breastfed infants continue to be breastfed after age 1 month.
Hmong	Extended family structure.	Do not touch children on the head. The head is considered sacred because it is where one's consciousness lies.	Seek shaman (a physician-priest) for treatment remedies and spiritual healing ceremonies.	Avoid praising an infant for fear that a spirit may overhear the praise and be tempted to steal the infant. Infants may wear colorful hats so they are disguised as "flowers" and the spirits will not notice them.
European				
Caucasian American	Nuclear family is highly valued. Divorce and remarriage are a common practice. Goal of individual often seen as more important than goal of the family. Success is measured in terms of financial wealth and status in society.	Pat children on head to show affection or approval. Uncomfortable with periods of silence. Expect people to look you in the eye when they are speaking to you. Avoiding eye contact can be considered an indication that a person is lying.	Rely on modern medicine and health care professionals to treat illness.	Style of parenting is authoritative. Children are encouraged to value individual differences, the future rather than the present, material well-being, competition, and to consider many options when making decisions. Adults readily praise the infant's and the child's behavior and appearance. Self-reliance is highly valued.

Continued

Table 15-2   Cultural Influences on the Family—cont'd

CULTURAL GROUP	FAMILY AND KINSHIP STRUCTURE	COMMUNICATION	HEALTH BELIEFS AND PRACTICES	FAMILY AND CHILD CARE PRACTICES
European, cont'd				
Irish American	Strong family bonds. Emphasis is placed on the well-being of family, not of individual members.	May communicate with flowery and sometimes exaggerated words. May be overly verbose in descriptions of their condition.	Health comes when person is goal oriented and nurtures a strong religious faith. Health is maintained with a great deal of sleep combined with fresh air, exercise, and balanced diet. Home remedies or treatments are first resort to treat illness. Medical assistance should be sought only in cases of emergency.	Strict followers of the church—typically Protestant or Catholic.
Italian American	Family roles are traditional. Father is head of household, and mother is heart of the household, although mother has powerful sway over internal family matters. Children are valued members and are showered with love and affection. Family is a source of comfort and pride for individual members. Members maintain close contact or close proximity with nuclear and extended family. Divorce is uncommon in traditional families. Large family size is attributed to adherence to Catholic beliefs and traditions.	Complaining loudly and making demands are often rewarded with attention.	Health is maintained by strong religious influence (primarily Catholic). Faith in God and saints will see them through illness. Beliefs about the cause of illness have been found to include winds and currents that bear diseases, contagion or contamination, heredity, supernatural or human causes, and psychosomatic explanations.	It is important to keep child warm in cold weather, stay out of drafts, and not go outside with wet hair. Maintain health with a nutritious diet of fruit, vegetables, pasta, hard cheese, and wine. Children are introduced to water-wine mixture at a young age.

Table 15-2 Cultural Influences on the Family—cont'd

CULTURAL GROUP	FAMILY AND KINSHIP STRUCTURE	COMMUNICATION	HEALTH BELIEFS AND PRACTICES	FAMILY AND CHILD CARE PRACTICES
European, cont'd				
Native American	Grandparents retain important role in parenting their grandchildren. Extended family network is valued. Many Native Americans have married into other tribes and other ethnic groups. Children respect elders.	Silence is critical during interactions. Strong need to sit quietly and think before responding to questions. Eye contact may be considered rude. May consider health practitioners to be loud and boisterous. Spokesperson may not be decision maker.	Wellness exists when there is harmony in body, mind, and spirit. Seek shaman (a physician-priest) for treatment remedies and spiritual healing ceremonies. High incidence of lactose intolerance. Eat nonperishable food items because of lack of refrigeration. Beans are the main source of protein. Frequent problems with obesity and alcoholism. Often feel that Western medicine places too much emphasis on medications. A holistic approach to healing is valued. Alcoholism is a major problem for many families.	High rate of breastfeeding. Mothers retain primary responsibility for childrearing and discipline. Medicine bag is often worn by ill person and must not be handled by caregivers.

From Bowden V, Dickey S, Greenberg C: *Children and their families: the continuum of care,* Philadelphia, 1998, Saunders; Lipson J, Dibble S: *Culture and nursing care,* ed 2, San Francisco, 2005, University of California–San Francisco Nursing Press; Leifer G, Fleck E: *Growth and development across the lifespan: a health promotion focus,* ed 2, St Louis, 2013, Saunders.

Erik Erikson, Sigmund Freud, Lawrence Kohlberg, Harry Stack Sullivan, and Jean Piaget are presented in Table 15-3. Other theorists are briefly contrasted within appropriate chapters devoted to specific age groups. Theories provide a framework for the practitioner; however, humans are not a gathering of isolated parts to be disassembled and reassembled according to some theoretical set of instructions, even when these parts must be examined for investigative purposes.

Cognitive Development

Cognition (*cognoscere,* "to know") refers to intellectual ability. Children are born with inherited potential, but the potential must be developed. Opportunities for successful exploration enhance the child's cognition development. The development of logical thinking and conceptual understanding is a complex process. One outstanding authority on cognitive development was **Piaget**, a Swiss psychologist. He proposed that intellectual maturity is attained through four orderly and distinct stages of development, all of which are interrelated: sensorimotor (up to 2 years), preoperational (2 to 7 years), concrete operations (7 to 11 years), and formal operations (11 to 16 years). The ages for each stage are approximate, and each stage builds on the preceding one.

Piaget believed that intelligence consists of interaction and coping with the environment. Infants begin their interaction by reflex response. As they grow older, their use of symbolism (particularly language) increases. Gradually they acquire a here-and-now orientation (concrete operations) and finally a fully abstract comprehension of the world (formal operations). Table 15-4 relates Piaget's theory to feeding and nutrition. It is a good example of how knowledge of development can help in understanding the behavior of a child at a particular time.

Moral Development

Lawrence **Kohlberg**, a childhood theorist, suggests that moral development in children is sequential. His theories on moral development are based on Piaget's cognitive development investigations. He describes three levels: *preconventional, conventional,* and *postconventional.* Each level contains two stages. In the preconventional stage (4 to 7 years), children try to be obedient to their parents because of fear of punishment. During the conventional phase (7 to 11 years), children show conformity and loyalty, and they focus on obeying rules. In the postconventional level (12 years and older), *moral values* are developed to solve complex problems. There is an emphasis on the conscience of the individual within the society. Although rules are still important, changing them to meet the needs of a culture is considered.

Table 15-3   Comparison of the Developmental Theories of Erikson, Freud, Kohlberg, Sullivan, and Piaget

DEVELOPMENTAL PERIOD	ERIKSON	FREUD	KOHLBERG	SULLIVAN	PIAGET
Infancy	*Trust/mistrust* Getting needs met Tolerating frustration in small doses Recognizing mother as distinct from others and self	*Orality*—understanding the world by exploring with the mouth	*Preconventional/ premoral*—cannot distinguish right from wrong	Security Patterns of emotional response Organization of sensation	*Sensorimotor stage* (birth to 2 years)—at birth, responses are limited to reflexes; begins to relate to outside events; concerned with sensations and actions that affect self directly
Toddler	*Autonomy/shame and doubt* Trying out own powers of speech Beginning acceptance of reality versus pleasure principle	*Anality*—learning to give and take	*Punishment/ obedience*—performance based on fear of punishment	Mastery of space and objects	*Preoperational* (2 to 7 years)—child is still egocentric; thinks everyone sees world as self does
Preschooler	*Initiative/guilt* Questioning Exploring own body and environment Differentiation of sexes	*Phallic/oedipal phase*—becoming aware of self as sexual being	*Morality*—rules are absolute; breaking rules results in punishment; behavior based on rewards	Speech and conscious need for playmates, interpersonal communication	*Perceptual* (4 to 7 years)—capable of some reasoning but can concentrate on only one aspect of a situation at a time
School-age	*Industry/inferiority* Learning to win recognition by producing things Exploring, collecting Learning to relate to own sex	*Latency*—focusing on peer relations; learning to live in groups and to achieve knowledge	*Conventional morality*—rules are created for the benefit of all; adhering to rules is the right thing to do (7 to 11 years)	Chumship, one-to-one relationship, self-esteem, compassion (homosexuality)	*Concrete operations* (7 to 11 years)—reasoning is logical but limited to own experience; understands cause and effect
Adolescence	*Identity/role diffusion* Moving toward heterosexuality Selecting vocation Beginning separation from family Integrating personality (e.g., altruism)	*Genitality*	*Principled morality* (autonomous stage) (12 years and older)—acceptance of right or wrong based on own perceptions of world and personal conscience	Capacity to love, empathy, partnership (heterosexuality)	*Formal operations* (11 to 16 years)—acquires ability to develop abstract concepts for self; oriented to problem solving

THE GROWTH AND DEVELOPMENT OF A PARENT

Table 15-5 shows the tasks of the parent as they relate to the child's developmental tasks in Erikson's system of stages, as well as some suggestions for nursing interventions that can aid the growth and development of a parent and a child.

Erikson's stages of child development demonstrate the various tasks that must be mastered at each age to achieve optimum maturity. Each stage builds on the successful completion of the previous stage. Achievement of the tasks of childhood does not occur in isolation. Parents must *interact* appropriately to assist

Table 15-4   Piaget's Theory of Cognitive Development in Relation to Feeding and Nutrition

DEVELOPMENTAL PERIOD	COGNITIVE CHARACTERISTICS	RELATIONSHIP TO FEEDING AND NUTRITION
Sensorimotor (birth to 2 years)	Progression is from newborn with automatic reflexes to intentional interaction with the environment and the beginning use of symbols.	Progression is made from sucking and rooting reflexes to the acquisition of self-feeding skills. Food is used primarily to satisfy hunger, as a medium to explore the environment, and to practice fine motor skills.
Preoperational (2 to 7 years)	Thought processes become internalized; they are unsystematic and intuitive. Use of symbols increases. Reasoning is based on appearances and happenstance. Approach to classification is functional and unsystematic. Child's world is viewed egocentrically.	Eating becomes less the center of attention than social, language, and cognitive growth. Food is described by color, shape, and quantity, but there is limited ability to classify food into "groups." Foods tend to be classed as "like" and "don't like." Child can identify food as "good for you," but reasons are unknown or mistaken.
Concrete operations (7 to 11 years)	Child can focus on several aspects of a situation simultaneously. Cause-effect reasoning becomes more rational and systematic. Ability to classify, reclassify, and generalize emerges. Decrease in egocentrism permits child to take another's view.	Child begins to realize that nutritious food has a positive effect on growth and health but has limited understanding of how or why this occurs. Mealtimes take on a social significance. Expanding environment increases the opportunities for, and influences on, food selection (peer influence rises).
Formal operations (11 to 16 years)	Hypothetic and abstract thought expands. Understanding of scientific and theoretic processes deepens.	The concept of nutrients from food functioning at physiological and biochemical levels can be understood. Conflicts in making food choices may be realized (knowledge of nutritious food versus preferences and nonnutritive influences).

From Mahan LK, Escott-Stump S: *Krause's food, nutrition and diet therapy*, ed 13, Philadelphia, 2012, Saunders.

the child to achieve successfully at his or her developmental level (Figure 15-5). For example, if the parent constructs a school project for a child, the child will not achieve a sense of industry. If the parent does not accept a positive attitude toward the pregnancy and unsuccessfully attempts to abort, the parent may become overly protective or abusive to the newborn infant, and bonding will not occur.

Parents should be guided not to attempt to prevent frustration in the lives of their children. Experiences in handling challenges and disappointments prepare the child to function independently in adulthood. Parents should encourage a child to manage successes and failures, should provide socially acceptable outlets, and should intervene only if the frustrations become overwhelming. The parent's task is to provide the child with the skills and tools appropriate at each age level to deal with events. Many websites provide tips concerning parenting skills.

NUTRITION

NUTRITIONAL HERITAGE

Good nutrition begins before conception. Nutritional needs during pregnancy are discussed in Chapter 4. The dependent child is fed for many years by adults whose eating habits may be based on misinformation, income level, folklore, fads, or religious, cultural, and ethnic preferences. Table 15-6 describes some common food patterns of various cultures found in the United States. Many families are poor, others have inadequate knowledge of how to prepare foods, and many rely on convenience foods to save time.

Some families do not consider food a priority in the home. However, optimum nutrition is essential for the child to reach his or her growth potential. A lack of adequate nutrition can lead to mental retardation. The obese child may be subject to decreases in motor skills and peer rejection, leading to low self-esteem.

The nurse is in a position to identify children at risk and to help families modify eating habits to ensure proper nutrition. An important resource for the nurse is the nutritionist in the community or on the staff of the health agency where the nurse is employed. Formula feeding and breastfeeding are discussed in Chapters 9 and 16.

FAMILY NUTRITION

The U.S. Department of Agriculture (USDA), in a joint effort with the U.S. Department of Health and Human Services (USDHHS), offers dietary guidelines for Americans; these were updated in 2011. Good nutrition is vital to good health and essential for normal growth and development. A healthy, balanced, nutrient-dense diet, combined with adequate physical activity, is the core of the new dietary guidelines. The 2011 Dietary

| Table 15-5 | The Growth and Development of a Parent |

CHILD'S TASKS (ERIKSON'S STAGES)	PARENTS' TASK	NURSING INTERVENTION
First Prenatal Trimester		
Growth	Develop attitude toward newborn: • Happy about child? • Parent of one disabled child? • Unwed mother? These factors and others will affect the developing attitude of the mother.	Develop positive attitude in both parents concerning expected birth of child. Use referrals and agencies as needed.
Second Prenatal Trimester		
Growth	Mother focuses on infant because of fetal movements felt. Parents picture what infant will look like, what future he or she will have, and other ideas.	Parents' focus is on child care and needs and providing physical environment for expected infant's arrival. Therefore information concerning care of the newborn should be provided at this time.
Third Prenatal Trimester		
Growth	Mother feels large. Attention focuses on how fetus is going to get out.	Detailed information should be presented at this time concerning the birth processes, preparation for birth, breastfeeding, and care of sibling at home.
Birth		
Adjust to external environment	Elicit positive responses from child and respond by meeting child's need for food and closeness. If parents receive only negative responses (e.g., sleepy infant, crying infant, difficult feeder, congenital anomaly), development of the parent will be inhibited.	Encourage early touch, feeding, and other practices. Explain behavior and appearance of newborn to allay fears. Help parents to identify positive responses. (Use infant's reflexes, such as grasp reflex, to elicit a positive response by placing mother's finger into infant's hand.)
Infant		
Develop trust	Learn "cues" presented by infant to determine individual needs of infant.	Help parents assess and interpret needs of infant (prevent feelings of helplessness or incompetence). Do not let in-laws take over parental tasks. Help parents cope with problems such as colic.
Toddler		
Autonomy	Try to accept the pattern of growth and development. Accept some loss of control but maintain some limits for safety.	Help parents cope with transient independence of child (e.g., allow child to go on tricycle but do not yell "Don't fall" or anxiety will be radiated).
Preschool-Age		
Initiative	Learn to separate from child.	Help parents show standards but "let go" so child can develop some independence. A preschool experience may be helpful.
School-Age		
Industry	Accept importance of child's peers. Parents must learn to accept some rejection from child at times. Patience is needed to allow children to do for themselves, even if it takes longer. Do not *do* the school project *for* the child. Provide chores for child appropriate to his or her age level.	Help parents to understand that child is developing his or her own limits and self-discipline. Be there to guide child, but do not constantly intrude. Help child get results from his or her efforts at performance.
Adolescent		
Establishing identity Accepting pubertal changes Developing abstract reasoning Deciding on career Investigating lifestyles Controlling feeling	Parents must learn to let child live his or her own life and not expect total control over the child. Expect, at times, to be discredited by teenager. Expect differences in opinion and respect them. Guide but do not push.	Help parents adjust to changing role and relationship with adolescent (e.g., as child develops his or her own identify, he may become a Democrat if parents are Republican). Expose child to varied career fields and life experiences. Help child to understand emerging emotions and feelings brought about by puberty.

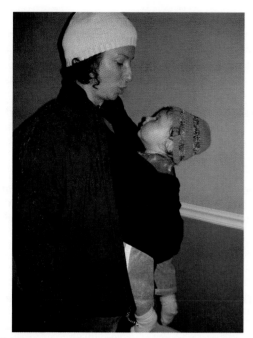

FIGURE 15-5 Infant carriers enable face-to-face interaction between young infant and parent. An older infant can be turned in the carrier to face outward and interact with the environment.

Guidelines can be designed to meet the individual needs of the consumer. Personalized, portion-sized diet plans that include advice on activity level can be found online, along with additional recommendations for specific populations.

Examples of culturally diverse food pyramids can be found in Chapter 4. The dietary guidelines are intended to help Americans make informed decisions about what they eat. Families who practice such principles are educating their children by good example. Figure 15-6 shows a suggested content of a food plate for children 2 to 6 years of age. Detailed information can be obtained by accessing www.choosemyplate.gov. Healthy food choices and appropriate portion size is an important part of weight control. One type of assistance available to parents and children is the "Portion Plate for Kids," a two-sided reusable placemat that shows the appropriate portion size for school-aged children expressed by common objects such as a yo-yo and an 8 pack of crayons and a softball; and for preschoolers, colorful cartoon characters representing a variety of healthy foods in each category that reinforces the latest USDA nutritional guidelines (Figure 15-7). The reverse side of the placemat offers tips on selection of foods and refers the parent to the Internet site.

Many families are vegetarian, and the use of teaching tools that respect the dietary limitations will encourage compliance. The nurse should assess restricted foods in the vegetarian diet and ensure that the diet is adequate in protein, vitamins, and minerals to promote growth and development in children. Children on vegetarian diets often consume large amounts of high-fiber foods.

High-fiber foods cause increased losses of calcium, zinc, magnesium, and iron in the stool and may necessitate the intake of supplements. A diet containing meat, poultry, or fortified foods lessens this nutrient deficiency (see Nutrition Considerations box).

Nutrition Considerations

Fiber Needs of the Young Child

The American Academy of Pediatrics recommends intake of 0.5 g of fiber per kilogram of body weight in childhood, gradually increasing to adult levels of 20 to 35 g/day by the end of adolescence. High-fiber foods can fill the small stomach capacity and provide few of the nutrients and calories needed by the active, growing child.

Different types of fiber are contained in foods (Table 15-7). The water-soluble fiber found in oats, apples, and citrus fruits delays intestinal transit and decreases serum cholesterol levels. The water-insoluble fiber found in whole-grain breads, wheat bran, and some cereals accelerates intestinal transit and slows starch digestion.

A well-balanced diet supplies all essential nutrients in the necessary amounts. Food provides heat and energy, builds and repairs tissues, and regulates body processes. A given food is a mixture of elements such as minerals (e.g., calcium, phosphorus, sodium, iron), compounds (carbohydrates, fats, proteins, some vitamins), and water. The body needs approximately 50 nutrients, which it absorbs at various sites (Figure 15-8). See the table on USDA Dietary Guidelines for Americans on the Evolve website.

Nutrition Considerations

Enhancing Absorption of Minerals

Foods containing essential minerals such as iron, zinc, and calcium should be combined with citrus, fish, or poultry to enhance absorption of the minerals. Vitamin D and lactose sugars also enhance mineral absorption in the body.

Children are susceptible to nutritional deficiencies because they are growing and developing. Infants require more calories, protein, minerals, and vitamins in proportion to their weight than do adults. Fluid requirements are also higher for infants. Eating a variety of foods selected from the basic food groups ensures good health for children. The *amount* and *size* of portions are important in maintaining a reasonable weight. There are no known advantages to consuming excessive amounts of any nutrients, and there are risks for overdoses.

NUTRITIONAL CARE PLAN

The nutritional care plan can be used in the hospital, home, or outpatient department. Other professionals may already have collected parts of the care plan,

Table 15-6	Culturally Diverse Food Patterns of Americans
CULTURE	**HISTORICAL DIETARY PATTERN***
African American	All meats, fish, and chicken; pork is often consumed (spareribs, bacon, and sausage). Vegetables are cooked in salt pork for long periods; grits and cornbread muffins. There is some lactose intolerance. Popular vegetables include collard greens, beet greens, and sweet potatoes.
Chinese American	Rich in vegetables (bean sprouts, broccoli, bamboo shoots, and mushrooms). Vegetables are cooked until crisp; meat is consumed in small portions with other food. Soy sauce, tofu, peanut butter; limited milk and cheese; fish baked with native spices; soups with egg, meat, and vegetables. Tea is China's national beverage. Rice is staple of diet.
Jewish American	Diet varies according to whether family is Orthodox, Conservative, or Reform. For an Orthodox family, food must be kosher (must conform to dietary laws); meat is soaked in salt water to remove blood; only meat eaten is that of divided-hoofed animals that chew a cud; fish without scales (shellfish) and pork are prohibited; milk and meat cannot be combined. Favorites are gefilte fish, lox (smoked salmon), herring, eggs, bagels, cream cheese, and matzo.
Laotian American	Numerous varieties of freshwater fish and shellfish (eaten fresh, dried, or salted); pork, beef, chicken, and rabbit, often mixed with vegetables and spices; eggs, peanuts, black-eyed peas; vegetables eaten raw, as juice, or cooked with meat or fish and preserved by drying or pickling; sticky rice, rice or bean thread noodles, and legumes often used in desserts; soybean drink, sugar cane drink, tea, and coconut juice. Popular seasonings include *padek,* chilies, curry, tamarind, and red and black pepper.
Italian American	All meats, fish, and chicken, including cold cuts (salami, mortadella) and Italian pork sausage; pasta (staple of diet), breads, olive oil, wine, cheese, and all varieties of fruits and vegetables.
Japanese American	Fish and seafood (fresh, smoked, and raw) and beef. Food is cut into small portions. Principal fruit is *nasi,* which tastes much like a pear. Many vegetables are eaten, such as seaweed, bamboo shoots, onions, beans, and dried mushrooms (shitake); enjoy pickled vegetables. Rice is national staple. Beverages include tea and sake. Little cheese, milk, butter, or cream is consumed. Chief cooking fat is soybean oil or rice oil.
Mexican American	Chicken, pork chops, wieners, cold cuts, hamburger, eggs (used frequently), beans (eaten mashed or refried with lard), potatoes (basic item, usually fried), chilies, fresh tomatoes, corn (maize—often used as basic grain), tortillas, packaged cereals; little milk because of lactose intolerance.
Native American	Acorn flour, a staple food made into mush or bread; salmon, fresh or dried; other varieties of fish, deer, duck, geese, and other small game; nuts such as buckeye and hazel; wild berries, seeds, and roots.
Puerto Rican American	Meat cooked in stews; poultry, pork, fish, dried beans or peas mixed with rice; milk in combination with coffee *(cafe con leche),* variety of fruits, starchy vegetables (plantains, cassava, sweet potatoes), salad, soft drinks.
Vietnamese American	Pork—most common meat; meats cut into small pieces and fried, boiled, or steamed; fish—all types of freshwater and saltwater fish and shellfish, often fried and dipped in fish sauce; eggs, soybeans, legumes, and wide variety of fruits and vegetables; rice often eaten with every meal; seasonings including oyster sauce, soy sauce, monosodium glutamate, ginger, garlic, *nuoc mam* sauce; tea, coffee, soft drinks, soybean milk.

*More diverse eating patterns occur as future generations of a culture become assimilated.
Data from Mahan LK, Escott-Stump S: *Krause's food, nutrition and diet therapy,* ed 13, Philadelphia, 2012, Saunders; Wetter AC, Goldberg JP, King AC, Sigman-Grant M, Baer R, Crayton E et al: How and why do individuals make food and activity choices? *Nutr Rev* 59(3):11-21, 2001; Booth S, Sallis J, Ritenbaugh C, Hill J, Birch L, Frank L et al: Environmental and societal factors affect food choice and physical activity: rationale, influences, and leverage points, *Nutr Rev* 59(2):S21-S39, 2001.

and the nurse should refer to the patient's chart for pertinent data. The nutritional care plan provides information and stores it in one place. It can also be put on a computer for easy retrieval.

NUTRITION AND HEALTH

The digestive system of the newborn is immature and functions minimally during the first 3 months. Saliva is minimal; hydrochloric acid and renin in the stomach and trypsin in the intestines aid in the digestion of milk. Amylase (a pancreatic enzyme) and lipase are not present in adequate quantity before age 4 months, and therefore complex carbohydrates and fats cannot be digested effectively. Excess fiber intake in the young infant results in loose, bulky stools. The ability of the liver to function is limited in the first year of life. The teeth are not present for chewing before 6 to 8 months of age.

 Safety Alert!

Raw fruits that contain seeds or some raw vegetables and nuts may not be appropriate foods for infants and young children because of the risk of choking. Beans and vegetables should be well cooked.

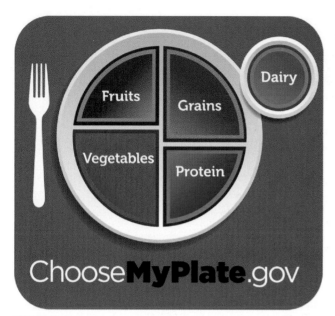

FIGURE 15-6 MyPlate is a guide to healthful eating. The colors represent the basic food groups in the diet with approximate recommended amounts to consume in relation to the total diet plan. Portion size can be individualized to the child by accessing the site www.choosemyplate.gov and entering information such as age, weight, and so forth.

Table 15-7	High-Fiber Foods for Relief of Mild Constipation in Children Older Than 12 Months	
TYPE OF FOOD	**SERVING SIZE**	**EXAMPLE***
Cereals	30 mL (1 oz)	Raisin Bran, Grape-Nuts, Shredded Wheat, Bran Chex
Bread	1 slice	Whole-grain bread
	1 medium	Bran muffin
	1-cm (2.5-inch) piece	Corn bread square
Fruits	120 mL (½ cup)	Cooked prunes
Vegetables	120 mL (½ cup)	Spinach
	1 medium	Corn on the cob
Meat substitute	120 mL (½ cup)	Beans (baked, black, garbanzo, kidney, lima, pinto, lentil)

*All products indicated are registered trademarks of their respective companies. From Baker S: Introduce fruits, vegetables, and grains but do not overdo high-fiber foods, *Pediatr Basics* 69(Summer):2-4, 1994; Mahon LK, Escott-Stump S: *Krause's food, nutrition and diet therapy,* ed 13, Philadelphia, 2012, Saunders.

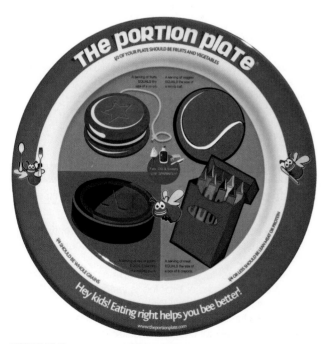

FIGURE 15-7 The Portion Plate for Kids is an educational placemat that can be used to guide portion amounts in terms school-age children can understand, such as, the portion of vegetables in one meal is about the size of a softball and the portion of protein is the size of an 8-pack of crayons. The reverse side of the mat offers tips on food selection. Preventing the supersizing of portions is important in preventing obesity. The plate designed for preschool age children features colorful characters representing a wide variety of healthy foods. (Courtesy beBetter Network, Charleston, W.Va.)

The physiology of digestion is the basis for food introduction in the first year of life. Breast milk or iron-fortified formula is the food of choice for the first 6 months to 1 year of life. Introducing baby food before age 4 to 6 months does not serve any nutritional purpose. Overnutrition and its link to obesity in adults have been explored. High sodium intake in children is a risk factor for developing high blood pressure as an adult. Counseling is a priority (Yang, 2012). The effects of childhood nutrition on adult health and illness patterns, such as heart disease, have been established. Home preparation of food for infants is discussed in Chapter 16.

NUTRITION AND HEALTH PROMOTION

Therapeutic diets, such as the diabetic diet, are well established in medical care. Some foods can promote dental caries, and others contain protective fibers that are known to prevent some diseases. Starting healthy dietary patterns in childhood can prevent atherosclerosis. However, restrictive diets are not advised for infants and young children. Fat and cholesterol are needed for calories and the development of the central nervous system. The sodium content of baby foods has been decreased because the average diet contains adequate sodium. Some food additives, such as aspartame (an artificial sweetener), may be harmful to children with phenylketonuria. Food additives that prolong the shelf life of foods and food dyes that make food look more attractive should be minimized in the child's diet. Fast-food chains, often depended on by working parents and preferred by adolescents, make available to the consumer the nutrient content of the foods they

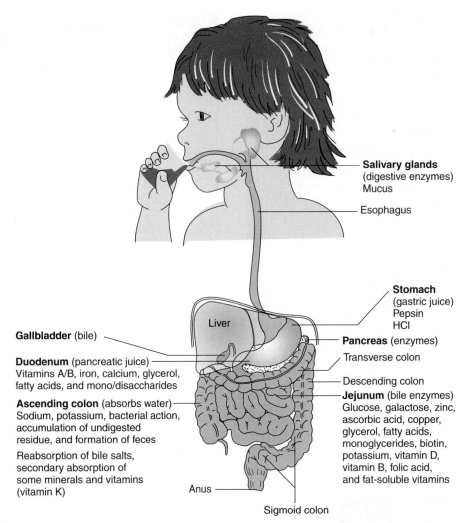

Salivary glands
(digestive enzymes)
Mucus

Esophagus

Stomach
(gastric juice)
Pepsin
HCl

Liver

Gallbladder (bile)

Pancreas (enzymes)

Duodenum (pancreatic juice)
Vitamins A/B, iron, calcium, glycerol,
fatty acids, and mono/disaccharides

Transverse colon

Descending colon

Jejunum (bile enzymes)
Glucose, galactose, zinc,
ascorbic acid, copper,
glycerol, fatty acids,
monoglycerides, biotin,
potassium, vitamin D,
vitamin B, folic acid,
and fat-soluble vitamins

Ascending colon (absorbs water)
Sodium, potassium, bacterial action,
accumulation of undigested
residue, and formation of feces

Reabsorption of bile salts,
secondary absorption of
some minerals and vitamins
(vitamin K)

Anus

Sigmoid colon

FIGURE 15-8 Nutrient digestion. The sites of absorption of major nutrients are shown in this illustration. Most nutrient absorption occurs in the duodenum and jejunum of the small intestine. Most water absorption occurs in the large intestine. Absorption of nutrients depends on adequate secretion of digestive enzymes, normal motility, and normal villi on the mucosal surface of the intestines. Portal circulation, lymphatic circulation, and hormones also play a role in the digestion and absorption of nutrients.

serve. The caloric content of the menu often depends on the foods selected and the toppings added. Therefore a "salad bar" is not necessarily synonymous with a low-calorie meal.

Height and weight should be plotted on a growth chart at each clinic visit to enable early identification of health problems related to dietary intake. The weight or triceps skinfold thickness greater than the 75th percentile or below the 3rd percentile indicates a need for further evaluation. The role of the grandparents in providing a diet that may lead to obesity must often be addressed, because the principles of good nutrition that were adhered to 20 or 30 years ago may no longer be valid. Concern is expressed regarding the level of cholesterol in children. Methods to reduce cholesterol in families are listed in the Health Promotion box, and the National Cholesterol Education Program's recommendations are cited in Box 15-4.

Health Promotion

Methods to Reduce Cholesterol in School-Age Children

- Exercise more with your children.
- Provide fresh fruits and vegetables rather than empty calories such as those found in doughnuts and store-bought pastries.
- Decrease trips to fast-food restaurants.
- Switch to low-fat foods; use vegetable oil cooking sprays in place of butter; bake or broil foods instead of frying them.
- Seek the advice of a nutritionist.
- If there is a family history of heart disease, have the child's as well as your levels of cholesterol tested.

Dietary supplements, formulas, and nutritional support techniques for preterm infants, children with cancer, and those with long-term disorders (e.g., cystic fibrosis) have become sophisticated and are used successfully. Total parenteral nutrition allows the physician to choose preparations ranging from amino acids

Box 15-4	National Cholesterol Evaluation Program (NCEP) Recommendations for Detecting and Managing Hypercholesterolemia in Children and Adolescents

The NCEP has made recommendations for managing hypercholesterolemia to be applied to adolescents and children greater than 2 years of age. For the general population of children and adolescents in the United States, NCEP recommends that eating patterns be adopted to meet the following criteria:

- Nutritionally adequate, varied diet
- Adequate energy intake to support growth and development and to maintain appropriate body weight
- Saturated fat—less than 10% of total calories
- Total fat—an average of no more than 30% of total calories
- Dietary cholesterol—less than 300 mg/day

To implement these patterns means involving the entire community—parents (in the selection and preparation of food), schools (by modification of school food service), health care clinics (by providing health education), government (by mandating improvement of food labeling), and the food industry (by developing low–saturated fat, low-fat foods that are appealing to children).

NCEP also aims to identify and treat individual children and adolescents who have hypercholesterolemia and a family history of premature cardiovascular disease or whose parents have hypercholesterolemia. For this group, NCEP recommends the following:

- Blood cholesterol screening of children and adolescents whose parents or grandparents (at age 55 years or younger) were found to have coronary atherosclerosis; suffered myocardial infarction, peripheral vascular disease, cerebrovascular disease, or sudden death; or underwent invasive cardiac therapy (balloon angioplasty or coronary artery bypass surgery)
- Blood cholesterol screening of offspring of a parent with a blood cholesterol of 240 mg/dL or greater
- Maintaining appropriate levels for total cholesterol and low-density-lipoprotein (LDL) cholesterol. For children with levels above these, dietary change is recommended:

CATEGORY	TOTAL CHOLESTEROL	LDL CHOLESTEROL
Acceptable	<170 mg/dL	<110 mg/dL
Borderline	170-199 mg/dL	110-129 mg/dL
High	>200 mg/dL	>130 mg/dL

A family history of high cholesterol is an indication for screening of the child. If there is insufficient blood lipid lowering after 6 months to 1 year of dietary therapy, drug therapy can be considered in children greater than 10 years of age.

Modified from Mahan LK, Escott-Stump S: *Krause's food, nutrition, and diet therapy*, ed 13, Philadelphia, 2012, Saunders.

and intravenous fats to complete multivitamins. Total parenteral nutrition and enteral feedings allow children who need nutritional support to be cared for at home, thus greatly enhancing the quality of life.

In the 1990s an oral rehydration solution (ORS) used by third-world populations for treating acute diarrhea in children gained acceptance and is now produced and distributed by the World Health Organization. It is composed mainly of electrolytes, glucose, and water. Health care workers are able to teach parents how to save the lives of their infants by using this simple solution. Medicine women, the respected leaders of some tribes, are being incorporated into the educational process. One example of a commercial preparation available in the United States is Pedialyte. See Chapter 28 for a detailed discussion of oral rehydrating solutions.

FEEDING THE HEALTHY CHILD

Table 15-8 specifies the nursing interventions that help to meet the nutritional needs of children from infancy to adolescence.

The Infant

Infants require more calories, protein, minerals, and vitamins in proportion to their weight than do adults. Their fluid requirements are also high. Breast milk is excellent in all these regards, and a nursing mother may continue this even when her infant is hospitalized. The nurse stresses that the mother should avoid fatigue, because it affects milk production. Breast milk can be manually expressed and refrigerated at the hospital and then given in the mother's absence.

Some infants cannot tolerate milk because of intestinal bleeding, allergy, or other negative reactions. Many milk substitutes are available for therapeutic use. Among these are soybean mixtures (such as ProSobee and Isomil) for infants with milk-protein sensitivity. Most products come in dry and liquid forms, and parents must be made aware of the concentrations that the physician recommends. Rice cereal is the first solid food introduced at age 6 months (Figure 15-9).

The nurse must be aware of the problems of underfeeding and overfeeding infants. Restlessness, crying, and failure to gain weight suggest underfeeding. Overfeeding is manifested by symptoms such as regurgitation, mild diarrhea, and too rapid weight gain. Diets high in fat delay gastric emptying and cause abdominal distention. Diets too high in carbohydrates may cause distention, flatus, and excessive weight gain. Constipation may be the result of too much fat or protein or a deficiency in bulk. Increased amounts of cereals, vegetables, and fruits can often correct this problem.

If the parents plan to prepare their own baby food at home, the nurse should discuss the choice of foods, their preparation, and safe storage. Blenders, strainers, and mashers are equipment often used, and ice cube trays may be used to freeze portions for storage. Spinach, broccoli, and beets should not be pureed at home for young infants because of their nitrite content, which can cause methemoglobinemia in infants (Akers and Groh-Wargo, 2005) but most fresh and frozen unsalted foods are appropriate. Water or juice used in cooking

Table 15-8	Nursing Interventions for Meeting the Nutritional Needs of Children
CHARACTERISTICS	**NURSING INTERVENTIONS**
Newborns and Infants	
High energy maintenance because of immature systems (e.g., heat loss)	Assist mother with breastfeeding. Assist family with bottle feeding. Teach formula preparation.
Immature digestive system	Burp infant frequently. Place infant on right side after feeding.
Nutrient requirements related to body size	Observe infant for tolerance to formula. Consider vitamin C and D supplementation. Anticipate iron deficiencies (particularly in preterm newborns).
Need for additional nutrients, satiety	Introduce solids when age-appropriate, at about 6 months, starting with rice cereal, which is the least allergenic. Fruits and then vegetables may be added one at a time in 1-week intervals to allow time to observe for adverse responses (consider variety, portions, and texture). Instruct parents not to add salt or sugar to baby foods to prevent high sodium and calorie intake.
Danger of choking decreases as swallowing matures	Anticipate allergies; as teething progresses, junior or chopped foods can be substituted for strained food. Explain selection and makeup of soy-based formulas if prescribed.
Prevention of dental decay	Encourage use of fluorides (after age 6 months) if fluoride content of community water supply is less than 0.6 ppm (parts per million). Encourage weaning as appropriate to prevent bottle-mouth caries. Rinse infant's mouth after feedings.
Continued requirements for basic food groups	Assess the educational and financial needs of the family. Use supplemental food programs (e.g., Women, Infants, and Children [WIC] program).
Toddlers and Preschoolers	
Slower rate of growth; although body needs are still high, energy requirements decrease	Emphasize that from a nutrition viewpoint, child can regulate intake if appropriate foods are offered.
Picky eater	Provide nutritional snacks. Respect need for independence; do not force child to eat. Use colored straws; if milk is refused, offer cheese, yogurt (not fortified with vitamin D); add milk to potatoes. Offer meat in bite-sized portions. Add fruit to cereal. Reduce sweets. Invite playmate to lunch. Relax at meals. Promote harmony.
School-Age Children	
Growth rate that continues to be slow but steady until puberty, some spurts and plateaus	Maintain education in nutrition. Introduce new foods when eating out. Assist child in preparing nutritious lunches. Provide fruits and raw vegetables for snacks. Encourage parents to include children's participation in meal planning and preparation and food shopping.
Adolescent Girls	
Girls' caloric requirements less than those of boys Concern with body image may lead to anorexia or bulimia	Emphasize that skipping meals can lead to decrease in essential nutrients. Encourage physical exercise to maintain body weight. Educate regarding proper nutrients to maintain body weight (e.g., skim milk, fruits). Avoid high-calorie fast foods. Consider emotional components related to foods (e.g., difficulty with peers, need for love and approval).
Athletic activities	See interventions for adolescent boys.

Table 15-8	Nursing Interventions for Meeting the Nutritional Needs of Children—cont'd
CHARACTERISTICS	**NURSING INTERVENTIONS**
Adolescent Girls, cont'd	
Oral contraceptives	Explain that oral contraceptives increase requirements for several nutrients (folic acid, vitamin B$_6$, ascorbic acid).
Adolescent pregnancy	Educate concerning increased nutritional needs to complete growth and nourish fetus.
Adolescent Boys	
Concern with body image, bodybuilding	Instruct regarding proper nutrition for sports. Avoid quack claims. Promote proper conditioning, well-balanced diet (increased calories), proper hydration without supplements—salt tablets unnecessary.
Overnutrition	Explain that this can lead to adult obesity. Teach that to lose weight, the following are advised: • Eat a variety of foods low in calories and high in nutrients. • Eat less fat and fewer fatty foods. • Eat less sugar and fewer sweets. • Drink less alcohol. • Eat more fruits, vegetables, whole grains. • Increase physical activity.

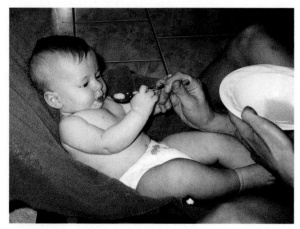

FIGURE 15-9 Spoon feeding. Solid foods should be introduced at age 6 months and fed by spoon to the infant. Cereal should not be mixed into the formula bottle when feeding the healthy infant.

can also be used to thin blended food, but overblending should be avoided because it can cause overoxidation of nutrients (Akers and Groh-Wargo, 2005). Prepared foods can be stored in the refrigerator for 48 hours or frozen for several months. Home-prepared foods are less expensive, contain less salt and sugar, and help the infant become familiar with the cultural tastes of the family.

Most infants naturally adapt to a schedule of three meals a day by the first birthday (Ionsdottir, 2012). At this time the appetite fluctuates as the growth rate slows somewhat. The child may not be interested in eating. Spills are frequent. At age 1 year, children cannot manipulate a spoon, but hand-to-mouth coordination is good enough that they enjoy holding a piece of toast while the nurse assists. In the hospital, children in highchairs are secured with safety belts. The nurse remains in constant attendance. Developmental advancements

that change eating patterns are explained to parents to prevent feeding difficulties.

> **Nursing Tip**
>
> Whole milk should not be introduced before 1 year of age. Low-fat milk should not be introduced before 2 years of age, as fats are needed to complete neurological development.

The Toddler

Toddlers can feed themselves by the end of the second year (Figure 15-10). This is important in developing a sense of independence. The toddler may be rebellious at times, and food may be pushed away or completely refused. Toddlers benefit from the caregivers' presence at mealtime. Feeding difficulties may result from the anxieties of parents and a lack of time planned for meals.

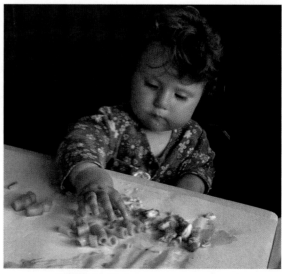

FIGURE 15-10 The self-feeding toddler.

The Preschool Child

Preschoolers and toddlers enjoy finger foods. Dawdling and regression are common in this age group. In general, preschoolers are more vulnerable to protein-calorie deficiencies; their younger siblings receive priority at home, and older brothers and sisters may receive the benefits of school lunch programs.

The School-Age Child

School-age children need food from the basic food groups but in increased quantities to meet energy requirements. Their attitudes toward food are unpredictable. Intake of protein, calcium, vitamin A, and ascorbic acid tends to be low. The intake of sweets decreases the appetite and provides empty calories.

Health Promotion

Nutrition Resources Within the Community

PROGRAM	ELIGIBILITY	PROGRAM CONTENT
Maternal and Child Health Bureau (Health Resources and Services Administration [HRSA])	Pregnant women and children of low-income families	Free or reduced-price food Improved health care services for mothers and children at a clinic affiliated with a specific hospital Free vitamins, immunizations
Special Supplemental Food Program for Women, Infants, and Children (WIC) Aid to Families with Dependent Children (AFDC)	*Individuals at nutritional risk:* • Pregnant women up to 6 months postpartum • Nursing mothers up to 1 year *Infants and children up to age 5 years identified as being at nutritional risk:* • Must live in geographically determined low-income area and be eligible for reduced-price or free medical care; must be certified by WIC staff member	Provision of supplemental foods: • *More than 1 year:* Iron-fortified formula and infant cereals, fruit juice high in vitamin C • *Women and children:* Whole fluid milk or cheese, eggs, iron-fortified hot or cold cereal, fruit or vegetables high in vitamin C • *Food distribution:* Directly from participating agency, via voucher system, or by home delivery
Program for Children with Special Health Needs (formerly Crippled Children's Services) (under Title V)	Periodic assessment of risk status Children with developmental disabilities	Nutrition education is an integral part of program Free nutrition counseling Funds available for equipment or supplies
Child Care Food Program (CCFP)	Preschool children in nonprofit facilities, Head Start, day care, after-school facilities	Year-round program Cash in lieu of commodities available as set by U.S. Department of Agriculture
School Breakfast Program	All public and nonprofit private schools Public and licensed nonprofit residential child care institutions For needy children or those who travel great distances to school	Breakfasts that meet nutritional standards Served free or at a reduced price to children from low-income families Costs to schools reimbursed by federal funds as set by U.S. Department of Agriculture
National School Lunch Program	All public and nonprofit private school pupils of high-school grades or lower, some residential institutions and temporary shelters	Nonprofit nutritious lunches offered free or at a reduced price for those who cannot pay Lunch follows specified guidelines and meets one third or more of daily dietary allowance
Summer Food Service Programs for children	Public agency–sponsored preschool and school-age recreation programs, summer camps	Schools reimbursed by federal and state funds Free lunch to children in summer programs Federal monetary support
Special Milk Program	Schools, child care centers, summer camps	Federal reimbursement for all or part of the milk served
Food Distribution (donated foods)	Supplemental programs for mothers and infants	Distribution of surplus food to eligible persons, schools, institutions
Food Stamps	Eligibility based on total income, expenses, number being fed in household Each applicant is considered on an individual basis	Patient should apply at local Food Stamp Office within the community, presenting wage slips, sources of income, rent receipts, utility bills Food Stamps are given free of charge depending on eligibility needs Used like cash to purchase food at authorized food stores (nonfood items and alcoholic beverages not allowed)

The Adolescent

Nutrition is particularly important during the adolescent years. Teenagers grow rapidly and expend large amounts of energy. Their food needs are great. The nurse attempts to involve the teenager in selecting foods that are nutritious and appetizing. Reviewing choices made on the daily menu may assist with this attempt. Sometimes it helps to stress how important good nutrition is to physical appearance and fitness. The need for peer approval is at its height during adolescence, and food fads and skipped meals may result in malnutrition, even in families of means. Fatigue is a common complaint at this age. If it is accompanied by a lack of appetite and irritability, anemia should be suspected. Some adolescents consult computer chat rooms for weight loss information, and this can lead to anorexic behavior. Parental guidance of computer use is necessary. The Health Promotion box on nutrition resources in the community lists nutrition services in the community that are available to children.

Childhood obesity has more than doubled the last 30 years, with obese children aged 6 to 11 increasing from 7% in 1980 to 18% in 2010. And obese adolescents increased from 5% in 1980 to 18% in 2010 (USDHHS, 2012). Excessive weight in childhood is related to obesity in adulthood. Obesity can cause health problems such as increased cholesterol, orthopedic problems, sleep apnea, high blood pressure, type 2 diabetes mellitus, and devastating social isolation that can lead to depression. The instrument to determine obesity is the body mass index (BMI) percentile (Skill 15-2).

A BMI over 18 in children aged 5 to 9 years, or more than 22 to 24 for 13- to 17-year-olds, evidences an overweight status (Ogden, 2012). The cause of obesity is most often related to diet and inactivity, although some causes can include illness syndromes. Monitoring, counseling, and follow-up are essential.

Parents and school-age children need guidance concerning appropriate portions of foods to provide at each meal. Supersized portions are advertised on TV in a positive way and are difficult to resist at the fast food restaurant or the store. Healthy food choices and appropriate portion sizes are an important part of weight control. One type of assistance available to parents and children is the Portion Plate for kids, a two-sided reusable placemat that compares the appropriate portion size for school-age children with common objects such as an 8-pack of crayons or a softball (see Figure 15-7).

FEEDING THE ILL CHILD

Children in the hospital continue in the process of growing. Well-nourished children can be characterized as follows:

- Nearly always show steady gains in weight and height
- Are alert
- Have shiny hair
- Have no fatigue circles beneath the eyes
- Have a skin color within normal limits
- Have a flat abdomen
- Have an erect posture
- Have well-developed muscles
- Have mouth and gum mucous membranes that are firm and pink, not swollen or bleeding
- Have no mouth or tongue lesions
- Have teeth that are erupting on schedule
- Have a generally good appetite and eliminate regularly
- Sleep well at night, have energy and vitality, and are not irritable

Calculating Body Mass Index (BMI)

PURPOSE

To estimate a healthy body weight for an individual based on height and to indirectly measure body fat percentage to determine obesity or underweight status

OBTAINING A BMI

A child greater than 2 years of age should be weighed and measured at every health checkup to determine growth and nutritional status. Any deviation from the trend that is plotted on the growth chart may indicate a developing health problem. The following formulas can be used to obtain a **BMI**:

$$BMI = \frac{Weight\ in\ kilograms}{(Height\ in\ meters)^2}\ OR$$

$$BMI = \frac{Weight\ in\ pounds}{(Height\ in\ inches)^2} \times 703$$

NOTE: Assistance in using formulas to obtain the BMI is available at www.cdc.gov/healthyweight/assessing/bmi/index.html. This site will calculate the BMI for individual data supplied. The nurse has the responsibility for measuring the growth of a child and understanding growth charts.

This picture changes somewhat during illness, but the child who is basically well nourished can easily be distinguished from one who is malnourished.

Many hospitalized children have poor appetites. This may be because of age, the nature of the illness, the type of diet, sudden exposure to strange foods and a strange environment, a reaction to hospitalization, or the degree of satisfaction obtained during mealtimes. The child may also refuse to eat in an attempt to manipulate the parents, particularly if lack of appetite was a concern in the past.

The nurse observes the patient's tray to determine if the food is the right consistency. Does the child have any teeth? Do lesions in the mouth prevent chewing? Can the child use a knife and fork? Children with bandaged limbs or those receiving intravenous fluids require assistance. The size of servings is important.

One should serve less food than one hopes will be eaten. A tablespoonful of food (not heaping) for each year of age is a good guide to follow. More is given if the patient appears hungry. One item at a time is placed before small children who feed themselves, so they do not become overwhelmed. The nurse avoids showing personal dislikes, because negative attitudes are easily transmitted. The nurse proceeds slowly with unfamiliar children to determine their level of mastery. Food is served warm, and sufficient time is allotted. Sweet drinks and snacks should not be served just before meals. Treatments such as chest physiotherapy should not be scheduled immediately after a meal.

Infants who are placed on "nothing by mouth" (NPO) status should be provided with a pacifier to meet their sucking needs. Some children prefer to use their thumb for nonnutritive sucking (Figure 15-11).

Food–Drug Interactions

Whenever a child is ill and treated with prescription medications, the nurse is responsible for monitoring drug–drug interactions, drug–food interactions, and drug–environment interactions. Monitoring drug–drug interactions involves knowledge of the side effects of each drug prescribed. Drug–environment interactions involve the effects of a drug on the response of the patient to his or her environment. For example, certain antibiotics have photosensitivity as a side effect. Nurses armed with this knowledge advise the patient or parent to avoid prolonged exposure to sunlight. Drug–food interactions are often overlooked but can have an impact on treatment and/or the growth and development of the child. The nurse should remain alert to food-drug interactions while dealing with the sick child.

THE TEETH

Deciduous Teeth

The development of the 20 **deciduous**, or baby, teeth begins at about the fifth month of intrauterine life. The health and diet of the expectant mother affect the soundness of the teeth. Primary teeth erupt during

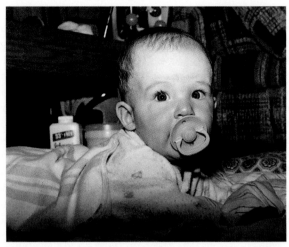

FIGURE 15-11 Nonnutritive sucking. Nonnutritive sucking involving the finger or a pacifier is common in infants less than 1 year of age and fulfills the needs of the oral phase of development. In general, malocclusion from nonnutritive sucking will not be a problem if the habit is discontinued by 3 years of age. *Frequency, duration,* and *intensity* of sucking influence the occurrence of malocclusion associated with finger or pacifier use. Behavior modification can help to decrease thumb sucking (e.g., a dental appliance or substances placed on the finger). The child must be physically and emotionally "ready" to discontinue thumb sucking, and appropriate rewards should be predetermined.

the first 2.5 years of life. It is a normal process and is generally accompanied by little or no discomfort. Wide individual differences in tooth eruption occur in normal, healthy infants. Occasionally an infant is born with teeth; neonatal teeth are removed to prevent the possibility of choking should they fall out. A delay in teething is significant if other forms of immaturity or illness are present. The physician evaluates the process of teething during the infant's regular health checkups.

The first tooth generally appears at about the sixth or seventh month. The 1-year-old has about six teeth, four above and two below. The order in which the teeth appear is almost always the same (Figure 15-12). They are shed in about the same order in which they appear (i.e., lower central incisors first, and so forth). Although the Academy of Pediatric Dentistry recommends that the first dental visit occur by 1 year, the majority of children begin seeing a dentist between ages 2 and 3 years. Tetracycline antibiotics stain developing teeth a yellowish brown and therefore are to be avoided during pregnancy and in the first 8 years of life.

Parents and nurses must not neglect baby teeth, thinking that they will eventually be lost. A 2-year-old who wants to brush his teeth when Mommy does is encouraged to do so. The deciduous teeth serve not only in the digestive process but also in the development of the jaw. When the deciduous teeth are lost early because of neglect, the permanent teeth become poorly aligned. The nurse checks that all patients ages 1 year and older have toothbrushes. Children sometimes must be reminded of oral hygiene at bedtime. Parental supervision of tooth brushing is necessary until 7 years of age.

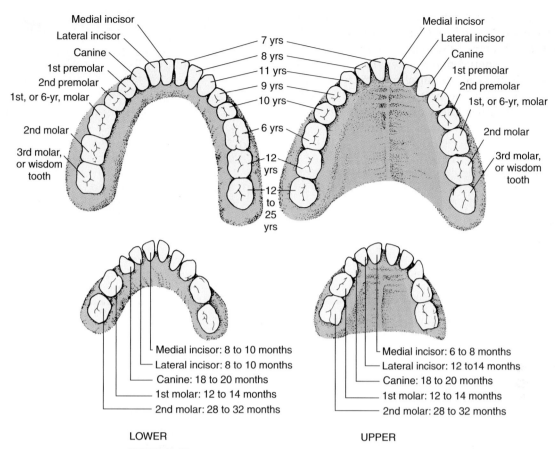

Medial incisor
Lateral incisor
Canine
1st premolar
2nd premolar
1st, or 6-yr, molar
2nd molar
3rd molar, or wisdom tooth

7 yrs
8 yrs
11 yrs
9 yrs
10 yrs
6 yrs
12 yrs
12 to 25 yrs

Medial incisor
Lateral incisor
Canine
1st premolar
2nd premolar
1st, or 6-yr, molar
2nd molar
3rd molar, or wisdom tooth

Medial incisor: 8 to 10 months
Lateral incisor: 8 to 10 months
Canine: 18 to 20 months
1st molar: 12 to 14 months
2nd molar: 28 to 32 months

Medial incisor: 6 to 8 months
Lateral incisor: 12 to14 months
Canine: 18 to 20 months
1st molar: 12 to 14 months
2nd molar: 28 to 32 months

LOWER   UPPER

FIGURE 15-12 Permanent and deciduous teeth and age of eruption.

Permanent Teeth

The 32 permanent teeth develop just before birth and during the first year of life. They do not erupt through the gums, however, until the sixth year. Nutrition and general health during the first year of life affect the formation of permanent teeth. This process is not completed until the wisdom teeth appear at about 18 to 25 years of age. The first permanent teeth do not replace any of the deciduous teeth but appear behind the deciduous molars. Cavities in them are often neglected because they are mistaken for baby teeth. The most common site of decay in children is the fissures of the molar teeth. These areas can be protected by the professional application of plastic sealants.

 Nursing Tip

To assess the number of teeth a child under age 2 years is expected to have, use the following formula:
Age in months − 6.
(Example: 20 months − 6 = 14 teeth.)

Oral Care in Health and Illness

Good dental care begins with a proper diet that supplies adequate nutrients while the teeth are developing in the jaws, especially during the prenatal period and the first year. The many essential elements found in milk include calcium, phosphorus, vitamins A and B complex, and protein. Vitamin D (the "sunshine vitamin") and vitamin C (found in citrus fruits) are also valuable. Dietary practices influence the development of cavities, and parents are encouraged to limit the frequency of fermentable carbohydrate intake.

In the past, total carbohydrate consumption was thought to be the most important dietary consideration for dental health. Today more attention is given to the frequency with which sweets are eaten and how long they stick to the teeth. Sticky foods have more potential to cause caries (cavities) than do sugared drinks that are quickly cleared from the mouth. Oral care after eating sticky foods is recommended. Recommended snack foods include cheese, peanuts, milk, sugarless gum, and raw vegetables. Items to be avoided include sugared gum, dried fruits, sugared soft drinks, cakes, and candy.

Of most importance in preventing caries is the administration of fluoride by mouth after age 6 months. Ideally, fluorides are present naturally in the water supply or are added to it. The fluoride content of city water or prepared formula may decrease the need for fluoride supplements. When necessary, systemic fluorides can be offered until the last permanent tooth erupts at about 13 years of age. Many fluoride preparations are available and are often incorporated with vitamins. These tablets are obtained by prescription and should not be interchanged among children of various ages, because too much fluoride may cause the teeth to become "mottled" (**fluorosis**). Fluoride may also be applied directly to the teeth by the dentist.

 ## Health Promotion

Developmental Dental Hygiene

FIRST YEAR OF LIFE

- Infant's gums are wiped daily after 2 months of age with a moist cloth or xylitol wipe.
- Gentle brushing is performed each night with a soft, small toothbrush.
- Use of anticaries fluoride toothpaste (amount equivalent to a grain of rice) is begun between 1 and 2 years of age.
- Child is not put to bed with bottle of milk or juice. If infant must have a bottle, water is used.

2 TO 3 YEARS

- Parents introduce toothpaste in addition to the soft toothbrush. Only a pea-sized amount of toothpaste is used to minimize fluoride ingestion.

3 TO 6 YEARS

- Deciduous teeth erupt, and baby teeth start to exfoliate (fall out) toward the end of this period.
- Parents assist children and remind them to brush and floss until at least age 8 years. A small, soft toothbrush is used.
- Bedtime routine of brushing is established, because salivary flow rates slow during sleep, reducing natural protective mechanisms.
- Parents are advised to brush for the child at least once a day and to clean teeth that are in contact with each other with dental floss.
- Sweets are limited to daytime meals, when saliva content is high.

6 TO 12 YEARS

- First permanent molars appear. The pits and fissures of molars make them the primary site for caries. Sealants (plastic coating) professionally applied to molars provide a mechanical barrier against bacteria.
- Parents continue with fluorides and flossing, and reducing *frequency* of exposure to fermentable carbohydrates. Adolescent gingivitis (*gingiv*, "gum," and *itis*, "inflammation of"), characterized by redness, swelling, and bleeding, is common in children and adolescents and may be aggravated by hormonal changes at puberty.
- Motivating the adolescent to assume responsibility for dental care may be complicated by rebellion against authority and some incapacity to appreciate long-term consequences.
- Topical fluorides and fluoride toothpastes are available.
- Orthodontic treatments place adolescents at high risk for gingivitis and caries around appliances or braces.
- Mouth protectors should be used to prevent dental injuries from contact sports.

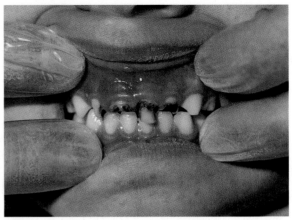

FIGURE 15-13 Nursing caries. During sleep, saliva production decreases and the teeth become more vulnerable to decay. When the infant is put to sleep with a bottle containing milk or sweetened juice, the sugar combines with the bacterial flora in the mouth to cause tooth decay. This is known as "milk caries." Parents should be taught to use unsweetened water as the only liquid in a bottle at bedtime. (From Swartz MH: *Textbook of physical diagnosis: history and examination,* ed 7, Philadelphia, 2013, Saunders.)

Another aspect of tooth care is the prevention of *bottle-mouth caries* (**nursing caries**) (Figure 15-13). This condition occurs when an infant falls asleep while breastfeeding or is put to bed with a bottle of milk or sweetened juice. Sugar pools within the oral cavity, causing severe decay. It is seen most often in children between 18 months and 3 years of age. Eliminating the bedtime bottle or substituting water in the bottle is recommended. Bottles and sippy cups, if used, should only contain water except at mealtimes. "Read, don't feed, at bedtime" should be the teaching motto (Hofman, 2008). Early childhood caries is defined, by the American Academy of Pediatric Dentistry, as one or more decayed or filled tooth surface in any primary tooth in a child less than 6 years of age (Wagner and Oskouians, 2008). Severe childhood caries is defined as smooth surface caries in a child younger than 3 years old. Signs of early decay include chalky white spots on tooth enamel near the gum line of maxillary incisors. Brown discoloration signals more advanced decay. Tooth decay can cause dental abscesses, which can result in serious complications.

The maintenance of good oral health is an integral portion of comprehensive care for a sick or disabled pediatric patient. Education, prevention, and referral in the home, school, or hospital setting must be part of the child's plan of care. Untreated dental caries or malposition of the erupting teeth can cause periodontal disease in later years if not treated promptly. Delayed or early eruption of teeth can be indicative of certain endocrine disorders or other pathological conditions and should be recorded and reported. Parents and caregivers should avoid "tasting" baby food fed to infants and young children, because the transmission of acid-producing bacteria from their mouths can be passed on to the food or feeding utensils and can contribute to tooth decay in the infant. The use of xylitol chewing gum by the parent can reduce cross-contamination of mouth bacteria with the infant. Regular tooth brushing can start with tooth eruption. Children should brush before bedtime because the protective bacteriocidal effects of saliva decrease during sleep, and bacterial growth can cause tooth decay. Fever (body temperature exceeding 38.1° C [100.6° F]) is not usually associated with teething and should be evaluated for other causes.

Parents and children should be educated concerning the care of the toothbrush to provide maximum effectiveness of the tooth brushing activity:

- Replace toothbrush every 3 months.
- Replace toothbrush after a viral illness.
- Avoid rinsing bristles in hot water.
- Do not use a closed container for toothbrush storage.
- Avoid sharing toothbrushes among children.

A properly sized toothbrush will aid in developing good tooth brushing technique. A soft brush with a small amount of toothpaste, about the size of a pencil eraser, is appropriate. Dental flossing should be done with an up-and-down motion. A back-and-forth "sawing" motion can cause injury to gingival tissues. Children need assistance and supervision with flossing until at least age 7 years.

Trauma to the teeth often occurs in school-age children. Appropriate protective devices can prevent injury during sports activities. If a primary tooth is knocked out (avulsed) because of trauma, the child should be referred to a dentist for a "spacer" that will maintain tooth alignment until the permanent tooth erupts. If a permanent tooth is avulsed because of trauma, the tooth should be immersed in milk and brought with the child to the dentist for immediate care. Open wounds to oral tissues may require tetanus prophylaxis or antibiotics. All tooth fractures should be referred to a dentist for evaluation and treatment.

Dental problems that often occur with adolescents include puberty gingivitis, gingivitis associated with oral contraceptive use, drug-related gingivitis, and hyperplastic gingivitis associated with orthodontic therapy. Temporomandibular joint problems (TMJ) and malocclusion caused by missing teeth necessitate a dental referral. Orthodontic appliances such as fixed braces can trap plaque and food and can increase tooth decay. Meticulous oral hygiene, brushing, flossing, and fluoride applications are part of comprehensive orthodontic care.

A team approach to dental care for the child receiving chemotherapy or radiation therapy includes the dentist, the physician, the nurse, the parent, and the patient. Brushing and flossing when the platelet count is more than 20,000/mm^3 and using moist gauze when the platelet count is less than 20,000/mm^3 are advised to prevent infection and bleeding. The use of chlorhexidine may be prescribed to reduce oral lesions. Table 15-9 reviews medical problems that have an effect on dental health.

Table 15-9	Medical Problems and Dental Health
MEDICAL PROBLEM	**EFFECT ON TEETH**
Asthma	Sucrose content of medication can cause decay
Hemophilia Cancer	Can cause oral bleeding, impaired healing
Seizure disorders	Causes decreased saliva; gingival overgrowth (use of phenytoin)
Medications that depress the central nervous system	Decrease salivary flow, increasing susceptibility to dental caries
Juvenile rheumatoid arthritis	Sucrose-containing medications increase risk of cavities
Bulimia	Erosion of teeth caused by acid contact during vomiting episodes
Chemotherapy	Oral ulcerations
Fluoride ingestion	Excess fluoride can cause fluorosis (mottling of teeth)

Disabled children can master independent tooth brushing by modifying the toothbrush. Using padded tongue depressors to visualize the oral cavity and an aspirating catheter attached to the toothbrush and connected to a suction machine can assist in providing dental care for a severely disabled child. Battery-operated toothbrushes can help to achieve optimum brushing technique.

In the year 2000, the U.S. Surgeon General issued a report concerning oral health in America (USDHHS, 2000). Preventive oral health was considered vital to the maintenance of general health. The principal goals established were to urge health care providers to integrate oral health concepts into education and general health care and to increase the accessibility of oral care for children. This continues to be a *Healthy People 2020* goal. Parents can find a local pediatric dentist by searching online.

Nursing Tip

When a tooth is "knocked out" or avulsed traumatically, the tooth should be gently cleansed of obvious dirt and placed in milk until dental care is obtained.

PLAY

Play is the business of children. Observing the child at play can aid in assessing growth and development and understanding the child's relationship with family members. Any plan of care for a hospitalized child of any age should include a play activity that either encourages growth and development or encourages the expression of thoughts and feelings. Playrooms in the hospital pediatric unit can be used for children who have conditions that are not communicable. Medications and treatments should not be administered in the playroom setting. Play can also be therapeutic and aid in the recovery process. An example of **therapeutic play** is the game of having the child "blow out" the light of a flashlight as if it were a candle to promote deep breathing. Table 15-10 reviews age-appropriate play behaviors.

Art is an appropriate play activity at almost any age and provides an avenue for experimentation as well as for creative expression and a feeling of accomplishment in the child. Computer programs are popular with all age groups, providing problem-solving games, manipulative skills, and opportunities for new learning. Both of these activities must be balanced with active play experiences.

Nursing interventions should focus on encouraging optimal play activities and experiences that are age appropriate. Parents need guidance concerning the value of play that may not always be a neat and clean activity. Helping parents to select appropriate toys that are safe as well as appropriate to the age and illness is essential. For example, a stuffed animal may not be the toy of choice for an asthmatic child. In the health care setting, a blood pressure cuff can give the child a "hug." Children can play with the equipment they see in their environment to provide stress relief.

ONGOING HEATH SUPERVISION

Children of all ages should receive ongoing health checkups. Specific health care recommendations for each age group are discussed in Chapters 16 through 20. The American Academy of Pediatrics, in partnership with the Academy of State Health Policy, supports a federally sponsored Children's Health Insurance Program (CHIP) for uninsured children. The program provides federally matching funds to the states that offer this kind of coverage. Information concerning CHIP for each state can be obtained online at www. medicaid.gov/Medicaid-CHIP-Program.

Table 15-10 Development of Play

AGE GROUP	TYPE OF PLAY	SUGGESTED PLAY ACTIVITY
Infants	Explore, imitate	Provide visual stimuli for newborns; touch stimuli for infants, and toys involving manipulation for 1-year-olds.
1 to 2 years	**Parallel play**	Children play next to each other but not with each other. Provide each child with toys that reflect activities of daily living.
3 to 5 years	**Cooperative play** Creative play	Children play with each other, each taking a specific role: "You be the mommy and I'll be the daddy." A simple box can become a train to a 3-year-old.
5 to 7 years	Symbolic group play; secret clubs	Secret codes, "knock-knock" jokes, and rhymes are popular at this age.
7 to 10 years	**Competitive play**	Children at this age start to accept competition with structured rules and highly interactive physical activity.
10 to 13 years	Group sports and explorative Internet activities, electronic or computer games	Monitored Internet contact.
13 to 18 years	Fantasy play; cliques	Leadership activities such as babysitting or tutoring are popular. Daydreaming occurs. Board games are popular. Interactive social activities in "cliques" occur at and after school.

Get Ready for the NCLEX® Examination!

Key Points

- Growth and development are orderly and sequential, although there are spurts and plateaus.
- Cephalocaudal development proceeds from head to toe.
- Children are susceptible to nutritional deficiencies because they are in the process of growth and development.
- Maslow depicted human development based on a hierarchy of needs.

- Freud's theories portrayed personality development as phases of psychosexual development.
- Piaget described phases of cognitive development.
- Erikson described eight stages of psychosocial development from birth to adulthood.
- Developmental theories can serve as guides to nursing intervention; however, each child grows and develops at an individual pace.
- A family is two or more persons that interact together.

- Parent–child interactions affect positive growth and development.
- Deciduous teeth are baby teeth. The proper care of the teeth depends on supervision by the caregiver according to the child's physical level of development and mastery.
- Optimal nutrition is essential to physical and neurological growth and development.
- Motor development follows a predictable sequence.
- Nutritional practices of early childhood tend to persist through adulthood.
- The nurse is responsible for counseling and teaching positive nutritional practices that are acceptable to the family's culture, religion, and lifestyle.
- The availability of age-appropriate toys enhances physical, emotional, and mental development in infants, children, and adolescents.
- Computer games can foster problem solving, cognitive development, and motor coordination but should be balanced with active play activities.
- Many hospitals have playrooms, which must be kept safe from painful or invasive experiences.
- A nurse is an advocate, educator, and collaborator in a family-centered care environment.

Additional Learning Resources

SG Go to your Study Guide for additional learning activities to help you master this chapter content.

evolve Go to your Evolve website (http://evolve.elsevier.com/Leifer) for the following learning resources:
- Animations
- Answer Guidelines for Critical Thinking Questions
- Answers and Rationales for Review Questions for the NCLEX® Examination
- Glossary with English and Spanish pronunciations
- Interactive Review Questions for the NCLEX® Examination
- Patient Teaching Plans in English and Spanish
- Skills Performance Checklists
- Video clips and more!

Online Resources
- 2000 CDC Growth Charts: www.cdc.gov/growthcharts
- American Academy of Pediatric Dentistry: www.aapd.org
- Children's Health Insurance Program (CHIP): www.ncsl.org/programs/health/chiphome.htm
- *Dietary Guidelines for Americans: www.healthierus.gov/dietaryguidelines*
- Gerber: www.gerber.com

- Inheritance and development: www.ncbi.nlm.nih.gov/omim
- Institute of Medicine: www.iom.edu
- www.choosemyplate.gov
- National Cholesterol Education Program: www.nhlbi.nih.gov/chd
- Parenting skills: http://store.parentsactionstore.org/prostores/servlet/storefront
- Portion Plate for kids: www.theportionplate.com

Review Questions for the NCLEX® Examination

1. How many erupted teeth would the nurse expect a healthy 8-month-old infant to have?
   1. 2
   2. 4
   3. 6
   4. 8

2. During the first week of life, the newborn's weight:
   1. increases about 5% to 10%.
   2. decreases about 5% to 10%.
   3. stabilizes.
   4. fluctuates widely.

3. The nurse should encourage the parent to introduce tooth brushing to the child by age:
   1. 6 months.
   2. 1 year.
   3. 3 years.
   4. 7 years.

4. To meet the needs (as described by Erikson) of a school-age child diagnosed with diabetes, the nurse should:
   1. explain carefully to the mother the need to adhere rigidly to dietary modifications.
   2. allow the child to eat whatever he or she wants and administer insulin to maintain optimum glucose levels.
   3. allow the child to perform his own Accuchecks and administer his own insulin.
   4. perform Accuchecks four times a day and at bedtime.

5. It is most appropriate to first introduce competitive games at age:
   1. 3 to 5 years.
   2. 5 to 6 years.
   3. 7 to 9 years.
   4. 12 to 15 years.

Objectives

1. Define each key term listed.
2. Describe normal vital signs for a 1-year-old infant.
3. Describe the physical and psychosocial development of infants from age 1 to 12 months, listing age-specific events and guidance when appropriate.
4. Discuss the major aspects of cognitive development in the first year of life.
5. Identify the approximate age for each of the following: posterior fontanelle has closed; central incisors appear; birth weight has tripled; child can sit steadily alone; child shows fear of strangers.
6. Relate the nursing responsibilities in health promotion and illness prevention of infants during the first year of life.
7. Discuss the approach to and the specifics of care of an infant with colic.
8. Discuss the development of favorable sleep patterns.
9. Examine nutritional counseling for the infant.
10. List four common concerns of parents about the feeding of infants.
11. Compare breastfeeding, bottle feeding, and the various infant formulas available.
12. Describe how to select and prepare solid foods for the infant.
13. Compare and contrast natural, organic, and processed foods.
14. Discuss the development of feeding skills in the infant.
15. Discuss the nutritional needs of growing infants.
16. Discuss safety issues in the care of infants.
17. Discuss principles of safety during infancy.
18. Identify age-appropriate toys and their developmental or therapeutic value.

Key Terms

colic (p. 395)
extrusion reflex (ĕks-TRŪ-zhŭn RĒ-flĕks, p. 397)
grasp reflex (p. 387)
milestones (p. 386)
norms (p. 386)
object permanence (p. 404)

oral stage (p. 387)
parachute reflex (p. 387)
pincer grasp (p. 387)
prehension (p. 387)
satiety (să-TĪ-ĕ-tē, p. 398)
weaning (p. 403)

Physical, emotional, and cognitive growth and the development of motor abilities occur rapidly during the first year of life. **Milestones** of growth and development describe general patterns of achievements at various stages of infancy. These milestones, or patterns, are referred to as **norms**. Norms can vary greatly for the individual child, but the nurse must understand the normal range for milestone achievement to assess the progress of growth and development of the infant and initiate early referral for follow-up care.

During the neonatal phase of development, the chief tasks mastered are the establishment of effective feeding patterns and a predictable sleep–wake cycle. Infants who have unmet hunger needs can become irritable, may not perceive feeding as pleasurable, and may fail to develop trust in the caregiver. Parental bonding and social interaction begin in the neonatal phase but heighten when the infant begins to respond with a social smile, making the caregiver feel "loved."

By the time the infant is age 4 to 6 months, the positive parental interaction with the infant should be obvious during clinic visits. If the parent does not appear to enjoy the developmental changes in the infant at this age or does not appear relaxed during interactions with the infant, further follow-up of possible family dysfunction or social or mental stresses should be initiated.

By age 9 months, control of feeding may become an issue of conflict between parent and infant. The parent needs to "let go" and introduce the infant to finger foods and initiate drinking from a cup. Offering limited choices can reduce conflict as the infant reaches toward autonomy. If the nurse notices an overly neat and orderly approach during feeding, parental guidance may be necessary. Separation anxiety (see Chapter 21) can be expected by the ninth-month clinic visit, and the nurse should expect to spend some time playing with the infant and getting to know the infant to establish the rapport necessary for a successful physical assessment.

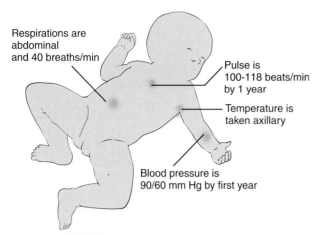

FIGURE 16-1 Average vital signs of the infant.

Respirations are
abdominal
and 40 breaths/min

Pulse is
100-118 beats/min
by 1 year

Temperature is
taken axillary

Blood pressure is
90/60 mm Hg by first year

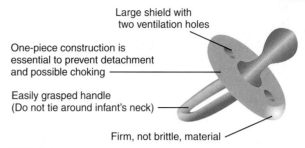

Large shield with
two ventilation holes

One-piece construction is
essential to prevent detachment
and possible choking

Easily grasped handle
(Do not tie around infant's neck)

Firm, not brittle, material

FIGURE 16-2 Pacifiers provide nonnutritive sucking to meet the needs of the oral phase of infancy. A safe pacifier is illustrated. Note the one-piece construction.

Repetition is the key to successful parent teaching and counseling by the nurse.

Children, unlike adults, are in the process of growing while they are hospitalized. To provide total patient care, the nurse must be able to recognize a patient's needs at various stages of growth and development. The pulse rate, respiration, and blood pressure measurements that are normal for an infant are not normal for the adult patient (Figure 16-1). The nurse must try to meet individual needs effectively and to administer the specialized nursing care required for the particular patient. The most common cause for concern about a child is a sudden slowing, not typical for age, of any aspect of development.

GENERAL CHARACTERISTICS

ORAL STAGE

Sucking brings the infant comfort and relief from tension. This **oral stage** of personality development is important for the infant's physical and psychological development. The nurse, knowing the importance of sucking to the infant, holds the infant during feedings and allows sufficient time to suck. Infants, who are warm and comfortable, associate food with love. The infant who is fed intravenous fluids is given added attention and a pacifier to ensure the necessary satisfaction of sucking (Figure 16-2). When the teeth appear, the infant learns to bite and enjoys objects that can be chewed. Gradually, the infant begins to put fingers into the mouth. When infants can use their hands more skillfully, they will not suck their fingers as often and will be able to derive pleasure from other sources. The need for close supervision to maintain safety increases as the child learns to use hands purposefully to grasp objects and put them into his or her mouth. Teaching parents about household safety should begin early.

MOTOR DEVELOPMENT

The **grasp reflex** is seen when one touches the palms of the infant's hands and flexion occurs. This reflex

disappears at about 3 months. **Prehension**, the ability to grasp objects between the fingers and the opposing thumb, occurs slightly later (age 5 to 6 months) and follows an orderly sequence of development (Figure 16-3).

The **parachute reflex** appears by age 7 to 9 months. This is a protective arm extension that occurs when an infant is suddenly thrust downward when prone. By age 1 year the **pincer grasp** coordination of index finger and thumb is well established.

EMOTIONAL DEVELOPMENT

Love and security are vital needs of infants. Babies require the continuous affection of their parents. If trust is to develop, consistency must be established. Parents are assured that they need not be afraid of spoiling their infants by attending promptly to their needs. Infants who are consistently picked up in response to crying show fewer crying episodes when they are toddlers and less aggressive behavior at 2 years of age. Loving adults affirm that the world is a good place in which to live. Each day the infant becomes impressed by parental actions and learns to imitate and trust caregivers. A sense of trust is vital to the development of a healthy personality. Many consider it to be the foundation of emotional growth. The child who does not develop a sense of trust learns to mistrust people, which could have a permanently negative effect on personality development.

Parents are taught to talk, sing, and touch their infants while providing care. Infants will easily accomplish various activities if they are not forced before they reach readiness. When an infant shows readiness to learn a task or skill, parents should provide encouragement.

🔷 Nursing Tip

Parental approval is important to the infant, and setting limits early is important (Anderson, 2008). Principles of discipline at this age include the following:
- Lowering the voice to say no firmly
- Removing the child from the situation
- Distraction
- Consistency

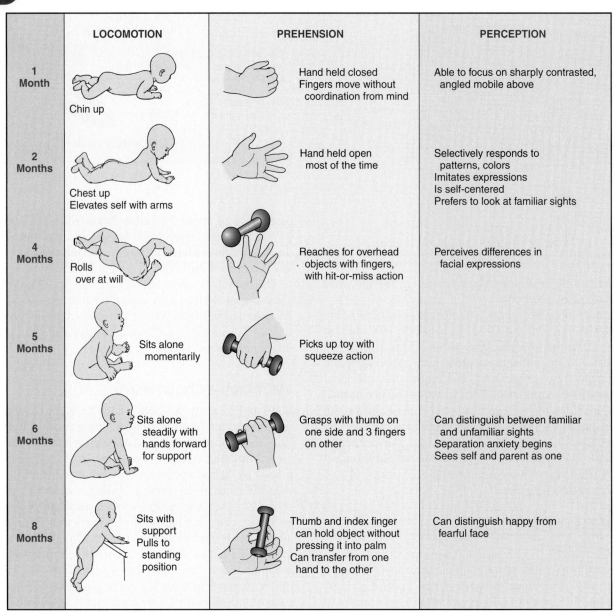

FIGURE 16-3 The development of locomotion, prehension, and perception.

NEED FOR CONSTANT CARE AND GUIDANCE

The full-time caregiver needs and deserves the understanding of and kind support from relatives at home and from the nurse in the hospital. Pediatrics involves family-centered care. A short break from pressures provides renewed energy with which to enjoy the infant. A trip to the store or a stroll with the infant in the carriage affords stimulation and a change of environment for the infant and the caregiver. The infant who is constantly left in a crib or playpen and is not introduced to a variety of learning experiences may become shy and withdrawn. Sensory stimulation is essential for the development of the infant's thought processes and perceptual abilities.

If a mother is unable to room-in with her hospitalized infant, personnel should try to imitate her care by promptly fulfilling the infant's physical and emotional needs. In the nursery the nurse first feeds the infant who appears hungry, rather than delaying feeding to adhere to a specific routine. Wet diapers are changed as soon as possible. The crying child is soothed. The exactness of time or method of bathing or feeding the infant is less important than the care with which it is done. The infant easily recognizes warmth and affection or the lack thereof.

DEVELOPMENT AND CARE

Box 16-1 is a guide to infant care from the first month to the first birthday. Some of the aspects of care (e.g., safety measures) are important throughout the entire year. The nurse explains to parents that physical patterns cannot be separated from social patterns and that abrupt changes do not take place with each new month.

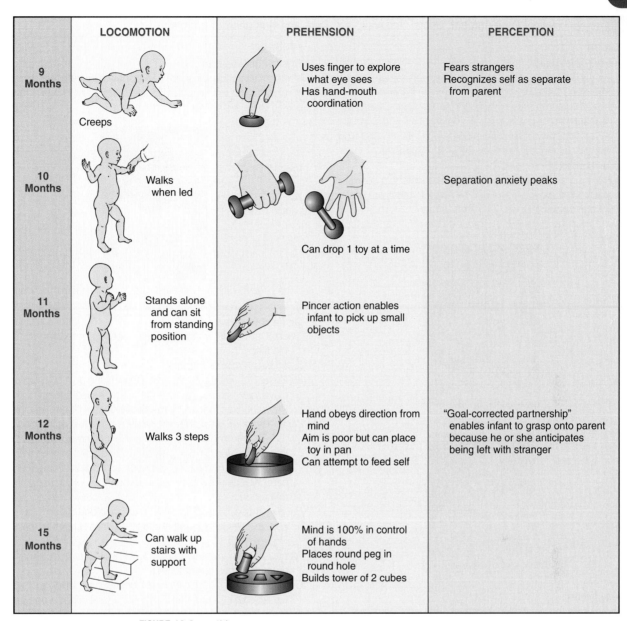

LOCOMOTION	PREHENSION	PERCEPTION
9 Months — Creeps	Uses finger to explore what eye sees / Has hand-mouth coordination	Fears strangers / Recognizes self as separate from parent
10 Months — Walks when led	Can drop 1 toy at a time	Separation anxiety peaks
11 Months — Stands alone and can sit from standing position	Pincer action enables infant to pick up small objects	
12 Months — Walks 3 steps	Hand obeys direction from mind / Aim is poor but can place toy in pan / Can attempt to feed self	"Goal-corrected partnership" enables infant to grasp onto parent because he or she anticipates being left with stranger
15 Months — Can walk up stairs with support	Mind is 100% in control of hands / Places round peg in round hole / Builds tower of 2 cubes	

FIGURE 16-3, cont'd The development of locomotion, prehension, and perception.

Human development cannot be separated into specific areas any more than the body's structure can be separated from its function.

No two infants are exactly alike at a certain age. Box 16-1 is just a guide. However, individual variations fall in a range about central norms that serve as guidelines in the evaluation of an infant's or child's progress. The addition of the various solid foods to the diet and the time of immunizations vary slightly, depending on the infant's health and the physician's protocol. See Table 15-5 for an outline of the parental tasks involved in guiding the infant through the stages of growth and development.

COMMUNITY-BASED CARE: A MULTIDISCIPLINARY TEAM

The prevention of disease during infancy is of the utmost importance and includes all measures that improve the physical health and psychosocial adjustment of the child. The concept of periodic health appraisal is not new. In the late 1800s, "milk stations" were established at various locations throughout the United States to provide safe water and milk for infants in an effort to reduce the number of deaths from infant diarrhea. Today there are many community resources for the health promotion of infants, including the following:

- The Special Supplemental Nutrition Program for Women, Infants, and Children (WIC) program assists parents to obtain formulas and foods.
- Public health and hospital clinics provide follow-up care.
- Head Start and The First Five offer varied support programs.

The social service worker and home health nurse are valuable links to community-based care resources.

Text continued on p. 394

Box 16-1   Physical Development, Social Behavior, and Care and Guidance of Infants

1 MONTH
Physical Development

Weighs approximately 3.6 kg (8 lb). Has regained weight lost after birth. Gains about 2.5 cm (1 inch) in length per month for the first 6 months. Lifts head slightly when placed on stomach. Pushes with toes. Turns head to side when prone. Head wobbles. Head lags when infant pulled from lying to sitting position. Clenches fists. Stares at surroundings.

Vaginal discharge in girls and breast enlargement in boys and girls from maternal hormones received in utero are not unusual and disappear without treatment.

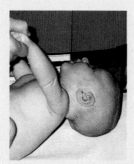

Note head lag of 1-month-old.

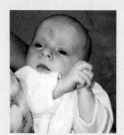

Infant keeps hands at midline.

Social Behavior

Makes small throaty noises. Cries when hungry or uncomfortable. Sleeps 20 of 24 hours. Awakens for 2 AM feeding.

Care and Guidance

Sleep: On back; if side-lying position, support back with blanket roll. Use a firm, tight-fitting mattress in a crib with bars properly spaced so that the infant's head cannot be caught between them. Raise crib rails. Do not use a pillow.

Diet: Breast milk every 2 to 3 hours or iron-fortified formula every 4 hours as infant indicates need. Vitamin D (400 international units/day) in dark-skinned infants, breastfed infants, or infants who are not regularly exposed to sunlight. Burp infant well.

Exercise: Allow freedom from the restraints of clothing before bath. Provide fresh air and sunshine whenever possible. (Protect the infant from sun and insects with sunscreen or protective clothing.) Support head and shoulders when holding infant. Attend promptly to physical needs. Provide colorful hanging toys out of infant's reach for sensory stimulation.

2 MONTHS
Physical Development

Posterior fontanelle closes. Tears appear. Can hold head erect in midposition. Follows moving light with eyes. Holds a rattle briefly. Legs are active.

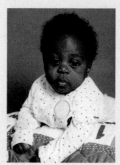

The 2-month-old can hold head erect in midline for brief periods.

Care and Guidance

Sleep: Develops own pattern; may sleep from feeding to feeding.

Diet: Breast milk or formula.

Exercise: Provide a safe, flat place to kick and be active. Do not leave infant alone, particularly on any raised surface. Physical examination by the family doctor or pediatrician.

Immunization: First diphtheria, tetanus, and whooping cough (DTaP), injectable polio vaccine (IPV), *Haemophilus influenzae* type b (Hib), and second hepatitis B virus (HBV) vaccine. Still completely depends on adults for physical care. Needs a flexible routine throughout infancy and childhood.

Pacifier: If used, select for safety. Choose one-piece construction and loop handle to prevent aspiration (see Figure 16-2).

Hiccups: Are normal and subside without treatment. Small amounts of water may help.

Colic: Consists of paroxysmal abdominal pain, irritable crying. Usually disappears after 3 months. Place infant prone over arms (see Chapter 22, Figure 22-4, *D*). Use pacifier. Massage back. Relieve caregiver periodically.

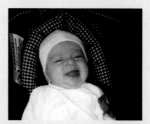

The smile of the 2-month-old delights parents.

3 MONTHS
Physical Development

Weighs 5.4 to 5.9 kg (12 to 13 lb). Stares at hands. Reaches for objects but misses them. Carries hand to mouth. Can follow an object from right to left and up and down when it is placed in front of face. Supports head steadily. Holds rattle.

Box **16-1** Physical Development, Social Behavior, and Care and Guidance of Infants—cont'd

3 MONTHS, cont'd

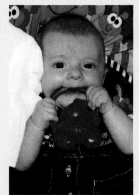

The 3-month-old carries hands to mouth.

Care and Guidance
Sleep: Yawns, stretches, naps in mother's arms.
Diet: Mother's milk or formula.
Exercise: May have short play period. Enjoys playing with hands.
Social Behavior
Cries less. Can wait a few minutes for attention. Enjoys having people talk to him or her. Takes impromptu naps.

4 MONTHS
Physical Development
Weighs about (5.9 to 6.8 kg (13 to 14 lb). Drooling indicates appearance of saliva and beginning of teething. Lifts head and shoulders when on abdomen and looks around. Turns from back to side. Sits with support. Begins to reach for objects he or she sees. Coordination between eye and body movements. Moves head, arms, and shoulders when excited. Extends legs and partly sustains weight when held upright. Rooting, Moro, extrusion, and tonic neck reflexes are no longer present.

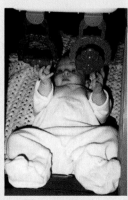

Visual stimulation is important to the growing infant.

Care and Guidance
Sleep: Stirs about in crib. Sleeps through ordinary household noises.
Diet: Mother's milk or formula.
Exercise: Plays with hand rattles and dangling toys. Start acquainting with a playpen, where infant can roll with safety.

Immunization: Second DTaP, IPV, and Hib.
Elimination: One or two bowel movements per day. May skip a day.

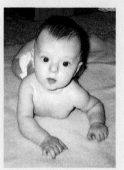

While on the abdomen the 4-month-old can lift the head and shoulders and look around.

5 MONTHS
Physical Development
Sits with support. Holds head well. Grasps objects offered. Puts everything into mouth. Plays with toes.
Social Behavior
Talks to self. Seems to know whether persons are familiar or unfamiliar. May sleep through 10 AM feeding. Tries to hold bottle at feeding time.

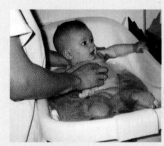

At 5 months the infant enjoys the bath. Firm head and shoulder support is essential for safety.

Care and Guidance
Sleep: Takes two or three naps daily in crib.
Diet: Mother's milk or formula.
Exercise: Provide space to pivot around. Makes jumping motions when held upright in lap.
Safety: Check toys for loose buttons and rough edges before placing them in playpen.
6 MONTHS
Physical Development
Doubles birth weight. Gains about 3 to 5 or 4 to 7 oz per week during the next 6 months. Grows about 1.3 cm (½ inch) per month. Sits alone momentarily. Springs up and down when sitting. Turns completely over. Hitches (moves backward when sitting). Bangs table with rattle. Pulls to a sitting position. Chewing more mature. First solid food introduced. Approximates lips to rim of cup.

Continued

| Box 16-1 | Physical Development, Social Behavior, and Care and Guidance of Infants—cont'd |

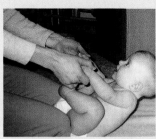

The infant can pull to sitting position without head lag at 6 months.

Social Behavior

Cries loudly when interrupted from play. Increased interest in world. Babbles and squeals. Sucks food from spoon. Awakens happy.

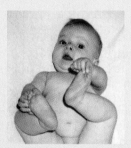

A 6-month-old discovers and plays with the feet.

7 MONTHS
Physical Development

Two lower teeth appear. These are the first of the deciduous teeth—the central incisors. Begins to crawl. Moves forward, using chest, head, and arms; legs drag. Can grasp objects more easily. Transfers objects from one hand to the other. Appears interested in standing. Holds an adult's hands and bounces actively while standing. Struggles when being dressed.

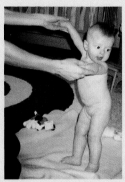

The infant enjoys standing position with assistance.

Social Behavior

Shifts moods easily—crying one minute, laughing the next. Shows fear of strangers. Anticipates spoon-feeding. Sleeps 11 to 13 hours at night.

Care and Guidance

Sleep: Fretfulness caused by teething may appear. This is generally evidenced by lack of appetite and wakefulness during the night. In most cases, merely soothing and offering a cup of water are sufficient.

Diet: Add fruit. Add finger foods, such as toast or zwieback.

Exercise: Primitive locomotion.

8 MONTHS
Physical Development

Sits steadily alone. Uses index finger and thumb as pincers. Pokes at object. Enjoys dropping article into a cup and emptying it.

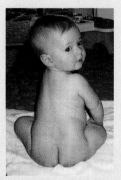

At 8 months the infant is able to sit steady with back straight.

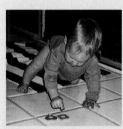

The pincer action is developed, and the infant can pick up small objects between the thumb and forefinger.

Social Behavior

Plays pat-a-cake. Enjoys family life. Amuses self longer. Reserved with strangers. Indicates need for sleep by fussing and sucking thumb. Impatient especially when food is being prepared.

Care and Guidance

Sleep: Takes two naps a day.

Diet: Add vegetables. Continue to add new foods slowly, observing for reactions.

Exercise: Enjoys jump chair. Rides in stroller. Stuffed toys or those that squeak or rattle are appropriate.

Safety: Remain with infant at all times during bath in tub. Protect from chewing paint from windowsills or old furniture. Paint containing lead can be poisonous. Use safety-lock doors to ovens, dishwashers, washing machines, dryers, and refrigerators.

| Box 16-1 | Physical Development, Social Behavior, and Care and Guidance of Infants—cont'd |

9 MONTHS
Physical Development

Can raise self to a sitting position. Holds bottle. Creeps (carries trunk of body above floor but parallel to it; more advanced than crawling). When standing, may move while holding onto furniture (cruise).

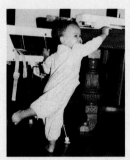

Infant cruises on furniture. Be sure it is stable!

Care and Guidance

Sleep: Has generally begun to sleep later in the morning.

Diet: Add meat, beans. Introduce chopped and mashed foods. Place newspaper beneath feeding table. Use unbreakable dishes. Allow infant to pick up pieces of food by hand and put them into mouth.

Safety: Know phone number of nearest poison control center. Avoid using tablecloths with overhangs infant could reach.

Exercise: Is busy most of the day exploring surroundings. Provide sufficient room and materials for safe play. Help infant to learn. Distract curious child from danger. In this way punishment is limited—avoid excessive spankings and "no's."

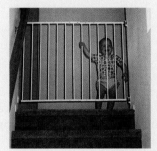

Stairway gates prevent falls. (Courtesy Pat Spier, RN-C.)

10 MONTHS
Physical Development

Pulls to a standing position in the playpen. Throws toys to floor for parent to pick up. Cries when they are not returned. Walks around furniture while holding onto it.

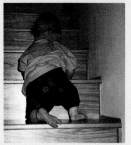

Infant is able to climb steps but needs supervision. (Courtesy Pat Spier, RN-C.)

Social Behavior

Knows name. Plays simple games such as peek-a-boo. Feeds self a cookie. May cry out in sleep without waking.

Care and Guidance

Sleep: Avoid strenuous play before bedtime. A nightlight is convenient for parent and makes infant's surroundings more familiar. Use pajamas with feet, because infant becomes uncovered easily.

Diet: Takes juice and water from cup. In general, solid foods are taken well.

Exercise: Tours around room holding adult's hands. Daytime clothing should be loose so as not to interfere with movement.

11 MONTHS
Physical Development

Stands upright holding onto an adult's hand.

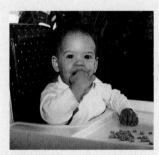

The 11-month-old can feed herself finger foods and drink from a "sippy cup."

Social Behavior

Understands simple directions. Impatient when held. Enjoys playing with empty dish and spoon after meals.

Care and Guidance

Sleep: Greets parents in morning with excited jargon.

Diet: Still spills from cup. Enjoys blowing bubbles.

Exercise: Plays with toys in tub. Enjoys gross motor activity. Kicks, pulls self up.

Safety: Cover electrical outlets. Put household cleaners and medicines out of reach if not previously done. Parent may need to sit infant down in playpen at times, because infant tends to stand to point of exhaustion.

Continued

Box **16-1**   Physical Development, Social Behavior, and Care and Guidance of Infants—cont'd

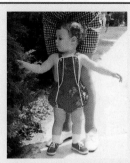

The 11-month-old is alert to surroundings and touches the leaves.

12 MONTHS
Physical Development
Pulse rate 100 to 140 beats/min. Respirations 20 to 40 breaths/min. Triples birth weight. Height is about 74 cm (29 inches). Stands alone for short periods. May walk. Puts arm through sleeve as an aid to being dressed. Six teeth (four above and two below). Drinks from a cup; eats with a spoon with supervision. Pincer grasp is well established. Handedness (the preference for the use of one hand), although not fully established, may be evidenced.

Social Behavior
Friendly. Repeats acts that elicit a response. Recognizes "no-no." Verbalization slows because of increased concentration about ambulation. Enjoys rhythmic music. Shows emotions such as fear, anger, and jealousy. Reacts to these emotions from adults. Plays with food and removes it from mouth.

Care and Guidance
Sleep: May take one long nap daily.
Diet: Gradually add egg white and fish (baked, steamed, or boiled). Add orange juice. Add well-cooked table foods. Interest in eating dwindles.
Exercise: Enjoys putting objects in a basket and then removing them. Places objects on head. Distraction is an effective way to handle the infant's determination to do what he or she wants regardless of outcome.

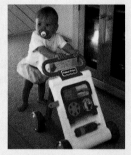

At 12 months the infant can stand alone and walk with assistance.

HEALTH PROMOTION
Role of the Nurse
Parenting skills can be impaired because of socioeconomic factors, as well as by physical and mental problems. A prime responsibility of the nurse in the community-based clinic is to guide the parents and assist in the development of the skills necessary to ensure the proper growth and development of their child. The nurse can provide encouragement and explanations of strategies that will enable parents to be successful in coping with various infant behaviors.

The nurse is the important link in the initiation of referral to the multidisciplinary health care team, follow-up of progress, and maintenance of communication between the family and members of the health care team. A home-based infant stimulation program can use a teacher, nurse, occupational or speech therapist, or physical therapist (depending on the specific need of the infant) to stimulate the infant directly and to teach the parents how to provide care.

Coping with the Irritable Infant. One of the goals of early parent–infant interaction is to promote a calm, alert infant who can respond to parents and the environment. Success in this area promotes a feeling of competence in the parent. Some infants cannot tolerate environmental stimulation and handling and start to cry during diaper changes, feeding, and rocking. Lights, sound, and movement cause some infants to become irritable. Techniques to cope with these problems include the following:
- Shield the infant's eyes from bright light.
- Sit quietly with the infant without talking or singing.
- Eliminate noise from radio, television, and computer.
- Talk in a soft voice.
- Change the infant's position slowly.
- Stop the interaction and reduce environmental stimuli if the infant turns away, squirms, grimaces, or puts the hands in front of the face.

- Swaddle the infant snugly in a lightweight blanket with extremities flexed and hands near the face.
- Provide nonnutritive sucking.
- Rock the infant slowly and gently.
- Avoid sudden movements.
- Cradle the infant firmly in the lap during feeding and remain still during sucking efforts.

Nursing Tip

An infant's repetitious banging of toys on a table may be perceived by the parent as an irritating type of behavior. Counseling may be required to help the parent to understand that this is a normal developmental phase of motor activity and should be encouraged!

Coping with Colic. **Colic** is characterized by periods of unexplained irritability and crying in a healthy, well-fed infant. Although the exact cause is unknown, it is thought to be a combination of infant, parental, and environmental factors. Colic can interfere with parent–infant interactions if the infant is not soothed by being held or carried, and parental fatigue and guilt develop. Providing periods of rest and "breaks" to parents of colicky infants can prevent a cycle that may lead to child abuse. See Figure 22-4 for an illustration of the "colic carry." Holding the infant face down and close to the body while supporting the abdomen and providing a gentle rocking motion often soothes the colicky infant. See Nursing Care Plan 16-1 for care of the infant with colic.

Coping with the Lethargic Infant. Stimulation, interaction, and nourishment are essential for optimal infant growth and development. Some infants respond to an excessively stimulating environment by "shutting down" and sleeping. Coping strategies for handling this infant include the following:

- Avoid bright lights.
- Move and handle the infant slowly and gently.
- Talk in a calm voice.
- Sit the infant upright at intervals.
- *Slowly* dress and undress the infant.

Developing Positive Sleep Patterns. Most newborns sleep at 4-hour intervals and increase their sleep intervals to 8 hours by age 4 to 6 months. Synchronizing the circadian rhythm of the infant to the family routine is a learned behavior. Parents must be alert to the infant's individual rhythm and promote activities that foster a stable synchronized pattern. Infants should be positioned for sleep on their backs on a firm mattress, both for their safety and to prevent sudden infant death syndrome (SIDS).

★ Nursing Care Plan 16-1 | The Family Care Plan When the Infant Has Colic

PATIENT DATA The parents of a 3-week-old infant state that they feel inadequate as parents because their infant is often fussy and irritable and does not respond to their efforts to calm him. They ask what they are doing wrong.

Selected Nursing Diagnosis: Interrupted family processes related to fussiness of infant

Goals	Nursing Interventions	Rationales
Parents will demonstrate increased coping behaviors by 1 week. Parents will verbalize feelings of increased confidence in caring for the infant.	Educate parents about common manifestations of colic.	No single cause has been established for colic. Infant appears otherwise healthy but demonstrates cramplike pain, drawing legs to abdomen and producing irritable cry. It is time-limited to about 3 months.
	Determine whether physician has ruled out other causes.	Intestinal obstruction and infection may mimic symptoms of colic. Bowel movements are not abnormal with colic.
	Review caregiver's history and usual day with infant.	This helps to determine if colic is related to type of feedings, diet of breastfeeding mother, passive smoking, milk allergy, activities of family members while infant is being fed, or other factors.
	Identify soothing measures used by parents and their effectiveness.	Environment may be overstimulating infant; parents may not know how to soothe the infant.
	Suggest abdominal massage, wind-up swing, and car rides.	These measures may help to relieve symptoms; burping before and after feedings and placing in an upright position after feedings may also decrease distress.
	Demonstrate "colic carry" (see Figure 22-4, *D*).	Position may comfort infant by applying a little extra pressure on abdomen.
	Suggest periods of free time for parents.	Constant crying by infants produces a great deal of frustration in family members; caution against shaking infant, which can be harmful to the head and neck.
	Emphasize that colic is not a reflection on parenting skills.	First-time parents may feel anxious and incompetent. Nurse provides reassurance and support and builds on their strengths.

When placing an infant in a car seat, care should be taken that the infant's chin does not rest on his or her chest as this can cause oxygen desaturation and hypoxia. For this reason, car seats should not be used as a prolonged sleeping arrangement for infants (Moon, 2011).

Many parents use "sling carriers" to carry their sleeping infants during the day. Care should be taken to ensure that the infant's head and face are above the fabric and that the nose and mouth are unobstructed. The use of pacifiers during sleep has a protective effect on preventing SIDS (Moon, 2011).

Until age 6 months, infants rely on parents to soothe them back to sleep when they awaken during the night. If the parent resorts to midnight pacing or car rides, the infant will learn to rely on the parent to get them back to sleep after age 6 months. The mother should assist the infant to develop "self-soothing" behaviors so the infant can roll over, grasp the pacifier, and return to sleep on his or her own. Helping the infant to achieve this ability will also make parents feel more confident in their parenting skills and less fatigued and frustrated.

> **! Safety Alert!**
>
> The American Academy of Pediatrics recommends a supine or back-lying position for infants to avoid sudden infant death syndrome (SIDS). Care should be taken to use a sturdy mattress and avoid soft pillows that can inhibit breathing. Comforters, quilts, loose bedding, and thick, pillowlike crib bumpers can be a danger to an infant in a crib.

Infants with Special Needs

All parents should be taught about normal growth and development and anticipated milestones for their children. When special needs are recognized, early intervention is essential in order to attain the best outcome.

Infants with special needs may require referral to community agencies for follow-up care. Early childhood education programs at colleges and in some day care centers can offer parent guidance concerning growth and development through their infant stimulation programs. A daycare nursery school can be used, and the public school system offers special classes and tutoring for children with special needs. A psychologist can provide counseling, behavior management techniques, and cognitive therapy. Neurodevelopmental therapy (NDT) can be provided by a professional therapist or by an occupational or physical therapist. Speech therapy and auditory testing are also available within the community. The social worker can assist with social and environmental problems.

ILLNESS PREVENTION

Skilled health services today encompass periodic health appraisal, immunizations, assessment of parent–child interaction, counseling in the developmental processes, identification of families at risk (e.g., for child abuse), health education and anticipatory guidance, referrals to various agencies, follow-up services, appropriate record-keeping, and evaluation and audit by peers. These services are provided in a variety of health care facilities. Ideally the infant is seen in the health care setting at least five times during the first year at specific intervals (2 months, 4 months, 6 months, 9 months, and 1 year). Private group practices, hospital-based clinics, and neighborhood health centers are examples of health care settings.

These visits are as important for the parents as they are for the infant. They provide caregiver support and reassurance as well as information and anticipatory guidance for the many developmental changes and health issues of the infant's first year. A common concern is diaper rash, which can cause discomfort to the infant. The mother should be taught the importance of frequent diaper changes, how to wipe from front to back, and the importance of exposing the skin in the diaper area to the air for periods of time. Some commercial diaper wipes may contain fragrance or other ingredients that can further irritate a diaper rash. Soiled areas can be washed with water and mild soap if needed. To prevent skin breakdown, A+D or another protective ointment such as Desitin can be applied when the skin in the diaper area appears pink and irritated. More serious physical or psychological concerns can be discussed with the health care provider and referral offered as appropriate.

A careful health history is obtained during routine clinic visits. Growth grids during infancy include measures of weight, length, and head circumference. The reading and recording of growth charts is described in Chapter 15. There are numerous developmental screening tests. In the 1986 Amendment to the Education of All Handicapped Children Act (PL99-457), all states are required to assess for developmental disabilities before age 5 years. Most pediatricians initiate their assessment at birth to enable early intervention. General screening tools are available to identify children in need of referral and further care. Some of the tests include the following:

- *Denver Developmental Screening Test (DDST):* This test is widely used and tests social, fine-motor adaptive, language, and gross-motor abilities from birth to age 6 years.
- *Denver Home Screening Questionnaire:* This tool provides information concerning the child-rearing environment.
- *Early Language Milestone Scale (ELM):* Because language is necessary for cognitive development, this test assesses expressive, receptive, and visual language from birth to age 3 years.
- *Clinical Linguistic and Auditory Milestone Scale (CLAMS):* This test assesses language milestones from birth to age 3 years.
- *Ages and Stages Questionnaire (ASQ):* This is administered between ages 4 and 48 months.
- *Brazelton Neonatal Behavioral Assessment Scale:* This scale is of particular value during the newborn

period, helping to describe the infant's emerging personality and evaluate infant reflexes, general activity, alertness, orientation to spoken voice, and response to visual stimuli.

The physical examination is adapted to the infant's needs. Routine assessments of hearing and vision are an integral part of the examination. In the newborn period, loud noises should precipitate the startle, or Moro, reflex. Standing behind the child who is seated on the mother's lap and ringing a bell or repeating voice sounds can roughly ascertain the infant's ability to localize sound. The infant's response is compared with the average for that age level. Vision is mainly assessed by light perception. The examiner shines a penlight into the eyes and notes blinking, following to midline, and other responses. Laboratory tests may include urinalysis and measurement of hemoglobin or hematocrit levels to detect anemia. Screening tests for various asymptomatic diseases are assuming greater importance; examples of these are the phenylketonuria (PKU), tuberculin, and sickle cell tests.

Immunizations

Health personnel must repeatedly stress to parents the importance of immunizations. A delay can lead to undue risks of serious illness, sometimes with fatal complications.

The nurse can stress to working parents that an unprotected child may become sick, making it necessary for them to lose valuable working hours. Immunization also prevents numerous physician and hospital expenses and is required before school entry. A delay or interruption in a series does not interfere with final immunity. It is not necessary to restart any series, regardless of the length of delay. Accurate records prevent confusion. See Chapter 32 for a detailed discussion of immunizations and common childhood communicable diseases.

Nutrition Counseling

The nutritional needs of infants reflect rates of growth, energy expended in activity, basal metabolic needs, and the interaction of the nutrients consumed (Mahan and Escott-Stump, 2012). The infant is born with a rooting reflex, which aids in finding the nipple. The sucking reflex is present at birth. There is a forward and backward movement of the tongue. As the infant grows, neuromaturation of the cheeks and tongue enables advancement to a more mature sucking pattern that uses negative pressure to obtain milk. At about the third to fourth month, the **extrusion reflex** (protrusion of the tongue), which pushes food out of the mouth to prevent intake of inappropriate food, disappears.

The digestive system continues to mature. By 6 months, it can handle more complex nutrients and is less susceptible to food allergens. The stomach capacity expands from 10 to 20 mL at birth to 200 mL by 12 months. This expansion enables the infant to consume more food at less-frequent intervals. As the pincer grasp becomes more developed, the infant can pick up food with tiny fingers and place it in the mouth. By age 2 years, the child masters spoon-feeding.

Taste cells develop during the eighth week of gestation, and the fetus begins to respond to flavors when swallowing amniotic fluid. At birth the infant demonstrates a preference for certain tastes, preferring sweet and rejecting sour. Breast milk may supply flavor experiences based on the mother's diet. Infants should be given an opportunity to develop their own personal tastes by being offered various foods when solids are introduced.

Parental Concerns. Parents have many concerns about feeding their infant during the first year of life. This is a period when readiness to receive nutrition education is usually high; therefore the nurse looks for opportunities to provide accurate information. Assessment of parental knowledge; infant development, behavior, and readiness; parent–child interaction; and cultural and ethnic practices is important. Nutritional care plans based on developmental levels assist parents in recognizing changes in feeding patterns. The components of a nutritional assessment are discussed in Chapter 15.

> ### 🔊 Nursing Tip
>
> Human milk or properly prepared formula supplies adequate fluid for the infant under normal conditions. The infant may require additional water during illness or hot, humid weather.

A suggested parental guide to determining the adequacy of the diet includes the following:

- The infant has gained 4 to 7 oz per week for the first 6 months.
- The infant has at least six wet diapers per day.
- The infant sleeps peacefully for several hours after feedings.

Monitoring of weight, height, head circumference, and skinfold thickness determines if the diet is adequate; therefore the value of periodic well-baby examinations is stressed. Bottle fed infants are usually fed at 3- to 4-hour intervals. Breastfed infants may require feedings at 2- to 3-hour intervals because breast milk is more easily digested. A flexible but regular schedule that provides a rest period between feedings is best for the parent and infant. The nurse reassures parents that most children eat enough to grow normally, although intake is seldom constant and varies in quantity and quality. Forced feedings are not appropriate.

Breastfeeding and Bottle Feeding. Infants, in proportion to their weight, require more calories, protein, minerals, and vitamins than adults. Their fluid requirements are also high. It is suggested that infants remain on human milk or iron-fortified formula for the first year of life (Table 16-1).

Human milk is the best food for infants younger than 6 months. It contains the ideal balance of nutrients in a

Table 16-1   Common Milk Preparations for the First Year

MILK PREPARATION	ADVANTAGES	DISADVANTAGES
Human breast milk	No preparation needed; nonallergenic; provides antibodies	Lifestyle or illness of mother may influence availability
Prepared, ready-to-feed formula	No preparation needed; no refrigeration needed before opening bottle	Expensive
Formula concentrate	Easy to prepare; can prepare one bottle at a time or a maximum of one day's feeding at a time	Must be refrigerated after preparation Must use accurate proportions; safe water supply necessary to dilute concentrate (water from a natural well may have a high mineral concentration)
Formula powder	Least expensive formula; lasts up to 1 month after opening	Necessitates accurate measurement; necessitates safe water supply and must be shaken thoroughly to dissolve powder

readily digestible form. Breastfeeding soon after birth helps to promote bonding and stimulates milk production. It has immunological properties that help to protect the infant from certain microorganisms, and allergic reactions are minimal.

Nutritious commercially prepared infant formulas are available (see Table 16-3). Many pediatricians recommend iron-fortified formulas because maternal iron stores decrease by 6 months of age. Whole cow's milk is not recommended for infants younger than 1 year because the tough, hard curd is difficult to digest. This type of milk may also contribute to iron-deficiency anemia by causing gastrointestinal blood loss.

Parents are sometimes unsure of when their infant has had enough formula. It is important to explain satiety (hunger satisfaction) behavior at the various ages (Table 16-2). Coaxing infants to finish the last drop in a bottle is unnecessary. Infants who are breastfed longer than 6 months gain less weight by age 1 year than bottle-fed infants and are less apt to be obese in later life.

Types of infant formula. The only recognized contraindications to breastfeeding are galactosemia or certain inborn errors of metabolism in the newborn (such as PKU), or mother with the following: positive human immunodeficiency virus (HIV) status; chemotherapy drug treatment; radioactive isotope therapy; illicit drug use; or active, untreated pulmonary tuberculosis.

When the mother cannot breastfeed, the American Academy of Pediatrics (AAP) recommends iron-

Table 16-2   Development of Mealtime Behavior and Implications for Caregivers

AGE	HUNGER BEHAVIOR	COMMUNICATION	FEEDING BEHAVIOR	SATIETY	PARENTAL GUIDANCE
Birth to 3 months	Cries; hands fisted; body tense	Roots in search of nipple	Strong suck reflex; needs to be burped	Falls asleep when full; hands relaxed; body relaxed; withdraws head from nipple	Burp frequently. Avoid overfeeding or underfeeding. Recognize signs of satiety.
3-5 months	Grasps and draws bottle to mouth; tongue protrudes in anticipation of nipple; fusses; mouths hands	Reaches with open mouth to receive nipple	Strong suck; holds nipple firmly; preference for tastes; pats bottle	Tosses head back; ejects nipple; distracted easily by surroundings; plays with nipple	Provide predictable eating routine. Allow infant to gain experience with textures of various foods.
6-9 months	Reacts to food preparation; reaches for bottle	Vocalizes hunger; pulls spoon to mouth; holds bottle	Picks up small food with raking, then pincer action; draws food from spoon with lips; chewing begins	Changes posture; closes mouth; plays with utensils; shakes head "no"	Offer one new food at a time at spaced intervals to assess responses. Include familiar favorites.
10-12 months	Vocalizes; grasps utensils; fussy	Attempts to feed self; purses lips to cup's edge	Skilled pincer action to pick up pieces of food and place in mouth; drinks from cup; chews food	Shakes head "no"; sputters food; throws food to floor	Allow infant to assist with feeding. Introduce foods with varied textures. Avoid foods that can be aspirated.

NOTE: Parents who are alert to infant's communication of hunger and satiety help the infant develop self-regulation and communication skills.

fortified cow's milk–based formula (Kliegman, 2011). The two major milk proteins are whey and casein. Human milk has a 60:40 ratio of whey to casein, whereas cow's milk has a 20:80 ratio. These ratios differ among various commercially prepared formulas. Whey is composed of amino acids that are very easily digested by stomach contents, but when unchanged whey reaches the small intestine, it may provoke symptoms of protein intolerance. Casein is more slowly digested, provides a slowly absorbed amino acid, and inhibits catabolic processes. Some formulas are 100% whey, such as Good Start Supreme cow's milk–based formula, whereas other commercially prepared formulas provide varied ratios of whey to casein (Table 16-3).

Docosahexaenoic acid (DHA), an omega-3 fatty acid, and arachidonic acid (ARA), an omega-6 fatty acid, are important for nervous system functioning and are added to most commercial infant formulas as a long chain polyunsaturated fatty acid (LC-PUFA), which will be noted on the label of the formula.

Probiotics have been defined by the World Health Organization (WHO) as live microorganisms (*Bifidobacterium* and lactobacilli) that, when administered in adequate amounts, offer a health benefit. Prebiotics are nondigestible food ingredients (oligosaccharides) that indirectly stimulate growth or activity of *Bifidobacterium* when it is present in the colon, ensuring a balance of bacteria is maintained. Probiotics are protective to the gastrointestinal (GI) tract and have been used to treat diarrhea with some success. Evidence of the value of routine use of probiotics in infant formulas is still being researched, but it is becoming a popular formula option.

Formulas such as Enfamil A.R. that contain rice starch thicken in the stomach and do not increase caloric value or clog nipples as does infant cereal added to the formula bottle. It is used for reflux or gastroesophageal reflux disease (GERD) problems in infants and often decreases loose stools. Lactose-free formulas such as ProSobee replace lactose with corn syrup as the carbohydrate source. Soy milk is used appropriately for infants with galactosemia, but infants allergic to cow's milk protein often do not do better with soy milk. Soy milk is often used temporarily during a bout of diarrhea, after which the infant returns to breastfeeding or milk-based formula. Extensively hydrolyzed formula and amino acid–based elemental formulas are used for infants with severe protein sensitivity. The nurse must know the difference between various commercial formulas. Feeding an infant the wrong infant formula is considered a medication error and must be reported according to facility policy.

Infants who screen positive for inborn errors of metabolism will require special nutritional formulas. Infants with some genetic problems such as phenylketonuria (PKU) require formula such as Mead-Johnson's *Lofenalac* or Ross Labs *Phenix* and cannot breastfeed exclusively. Current research has shown there is some

evidence that some illnesses may be associated with feeding patterns (Jonsdottir, 2012). Children less than 4 months of age who are fed gluten-containing foods may be at increased risk of developing gastrointestinal problems later in life, and the risk may decrease if gluten is withheld until 6 months of age (Jonsdottir, 2012). The clinical decision about which formula is best for a specific infant should be made in partnership between the health care provider and the parent (Bartram, 2013).

The practice of feeding breast milk and then immediately supplementing with commercially prepared formula may be counterproductive, because substances in the formula may compete for binding or absorption sites in the intestine, thus preventing absorption of some nutrients from the breast milk. Supplemental commercially prepared formula given at a different time of day (separated by several hours) might not have this interaction with breast milk, but research is ongoing. Formula preparation and breast milk storage are discussed in Chapter 9. Table 16-1 shows a review of the advantages of the various forms of milk available. Table 16-3 discusses the various commercially prepared infant formulas that are available.

Safe bottle feeding. The nurse should teach parents the basic principles of safe bottle feeding to prevent problems that can result in illness or injury:

- Always check the expiration date on the formula container; do not buy formula that has expired.
- Wash hands thoroughly before preparing formula.
- Wash top of can with detergent and hot water before opening it.
- Use a clean can opener to open can, and wash it between uses. Check the can opener for food or rust spots before using it again.
- Have a clean container (dishpan) reserved for washing all things used for feeding newborn. Squeeze soapy water through nipple holes, then rinse several times.
- Follow the product directions precisely when mixing formula.
- Heat bottle of formula if necessary by running warm water over it. (Most newborns are just as content with their formula unheated. Be consistent in your choice.)
- Test formula temperature by shaking a few drops on your inner wrist, not just feeling the bottle.
- Do not heat bottle in a microwave oven; the liquid often warms unevenly unless stirred. The container may remain cool when the formula inside is hot enough to burn the newborn.
- Keep prepared bottles of formula refrigerated until ready to use.
- Opened containers of liquid formula should be tightly covered and stored in the refrigerator for no longer than is designated on the label.
- After a formula can is opened or a formula is mixed, use it right away or refrigerate it, because bacteria multiply rapidly at warm temperatures.

Table 16-3 Commercially Prepared Infant Formulas

TYPE OF FORMULA	BRAND NAME OF FORMULA	PROTEIN/NUTRIENT CONTENT
Infant Formulas		
		Whey/Casein Ratio
Standard formula	Enfamil Lipil	60 : 40
Iron fortified cow's milk–based formula with DHA and ARA	Good Start Supreme	100 : 0
	Similac Advance	48 : 52
Modified cow's milk–based protein (partially hydrolyzed)	Enfamil Gentlease-Lipil	60 : 40
	Good Start Supreme	100 : 0
	Gentle Infant Formula	60 : 40
	Similac Sensitive (kosher)	48 : 52
Organic cow's milk–based	Similac organic, Bright Beginnings organic	48 : 52
Specialty Formulas		
Cow's milk–based with rice starch added	Enfamil A.R. Lipil Similac Sensitive R.S.	
Lactose free	Similac Isomil Enfamil ProSobee Good Start Soy	
With prebiotics or probiotics	Similac EarlyShield Bright Beginnings	Contains prebiotics (oligosaccharides)
	Nestle Good Start Natural Cultures (100% whey protein)	Contains *Bifidobacterium* (*Bifidobacterium animalis* subsp lactis) cultures; probiotics
Iron-fortified soy-based	Bright Beginnings Soy	Soy protein isolate
	Enfamil ProSobee Lipil	Soy protein and methionine
	Isomil Advance	Soy protein isolate
Extensively hydrolyzed milk protein formulas	Similac Alimentum	Casein hydrolysate
	Nutramigen	Lactose and sucrose free
	Pregestimil	Casein hydrolysate and free amino acids
Amino acid–based	Elecare	Free L-amino acids
Elemental formula amino acid–based	Neocate	Free L-Amino acids Corn syrup solids
Electrolyte solution	Pedialyte Lytren Enfalyte	Electrolytes and rice syrup as carbohydrate source 115 mg sodium, 98 mg potassium
Toddler Formulas		
For poor eaters	Enfamil Next Step	Nonfat milk 20 : 80 whey/casein ratio 20 calories/oz
	Similac Go and Grow (kosher) milk or soy based	48 : 52 whey/casein ratio 20 calories/oz
	Nestle Good Start	100% whey protein milk–based protein
	Nestle Good Start Natural Cultures	Contains 100% whey proteins with *Bifidobacterium* culture, or *Bifidobacterium lactis* probiotics
Full nutrient formula for failure to thrive (FTT) or tube feedings	Ross PediaSure	Nonfat milk base and vegetable oils
	Bright Beginnings 2 (follow-on)	
	Mead-Johnson Kindercal	

NOTE: Other formulas are available for specific conditions such as maple syrup urine disease, homocysteinuria, phenylketonuria (PKU), and others.
ARA, Arachidonic acid; *DHA,* docosahexaenoic acid.
Data from Abbot Laboratories: http://abbotnutrition.com/products; Bright Beginnings: www.brightbeginnings.com/professionals; Mead Johnson: www.meadjohnson.com; Nestle: www.nestle-infantnutrition.com; Ovewehand A: Antibacterial effects of probiotics, *J Nutr* 137(1):7945-7975, 2011; Gottesmen M: Choosing the right infant formula, *Adv Nurs Practitioner* 16(5):47-51, 2008; Rojas M, Lozano J, Rojas M, Rodriguez V, Rondon M, Bastidas J, Perez C: Prophylactic probiotics to prevent death and nosocomial infection in preterm infants, *J Ped* 730(5):1113-1120, 2012; Mugambi M, Musekiwa A, Lombard M, Young M, Young T: Synbiotics, probiotics or prebiotics in infant formula for full term infants: a systematic review, *Nutr J* 11:81-88, 2012, Bartram J, Montoya C: Infant formulas: partnering with parents for rational decision making, *Advance for NPs and PAs* 4(7):31-36, 2013.

- Carry filled bottles away from home in an insulated bag or cooler with ice packs inside.
- Milk should not be saved for the next feeding if the newborn does not empty the bottle. Microorganisms will grow, and the newborn can develop diarrhea (infection).
- Note that hard, clear plastic bottles made of polycarbonate may contain bisphenol-A (BPA), phthalates, and PVC, and they may be toxic. Plastic bottles with the numbers 3, 6, or 7 stamped inside a triangle on the bottom of the bottle are not safe to reuse (Morin, 2008).
- New bottles made of tritan copolyester have no BPA. Polyethylene or polypropylene is considered safe. All bottles, sippy cups, and pacifiers should be labeled BPA free; those that are not should not be used. Microwaving food or fluids in plastic containers may allow chemicals to leach into the food or fluid and is considered unsafe.

> **Nursing Tip**
>
> Whole milk and "imitation milk" should not be given to infants until after 1 year of age.

Adding Solid Foods. Parents often wonder when to begin adding solid foods. The addition of solid food at about 4 to 6 months is recommended because this is when the tongue extrusion reflex has completely disappeared and the gastrointestinal tract is mature enough to digest the foods. There are a number of commercially prepared brands of baby foods. Parents should be instructed to read the labels on the jars to obtain nutrition information. Home-prepared foods may also be used.

> 🚶 **Health Promotion**
>
> **Directions for Home Preparation of Infant Foods**
>
> - Select fresh, high-quality fruits, vegetables, and meats.
> - Be sure all utensils, including cutting boards, grinder, and knives, are thoroughly clean.
> - Wash hands before preparing the food.
> - Clean, wash, and trim the food in as little water as possible.
> - Cook the foods until tender in as little water as possible. Prevent overcooking, which may destroy heat-sensitive nutrients.
> - Do not add salt. Add sugar sparingly. Do not add honey to food for infants less than age 1 year. (Botulism spores have been reported in honey, and young infants do not have the immune capacity to resist this infection.)
> - Add enough water so that the food can be easily pureed.
> - Strain or puree the food with an electric blender, food mill, baby food grinder, or kitchen strainer.
> - Pour the pureed food into an ice cube tray and freeze.
> - When food is frozen hard, remove the cubes and store in freezer bags.
> - In a serving container unfreeze and heat (in water bath or microwave oven) the amount of food that will be consumed at a single feeding (Mahon and Escott Stump, 2012).

Between 4 and 6 months of age, sucking becomes more mature, and munching (up-and-down chopping motion) commences. Rice cereal is often recommended as the first solid food because it is less allergenic. Figure 16-4 illustrates how feeding skills develop in infants and toddlers.

> **Nursing Tip**
>
> Cereal and baby food should *not* be mixed in a bottle with formula.

Only small amounts are offered at first (1 teaspoonful). A small amount of food is placed on the back of the tongue. Cereal may be diluted with formula or water. The consistency is thickened, and amounts of solid foods are gradually increased as the infant becomes more familiar with them. A small bowl and a spoon with a long, straight handle are suggested. Single-ingredient foods are introduced (green beans rather than mixed vegetables), because it is easier to determine food allergies this way. To determine tolerance, only one new food is offered in a 4-day to 1-week period.

If the infant refuses a certain food, it is temporarily omitted. Mealtime is kept pleasant. The infant is allowed to try new foods, even ones that the parents dislike. New foods should not be introduced when the infant is ill, because adverse responses might not be effectively assessed. The amount of food consumed varies with the child. Fruit juices are generally offered at about 5 to 6 months of age, when the infant begins to drink from a cup. An exception is the addition of orange juice, which is withheld until the infant is 1 year old, especially when family members have known allergies. Other highly allergenic foods that may be delayed include fish, nuts, strawberries, chocolate, and egg whites.

> **Nursing Tip**
>
> New solid foods should be introduced *before* the milk feedings to encourage the infant to try the new experience. As solid food intake increases, the amount of formula or milk should be decreased to avoid overfeeding.

A children's plastic "sipper" or "sippy" cup is helpful at first. The juice is initially diluted. The National Research Council (NRC) recommends a daily *liquid* intake of 140 to 160 mL/kg/day for a 3-month-old, 130 to 155 mL/kg/day for a 6-month-old, 120 to 135 mL/kg/day for a 1-year-old, and 90 to 100 mL/kg/day for a 6-year-old (Kliegman, 2011). Baby food can be prepared in a food grinder, electric blender, or food mill or by mashing the food to the desired texture.

> ❗ **Safety Alert!**
>
> To prevent the development of botulism, honey should not be included in the diet of infants younger than 1 year.

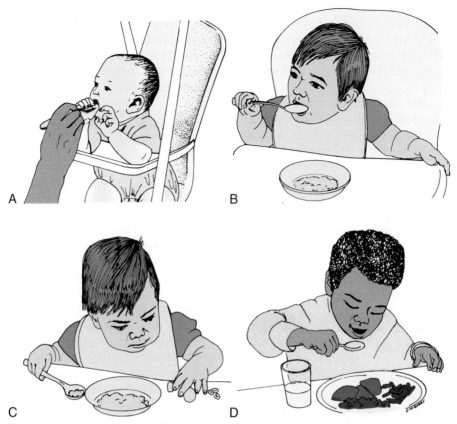

FIGURE 16-4 Development of feeding skills in infants and toddlers. **A,** At 7 months, this child begins to reach for the spoon. **B,** At 9 months, this little girl begins to use her spoon independently, although she is not yet able to keep food on it. **C,** The 9-month-old shows a refined pincer grasp to pick up food. **D,** The 2-year-old is much more skilled at self-feeding and has the ability both to rotate the wrist and to elevate the elbow to keep food on the spoon. (Modified from Mahan LK, Escott-Stump S: *Krause's food, nutrition and diet therapy,* ed 9, Philadelphia, 1996, Saunders.)

Research has shown that early introduction of allergenic foods such as wheat, egg, nuts and seafood may reduce the risk of developing food allergies (Fleischer, 2013). Acidic foods such as berries and tomatoes rarely cause systemic reactions.

Recommended Fat Intake During Infancy. Fat contains more calories than carbohydrates and proteins. Because infants have a limited stomach capacity and a high caloric need, fats in easily digestible forms are needed for meeting their caloric needs for growth and development and for brain development. Infants have a high basal metabolic rate (BMR) and require almost three times more calories per kilogram of weight than adults do to maintain their rapid growth and development in the first year of life. In the young infant, breast milk and infant formulas provide the necessary fats that the infant is able to digest. Feeding a low-fat diet to infants younger than 2 years will compromise their growth and development.

The fat and cholesterol content may not be designated on the label of many baby foods. By age 6 months, amylase and lipase are present in the digestive tract to aid in digesting the fat present in solid foods. A well-balanced diet provides appropriate fat and cholesterol intake. Whole cow's milk can be introduced after age 1 year, and low-fat milk can be introduced after age 2 years. Evaluating the height and weight of infants on a growth chart during clinic visits is an essential part of the assessment of growth and development.

Buying, Storing, and Serving Foods. Baby foods stored in jars are vacuum-packed. Parents are taught to check safety seals before purchase. Directions are generally indicated on the jar (e.g., to reject product if safety button is up). The expiration date of the product should be checked. Dates are usually found on the caps of jars and on the sides of cereal and bakery items. Unopened jars of baby food and juices are stored in a dry, cool place. Jars are rotated, and those on hand the longest are used first.

When a jar is opened, a definite "pop" is heard when the vacuum seal is broken. Food is transferred to a serving dish. The infant should not be fed out of the jar, and leftovers should not be returned to the jar, because saliva may turn certain foods to liquid by digesting them in the jar. Unused portions may be stored in the refrigerator in the original jar. Special precautions are taken when food is heated in the microwave, because food sometimes heats unevenly.

Nursing Tip

- Encourage breastfeeding.
- Discourage overfeeding.
- Teach recognition of satiety signs.
- Prevent early introduction of solid foods.

Weaning. **Weaning** is defined as substituting a cup for a bottle or breastfeeding. Because sucking is a major source of pleasure in the first year of life, weaning is a major step in growth and development. Signs of readiness to wean can be seen in the infant who eagerly looks forward to new tastes and textures found on the spoon. The infant may not want to be held close during feedings and may start to "bite" the nipple as teeth erupt. The approaching stage of autonomy provides the child with motivation to manipulate the cup. Imitation of older siblings or parents also contributes to readiness. Weaning should be very gradual and start with daytime feedings. Weaning is usually completed by 2 years of age but may continue longer in some cultures.

Organic and Natural Foods. Natural foods are defined as those foods that do not contain any additives and that have been altered as little as possible during production. Organic foods are considered to be natural foods whose production is governed by strict regulations. In the case of plants, regulations concern soil, fertilizers, herbicides, and pesticides used for plant growth. In the case of meats, the animal must not have been treated with drugs or hormones before processing (USDA, 2011). Although appearance and taste of organic foods may vary because of production techniques, their nutritive value has not been shown by evidence-based research to be superior to that of nonorganic foods. Parents should be encouraged to read the product labels, because organic foods may not contain recommended dietary allowances for some nutrients and may contain more salt, sugar, or fat than nonorganic foods. Seasonal fruits and vegetables provide the best nutritive value at the lowest cost, and meeting the nutritional needs of the infant should be the primary focus of food selection.

 Nursing Tip

The nutritive value of the food and the nutritional needs of the infant should be the primary focus of food selection.

INFANT SAFETY

CAR SAFETY

Infant seats should be used for all infants traveling in automobiles. A rear-facing infant seat should be used for infants less than 1 year old and weighing less than 22 lb (10 kg), and it should be located in the center of the rear seat of the automobile. Cars with passenger-side safety air bags pose a danger to infants in infant seats that are placed in the front seat. The infant seat should be firmly anchored to the vehicle by the car seat belt (see Chapter 17). Infant car seats are not recommended for use other than for automobile safety. Infants left to sleep in car seats for prolonged periods tend to flex their necks so that the chin rests on the chest, and this can cause oxygen desaturation and hypoxia (Moon, 2011).

FALL PREVENTION

An infant should never be left unattended on a flat surface, such as a changing table. Newborn infants have crawling reflexes that can cause them to fall off a changing table. Infants younger than 4 months have rounded backs and can accidentally roll off a flat surface. Infants older than 4 months can voluntarily roll over. Crib rails should be raised and securely locked. Infants should be secured in high chairs or swings. An infant seat should not be placed on a table or high surface. Crawling infants should be protected from stairways, and neither heavy nor unsteady furniture should be available for them to use to pull themselves to a standing position.

A safe environment for a crawling infant includes storage of poisonous items out of the infant's sight and reach. Cabinet locks are available for purchase. Plants, batteries, pool areas, plugs, loose hanging wires, and pets can be hazardous to an infant. Close supervision at all times is essential to safety in any environment. Resource consultants are available in most communities for information concerning "childproofing" the home.

TOY SAFETY

Toys should be appropriate for developmental level and diagnosis of the child, but safety is the most important feature involved in toy selection. Infants put everything into their mouths, and therefore choking is a major problem if a toy has small or removable parts. When the pincer skill is developed, infants will be able to pick up small objects such as pins and put them in their mouths. Toys appropriate for older siblings can be dangerous to infants. For example, the glue from a model airplane that an older sibling is playing with can be deadly if an infant drinks it. Constant supervision is essential. Toys should nurture growth and development (Table 16-4). A child's response to a toy can indicate readiness to learn new skills. An infant who is able to reach for and pick up a toy shows readiness for communication.

SUMMARY OF MAJOR DEVELOPMENTAL CHANGES IN THE FIRST YEAR

- Weight doubles by age 6 months and triples by age 1 year.
- Height increases by 1 inch per month for first 6 months to reach 74 cm (29 inches) by age 1 year (increase is mainly in the trunk of the body).

Table 16-4   Toys for the First Year

AGE	VISUAL STIMULATION	AUDITORY STIMULATION	SENSORIMOTOR STIMULATION
0-2 months	Black-and-white contrasting mobiles placed at midline of infant's vision	Talk Music Ticking clock	Cuddle, rock
3-5 months	Unbreakable mirrors Infant seat positioned to view room	Talk to infant, provide rattles	Cradle gym, infant swing
6-9 months	Peek-a-boo (teaches object permanence) Encouraging imitation of facial expression	Use appropriate names for objects Speak clearly	Introduce various textures for infant to touch Use teething toys
10-12 months	Large picture books Shopping trips Soft blocks Nested boxes	Reading, singing nursery rhymes Imitating sounds of animals	Push-pull toys Activity boxes

NOTE: Toys for each age group should be varied to stimulate vision, touch, hearing, and movement. Safety for age and diagnosis is of utmost importance in selection of a play activity or toy.

- Head circumference increases 1.5 cm (0.6 inch) each month for the first 6 months and is 46 cm (18 inches) by age 12 months.
- Head circumference and chest circumference are equal by age 1 year.
- Closure of the posterior fontanelle occurs by age 2 months.
- Closure of the anterior fontanelle occurs by age 18 months.
- Voluntary movements replace primitive reflexes.
- Maternal iron stores decrease by age 6 months.
- Digestive processes increase functioning by age 3 months. Amylase and lipase are deficient until age 4 to 6 months, which decreases the ability to digest the fats found in solid foods.
- Tooth eruption begins at age 6 months, when "biting" activities start.
- Binocular vision is established by age 4 months.
- Depth perception begins to develop at age 9 months.
- Infants older than 4 months can voluntarily roll over.
- By age 1 year, infants can take some independent steps.
- *Separation* (of self from others), **object permanence** (objects exist even if they are out of visual field), and *symbols* (saying "bye-bye" means someone is leaving) are major aspects of cognitive development in the first year of life.

Get Ready for the NCLEX® Examination!

Key Points

- The development of a sense of trust begins in infancy and is vital to a healthy personality.
- Sensory stimulation is essential for the development of the infant's thought processes and perceptual abilities.
- Health maintenance visits are essential during the first year to detect variations from normal growth patterns, to provide immunizations, and to educate and support parents.
- For safety and to prevent sudden infant death syndrome (SIDS), infants should be positioned for sleep on their backs on a firm mattress. The infant can be placed on his or her abdomen during playtime.
- An appropriate car seat should be used for automobile safety. The car seat should not be used as a prolonged sleeping arrangement outside of the automobile.
- When using a "sling carrier," care should be taken that the infant's face is above the fabric and that the nose and mouth are unobstructed.
- The nurse must stress to parents the value of immunizations for infants and children.
- Breast milk or formula is the most desirable food for the first 6 months of the infant's life, and it is followed by the gradual introduction of a variety of solid foods.
- Human milk and properly prepared formula supply an adequate fluid intake for the infant under normal conditions. The infant may require additional water during illness or in very hot, humid weather.
- Various commercially prepared infant formulas are available for infants with special dietary needs.
- Seasonal fruits and vegetables provide the best nutritive value at the lowest cost.

- Parents should be encouraged to read food labels, because some foods may not contain recommended dietary allowances for some nutrients.
- Feeding an infant a low-fat diet before age 2 years will compromise growth and development.
- The most common cause of concern is an atypical-for-age slowing of any aspect of development.

Additional Learning Resources

SG Go to your Study Guide for additional learning activities to help you master this chapter content.

evolve Go to your Evolve website (http://evolve.elsevier.com/Leifer) for the following learning resources:
- Animations
- Answer Guidelines for Critical Thinking Questions
- Answers and Rationales for Review Questions for the NCLEX® Examination
- Glossary with English and Spanish pronunciations
- Interactive Review Questions for the NCLEX® Examination
- Patient Teaching Plans in English and Spanish
- Skills Performance Checklists
- Video clips and more!

 Online Resources
- American Association of Poison Control Centers: www.aapcc.org
- Forum on Child and Family Statistics: www.childstats.gov
- Immunization Action Coalition: www.immunize.org
- Recommendations of the Advisory Committee for Immunization Practices (ACIP): www.cdc.gov/vaccines/pubs/ACIP-list.htm
- Vaccines and immunizations: www.cdc.gov/vaccines

Review Questions for the NCLEX® Examination

1. The startle reflex is also known as the:
   1. Moro reflex.
   2. rooting reflex.
   3. pincer reflex.
   4. grasp reflex.

2. A car seat for an infant less than 1 year of age:
   1. is not needed if the infant is held securely in the lap of an adult.
   2. should be placed close to the driver in the front passenger seat.
   3. should face the rear and be placed in the center of the back seat.
   4. should face forward and be placed on the driver's side of the back seat.

3. To detect allergies when feeding new foods:
   1. introduce single-ingredient foods.
   2. mix the food with one the infant likes.
   3. mix the food with formula.
   4. offer two new foods at a time.

4. The nurse is discussing home safety with the mother of a 4-month-old infant. Which of the following is a priority topic?
   1. Placing locks on cabinet doors that contain cleaning supplies
   2. Covering electrical outlets
   3. Raising and securing crib side rails
   4. Encouraging reading and talking to infant

5. A mother expresses concern that her 1-year-old infant is overweight. She states that her family has a tendency to be overweight and wishes to discontinue formula feedings and start the infant on low-fat milk. The nurse assesses that the present weight of the infant is 24 lb. The infant's birth weight was 8 lb, 2 oz. The best response of the nurse would be:
   1. to place the infant on low-fat milk because the infant is slightly overweight at this time.
   2. to place the infant on regular whole milk because the infant's weight is appropriate for his age.
   3. to indicate that the infant is underweight for his age and needs to have supplemental formula added to the diet.
   4. to note that infancy is a period of rapid growth and weight loss will occur as the infant becomes more active.

Critical Thinking Question

1. A mother brings her 8-week-old infant to the clinic and complains that the infant is fussy and acting as if he has colic. What information does the nurse need to obtain from the parent to develop a teaching plan?

Objectives

1. Define each key term listed.
2. Describe the physical, psychosocial, and cognitive development of children from 1 to 3 years of age, listing age-specific events and guidance when appropriate.
3. Describe the task to be mastered by the toddler according to Erikson's stages of growth and development.
4. List two developmental tasks of the toddler period.
5. Discuss speech development in the toddler.
6. Discuss the principles of guidance and discipline for a toddler.
7. Discuss how adults can assist small children in combating their fears.

8. Identify the principles of toilet training (bowel and bladder) that will help guide parents' efforts to provide toilet independence.
9. Describe the nutritional needs and self-feeding abilities of a toddler.
10. List two methods of preventing the following: automobile accidents, burns, falls, suffocation and choking, poisoning, drowning, electric shock, and animal bites.
11. Describe the characteristic play and appropriate toys for a toddler.

Key Terms

autonomy (p. 406)
cooperative play (p. 418)
egocentric thinking (p. 418)
negativism (p. 406)
object permanence (p. 406)

parallel play (p. 418)
ritualism (p. 406)
temper tantrums (p. 410)
time-out (p. 410)
toddlers (p. 406)

GENERAL CHARACTERISTICS

Children between 1 and 3 years of age are referred to as **toddlers**. They are able to get about by using their own powers and are no longer completely dependent persons. By 1 year of age, they have generally tripled their birth weight and gained control of their head, hands, and feet. The remarkably rapid growth and development that took place during infancy begins to slow down. The toddler period presents different challenges for the parents and the child.

The toddler is in Erikson's stage of **autonomy** versus shame and doubt, which is based on a continuum of trust established during infancy (see Chapter 15). Along with the toddler's increasing independence and curiosity to explore the widening environment come many challenging tasks to be mastered, including toilet training, self-feeding, self-dressing, and speech development. One major parental responsibility is to maintain safety while allowing the toddler the opportunity for social and physical independence. Another major parental responsibility is to maintain a positive self-image and body image in the child whose behavior is inconsistent and often frustrating. Toddlers alternate

between dependence and independence. They test their power by saying "no" frequently. This is called **negativism**. Offering limited choices and making use of distraction can be helpful strategies in handling toddlers (too many choices can cause confusion). Developing self-control and socially acceptable outlets for aggression and anger are important factors in the formation of personality and behavior. **Ritualism** is another characteristic of toddler behavior. Toddlers increase their sense of security by making compulsive routines of simple tasks, and therefore their rituals should be respected. Table 17-1 summarizes the toddler's physical development, social behavior, and abilities at various ages.

PHYSICAL DEVELOPMENT

The toddler's body changes proportions (Figure 17-1). The legs and arms lengthen through ossification and growth in the epiphyseal areas of the long bones. The trunk and head grow more slowly. The toddler gains 1.8 to 2.7 kg (4 to 6 lb) per year. The birth weight has quadrupled by 2.5 years of age. The toddler grows 10 cm (4 inches) per year in height. The height of a 2-year-old is thought to be one half of the potential

Table 17-1   Physical Development, Social Behavior, and Abilities of Toddlers

	SOCIAL	FINE MOTOR	GROSS MOTOR	LANGUAGE	COGNITION
12-16 months	Imitates adults' activities Seeks alternate methods of achieving solitary play	Drinks from cup, holds spoon Builds tower of two blocks Prefers finger feeding	Begins to walk	Uses words Is activity oriented Follows simple commands	Classifies objects with function Object permanence begins to develop
16-18 months	Curious Parallel play	Places objects in appropriately shaped openings Improved self-feeding	Walks alone Can walk backward	Uses symbolic language ("bye-bye") Is able to point to familiar objects	Can imitate from memory Begins to realize cause and effect
24 months	Increased independence Egocentric—everything is "mine" Increased autonomy, often says "no"	Builds tower of six to seven blocks Turns pages of book Can undress self	Runs, throws ball Climbs steps Imitates oral hygiene Jumps with both feet	Uses plural words Uses words to tell story Names familiar objects	Continuous investigation and exploring Develops likes and dislikes
36 months	Establishes toilet independence Identifies sexual roles Begins to share May have imaginary playmate Ritualistic behavior	Holds cup by handle and spoon with two fingers Copies a circle	Balances (hops) Jumps on one foot Uses tricycle Climbs stairs using alternate feet	Can hold conversation Frequently asks why and how Says full name	Can understand one idea or concept at a time Knows two colors Imitates parental roles

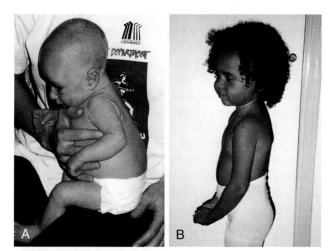

FIGURE 17-1 Change in body contour. **A,** The back of the infant is rounded. **B,** In the toddler, the exaggerated lumbar lordosis makes the abdomen protrude.

adult height of that child. The height and weight are plotted carefully on a growth chart during each clinic visit to reflect what should be a steady pace of growth and development (see Figure 15-3).

The rate of brain growth decelerates. The increase in head circumference during infancy is 10 cm (4 inches), whereas during the second year of life it is only 2.5 cm

(1 inch). Chest circumference continues to increase. After the second year the child appears leaner because the chest circumference begins to exceed the abdominal circumference. The protuberant abdomen flattens when the muscle fibers increase in size and strength.

Myelination of the spinal cord is practically complete by 2 years of age, allowing for control of anal and urethral sphincters. Bowel and bladder control is usually complete by 2.5 to 3 years of age.

Respirations are still mainly abdominal but shift to thoracic as the child approaches school age. The toddler is more capable of maintaining a stable body temperature than is the infant. The shivering process, in which the capillaries constrict or dilate in response to body temperature, has matured.

The skin becomes tough as the epidermis and dermis bond more tightly, which protects the child from fluid loss, infection, and irritation. The defense mechanisms of the skin and blood, particularly phagocytosis, work more effectively than they did during infancy. The lymphatic tissues of the adenoids and tonsils enlarge during this period. The eustachian tubes continue to be shorter and straighter than in the adult. Tonsillitis, otitis media, and upper respiratory infections are common problems. Eruption of deciduous teeth continues until completion at about 2.5 years of age (see Figure 15-12).

The blood pressure of a toddler may average 90/56 mm Hg; the respiratory rate slows to 25 breaths/min, and breathing continues to be abdominal. The pulse of a toddler slows to a range of 70 to 110 beats/min. Digestive processes and the volume capacity of the stomach increase to accommodate a three-meal-a-day schedule.

SENSORIMOTOR AND COGNITIVE DEVELOPMENT

The senses and motor abilities of the toddler do not function independently of one another. Two-year-old toddlers reach, grasp, inspect, smell, taste, and study objects with their eyes. Their attention becomes centered on characteristics of their surroundings that capture their interest. Binocular vision is well established by age 15 months. Visual acuity is about 20/40 by 2 years of age.

As memory strengthens, toddlers can compare present events with stored knowledge. They assimilate information through trial and error plus repetition. They try alternative methods of accomplishing a goal. Thought processes advance, preparing the way for more complex mental operations. The sensorimotor and preconceptual phase of development described by Piaget develops rapidly between 1 and 3 years of age, and the toddler's behavior reflects this.

Separation anxiety, which consists of *protest, despair,* and *detachment,* develops in infancy and continues throughout toddlerhood. Toddlers are able to tolerate longer periods of separation from parents to explore their environment. They become aware of cause and effect. Often they correlate a type of object with its function. For example, if their toys are stored in a paper bag, they will gleefully open any paper bag they see, expecting to find toys. If the bag contains garbage or drugs, they can be injured or may be punished. This can be confusing to the toddler and frustrating to the parents.

The concept of spatial relationships develops, and toddlers are able to fit square pegs in a square hole and round pegs in a round hole. Toys should be selected to promote this ability. **Object permanence** continues to develop, and the toddler becomes aware that there may be fun items behind closed doors and in closed drawers. The toddler's curiosity and ability to explore make it important to educate parents to keep dangerous objects out of their reach. The toddler begins to internalize standards of behavior as evidenced by saying "no-no" when tempted to touch a forbidden object.

The toddler copies the words and the roles of the models seen in the home. The toddler may "help Mommy clean" or "help Daddy shave." By 2 years of age there is recognition of sexual differences.

Toddlers may confuse essential with nonessential body parts. Expelling feces and flushing them down the toilet can be upsetting to some toddlers, because they may feel they expelled a part of themselves that has disappeared. Toddlers' body image and self-esteem may be impaired if they are scolded in a way that makes them feel *they* are bad rather than their *behavior* being bad. The nurse must help the parents develop skills that will enable toddlers to feel they are loved even though the specific behavior is unacceptable.

SPEECH DEVELOPMENT

Language development parallels cognitive growth. The increase in the level of comprehension is particularly striking and exceeds verbalization. By 3 years of age the child has a rather extensive vocabulary of about 900 words. Speech is more than 90% intelligible (Table 17-2). At about the end of the first year, the infant begins to make noises that sound like "bye-bye," "mama," and "da-da." When toddlers see the happy response to these sounds, they repeat them. This is true throughout the toddler period. To want to learn to talk, small children must have an appreciative audience.

Children first refer to animals by the sounds the animals make. For example, before saying "dog," the toddler repeats "bow-bow." Soon the child can say short phrases such as "Daddy gone car." Toddlers also respond to tone of voice and facial expression. If an adult sounds threatening, the toddler may answer "no" and then repeat it in a louder voice.

Sometimes adults scold the child merely for being too young to understand what is requested. However, imagine being punished in a foreign country because you could not speak or comprehend the language well enough to defend yourself. Adults who show empathy to the small child can help to minimize their frustrations.

Parents who are concerned about their child's delayed speech can discuss it with their health care provider during a routine physical examination so it can be evaluated in light of total physical growth and development (Table 17-3). Many late talkers are perfectly normal children who prefer listening rather than active participation. Lead poisoning and hearing deficits should be ruled out before screening for other developmental problems such as autism (Box 17-1). Many common household items, such as vertical window blinds and decorative metal vases, contain lead. Autism Spectrum Disorder is discussed in Chapter 33.

GUIDANCE AND DISCIPLINE

Discipline for the toddler involves guidance. The goal is to teach, not to punish. Teaching the toddler self-control with positive self-esteem is more desirable than encouraging a completely submissive, "obedient" child. The toddler who scribbles on the wall must be given the opportunity to scribble on paper, a more socially acceptable outlet.

Nursing Tip

The toddler is beginning to exercise autonomy and independent functioning. Gentle guidance, positive discipline and patience will help the toddler master the stage of autonomy and maintain a positive self-image.

Table 17-2   Language Milestones

EXPRESSIVE LANGUAGE	AGE (MONTHS)	RECEPTIVE LANGUAGE	AGE (MONTHS)
Social smile	2	Becomes alert	1
Coos	3	Recognizes mother	2
Laughs	4	Orients to voice	4
Razzes	5	Orients to bell	5
"Ah-goo"	5	Looks directly at bell	9
Babbles	6	Understands "no"	9
Dada, mama		Plays gesture games	9
Nonspecific	8	Follows one-step command:	
Specific	10	With gesture	12
First word	11	Without gesture	16
Second word	12	Knows one body part	18
Jargon	15	Points to one picture	18
Four to six words	16	Follows two-step command	24
Two-word phrases	21	Points to seven pictures	24
Two-word sentences	24	Follows prepositional commands	36
Pronouns	36		
Plurals	36		

NOTE: This table of language milestones is a guide to assessing normal language development. Although most mentally handicapped children are language delayed, not all language-delayed children are mentally retarded. Some normal children also are late talkers.
Modified from Montgomery T: When not talking is the chief complaint, *Contemp Pediatr* 11(9):49, 1994; Kliegman R et al: *Nelson's textbook of pediatrics,* ed 19, Philadelphia, 2011, Saunders/Elsevier.

Table 17-3   When a Child with a Communication Disorder Needs Help

AGE	BEHAVIOR INDICATING HELP IS NEEDED
0-11 months	Before 6 months the child does not startle, blink, or change immediate activity in response to sudden loud sounds. Before 6 months the child does not attend to the human voice and is not soothed by his or her mother's voice. By 6 months the child does not babble strings of consonant and vowel syllables or imitate gurgling or cooing sounds. By 10 months the child does not respond to his or her name. At 10 months the sounds the child makes are limited to shrieks, grunts, or sustained vowel production.
12-23 months	At 12 months the child's babbling or speech is limited to vowel sounds. By 15 months the child does not respond to "no," "bye-bye," or "bottle." By 15 months the child will not imitate sounds or words. By 18 months the child is not consistently using at least six words with appropriate meaning. By 21 months the child does not respond correctly to "Give me...," "Sit down," or "Come here," when spoken without gestural cues. By 23 months, two-word phrases have not emerged that are spoken as single units (e.g., "Whatzit," "Thank you," "All gone").
24-36 months	By 24 months, familiar listeners do not understand at least 50% of the child's speech. By 24 months the child does not point to body parts without gestural cues. By 24 months the child is not combining words into phrases ("Go bye-bye," "Go car," "Want cookie"). By 30 months the child does not demonstrate understanding of *on, in, under, front, back.* By 30 months the child is not using short sentences ("Daddy went bye-bye"). By 30 months the child has not begun to ask questions, using where, what, why. By 36 months unfamiliar listeners do not understand the child's speech.

NOTE: At any age the child is consistently dysfluent (not clear) with repetitions, hesitations, or blocks, or struggles to say words. Struggle may be accompanied by grimaces, eye blinks, or hand gestures.
Data from Kliegman R, Marcdante K, Jenson H, Behrman R: *Nelson's essentials of pediatrics,* ed 5, Philadelphia, 2011, Saunders; Kliegman R et al: *Nelson's textbook of pediatrics,* ed 19, Philadelphia, 2011, Saunders/Elsevier; American Speech and Language Association: *How does your child hear and talk?* 2011. Accessed 5/13 at www.ASHA.org/public/speech/devel/chart.htm.

Box 17-1	Screening for Signs of Autism

- No pointing, gesturing (bye-bye) by 12 months
- No single words by 16 months
- No spontaneous two-word phrases by 24 months
- Loss of achieved language or social skills

NOTE: These are preliminary symptoms. Lead poisoning or hearing deficits should be ruled out.
Data from Kantz B: Autism spectrum disorders: early screening for early intervention, *Nurseweek* 21(3):38-39, 2008; Inglese M: Caring for children with autism spectrum disorder: screening, diagnosis and management, *J Ped Nurs* 24:49-59, 2009; Golnik A, Maccabee-Ryboy N: Autism: clinical pearls for primary care, *Contemp Ped* 42:60, 2010.

Temper tantrums (uncontrolled anger reactions) often occur during the toddler years, and parent responses reinforce to the child either the desirability or the risks involved with such behavior. Expectations must be commensurate with the child's physical and cognitive abilities. Toddlers get into many situations that are over their heads. When adults make firm decisions, the problem is resolved, at least for the time being. The child feels secure.

Setting limits should include praise for desired behavior as well as disapproval for undesired behavior. A **time-out** period in a safe place helps the child to develop the ability to tolerate delayed gratification and self-regulation. Timing should not begin until the child has settled down. The child is praised after he or she is calm. Timing for time-out is usually based on 1 minute per year of age.

Children, like adults, seek approval. It is effective and helps to increase their self-confidence. The positive approach should be taken as often as possible. One assumes that the toddler is going to be good rather than bad. "Thank you, Johnny, for giving me the matches" will make them arrive in your hand more quickly than "Give me those matches right now," said in a threatening tone. The use of fear or physical aggression should not be a part of discipline, because it does not foster self-control and can lead to physical or mental abuse of the child.

Fear is a valuable emotion to the child if it does not become too intense. Unfortunately, many children fear situations that are not in themselves dangerous, and this sometimes deprives them of activities that otherwise would be enjoyable. If the parent warns, "Be careful, don't fall," when a toddler begins to ride a tricycle, the toddler may develop a fear of taking risks that may be involved when experiencing new activities.

The physical and mental health of the child at the time of a fear-provoking experience affects the extent of the reaction. If the child is alone, fear may be greater than if someone such as a parent or nurse is present. After a fear has been learned, it is more difficult to eliminate. Clinging to favorite possessions and repetitive rituals are self-consoling behaviors for the toddler, particularly at bedtime and during separation from parents.

Stress increases fear of separation. Adults should attempt to control their own fears while in the presence of young children. Respect and understanding should always be accorded to children who are afraid. Making fun of the fear or shaming the child in front of others is detrimental to self-esteem.

Many toddlers who independently explore the clinic examining room while waiting to be examined may cling to the parent when the stranger (the health care provider) enters the room and approaches the child. The toddler who does not seek the parent during stressful situations or turns to a stranger for comfort reflects a need for closer evaluation of the parent–child relationship.

The "terrible twos," during which negativistic behavior is predominant, begin the disciplinary pattern of the family that will carry throughout childhood and affect the child's personality. Corporal punishment, involving spanking, is accepted in many traditional cultures as the mainstay of discipline. However, regular spanking reflects a desperate effort by the parent to gain control over a toddler who is exercising his or her beginning autonomy (independent functioning) and developing negativism. Potential injury, child abuse, and reciprocal aggressive behavior in the child can be avoided with careful parental guidance concerning alternative techniques of discipline. Time-out, limit setting, clear communication, and frequent rewards and approval for positive behavior are effective noncorporal techniques of discipline.

Communicating love and respect to the child with a clear message that it is the behavior, not the child, that the adult disapproves of are the keys to effective discipline. Behavior problems that can occur during early childhood are detailed in Table 17-4.

⌂	Nursing Tip

Caregivers must provide safe areas for the toddler to explore. They need to watch carefully before saying "no."

DAILY CARE

Nutrition, dentition, and oral care are discussed in Chapter 15. When talking to the toddler, the adult should be at eye level with the child so the adult seems less overwhelming. This is of particular importance when the child is in a fear-provoking environment, such as the hospital. A flexible schedule organized around the needs of the entire household is best for the toddler. The toddler needs a consistent routine, but it can differ for special occasions.

The clothing of toddlers should be simple and easy for them to put on and take off. Pants with elastic waists are convenient for them to pull down when they use the toilet. All clothing must be fairly loose to provide freedom of movement for jumping and other strenuous activities. Sunburn protection with clothing or sunscreen is necessary to prevent skin damage.

Table 17-4   Behavior Problems During Early Childhood, Normal Expectations, and Parental Guidance

BEHAVIOR	NORMAL EXPECTATIONS	FACTORS CONTRIBUTING TO PROBLEM	PARENTAL GUIDANCE
Sleep disorders	Occasional nightmares begin at about 36 months. Ritual bedtime routine begins; attempt to delay sleep peaks between 2 and 3 years. Head banging and rocking between 1 and 4 years provide a release of tension.	Excessive napping during the day Insufficient adult interaction during the day, leading to the use of bedtime as opportunity to gain adult attention Unusual fears related to darkness, being left alone Discomfort of wet diapers Illness	Provide one nap a day until end of second year, when naps can be eliminated. Use of bedtime rituals, such as a quiet activity or bedtime stories, is helpful. Use of favorite toy or blanket in the bed can ease insecurities involved in separation. Provide environment conducive to sleep. Avoid scary television shows. Restrict fluids before bedtime.
Temper tantrums	Tantrums peak at 2 years of age, decreasing in frequency and intensity until they rarely occur by about 4 years of age. Tantrums usually occur in response to the frustrated desires of a child, such as wanting a toy that cannot be purchased.	Used as a manipulative device to gain control of parental behavior Insufficient positive interaction with adults, leading to use of tantrums to gain attention	Use simple explanations of behavior expectations. Use "time-out" responses (1 minute per year of age). Maintain consistency of expectations from both parents. Reward good behavior.
Toilet training and bed wetting	Child has full physiological capacity for day control by age 3 years, night control by age 4 years. Daytime and nighttime "accidents" occur throughout early childhood, decreasing in frequency by age 4 years. Regression occurs with environmental or social changes, such as arrival of sibling, moving, or divorce.	Fears and anxiety in response to negative toilet training Used as an attention-getting device if positive means of gaining attention are lacking May use constipation as a control mechanism Excessive fluid intake before bedtime	Use positive rewards for successful toileting and do not criticize child for accidents. Recognize signals of need to use toilet. Restrict fluids before bedtime. Use clothing that toddler can easily remove for self-toileting.
Aggressive or quarrelsome behavior, sibling rivalry	Ability to play cooperatively begins to emerge at 3-5 years. Before this age, the child is seldom able to share toys and often wants toys that another child has. There is a predominant use of physical hitting and shoving to express displeasure; verbal abilities begin to emerge.	Insufficient positive adult attention, leading to deliberate use of aggression to gain adult attention May arise from actual or perceived adult preference for sibling or playmate	Prepare toddler for the separation and change involved in the arrival of a new sibling. Provide for any changes involved 1-2 months before arrival of sibling (e.g., change to a new bed or room). Provide toddler with doll to imitate parental behaviors. Provide for special individual time with toddler each day.
Inability to separate, excessive shyness	Child can separate easily by age 3 years if surroundings are consistent, predictable, and positive. Child continues to protest separation if environment changes or if confronted by total strangers. Child is shy in new and strange surroundings but relaxed and spontaneous in familiar surroundings.	Inadequate establishment of self-concept, leading to lack of confidence, even in familiar surroundings Uses protest of separation as a manipulative control device Fear of being abandoned	Prepare toddler for anticipated separation. Refer to time using concrete terms ("I will return after lunch" rather than "I will return at 1 PM"). Avoid radiating parental anxiety at the planned separation. Spend time with toddler and in new environment or with new caregiver before leaving.

Data from Chinn P, Leitch C: *Child health maintenance,* ed 2, St Louis, 1979, Mosby; Mundy P, Jarrold W: Infant joint attention, neural networks and social cognition, *Neural Networks* 23(8-9):985-997, 2010; Santrock J: *Child development,* ed 13, New York, 2011, McGraw Hill.

The toddler wears shoes mainly for protection. They should fit the shape of the foot and be half an inch longer and a quarter of an inch wider than the foot. They must fit securely at the heel. Children should wear their usual shoes at their periodic checkups, because these show how the shoes have been worn, which indicates to the health care provider how the children are using their bodies. The toddler may go barefoot whenever it is safe and possible, because this strengthens the foot muscles. Socks must be large enough that they do not flex the toes. The toddler should be taught to pull socks free from the toes before putting on shoes.

Good posture is the result of proper nutrition, plenty of fresh air and exercise, and sufficient rest. The toddler's mattress must be firm. The chair and play table are adapted to size. In some cases, this can be easily accomplished by placing a rolled-up blanket or pad in the seat of the chair. A small, sturdy stool placed in the bathroom will bring the child to the proper height for brushing the teeth. As in all areas of learning, the child's posture is greatly influenced by that of other members of the family. The toddler who is happy and is allowed gradually increasing independence develops a sense of security, which is reflected in the posture. Slouching is sometimes seen in children who are insecure and lack self-confidence.

TOILET INDEPENDENCE

There are many approaches to toilet training. Much depends on the temperament of both the individual child and the person guiding the child. Readiness is important. Voluntary control of anal and urethral sphincters begins at about 18 to 24 months. If the child wakes up dry in the morning or after naptime, it is an indication of maturity. Children must be able to communicate in some fashion that they are wet or need to urinate or defecate. They must be willing to sit on the potty for several minutes at a time.

Toddlers seek approval and like to imitate the actions of parents. They wander into the bathroom and are curious about what is taking place there. If a parent feels that the child will respond to training at this time, the parent might first put the child in training pants or pull-up diapers. These can be removed quickly and easily, and the child becomes more aware of being wet.

The use of a child's potty chair or a device that attaches to an adult toilet seat is a matter of personal preference (Figure 17-2). A potty chair may make the toddler feel more secure because it is small. It should support the back and arms of the child. The child's feet should touch the floor. If a potty chair is not available, the child can be placed on the standard-size toilet, facing the toilet tank. This method may increase feelings of security. The toddler can use a regular toilet with a bench to support the child's feet.

Bowel training is generally attempted first; however, some toddlers become bladder trained during the day

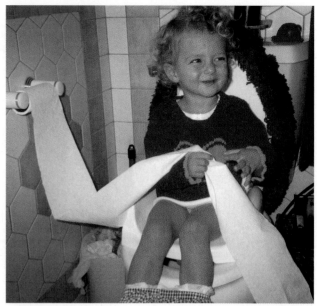

FIGURE 17-2 Toilet training. Toilet training should be a nonstressful experience for the toddler. Nurses can help parents identify readiness for toilet independence. The nurse assesses the parents' expectations, family and cultural preferences, and developmental readiness of the child when instructing parents. Sitting on the potty too long without supervision may result in bathroom playtime!

because they enjoy listening to the "tinkle" in the potty. If toddlers have bowel movements at the same time each day, they may progress fairly rapidly. They should not be left on the potty chair for more than a few minutes at a time.

Bladder training is begun when the toddler stays dry for about 2 hours at a time. The parent may discover that the toddler has gone the entire night without wetting. It is then logical to put the child on the potty chair and to praise success. Bladder training varies widely, particularly during the night. Restricting fluids before bedtime may help. Placing the half-asleep child on the potty chair accomplishes little.

Most children continue to have occasional accidents until age 4 years. If the toddler has a mishap, parents should accept it matter-of-factly and merely change the clothes. Children benefit when adults show continuous affection to them and accept both bad and good days.

The word that toddlers use to signal defecation or urination should be one that is recognized by others besides the immediate family. Sometimes a parent may forget to inform the babysitter or nursery school teacher of the word that the child uses. This causes toddlers unnecessary frustration because those around them cannot understand what they are trying to say.

Toddlers who are toilet trained at home should continue to use the potty in the hospital setting. Wetting the bed may acutely embarrass them. Although regression of bowel and bladder training is common during hospitalization, personnel often contribute to it by not taking time to investigate the child's needs. Nurses regularly consult the child's nursing care plan to maintain continuity of care as well as to promote growth and development of the toddler.

Demands and threats do more damage than good. Life is smoother for all if the parent remains patient and keeps this new adventure pleasant. Training should not be undertaken when the family or child is under stress, such as during illness or a move to a new location.

 Nursing Tip

Nurses can help parents identify readiness for toilet independence.

NUTRITION COUNSELING

Caloric requirements per unit of body weight decline from 120 calories/kg per day during infancy to 100 calories/kg per day in the toddler. Children need an adequate protein intake to cover maintenance needs and to provide for optimum growth. Milk should be limited to no more than 720 mL (24 oz) a day. Too few solid foods can lead to dietary deficiencies of iron. Children between 1 and 3 years of age are high-risk candidates for anemia.

The toddler who is well nourished shows steady proportional gains on height and weight charts and has good bone and tooth development. The diet history should be adequate, avoiding excessive calories and large amounts of vitamins.

The toddler normally has a fluctuating appetite with strong food preferences. The nurse reminds parents that any nutritious food can be eaten at any meal; for example, soup for breakfast and cereal for dinner are acceptable. Serving size is important (Table 17-5). Too-large servings are discouraged, because they may overwhelm the child and can lead to overeating problems. One tablespoon of solid food for each year of the child's age serves as a measurement guide. A quiet time before meals provides an opportunity for the child to "wind down." The toddler's refusal to eat may result from fatigue or not being particularly hungry. The toddler might eat one food with vigor one week and refuse it the next. The individual family must work out a flexible schedule designed to meet the needs of the toddler and the rest of the family. Forcing toddlers to eat only creates further difficulties. They are quick to sense parents' frustration and may use mealtime to obtain attention by behaving poorly and refusing to eat. Discipline and arguments during mealtime only upset everyone's digestion.

Toddlers are fond of ritual. This is often seen at mealtime. They want a particular dish, glass, and bib. It is best to go along with their wishes as long as they do not become too pronounced. It gives them a sense of security and, in the long run, saves time and energy for the adult.

Toddlers have brief attention spans. They rarely sit at the table or stay in the high chair for long periods. They may try to stand in the high chair or may wander away from the table. They may be excused if they have eaten a fair amount of the meal; otherwise distraction of some type may be necessary. Toddlers who regularly feed themselves may enjoy being helped by mommy or daddy. Some restaurants that cater to families provide crayons and special place mats to keep the small child occupied until the adults finish their dinners. In the hospital, the toddler who is fed in a high chair wears an appropriate safety restraint, and the nurse remains with the child during the meal.

The toddler's food is chopped into fine pieces. Various foods are offered, and one should try to plan contrasts of colors and textures. A 2-year-old likes finger foods. Foods are served at moderate temperatures. Candy, cake, and soda between meals should be avoided. (See Chapter 15 for a food guide.)

Children like to eat from colorful dishes, which must be made of an unbreakable substance. Washable plastic bibs, place mats, and protection for the floor around the high chair are advisable. Eating utensils should be small enough that they can be handled easily. Seating equipment should be adjusted so the child is comfortable and maintains good posture.

 Nursing Tip

When determining the size of portions, toddlers and young children should be offered 1 tablespoon of solid food per year of age.

Table 17-5 Approximate Serving Sizes per Meal

	AGE 1 YEAR	AGE 2-3 YEARS
Bread	1 slice	1 slice
Cereal	1 oz	1 oz
Rice or pasta	1 cup	1 cup
Vegetables	2 tablespoons	3 tablespoons
Fruit	1 cup	1 cup
Milk	1 cup	1 cup
Meat, beans	2 tablespoons	3 tablespoons

NOTE: Approximate serving sizes per meal for a toddler (see Figure 15-7).

THE PICKY EATER VERSUS A FEEDING DISORDER

A "picky eater" is one who is selective about foods and their color, taste, texture, or smell but eats sufficient foods and fluids to maintain growth and development. A child who refuses to eat or drink a variety of foods or liquids to maintain adequate growth and development may have a feeding disorder. A feeding disorder results in weight loss for more than 1 month. According to *DSM-5*, a "feeding disorder" is relabeled as an "avoidance/resistance to food intake" that occurs before 6 years of age. A study of the GI tract for anomalies should be performed before using strategies to increase appetite.

Orexigenic medication to increase appetite, uniform feeding expectations and feeding environment, and gradually exposing the child to the smell, textures, and taste of new foods can increase the acceptance and intake of new foods (Kreipe, 2012).

DAY CARE

Family life has changed dramatically since the 1970s. Today many more children are cared for in community settings outside of the home. From 2000 to 2010, the fastest-growing group of persons in the labor force has been women with infants. Not only were more mothers working, but they were also returning to the work force sooner after the child was born. It was clear that alternative methods of child care were necessary. These arrangements must meet families' personal preferences, cultural perspectives, and financial and special needs. Parents must take an active role in ensuring high-quality care. Nurses need to be resource persons and family advocates, because finding adequate day care can be stressful.

The decision to place a toddler in the care of others while parents work can be difficult and produce feelings of guilt in the parent. The concept of such care is not new. Many cultures have some type of arrangement, for example the Israelis, who have traditionally placed toddlers in day care while working on a "kibbutz." The hours of care extend from early morning to the dinner hour. Successful alternative child care arrangements depend on specific guidelines in selecting the facility (see Chapter 18), frequent visits to the facility, and close communication and conferences with the staff in the facility. Day care for the toddler differs somewhat from what is appropriate for the preschool child because of the toddler's shorter attention span, the tendency to engage in *parallel play* rather than group play, and the need for closer supervision to maintain safety (Figure 17-3).

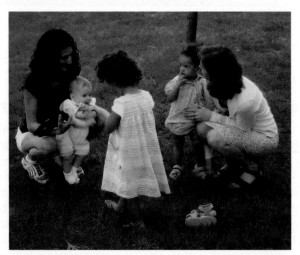

FIGURE 17-3 Beginning social skills, parallel play, and short attention spans of toddlers require them to have close supervision in day care settings.

There are various types of child care. Relatives, friends, neighbors, or those who have advertised such services can care for many children today. However, there is little research on these types of home arrangements and few standards of quality control. Most licensed day care centers are private businesses run for profit. They are subject to state regulations about physical layout, number of children per caretaker, education of personnel, and other factors. Parents must plan ahead for times when the child is sick and unable to attend. A few innovative programs for the in-home care of sick children have been developed. Employer-supported child care is a rapidly growing area, and these programs are very diverse. Some companies provide family day care (care of the child in the provider's home). Other employers assist parents through reimbursement, referral programs, or support of existing child care programs in the community.

For low- and some middle-income families, the cost of child care is difficult if not impossible to maintain. Some form of continued or expanded government assistance or private funding is necessary. Inspection and monitoring of child care facilities to ensure compliance with health (physical and mental) and safety standards are paramount. Ideally, all day care programs would include comprehensive health services and health education programs. Criteria for selecting a day care center are similar to those discussed for nursery schools (see Chapter 18).

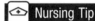

Nursing Tip

It is a major task for parents to "let go" and allow the toddler to interact with influences outside the family in day care centers or preschools.

INJURY PREVENTION

Accidents kill and cripple more children than any disease known and are the leading cause of death in childhood. The best prevention is knowledge of age-appropriate risks and anticipatory guidelines. If parents understand their child's activities at certain ages, they can prevent many serious injuries by taking necessary precautions (see Health Promotion box).

Nurses have an important responsibility to review injury prevention with parents during each clinic visit. The normal behavior characteristics of a toddler, including curiosity, mobility, and negativity, make the toddler prone to injuries that often occur in and around the home (Figure 17-4).

Car safety is important. The use of seat belts is effective if they are worn properly. A shoulder strap that extends across the neck or a lap belt that fits high on the abdomen or waist area can be harmful rather than helpful. A child seat placed in the front car seat close to the passenger air bag can be dangerous.

Health Promotion

How to Prevent Hazards Caused by the Behavioral Characteristics of Toddlers

BEHAVIORAL CHARACTERISTICS	HAZARD AND PREVENTION STRATEGIES
TRAFFIC AND AUTOMOBILE Impulsive Unable to delay gratification Increased mobility Egocentric	Teach child street safety rules. Teach child the meaning of red, yellow, and green traffic lights. Caution children not to run from behind parked cars or snow banks. Use car seat restraints appropriately. Hold toddler's hand when crossing the street. Supervise tricycle riding. Do not allow children to play in the car alone. Driver must look carefully in front and behind vehicles before accelerating. Teach children what areas are safe in and around the house. Supervise child under age 3 years at all times.
BURNS Fascination with fire Can reach articles by climbing Pokes fingers in holes and openings Can open doors and drawers Unaware of cause and effect	Teach the child the meaning of "hot" (one mother taught this by allowing the child to touch beach sand warmed by the sun). Put matches, cigarettes, candles, and incense out of reach and sight. Turn handles of cooking utensils toward the back of the stove. Beware of hot liquids; avoid using tablecloths with overhang. Keep appliances such as coffee pots, electric frying pans, and food processors and their cords out of reach. Test food and fluids heated in microwave ovens to ensure that center is not too hot. Beware of hot charcoal grills or gas barbecues. Use snug fireplace screens. Mark children's rooms to alert firefighters in emergency. Keep a pressure-type fire extinguisher available, and teach all family members who are old enough how to use it. Practice what to do in case of fire in the home. Install smoke detectors. Cover electrical outlets with protective caps. Check bath water temperature before placing child in water. Do not allow child to handle water faucets.
FALLS Like to explore different parts of the house Can open doors and lean out open windows Have immature depth perception Capabilities change quickly May seem quite grown up at times but still require constant supervision at home and on the playground	Teach children how to go up and come down stairs when they show a readiness for this task. Fasten crib sides securely and leave them up when child is in the crib. Use side rails on a large bed when child graduates from crib. Lock basement doors or use gates at top and bottom of stairs. Mop spilled water from floor immediately. Use window guards. Use car seat restraints appropriately. Keep scissors and other pointed objects out of the toddler's reach. Use childproof doorknobs and drawer closures. Secure child in shopping cart at store. Supervise climbing child in playground. Keep clothing and shoelaces appropriate to prevent tripping.
SUFFOCATION AND CHOKING Explores with senses; likes to bite on and taste things Eats on the run	Do not allow small children to play with deflated balloons; these can be sucked into airway. Inspect toys for small or loose parts. Remove small objects such as coins, buttons, and pins from reach. Avoid popcorn, nuts, small hard candies, chewing gum, or large chunks of meat, such as hot dogs. Debone fish and chicken. Learn the Heimlich maneuver and cardiopulmonary resuscitation (CPR). Inspect width of crib and playpen slats. Keep plastic bags away from small children; do not use as mattress cover. If child is vomiting, turn him or her on side. Do not use nightclothes with drawstring necks. Discard old refrigerators and appliances, or remove doors.

Continued

Health Promotion—cont'd

BEHAVIORAL CHARACTERISTICS	HAZARD AND PREVENTION STRATEGIES
POISONING	
Ingenuity increases, can open most containers	Store household detergents and cleaning supplies out of reach and in a locked cabinet.
Increased mobility provides child access to cupboards, medicine cabinets, bedside stands, interior of closets	Do not put chemicals or other potentially harmful substances into food or beverage containers.
Looks at and touches everything	Keep medicines in a locked cabinet; put them away immediately after use.
Learns by trial and error	Use child-resistant caps and packaging.
Puts objects in mouth	Flush old medicine down toilet.
	Follow health care provider's directions when administering medication.
	Do not refer to pills as "candy."
	Explain poison symbols to child and to parents not fluent in English.
	Keep telephone number of poison control center available.
	When painting, use paint marked "for indoor use" or one that conforms to standards for use on surfaces that may be chewed on by children.
	Wash fruits and vegetables before eating.
	Obtain and record name of any new plant purchased.
	Alert family to location and appearance of poisonous plants on or around property or frequently encountered when camping.
	Use childproof locks on cabinets.
	Use dishes that do not have high lead content.
DROWNING	
Lacks depth perception	Watch child continuously while at beach or near a pool.
Does not realize danger	Empty wading pools when child has finished playing.
Loves water play	Cover wells securely.
	Wear recommended life jackets in boats.
	Begin teaching water safety and swimming skills early.
	Lock fences surrounding swimming pools.
	Supervise tub baths; be aware that a young child can drown in a very small amount of water.
ELECTRIC SHOCK	
Pokes and probes with fingers	Cover electrical outlets.
	Cap unused sockets with safety plugs.
	Water conducts electricity; teach child not to touch electrical appliances when hands are wet; keep appliances out of reach.
	Keep electrical appliances away from tub and sink area.
ANIMAL BITES	
Has immature judgment	Teach child to avoid stray animals.
	Do not allow toddler to abuse household pets.
	Supervise closely.
SAFETY	
Easily distracted	Teach toddler stranger safety.
Trusting of others	Do not personalize clothes.
Falls frequently	Do not allow toddler to eat or suck lollipops while running or playing.
	Keep sharp-edged objects out of reach.
	Keep sharp-edged furniture out of play area.

NOTE: Keep first aid chart and emergency numbers handy. Know location of and how to get to nearest emergency facility.

Nurses demonstrate safety measures to their patients and their families. This is most effectively done by good example. Safety measures pertinent to the pediatric unit are discussed in Chapter 22. Nurses in the community can often contribute indirectly to the welfare of others by the example they set and by being aware of emergency medical facilities available in the community.

CONSUMER EDUCATION

The federal government and concerned private agencies have attempted to regulate some of the variables that cause injuries. A few examples are ensuring the use of non-flammable material for children's sleepwear, mandating childproof caps on medicine bottles and certain household products, and establishing maximum temperatures for

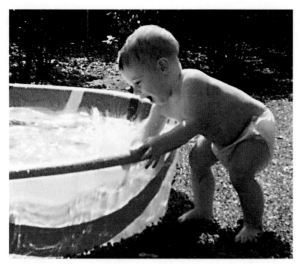

FIGURE 17-4 The playful toddler needs close supervision during water play. Falling into a kiddie pool can result in serious injury.

The use of car seats begins with the first ride home from the hospital. The car seat should be rear facing for children less than up to 2 years of age with a 5-point restraint harness. A booster seat can be used when the child outgrows the car seat until the automobile safety belt restraints fit properly. After a child is large enough for a car safety belt to fit correctly (usually heavier than 36.3 kg [80 lb] and taller than 142.5 cm [57 inches]), a shoulder and lap belt system is ideal. Incorrectly used safety belts can cause injury to a child (AAP, 2011).

New homes are required to have smoke and carbon monoxide detectors when they are built. Consumers who live in older homes and apartment complexes are also encouraged to install them. Various other safety codes are mandatory for public buildings, with additional measures required for buildings specifically for the disabled. Nevertheless, the problems of surveillance and upkeep are considerable. Many children live in substandard housing with little supervision. The education of parents is of monumental importance in decreasing death and disability.

home hot-water heaters. Smoke detectors in homes and public places are commonplace. The United States Consumer Product Safety Commission has established regulations for crib slats, locks and latches, and crib mattress size and thickness. Safety warnings on the crib's carton advise buyers to use a snug mattress only. The nurse should reinforce this type of information.

Laws have been passed in virtually all states that require infants and small children to be restrained while riding in automobiles (Figure 17-5). These restraints must follow standards established by the Federal Motor Vehicle Safety Department and follow American Academy of Pediatrics (AAP) guidelines. Rental car companies also lend child seat restraints to their customers.

TOYS AND PLAY

In 1970 the Child Protection and Toy Safety Act was passed in an effort to halt the distribution of unsafe toys. In addition, parents must be taught to inspect toys routinely for damage and to buy toys suitable for the age, skills, and abilities of the individual child. Some labels now provide safety information and age guidelines for the intended user. In general, notification of recall for a specific toy is announced on radio and television and is published in newspapers and consumer journals.

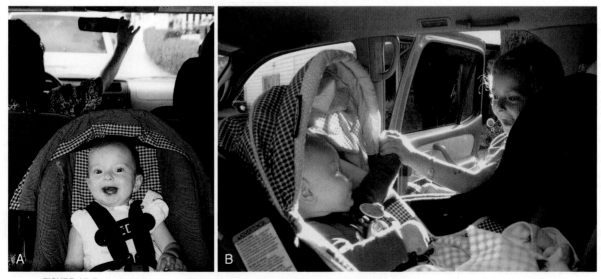

FIGURE 17-5 A, The infant's car seat faces the rear of the car to prevent the infant's large and heavy head from falling forward when the car stops suddenly or in case of an accident. The driver can look through the rearview mirror of the car toward a mirror mounted on the rear window or the seat back to see the face of the infant in a rear-facing car seat. Note that the metal clip or lock of the car seat belt is not under the chin of the infant, but rests firmly on the chest. **B,** The toddler's car seat can face front in the center of the rear seat of the car and secured by the car's seat belt. The infant's car seat remains rear facing behind the driver.

Toy boxes and toy chests are another potential hazard. The most serious injuries caused by a box or chest are the result of the lid falling on a child or a child being trapped inside. A parent can report a product hazard by writing to the United States Consumer Product Safety Commission, Washington, DC, 20207.

Play is the work of a toddler. Through play, toddlers learn how to manipulate and understand their environment, socialize, and explore their world. High-priced toys are not necessary. Toddlers prefer pots and pans from the kitchen, supervised water play, dancing to music, and crayons or finger paint and paper. A picture book reviewed while on the lap of a family member can often be enjoyed over and over again. Tricycles can be adapted to the size and ability of the toddler. Objects that can be pushed or pulled are preferred to wind-up toys for this age group, because walking and running are the developmental tasks at hand. Providing materials such as fur, sandpaper, felt, and nylon can stimulate the sense of touch. Colors can be taught while having the toddler help to sort the laundry. Pointing to familiar pictures in a book, newspaper, or magazine can stimulate memory. Counting can be taught while climbing stairs. Supervision and maintenance of safety are the keys to a positive play experience for the toddler. Particular attention should be given whenever a pet is part of the environment (Figure 17-6).

As toddlers become aware of their expanding environment, their social development takes form. **Egocentric thinking**, in which children relate everything to themselves, predominates. They engage in **parallel play**, playing next to, but not with, their peers. They gradually develop **cooperative play**, which involves imagination and sharing skills. Toddlers do not yet understand property rights and therefore believe all toys are theirs to play with. Frequent frustrations can lead to temper tantrums. It is important to calm and distract the child when he becomes frustrated rather than just removing him abruptly from the play area.

Nurses must closely assess children with special needs for safety precautions. Caregivers of children with disabilities require extended instruction according to the child's particular needs; these children include those with visual, motor, or intellectual impairments, convulsive disorders, or diabetes mellitus. Immobile children must be protected from sunburn and wind or rainy weather. Adults must also guard these children

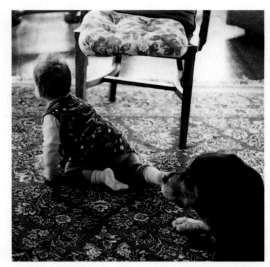

FIGURE 17-6 Close supervision is necessary when a child plays in any home where there is a pet, whether large or small. Both the toddler and the pet have unpredictable behavior.

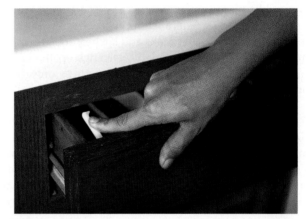

FIGURE 17-7 Childproofing the home. A simple drawer or cabinet latch prevents access to the contents by the young child while the contents still remain accessible to the adult, who can press and release the latch with one finger. (From Harkreader H, Hogan MA: *Fundamentals of nursing: caring and clinical judgment*, ed 3, Philadelphia, 2007, Saunders.)

from mosquitoes and other disease vectors. Injury prevention involves some of the methods mentioned in the discussion of consumer education: the use of items such as electric outlet covers, cabinet locks, drawer locks, and the creation of a hazard-free or "childproof" environment for the child (Figure 17-7).

Get Ready for the NCLEX® Examination!

Key Points

- The birth weight has quadrupled by age 2.5 years.
- Physical changes of the toddler include the acquisition of fine and gross motor skills, among which are increased mobility and increased eye–hand coordination.
- The digestive volume and processes of the toddler increase to accommodate a three-meal-a-day schedule.
- Complete bowel and bladder control is usually achieved by age 2.5 to 3 years.
- Erikson refers to the toddler stage as one in which the child's task is to acquire a sense of autonomy (self-control) while overcoming shame and doubt.
- The most evident cognitive achievements of the toddler involve language and comprehension.

- Some important self-regulatory functions mastered by the toddler include toilet independence, self-feeding, tolerating delayed gratification, separation from parents, and perfecting newfound physical skills and speech.
- Separation anxiety includes the stages of protest, despair, and detachment.
- Parental guidance is needed to handle the negativism, temper tantrums, and sibling rivalry that are characteristic of this age group.
- Discipline for the toddler should be designed to teach rather than punish.
- Some methods of dealing with the inconsistencies of the toddler include distraction, reward and praise, and time-out in a safe place.
- Accidents and poisoning are the leading causes of death in the toddler age group.
- Infants and young children should ride in a car safety seat for all car trips.

Additional Learning Resources

SG Go to your Study Guide for additional learning activities to help you master this chapter content.

evolve Go to your Evolve website (http://evolve.elsevier.com/Leifer) for the following learning resources:
- Animations
- Answer Guidelines for Critical Thinking Questions
- Answers and Rationales for Review Questions for the NCLEX® Examination
- Glossary with English and Spanish pronunciations
- Interactive Review Questions for the NCLEX® Examination
- Patient Teaching Plans in English and Spanish
- Skills Performance Checklists
- Video clips and more!

 Online Resources
- Alliance for Children and Families: www.alliance1.org
- American Academy of Family Physicians: www.aafp.org
- *Car Safety Seats: Information for Families:* www.aap.org/family/Carseatguide.htm
- Resources for toddler development: www.zerotothree.org

Review Questions for the NCLEX® Examination

1. A parent states she is having a conflict with her toddler who seems to "always want to do things his way." He insists on putting on his right sock and shoe before his left and has a tantrum if the parent tries to put on the left sock and shoe first. The parent asks the nurse why the child is acting this way. The best response of the nurse would be to:
   1. explain to the child that it really doesn't matter which sock and shoe is donned first.
   2. put the child in a "time-out" for the appropriate time.
   3. explain that this is normal ritualistic behavior at this age and should be respected.
   4. let the child walk barefoot and take the shoes away.

2. The nurse assesses the vital signs of a 2-year-old. A normal respiratory rate (per minute) would be:
   1. 18 to 20.
   2. 25 to 30.
   3. 35 to 40.
   4. 45 to 50.

3. Which statement by the parent would indicate a need for further guidance?
   1. I use a car seat for my toddler whenever we are in the car, and he is right beside me as I drive so I can keep an eye on him.
   2. I use a car seat for my toddler whenever we are in the car and secure it onto the rear seat of the car.
   3. I use a car seat for my toddler that is designed to hold children up to 40 lb.
   4. I use a car seat for my toddler that is designed to fasten with the seat belt.

4. A mother tells the nurse that her 2-year-old toddler often has temper tantrums at the family dinner table and asks how to handle the behavior. The best response of the nurse would be:
   1. temper tantrums are normal for a 2-year-old, and the child will grow out of it.
   2. the toddler should be removed from the family dinner table until he or she is old enough to behave.
   3. strict discipline and corporal punishment are appropriate to help the child to gain self-control.
   4. parents should agree on a method of discipline, such as time-out, and use it when the child misbehaves.

5. One of the developmental hallmarks of the toddler that most frequently gives rise to safety hazards is:
   1. brief attention span.
   2. need for ritual.
   3. fluctuating appetite.
   4. need to explore.

Critical Thinking Question

1. The parents of a toddler discuss safety in the home with the nurse. The parents state that they will use a car seat as required by law and safety gates on the stairs to prevent accidental falls. However, they believe no other safety "childproofing" is necessary, because their child is a good child and they plan to teach him to be obedient so he will learn not to touch certain items. What is the best response of the nurse?

Objectives

1. Define each key term listed.
2. List the major developmental tasks of the preschool-age child.
3. Describe the physical, psychosocial, and spiritual development of children from age 3 to 5 years, listing age-specific events and guidance when appropriate.
4. Describe the development of the preschool child in relation to Piaget's, Erikson's, and Kohlberg's theories of development.
5. Describe the speech development of the preschool child.
6. Discuss the development of positive bedtime habits.
7. Discuss one method of introducing the concept of death to a preschool child.
8. Discuss the value of the following: time-out periods, consistency, role modeling, and rewards.
9. Discuss the approach to problems such as enuresis, thumb sucking, and sexual curiosity in the preschool child.
10. Designate two toys suitable for the preschool child, and provide the rationale for each choice.
11. Describe the developmental characteristics that predispose the preschool child to certain accidents, and suggest methods of prevention for each type of accident.
12. Discuss the characteristics of a good preschool.
13. Discuss the value of play in the life of a preschool child.
14. Explain the use of therapeutic play with a handicapped child.

Key Terms

animism (p. 421)
art therapy (p. 432)
artificialism (p. 421)
associative play (p. 424)
centering (p. 421)
echolalia (ĕk-ō-LĀ-lē-ă, p. 422)
egocentrism (p. 421)
enuresis (ĕn-yū-RĒ-sĭs, p. 428)

modeling (p. 427)
parallel play (p. 424)
play therapy (p. 432)
preconceptual stage (p. 421)
preoperational phase (p. 421)
symbolic functioning (p. 421)
therapeutic play (p. 432)
time-out (p. 426)

GENERAL CHARACTERISTICS

The child from age 3 to 5 years is often referred to as the *preschool child*. Slowing of the physical growth process, and mastery and refinement of the motor, social, and cognitive abilities that mark this period will enable the child to be successful in his or her school years.

The major tasks of the preschool child include preparation to enter school, development of a cooperative type of play, control of body functions, acceptance of separation, and increase in communication skills, memory, and attention span.

PHYSICAL DEVELOPMENT

The infant, who tripled his or her birth weight at 1 year, has doubled the 1-year weight by the age of 5 years. For instance, the infant who weighs 9 kg (20 lb) on the first birthday will probably weigh about 18 kg (40 lb) by the fifth birthday. The child between 3 and 6 years of age grows taller and loses the chubbiness seen during the toddler period. Between 3 and 5 years of age, there will be an increase of 7.6 cm (3 inches) in height, mostly in the legs, which contributes to the development of an erect, slender appearance. Visual acuity is 20/40 at 3 years of age and 20/30 at 4 years of age. The achievement of 20/20 vision may be accomplished by school age. All 20 primary teeth have erupted. Hand preference develops by 3 years of age, and efforts to change a left-handed child to a right-handed child can cause a high level of frustration. Appetite fluctuates widely. The normal pulse rate is 90 to 110 beats/min. The rate of respirations during relaxation is about 20 breaths/min. The systolic blood pressure is about 85 to 90 mm Hg, and the diastolic blood pressure is about 60 mm Hg.

Preschool children have good control of their muscles and participate in vigorous play; they become more adept at using already familiar skills as each year passes. They can swing and jump higher. Their gait resembles that of an adult. They are quicker and have more self-confidence than they did as toddlers.

COGNITIVE DEVELOPMENT

The thinking of the preschool child is unique. Piaget calls this period the **preoperational phase**. It comprises children from 2 to 7 years of age and is divided into two stages: the **preconceptual stage** (2 to 4 years of age) and the intuitive thought stage (4 to 7 years of age). Of importance in the preconceptual stage is the increasing development of language and symbolic functioning. **Symbolic functioning** is seen in the play of children who pretend that an empty box is a fort; they create a mental image to stand for something that is not there.

Another characteristic of this period is **egocentrism**, a type of thinking in which children have difficulty seeing any point of view other than their own. Because children's knowledge and understanding are restricted to their own limited experiences, misconceptions arise. One misconception is **animism**. This is a tendency to attribute life to inanimate objects. Another is **artificialism**, the idea that people created the world and everything in it.

The intuitive stage is one of prelogical thinking. Experience and logic are based on outside appearance (the child does not understand that a wide glass and a tall glass can both contain 4 oz of juice). A distinctive characteristic of intuitive thinking is **centering**, the tendency to concentrate on a single outstanding characteristic of an object while excluding its other features.

More mature conceptual awareness is established with time and experience. This process is highly complex, and the implications for practical application are numerous. Interested students are encouraged to explore these concepts through further study. Table 18-1 summarizes some major theories of personality development for the preschooler.

EFFECTS OF CULTURAL PRACTICES

Cultural practices can influence the development of a sense of initiative in families who practice authoritarian types of parenting styles that put a great value on obedience and conformity. Parents and older siblings are models for language development, and the mastery of sounds proceeds in the same order around the world. Some parents speak both English and a native language in the home. Studies have shown that young children adapt quickly to a bilingual environment and cultural practices (Figure 18-1). Cultural preferences related to dietary practices are discussed in Chapter 15.

LANGUAGE DEVELOPMENT

The development of language as a communication skill is essential for success in school (Figure 18-2). Physiological, psychological, or environmental stressors can cause delays or problems in language expression. Typically, in the preschool period between 2 and 5 years of

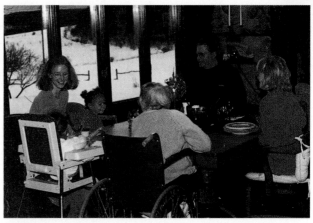

FIGURE 18-1 The family meal. The multigenerational family enjoys a meal together. Cultural traditions and family bonding occur here.

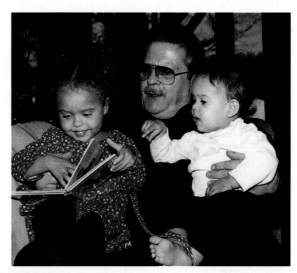

FIGURE 18-2 Grandpa reads to the children. Preschool language development depends on exposure to the written word and picture familiarity. In interactive reading, the child is asked questions about the pictures she sees and she receives immediate feedback. It is the ideal way to optimize the mastery of language.

age, the number of words in the child's sentence should equal the child's age (e.g., two words at 2 years of age). By 2½ years of age, most children evidence possessiveness (*my* doll). By 4 years of age they can use the past tense, and by 5 years of age they can use the future tense. The development of language skills includes both the understanding of language and the expressing of oneself in language. Children who have difficulty expressing themselves in words often exhibit tantrums and other acting-out behaviors.

Table 18-2 lists the language, cognitive, and perceptual abilities required for success in school. Problems detected and treated during the preschool years can prevent many school problems in later years. Table 18-3 describes the clinical symptoms of typical language disorders. Evaluation of language development must be performed together with an assessment of problem-solving skills.

Table 18-1 Preschool Growth and Development

	INTELLIGENCE	EMOTIONAL ASPECTS	LANGUAGE	PLAY	PARENTAL GUIDANCE
3 years	Piaget's preoperational phase Understands time in relation to concrete activities Knows own sex Has attention span of approximately 15 minutes; is easily distracted	Freud's phallic stage Oedipus complex may develop in boys Erikson's stage of initiative vs. guilt Wishes to please parents Ritualism provides security (see Chapter 17) Egocentric (unable to see viewpoint of others)	Has vocabulary of approximately 300-800 words Uses plurals Forms three-word sentences Can repeat three numbers Understanding occurs before expressive ability	Kohlberg: beginning moral development Identifies with same-sex parent Develops understanding of good/bad Explains different emotions in pretend play Starts to engage in group play Is highly imaginative	Child usually wants to please parents. Guidance techniques are based on this principle. Overprotection during this stage of initiative can frustrate the development of a coping mechanism in the child. Having the child "help" the parent will enhance self-esteem.
4 years	Can count to 5 Knows simple songs Sexual curiosity is high Has attention span of approximately 20 minutes Adds logic to thinking Understands that feelings are connected to actions	May use tantrums to relieve frustrations and, if successful, these may become a coping mechanism Has mood swings Is highly imaginative Asks many questions Likes to "show off" accomplishments Experiments with masturbation	Has vocabulary of 1500 words Uses four- to five-word sentences Experiments with language and words May use offensive words without understanding the meaning	Engages in rough-and-tumble play Learns how much he or she can control Demonstrates sibling rivalry	Minimize passive activity, such as doing puzzles, for the child. Repetition of words without comprehension (**echolalia**) should be referred for follow-up care. Teach self-control through setting limits. Guide parent in discipline techniques. Provide nutritious snacks. Answer questions truthfully.
5 years	Beginning concept of past, present, and future, although time is evidenced in activity rather than hours Knows the days of the week Attention span reaches 30 minutes Can count to 10 Knows name and address Behaviors that result in rewards are considered right; behaviors that result in punishment are considered wrong	Is less egocentric and has beginning awareness of the outside world Enjoys activities with parent of the same sex	Has vocabulary of 2000 words Can name four colors Uses six- to eight-word sentences with pronouns	Wants to play "by the rules" but cannot accept losing Can copy sample shapes and print first name Establishes preference for hand use	Child can participate in own care. Teach front-to-back wiping after bowel movements. Provide information concerning vision and hearing assessment facilities in community. Review immunization status. Prepare parent for separation and entrance of child into school.

Table 18-2	Selected Perceptual, Cognitive, and Language Processes Required for Elementary School Success	
PROCESS	**DESCRIPTION**	**ASSOCIATED PROBLEMS**
Perceptual		
Visual analysis	Ability to break a complex figure into components and understand their spatial relationships	Persistent letter confusion (e.g., between *b*, *d*, and *g*); difficulty with basic reading and writing and limited "sight" vocabulary
Proprioception and motor control	Ability to obtain information about body position by feel and unconsciously program complex movements	Poor handwriting, requiring inordinate effort, often with overly tight pencil grasp; special difficulty with timed tasks
Phonological processing	Ability to perceive differences between similar-sounding words and to break down words into constituent sounds	Delayed receptive language skills; attention and behavior problems secondary to not understanding directions; delayed acquisition of letter-sound correlations (phonetics)
Cognitive		
Long-term memory, both storage and recall	Ability to acquire skills that are "automatic" (i.e., accessible without conscious thought)	Delayed mastery of the alphabet (reading and writing letters); slow handwriting; inability to progress beyond basic mathematics
Selective attention	Ability to attend to important stimuli and ignore distractions	Difficulty following multistep instructions, completing assignments, and behaving well; peer interaction problems
Sequencing	Ability to remember things in order; skill with time concepts	Difficulty organizing assignments, planning, spelling, and telling time
Language		
Receptive language	Ability to comprehend complex constructions, function words (e.g., if, when, only, except), nuances of speech, and extended blocks of language (e.g., paragraphs)	Difficulty following directions; wandering attention during lessons and stories; problems with reading comprehension; problems with peer relationships
Expressive language	Ability to recall required words effortlessly (word finding), control meanings, and vary position and word endings to construct meaningful paragraphs and stories	Difficulty expressing feelings and using words for self-defense, with resulting frustration and physical acting out; struggling during "circle time" and in language-based subjects (e.g., English)

Adapted from Kliegman R et al: *Nelson's textbook of pediatrics*, ed 19, Philadelphia, 2011, Saunders.

Table 18-3	Not Talking: A Clinical Classification	
WHEN PARENTS SAY	**CLASSIFY THE SYMPTOMS AS**
"I'm the only one who understands what she says."	Articulation disorder
"She'll do what I say, but when she wants something, she just points."	Expressive language delay
"He can't play 'show me your nose,' and the only word he says is 'mama.'"	Global language delay
"He never made those funny baby sounds or said 'mama' and 'dada,' and now he just repeats everything I say."	Language disorder
"He used to say things like 'Joey go bye-bye,' but now he doesn't talk at all."	Language loss

Data from Montgomery T: When children do not talk, *Contemp Pediatr* 11(9):49, 1994; Kliegman R et al: *Nelson's textbook of pediatrics*, ed 19, Philadelphia, 2011, Saunders.

DEVELOPMENT OF PLAY

Play activities in the preschool child increase in complexity. At 2 to 3 years of age, the child imitates the activities of daily living of the parents (hammering, shaving, feeding the doll). By 4 years of age, the child may develop broader themes such as a trip to the zoo. By 5 years of age, a trip to the moon demonstrates the child's imaginary abilities. Play enables the child to experience multiple roles and emotional outlets, such as the aggressor, the victim, the superpower, or the acquisition of toys or friends they desire. Appealing to the child's magical thinking is the best approach to communication.

SPIRITUAL DEVELOPMENT

Preschoolers learn about religious beliefs and practices from what they observe in the home. Preschoolers cannot yet understand abstract concepts; their concept of God, sometimes treated as an invisible friend, is concrete. Preschool children can memorize Bible stories and related rituals, but their understanding of the concepts is limited. Observing religious traditions practiced in the home during a period of hospitalization (e.g., before-meal or bedtime prayers) can help the preschool child manage stressors.

SEXUAL CURIOSITY

When guiding parents concerning the sexual education of young children, the nurse should use the following common principles of teaching and learning:

- First assess the knowledge base of the child; then assess what specific information the child is seeking.
- Be honest and accurate in providing information at the child's level. Although the child may not understand completely at first, the child's repeated questions and explanations will form the basis of later learning and understanding.
- Use correct terminology so that misinformation or misinterpretation can be avoided.
- Provide sex education at the time the child asks the question. The asking of the question often indicates readiness to learn.
- Parents must understand that sexual curiosity starts as an inquiry into anatomical differences. Differences in how urination occurs may later become the focus. A general understanding of infants coming from "Mommy's tummy" precedes the more mature concept of sexual organs and functioning.

Preschool children are as matter-of-fact about sexual investigation as they are about any other learning experience and are easily distracted to other activities. Sexual curiosity displayed in the form of masturbation or "playing doctor" should be approached in a positive manner. The appropriate touch or dress can be taught without generating a "bad" or "dirty" concept of the activity. Teaching socially acceptable behavior must be in the form of guidance rather than discipline.

Masturbation

Masturbation is common in both genders during the preschool years. The child experiences pleasurable sensations, which lead to a repetition of the behavior. It is beneficial to rule out other causes of this activity, such as rashes or penile or vaginal irritation. Masturbation in the preschool child is considered harmless if the child is outgoing, sociable, and not preoccupied with the activity.

Education of the parents consists of assuring them that this behavior is a form of sexual curiosity and is normal and not harmful to the child, who is merely curious about sexuality. The cultural and moral background of the family must be considered in assessing the degree of discomfort about this experience. A history of the time

and place of masturbation and the parental response is helpful. Punitive reactions are discouraged. Parents are advised to ignore the behavior and distract the child with some other activity. The child should know that masturbation is not acceptable in public, but this must be explained in a nonthreatening manner. Children who masturbate excessively and who have experienced a great deal of disruption in their lives benefit from ongoing counseling.

BEDTIME HABITS

The development and reinforcement of optimal bedtime habits are important in the preschool years. Parents should be guided to engage the child in quiet activities before bedtime, to maintain specific rituals that signal bedtime readiness (such as storytelling), and to verbally state "after this story, it will be bedtime." The use of a night-light, a favorite bedtime toy, or a glass of water at the bedside is an option. Attention-getting behavior that results in taking the child into the parent's bed should be discouraged, because it rewards the attention-getting behavior and defeats the objectives of the bedtime ritual. The nurse should be aware that specific cultures encourage "family beds," where children regularly sleep with siblings and parents. Understanding cultural practices is essential before preparing a teaching plan.

PHYSICAL, MENTAL, EMOTIONAL, AND SOCIAL DEVELOPMENT

THE THREE-YEAR-OLD

Three-year-olds are a delight to their parents. They are helpful and can assist in simple household chores. They obtain articles when directed and return them to the proper place. Three-year-olds come very close to the ideal picture that parents have in mind of their child. They are living proof that their parents' guidance during the trying 2-year-old period has been rewarded. Temper tantrums are less frequent, and in general the 3-year-old is less erratic. They are still individuals, but they seem better able to direct their primitive instincts than previously. They can help to dress and undress themselves, use the toilet, and wash their hands. They eat independently, and their table manners have improved.

Three-year-olds talk in longer sentences and can express thoughts and ask questions. They provide more company to their parents and to other adults because they can talk about their experiences. They are imaginative, talk to their toys, and imitate what they see about them. Soon they begin to make friends outside the immediate family. **Parallel play** (playing independently within a group) and **associative play** (playing in loosely associated groups) are both typical of this period. Because they can now converse with playmates, they find satisfaction in joining their activities. Three-year-olds play cooperatively for short periods. They can ask others to "come out and play." If 3-year-olds are placed in a strange situation with children they do not know, they commonly revert to parallel play because it is more comfortable.

Preschoolers begin to find enjoyment away from Mom and Dad, although they want them nearby when needed. They begin to lose some of their interest in their mother, who up to this time has been more or less their total world. The father's prestige begins to increase. Romantic attachment to the parent of the opposite sex is seen during this period. A daughter wants "to marry Daddy" when she grows up. Children also begin to identify themselves with the parent of the same sex.

Preschool children have more fears than the infant or older child because of increased intelligence (which enables them to recognize potential dangers), memory development, and graded independence (which brings them into contact with many new situations). Toddlers are not afraid of walking in the street because they do not understand its danger. Preschool children realize that trucks can injure, and they worry about crossing the street. This fear is well founded, but many others are not.

The fear of bodily harm, particularly the loss of body parts, is unique to this stage. The little boy who discovers that his infant sister is made differently may worry that she has been injured. He wonders if this will happen to him. Masturbation is common during this stage as children attempt to reassure themselves that they are all right. Other common fears include fear of animals, fear of the dark, and fear of strangers. Night wandering is typical of this age group.

Preschool children become angry when others attempt to take their possessions. They grab, slap, and hang onto them for dear life. They become very distraught if toys do not work the way they should. They resent being disturbed from play. They are sensitive, and their feelings are easily hurt. Much of the unpleasant social behavior seen during this time is normal and necessary to the child's total pattern of development.

THE FOUR-YEAR-OLD

Four-year-olds are more aggressive and like to show off newly refined motor skills. They are eager to let others know they are superior, and they are prone to pick on playmates. Four-year-olds are boisterous, tattle on others, and may begin to swear if they are around children or adults who use profanity. They recount personal family activities with amazing recall but forget where they left their tricycle. At this age, children become interested in how old they are and want to know the exact age of each playmate. It bolsters their ego to know that they are older than someone else in the group. They also become interested in the relationship of one person to another, such as Timmy is a brother but is also Daddy's son.

Four-year-olds can use scissors with success. They can lace their shoes. Their vocabulary has increased to about 1500 words. They run simple errands and can play with others for longer periods. Many feats are done for a purpose. For instance, they no longer run just for the sake of running. Instead, they run to get someplace or see something. They are imaginative and like to pretend they are doctors or firefighters. They begin to prefer playing with friends of the same sex.

The preschool child enjoys simple toys and common objects. Raw materials are more appealing than toys that are ready-made and complete in themselves. An old cardboard box that can be moved about and climbed into is more fun than a dollhouse with tiny furniture. A box of sand or colored pebbles can be made into roads and mountains. Parents should avoid showering their children with ready-made toys. Instead, they can select materials that are absorbing and that stimulate the child's imagination.

Stories that interest young children depict their daily experiences. If the story has a simple plot, it must be related to what they understand to hold their interest. They also enjoy music they can march around to, enjoy music videos, and like simple instruments they can shake or bang. (Make up a song about their daily life, and watch their reaction.)

The Concept of Death

Children between 3 and 4 years of age begin to wonder about death and dying. They may pretend to be the hero who shoots the intruder dead, or they may actually witness a situation in which an animal is killed. Their questions are direct. "What is 'dead'? Will I die?" The view of the family is important to the interpretation of this complex phenomenon.

Children may become acquainted with death through objects with no particular significance to them. For instance, the flower dies at the end of the summer and does not bloom anymore. It no longer needs sunshine or water, because it is not alive. Usually young children realize that others die, but they do not relate death to themselves. If they continue to pursue the question of whether or not they will die, parents should be casual and reassure them that people do not generally die until they have lived a long and happy life. Of course, as they grow older they will discover that sometimes children do die.

The underlying idea is to encourage questions as they appear and gradually help them to accept the truth without undue fear. There are many excellent books for children about death. Two that are appropriate for the preschool child are *Geranium Mornings* by S. Powell and *My Grandpa Died Today* by J. Fassler. The dying child is discussed in Chapter 27.

THE FIVE-YEAR-OLD

Five is a comfortable age. Children are more responsible, enjoy doing what is expected of them, have more patience, and like to finish what they have started. Five-year-olds are serious about what they can and cannot do. They talk constantly and are inquisitive about their environment. They want to do things correctly and seek answers to their questions from those whom they consider to "know" the answers. Five-year-old children can play games governed by rules. They are less fearful, because they believe that authorities control their environment. Their worries are less profound than at an earlier age.

The physical growth of 5-year-olds is not outstanding. Their height may increase by 5 to 7.6 cm (2 to 3 inches), and they may gain 1.4 to 2.7 kg (3 to 6 lb). They may begin to lose their deciduous teeth at this time. They can run and play games simultaneously, jump three or four steps at once, and distinguish a penny from a nickel or a dime. They can name the days of the week and understand what a weeklong vacation is. They usually can print their first name.

Five-year-olds can ride a tricycle around the playground with speed and dexterity. They can use a hammer to pound nails. Adults should encourage them to develop motor skills and should not continually remind them to "be careful." The practice children experience will enable them to compete with others during the school-age period and will increase confidence in their own abilities. As at any age, children should not be scorned for failure to meet adult standards. Overdirection by solicitous adults is damaging. Children must learn to do tasks themselves for the experience to be satisfying.

The number and type of television or computer programs that parents allow the preschool child to watch is a topic for discussion. Although children enjoyed television at age 3 or 4 years, it was usually for short periods. They could not understand much of what was occurring. The 5-year-old, however, has better comprehension and may want to spend a great deal of time watching television or playing computer games. The plan of management differs with each family. Whatever decision is made must be discussed with the child. For example, television and computers should not be allowed to interfere with good health habits, sleep, meals, and physical activity. Most parents find that children do not insist on watching television if there is something better to do.

GUIDANCE

DISCIPLINE AND LIMIT SETTING

Much has been written on the subject of discipline, views of which have changed considerably over time. Today, authorities place much importance on the development of a continuous, warm relationship between children and their parents. They believe this helps to prevent many problems. The following is a brief discussion that may help the nurse in guiding parents.

Children need limits for their behavior. Setting limits makes them feel secure, protects them from danger, and relieves them from making decisions that they may be too young to formulate. Children who are taught acceptable behavior have more friends and develop good self-esteem. They live more enjoyably within the neighborhood and society. The manner in which discipline or limit setting is handled varies from culture to culture. It also varies among different socioeconomic groups. Individual differences occur among families and between parents and vary according to the characteristics of each child.

The purpose of discipline is to teach and to gradually shift control from parents to the child, that is, to develop self-discipline or self-control. Positive reinforcement for appropriate behavior has been cited as more effective than punishment for poor behavior. Expectations must be appropriate to the age and understanding of the child. The nurse encourages parents to try to be consistent, because mixed messages are confusing for the learner.

Timing the Time-Out

Most researchers agree that to be effective, discipline must be administered at the time the incident occurs. It should also be adapted to the seriousness of the infraction. The child's self-worth must always be considered and preserved. It may be helpful to warn the preschool child who appears to be getting into trouble. However, too many warnings without follow-up lead to ineffectiveness. For the most part, spankings are not productive and can be physically and psychologically damaging. The child associates the fury of the parents with the pain rather than with the wrong deed, because anger can be the predominant factor in the situation. Therefore there is no real positive outcome in spanking children. Spanking in anger administered by parents as a release for their own pent-up emotions is totally inappropriate and can lead to child abuse charges. In addition, the parent serves as a role model of aggression. Whether a parent is affectionate, warm, or cold (uncaring) also plays a role in the effectiveness of child rearing and the development of personality responses in the child.

Time-out periods, usually lasting 1 minute per year of age, with the child sitting in a straight chair facing a corner are considered an effective discipline technique. There should be no interaction or eye contact during the time-out period, and a timer with a buzzer should be used to signal the end of the time-out. Often a child will attempt interaction during this period by asking, "How much more time is left?" The child should learn that any interaction restarts the timer at zero. Using the child's room or a soft comfortable chair for time-out is not effective, because the child will either fall asleep or engage in another activity, and the objective of time-out is defeated. Time-out should be preceded by a short (no longer than 10-word) explanation of the reason and followed by a short (no more than 10 words) restatement of why it was necessary. Longer explanations are not effective for young children. If the child knows the rules and the behavior that will precipitate a time-out and receives no more than one warning that there will be a time-out if the undesirable behavior continues, he or she will learn self-control. Consistency is the key to helping the child learn acceptable behavior. Parents must be taught to resist using power and authority for their own sake. As the child matures and understands more clearly, privileges can be withheld as a consequence for undesirable behavior. The reasons for such actions are carefully explained.

Reward

Rewarding the child for good behavior is a positive and effective method of discipline. This can be done with hugs, smiles, tone of voice, and praise. Praise can always be tied with the act, such as "Thank you, Zoe, for picking up your toys," or "I appreciate your standing quietly like that." The encouragement of positive behavior eliminates many of the undesirable effects of punishment.

Rewards should not be confused with bribes. The parent may offer a child a reward if he or she behaves well in a specific situation *before* an incident occurs. For example, the parent may say, "You may pick out one small toy after we are finished shopping if you behave during this trip." If this agreement is not made *before* an incident and the child misbehaves and *then* is offered one small toy to behave, this is a bribe that serves to reinforce the bad behavior and is not a desirable technique of behavior management.

Consistency and Modeling

Being consistent is difficult for parents. Realistically, it is only an ideal for which to strive—no parent is consistent all the time. Consistency must exist *between* parents as well as within each parent. It is suggested that parents establish a general style for what, when, how, and to what degree punishment is appropriate for misconduct. Parents who are lax or erratic in discipline and who alternate it with punishment have children who experience increased behavioral difficulties.

The influence of **modeling**, or good example, has been widely explored. Studies show that adult models significantly influence children's education. Children identify and imitate adult behavior, both verbal and nonverbal. Parents who are aggressive and repeatedly lose control demonstrate the power of action over words. Those who communicate well, show respect and encouragement, and set appropriate limits are more positive role models. Finally, parents need assistance in reviewing parental discipline during their own childhood to recognize destructive patterns that they may be repeating. Modeling also involves teaching a child how to be self-sufficient and responsible. Asking children to do simple chores around the house is a good way to make them feel good about themselves; it gives them an opportunity to please the parent and to learn at

the same time, as long as the chore is not expected to be performed with expertise! Some chores a preschooler can perform include setting the table, sorting colored and white laundry, and picking up toys. If the chore is associated with a positive outcome, the concept of consequences can be learned. For example, "If we pick up the toys quickly, then we will have time to read a story before bedtime."

JEALOUSY

Jealousy is a normal response to actual, supposed, or threatened loss of affection. Both children and adults may feel insecure in their relationship with the person they love. The closer children are to their parents, the greater is their fear of losing them. Children envy the newborn. They love the sibling but resent his or her presence. They cannot understand the turmoil within themselves (Figure 18-3). Jealousy of a new sibling is strongest in children less than 5 years of age and is shown in various ways. Children may be aggressive and may bite or pinch, or they may be rather discreet and may hug and kiss the infant with a determined look on their faces. Another common situation is children's attempts to identify with the infant. They revert to wetting the bed or want to be powdered after they urinate. Some 4-year-olds even try the bottle, but it is usually a big disappointment to them.

Preschool children may be jealous of the attention that their mother gives to their father. They may also envy the children they play with if they have bigger and better toys. There is less jealousy in an only child, who is the center of attention and has a minimum number of rivals. Siblings of varied ages are apt to feel that the younger ones are "pets" or that the older ones have more special privileges.

Parents can help to reduce jealousy by the early management of individual occurrences. Preparing young children for the arrival of the new brother or sister minimizes the blow. They should not be made to think that they are being crowded. If the newborn is going to

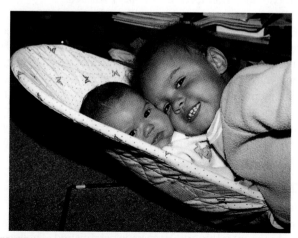

FIGURE 18-3 Child and new sibling. A new sibling is welcomed into the home. Both children need attention to minimize the development of jealousy.

occupy their crib, it is best to settle the older child happily in a large bed before the infant is born. Children should feel that they are helping with care of the infant. Parents can inflate their egos from time to time by reminding them of the many activities they can do that the infant cannot.

If it is convenient, the newborn is given a bath or a feeding while the older child is asleep. In this way, the older sibling avoids one occasion in which the mother shows the newborn affection for a relatively long time. Some persons think that it helps to give the child a pet to care for. Many hospitals offer sibling courses that assist parents in helping their children to overcome jealousy.

If the child tends to hit the infant or another child, both children must be separated. The child who has caused or is about to cause the injury needs as much attention as the victim, if not more. Similar aggressiveness is seen when the child is made to share toys. It is even more difficult to learn to share Mother, so the child must be given time to adjust to new situations. Children are assured that they are loved but are told that they cannot injure others.

THUMB SUCKING

Thumb sucking is an instinctual behavioral pattern and is considered normal. It is seen by sonogram about the twenty-ninth week of embryonic life. Although the cause is not fully understood, it satisfies and comforts the infant. Nonnutritive sucking in the form of thumb sucking or use of a pacifier has several documented benefits in the first year of life—when the infant is in the oral phase of development. Increased weight gain, decreased crying, the development of self-consoling ability, and increased behavioral organization have been documented in infants who have been allowed to suck unrestrained. If a pacifier is used, safe construction is essential (see Figure 16-2). The pacifier causes fewer dental problems than the rigid finger and is more easily relinquished. Parents need guidance in the safe use of pacifiers. Cleanliness is essential, because the pacifier often falls onto a dirty surface.

Finger or thumb sucking will not have a detrimental effect on the teeth as long as the habit is discontinued before the permanent teeth erupt. Most children give up the habit by the time they reach school age, although they may regress during periods of stress or fatigue. Management includes education and support of the parents to relieve their anxiety and prevent secondary emotional problems in their children. The child who is trying to stop thumb sucking is given praise and encouragement.

ENURESIS

Pathophysiology

Enuresis is involuntary urination after the age at which bladder control should have been established. The term *enuresis* is derived from the Greek word *enourein*, "to void urine." Bed-wetting has existed for generations and affects many cultures. There are two types: primary and secondary. Primary enuresis refers to bed-wetting in the child who has never been dry. Secondary enuresis refers to a recurrence in a child who has been dry for a period of 1 year or more. *Diurnal,* or daytime, wetting is less common than *nocturnal,* or nighttime, episodes. It is more common in boys than in girls, and there may be a genetic influence. In many children a specific cause is never determined.

Approximately 92% of children achieve daytime dryness by 5 years of age. By 12 to 14 years of age, approximately 98% of children remain dry during the night. Sometimes enuresis is the result of inappropriate toilet training. Parents who demand early toilet training can cause a child to rebel and defy them by continuing to wet the bed. Parents who are not alert to the needs of the child may not recognize readiness to toilet train and therefore frustrate the child's efforts to master this developmental task. Stressful events can precipitate bed-wetting.

In some cases, organic causes of nocturnal enuresis include urinary tract infections, diabetes mellitus, diabetes insipidus, seizure disorders, obstructive uropathy, abnormalities of the urinary tract, and sleep disorders. Maturational delays of the nervous system and small bladder capacity have also been suggested as causes.

Treatment and Nursing Care

A detailed physical and psychological history is obtained. Factors such as the pattern of wetting, number of times per night or per week, number of daytime voidings, type of stream, dysuria, amount of fluid taken between dinner and bedtime, family history, stress, and reactions of parents and child are documented. The nurse also investigates any medications that the child may be taking and determines the extent to which the child's social life is inhibited by the problem, such as the inability to spend the night away from home. Developmental landmarks, including toilet training, are reviewed. If there appears to be an organic cause, appropriate blood and urine studies are undertaken. In most cases, the physical findings are negative.

Education of the family is crucial to prevent secondary emotional problems. Parents are reassured that many children experience enuresis and that it is self-limited. Power struggles, shame, and guilt are fruitless and destructive. Reassurance and support by the nurse are of great help.

It is essential that the child be the center of the management program. The positive approach of rewarding dry nights and charting the progress is very helpful. Liquids after dinner should be limited, and the child should routinely void before going to bed.

When the child does not respond to routine management, other techniques include counseling, hypnosis, behavior modification, and pharmacotherapy. Moisture-activated conditioning devices are also commercially available (e.g., an alarm rings when the child wets). These have had limited success. Bladder-training exercises in which the child is asked to hold the urine for as long as possible may stretch the bladder and increase its size. The child's bedroom should be as close to the bathroom as possible, and a night-light should be used.

The nurse prepares the parents for relapses, which are common. The response to various therapies is highly individual. Overzealous treatment is to be avoided. A nonpunitive, matter-of-fact attitude is most prudent. Imipramine hydrochloride (Tofranil) has been found to decrease enuresis. It is administered before bedtime. Imipramine has a variety of side effects, including mood and sleep disturbances and gastrointestinal upsets. Overdose can lead to cardiac dysrhythmias, which may be life threatening. Dosage and administration should be closely supervised. It is not recommended for children less than 6 years of age. Desmopressin (DDAVP) nasal spray has been used with some success, but it is expensive.

PRESCHOOL

The change from home to nursery school or preschool is a big step toward independence. At this age, children are adjusting to the outside world as well as to the family. Some children have the complicating factor of a new brother or sister in the house.

Many parents work outside the home and find it necessary to provide alternative care settings for their children. Some parents who have only one child seek preschool experiences for their child to enhance growth and development by providing experience with playmates. Nurses can provide guidance to parents in selecting an appropriate preschool to meet their child's needs. A *family day care center* provides child care for small groups of children for 6 or more hours of a 24-hour day. Some employers may provide work-based group care as a convenience to their employees. Preschool programs provide structured activities that foster group cooperation and the development of coping skills. The child can gain self-confidence and positive self-esteem in a good preschool program. Qualified preschool teachers are objective in their interaction with the child and often can detect problems that can be followed up before the child enters kindergarten. Parents may need guidance in selecting a preschool for their child.

The following list of suggestions can guide the nurse in helping parents to select a facility appropriate for their child:

- The facility should be licensed by the state; contact a state-licensing agency for a list of local day care centers or preschools.
- The accreditation criteria for preschools can be obtained by writing the National Association for the Education of Young Children, 1834 Connecticut Avenue NW, Washington, DC 20009, or accessing http://families.naeyc.org/accredited-article/10-naeyc-program-standards online.
- Teachers prepared in early childhood education should staff the preschool.
- The student-to-staff ratio should be reviewed.
- The philosophies of the facility, including discipline procedures, environmental safety, sanitary provisions, fee schedules, and facilities for snacks, meals, and rest time, should be reviewed.
- Schedules and facilities for active/passive and indoor/outdoor play should be reviewed.
- The school should routinely require a personal and health history of the child before admission to the program.
- The parent should visit the preschool and personally observe the environment. Talking with the parents of other children attending the school is helpful. Children are accepted into nursery schools between ages 2 and 5 years. Most sessions last about 3 hours.

DAILY CARE

The child between ages 3 and 6 years does not require the extensive physical care given to an infant but still needs a bath each day and a shampoo at least twice a week. It is best to keep hairstyles simple. Dental hygiene and nutrition are discussed in Chapter 15.

CLOTHING

Clothes should be loose enough so they don't restrict movement but allow for active play without hems getting stepped on or tripped over. Clothes should be washable. Simple clothes make it easy for preschoolers to dress themselves. A hook within reach, nailed to the door perhaps, is helpful. Preschool children should dress and undress themselves as much as they can. The child's mother or father can assist but should not take over.

Shoes should be sturdy and supportive. Protective gear such as helmets for bicycling should be a natural part of dressing for play activities. Dressing appropriately for the weather that will be encountered is essential. Flame-retardant sleepwear is available in most stores.

ACCIDENT PREVENTION

Accidents are still a major threat during the years from 3 to 5. At this age, children may suffer injuries from a bad fall. Preschool children hurry up and down stairs. They climb trees and stand up on swings. They play hard with their toys, particularly those they can mount. Stairways must be kept free of clutter. Shoes should have rubber soles, and new ones should be purchased when the tread of older shoes becomes smooth. When buying toys, parents must be sure they are sturdy and age appropriate. Preschool children should not be asked to do anything that is potentially dangerous,

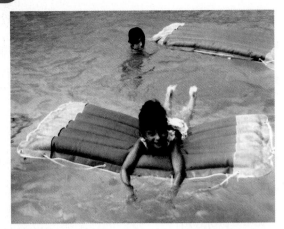

FIGURE 18-4 Unsupervised water play can quickly lead to unexpected injuries.

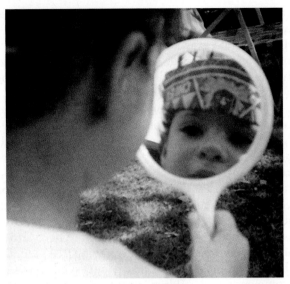

FIGURE 18-5 A self-image begins to develop during the preschool years with imaginative play.

such as carrying a glass container or sharp knife to the kitchen sink.

Automobiles continue to be a threat. Children are taught where they can safely ride their tricycles and where they can play ball, and they should not be allowed to use sleds on streets that are not blocked off for this purpose. They must not play in or around the car or be left alone in the car. The use of *car seats* or *seat belt restraints* continues to be important.

Burns that occur at this age often result from the child's experimentation with matches or lighters. Burns from hot coffee are also common. These items are common hazards for this age group; they should be kept well out of reach, and their dangers should be explained to the child.

Poisoning is still a danger. Children try to imitate adults and are apt to sample pills, especially if they smell good. Their increased freedom brings them into contact with many interesting containers in the garage or basement.

Preschool children are also taught the dangers of talking to or accepting rides from strangers. If a driver stops them, they should run to the house of people they know. Parents should make it clear to children in nursery school that they will never send a stranger to call for them. Children must know the dangers of playing in lonely places and of accepting gifts from strangers. Children should always know where to go if Mother or Father or the babysitter cannot be found. Preschool children still require a good deal of indirect supervision to protect them from dangers that arise from their immature judgment or social environment (Figure 18-4).

PLAY DURING HEALTH AND ILLNESS

VALUE OF PLAY

Play is important to the physical, mental, emotional, and social development of both healthy and sick children (Figure 18-5). Children climbing on a jungle gym develop muscles and coordination as they exercise all parts of their bodies. They use energy and develop self-confidence. Their imagination may take them to the jungle, where they swing from limb to limb. They may face imagined fears and solve problems that would be much more trying, if not impossible, in reality. They communicate with other children and take a further step in developing moral values, that is, taking one's turn and considering others. Other types of play help children learn colors, shapes, sizes, and textures and can teach creativity. Nursing and health care personnel must tap this natural and readily available outlet. Children may be unfamiliar with every facet of the hospital, but they know how to play, and playing is a good way for the nurse to establish rapport with the children.

THE NURSE'S ROLE

Some hospitals have well-established playroom programs supervised by play therapists. Play therapy is an important part of every pediatric nursing care plan. It is not necessary to be an expert in manual dexterity, art, or music; rather, one must understand the needs of the child. Play is not just the responsibility of those assigned to it, nor is it confined to certain times or shifts.

Many factors are involved in providing suitable play for children of various ages in the hospital. The patient's state of health affects the amount of activity in which he or she can participate. The nurse can facilitate many activities that relieve stress and provide enjoyment for the child who has been prescribed bed rest. Overstimulation would be hazardous for some severely ill children. Nurses are always on guard for signs of fatigue in patients and use their judgment accordingly.

The diagnosis of the hospitalized child should also be considered when choosing an appropriate toy. For example, a friction toy is inappropriate for a child in an oxygen-rich environment. Sparks from the toy could cause an explosion. A stuffed animal may not be an appropriate toy for a child with asthma, who may be allergic to the contents of the stuffing.

Safety must be considered in selecting an appropriate toy. Toys should be safe, durable, and suited to the child's developmental level. Toys should not be sharp or have parts that are easily removed and swallowed. Providing too many toys at one time to the child can be confusing. Complicated toys are frustrating and disappointing. Well-selected toys such as crayons, blocks, and dolls are useful throughout the years. A washable laundry bag tied to a hospitalized child's bed can be used to store the child's own toys neatly and safely. Toys may be taken home with the child or discarded after he or she is discharged from the hospital.

Each child needs sufficient time to complete an activity. In general, quiet play should precede meals and bedtime for both well and sick children. Investigations have shown that the toys enjoyed by boys and those enjoyed by girls are more similar than dissimilar.

During routine procedures the nurse can entertain the child with nursery rhymes, stories, nonsense games, songs, finger play, or puppets. Often the other children on the unit can be included in the game "I'm thinking of something blue, red, and green," and so forth. Simple crafts are fun. The nurse may find various instructions from children's magazines or the local public library. Scrapbooks are entertaining. Children may even enjoy making a storybook about their hospital experience. The nurse involved in enrichment programs for children can definitely make a positive contribution. Surprise boxes in which a gift is opened daily provide a sense of anticipation for the patient. Collections of scraps can be started consisting of bright ribbons, bits of string, pipe cleaners, paper bags, newspapers, or bits of cotton. Because the turnover of patients is rapid, many projects can be repeated with different children.

Radios, CDs, MP3 players, computers, iPads, iPods, and instruments provide music. Older children enjoy sending e-mails and text messages to friends. Special children's recordings and videos are available. The services of a music therapist are available in some institutions. Drawing materials, finger paints, and modeling clay foster expression and creativity. They require only a flat surface, such as the overbed table, and a particular medium. The bedridden child can participate in messy projects, too. The bed is simply protected with newspapers or plastic. Children in cribs require adequate back support for such projects. This is done by elevating the mattress or using pillows. Simple computer games may be available in the hospital setting.

Playmates may be limited in the hospital setting if the child has a condition that is communicable. However, surgical and orthopedic patients can play together in a playroom with appropriate supervision. The nurse should guide the parents in how to play *for* a child who is fatigued or weakened by illness. The child can maintain the role of observer.

TYPES OF PLAY

Preschool children need playmates to promote social development. The play characteristics of each age group are shown in Table 15-10. The preschool-age child gradually moves from parallel and associative play to cooperative play with playmates.

The play of preschool children should be noncompetitive. The healthy preschool child requires active play activities that are supervised for safety. Large construction sets, number or alphabet games, crayons, play tools, housekeeping toys, musical toys, pop-up books, large puzzles, and clay are examples of suitable toys for the preschool-age child. Active play can involve simple climbing, sliding, and running activities. Imaginary friends are common to the preschool-age child. They serve many purposes in helping the child adjust to an expanding world and increased independence. Parents can acknowledge the presence of the imaginary friend as part of pretend play, but the responsibilities of reality do not include the pretend friend. Parents should not intervene in playgroups. Allowing the child to master frustration and develop social skills is essential to growth and development.

> **Nursing Tip**
>
> Imaginary playmates are common and normal during the preschool period and serve many purposes, such as relief from loneliness, mastery of feats, and provision of a "scapegoat."

Play and the Child with a Neurodevelopmental, Sensory, or Motor Disorder

The child with a neurodevelopmental, sensory, or motor disorder needs more stimulation through play than the child who is not challenged by these conditions. The nurse must consider the mental age and motor ability of the child rather than the chronological age when guiding parents about the selection of toys. The environment should be as colorful and bright as possible. The child may be introduced to objects of various sizes and textures. Play with other children must be supervised, because the poorer judgment of neurodevelopmentally impaired children may lead them into difficulty. They may be aggressive and unaware of their own strength. Adequate space is necessary in which the children can run. These children should be brought into group play gradually. Materials are presented one at a time.

Neurodevelopmentally or motor-impaired children may need to be taught how to play, because they may not have had the preschool play experience of the nonhandicapped child. Repetition of play experiences is necessary. Equipment and play materials must be altered to accommodate the child's size and yet be suitable for the mental age. The nurse or teacher should improvise games and songs to meet the special needs of this group. (See Chapters 23 and 33 for a more complete discussion of the growth, development, and care of the neurodevelopmentally, sensory, or motor-impaired child.)

Therapeutic Play

Play and toys can be of therapeutic value in retraining muscles, improving eye–hand coordination, and helping children crawl and walk (push-pull toys). A musical instrument such as the clarinet promotes flexion and extension of the fingers. Blowing is an excellent prerequisite for speech therapy. Therapists supervise such activities. They leave specific instructions if they wish their work to be reinforced on the unit. Blowing out the light of a flashlight as if it were a candle is **therapeutic play** for a postoperative preschool child.

Play Therapy

The nurse may also hear the term **play therapy**. This technique is used for the child under stress. A well-equipped playroom is provided. Children are free to play with whatever articles they choose. A counselor may be in the room observing and talking with the child, or the child may be observed through a one-way glass window. By using these as well as other methods, the therapist obtains a better understanding of the patient's struggles, fears, resentments, and feelings toward self and others. When children act out their feelings through "dramatic play," the feelings are externalized, which relieves tension. The interpretation of child behavior is complex, and a great deal of time, study, and sensitivity is required for full understanding.

Art Therapy

Art therapy is useful in communicating with children and adults. It is becoming more widely used. The art therapist is especially trained to assist children to express their feelings and communicate through drawings, clay, and other media. Some hospitals with inpatient mental health units have art therapy departments.

NURSING IMPLICATIONS OF PRESCHOOL GROWTH AND DEVELOPMENT

The nurse should anticipate parental concern with nutritional problems in the preschool child. Daily appetites may fluctuate widely, but the weekly pattern will probably show stability to meet the child's growth needs. During clinic visits the parents should be guided to provide age-appropriate foods at mealtimes in appropriate portions. The child's developing self-regulatory mechanism will determine how much he or she will eat based on feelings of hunger or satiety. Efforts to control the preschool child's intake may result in power struggles or patterns of overeating or undereating.

Safety is a high priority in this active age range. "Childproofing" the home and the need for adequate supervision and safety equipment during sports activities should be emphasized. Preschoolers, who will be given immunizations via a "shot," can be calmed by giving pretend "shots" to their doll and having a parent present to comfort the doll. Explanations such as "the shot will hurt just a little but will prevent you from getting sick" are beyond the Piaget preoperational level of understanding of the preschool child. The ability to understand detailed explanations is not yet present in preschool-age children, even if verbal ability is high. The preschool-age child may have unfounded fears that respond best to reassurance and "protection" by parents, rather than reasoning about why the fear is unfounded.

The nurse should provide parental guidance concerning the changing behavior patterns of the preschool-age child. The characteristic alternating dependence and independence can be frustrating for parents. Parents who do not volunteer any positive comments about their child during conversations may require further investigation and interview. Problems with day care and discipline must be discussed. The use of corporal punishment (spanking) as a major disciplinary technique can lead to child abuse. The use of time-out and alternative methods of discipline should be emphasized.

Hospitalization can be frightening to a preschool child who is egocentric and prone to magical thinking. Because the preschool child cannot fully understand cause and effect, he or she may perceive hospitalization as punishment for behavior. The preschool child may feel abandoned by the parents and continues to be subject to separation anxiety. Separation anxiety (see Chapter 21) is manifested by the stages of *protest, despair, detachment,* and *regression* to earlier behaviors. Bed-wetting is common in the hospitalized preschool-age child, and parents should be encouraged to be patient and positive. Assigning a consistent caregiver and providing age-appropriate diversional activities are essential for a hospitalized preschool-age child.

The nurse who is with children daily can describe their behavior. It is important to describe good and poor behavior, conversations that seem pertinent, and the child's relationships with other children in the hospital. What is the child's approach to play? Does the child join in freely or linger outside the group? Does the child prefer active or quiet activities? Does the child seem to tolerate frustrations? Can the child talk with his or her playmates and convey ideas? What type of attention span does the child have? These observations and charting are meaningful and promote better understanding and appropriate interventions by nurses and other personnel.

Get Ready for the NCLEX® Examination!

Key Points

- The child aged 3 to 5 years is often referred to as the "preschool child." During this period, the child grows taller and loses the chubbiness of the toddler period.
- The major tasks of the preschool child include preparation to enter school, the development of a cooperative type of play, control of body functions, acceptance of separation, and increase in communication skills, memory, and attention span.
- Gross and fine motor skills become more developed, as evidenced by participation in running, skipping, and drawing pictures.
- Piaget refers to the preschool period as one in which symbolic thought processes and language emerge.
- Erikson's preschool stage involves the development of initiative. Kohlberg's theory concerning preschoolers refers to the moral development and the beginning awareness of the needs of others.
- Language ability develops rapidly, and the child is able to construct rather complicated sentences by the end of this period.
- The many questions of the preschool child must be listened to carefully and answered thoughtfully and truthfully.
- Play is the business of children. It contributes to physical and mental well-being by encouraging communication, socialization, and outlets for energy.
- Cooperative and highly imaginative play is characteristic of the preschool child.
- Social issues of the preschool period include learning to share and to control impulses.
- Common concerns of parents during this period include how to set limits, handle jealousy, and respond to thumb sucking and masturbation.
- Corporal punishment of the preschool child can nurture rebellion and aggression. Appropriate discipline techniques can assist the child to develop self-control.
- Careful evaluation of day care and nursery school programs is important to ensure high-quality care.
- Accidents are still a major hazard for preschool children because of the child's immature judgment and increased locomotive skills.
- During the preschool years, the parents need guidance to understand the developmental road map of physical, emotional, and cognitive growth to help the child to meet life's challenges and goals and to enrich family interaction.
- Primary enuresis refers to bed-wetting in a child who has never been dry. Secondary enuresis refers to bed-wetting in a child who has been dry for a period of 1 year or more.

Additional Learning Resources

SG Go to your Study Guide for additional learning activities to help you master this chapter content.

evolve Go to your Evolve website (http://evolve.elsevier.com/Leifer) for the following learning resources:
- Animations
- Answer Guidelines for Critical Thinking Questions
- Answers and Rationales for Review Questions for the NCLEX® Examination
- Glossary with English and Spanish pronunciations
- Interactive Review Questions for the NCLEX® Examination

- Patient Teaching Plans in English and Spanish
- Skills Performance Checklists
- Video clips and more!

 Online Resources
- American Academy of Pediatrics, Children's Health Topics: www.aap.org/topics.html
- Sexuality Information and Education Council of the United States: www.siecus.org

Review Questions for the NCLEX® Examination

1. When selecting play activities for a healthy 4-year-old, the parent should be guided to understand that the 4-year-old enjoys:
   1. solitary play, sitting next to a friend.
   2. cooperative play with friends.
   3. competitive play with teams.
   4. observing rather than participating.

2. An example of a therapeutic play activity for a preschool child who is recovering from an appendectomy would be:
   1. a Wii game of bowling.
   2. blowing bubbles.
   3. reading a storybook.
   4. coloring with crayons.

3. The nurse is guiding a parent concerning techniques of handling a child with enuresis. The most appropriate suggestion by the nurse would be to:
   1. wake the child often during the night and take him to the bathroom to void.
   2. limit liquids after dinner and have the child void before going to bed.
   3. use a consistent technique of discipline whenever the bed is wet.
   4. keep the child in diapers until bed-wetting is no longer a problem.

4. The appropriate amount of time to use in a time-out period for a 3-year-old child is:
   1. 1 minute.
   2. 3 minutes.
   3. 5 minutes.
   4. 10 minutes.

5. A 4-year-old child is in Erikson's stage of:
   1. autonomy.
   2. industry.
   3. initiative.
   4. identity.

Critical Thinking Question

1. The parents of a preschool child discuss the typical play activities of their child. They express concern that they have seen their child choose to play the role of "the aggressive bad guy" in play scenarios and are concerned that he may be developing aggressive behavior. They ask if they should stop him from assuming roles in play that are not acceptable behaviors. What is the best response of the nurse?

Objectives

1. Define each key term listed.
2. Contrast two major theoretical viewpoints of personality development during the school years.
3. Describe the physical and psychosocial development of children from 6 to 12 years of age, listing age-specific events and type of guidance where appropriate.
4. Discuss how to assist parents in preparing a child for school.
5. List two ways in which school life influences the growing child.
6. Discuss accident prevention in this age group.
7. Discuss the role of the school nurse in providing guidance and health supervision for the school-age child.
8. Discuss the value of pet ownership for the healthy school-age child and the family education necessary for the allergic or immunocompromised child.

Key Terms

androgynous (ăn-DRŎJ-ĭ-nŭs, p. 435)
concrete operations (p. 434)
latchkey children (p. 439)
preadolescent (prē-ăd-ō-LĔS-ĕnt, p. 441)

Sexuality Information and Education Council of the United States (SIECUS) (p. 436)
sexual latency (p. 434)
stage of industry (p. 434)

GENERAL CHARACTERISTICS

School-age children (6 to 12 years of age) differ from preschool children in that they are more engrossed in fact than in fantasy and are capable of more sophisticated reasoning. School-age children develop their first close peer relationships outside of the family group and their first affiliation with adults outside of their family who will influence their lives in a significant way.

As a result of the increased contact with the outside world and increased cognitive abilities, school-age children begin to understand how others evaluate them. School-age children are often judged by their performance—good grades or athletic feats. Their sense of industry and the development of positive self-esteem are directly influenced by their ability to become an accepted member of a peer group and meet the challenges in the environment.

The school-age child must be able to pay attention in class (with at least a 45-minute attention span), understand language, and progress from the *skill* of writing or reading to *understanding* what is written or read. To succeed in school, the child must work toward a delayed reward and must risk being unsuccessful in his or her efforts. However, parents must be guided to understand that multiple unsuccessful experiences for their child can lead to the development of a fear of trying in the future. New experiences for the school-age child include the first night sleeping away from home at a friend's house or camp, successes that are formally celebrated, chores that are dependably performed, conflict resolution with peers, and the selection of adult role models.

School-age children have an ardent thirst for knowledge and accomplishment. They tend to admire their teachers and adult companions. They use the skill and knowledge they obtain to attempt to master the activities they enjoy, including music, sports, and art. Thus, Erikson refers to this phase as the **stage of industry**. Unsuccessful adaptations at this time can lead to a sense of inferiority. Participation in group activities heightens. Romantic love for the parent of the opposite sex diminishes, and children identify with the parent of the same sex. Freud refers to this period as a time of **sexual latency**. The type of acceptance that school-age children receive at home and at school will affect the attitudes they develop about themselves and their role in life. Piaget refers to the thought processes of this period as concrete operations.

Concrete operations involve logical thinking and an understanding of cause and effect. The egocentric view of the preschool child is replaced by the ability to understand the point of view of another person. The child can understand the origin or consequence of an event he or she is experiencing. By 10 years of age, the child understands that people do not always control events in life, such as death, spirituality, or the origin of the world (Box 19-1).

| Box 19-1 | Features of Major Theories of Development During Later Childhood |

SIGMUND FREUD

The child is in a period of sexual latency.

The child's repression of sexuality makes it possible to form same-sex friendships; the child assumes the role of leader or follower.

The child is heavily influenced by parents and teachers, who can bolster his or her self-image or more deeply repress sexuality.

ERIK ERIKSON

Other people heavily influence the child's development.

The child's leadership abilities and popularity depend on successfully controlling the environment.

By learning to be productive, self-directing, and accepted at school and in society, the child gains a positive self-concept.

JEAN PIAGET

The child can concentrate on more than one aspect of a situation at a time.

The child becomes capable of abstract reasoning, but thought is still limited to his or her own experience.

The child understands cause and effect.

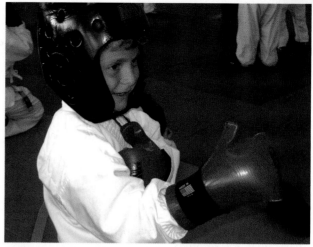

FIGURE 19-1 School-age children are often evaluated by their peers according to their performance, such as achieving good grades or demonstrating their ability to spar by earning a "yellow belt" in karate.

Between 6 and 12 years of age, children prefer friends of their own sex and usually prefer the company of their friends to that of their brothers and sisters. Outward displays of affection by adults are embarrassing to them. Although they are now too big to cuddle on their parents' laps, they still require much love, support, and guidance.

Between 6 and 12 years of age, self-esteem becomes very important in the developmental process. Children are evaluated according to their social contribution, such as the ability to attain good grades, hit home runs, or earn a "yellow belt" in karate class (Figure 19-1). Children's feelings about themselves are very important and should be assessed.

PHYSICAL GROWTH

Growth is slow until the spurt directly before puberty. Weight gains are more rapid than increases in height. The average gain in weight per year is about 2.5 to 3.2 kg (5.5 to 7 lb). The average increase in height is approximately 5.0 cm (2 inches). Growth in head circumference is slower than before, because myelinization within the brain is complete by 7 years of age. Head circumference increases from 20 to 21 inches between 5 and 12 years of age. At the end of this time, the brain has reached approximately adult size. (Dentition and nutrition are discussed in Chapter 15.)

Muscular coordination is improved, and the lymphatic tissues become highly developed. The skeletal bones continue to ossify, and the body has a lower center of gravity. The body is supple, and skeletal growth is sometimes more rapid than growth of muscles and ligaments. The child may appear "gangling." There is a noticeable change in facial structures as the jaw lengthens. The sinuses are often sites of infection. The 6-year molars (the first permanent teeth) erupt. The loss of primary teeth begins at about age 6 years, and about four permanent teeth erupt per year. The gastrointestinal tract is more mature, and the stomach is upset less often. Stomach capacity increases, and caloric needs are less than in preschool years. The heart grows slowly and is now smaller in proportion to body size than at any other time of life.

The shape of the eye changes with growth. The exact age at which 20/20 vision occurs, once believed to be about 7 years of age, is now believed to be sometime during the preschool years. The capabilities of the child's sense organs, including hearing, have an important bearing on learning abilities.

The vital signs of the child of school age are near those of the adult. The temperature is 37° C (98.6° F), the pulse is 85 to 100 beats/min, and respirations are 18 to 20 breaths/min. The systolic blood pressure ranges from 90 to 108 mm Hg; the diastolic blood pressure ranges from 60 to 68 mm Hg. Boys are slightly taller and somewhat heavier than girls until changes indicating puberty appear. The differences among children are greater at the end of middle childhood than at the beginning.

The changes in body proportions help the child prepare for activities commonly enjoyed in school. However, size is not correlated with emotional maturity, and a problem is created when a child faces higher expectations because he or she is taller and heavier than peers. Sedentary activities and habits in the school-age child are associated with a high risk of developing obesity and cardiovascular problems later in life.

SEXUAL DEVELOPMENT

Gender Identity

The sex organs remain immature during the school-age years, but interest in gender differences increases as the child progresses to puberty. Gender role development is greatly influenced by parents through differential treatment and identification. These two interdependent processes are at work in the family and in society. In infancy, boys and girls are often wrapped in blue or pink blankets. Later, their dress, the types of toys and games chosen for them, television, and the attitudes of family members may serve to fortify gender identity, although unisex dress and play are currently popular.

The influence of the school environment is considerable. The teacher can directly foster stereotyping in the assignment of schoolroom tasks, the choice of textbooks, and the disapproval of behavior that deviates from the child's gender role. Aggressive behavior is sometimes overlooked in boys but is discouraged in girls.

Some adults develop a gender role concept that incorporates both masculine and feminine qualities, sometimes termed **androgynous**. Because healthy interpersonal relationships depend on both assertiveness and sensitivity, the incorporation both of traditionally masculine and traditionally feminine positive attributes may lead to fuller human functioning.

Sex Education

Sex education is a lifelong process. Parents convey their attitudes and feelings about all aspects of life, including sexuality, to the growing child. Sex education is accomplished less by talking or formal instruction than by the whole climate of the home, particularly the respect shown to each family member.

Children's questions about sex should be answered simply and at their level of understanding. Correct names should be used to describe the genitalia. All people understand the hospitalized child who complains, "My penis hurts." Private masturbation is normal and is practiced by both males and females at various times throughout their lives. It does not cause acne, blindness, insanity, or impotence. The young boy must be prepared for erections and nocturnal emissions ("wet dreams"), which are to be expected and are not necessarily the result of masturbation. The young girl is prepared for menarche and is provided with the necessary supplies. This is particularly important to the early maturer because an elementary school may not provide dispensing machines for supplies in the restrooms. (See the discussion of the menstrual cycle in Chapter 2.)

Both sexes are concerned during the school years with the disproportion of their bodies, and they may be self-conscious when undressing. They may compare themselves with their friends. They need reassurance about their awakening sexuality, which affects their thoughts and behavior.

Factual knowledge concerning sex and drugs is an essential component of sex education both in the home and at school. School nurses can assist in preparing sex education programs, but the participation of parents

is valuable. Sex education can be taught in the context of the normal process and function of the human body. Facts must be provided. Values clarification can be added and influenced by parents in the home. If children realize that their parents are uncomfortable with discussing the subject, they may turn to peers, who often supply erroneous and distorted information. The **Sexuality Information and Education Council of the United States (SIECUS)** maintains that every sex education program should present the topic from six aspects: biological, social, health, personal adjustment and attitudes, interpersonal associations, and establishment of values.

Regardless of the practice setting, nurses can help parents and children with sex education through careful listening and anticipatory guidance (Table 19-1). They can teach decision-making skills and responsibility. Nurses should review normal developmental behavior and explain age-specific information. They provide families with useful written information that stresses sexuality as a healthful rather than as an illness-related concept. The nurse should always consider cultural differences when counseling.

Sexually Transmitted Infections. Education concerning sexually transmitted infections (STIs) and human immunodeficiency virus (HIV) prevention should be presented in simple terms. The school nurse is a vital link in the education of the child and the parents.

Table 19-1   Using the Nursing Process in Sex Education of the School-Age Child

INTERVENTION	OBSERVATION
Data collection, history taking	Readiness to learn is indicated by asking questions concerning sex, menstruation, "wet dreams," and pregnancy.
Analysis	Observe parent–child interactions and determine level of communication. Observe peer interaction to determine the child's self-image, self-confidence, and ability to communicate. Observe parent's knowledge and ability to discuss issues pertaining to sex education. Determine child's understanding of sexual development and body changes.
Planning and implementation	Discuss growth and development with the parent and the child. Reinforce teaching techniques and opportunities with parents.
Evaluation	With each clinic or home visit, evaluate the results of parent–child interaction concerning sex education.

There are audiovisual materials designed for the school-age child. Factual information about STIs and concrete information on how to say "no" to sexual intercourse and drugs are essential components in the sex education of the preadolescent. The nurse can help to implement educational programs in the school, the clinic, the church, and other community organizations. The facts concerning the harmful effects of drugs and unprotected sex should be communicated to the child without using scare tactics.

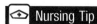 **Nursing Tip**

When discussing sexuality with school-age children, it is necessary to review slang or street terms. Most children hear the terms but may be confused about their meanings.

INFLUENCES FROM THE WIDER WORLD

SCHOOL-RELATED TASKS

The home, the school, and the neighborhood each have an impact on the growth and development of the child. Schools have a profound influence on the socialization of children, who bring to school what they have learned and experienced in the home. Although some children come from healthy, intact, and financially secure families, many do not. A child may be disabled or abused or may suffer from a chronic illness. Parents may be alcoholics, substance abusers, unemployed, or suffering from numerous other physical or stress-related conditions. Nurses must remember these factors, because they surface continually with this age group. Moral development occurs as they have experience with, and understand, rules and fairness. The understanding of what is right and wrong and the development of values occurs as a result of their experience.

Children may be unable to verbalize their needs; therefore caretakers must become particularly astute in their observations. Table 19-2 reviews the expected growth and development abilities related to required school tasks. Success in school requires an integration of cognitive, receptive, and expressive (language) skills. Repeating a grade in school can seriously impair self-image, and therefore it is important to identify deficits or health problems that affect learning as early as possible.

A holistic attitude toward child care must focus not only on intellectual achievement and test scores but also on such qualities as artistic expression, creativity, joy, cooperation, responsibility, industry, love, and other attributes. The sensitive nurse can assist parents by affirming the individuality of children and by encouraging parents to share with their children the pride they are experiencing as the children learn and progress through the elementary grades. The Patient Teaching box summarizes parental guidance that the nurse may find useful in preparing children for the beginning of school.

Table 19-2 Growth and Development of the School-Age Child in School-Related Tasks

CHILD'S TASK	PARENT'S TASK	NURSING INTERVENTIONS
Adapt to differences in expectations of teachers.	Communicate with teacher to maintain consistency in expectations and discipline.	School nurse should be contacted to facilitate parent–teacher–child interaction.
Compete with 30 or more peers for adult attention.	Praise child's accomplishments. Avoid making comparisons to other children.	Evaluate parent–teacher interactions, and provide guidance and positive support.
Learn to accept criticism from peers and teachers without losing self-esteem.	Supervise peer activities. Provide constructive activities.	Provide teacher–parent guidance.
Assimilate peer values, and integrate with family values.	Maintain open communication. Encourage peer activity. Introduce and accept other cultures in the community.	Provide anticipatory guidance in handling behavior problems. Observe and respond to signs of prejudice.
Find satisfaction in achievements at school.	Allow children to achieve. Do not complete tasks for them.	
Participate in group activities.	Encourage child to join a group or club and actively participate as a member.	Refer to community agencies such as churches, organizations, and club activities as needed.
Learn self-control. Handle prejudice from others in a positive way.	Encourage participation in activities away from home and with peers. Have faith in child's problem-solving abilities. Discuss coping with prejudices of others.	Encourage parents to "let go" and provide guidance while encouraging independence.

Parental Guidance for Children Starting School

Encourage parents to do the following:
- Review normal growth and development of 5- to 6-year-olds.
- Anticipate regression such as thumb sucking, clinging behavior, and occasional soiling.
- Encourage children to express what they think school will be like.
- Arrange for children to meet others who will be entering school with them.
- Tour the school with the child.
- Introduce the child to the school crossing guard and the bus driver.
- Teach the child his or her family name and telephone number.
- Teach safety precautions about crossing the street, strangers, and "blue star" homes (community-established "safe homes" for children in an emergency; such houses are designated by a blue star or other symbol).
- Allow sufficient time in the morning to prepare for school.
- Provide a cheerful send-off.
- Instruct the child about where to go in case of an emergency at home, such as to a neighbor or a relative.
- Walk with the child to school until the child understands the route, or designate a bus stop.
- Listen to the child at the end of the day; take an interest in his or her school life.
- Get to know the child's teacher; take an interest in the school.
- Inform the teacher of sudden or unusual stress in the child's life.

Data from Rogers F, Head B: *Mister Rogers talks with parents*, New York, 1983, Berkley Books; Kliegman RM, et al: *Nelson's textbook of pediatrics*, ed 19, Philadelphia, 2011, Saunders.

The nurse observes patterns of communication between parents and child and assists with specific behavioral problems. In general, the transition to junior high school or "middle school" means multiple classrooms, a series of teachers, and a change of buildings. The child is developing adult characteristics and has new feelings about his or her body, parents, teachers, and peers. Anticipatory guidance includes a review of normal physiology and how it changes with puberty. Information concerning sexuality is reviewed, and the child is encouraged to ask questions at the time they arise.

A warm, ongoing relationship between the parents and child helps to provide a safe atmosphere of caring. Adults should develop a heightened awareness for things such as school attendance problems, tardiness, and signs of loneliness or depression. They should continue to encourage children to discuss their school problems, feelings, and worries. Parents and children must set realistic goals. A good question for adults to contemplate periodically is, "When was the last time this child had a success?" Homework should be the child's responsibility, with a minimum of assistance from parents. For some children, visits to the nurse's office may be their only continuous contact with a health care worker. The nurse may be instrumental in establishing positive health patterns that may be carried into adulthood.

The school nurse can guide the parents in determining health care requirements for the school-age child.

Schools provide some health screening, but the financial resources of the family may prevent adequate follow-up care, clothing, or transportation. School lunch programs are available in most schools for the child identified as being in need.

Safety is an important issue for the school-age child. The rules of the road should be taught before the child walks or rides a bike to school. Car safety and the use of seat belts must be a regular ritual. Caution in play is essential, but a child must not be made to feel afraid to try new activities or skills.

PLAY

Play activities for the school-age child involve increased physical and intellectual skills and some fantasy. The sense of belonging to a group is very important, and conformity to "be just like my friends" is of vital importance to the child. The culture of the school-age child involves membership in a group of some type. If parents do not provide a club, scout, or church group, the child may find a group of his or her own, which may be a gang.

Teams are important to growth and development, and competition is a new challenge. Rituals such as collecting items and playing board games are enjoyable quiet activities for the school-age child. Television is often considered to be a "babysitter" when overused, but many educational and exciting programs are offered during prime-time hours. Computer and video games challenge intellect and skill and are healthy outlets as long as they do not completely replace active physical play. Play enables the child to feel powerful and in control. Mastering new skills helps the child to feel a sense of accomplishment, which is necessary to achieve Erikson's phase of industry successfully (Figure 19-2). Participation in organized sports can develop skill, teamwork, and fitness, but excessive pressure and unrealistic expectations can have negative effects. High-stress and high-impact sports such as football are not desirable sports activities for the school-age child because of the risk of injury to the immature skeletal system.

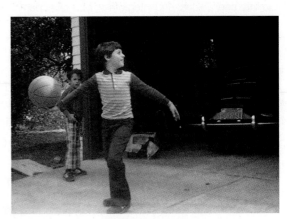

FIGURE 19-2 Developing the skills of a team sport is important to the school-age child.

Emergency Treatment of an Avulsed Tooth

When a permanent tooth is accidentally knocked out of the socket, the tooth should be picked up by the crown to avoid damaging the root area. Place the tooth in milk until the child and tooth arrive at a dentist's office.

Observing Play

Play is an essential tool to promote growth and development in children. Play is essential to a healthy lifestyle that includes a feeling of wellbeing and fitness. Play provides a link between the spontaneity of childhood and the disciplined activities of adulthood. Elements of play that should be assessed include the following:

- Motivation and intensity of engagement
- Whether the child initiated it or the child joined the group
- Relation to reality or creativity
- The element of choice in how to play
- Self-control
- Following or changing rules
- Sharing—giving and receiving cues from others
- Skills used in the play activity

Factors that may limit play effectiveness are adult intervention, limited space, and an older dominant player or younger players that interfere with action.

LATCHKEY CHILDREN

In the United States, **latchkey children** are those who are left unsupervised after school because parents are away from home or at work and extended family is not available to care for them. Local after-school programs and clubs have decreased the number of children left home alone since 1990, but there are still many children who do not have these options available, and babysitters are expensive. Children left home alone are subject to a higher rate of accidents and are at risk of feeling isolated and alone. Some children, however, enjoy the independence and become skilled in problem solving and self-care. A back-up adult should be available to the child in case of emergencies. Many latchkey children do not participate in after-school social and sports activities and may be slower to identify themselves as belonging to a group. The school nurse can be a key source for providing information about the needs of the school-age child and quality after-school care programs that may be available in the community.

 Safety Alert!

Caution parents about the safe storage of firearms. Many deaths caused by firearms occur in the home, not on the streets.

Nurses should be aware of local resources, such as the National Boy Scouts and Girl Scouts of America, Boys & Girls Club of America, and Young Men's Christian Association (YMCA) and Young Women's Christian Association (YWCA) after-school activities. They can also assist

 Health Promotion

Guidance for Children at Home Alone

TEACH CHILD ABOUT SAFETY

Do not enter the house if the door is ajar or if anything looks unusual.
Do not leave the house or yard without permission.
Never admit a stranger into the house.
Never agree to meet with someone you met online.
Never respond to messages on the computer that sound weird.
Do not display keys; keep the door locked.
Answer the telephone according to parents' teaching (parents are busy, not "out").
Do not take shortcuts to school through alleys or across train tracks.
Walk to and from school with friends.
Never accept rides with strangers.
Know how to reach a trusted adult.
Follow first aid techniques taught by parents; know how to call 911.
Review fire safety rules and the route of escape; walk through the procedure with your parents.
Know and obey basic safety rules.

TEACH PARENTS

List emergency numbers and post them near the telephone.
Designate a neighbor who is usually home for help in emergencies.
Teach the child his or her own name, telephone number, address, and parents' name.
Leave work number with the child.
Lock up firearms or remove them from the house.
Prepare a first aid kit and designate its location.
Review fire safety rules and the route of escape; walk through the procedure with the child.
Address street safety with the child when returning from school; include precautions with strangers.
Consider obtaining a pet for the child.
Be home on time or call the child.
Leave a recorded message to decrease the loneliness of the child; recommend specific activities rather than television.
Help the child to feel successful and appreciated.
Assess the home and the neighborhood for hazards specific to their locale.
Teach child safe telephone behavior.

Data modified from 2013 *Times Dispatch:* "Latch key kids drop sharply since 1990's," *National and World News; Bloomberg News* Times dispatch.com, and State of California Office of Criminal Justice Planning, Sacramento, Calif, 95814.

in developing innovative programs such as cooperative babysitting, in which parents exchange child care services. The nurse must spend time with parents, lend support, and help them to explore their options.

PHYSICAL, MENTAL, EMOTIONAL, AND SOCIAL DEVELOPMENT

THE SIX-YEAR-OLD

At 6 years of age, children burst with energy and are on the go constantly. They soon become overtired, and it is necessary to limit their activities. They like to start tasks but do not always finish them, because their attention span is fairly brief. They tend to be bossy, are sometimes rude, and experiment with language, but they

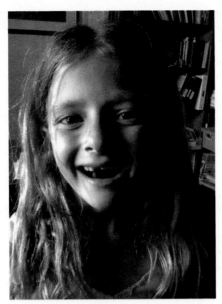

FIGURE 19-3 One of the most obvious physical changes of the 6-year-old is the loss of primary teeth. The loss of primary teeth starts at 6 years of age, and about four permanent teeth erupt each year.

are very sensitive to criticism. Their conscience is active, and they find it difficult to make decisions.

One of the most obvious physical changes at this age is the loss of the temporary teeth (Figure 19-3). The important 6-year molars also erupt. Children can jump rope, throw and catch a ball, tie shoelaces, and perform numerous other feats that require muscle coordination. Their language differs from that of the preschool child. They use it for a purpose rather than for the pure joy of talking. Their vocabulary consists of about 2500 words. They require 11 to 13 hours of sleep a night.

Boys and girls play together at this age, although they begin to prefer to associate with children of their own gender. Most children enjoy collecting objects such as shells, leaves, or stones. Play at this time usually reflects events that occur in the immediate environment.

Six-year-old children need time and support to help them adjust to school. The transition may be more comfortable if they have nursery school or kindergarten experience. Most children go to school expecting the same reception they are accustomed to at home. If parents are critical or overly protective, children will assume that the teacher will be also. When the teacher's response differs markedly from the child's expectations, they feel insecure and may even be hostile toward the teacher. Parents must observe children for signs of fatigue and stress. Not all children are ready for school merely because they reach the proper age. Even those who are ready need time and support from parents and teachers before they can settle down to the job at hand. Being in school exposes the child to infection more frequently than being at home. Preschool immunizations and a physical examination are indicated (see Chapter 32).

THE SEVEN-YEAR-OLD

The 7-year-old is a quieter child, and some educators have noted that second-graders are the easiest children

to teach. They set high standards for themselves and for their families. They have a good sense of humor, tend to be somewhat of a "tease" (wiggle loose teeth to annoy adults), and are a little more modest than at an earlier age. They enjoy being active but also appreciate periods of rest. The second-grader may have a "crush" on a friend of the opposite sex.

These children know the months and seasons of the year and begin to tell time. They have a beginning concept of arithmetic, can count by twos and fives, and know that money is valuable. Their hands are steadier. Their interest in God or heaven may be heightened.

Active play is still important to both sexes. The boys are more apt to tease the girls than to participate in games such as jump rope or tag. Both sexes enjoy bike riding and table games. Realistic toys, such as dolls that can be bathed and fed and video games or radio-controlled cars, appeal to the 7-year-old. Graphic novels are also popular especially if they can be read on the Kindle. Becoming increasingly independent, the children imagine themselves accomplishing feats more adventurous than those of their parents. They keep busy on their "smart phones" and they cannot understand how Mom and Dad ever chose to lead such "dull lives."

THE EIGHT-YEAR-OLD

The 8-year-old wants to do everything and can play alone for a longer period than can the 7-year-old. The work of an 8-year-old is usually creative. These children enjoy group activities, such as Brownies and Cub Scouts, and prefer companions of the same sex. They become interested in group fads. Eight-year-olds like to be considered important, particularly by adults. They may behave better for company than for the family. Hero worship is evident.

The arms and hands of the 8-year-old seem to grow faster than the rest of the body. The large and small muscles are better developed, and movements are smoother and more graceful. The child can write rather than print and understands the number of days that must pass before special events such as Christmas, birthdays, and discharge from the hospital.

The 8-year-old enjoys competitive sports but is generally a poor loser (Figure 19-4). Long, involved arguments often occur. A healthy way to teach a child to express anger is to have the child pound on a pillow (Figure 19-5). Wrestling is common, and dramatic play is popular. Most children like to be the hero or heroine of their favorite program. Neighborhood secret clubs are organized, and all members must strictly adhere to the rules.

THE NINE-YEAR-OLD

Nine-year-olds are dependable, show more interest in family activities, assume more responsibility for personal belongings and for younger brothers and sisters, and are more likely to complete tasks. They resist adult authority if it does not coincide with the opinions or

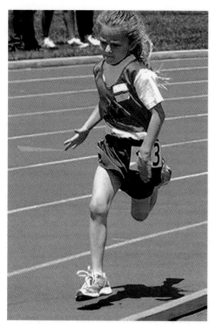

FIGURE 19-4 Competitive sports. The 8-year old is ready for competitive sports.

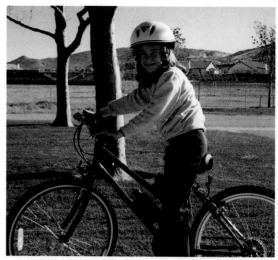

FIGURE 19-6 Protective clothing is necessary for potentially hazardous play. Providing protective equipment appropriate for any sport the child plays is an important parental responsibility (e.g., helmets for bicycling, skateboarding, or ice hockey).

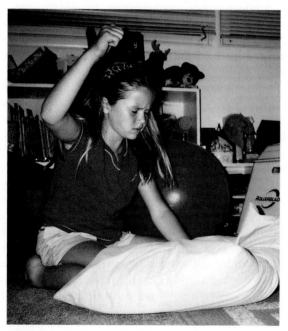

FIGURE 19-5 A healthy outlet for feelings of anger is pounding on a pillow. (Courtesy Pat Spier, RN-C.)

ideals of the group. However, they are more able to accept criticism for their actions. Individual differences are pronounced.

Worries and mild compulsions are common. Nervous habits, sometimes referred to as tics, may appear and may vary widely. Eye blinking, facial grimacing, and shoulder shrugging are but a few examples. The child cannot help such actions and should not be scolded for them, because they are mainly caused by tension; they usually disappear when home and social life become more relaxed.

Hand and eye coordination is well developed, and manual activities are managed with skill. The child works and plays hard and can become overly tired. About 10 hours of sleep a night are needed. The permanent teeth are still erupting.

Competitive sports are still popular, as are reading, listening to music, watching television, playing online computer games, and texting. Sports programs that take into consideration the limitations of children at various ages should be encouraged. Teaching proper techniques and the use of adequate safety devices is essential (Figure 19-6). Boys develop more muscle mass than girls as puberty approaches; therefore competitive contact sports should have separate teams for boys and girls.

An interest in music is shown, and the child may desire to take lessons. Children know the date, can repeat months of the year in order, can multiply and do simple division, and are ready for more complex math. They take care of their body needs, and by now their table manners have improved considerably.

PREADOLESCENCE

The Ten-Year-Old

Age 10 marks the beginning of the **preadolescent** years. Girls are more physically mature than boys. The child begins to show self-direction, is courteous to adults, and thinks clearly about social problems and prejudices. The 10-year-old wants to be independent and resents being told what to do but is receptive to suggestions. The ideas of the group are more important than are individual ideas. Interest in sex and sexual curiosity continue.

In general, girls are more poised than boys. Both sexes are fairly reliable about household duties (Figure 19-7). Slang terms are used. The 10-year-old can write for a

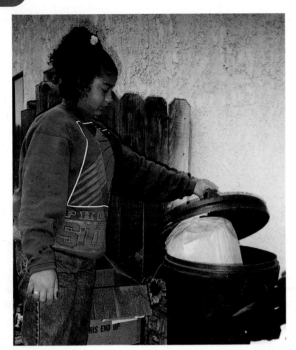

FIGURE 19-7 Household chores. The school-age child contributes to the smooth running of the household by performing household chores. (Reminders may be needed!)

relatively long period of time and maintains good writing speed. The child uses fractions and knows abstract numbers. Boys and girls begin to identify themselves with skills that pertain to their sex roles. They are intolerant of the opposite sex. The play enjoyed by the 10-year-old is similar to that enjoyed by the 9-year-old. In addition, the child takes more interest in personal appearance. Sending texts to friends is important.

Eleven- and Twelve-Year-Olds

Adjectives that describe 11- and 12-year-olds include intense, observant, all-knowing, energetic, meddlesome, and argumentative. This period before the onset of puberty is one of complete disorganization. It begins earlier in some children; the onset and rate of physical maturity vary greatly. Before the end of this period the hormones of the body begin to influence physical growth. Posture is poor. There are 24 to 26 permanent teeth.

The child has an overabundance of energy and is on the go every minute. Girls become "tomboyish" in their actions. Table manners are a thing of the past, and the refrigerator is constantly emptied. Children at this age are less concerned with their appearance. They often seem to be preoccupied; this, along with physical activities and numerous anxieties, accounts for some of the decline seen in school grades. The ability to concentrate decreases, and parents complain that the child "never hears anything." When asked to do a new task, these children moan and groan.

Group participation is still important. They enjoy being team players. Preadolescent children are not ready to stand alone, but they cannot bear the thought of depending on parents. They must overcome the problems they confront without parental help. Their attitude implies, "Can't you see that I'm not a child anymore?"

During preadolescence, children are interested in their bodies and watch for signs of growing up. Girls look forward to menstruation and wearing their first bra. Boys and girls tend to "ignore" those of opposite sex, but really they are very much aware of them. There is a tendency to tease one another. Their descriptions of each other are far from complimentary: "stupid," "crazy," and "nerd." At this age, words are often used without full understanding of their true meaning. Both genders enjoy earning money by obtaining odd jobs. The preadolescent often seeks an adult friend of the same sex to idolize.

Guiding preadolescents is not easy. They need freedom within limits and recognition that they are no longer infants. They should know why parents make a decision. They should not be expected to follow household rules blindly. Their conscience enables them to understand and accept reasonable discipline. They ignore constant verbal nagging. They should be provided constructive opportunities to release pent-up emotions and energy. One can more easily accept their irritating behavior by realizing that much of it is indeed "just a phase." Texting friends occurs in regular spurts throughout the day.

The American Academy of Pediatrics Committee on Sports Medicine and School Health recommends teaching motor skills and fitness exercises in the school setting to promote positive attitudes toward exercise in later life. The focus should be on mastering the skill of the sport and enjoying the exercise rather than winning a game. Selecting students for teams based on athletic prowess is inappropriate for the preadolescent child. Ceremonies should recognize all participants rather than star players. In the physical education or gym class, discipline for misbehavior should not be in the form of assigned extra pushups or extra laps of running on the track. Such discipline measures foster a negative attitude toward healthy exercise.

Chores as Teaching Tools

Chores help children do a job, take responsibility, feel that they are an important part of a family, and develop self-esteem. Age-appropriate chores for a preschooler may include setting the table, sorting colored and white laundry, making beds, or watering plants. Age-appropriate chores for the school-age child may include loading the washer or dryer, taking out the garbage (see Figure 19-7), and caring for pets. Teens can mow or rake the lawn for the family or others. The nurse can refer the parent to various websites for suggestions concerning age-appropriate chores.

GUIDANCE AND HEALTH SUPERVISION

HEALTH EXAMINATIONS

A physical examination is given in the spring preceding school admission. This allows time to correct any problems that are found. Booster immunizations are provided as needed (see Chapter 32); also the child's teeth are examined, and dental work is completed. Good dental hygiene and regular professional dental care are essential as the permanent set of teeth erupts. Dental health and nutrition are discussed in Chapter 15.

School health programs aimed at maintaining and promoting health are provided in most school systems. Nurses and other professional persons who take part in such programs can play an important role in counseling parents. They also help to meet the needs of disabled children enrolled in their schools. A carefully obtained health history provides the nurse with much-needed information. Table 19-3 reviews the development of the school-age child.

The eating habits of a child of this age should be basically sound, as long as a variety of nutritious foods are offered. Food preferences occur. A nutritious breakfast is important. The federal government has established the school breakfast program in many areas. The National School Lunch Program has been ongoing. Summer lunch programs are also available. These lunches must provide certain nutritional standards (the goal is to provide one third of the recommended daily allowance of foods).

Children who are inattentive at school should be screened for vision or hearing deficits and language or learning disabilities before being worked up for attention-deficit hyperactivity disorder (ADHD). Increasing structure and decreasing distractions are the first steps in helping any child with a school problem. Emphasis should be placed on producing successful experiences and increasing complexity slowly. Realistic demands must be balanced by unconditional support during the successes and failures of the developing child. If the development of behavior problems is to be averted, the school nurse should be aware of parenting styles that demonstrate difficulty in "letting go" and parenting styles that demonstrate excessive pressure.

Active play with family members is important to the school-age child. Divorce, separation, domestic violence, and neighborhood gangs can negatively affect the progress of development in the school-age child. The school nurse can initiate appropriate referrals to community agencies.

Health supervision should include the assessment of physical activity and school performance. A child who avoids activities that may reveal his physical appearance, such as changing into gym clothes or cooperating in health examinations, may have a negative perception of his or her own physical appearance. Parents need guidance to understand the difference between participation in sports activities that help to develop skill, teamwork, and fitness, and participation in high-stress activities that increase the risk of skeletal injury and focus on winning as a central theme. Often a 6-year-old with advanced athletic ability who is guided into early competition and who experiences outstanding commendations loses his or her self-esteem on reaching 12 years of age—when the ability of peers reaches or exceeds his or her level and he or she no longer experiences the spotlight. The school-age child can understand simple explanations of his or her illness but sometimes can revert to believing illness is "punishment" for bad behavior or thoughts.

School-age children need time and a place to study. They require a desk in their own room or at least a private area of the house where they can concentrate. Their furniture should be of the proper size; lighting should be adequate. They must learn to take responsibility for their assignments and school supplies. Parents can encourage school children by showing interest in what they are learning, by joining parent–teacher organizations, and by visiting periodically with the teacher. Parents should be encouraged to vote on civic matters that will benefit the school system in their community.

At this age an allowance or at least a means of earning money provides children with opportunities to learn money's value. It takes time and encouragement for them to learn to spend money wisely. Such experiences aid in making the school-age child a more responsible person.

Nursing Tip

Tips to help prevent obesity:
- Use appropriate serving sizes for age.
- Limit intake of soda and/or juice drinks that are not 100% juice (empty calories).
- Replace whole milk with skim milk.
- Eat breakfast every day.
- Encourage family meal times.
- Parents should role model healthy eating and activity.
- Encourage physical activity.
- Decrease computer and TV time.

Nursing Tip

Mutual respect involves accepting the child's feelings. When helping children to identify feelings, start with the terms *mad*, *glad*, *sad*, or *scared*.

PET OWNERSHIP

Pet ownership is a common practice in families with children. After 7 years of age, children can be responsible for caring for the needs of a family pet. Pets that have close contact with children have the potential of transmitting disease (Table 19-4). Studies have documented the positive influence of pet ownership on improving the medical and psychological outcome

Text continued on p. 447

Table 19-3 Summary of Growth and Development and Health Maintenance of School-Age Children

AGE (YEARS)	PHYSICAL COMPETENCY	INTELLECTUAL COMPETENCY	EMOTIONAL-SOCIAL COMPETENCY	NUTRITION	PLAY	SAFETY
General: 6-12 years	Gains an average of 2.5-3.2 kg/year (5.0 to 7 lb/year) Has overall height gains of 5.0 cm/year (2 inches/year); growth occurs in spurts and mainly in the trunk and the extremities Loses deciduous teeth; most permanent teeth erupt Progressively more coordinated in both gross and fine-motor skills Caloric needs increase during growth spurts	Masters concrete operations Moves from egocentrism; learns that he or she is not always right Learns grammar and expression of emotions and thoughts Vocabulary increases to 3000 words or more Handles complex sentences	Central crisis; industry versus inferiority; wants to do and make things Progressive sex education needed Wants to be like friends; competition is important Fears body mutilation, alterations in body image; earlier phobias may recur; fears death Nervous habits are common	Fluctuations in appetite because of uneven growth pattern and tendency to become involved in activities Tendency to neglect breakfast in rush of getting to school Although school lunch is provided in most schools, child does not always eat it	Plays in groups, mostly of same gender; gang activities predominate Books important for all ages Bicycles important Sports equipment, cards, board and computer games Most play consists of active games requiring little or no equipment	Enforce continued use of seat belts during car travel. Bicycle safety must be taught and enforced. Teach safety related to hobbies, handicrafts, and mechanical equipment.
6-7 years	Gross motor skill exceeds fine motor coordination Has good balance and rhythm—runs, skips, jumps, climbs, gallops Throws and catches ball Dresses self with little or no help	Has vocabulary of 2500 words Learning to read and print Begins concrete concepts of numbers, general classification of items Knows concepts of right and left; morning, afternoon, and evening; and coinage Has intuitive thought process Is verbally aggressive, bossy, opinionated, argumentative Likes simple games with basic rules	Boisterous, outgoing, and a know-it-all Whiny; parents should sidestep power struggles, offer choices Becomes quiet and reflective during seventh year; very sensitive Can use telephone Likes to make things; starts many projects, finishes few Give some responsibility for household duties	Persistence of preschool food likes and dislikes Tendency for deficiencies in iron, vitamin A, and riboflavin; needs 100 mL/kg of water per day, 3 g/kg protein daily	Still enjoys dolls, cars, and trucks Plays well alone but enjoys small groups of both sexes; begins to prefer same-sex peers during seventh year Ready to learn how to ride a bicycle Prefers imaginary, dramatic play with real costumes Begins collecting for quantity, not quality Enjoys active games such as hide-and-seek, tag, jump rope, roller skating, kickball	Teach and reinforce traffic safety. Child needs adult supervision of play. Teach child to avoid strangers and never to take anything from strangers. Teach illness prevention and reinforce continued practice of other health habits. Restrict bicycle use to home grounds and no-traffic areas; teach bicycle safety. Child should wear helmet. Teach and set examples about harmful use of drugs, alcohol, and smoking.

| 8-10 years | Myopia may appear Secondary sex characteristics begin in girls Hand-eye coordination and fine motor skills are well established Movements are graceful, coordinated Cares for own physical needs completely Is constantly on the move; plays and works hard | Learning correct grammar and expression of feelings in words Likes books he or she can read alone; will read funny papers and scan newspaper Enjoys making detailed drawings Mastering classification, seriation, spatial, temporal, and numerical concepts Uses language as a tool; likes riddles, jokes, chants, word games Rules are a guiding force in life now Very interested in how things work and how what and how weather, seasons, and the like are made | Strong preference for same-sex peers Antagonizes opposite-sex peers Self-assured and pragmatic at home; questions parental values and ideas Has a strong sense of humor Enjoys clubs, group projects, outings, large groups, camp Modesty about own body increases with time; sex-conscious Works diligently to perfect the skills he or she does best Happy, cooperative, relaxed, and casual in relationships Increasingly courteous and well mannered with adults Gang stage at a peak; secret codes and rituals prevail Responds better to suggestion than to dictatorial approach | Needs about 2100 calories/day; nutritious snacks Tends to be too busy to bother to eat Tendency for deficiencies in calcium, iron, and thiamine Problem of obesity may begin now Has good table manners Able to help with food preparation | Ready for lessons in dancing, gymnastics, music Restrict television time to 1-2 hours each day Likes hiking, sports Enjoys cooking, woodworking, crafts Enjoys cards and computer games Likes radio and music Begins qualitative collecting | Stress safety with firearms. Keep them out of reach, and allow their use only with adult supervision. Know who the child's friends are; parents should still have some control over friend selection. Teach water safety; an adult should supervise swimming. Enforce balance in rest and activity. |

Continued

Table 19-3   Summary of Growth and Development and Health Maintenance of School-Age Children—cont'd

AGE (YEARS)	PHYSICAL COMPETENCY	INTELLECTUAL COMPETENCY	EMOTIONAL-SOCIAL COMPETENCY	NUTRITION	PLAY	SAFETY
11-12 years	Vital signs approximate adult norms Growth spurt for girls Inequalities between sexes increasingly noticeable, with boys having greater physical strength Eruption of permanent teeth complete except for third molars Secondary sex characteristics begin in boys Menstruation may begin	Able to think about social problems and prejudices; sees others' points of view Enjoys reading mysteries, love stories Begins playing with abstract ideas Interested in whys of health measures and understands human reproduction Very moralistic; religious commitment often made during this time	Intense team loyalty; boys begin teasing girls, and girls flirt with boys for attention Best-friend period Wants unreasonable independence; is rebellious about routines; has wide mood swings; needs some time daily for privacy Very critical of own work Hero worship prevails Facts-of-life chats with friends prevail Masturbation increases Appears under constant tension	Male needs 2500 calories/day; female needs 2250 (70 calories/kg/day), both need 75 mL/kg of water/day and 2 g/kg protein daily	Enjoys projects and working with hands Likes to do errands and jobs to earn money Very involved in sports, dancing, talking on phone Enjoys all aspects of acting and drama	Continue monitoring friends. Stress bicycle and roller blade safety on streets and in traffic and the use of helmets and other protective gear.

Data from Betz C, Hunsberger M, Wright S: *Family-centered nursing care of children*, ed 2, Philadelphia, 1994, Saunders; Craig G: *Understanding growth and development*, ed 3, Englewood Cliffs, N.J., 2010, Pearson, Prentice-Hall; Lester B, Sparrow J, ed: *Nurturing children and families: building on the legend of T. Berry Brazelton*, Hoboken, N.J., 2010, Wiley Blackwell.

Table 19-4	Diseases That Can Be Transmitted by Pets to Humans
VECTOR	**DISEASE**
Dog bites	Cellulitis, septicemia
Geckos, reptiles	Salmonella
Dogs, cats, birds, farm animals	*Campylobacter pylori* (gastroenteritis, Guillain-Barré syndrome)
Cats, dogs, ferrets, raccoons, skunks, bats, foxes, wolves	Rabies
Reptiles, rodents, cats, dogs	Cryptosporidiosis (gastroenteritis) and skin infections
Dogs, cats	Parasites, pneumonia, hypereosinophilia, toxocariasis, fungal skin infections
Dogs, cats, reptiles, turtles	Leptospirosis
Blood contact during birth of animals	Brucellosis, Q fever
Kitten	Cat scratch disease (lymphadenopathy and preauricular adenitis)
Cats	Toxoplasmosis*
Birds, farm animals, cats	Q fever
Birds	Psittacosis, histoplasmosis, avian flu
Fish	Fish tank granuloma (related to *Mycobacterium tuberculosis* organism that causes ulcerated skin lesions after cleaning the fish tank)
Petting zoo	*E. coli, Giardia, Campylobacter,* and sensitivity to animal dander, scales, fur, and feathers

*Toxoplasmosis can cause congenital malformations in the fetus. Pregnant females are urged to avoid contact with litter boxes.
Data from Neumann B: Management of dog and cat bites, *Adv Nurs Pract* 17(3):53-55, 2009; Pickering L: Exposure to non-traditional pets at home and to animals in public settings: risks to children, *Pediatrics* 122:876-878, 2008; Behravesch C: *Pets can make people sick,* Atlanta, 2011, CDC; Compendium of measures to prevent diseases associated with animals in public settings: recommendations and reports of the National Association of State Public Health Veterinarians, Inc., *MMWR* 60(RR04):1-24, 2011; National Center for Infectious Diseases, 2013. Accessed Dec 2013 at www.cdc.gov/mmwr/preview/mmwrhtml/rr6004Al.htm.

after illness or surgery. Disabled children especially benefit from interacting with pets. The interaction with animals can lower blood pressure and heart rate, reduce loneliness and feelings of isolation, improve communication, foster trust, and motivate participation in physical therapy (Ernst, 2012). Pets allow the ill child who feels separated from other people to feel companionship and acceptance. Shy children often find pet ownership eases the path to socialization with others who initiate contact because of the pet.

The age of the child, the presence of allergies, and an immunocompromised family member are major factors that influence the desirability of pet ownership. Toddlers and young children may not understand the limitations in handling pets that can respond by biting or scratching. Certain breeds of dogs have a greater tendency to bite, such as pit bulls, German Shepherds, Rottweilers, Doberman Pinschers, and Chihuahuas. These breeds are involved in 50% of bite injuries with 75% of the attacks being from unaltered male dogs (Kliegman, 2011). Pregnant women should not handle cat litter boxes because the risk for toxoplasmosis affecting the fetus is high.

Immunocompromised children are at risk for contracting illness that is spread by some animals. Birds,

Health Promotion

Ways to Protect Immunocompromised Children from Pet-Transmitted Disease

- Choose a healthy animal (preferably a dog or cat) older than age 1 year to reduce the likelihood of colonization with human pathogens.
- Neuter the pet at an early age to minimize roaming activity and interaction with animals in the wild.
- Feed pets only cooked meat and foods unlikely to be contaminated with animal feces to minimize gastrointestinal colonization with potential pathogens.
- Keep the animal indoors as much as possible to limit interaction with other animals and reduce exposure to disease.
- Treat the animal for fleas during flea season to prevent transmission of disease by these ectoparasites.
- Do not keep birds, reptiles, turtles, or rodents as pets, because they are more likely to carry unusual human pathogens, cannot be immunized, and are difficult to screen for transmissible diseases.

- Make sure a pet dog or cat receives booster immunizations for rabies, distemper, canine hepatitis, leptospirosis, parvovirus, and feline leukemia virus.
- Have a veterinarian test the pet's stools annually for *Salmonella, Campylobacter, Giardia,* and *Cryptosporidium* species, and screen the animal for dermatophytes (which are transmissible to humans).
- Have cats tested annually for feline leukemia, because cats with this disease are more likely to acquire human infectious agents such as cryptosporidiosis.
- Prevent exposure to farm animals and petting zoos unless the animals have been carefully screened for human pathogens.
- Educate concerning adequate hand hygiene and proper disposal of animal waste.

Data from Pickering L: Exposure to non-traditional pets at home and public settings: risks to children, *Pediatrics* 122:876, 2008; Ehravesch C: Pets can make people sick, Atlanta, 2011, CDC, CDC.org; Compendium of measures to prevent diseases associated with animals in public settings: recommendations and report of National Association of State Public Health Veterinarians, Inc., *MMWR* 60(RRo4):1-24, 2011.

rodents, turtles, and reptiles are not recommended as pets because they cannot be screened for potential pathogens, have few vaccines, and are most likely to transmit disease. Infection can occur via contact with the pet's saliva, feces, or urine or by inhalation or skin contact with organisms. Risk factors in pet ownership of cats and dogs can be further reduced if children are cautioned not to kiss pets, if pets are not allowed to sleep in bed with the child, if exposure to animal feces is avoided, and if hand washing after handling a pet is encouraged. Families and pets can benefit by taking the pet to an obedience course. These courses are available at low cost in many communities.

Having an allergy to animal dander does not always rule out having a pet. Parent education concerning pet selection and hygiene can assist the family in making a decision that is best for all family members. Toddlers who spend most of their time indoors and infants born in winter months are more likely to have a cumulative exposure to allergens that increases a sensitivity response. Cats are most often the allergen offender because allergens are secreted in the saliva and by sebaceous glands onto the cat hair and skin. Cats shed their hair and dander, and electrostatic properties enable the allergens to adhere to carpets and walls, making allergy-proofing the house a difficult challenge. The poodle breed of dog does not have a shed cycle and therefore may be the least offensive pet for the allergic child. Shar Peis, terriers, Labrador retrievers, and pit bulls may release more allergens, because they are very susceptible to atopic conditions that cause scratching. Young, neutered female dogs produce fewer allergens than older, unneutered males.

If an allergenic pet is already part of the family, the risks can be minimized by frequent bathing and by keeping the pet outdoors or at least out of the child's bedroom. A 3% tannic acid spray to carpets and furniture can reduce the allergen potential of cat dander. Desensitization of the child by an allergist is also an option. Except for bite injuries, where secondary infection is common, the benefits of pet ownership often outweigh the risks. Education concerning the approach to and handling of pets is beneficial to children whether or not they own pets, because they are likely to come in contact with pets in their neighborhood or at their friends' houses.

Get Ready for the NCLEX® Examination!

Key Points

- School age (6 to 12 years of age) is a time of increased independence and a time in which the child begins to incorporate, perfect, and process the skills and information gained in earlier years.
- Erikson calls this stage the *stage of industry* or accomplishment.
- Freud describes this period as the *sexual latency stage*, when the child's energy is directed toward cognitive and physical skills.
- Major changes occur in the child's cognitive-perceptual patterns. Piaget refers to this stage as the *concrete operations stage*.
- Growth is slow until the spurt that occurs directly before puberty.
- School has an important influence on the socialization of children.
- The child acquires a positive self-concept from the ability to be productive, self-directed, and accepted.
- Peers range from same-sex friends in the early years to opposite-sex friends around puberty.
- Group acceptance is important.
- Both sexes need accurate information and reassurance in advance about changes of puberty and reproduction.
- The availability of junk food hampers efforts to provide proper nutrition. Meals may be sporadic because of the child's activities and the parents' working schedules.
- Accident prevention is still extremely important. School-age children are prone to injuries from motor vehicles, bicycles, skateboards, swimming, and their tendency to be overactive and distracted.

- Language development during the school-age years develops and expands the ability to communicate. The school-age child experiments with words without fully understanding their meanings.
- Moral development includes an understanding of rules, fairness, and values, and a knowledge of right and wrong.
- After-school day care and its relation to developmental needs is a concern for working parents.
- Pet ownership can nurture a sense of responsibility and encourage socialization in a shy child.
- Selection of an appropriate pet for the child and family is essential.
- The school nurse plays an important role in providing anticipatory guidance, health assessment, and community referral.

Additional Learning Resources

SG Go to your Study Guide for additional learning activities to help you master this chapter content.

evolve Go to your Evolve website (http://evolve.elsevier.com/Leifer) for the following learning resources:
- Animations
- Answer Guidelines for Critical Thinking Questions
- Answers and Rationales for Review Questions for the NCLEX® Examination
- Glossary with English and Spanish pronunciations
- Interactive Review Questions for the NCLEX® Examination
- Patient Teaching Plans in English and Spanish
- Skills Performance Checklists
- Video clips and more!

Online Resources:

- Alliance for Children and Families: www.alliance1.org
- American Medical Association: www.ama-assn.org
- Animal safety tips: www.cdc.gov/healthypets/child.htm
- Boys & Girls Club of America: www.bgca.org
- Family education: www.familyeducation.com
- Latchkey Kids Calling Program: www.latchkey-kids.com
- National Institute of Child Health and Human Development: www.nichd.nih.gov
- Parents Without Partners: www.parentswithoutpartners.org
- Sexuality Information and Education Council of the United States (SIECUS): www.siecus.org

Review Questions for the NCLEX® Examination

1. The pulse of the school-age child is approximately:
   1. 100 to 120 beats/min.
   2. 95 to 120 beats/min.
   3. 85 to 100 beats/min.
   4. 60 to 80 beats/min.

2. A parent asks the nurse if it is healthy to allow her school-age child to play computer games after school every day. The best response of the nurse would be that computer and video games:
   1. interest the school-age child and they will keep him off the streets.
   2. can challenge the intellect but should be balanced with active play activities.
   3. should only be played on weekends and not on school days.
   4. can teach new skills and are appropriate for school-age children.

3. While playing in school, a 9-year-old child suffers an injury that knocks his tooth out of his mouth. What should the teacher or school nurse do?
   1. Place the tooth in a cup of clean water, and send the child home.
   2. Place the tooth in a cup of milk, and call the parent to take the child to the dentist.
   3. Wrap the tooth in a clean cloth, and call the parent to take the child to the dentist.
   4. Rinse the child's mouth, and place the tooth in an envelope for the child to show his parent.

4. The parent of an 8-year-old child seeks advice from the nurse because her child is overweight. What would the nurse advise the parent to do?
   1. Provide a reward for the child when he avoids between-meal snacks for a full week.
   2. Limit privileges when the child eats sweets or junk food.
   3. Include the child in meal planning and preparation.
   4. Limit party-going activities where sweets will be served.

5. A 9-year-old practicing the piano continues to have difficulty in playing the theme song from a popular movie. She starts to pound on the piano keys in frustration. The best response would be to enter the room and say:
   1. "Just what do you think you're doing? That piano cost money!"
   2. "That's not difficult. Pull yourself together or you'll never amount to anything."
   3. "That piece sounds hard. I can see how you could be discouraged."
   4. "Here, let me show you how to play that."

Critical Thinking Question

1. Parents discuss their child's behavior with the nurse. They state that they are anxious for their child to succeed in school so he can have all the advantages of a good education. However, the child does not seem to want their help, nor does he appreciate their efforts to help him. They give the example of a science project that was due for school last week. His father, an engineer, built the best-looking project for his child to take to school. "It earned an easy 'A' grade for him." However, the boy didn't appreciate the help given to him and didn't seem to care about the "A" grade received. They are worried that school may not have the same meaning for the child as it does for them. What is the best response of the nurse?

Objectives

1. Define each key term listed.
2. Discuss three major theoretical viewpoints on the personality development of adolescents.
3. Discuss two main challenges during the adolescent years to which the adolescent must adjust.
4. List major physical changes that occur during adolescence.
5. Identify two major developmental tasks of adolescence.
6. Describe menstruation to a 13-year-old girl.
7. Describe Tanner's stages of breast development.
8. List five life events that contribute to stress during adolescence.
9. Identify two ways in which a person's cultural background might contribute to behavior.
10. Discuss the importance of peer groups, cliques, and best friends in the developmental process of an adolescent.
11. List a source for planning sex education programs for adolescents.
12. Summarize the nutritional requirements of the adolescent.
13. List three guidelines of importance for the adolescent participating in sports.
14. Discuss the common problems of adolescence and the nursing approach.

Key Terms

abstract reasoning (p. 451)
adolescence (p. 450)
asynchrony (p. 451)
cliques (p. 457)
epiphyseal closure (ĕp-ĭ-FĬZ-ē-ăl CLŌ-zhŭr, p. 456)
formal operations (p. 459)
gay (p. 460)
gender roles (p. 451)

growth spurt (p. 451)
homosexual (p. 460)
intimacy (p. 450)
lesbian (p. 460)
menarche (p. 453)
puberty (p. 451)
self-concept (p. 456)
sexual maturity ratings (SMRs) (p. 454)

GENERAL CHARACTERISTICS

Adolescence is defined as the period of life beginning with the appearance of secondary sex characteristics and ending with cessation of growth and with emotional maturity. The term comes from the Latin word *adolescere*, meaning "to grow up." Adolescence is often divided into early, middle, and late periods, because the 13-year-old adolescent differs a great deal from the 18-year-old adolescent. Middle adolescence appears to be the time of greatest turmoil for most families. Perhaps one of the most characteristic features of adolescence is its uncertainty. It is a period of life that in our culture lasts a comparatively long time and involves a great number of adjustments. The major tasks of adolescence include establishing an identity, separating from family, initiating intimacy, and developing career choices for economic independence. Some of the major theories of development are summarized in Box 20-1. Life is never dull when there are adolescents in the family. The surge toward independence becomes more and more pronounced, making it

practically impossible for adolescents to get along with their parents, who represent authority. When adolescents submit to parental wishes, they may feel humiliated and childish. If they revolt, conflicts arise within the family. Parents and adolescents must weather the storm together and try to discover solutions that are relatively satisfactory to all.

Numerous other factors account for the restlessness of adolescents. Their bodies are rapidly changing, and they experience intense sexual drives. They want to be accepted by society, but they are not sure how to attain this goal. Adolescents question life and search to find what psychologists call their sense of identity; they ask, "Who am I?" "What do I want?" This is followed by the **intimacy** stage, in which adolescents must learn to avoid emotional isolation. They must face the fear of rejection in shared activities such as sports, in close friendships, and in sexual experiences. The older adolescent thinks about the future and is generally idealistic. Jean Piaget and other investigators indicate that during this time adolescents reach the final stages of

Box **20-1**	Features of Major Theories of Development During Adolescence

SIGMUND FREUD

Adolescent is in the genital stage, the final stage of psychosexual development.

Self-love (narcissism) diminishes; love for others (altruism) develops.

Peers and parents are less influential than before but still provide love and support.

ERIK ERIKSON

The adolescent's main concerns are self-definition and self-esteem.

The adolescent experiences an identity crisis brought on by physical (including sexual) changes and conflict about future choices and expectations of others.

The adolescent must adapt to these changes and develop a new self-concept and appropriate vocational choices.

The adolescent learns to understand self in relation to others' perceptions and expectations.

JEAN PIAGET

The adolescent is in the stage of formal operations and therefore has the ability to reason logically and abstractly.

The adolescent is oriented toward problem solving.

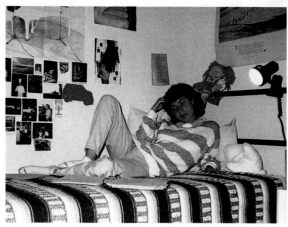

FIGURE 20-1 Adolescents need privacy.

abstract reasoning, logic, and other symbolic forms of thought, which increases sophistication in moral reasoning.

These facts sound complicated in themselves, but they are intensified by a world that is constantly changing. **Gender roles** are less defined in many households, and parents may not act as traditional role models for their children. Many adolescents live in single-parent homes or with working relatives where little, if any, supervision is available.

Conformity is one of the strongest needs of the adolescent in society. Today, with electronic technology bringing common experiences to people all over the world via radio, television, and computers, the combined pressure to conform often overrides cultural or traditional practices. Assimilation is beginning to occur via technology.

The needs of the family often compete with the needs of the adolescent when parents try to push the adolescent into an activity or career that meets the parent's own personal need or dreams. Parents must be guided to enjoy the interests and activities of the adolescent without imposing their personal desires. The main challenges of the adolescent years include adjusting to rapid physical and physiological changes, maintaining privacy, coping with social stresses (Figures 20-1 and 20-2) and pressures, maintaining open communication, and developing positive health care practices and lifestyle choices.

GROWTH AND DEVELOPMENT

PHYSICAL DEVELOPMENT

Preadolescence is a short period immediately preceding adolescence. In girls it comprises the ages of 10 to 13 years and is marked by rapid changes in the structure and function of various parts of the body. It is distinguished by **puberty**, the stage in which the reproductive organs become functional and secondary sex characteristics develop. Both sexes produce male hormones (*androgens*) and female hormones (*estrogens*) in comparatively equal amounts during childhood. During puberty the hypothalamus of the brain signals the pituitary gland to stimulate other endocrine glands—the adrenals and the ovaries or testes—to secrete their hormones directly into the bloodstream in differing proportions (more androgens in the boy and more estrogens in the girl).

The age of puberty varies and is somewhat earlier for girls than for boys. The final 20% of mature height that is achieved during adolescence is called the **growth spurt** and usually occurs by 18 years of age. The major cause of weight gain is the increase in skeletal mass. The implications of growth and development for nursing assessments are illustrated in Figure 20-3.

The general appearance of the adolescent tends to be awkward, that is, long-legged and gangling; this growth characteristic is termed **asynchrony**, because different body parts mature at different rates. The sweat glands are very active, and oily skin and acne are common. Both sexes mature earlier and grow taller and heavier than in past generations. Because of the gross motor development that occurs during adolescence, teenagers can gain satisfaction from sports. Table 20-1 outlines the growth and development of adolescents.

 Nursing Tip

A *growth spurt* is a rapid period of growth in which the body reaches adult height and weight before age 18 years.

Boys

During fetal life the placental chorionic gonadotropin stimulates Leydig cells to secrete testosterone. Thus weeks 8 to 12 of fetal life are important in the sexual development of the male (XY) child. Luteinizing hormone (LH) maintains testosterone levels. Serum levels

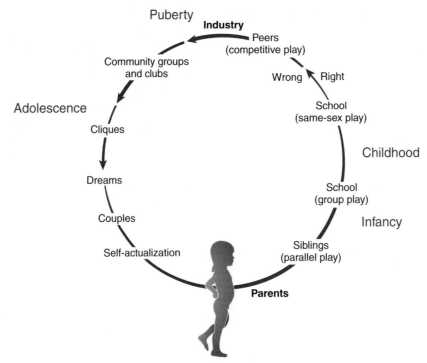

FIGURE 20-2 Roadmap of social interaction. In infancy and early childhood the child's focus is on parents. As the child grows, peers replace parents in importance. When adolescents mature, they return to the family with new respect, independence, and cooperation.

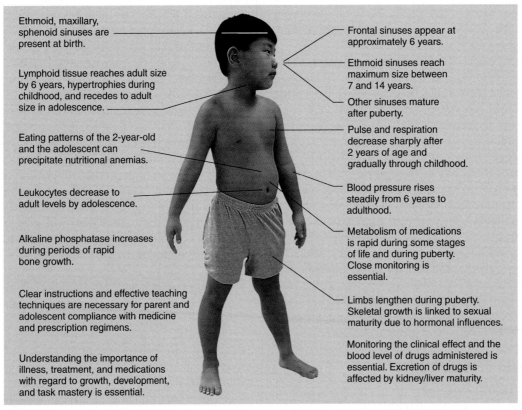

FIGURE 20-3 Many developmental changes occur between infancy and adolescence. The nurse must understand the implications of growth and development for nursing assessments. (Art overlay courtesy Observatory Group, Cincinnati, Ohio.)

Table 20-1 Growth and Development of the Adolescent

	EARLY (10-13 YEARS)	MIDDLE (14-16 YEARS)	LATE (17-21 YEARS)
Physical growth	Appearance of secondary sex characteristics	Growth spurt in height	Growth slows
Body image	Self-conscious Adjusts to pubertal changes	Experiments with different "images" and "looks"	Accepts body image Personality emerges
Self-concept	Low self-esteem Denial of reality	Impulsive Impatient Identify confusion	Positive self-image Empathic Independent thinker
Behavior	Behaves for rewards	Behaves to conform	Shows responsible behavior
Sexual development	Sexual interest	Sexual experimentation	Sexual identity emerges Develops caring relationships
Peers	Cliques of unisex friends Has "best friend" Hero worship Has adult "crushes"	Begins dating Has need to please significant peer Develops heterosexual peer group	Values individual relationships Partner selection
Family	Is ambivalent to family Strives for independence	Struggles for autonomy and acceptance Rebels/withdraws Demands privacy	Achieves independence Reestablishes family relationships
Cognitive development	Concrete thinking Here and now is important	Early abstract Daydreams, fantasizes Starts inductive and deductive reasoning	Abstract thinking Idealistic
Goals	Socializing is priority Goals are unrealistic	Identifies skills and interests Becomes superachiever or dropout	Identifies career goals Enters work or college
Health concerns	Concerned about normalcy	Concerned about experimenting with drugs or sex	Idealistic Decision making for lifestyle choice
Nursing interventions	Convey limits Encourage verbalization	Help them solve problems by providing choices Use peer group sessions Provide privacy	Discuss goals Allow participation in decisions Provide confidentiality

of LH increase during sleep 1 to 2 years before puberty. The secretion of gonadotropin stimulates gonad enlargement and the secretion of sex hormones. The interaction among the hypothalamus, pituitary, and gonads supports the development of puberty.

In boys, puberty begins with hormonal changes between 10 and 13 years of age. The shoulders widen, the pectoral muscles enlarge, and the voice deepens. Hair begins to grow on the face, chest, axillae, and pubic areas (Figure 20-4 and Box 20-2). Enlargement of the testicles and of internal structures and pigmentation of the scrotum are followed by enlargement of the penis. Erections and nocturnal emissions take place. The production of sperm begins between 13 and 14 years of age. An athletic scrotal support device (jockstrap) is necessary for boys participating in sporting events or for any activity in which support and protection of the genitalia are required. Athletic supporters not only support and protect the genitalia but also prevent embarrassment from exposure. Athletic

supporters are purchased by size. Good personal hygiene is necessary, because heat and friction may lead to jock itch, a fungal infestation of the groin. Sharing athletic supporters is discouraged.

Some experts recommend that after puberty boys examine their testes during or after a hot bath or shower. Each testicle is examined using the index and middle fingers of both hands on the underside of the testicle and the thumbs on the top of the testicle. The testicles are gently rolled between the thumb and the fingers to feel for abnormalities. Testicular and scrotal self-examinations are performed once a month. If a lump is discovered, it should be reported immediately to a health care provider (American Cancer Society, 2010).

Girls

Pubertal changes in girls occur 6 months to 2 years before they occur in boys. Puberty is easily recognized in girls by the onset of menstruation (Figure 20-5). The first menstrual period is called the **menarche**.

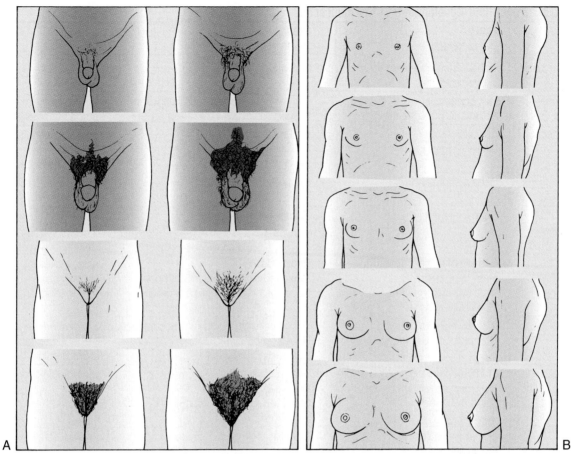

A   B

FIGURE 20-4 A, Sexual maturity ratings (SMRs) of pubic hair changes in adolescent boys and girls. **B,** SMRs of breast changes in adolescent girls. Bone growth is closely correlated with SMR, because hormones control epiphyseal closure. (Redrawn from photographs of J.M. Tanner, MD, Institute of Child Health, Department of Growth and Development, University of London, London, England.)

Box 20-2 Tanner's Stages of Sexual Maturity

Sexual maturity ratings (SMRs) range from 1 to 5. A score of 1 represents the prepubertal child; 5 corresponds to adult status.

BOYS: GENITAL DEVELOPMENT
Stage 1: Preadolescent; testes, scrotum, and penis about the same size and proportion as in early childhood
Stage 2: Enlargement of scrotum and testes; skin of scrotum reddens and changes in texture; little or no enlargement of penis at this stage
Stage 3: Enlargement of penis, which occurs at first mainly in length; further growth of testes and scrotum
Stage 4: Increased size of penis with growth in breadth and development of glands; testes and scrotum larger; scrotal skin darkened
Stage 5: Genitalia adult in size and shape

GIRLS: BREAST DEVELOPMENT
Stage 1: Preadolescent: elevation of papilla only
Stage 2: Breast bud stage: elevation of breast and papilla as small mound; enlargement of areolar diameter
Stage 3: Further enlargement and elevation of breast and areola, with no separation of their contours

Stage 4: Projection of areola and papilla to form a secondary mound above the level of the breast
Stage 5: Mature stage; projection of papilla only because of recession of the areola to the general contour of the breast

BOTH SEXES: PUBIC HAIR
Stage 1: Preadolescent; vellus over the pubes is not further developed than that over the abdominal wall, that is, no pubic hair
Stage 2: Sparse growth of long, slightly pigmented, downy hair, straight or curled, chiefly at the base of the penis or along the labia
Stage 3: Considerably darker, coarser, and more curled hair; hair spreads sparsely over the junction of the pubes
Stage 4: Hair now adult in type, but area covered is considerably smaller than in the adult; no spread to the medial surface of thighs
Stage 5: Adult in quantity and type with distribution of the horizontal (or classically "feminine") pattern; spread to medial surface of thighs but not up linea alba or elsewhere above the base of the inverse triangle (spread up linea alba occurs and is rated stage 6)

Data from Tanner JM: *Growth of adolescence,* ed 2, Oxford, 1962, Blackwell Scientific; Kliegman R et al: *Nelson's textbook of pediatrics,* ed 19, Philadelphia, 2011, Saunders.

1. The *pituitary gland* is a small gland at the base of the brain. It sends chemical messengers through the blood to various parts of the body. These messengers, or hormones, are responsible for many steps of growth and change as we develop. When a girl reaches the age of puberty, the pituitary gland sends out a new hormone that affects the functions of a group of organs concerned with menstruation.

3. The *ovaries* are two small female organs that manufacture human egg cells. When a girl reaches the age of puberty, these little cells receive a signal from the pituitary gland and begin to grow. Each month a cell escapes from an ovary and starts to travel along a passageway—one of the fallopian tubes. This movement of the egg cell is called ovulation. If one of these cells becomes fertilized by a male cell, it can develop into a baby.

4. The *fallopian tubes*, into which the egg cells pass, lead toward the uterus.

5. The *uterus* is also called the womb. This is where the egg cell develops if it has been fertilized. Each month a soft, thick lining (the endometrium) of tissue and blood vessels forms inside the uterus.

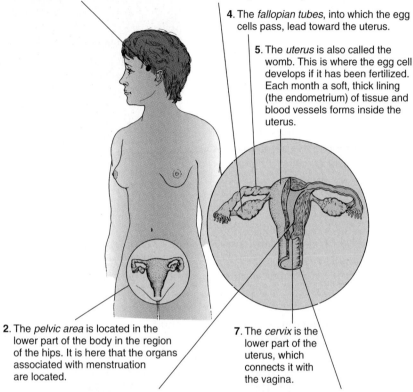

2. The *pelvic area* is located in the lower part of the body in the region of the hips. It is here that the organs associated with menstruation are located.

7. The *cervix* is the lower part of the uterus, which connects it with the vagina.

6. The *endometrium*, or uterus lining, serves as a warm nest to shelter and nourish the unborn child until it has grown enough to be ready to come into the world as a baby. But unless an egg cell has been fertilized and a baby started on its way toward birth, there is no need for the cell or for the blood and tissues of the endometrium. Therefore they are passed from the body.

8. The *vagina*, a passageway leading to the outside of the lower part of the body, carries away these materials in a flow of blood. This is called menstrual flow. When it occurs, it lasts for several days each month and is known as menstruation.

FIGURE 20-5 Menstruation.

It commonly occurs about age 12 or 13 years, but this varies. It may occur as early as age 10 years or as late as age 15 years. Secondary sex characteristics become more apparent before the menarche. Fat is deposited in the hips, thighs, and breasts, causing them to enlarge (see Box 20-2).

At this time the adolescent girl may need to be fitted for a bra. Measurements must be ascertained and various styles tried on for comfort. Straps should fit so that they do not continually fall from the shoulders. Cups need to be large enough to support fullness near the underarms. The garment must fit across the back so that it is not uncomfortably tight. Adolescents generally like attractive undergarments that have some type of lace

trim. Sports bras are available for girls who participate in active sports. Puberty is a good time to begin teaching breast self-examination (see Skill 11-1). Instructional materials are available through the American Cancer Society.

The external genitalia grow. Hair develops in the pubic area (see Figure 20-4 and Box 20-2) and the underarms. It is important to note that in ballet dancers, runners, gymnasts, and adolescents engaged in other athletic activities that involve a lean body and high level of physical activity, the mechanisms affecting puberty can be altered and cause a delay in the onset of menarche. Energy balance, activity, and nutrition are important factors to evaluate when menstruation is delayed. Further growth can no longer take place when the ends of the long bones knit securely to their shafts (**epiphyseal closure**). See Chapter 2 for a detailed discussion of the physiology of reproductive organs.

> ### ☝ Nursing Tip
>
> Young women are taught breast self-examination, and young men are instructed in self-examination of the testes.

PSYCHOSOCIAL DEVELOPMENT

Sense of Identity

Physical growth and sexual interest correlate with sexual maturity. Cognitive growth and social changes correlate with chronological age and placement in school. Stress can increase when physical growth and cognitive growth occur at different rates in the same adolescent. Although the early-maturing male often finds positive social adjustment and acceptance, early-maturing females are often embarrassed and develop low self-esteem. The adolescent's desire for freedom and independence is extremely important and necessary for developing individuality. To accomplish this, young persons must reject their childhood self and often the people most closely associated with it. Erikson identifies the major task of this group as *identity versus role confusion*. Emancipation is a critical element in the establishment of identity.

Adolescents want to be people in their own right, and they "try on" different roles. **Self-concept** (one's view of oneself) fluctuates during this time and is molded by the demands of parents, peers, teachers, and others. Interaction with others helps adolescents determine who they are and in what direction they want to proceed. This process is more difficult for low-income minorities and is complicated by many factors, such as illness, broken homes, and the extent of formal education. Young persons who are unable to master confusion and establish an identity may become rigid in their actions, bewildered, or depressed, or they may cling to the conformity of peer groups long after the need should have passed. Some show an inordinate need for something "new and exciting." They may experience low self-esteem and alienation, and they may confront many other difficulties on entering the adult world.

> ### ☝ Nursing Tip
>
> In adolescence, dependency creates hostility. Parents who foster dependence invite unavoidable resentment. Wise parents make themselves increasingly dispensable. Their language is sprinkled with such statements as "The choice is yours," "You decide about that," "If you want to," and "It's your decision."

Sense of Intimacy

Developing intimacy is closely entwined with the resolving of a person's sense of identity. As adolescents move toward young adulthood, they become ready to take the

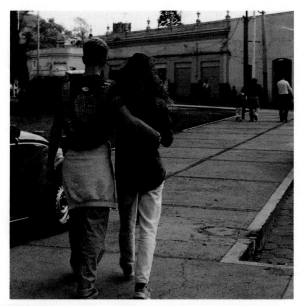

FIGURE 20-6 As adolescents move toward young adulthood, they become ready to take the risks of close affiliations and friendship and to establish relationships with members of the opposite sex.

risks of close affiliations and friendships and to establish relationships with the opposite sex (Figure 20-6). Avoidance of building these relationships may lead to a deep sense of isolation. Adolescence is a period of trying and testing. Disagreements with parents often revolve around dating, the family car, money, chores, school grades, choice of friends, smoking, sex, and the use of illicit drugs. The young person questions parental values and morals and is particularly sensitive to hypocrisy.

Adults who associate with adolescents should try to create an atmosphere of interest and understanding. Adolescents must know that adults care. Adolescents need practice in making decisions that must be respected even if they have made a mistake. Parents should set limits and expect them to be challenged but not exceeded. Parents and nurses who see other people's intrinsic worth, feel good about themselves, and do not see the adolescent's behavior as a reflection on their parenting or nursing provide a more secure environment for growth. Loving detachment is not easy, but it is an effective tool when interacting with adolescents.

Cultural and Spiritual Considerations

Americans are multiethnic, multicultural, and multilingual. All may not adopt the value of independence as a goal of maturational and emotional development. The traditional Chinese do not recognize the period of adolescence; there is no word for it in their language. Many immigrants and Americans of Asian descent come from societies that are patriarchal and highly structured and have distinct social roles. The good of the family takes precedence over personal goals. The protection of family image and neighborhood reputation is essential.

As part of a search for their identity, adolescents focus on the values and ideals of the family and decide either to embrace them or to separate from them. Adolescents often perceive their feelings and thoughts as unique and therefore do not express their feelings freely. Adolescents can understand abstract concepts and symbols, and exposure to religion and religious practices other than those experienced within their own traditional family can help them stabilize their group identity (Figure 20-7). The nurse's awareness of these and other cultural influences on the adolescent's behavior will help in the effort to provide holistic care.

> ### 👁 Nursing Tip
>
> Every culture is unique. Adolescent behavior problems and expectations differ in other areas of the world and must be respected.

Body Image

In early adolescence the young person must adjust to the dramatic changes of puberty. Focusing on body development during early and middle adolescence is one factor that contributes to egocentrism, or self-centeredness. Young persons create what has been termed an "imaginary audience." They believe that everyone is looking at them. This preoccupation with self is normal and accounts for the constant hair combing and makeup repairing often observed in a group of adolescents. Young adolescents may try to hide their changing body or may advertise it. They may take pride in their abilities or feel frustrated when their actual abilities do not match their perceived abilities.

In early adolescence, teens make every effort to be just like their peers. A pimple on the skin or a disability is disastrous to the young adolescent. By late adolescence, most have completed their growth, are less self-conscious, and enjoy their individual skills, abilities, and interests. Chronic illness or eating disorders (see Chapter 33) may complicate or exacerbate unresolved problems of body image.

Peer Relationships

Peer groups help adolescents to feel that they "belong" and make it possible to experiment with social behaviors (Figure 20-8). School assumes an important role in the psychological development of the adolescent by providing the focus for initiating social interaction. Small, exclusive groups form, which are called **cliques**. These unisex groups are made up of adolescents with similar interests, values, and tastes. Belonging to the group is of utmost importance to the young adolescent.

Within the clique, the adolescent often develops a close personal relationship with one peer of the same sex. This best friend interaction supports social development by enabling adolescents to experiment with behaviors together and listen to and care about each other (Figure 20-9). Stable "best friend" experiences often precede successful heterosexual relationships in later life.

The peer group serves as a mirror for "normality" and helps to determine where one "fits in." It is vitally important in helping adolescents define themselves. Acceptance by one's friends helps to decrease the

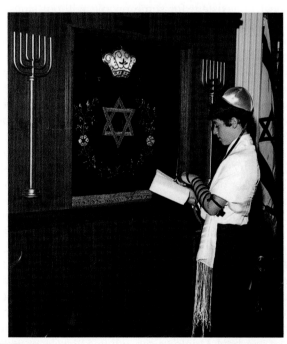

FIGURE 20-7 Adolescents can understand abstract concepts and symbols, and religious traditions can help to stabilize identity. The bar mitzvah is a spiritual rite of passage into adulthood.

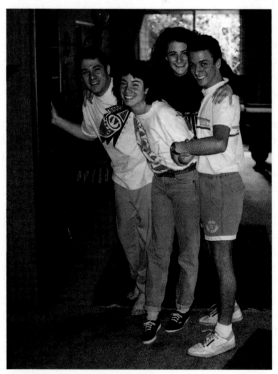

FIGURE 20-8 Immersion into a peer group helps adolescents free themselves from childhood dependence.

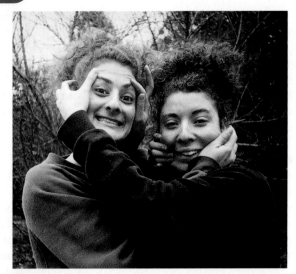

FIGURE 20-9 Adolescents practice facial expressions and try out new hairstyles. "Best friend" interaction supports social development by enabling the adolescent to experiment with behavior and to care about others.

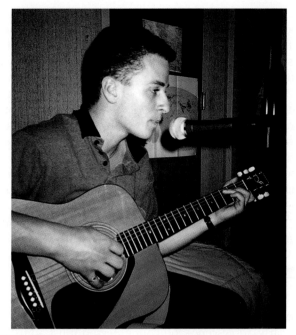

FIGURE 20-10 Parents should encourage adolescents to take advantage of their talents. Singing, playing a musical instrument, or developing mechanical skills is part of adolescent life.

loneliness and sense of loss many adolescents experience on the road to adulthood.

The social norms and pressures exerted by the group may cause problems. The selection of friends and allegiance to them may bring about confrontations within the family. Parents need help in understanding that the adolescent's exaggerated conformity is necessary to moving away from dependence and obtaining approval from persons outside the nuclear family. Failure to develop social competence may produce feelings of inadequacy and low self-esteem.

Nurses can assist the family by supporting and educating them in the dynamics of this age group. Parents can be directed to groups such as peer helpers (for the adolescent) and community educational programs sponsored by various agencies. Organizations such as *Parents Without Partners* might be another resource to consider.

Career Plans

Some adolescents graduate from high school with a definite idea of what they would like to do. Many, however, are unsure of what they want. To choose a career that is best suited for them, adolescents must first know themselves. What particularly interests them? What are they good at? What are their shortcomings?

By this time, adolescents have already taken some definite steps toward a goal. Choice of high school curriculum and grades determine eligibility for college or preparation for a specific vocation. Parents should observe the interests of their children and encourage them to take advantage of their talents (Figure 20-10). Whenever possible, an adolescent should investigate various fields by talking to people who are involved in those areas of interest.

Valuable information can also be obtained by career exploration, which is available at most colleges, and by

pamphlets from professional organizations, the government, Internet sites, and other sources. The school guidance counselor administers aptitude tests as an additional guide and can work with adolescents to expose them to as wide a selection of careers as possible. The adolescent must make the final decision. To be happy in a career, the adolescent must choose it of his or her own free will and not because parents expect him or her to follow in their footsteps.

The job market today is extremely competitive and almost nonexistent for some people without skills or higher education. Productive employment must fit young people's life framework and offer an opportunity for personal growth. Some positive aspects of employment include helping to build self-esteem, promoting responsibility, testing new skills, constructively channeling energies, providing money for increased independence, engaging the young person in interactions with adults, and allowing the adolescent to assume an active rather than a passive role. In contrast, when adolescents are forced to take a job because of economic or personal pressures, they may need to drop out of school. With few skills and no experience, they may remain locked into low-level employment. This is often perpetuated from one generation to another.

Responsibility

Adolescents look forward to challenges. Parents must encourage their children to take on new responsibilities. The adolescent is often humiliated by being placed in a dependent role, such as when a parent or sibling drives them to school. Driving a car, riding a bicycle, or walking provides a sense of independence and responsibility. Even routine jobs can be made more inspiring if youths are taught to see them in relation to a longer-term objective.

Young adolescents must also be taught the value of money. An allowance helps them to learn financial management. If money is simply handed out as requested, it is more difficult to develop responsibility for finances. Allowances should be increased from time to time to comply with the age and needs of the adolescent.

Middle and older adolescents who have jobs can be taught to use a checkbook and a savings account. Many find satisfaction in purchasing their own clothes. An adolescent who buys an old car soon discovers that it takes money to insure, run, and repair it. Such experiences provide valuable lessons in finance. Babysitting is a common means of earning money among younger adolescents. Many boys and girls begin to assist with babysitting at about 12 or 13 years of age. Babysitting courses are valuable because young people need to be prepared for this important responsibility.

COGNITIVE DEVELOPMENT

Piaget's theory of cognitive development states that development is systematic, sequential, and orderly. Young adolescents are still in the *concrete phase* of thinking. They take words literally. A young adolescent girl, if asked by the nurse, "Have you ever slept with anyone?" may not connect the question with a vaginal infection or sexual intercourse. By middle adolescence the ability to think abstractly has increased. Piaget calls this the stage of **formal operations**. Older adolescents can see a situation from many viewpoints and can imagine or organize unseen or unexperienced possibilities. *Abstract thinking* and reasoning emerges.

Therefore when teaching early adolescents about menstruation, the nurse focuses on concrete issues and concerns. When abstract thinking emerges in later adolescence, the abstract meaning of menstruation relating to womanhood or motherhood can be discussed. Empowering young adolescent girls by educating them according to their intellectual and emotional developmental level can increase their self-image. Adolescents are able to sympathize and empathize. They can understand their own values and actions and can also understand and accept the differing values and actions of people from other cultures.

Daydreams

Adolescents spend a lot of time daydreaming in the solitude of their rooms or during a class lecture. Most of this behavior is normal and natural for this age group. Daydreaming is usually considered harmless if the young person continues the usual active pursuits. It also serves several purposes. Adolescence is a lonely, in-between age; daydreaming helps to fill the void. Imaginatively acting out what will be said or done in various situations prepares adolescents to interact with others so they can better cope with real situations. Daydreams are also a valuable safety valve for the expression of strong feelings.

SEXUAL DEVELOPMENT

Sexual Behavior

Adolescents must meet and become acquainted with members of the opposite sex. This may begin with admiration from afar, which is accompanied by daydreams as the young person attempts to attract the other's attention.

Group dates during structured school or church functions are followed by double dating and then single-couple dating. Dancing provides an opportunity for the symbolic expression of sexual urges without physical contact. Slow dancing provides a mode of close physical contact in public that is socially acceptable. When adolescents are at home or feeling alone, long telephone or text messaging conversations link the adolescent to peers. "Crushes"—feelings of attachment to a person of the opposite sex who is popular or possesses qualities important to the adolescent—are a common occurrence. Competition and rivalry may be keen, but long-term commitment and deep romantic attachments are not often present.

Sexual experimentation often occurs as a response to peer pressure, as a means for momentary pleasure, as a learning experience to satisfy curiosity, or as a means of gaining a feeling of being loved and cared about. Sexual behavior can affect the growth and development of the adolescent. Unplanned pregnancies or sexually transmitted infections (STIs) are two major complications of adolescent sexual interaction, because few adolescents responsibly use protection (Kliegman et al, 2007).

The adolescent's cultural background influences patterns of dating. Conflict often arises when the adolescent wants to be independent and quickly adopts American norms of dating while parents are insisting on strict traditional values. This is particularly noticeable with daughters.

Dating is one of the early social aspects of growing up. Attending the high school prom is a rite of adolescence. As such, it may become a battleground for the struggle for independence. Parents' opposition is often based on their unspoken fears. Parents may also fear sexual experimentation, pregnancy, or acquired immunodeficiency syndrome (AIDS). They may respond by imposing strict restrictions, such as curfews, chaperones, and limitations on use of the car. When these problems are not discussed openly, the adolescent may react by rebelling sexually or by other means to test general parental control, rather than for the sake of the prohibited act itself.

Sexual curiosity and masturbation are common among adolescents. There is also a need for the intimacy of close personal friendships. Seeking one person of the opposite sex to share confidences and feelings may lead to sexual intimacies. This may produce guilt feelings and can lead to isolation from friends and family.

The breaking up of such romances is often a source of great emotional pain.

Most of our knowledge about the sexual behavior of Americans comes from the pioneering efforts of Alfred Kinsey. Although his studies included flaws, they provided much in-depth information. A wide variety of sexual behavior is freely discussed and depicted in movies, in magazines, online, and on television. Music directed toward young people often centers on sexual themes. Premarital sexual activity has become much more widespread, and adolescents are initiating their sexual activity at increasingly younger ages. Thirty percent of girls and 48% of boys report having had sexual intercourse by 18 years of age (Kliegman et al, 2011).

Sex Education

Sex education for the adolescent is a challenge. Nurses must put aside their own attitudes and biases; understand society, cultural, and moral values; and incorporate a broad understanding of physical and psychological growth and development to prepare an effective school or clinic program. Television, movies, magazines, and computer chat rooms or websites provide a source of information for sex education for the adolescent that may or may not be accurate and helpful to the young adult.

The prevalence of human immunodeficiency virus (HIV) exposure, AIDS, and other STIs was a factor that resulted in the formalized incorporation of sex education in schools. This education focuses on the physiology of sex, the reproductive systems, and STIs as well as personal values concerning sexuality, facts about contraception, safe sex, and peer pressure. Formal structured comprehensive sex education programs are available from the Sexuality Information and Education Council of the United States (SIECUS) and other community agencies. These types of programs are geared to kindergarten through grade 12 and present information about all aspects of health, such as nutrition, dental care, avoidance of drugs, and STIs. These courses should be presented as age appropriate. The physiology of the reproductive systems can be taught at about grade 5. By grade 8, topics such as coping skills for dating and sexuality, pregnancy, and birth can be reviewed. Abstinence and contraception are also discussed.

Decision making is emphasized. Flowcharts should show the possible consequences of certain actions. The high school units can include how to handle adolescent pregnancy, prenatal and postnatal care, and effective parenting techniques. A unit on intimate relationships can be presented as a series of discussions and activities designed to help students think about the nature of love. It can cover ideas such as compromise, problem solving, and communication skills. It should emphasize the many reasons why adolescents should say "no" to casual sex.

Factual and sensitive information provided by concerned parents is, of course, the ideal. However, too often peers provide erroneous material or parents postpone education until a crisis arrives. Children must be told what body changes to expect and why these changes occur. **Two years too soon is better than 1 day too late!** Parents who have answered their children's questions truthfully throughout childhood offer a secure and natural foundation on which to build. Studies have shown that adolescents who obtain early sex education information from caring parents or well-informed adults do *not* have a higher rate of sexual activity.

Concerns About Being "Different"

Adolescents have certain concerns that are specific to puberty. The girl who begins to experience physical changes at about 10 years of age may feel self-conscious because she towers over her friends or needs to wear a bra. She may be teased because she is different. The other extreme is the latecomer who feels abnormal and unattractive because her friends look more feminine.

Such problems are not limited to girls. Of particular concern is the boy on a slow schedule of development. Still short at 15 years of age, he is unable to compete for placement on school teams because of his size. He sees his male friends being admired for their height and strength, and this is a threat to him. Such fears are natural and usually are alleviated by reassurances that, although boys begin to grow later than girls, their growth spurt lasts longer. During data collection, the nurse has an opportunity to support the adolescent who is concerned about normal growth and development.

Traditional gender stereotypes define being "male" by activity and achievement and being "female" by sensitivity and interpersonal competence. Society's current trends toward equality of the sexes may affect these roles. Nevertheless, few adolescents escape the social pressures that dictate acceptable sexual attitudes and behavior for each gender.

Homosexuality

When a person has an attraction for a person of his or her own sex, that person is referred to as **homosexual**. A **lesbian** is a female who prefers other females as sexual partners. A male is referred to as **gay** when he prefers another male as his sexual partner. Homosexual behavior in adolescence is not uncommon. **This experimentation with homosexuality is not a positive predictor of adult sexual preference;** it may merely indicate a desire to explore alternative lifestyles. About 1.1% of high school students declare themselves as homosexual, but 2.8% have had homosexual experiences (Kliegman, 2011). It is thought that a combination of cultural, biological, and psychological factors contributes to sexual orientation and development. The nursing role is not to change homosexual behaviors but to help the child understand how to cope with the reaction of others.

Table 20-2	Using the Nursing Process in Planning Sex Education for the Adolescent
NURSING PROCESS STEP	**NURSING ACTIONS**
Data collection	Determine the level of knowledge concerning puberty and body changes. Discuss peer acceptance. Determine sexual practices and outlets, such as masturbation. Discuss the use of drugs, alcohol, and cigarettes.
Analysis	Review body image and understanding concerning body changes. Observe for signs of abuse. Determine risk factors involving sexual behavior and substance abuse. Clarify sexual practices, including contraception. Review for sexual variation or deviation.
Planning and implementation	Provide a private area and nonjudgmental environment for teaching. Discuss safe sex practices and personal views and values of the adolescent. Teach techniques and the value of breast or testicular self-examination. Discuss contraceptive choices, if appropriate. Teach the need for regular follow-up health care.
Evaluation	Follow-up during scheduled home or clinic visits concerning problems identified or teaching completed.

Nurses must be sensitive to these issues when obtaining histories and working with young adolescents. They must also be aware of their personal biases to determine their potential effectiveness with this population. Support groups for parents and friends of gays and lesbians are available. Those who question their sexual orientation are referred to counselors and health agencies that can respond to their needs. Table 20-2 provides an example of the use of the nursing process in planning sex education for the adolescent.

PARENTING THE ADOLESCENT

The media have an increasing influence on the growth and development of the adolescent. Over ½ of high school students have a TV in their bedroom and a computer in their house, and 75% frequent the Internet by computer, iPad, or smartphone. Social networking is the norm. Parenting an adolescent requires major adaptations on the part of the parents. At times it is difficult for parents to cope with adolescents. The shift in parenting philosophies from the rigid rules of discipline to permissiveness or the current middle-of-the-road

position often leads to confusion. Negotiation is a more successful strategy in managing adolescents than an authoritarian approach. Some parents are unsure of their own opinions and may hesitate to exert authority. Others refuse to "let go" or to change any of their beliefs to accommodate today's youth. Issues of privacy and trust abound, and conflict occurs as the adolescent desires more adult liberties. Adolescents may need time alone to separate themselves from family and search for their identity.

Adolescents need to talk about their fears, such as school examinations or how they will look with a certain haircut. They need assistance in sorting out confused feelings. A confidential, accepting atmosphere will promote quality communications (Figure 20-11). Physical symptoms, such as stomachaches, insomnia, and headaches, surface in relation to anxiety. Bizarre behavior may be a call for long-overdue help.

Nursing Tip

Adolescent warning signs indicating need for psychosocial intervention and follow-up:
- Spends time on computer in early hours of the morning
- Changes screen on computer when parent enters room
- Has pornographic material on the computer
- Makes frequent long-distance calls

Some approaches to such problems are presented in the Health Promotion box that follows. As adolescents try to separate themselves from their family, they may reject some family traditions such as family outings or dress codes. When parents respond to this behavior negatively, the separation widens and tension grows. Often adolescents search for adults outside of the family as role models and confidants. Coaches or scout leaders can fulfill this role and serve as positive outlets for gaining a sense of "belonging" when there are conflicts at home.

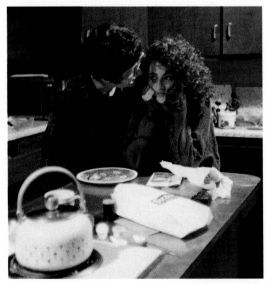

FIGURE 20-11 Listening is an important tool for establishing rapport. A confidential, accepting atmosphere will promote good communication.

Health Promotion

Effective Approaches to Problems

APPROACH	PURPOSE	EXAMPLE
Reflective listening	Showing you understand adolescent's feelings; used when adolescent "owns" problem	"You're very worried about the semester exam." "Sounds like you're feeling discouraged because the job's so difficult."
"I" message	Communicating your feelings about how adolescent's behavior affects you; used when you own problem	"When I'm ill and the dishes are left for me to do, I feel disrespected because it seems no one cares about me." "When you borrow tools and don't return them, I feel discouraged because I don't have the tools I need when there's a job to do."
Exploring alternatives	Helping adolescents decide how to solve problems they own Negotiating agreements with adolescent when you own problem	"What are some ways you could solve this problem?" "Which idea appeals to you most?" "Are you willing to do this until...?" "What can we do to settle this conflict between us?" "Are we in agreement on that idea?" "What would be a fair consequence if the agreement is broken?"
Natural and logical consequences	Permitting adolescents, within limits, to decide how they will behave and allowing them to experience consequences Natural consequences apply when adolescent owns problem Logical consequences apply when either parent or adolescent owns problem	*Natural:* Adolescent who forgets coat on cold days becomes cold; adolescent who skips lunch becomes hungry. *Logical:* Adolescent who spends allowance quickly will not receive any more money until next allowance day; adolescent who neglects to study for a test receives low grade.

From *Systematic training for effective parenting of teens: parenting teenagers.* Circle Pines, Mich., 1990, American Guidance Service. Copyright © 1990 by Don Dinkmeyer and Gary D. McKay.

Nurses should help parents keep the lines of communication open, promote respect and trust, and provide confidentiality and a sense of privacy. Despite the problems parents face with their adolescents, the family continues to play a major role in socialization.

Nursing Tip

Privacy and confidentiality are essential when communicating with adolescents.

HEALTH PROMOTION AND GUIDANCE

NUTRITION

Adolescents grow rapidly; therefore they need foods that provide for their increase in height, body cell mass, and maturation. Adolescents appear to be "always hungry" because their stomach capacity is too small to meet the increased caloric and protein requirements of their rapid growth spurt. Frequent meals are needed. Dietary deficiencies are more likely to occur at this age because of this growth acceleration and because eating patterns become more irregular. Nutritional requirements are more strongly correlated with sexual maturity ratings (SMRs) (see Box 20-2) than with age. For example, girls at SMR 2 and boys at SMR 3 are close to their peak growth velocities. They require adequate intake of nutrients and calories, regardless of their chronological age.

The most noticeable changes in the adolescent's eating habits are skipped meals, more between-meal snacks, and eating out more often. Breakfast and lunch are often omitted. Part-time jobs, school activities, and socialization may result in the adolescent eating little or nothing during the day and then "catching up" in the evening. Fast-food restaurants are inexpensive and provide food quickly for the busy adolescent. These foods tend to be high in calories, fat, protein, sugar, and sodium and low in fiber. In general, to determine the dietary fiber intake needs in children, add 5 g (0.2 oz) to the age in years (Dartmouth-Hitchcock, 2010). Most food chains have added salads and other healthier foods, which is applauded. Carbonated drinks often replace milk, resulting in low intakes of calcium, riboflavin, and vitamins A and D.

Foods should be selected from the basic food MyPlate (see Figure 4-7). In estimating calories, variables such as physical activity and sex must also be considered. The elements most likely to be inadequately supplied in the adolescent's diet are calcium, iron, and vitamin B_{12}. Zinc is known to be essential for growth and sexual maturation and is therefore of great importance in adolescence. The recommended dietary allowances (RDAs) for adolescents are listed in the Evolve resources for Chapter 15.

Vegetarian Diets

Foods and eating fads are often the main conflict between adolescents and their parents. However, adolescents are now a growing segment of the vegetarian population. Ninety percent of adolescent vegetarian diets include eggs and milk. Iron-rich foods include fortified grain products. However, a high intake of whole grains, bran, and foods rich in oxalic acid (e.g., spinach) can impair the absorption of iron. Tofu, nuts, wheat germ, and legumes can provide the zinc necessary for cognitive development. If animal products are totally excluded from the diet, a vitamin B_{12} supplement may be necessary. The nursing role is to understand the eating pattern, identify fad diets, and understand the reason the diet was selected, and then evaluate and discuss any deficiencies or needs within that diet. Developing a partnership with the adolescent in meeting growth needs and allowing the adolescent to take responsibility for meeting his or her own health needs are the cornerstones for success in nutritional education.

Vegetarians who eat no animal protein, eggs, or dairy products (vegans) are at particular risk of developing deficiencies in protein, vitamin B_{12}, calcium, iron, iodine, and possibly zinc. A total vegetarian diet is adequate only if it is carefully planned.

Sports and Nutrition

The best training diet is one that contains foods from each of the basic food groups in sufficient quantities to meet energy demands and nutrient requirements. What to eat and when to eat it in relation to muscle exercise are vital to successful athletic performance. Athletes exhaust reserves of muscle glycogen. Carbohydrates that can be rapidly converted to blood glucose and transported to muscles will provide the rapid recovery of muscle glycogen necessary for maintaining prolonged intense muscle activity. Eating a slowly absorbed glucose source will prevent the development of chronically low muscle energy stores. To hasten muscle energy recovery, the young athlete should consume at least 50 g of a rapidly used carbohydrate within 4 hours after exercise (see Table 31-5). Foods high in fat and protein will prolong carbohydrate metabolism.

Carbohydrates that provide both energy and other nutrients are best for athletes. Therefore fruits and fruit juices are a better choice than sugar-rich soft drinks and candy. The fat content in candy will slow carbohydrate absorption. Some foods that provide a rapid supply of carbohydrates to muscles include corn flakes, bagels, raisins, maple syrup, potatoes, and rice. Some foods that supply a slow release of carbohydrates to muscles include apples, pears, green peas, chickpeas, skim milk, and plain yogurt.

Fluids lost by sweat must be replaced by drinking small amounts of fluid during a workout. Thirst is one guide for intake. Caffeine and alcohol deplete body water and are to be avoided.

Anabolic steroids, used by some athletes to gain weight and increase strength, are detrimental to bone growth. Iron is particularly necessary for female athletes, who may be borderline or deficient in their intake of this mineral.

Nutrition and School Examinations

The role of diet in the management of illness has become traditional practice. The role of diet in maintaining health is becoming prominent in health education today. Nutritional practices are the focus of weight control programs, and special nutritional supplements are available for athletes, pregnant women, and older adults. Studies have shown that foods can affect behavior, moods, and alertness.

For the adolescent who is scheduled to take an important school examination, the nurse can offer nutritional guidance as part of the examination preparation. Carbohydrates such as pancakes and syrup, breakfast pastries, or a muffin and jelly increase serotonin in the brain, resulting in a soothing, sleepy response. Bacon and eggs are high in fat and cholesterol and are therefore slow to digest, diverting blood from the brain during the digestion process and causing decreased alertness. Drinking more than 4 cups of a caffeine-containing beverage such as coffee can cause overstimulation and nervousness. However, protein-rich meals increase amino acids and tyrosine, which will break down into norepinephrine in the brain and result in increased alertness. Fish, soy, peanuts, and rice increase choline and acetylcholine in the brain, which result in increased memory. Therefore a "proper" meal before a big school test may help the adolescent's achievement as well as his or her health.

PERSONAL CARE

Hygiene

The adolescent needs personal hygiene information, because body changes require more frequent bathing and the use of deodorants. The nurse can help the young person sort out the various claims of reliability for hair removal, menstrual hygiene, and cosmetic products and procedures. Body piercing, a popular adolescent fad, should be performed only by an experienced person using sterile instruments. The skin around the point of insertion of the body ring should be regularly inspected for signs of infection. Swapping body rings is discouraged. Adolescents are warned not to use another's razor or toothbrush, particularly in light of the risk of HIV infection.

Dental Health

The prevalence of tooth decay has substantially decreased. This is believed to result from the widespread use of fluorides, including community fluoridation, dental sealants, and dental products containing fluorides. Adolescents are nonetheless at risk for dental caries because of inadequate dental maintenance and frequent snacking on sucrose-containing candies and beverages. When dental hygiene is neglected, the period of greatest tooth decay in the permanent teeth is from ages 12 to 18 years. Lack of oral hygiene (inadequate brushing, flossing, and rinsing, particularly after meals) fosters the accumulation of plaque and food debris. Missing, aching, or decayed teeth contribute to poor nutrition. Young people with unattractive teeth may suffer from low self-esteem. Corrective orthodontic appliances are often worn during adolescence, and meticulous oral hygiene is essential to prevent discoloration of tooth enamel and other complications.

According to media hype, healthy, white teeth are synonymous with popularity and sex appeal. Regular dental visits during adolescence must be maintained as a priority in the health care teaching of adolescents and their families. See Chapter 15 for a detailed discussion of dental health.

Sunbathing

Adolescents respond to movie and magazine pictures of the ideal "healthy suntanned body" as an attractive aspect of a body image. The young adult looks forward to sunbathing on the beach or at the pool during summer vacations and often prepares his or her body by trying to obtain a tanned appearance using artificial means. The nurse plays a vital role in educating the adolescent concerning the danger of the sun's rays and the need for skin protection with a sun protective factor (SPF) of at least 15. Protection of the eyes from the sun is also essential. Excessive sunlight and the use of artificial tanning machines can cause serious long-term reactions such as early aging of the skin or skin cancer (see Chapter 30).

SAFETY

The chief hazard to the adolescent is the automobile (Figure 20-12). Road and off-road vehicle accidents kill and cripple adolescents at alarming rates. Some schools now offer driver-training courses as an integral part of the educational program. Students learn how to drive and learn the accompanying responsibilities; however, this does not ensure compliance. Preventing motor vehicle accidents is of utmost importance to every community. Adolescents who ride motorcycles, motor scooters, or motorbikes should know the rules of the road and should wear special safety equipment, such as helmets.

Young people should learn how to swim and practice swimming safety. Accidents result from diving into unsafe areas, from using alcohol or drugs while swimming, and from unsafe use of jet skis. If adolescents are interested in hunting or similar sports that require a gun, they must be instructed in the proper safeguards.

Sports Injuries

Sports involving body contact can be hazardous to the adolescent. Sports teams separated by age only are a special problem, because adolescents of one specific age group can vary in size, weight, and muscle strength. Protective gear should be worn by all team players in any contact sport. The feeling of strength and the need to show off can motivate the adolescent to participate in risky behavior. Assessment of the female athlete in training should include identification of the "female athlete triad," which includes an eating disorder, amenorrhea, and osteoporosis. Coaches, parents, and health care providers must be vigilant for this condition, which has serious long-term complications (Loman, 2009).

All student athletes should have comprehensive cardiovascular screening before participating in competitive sports activities. Each year, many high school athletes die in nontraumatic sports-related deaths. Most deaths result from cardiac problems that were not obvious. The American Academy of Pediatrics Committee on Sports Medicine has established guidelines for medical clearance for sports activities (Saglimbeni, 2010). There may be a future role for genetic testing for cardiac disease in athletes with a family history of cardiac problems. The school nurse can play a key role in safety education by working closely with school coaches and parents.

> **Nursing Tip**
>
> Obtaining a driver's license, graduating from high school, and reaching the legal drinking age are American rites of passage through adolescence. Other cultures offer specific ceremonies to mark phases of development.

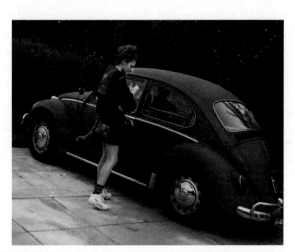

FIGURE 20-12 Adolescents look forward to obtaining their driver's license. The search for independence also brings responsibilities.

COMMON PROBLEMS OF ADOLESCENCE

School-age children begin an exposure to the outside world, where peers gradually become more important to them than their family contacts and they begin to spend more time in outside experiences and less time with family activities. During adolescence, more complex social tasks include entering high school where new friendships are formed, interacting with multiple teachers in one day, increasing academic rigor that must be mastered, and romantic experiences that are introduced. Social anxiety disorders affect 1 in 10 adolescents, although only 1 in 5 are ever recognized or treated (Burstein, 2012). Many adolescents are shy, and basic shyness is a totally normal characteristic for an adolescent and should not be confused with a social anxiety disorder, which most often involves distress that impairs functioning. However, the adolescent that has few personal friends and displays impaired social skills may be at risk and may drop out of high school. The at-risk adolescent should be referred for professional care where diagnostic tools and therapy are available. Contact information concerning licensed mental health professionals may be obtained at www.adaa.org (Anxiety and Depression Association of America or the American Psychiatric Association at www.psych.org). The child with an emotional or behavioral condition is discussed in more detail in Chapter 33.

DRUG USE

Drugs are often made available in the schools and in the streets of the neighborhood where emotional depression often occurring in the turmoil of adolescent adjustments are strong influences promoting drug use.

Inhalants: Common household products whose vapors can be inhaled to produce a psychoactive response. Abuse of inhalants is popular in the teen who does not have the money for street drugs. Inhalants such as glue, spray paint, and shoe polish are popular. The practice of *huffing* is the inhaling via a paper bag filled with a rag that is soaked with the product. Some common products used as inhalants include:

- *Benzene:* Found in gasoline and can cause reproductive toxicity and bone marrow injury.
- *Propane* or *butane:* Found in lighter fluid and hair sprays, Can cause sudden death and high risk of burns.
- *Freon:* Found in refrigerants and aerosols. Can cause sudden death by cold stress to respiratory tissues.
- *Toluene:* Found in paint removers, paint thinners, and gasoline and can cause impaired cognition and loss of coordination.
- *Trichlorethylene:* Found in spot removers and can cause hearing and vision damage and liver failure.

Education concerning the dangers of drug experimentation and use is essential in the home and in the school. See Chapter 33 for a detailed discussion of substance abuse.

Adolescents are prone to mood swings as they try to adjust to the many physical and psychological changes occurring in their lives. The present may feel overwhelming, and the future blurs. The PACE interview (Schwartz, 1997) can assist in distinguishing the drug-free adolescent from one who may be experimenting with drugs and requires a follow-up referral.

Memory Jogger

P—Parents, peers, and pot: Question the adolescent concerning his or her parents, relationships with peers, and attitude toward and exposure to marijuana.
A—Alcohol, automobiles: Question the adolescent concerning alcohol use (e.g., alcohol at parties) and his or her driving record.
C—Cigarettes: Discuss the adolescent's smoking history.
E—Education: Discuss the adolescent's attitude and performance in school.

If two or more of the PACE letters are problem areas, the adolescent may be at high risk for drug abuse and require a professional referral. Follow-up care may involve making a contract with the adolescent to be drug free, educating the adolescent, teaching coping skills, and referring the parents to a support group such as Tough Love groups or the National Family Partnership.

DEPRESSION

Sometimes an adolescent who appears to be adjusted and performing well in school may become depressed. Drug use can precede the development of depression. Working parents and busy teachers can easily overlook behaviors that are slowly changing. A change in school performance, in appearance, or in behavior can be a warning sign of depression, which can lead to suicide if left untreated. A threat of suicide is a call for help that must be taken care of without delay. Suicide is the third leading cause of death in the adolescent group age 15 to 19 years (Centers for Disease Control and Prevention, 2013). The school nurse can help the adolescent by recognizing the depression, encouraging open communication, posting the numbers of available hotlines, identifying appropriate coping mechanisms, and providing professional referrals. See Chapter 33 for details concerning suicide and other behavioral problems.

ADOLESCENT PREGNANCY

Adolescent pregnancy continues to be a social and health concern in the United States. Nurses must be familiar with the tasks of the adolescent years and recognize that adolescent pregnancy occurs while the adolescent is still struggling to manage developmental issues. There are many psychosocial factors that influence sexual activity during the adolescent years. The developmental and physiological impact of pregnancy on the adolescent, the tasks and adolescent responses, and the appropriate nursing interventions are described in Tables 20-3 and 20-4. Nutritional needs and nursing care of the pregnant adolescent are discussed in Chapter 4, and nursing care during labor and delivery is discussed in Chapters 7 and 9.

THE NURSING APPROACH TO ADOLESCENTS

The nurse must open the lines of communication with adolescents and enable them to feel at ease before

Table 20-3 Developmental and Physiological Impact of Pregnancy on the Adolescent

FACTOR	RISK	EFFECT
Age at which pregnancy occurs	At menarche, the first menstrual cycles are irregular and anovulatory. Young adolescents have immature vascular development in the uterus.	"Natural" methods of birth control are ineffective in young adolescents. Condition may lead to gestational hypertension and fetal perfusion problems that result in poor pregnancy outcome, such as prematurity and low birth weight.
	Long bone growth is incomplete until 2 years after menses start.	Pregnancy before long bone growth is complete can cause early closure of epiphysis because of increase in estrogen levels.
	Pelvis does not reach adult size and dimensions until 3 years after menarche.	A small pelvis increases problems during labor and delivery and increases need for cesarean section.
Nutritional intake	Dietary intake often contains "empty" calories and consists of fad diets; eating disorders may be present; dieting to control weight and meet media definition of a beautiful body is common.	Inadequate nutrition, especially in early months of pregnancy, results in negative pregnancy outcome and birth defects. Poor nutrition can result in gestational hypertension, low-birth-weight newborn, and prematurity.
Sexual activity	Multiple partners or unprotected sex can result in sexually transmitted infections (STIs).	STIs increase risk to fetus and newborn.
Limited access to health care	Adolescent may fear revealing pregnancy to parents.	Delayed prenatal care can result in problems for mother and fetus.

NOTE: Studies have shown that pregnancy in late adolescence accompanied by good prenatal care does not pose as high a risk for physiological problems as it does in early and middle adolescence. A multidisciplinary approach is essential, because teen pregnancy is a complex problem.
From Leifer G: *Maternity nursing,* ed 11, St Louis, 2012, Saunders.

Table 20-4 Nursing Care and the Effect of Adolescence on the Tasks of an Unplanned Pregnancy

STATE OF PREGNANCY	TASK	ADOLESCENT RESPONSE	NURSING INTERVENTION
First trimester	Confirmation of pregnancy	Fear of disclosing pregnancy may result in delayed confirmation, hidden pregnancy, and delayed prenatal care	Educate concerning signs and symptoms of pregnancy so as not to confuse with other conditions. Discuss health behaviors required for healthy fetus.
Second trimester	Focus on newborn as real	Family chaos may result when parents, baby's father, and friends see reality of pregnancy; may try to maintain control by dieting and continuing to conceal pregnancy Egocentric phase may prevent full focus on baby as being real	Preserve adolescent image by wearing appropriate clothes. Discuss disclosure to parents and friends. Discuss prenatal needs; show attractive pictures of fetus at various gestational ages.
Third trimester	Preparation for newborn and birth process	Focuses on ending experience but may fear labor; may not wish to bond or consider needs of newborn	Initiate discussions of child care; tour birthing facility and refer to community agencies as needed; provide education regarding birth process.

From Leifer G: *Maternity nursing,* ed 11, St Louis, 2012, Saunders.

initiating care or teaching. A sense of humor is helpful. Providing privacy and ensuring confidentiality and respect are basic to adolescent communication. The nurse must be careful not to behave like an adolescent, because the adolescent may perceive that behavior as "phony." Adolescent hostility may be evidence of fear of the unknown, and rebellion may be an effort to grasp

independence. The nurse should guide the parents concerning the need to listen, understand, and share with adolescents. Helping parents distinguish between normal problems of adolescence and problems that necessitate referral and follow-up is essential. For example, demands for privacy are normal, but overall withdrawal necessitates referral and follow-up care.

Health care teaching should include nutrition, dental care, personal care, body piercing, accident prevention, substance abuse, self-control, risk-taking behavior, money, and time management. Open-ended questions concerning common problems of adolescence may encourage the discussion of a topic that adolescents may not initiate by themselves.

Graduation from high school is self-actualization for the adolescent (Figure 20-13). Getting a job that will provide for self-support or going to college, which may involve leaving home, is the first step of entrance into independent adulthood (Figure 20-14).

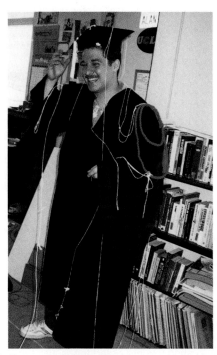

FIGURE 20-13 Graduation from high school is the self-actualization of the adolescent. Peers and family share the joy with the new graduate.

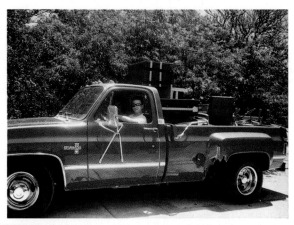

FIGURE 20-14 Moving away from home and going away to college mark the entrance into adulthood.

Get Ready for the NCLEX® Examination!

Key Points

- Adolescence is defined as the period of life that begins with the appearance of secondary sex characteristics and ends with emotional maturity and the cessation of growth.
- According to Erikson, the major developmental task of adolescence is to establish a sense of identity. Other major tasks of adolescence include separating from family, initiating intimacy, and making career choices.
- Freud considered adolescence as the last stage of psychosexual development. He termed this the *genital stage*.
- Jean Piaget suggests that the cognitive development during adolescence reflects abstract reasoning and logic. He calls this stage the *period of formal operations*.
- The physical development seen during this period is distinguished by puberty, the stage at which the reproductive organs become functional and secondary sex characteristics develop.
- Adolescents vary in their rate of physical and social maturation and their ability to resolve conflicts concerning self-esteem and autonomy.
- A nonjudgmental adult role model who can maintain confidentiality can help avoid a crisis for the adolescent.
- The Sexuality Information and Education Council of the United States (SIECUS) is an example of a national organization that assists in the development and implementation of sex education programs.
- Some primary challenges of the adolescent years include adjusting to rapid physical changes, maintaining privacy, coping with stresses and pressures, maintaining open communication, and developing positive lifestyle choices.
- Peer groups help the adolescent to separate from the family and experiment with social behaviors.
- A clique affords the adolescent the opportunity to "belong" and to develop close personal relationships with others who have similar interests and values.
- The first menstrual period is called *menarche*.
- The adolescent struggles with the development of a realistic body image.
- Accurate, safe, and timely sex education can help prevent STIs and HIV.
- Adolescence is a time of conflict with parental authority and values. The influence of peers and heterosexual relationships increases.
- Motor vehicle accidents, homicide, and drownings are the leading causes of mortality in the adolescent age group.

Additional Learning Resources

 Go to your Study Guide for additional learning activities to help you master this chapter content.

evolve Go to your Evolve website (http://evolve.elsevier.com/Leifer) for the following learning resources:

- Animations
- Answer Guidelines for Critical Thinking Questions
- Answers and Rationales for Review Questions for the NCLEX® Examination
- Glossary with English and Spanish pronunciations
- Interactive Review Questions for the NCLEX® Examination
- Patient Teaching Plans in English and Spanish
- Skills Performance Checklists
- Video clips and more!

 Online Resources

- American Academy of Pediatrics: http://aappolicy.aappublications.org/cgi/reprint/pediatrics; 108/4/1030.pdf
- Bicycle Helmets: www.aap.org/policy/0103.html
- MTV, It's Your Sex Life: www.itsyoursexlife.com
- National Family Partnership: http://cmnfp.pictco.org/default.asp
- Parents Without Partners: www.parentswithoutpartners.org
- Sexuality Information and Education Council of the United States (SIECUS): www.siecus.org
- Suicide prevention: www.cdc.gov/ncipc/dvp/Suicide/youthsuicide.htm

Review Questions for the NCLEX® Examination

1. One of the tasks of adolescence as defined by Erikson is:
   1. finding an identity.
   2. sexual latency.
   3. heterosexuality.
   4. concrete operations.

2. When communicating with an adolescent about safety concerns, which concept of adolescent behavior should be considered?
   1. The typical adolescent understands teaching and respects and usually follows the advice of adults.
   2. Growth and development are complete in the adolescent, and muscle coordination and skills lessen the risks for injury.

3. Safety concerns at this age mostly focus on sports injuries.
   4. Adolescents are risk takers and tend to experiment with potentially dangerous outcomes.

3. Puberty can most accurately be defined as the period of life characterized by the:
   1. occurrence of sexual maturity and appearance of secondary sex characteristics.
   2. substitution of adult interests and value systems for child interests.
   3. most rapid rate of physical and mental growth and development.
   4. awakening of sexual feelings and the initiation of sexual experience.

4. A 16-year-old female towers over her companions, which bothers her. She confides to the nurse and says, "I just hate school—everyone is always staring at me." The nurse's best response would be:
   1. "Don't pay any attention to it."
   2. "You just don't know how lucky you are to be tall."
   3. "This will resolve itself in time. Don't worry."
   4. "Tell me more about how this embarrasses you."

5. Which action is most important when planning nutrition management for the adolescent?
   1. Planning a low-calorie diet
   2. Incorporating favorite or fad foods into the diet
   3. Encouraging a positive attitude toward obesity
   4. Skipping a meal to reduce caloric intake

Critical Thinking Question

1. A high school senior expresses her concern to the nurse about taking her college entrance examination. The examination is given early in the morning, which is when she often feels sleepy and less alert and has trouble concentrating. She states that she usually studies hard the night before an examination and tries to eat a good breakfast on the day of the test. The breakfast usually consists of bacon and eggs, a muffin, and chocolate milk. What is the appropriate response of the nurse?

The Child's Experience of Hospitalization

http://evolve.elsevier.com/Leifer

Objectives

1. Define each key term listed.
2. Identify various health care delivery settings.
3. Describe three phases of separation anxiety.
4. Discuss the management of pain in infants and children.
5. List two ways in which the nurse can lessen the stress of hospitalization for the child's parents.
6. Identify two problems confronting the siblings of the hospitalized child.
7. Organize a nursing care plan for a hospitalized child.
8. Interpret a clinical pathway for a hospitalized child.
9. Describe two milestones in the psychosocial development of the preschool child that contribute either positively or negatively to the adjustment to hospitalization.
10. Contrast the problems of the preschool child and the school-age child facing hospitalization.
11. List three strengths of the adolescent that the nurse might use when formulating nursing care plans.
12. Recognize the steps in discharge planning for infants, children, and adolescents.

Key Terms

clinical pathway (p. 478)
conscious sedation (p. 474)
emancipated minor (ē-MĂN-sĭ-pā-ĭd MĪ-nŭr, p. 483)
narcissistic (năhr-sĭ-SĬS-tĭk, p. 482)
personal space (PŬR-sŭn-ŭl spās, p. 476)

pictorial pathways (p. 479)
regression (rē-GRĔSH-ŭn, p. 474)
respite care (RĔS-pĭt kār, p. 484)
separation anxiety (sĕpă-RĀ-shŭn ăng-ZĪ-ĭ-tē, p. 471)
transitional object (trăn-ZĬSH-ŭn-ŭl ŎB-jĕkt, p. 480)

HEALTH CARE DELIVERY SETTINGS

OUTPATIENT CLINIC

Many hospitals today have well-organized outpatient facilities, satellite clinics for preventive medicine and urgent care centers for the care of the child who is ill. The advent of Medicaid and other such programs has made these services available to low-income families. Within clinics, there may be specialty areas (particularly at children's facilities) such as well-child clinics, asthma clinics, cardiac clinics, and orthopedic clinics. In some institutions, information is distributed and brief classes are held for waiting parents.

In many private medical offices the pediatricians or their nurses are available at certain hours of each day to answer telephone inquiries. The pediatric nurse practitioner may visit patients in the home, give routine physical examinations at the clinic, and otherwise work with the physician so that a higher quality of individual care may be attained. The nurse practitioner is often the primary contact person for children in the health care system.

Types of Outpatient Clinics

Satellite clinics are convenient and offer families flexible coverage. Some are located in shopping malls. Parents may walk with children and be contacted by a beeper when it is their turn to see the health care provider. This eliminates confining children in a small area and is less frustrating to caregivers. In many cities, a group of pediatricians practice in an office removed from the hospital, which aids in the distribution of health services and provides evening and weekend health coverage.

Another area of outpatient care is the pediatric research center, such as the one at St. Jude's Hospital in Memphis, Tennessee. This type of institution offers highly specialized care for patients with particular disorders, often at little or no expense to the patient. In the outpatient clinic, as in all other settings, documentation and record review are important parts of data collection.

For patients with uncomplicated conditions, elective surgery at an outpatient surgery clinic offers the advantage of lower cost, reduced incidence of health care–associated infection, and recuperation at home in familiar surroundings (e.g., herniorrhaphy or tonsillectomy). These outpatient clinics eliminate the need to separate the child from the family and reduce the extent of treatment and the emotional impact of the illness. Careful preparation must be provided, and assurance must be obtained that the child's home environment is adequate to meet recovery needs.

Promoting a Positive Experience

The attitude of nurses, receptionists, and other personnel in the clinic, office, or hospital unit is of the utmost importance. It can make the difference between an atmosphere that is warm and friendly and one in which the child is made to feel dehumanized. As more and more medical care is offered in outpatient clinics, there will be an even greater reduction in the number of children who require hospitalization. For many, the only exposure to medical personnel is through brief clinic appointments. Therefore it is very important that these encounters are positive ones for children and their families.

Preparing the Child for a Treatment or Procedure.

Whenever possible the parent should be involved in the preparation for and initiation of a treatment or procedure, and the child should be prepared according to his or her developmental level (Box 21-1). For example, for infants, keep a familiar object with the infant, restrain as needed, and cuddle and hug the infant following the procedure. For a toddler, model the behavior desired (e.g., opening the mouth), tell the child it is

Box **21-1**	Preparing a Child for Treatments or Procedures

The developmental stage of the child guides the type of preparation needed.

INFANTS
Involve parents
Include familiar object
Soothe, distract, and hug after treatment or procedure

TODDLERS AND PRESCHOOLERS
Involve parents
Offer simple explanations
Give permission to express discomfort
Offer one direction at a time
Allow for choices, if possible
Use distraction
Hug after treatment or procedure

SCHOOL-AGE CHILD
All of the aforementioned, plus the following:
• Let child examine equipment
• Encourage verbalization of fears
• Offer small reward after treatment or procedure, for example, a sticker

ADOLESCENT
Provide privacy
Involve adolescent in treatment or procedure
Explain treatment or procedure and equipment
Suggest coping techniques

okay to yell if the treatment or procedure is uncomfortable, and use distractions. For a preschooler, explain the treatment or procedure in simple terms, allow the child to handle some of the equipment, and keep other equipment out of sight. For a school-age child, explain in advance what the treatment or procedure is and the reason it is needed, and allow the child responsibility for simple tasks, such as applying tape. For adolescents, explain the treatment or procedure in more detail, and encourage questioning. Involve them in decision making and planning, such as who should be in the room. Proper preparation decreases anxiety, increases cooperation, and assists the child in coping with the experience.

HOME

Because hospitalization is now brief for most children, the choice is not either hospital or home care but a combination of the two. They are becoming interdependent. Dramatic technical improvements and research in specific disease entities are also helping to advance the movement to home care (e.g., cryoprecipitate for hemophiliacs, Broviac catheters for chemotherapy, heparin locks for intravenous access, glucometers for monitoring blood glucose). However, home care is broader than in years past. It is not merely a matter of supplying appliances and nursing care, but it also includes assessment of the total needs of children and their families. Families need to be linked to a wide variety of network services. This ideally involves a multidisciplinary approach spearheaded by the health care provider.

The hospice concept for children has received accolades from parents who have benefited from its service. Local and national support groups for specific problems afford opportunities for families to share and support one another and to learn from others' successes and failures. Special groups and camps for children with chronic illnesses are also well established. Group therapy for children under stress is equally important in preventing mental health problems (e.g., groups for children whose parents are divorced, Alateen for children of alcoholics). These and other programs not only have the potential for improving life for the child and family but also may help to reduce the high cost of medical care. There have been dramatic changes in the delivery of health care to children and families. These changes affect the role and responsibilities of the nurse working both in wellness centers providing preventive care and in hospitals or homes treating illness.

CHILDREN'S HOSPITAL UNIT

The children's hospital unit differs in many respects from adult divisions. The pediatric unit or hospital is designed to meet the needs of children and their parents. A cheerful, casual atmosphere helps to bridge the gap between home and hospital and is in keeping with the child's emotional, developmental, and physical needs. Nurses wear colorful uniforms, and colored bedspreads and wagons or strollers for transportation provide a more homelike atmosphere.

The physical structure of the unit includes furniture of the proper height for the child, soundproof ceilings, and color schemes with eye appeal. There is a special treatment room for the health care provider to examine or treat the child. In this way the other children do not become disturbed by the proceedings. Some hospitals have a schoolroom. When this is not available, it is necessary for the home-school teacher to visit each school-age child individually. Today's modern general hospitals have separate waiting rooms for children. This is more relaxing for parents, because they do not need to worry about whether their child is disturbing adult patients, and it is less frightening to the child.

Most pediatric departments include a playroom. It is generally large and light in color. Bulletin boards and whiteboards are within reach of the patients. Mobiles may be suspended from the ceiling. Some playrooms are equipped with an aquarium of fish because children love living things. Various toys suitable for different age groups are available. This room may be under the supervision of a child–life specialist or a play therapist. Parents usually enjoy taking their children to the playroom and observing the various activities. The playroom is considered an "ouch-free" area, or a safe haven from painful treatments.

When the child cannot be taken to the playroom because of the diagnosis or physical condition, bedside play activities appropriate to the developmental level and diagnosis of the child should be provided. The daily routine of the pediatric unit emphasizes parent rooming-in, the provision of consistent caregivers, and flexible schedules designed to meet the needs of growing children.

THE CHILD'S REACTION TO HOSPITALIZATION

The child's reaction to hospitalization depends on many factors such as age, amount of preparation given, security of home life, previous hospitalizations, support of family and medical personnel, and child's emotional health. Many children cannot grasp what is going to happen to them even though they have been well prepared. At a time when children need their parents most, they may be separated from them, placed in the hands of strangers, and even fed different foods. Add to this a totally new environment and physical discomfort, and the result is one frightened and unhappy child.

Each child reacts differently to hospitalization. One may be demanding and exhibit temper tantrums, whereas another may become withdrawn. The "good" child on the unit may be going through greater torment than the one who cries and shows feelings outwardly. The best-prepared nurse cannot replace the child's parents. However, hospitalization can be a period of growth rather than just an unpleasant interlude. Children may see the nurse as someone who cares for

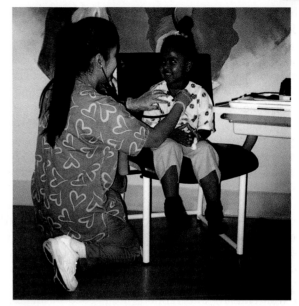

FIGURE 21-1 The nurse greets the child at eye level in a nonthreatening manner. This child views the nurse as a person who cares for her physically and is a source of security and comfort. (Courtesy Pat Spier, RN-C.)

them physically, as their parents would, and as a source of security and comfort (Figure 21-1).

The major causes of stress for children of all ages are separation, pain, and fear of body intrusion. This is influenced by the child's developmental age, the maturity of the parents, cultural and economic factors, religious background, past experiences, family size, state of health on admission, and other factors.

Nursing Tip

Familiar rituals and routines must be incorporated into the plan of care for a hospitalized child.

SEPARATION ANXIETY

Separation anxiety occurs in infants age 6 months and older and is most pronounced at the toddler age. There are three stages of separation anxiety: *protest, despair,* and *denial* or *detachment.* Unless infants are extremely ill, their sense of abandonment is expressed by a loud *protest.* Toddlers may watch and listen for their parents. Their cry is continuous until they fall asleep in exhaustion. Toddlers may call out, "Mommy," repeatedly, and the approach of a stranger only causes increased screaming. The crying gradually stops, and the second stage of *despair* sets in. Children appear sad and depressed. They move about less and withdraw from strangers who approach. They do not play actively with toys. In the third stage, *denial* or *detachment,* children appear to deny their need for the parent and become detached or disinterested in their visits. They become more interested in their surroundings, their toys, and their playmates. On the surface, it appears the child has adjusted to the separation. However, it is important for the nurse to understand that the child is using a coping mechanism to detach and reduce the emotional pain.

If the detachment stage is prolonged, an irreversible disruption of parent–infant bonding may occur. Health care workers who do not understand the stages of separation anxiety may label the crying, protesting child as "bad," the withdrawn depressed child in despair as "adjusting," and the child who is in the detachment phase as a "well-adjusted" child. This misinterpretation can prevent health care workers from providing desperately needed assistance and guidance to the child and family.

The nurse must understand that the child who is in despair reverts back to the protest stage when the parent arrives for a visit. Rather than showing joy, the child cries loudly when the parent appears at the door. This is good! The child who has reached the detached phase appears unmoved and uninterested in the parent's arrival. Nursing interventions are needed in this case to preserve and heal parent–child relationships. Optimally the nurse helps the parents to understand they should not deceive the child into believing they will stay and then "sneak out" while the child is distracted. This can tear the bond of trust.

 Nursing Tip

The stages of separation anxiety include protest, despair, and detachment or denial.

PAIN

The accepted definition of pain is that "pain is whatever the experiencing person says it is, existing whenever the experiencing person says it does" (American Academy of Pediatrics [AAP], 2012). This includes verbal and nonverbal expressions of pain. Freedom from pain is a basic need and right of the infant and child. To increase awareness of pain during patient assessment, pain has come to be considered a "fifth vital sign." An assessment for pain is recorded with routine vital sign documentation.

The negative physical and psychological consequences of pain are well documented. Patients in pain secrete higher levels of cortisol, have compromised immune systems, experience more infections, and show delayed wound healing. Nurses must maintain a high level of suspicion for pain when caring for children. Infants cannot show the nurse where it hurts, and often a child's report of pain is not given the credibility of an adult's report. In addition, children may not realize they are supposed to report pain to the nurse.

The nurse should ask the child about pain using a pain rating scale. See Figure 21-2 for sample pain assessment tools. Children may sometimes refrain from complaining if they believe they will receive an injection to relieve the pain. In infants, pain may be assessed according to a behavior scale that includes tightly closed eyes, clenched fists, and a furrowed brow (see Figure 12-8). An example of a pain assessment tool for preverbal children is the Neonatal/Infant Pain Scale (NIPS) which can be used for infants under 1 year of age (Figure 21-2, E). In toddlers, crying may be caused by anxiety and fear rather than by the degree of pain. On the other hand, chronically ill children may not grimace or cry when in pain, but withdraw from interacting with their surroundings.

A pain indicator for communicatively impaired children (PICIC) has been developed and includes observations rated on a 4-point scale including the following:

- Crying with or without tears
- Screaming or groaning
- Distressed facial expression
- Tense body
- Irritability to touch

The FLACC scale is a pain indicator that can be used with nonverbal children and is rated on a 0 to 2 scale for each observation, with 10 being the highest level of pain; it includes the following:

- *F*ace: grimace
- *L*egs: restless → kicking
- *A*ctivity: quiet → arched
- *C*ry: moan → scream
- *C*onsolability: touch → inconsolable

All factors relating to pain assessment should be considered. Family members also experience emotional pain when they see their child in pain.

Nonpharmacological techniques such as drawing, distraction, imagery, relaxation, and cognitive strategies may enhance analgesia to provide necessary relief from pain symptoms. The child may draw "how the pain feels" and where it is located. Distractions such as storytelling, quiet conversation, and puppet play are effective. Imagery techniques, such as having children imagine themselves in a safe place, relieves anxiety. Slowing down breathing and listening to relaxation tapes are effective in reducing pain in adolescents. Cognitive (thinking) techniques such as "thought stopping" are also helpful in older patients. In this technique, the patient is instructed to repeat the word "stop" in response to negative thoughts and worries. A backrub or hand massage is also relaxing, depending on the child's age and diagnosis. In newborns and infants undergoing brief painful procedures, oral sucrose may provide some analgesia. Pain medications should not be withheld from infants and children when needed.

RESPONSE TO DRUGS

Infants and children respond to drugs differently than adults. Elimination of the drug from the body may be prolonged because of an immature liver enzyme system. However, the renal clearance of drugs may be greater in toddlers than in adults. A decreased protein-binding capacity in the blood of small newborns may allow a greater proportion of free unbound

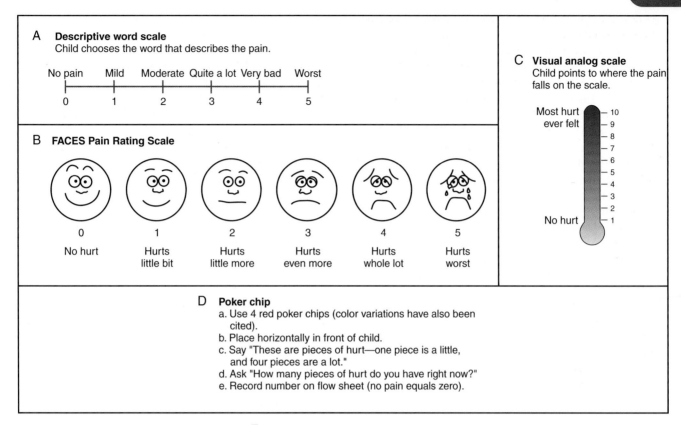

A   Descriptive word scale
Child chooses the word that describes the pain.

No pain	Mild	Moderate	Quite a lot	Very bad	Worst
0	1	2	3	4	5

C   Visual analog scale
Child points to where the pain falls on the scale.

Most hurt ever felt — 10, 9, 8, 7, 6, 5, 4, 3, 2
No hurt — 1

B   FACES Pain Rating Scale

0	1	2	3	4	5
No hurt	Hurts little bit	Hurts little more	Hurts even more	Hurts whole lot	Hurts worst

D   Poker chip
a. Use 4 red poker chips (color variations have also been cited).
b. Place horizontally in front of child.
c. Say "These are pieces of hurt—one piece is a little, and four pieces are a lot."
d. Ask "How many pieces of hurt do you have right now?"
e. Record number on flow sheet (no pain equals zero).

E   Neonatal/Infant Pain Scale (NIPS)
(Recommended for children less than 1 year old)—A score greater than 3 indicates pain

Pain Assessment		Score
Facial Expression 0 – Relaxed muscles 1 – Grimace	Restful face, neutral expression Tight facial muscles; furrowed brow, chin, jaw, (negative facial expression—nose, mouth and brow)	
Cry 0 – No Cry 1 – Whimper 2 – Vigorous Cry	Quiet, not crying Mild moaning, intermittent Loud scream; rising, shrill, continuous (Note: Silent cry may be scored if baby is intubated as evidenced by obvious mouth and facial movement)	
Breathing Patterns 0 – Relaxed 1 – Change in Breathing	Usual pattern for this infant Indrawing, irregular, faster than usual; gagging; breath holding	
Arms 0 – Relaxed/Restrained 1 – Flexed/Extended	No muscular rigidity; occasional random movements of arms Tense, straight legs; rigid and/or rapid extension, flexion	
Legs 0 – Relaxed/Restrained 1 – Flexed/Extended	No muscular rigidity; occasional random leg movement Tense, straight legs; rigid and/or rapid extension, flexion	
State of Arousal 0 – Sleeping/Awake 1 – Fussy	Quiet, peaceful, sleeping or alert, random leg movement Alert, restless, and thrashing	

FIGURE 21-2 Pain assessment tools for children. **A,** Data from Tesler MD, Savedra MC, Holzemer WL: The word-graphic rating scale as a measure of children's and adolescents' pain intensity. *Res Nurs Health*, 14, 1991, 361–371. **B,** From Hockenberry MJ, Wilson D: *Wong's essentials of pediatric nursing*, ed 9, St Louis, 2013, Mosby. Used with permission. Copyright © Mosby. **C,** Data from Cline ME, Herman J, Shaw ER: Standardization of the visual analogue scale. *Nurs Res*, 41(6), 1992, 378–380. **D,** Data from Hester NO, Foster RL, Jordan-Marsh M: Putting pain measurement into clinical practice. In Finley GA, McGrath PJ (eds): *Measurement of pain in infants and children*, vol 10, 1998, International Association for the Study of Pain Press, Seattle. **E,** Copyright 1989, Children's Hospital of Eastern Ontario, Ottawa, Ontario, Canada. From Lawrence J, Alcock D, McGrath P, Kay J, MacMurray B, & Dulberg C (1993). The development of a tool to assess neonatal pain. *Neonatal Network*, 12(6), 59–66.

drug to remain in the body of the small infant. Dosages are influenced by weight and differences in expected absorption, metabolism, and clearance. The nurse must calculate every medication to determine the safety of the dose before the medication is administered. See the dosage calculation technique in Chapter 22.

Drugs Used for Pain Relief in Infants and Children

Acetaminophen is commonly used for the relief of mild to moderate pain in infants and children. The maximum dose is 15 mg/kg/dose for infants and children, with a maximum of 5 doses in 24 hours. Toxicity involves liver failure.

Nonsteroidal antiinflammatory drugs (NSAIDs), such as ibuprofen (Motrin), are given in a maximum dosage of 8 to 10 mg/kg every 6 hours (q6h). Ketorolac is a parenterally administered NSAID given for a maximum of 5 days.

Opioids are used for moderate to severe pain such as postoperative pain, sickle-cell crises, and cancer and should be administered with stool softeners to prevent constipation. If used for long periods, tolerance to the pain-relieving effect as well as respiratory depression effects can develop. The right dose of an opioid drug is the amount that relieves pain with a margin of safety for the child. The dose should be repeated before the pain recurs. Addiction is rare in children and adults receiving opioids for pain (Kliegman, 2011). Providing adequate pain relief enables patients to focus on their surroundings and other activities, whereas inadequate pain relief causes the patient to focus on the pain and the time when more medication will be given to stop the pain.

Fentanyl is a potent analgesic given for short surgical procedures. It has a rapid onset with a short duration of action.

Naloxone should be available for use in case of opioid overdose. Flumazenil (Romazicon) should be on hand for a midazolam (Versed) or diazepam (Valium) overdose.

Local anesthetics are used with safety and effectiveness in children. *Topical anesthetics* are used for skin sutures, intravenous (IV) catheter placement, and lumbar punctures. *EMLA cream* is a mixture of lidocaine and prilocaine (eutectic mixture of local anesthetics) that is applied topically to the intact skin (Figure 21-3) and can be used with neonates. "Numby Stuff" uses a

mild electrical current (iontophoresis) to push a topical preparation of Lidocaine and epinephrine into the skin providing local anesthesia within 10 minutes of the application of the patch. "LMX4" is a nonprescription topical anesthetic that is similar to *EMLA*. A vapocoolant spray can provide superficial skin anesthesia for short periods of time. Preoperative and postoperative care are discussed in Chapter 22.

Patient-controlled analgesia (PCA) allows the patient to press a button attached to an IV analgesic infusion to self-administer a bolus of medication. Parents and children as young as 7 years old can be taught to use PCA. A built-in lockout interval prevents accidental overdosing. Any child receiving opioid analgesic drugs should be observed closely for side effects, such as respiratory depression.

More effective pain relief at lower dosages may be achieved when a low-dose analgesic is administered around-the-clock on a regular schedule rather than as needed (PRN). However, "breakthrough pain" can occur, and additional doses of an analgesic may have to be administered. This type of pain management is called preventive pain control.

Conscious Sedation

Conscious sedation is the administration of IV drugs to a patient to impair consciousness but retain protective reflexes, the ability to maintain a patent airway, and the ability to respond to physical and verbal stimuli. Conscious sedation is used to perform therapeutic or diagnostic procedures outside the traditional operating room setting. A skilled registered nurse is required to continuously monitor the patient in an area where emergency equipment and drugs are accessible for resuscitation.

A 1:1 nurse–patient ratio is continued until there are stable vital signs, age-appropriate motor and verbal abilities, adequate hydration, and a presedation level of responsiveness and orientation. Parents are instructed concerning diet, home care, and follow-up visits.

FEAR

Intrusive procedures, such as placing IV lines and performing blood tests, are fear provoking. They disrupt the child's trust level and threaten self-esteem and self-control. They may make it necessary to restrict activity. Care must be taken to respect the modesty, integrity, and privacy of each child. Hospital personnel can provide an environment that supports the child's need for mastery and control. These interventions are discussed according to age in this chapter and throughout the text. Selected nursing diagnoses for the hospitalized child and family are presented in Nursing Care Plan 21-1.

REGRESSION

Regression of growth and development during hospitalization can be expected. **Regression** is the loss of an achieved level of functioning to a past level of behavior

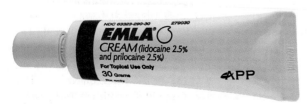

FIGURE 21-3 EMLA cream, a topical anesthetic used before an invasive procedure to reduce pain involved in piercing the skin. (Courtesy APP Pharmaceuticals, Schaumburg, Ill.)

★ Nursing Care Plan 21-1   The Hospitalized Child and Family

PATIENT DATA A 5-year-old girl is admitted to the hospital with a diagnosis of a compound fracture of the right tibia. She cries whenever her parents leave or return to her room, and she has had episodes of bedwetting since admission.

Selected Nursing Diagnosis: Anxiety related to hospitalization of the child as evidenced by restlessness, facial tension, insomnia, crying, clinging behavior, regression to previous stage of growth and development, or maladaptive behaviors

Goals	Nursing Interventions	Rationales
Child and family will experience decreased anxiety as demonstrated by ability to relax, present a calm demeanor, and effectively participate in child's care.	Determine the child's and the family's knowledge regarding reason for hospitalization.	Provides information to the nurse as to which areas need clarification and which need reinforcement of correct information.
	Explain routines usually followed on unit and orient the child and the parent to the unit, including playroom.	Helps to decrease level of anxiety for the child and the parents.
	Suggest that parents or family members bring in a photograph, favorite toy, or favorite DVD or CD for child.	These items help to provide a link to home and help to promote a sense of security in the child.
	Recognize and teach the parent about age-appropriate separation anxiety.	The age of the child is a major factor to consider in the adjustment to separation from familiar people and surroundings.
	Instruct parents to explain to the child when they will return in an age-appropriate manner (e.g., "after your TV program is over" or "after lunch" or "before dinner").	Establishes a sense of trust that the child has not been abandoned. Also, toddlers and young children do not fully understand the concept of time. Using a favorite show or a mealtime as a marker helps to lessen the degree of anxiety the child may feel.
	Provide for consistency in personnel assigned to child as much as possible.	Consistency is necessary to develop a sense of trust. Maladaptive behaviors may be normal in unfamiliar circumstances. However, if consistency and support are not provided, coping abilities decrease.
	Support parents by showing a willingness to be available to them to listen and/or to answer questions.	Nurse's availability to answer questions shows concern and interest for parents' concerns, prevents the potential for misunderstanding of prescribed treatments, and helps to lessen the anxiety of family members.
	Maintain child's contact with family; involve family in child's care when appropriate.	Increases sense of security in child and provides a sense of purpose for the family.

that was successful during earlier stages of development. Examples of regression include demanding a bottle in a child who usually drinks from a cup, refusal to use a potty chair in a child who has achieved bowel and bladder control, or demanding to be carried by a child who had been walking independently. An accurate nursing assessment of the child's abilities, and the planning of care to support and maintain growth and development, can minimize regression. However, regression should not be punished. Nurses can guide parents to praise appropriate behavior and ignore regressions. When the child is free of the stress that caused the regression, praise will motivate the achievement of appropriate behavior.

CULTURAL RESPONSE

Showing culturally sensitive attitudes toward families with hospitalized children decreases anxiety. Flexibility and careful listening are necessary to understand cultural needs. Studies of children in many different societies show that the childhood environment typical in American culture is different from environments deriving from other traditions. Nurses must also be aware of their own cultural biases and how these might affect their assessments. In some cases a translator may be required.

The nurse must create a bridge between the health care system of the United States and the diverse people that system serves. Effective use of health care services and compliance with treatment plans is enhanced when the nurse's approach is compatible with cultural needs and beliefs. Teaching will be effective only if the parents or child understand the language used. Interpreters should be used as needed. Nonverbal cues and body language are important in intercultural communication. Nurses should take the time to learn what their gestures and movements mean to the family from another culture.

In some developing countries, the energies of parents are focused on survival rather than on promoting growth and development or intellectual skills. These practices become ingrained in the childrearing practices handed down from generation to generation. For example, within these cultures, parents may believe that an ill infant must be near the caregiver's body at all times.

Therefore, in the Western hospital, the nurse may find it a challenge to coax parents to allow the infant to remain in the crib, enveloped by an oxygen tent and separated from them.

Crying may be interpreted by some cultures as a signal of an organic upset or illness. Because diarrhea is a common cause of infant death in developing countries, frequent feeding in response to crying is a survival response. When families from developing countries that use these survival practices move to the United States (where survival threats decrease), it may take generations to change the child care practices and focus on promoting optimum growth and development.

One cultural group may prize autonomy and initiative in their children, whereas another may tolerate only complete obedience. Protective amulets or charms placed on the wrists or clothing of infants must be respected. In the gypsy culture, the color red and the number three are positive symbols. Therefore a red-colored medicine to be given 3 times a day will receive more compliance than a white-colored medication prescribed 2 times a day. Respecting cultural and religious beliefs will enhance compliance.

The nurse must be careful to separate survival practices from cultural beliefs. It may be advantageous to change care practices based on survival when the threat to survival is no longer present. If the practice is based on cultural belief, however, the practice must be respected and no attempt should be made to change it. The nurse must assess the family through the eyes of its culture to avoid labeling a family who is *different* as *dysfunctional*.

INTERCULTURAL COMMUNICATION: RESPONSES TO HOSPITALIZATION

Personal Space

Personal space is defined as an imaginary circle that surrounds us. The size of that space and how securely it is guarded is largely determined by culture. We can observe the space by watching two friends of the same culture talk to each other. Some people stand close to each other. Nurses, who often must invade that personal space in carrying out their duties, can be perceived as "pushy" or suspect, and the parent who retreats to protect it can be thought of by the nurse as "cold."

Smiling

A smiling nurse may not be received in all cultures as a "friendly" nurse. In Russia a smile indicates happiness and is inappropriate in a serious or sad situation. Nurses may interpret a nonsmiling Russian as "unfriendly" if they are unaware of this cultural difference. Members of some cultures, however, smile in all circumstances. Their smile is a show of respect. When they are reprimanded, they smile to show they did not mind being reprimanded.

Eye Contact

In the United States, establishing eye-to-eye contact with the person with whom one is communicating is considered a show of respect and attention. In some Asian cultures, however, eye-to-eye-contact is seen as disrespectful. Native Americans consider it rude to stare at a speaker. Eye contact is acceptable for short periods only. The cultural term *evil eye* originates from cultures that interpret eye-to-eye contact as disrespectful.

Touch

In the United States, touch is often considered a gesture of friendliness. However, touch can give misleading messages. A pat on the head may imply superiority of the person touching the head. In the Vietnamese culture, touching the head is thought to rob those being touched of their souls.

Focus

Some cultures are receptive to communication or teaching if the focus is on the problem. Some cultures deal with the problem by focusing on its future impact on the family or the life of the child. Teaching strategies must be designed to approach the topic from the perspective appropriate to that culture.

When teaching infant care and child care, the nurse must always determine the values of the cultural practice of the family before imposing a standardized process. Avoiding cultural conflict is essential to the successful outcome of parent and child teaching. Culture evolves and is not static. However, most families from varying cultures strive to maintain their cultural identities while adapting to Western practices. The nurse should support maintaining the individual cultural identity of each family. Culturally sensitive health care is also discussed in Chapter 15.

THE PARENTS' REACTIONS TO THE CHILD'S HOSPITALIZATION

When children are hospitalized, the entire family is affected. The parents of the hospitalized youngster need others to show interest in their physical and emotional needs. If they are frightened and tense, the child soon senses it.

Parents may believe they are to blame for the child's illness; they may believe they should have recognized the symptoms earlier or could have prevented an accident by closer supervision. Immunizations and other types of preventive care may also have been neglected. These feelings can cause a sense of guilt, helplessness, and anxiety.

Parents seldom are the direct cause for hospital admission of a child. Even in cases of child abuse or neglect, nothing is gained by blaming the parents. The nurse must remain objective and empathic. The nurse listens carefully to parental concerns and acknowledges the legitimacy of their feelings, for example, "It is understandable that you feel this way; everything happened so fast." Parents also commonly express feelings of helplessness at the loss of the parental role as protector. The nurse encourages and supports parents and other family members, stresses their importance to the child's recovery, and encourages their participation in the care of the child. The admission of a child to the hospital produces anxiety. The uncertainty of the situation can become overwhelming, causing feelings of panic. However, these feelings are usually temporary. The nurse should remain relaxed, reassure the parents, and reinforce positive parenting. Information about the child's condition and the treatment plan are given. Needs are assessed, and interventions are planned to meet specific needs.

> **Nursing Tip**
>
> Many hospitals allow parents to be with their child during painful or stressful procedures and during the recovery phase postoperatively.

Poor communication results in unnecessary fears. The nurse should explain in simple terms some of the equipment being used and facilities available on the unit. The nurse listens attentively and tries to clear up misconceptions. Rooming-in may alleviate some anxieties of parents. However, the nurse must continue promptly and cheerfully to tend to the needs of the child to indicate to the parents that their child is in good hands. Parental involvement in a child's care offers the nurse the opportunity to assess the relationship and to provide guidance and teaching as needed.

Parents may need to take time away from work, especially if treatment involves travel to special centers. Ronald McDonald homes offer lodging and other homelike amenities for parents of patients with life-threatening illnesses. The availability of these facilities is explored with the family. The social service worker may be of help in such instances. The care and welfare of other children at home while one parent is at work and the other is rooming-in with the ill child should be discussed. Parents should be advised that pain-control techniques are available and will be used to minimize painful experiences for the ill child.

Parents may ventilate their feelings and stresses through anger, crying, or body language. Behavior is not only a response to the current situation but often involves attitudes resulting from early childhood experiences. The nurse must not pass judgment on individuals whose behavior may seem demanding or unreasonable. An understanding and acceptance of people and their problems is essential for the successful pediatric nurse.

Siblings are also affected when a brother or sister is hospitalized. They may be afraid or feel left out, guilty, or resentful of the attention focused on the ill child. Suitable interventions by the nurse include directing some attention to the siblings, supporting their efforts to comfort the family member, and engaging them in play or drawing pictures, such as "How it feels to have an ill brother or sister." They may also make cards and pictures for the patient.

> **Nursing Tip**
>
> When a child is admitted to the hospital, every family member is affected.

THE NURSE'S ROLE IN THE CHILD'S HOSPITALIZATION

ADMISSION

Nurses are responsible for admitting new patients to the hospital unit. Besides performing the procedure skillfully, they must be prepared to meet the emotional needs of those involved. The impression the nurse gives, whether good or bad, definitely affects the child's adjustment. Empathy in responding to the fears of the child and family members makes the admission procedure stimulating and educational—a positive experience for all.

A child should be prepared for hospitalization when possible. Ideally, the child and parents should tour the pediatric unit before admission. This enables the parents to meet some of the people who will care for their child. Children and their families may be overwhelmed by the size of the institution and the fear of becoming lost.

Between 1 and 3 years of age, children are worried about being separated from their parents. After 3 years of age, children may become more fearful about what is going to happen to them. Parents should try to be as matter-of-fact as possible about this new experience. Unless they have been hospitalized before, children can only try to imagine what will happen to them. It is not necessary to go into much detail; the child's imagination is great, and giving information that is beyond comprehension may create unnecessary fears. It is logical to dwell on the more pleasant aspects, but not to the extent of saying that hospitalization involves no discomforts. For example, one might mention that meals will be served on a tray, that baths will be taken from a basin at the bedside, and that the child will be with other children. The fact that there is a buzzer for calling the nurse may add to the child's sense of security. The parents may plan with the child what favorite toy or book to bring.

Perhaps listening to how the child feels and encouraging questions is more important than explaining certain occurrences. Parents should prepare children for a few days, but not weeks, in advance. Parents should never lure children to the hospital by pretending that it is some other place. In emergency situations, there is little time for preparation. In such cases the entire medical team must try to give added emotional support to the child. The initial greeting should show warmth and friendliness—smile and introduce yourself.

Some hospitals allow the patient to be taken to the playroom for a short time before going to the room where the patient will stay. When the parent tells the nurse the child's name, associating it with a familiar person who has the same name will help the nurse to remember it. It creates a much warmer feeling to speak of "John" or "Suzy" than "your little boy" or "your daughter."

The parent is encouraged to do as much for the child as possible, for example, removing clothes. The nurse tries not to appear rushed. A matter-of-fact attitude must be maintained regardless of the patient's condition. A soft voice and quiet approach are less frightening to the child. A nurse who looks anxious causes unnecessary worry for everyone concerned. A troubled look may have nothing to do with the child. Taking one step at a time is advised. Calmness is catching. The nurse remains available to answer questions that might arise. When there is a good relationship between the parent and nurse, the child benefits from higher quality care.

When children are hospitalized, the nurse should be aware of the developmental history as well as the medical history. A developmental history includes the following:

- Family relationships and support systems
- Cultural needs that may affect care and hospital routine
- Nicknames, rituals, routines
- Developmental level and abilities
- Communication skills
- Personality, adaptability, coping skills
- Past experiences, divorce, new siblings, extended family
- Previous separation experiences—vacations or hospitalizations
- Impact of current health problem on growth and development
- Preparation given the child
- Previous contact with health care personnel

 Nursing Tip

When explaining procedures to children, it is helpful to identify the child's role in the event, for example, "You will be asked to step on the scale."

DEVELOPING A PEDIATRIC NURSING CARE PLAN

Developing the pediatric nursing care plan is similar to developing an adult care plan. The care plan is the result of the nursing process. It states specifically what is to be done for each child and keeps the focus on the child—not on the condition or the therapy. An established list of accepted nursing diagnoses is available and in use. These serve as a standard for organizing data collection. They

also serve as a vehicle by which one nurse can communicate with another. A nursing diagnosis for a pediatric patient may require some modification. A survey of the child includes knowledge of growth and developmental processes. It also includes evaluating the primary caregiver, who has a direct role in the safety and maintenance of the child's health. Nursing care plans are guides, and continual evaluation and reevaluation are called for to determine whether the goals for the individual child are being met. A Kardex system consisting of an 8-inch by 10-inch card summarizing pertinent medical and nursing orders, formerly used by many hospitals, has been replaced by electronic (paperless) charting. Figure 21-4 shows a nurse entering data in the unit computer, which may be located at the nursing desk or at the individual patient's bedside.

 Nursing Tip

Play is an important part of a nursing care plan for children.

 Nursing Tip

The achievement of developmental tasks should be part of the plan of care for the hospitalized child.

CLINICAL PATHWAYS

Clinical pathways are used in acute care settings as well as in alternate care settings. The **clinical pathway** is an interdisciplinary plan of care that displays the progress of the entire treatment plan for the patient. The main difference between a clinical pathway and a nursing care plan is that the nursing care plan focuses on the nurse's role in the care of the patient, whereas the clinical pathway focuses on the broader view of the entire multidisciplinary health care team and general outcome goals of care with specific timelines. Understanding the nursing process and the nursing care plan is essential to understanding the nurse's role in the clinical

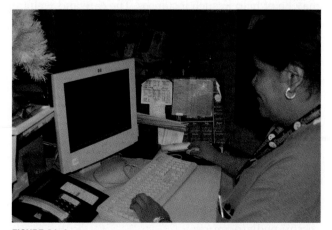

FIGURE 21-4 The nurse enters data and retrieves information about the patient's progress on the unit computer. (From Leifer G: *Maternity nursing*, ed 11, St Louis, 2012, Saunders.)

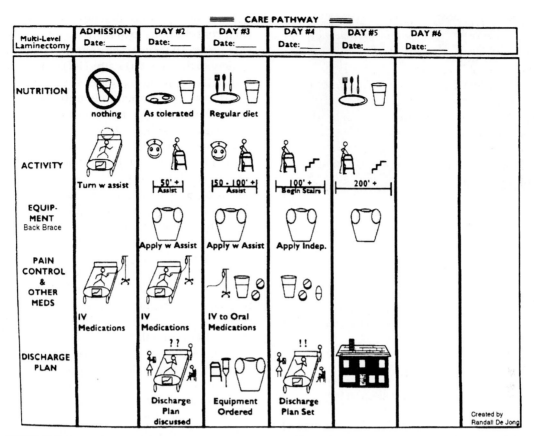

FIGURE 21-5 Pictorial pathway. Pictorial pathways are especially valuable in patient education and anticipatory guidance. (Courtesy Providence General Medical Center, Everett, Wash. Created by Randall De Jong.)

pathway. See Chapters 1, 12 and 25 for details and examples of clinical pathways.

Clinical pathways for children with specific conditions are presented in various chapters of this text. **Pictorial pathways** (Figure 21-5) have been used and are especially valuable in patient education and anticipatory guidance.

MEETING THE NEEDS OF THE HOSPITALIZED CHILD

The Hospitalized Infant

Hospitalization is frustrating for infants. During infancy, rapid physical and emotional development takes place. Infants are accustomed to receiving what they want when they want it, and they show their displeasure quickly when illness restricts the satisfaction of their desires. Infants who were breastfed at home may be unable to continue this regimen. They miss the continuous affection of their parents. Their daily schedule is upset. The infant who drinks well from a cup at home may refuse it entirely at the hospital.

Nursing personnel must try to meet the needs of these patients by protecting them from excess frustration. It is not wise to expect infants to develop new habits when they need energy to cope with their illness and the strange environment. One of the nurse's major goals during this period is to assist with the parent–infant attachment process and to promote sensorimotor activities. This can be fostered by providing means for the infant and significant caregiver to interact and by attempting to ease the tension of the parents. The nurse can serve as a role model by performing activities with the infant, such as cuddling, rocking, talking, and singing. A swing, a bath with squeeze toys, a pacifier, and a hanging mobile are also appropriate as the infant's condition permits.

Because the infant cannot understand explanations, the nurse administers uncomfortable procedures as gently as possible and returns the infant to the parents for consolation. Liberal visiting hours are essential (Figure 21-6). When parents are not available, soothing support and gentle touch are provided; otherwise the infant may learn to associate only pain with nursing care. Consistency in caregivers is also important at this stage of development.

The Hospitalized Toddler

The toddler's world revolves around the parents, particularly the mother (or significant caregiver). Hospitalization is a painful experience for toddlers. They cannot understand why they are separated from their mothers, and they become very distressed. Toddlers who have a continuous, secure relationship with their mothers react more violently to separation because they have more to lose. Nursing goals in the care of the hospitalized toddler are presented in Box 21-2.

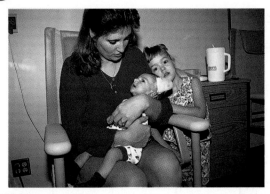

FIGURE 21-6 Liberal visiting hours enable the parent to meet the needs of the hospitalized infant. Family-centered hospital care allows the sibling to maintain contact with the parent while visiting in the hospital. (Courtesy Children's Medical Center, Dallas, Tex.)

Box 21-2	**Nursing Goals in the Care of Hospitalized Toddlers**

- Reassure parents, particularly the child's primary caregiver.
- Maintain the toddler's sense of trust.
- Incorporate home habits of the child into nursing care plans, for example, transitional objects.
- Allow the child to work through or master threatening experiences through soothing techniques and play.
- Provide individualized, flexible nursing care plans in accordance with the child's development and diagnosis.

Separation anxiety is at its peak in the toddler (see Chapter 17). The nurse who comprehends the various separation stages sees parental visits as necessary, even though the process of separation and reunion is painful. A cohesive staff is essential to meet the needs of the children and their parents. Educating parents helps to promote their continued visits and to decrease feelings of inadequacy. Ritualistic patterns of care create a sense of structure and are appropriate for children in this age group.

Repetitive games involving disappearance and return are helpful. Peek-a-boo and hide-and-seek serve such purposes. The use of a **transitional object**, such as a blanket or a favorite toy from home, promotes security. Pictures of the family and tape recordings of favorite stories are other tools that help the child remain connected with the family. When the nurse or parent leaves, he or she explains when he or she will return in terms that the toddler can understand by experience (e.g., after naptime or lunch) and then the nurse or parent returns promptly at that time. A loving hug, good-bye, and prompt exit are then necessary. The continued reappearance of the parents as promised is of value in reducing the child's anxiety and reestablishing his or her sense of trust. The parent should not wait until a child falls asleep to depart. This prevents confrontation, but it disturbs the child's sense of trust. The nurse assures the parents that he or she will remain with the child for comfort.

Rooming-in is highly desirable. When rooming-in is impossible, consistent caregivers should be assigned to care for the child and the parent. The nurse indicates by his or her approach that he or she considers the parent's contributions extremely important to the child's well-being. The nurse interprets the stages of separation anxiety to the parent (Figure 21-7). The nurse must also realize that parents are under stress and should not be asked to assume responsibilities beyond their capabilities. The nurse observes parents for signs of fatigue and suggests appropriate interventions.

Occasionally parents do not choose to care for their child; for example, "We feel that since we are paying for this, we should just be able to entertain him." In such instances, the parents' wishes are respected. Referral to the clinical nurse specialist might also be appropriate to facilitate communication and to understand better the underlying dynamics of the situation.

The home habits of the toddler are recorded and used as a basis for everyday routine. A potty chair is provided if the child is trained. Some regression in behavior is to be expected. If the toddler still prefers bottles to cups, there should be no attempt to change this in the hospital. Familiar toys and books are important. A steady, calm voice communicates safety. Toddlers are in the stage of autonomy. Loss of a small amount of the self-control they have achieved usually results in resistance and negativism.

Children are forewarned about any unpleasant or new experiences that they may need to undergo while in the hospital. These are communicated in keeping with their level of understanding. Being truthful about things that may hurt prevents the child from feeling betrayed. Preparation and explanation are provided immediately before a procedure so that the child does not worry needlessly for an extended period. Crying and protesting when told about certain procedures are healthy expressions of feelings and relieve tension. Distractions such as blowing bubbles, looking through a kaleidoscope, and playing with pop-up toys may help to reduce anxiety and pain.

Supervised playroom activity contributes to intellectual, social, and motor development. Treatments in the playroom are avoided. Toddlers are encouraged to play with safe equipment used in their care, such as bandages, tongue blades, and stethoscopes. Whenever possible, they are allowed out of their cribs, because confinement is frustrating for little ones who have just begun to enjoy walking. Playtime establishes rapport and is an important part of the nursing care of children.

There are indications that restricting the child's mobility for surgical and medical procedures involving splints, IV therapy, burn dressings, and so on may contribute to the development of emotional or personality problems or to speech and learning difficulties (Kliegman et al, 2011). Therefore, when restraint is required, it must be accompanied by increased emotional support such as rooming-in, additional attention from nurses, and suitable diversion.

It is common for children to experience changes in behavior on their return home. They may be demanding and may cling to the parent every minute.

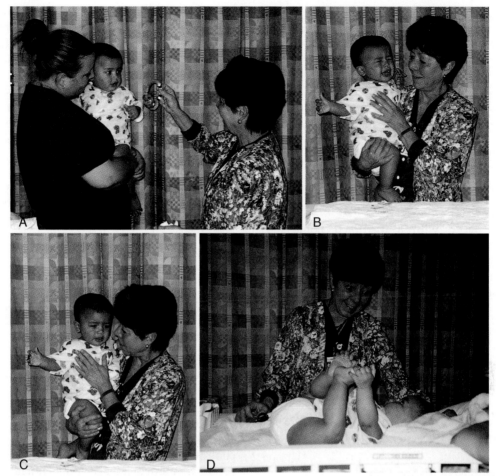

FIGURE 21-7 **A,** The clinical nurse specialist (CNS) approaches the small child calmly, slowly, at eye level, and with the parent present. **B,** The infant shows apprehension and anxiety when carried by the CNS. **C,** Beginning trust is established. **D,** After trust is established, general assessment can begin. (Courtesy Pat Spier, RN-C.)

"He just won't let me out of his sight" is a common description. The parent should give the toddler extra attention and reassurance until trust is regained.

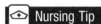 **Nursing Tip**

Toddlers experience some degree of separation anxiety any time their parent or primary caregiver leaves, such as when the child is left with day care personnel, babysitters, or relatives.

The Hospitalized Preschooler

The experience of hospitalization may be easier for preschool children who have already had outside contact (e.g., nursery school and kindergarten) than for those who have never been separated from their parents. Because children of this age operate with concrete thinking, they can understand more and they can be better prepared for hospitalization. Explanations must be made in realistic terms, because preschool children cannot understand abstract explanations. When explaining procedures the nurse should be careful to use nonthreatening words (Table 21-1). They are made to realize that hospitalization is not a punishment for something they have done wrong. Children may feel guilty, particularly

if an accident happens because of some mischief on their part, such as in the case of burns or falls.

Preschool children are distressed when their parents prepare to leave them but, unlike the toddler, they can understand time relationships through activities—at breakfast, after lunch, and the like. The nurse and parents must not tell the child that they will return unless they intend to do so.

At this age the child is afraid of bodily harm, particularly invasive procedures. The surgical patient must be shown the part of the body that requires surgery. The nurse can sketch a body outline and draw a circle around the operative site, giving simple information about the system that will be affected. It is stressed that only this area of the body will be involved. Children in this age group engage in magical thinking and fantasy. Fantasizing about the unknown can be frightening to a young child. The preschooler needs clear, understandable, and truthful explanations. Children who ask questions should be complimented and listened to; any misinterpretations should be corrected. Praise helps to increase the child's self-esteem. The child relieves tension through role-playing. The sick child relishes tongue depressors, adhesive bandages, and other materials related to everyday hospital life.

Table 21-1   Words to Avoid and Words to Use

AVOID	USE INSTEAD
Shot	Medicine under the skin
Incision	Special opening
Put to sleep, anesthesia	Special sleep
Electrodes	Stickers
X-ray	Special picture
Stretcher, gurney	Rolling bed
Catheter	Tube
Take "your temperature"	Check "your temperature"

Parents are faced with a disrupted home life throughout the child's hospitalization. Parents often have trouble coping with everyday tasks when they are lonely for and worried about their children. The frequent trips to the hospital interfere with the daily routine, and other children in the family may resent the ill child. Contact with the physician is needed. Parents have a legal and ethical right to be informed of the benefits and risks of therapy and to be included in the decision-making process. When the child is finally discharged, he or she may be demanding and irritable. Parents need the kind support of hospital personnel to enable them to make informed decisions and to handle these added strains.

The Hospitalized School-Age Child

Children of school age can endure separation from their parents if it is not prolonged. Children who have been cherished from birth can tolerate brief interruptions in their lives more easily than can those who have been denied a secure environment. The school-age child is in a stage of industry and independence. Forced dependency in the hospital (such as immobilization) can result in a feeling of loss of control and loss of security. School-age children need to feel "grown up." They can participate in their care and be offered simple choices to foster their feeling of independence. They can choose their menus within appropriate restrictions, "help the nurse" in various activities, and keep busy with age-appropriate toys.

Knowledge of growth and development in the school-age child helps the nurse provide anticipatory guidance. Nurses can also enlist parents to determine what, if any, successful approaches they use in guiding the child. Behavioral problems may be addressed by a team conference. Nurses who work with children should keep abreast of current trends and guidance approaches. Positive direction and consistency are tools of particular importance to the pediatric nurse.

The education of the school-age child must continue throughout any illness. This gives the child a sense of continuity with the outside world, provides periods of socialization, reinforces weak academic areas, and reassures the child that he or she can return to his or her peers after discharge. The parents may act as liaisons between school and hospital. To be effective at his or her job, the teacher must be informed of the child's physical and emotional health. The nurse provides children with opportunities to study undisturbed so that they will be prepared for classes. Diagnostic tests and treatments should be scheduled around established school routines whenever possible. Many school districts have individual tutors for homebound or hospitalized school-age children.

It is common for school-age children to be "brave" and to show little, if any, fear in situations that actually upset them a good deal. Observation of body language may provide some clues to emotional states. The nurse's presence during unfamiliar procedures is comforting. Following treatments, the nurse should encourage children to draw and talk about their drawings or to act out their feelings through puppet play.

> **!** **Safety Alert!**
>
> Observation of nonverbal clues such as facial grimaces, bodily squirming, and finger tapping is important in determining the need for pain relief and support for the child.

The Hospitalized Adolescent

Adolescents, in particular, experience feelings of loss of control during hospitalization. Daily routines are disrupted, and dependence–independence issues come to the foreground. When feelings of independence, self-assertion, and identity are threatened, the adolescent may respond by withdrawal, noncompliance, or anger. Care plans must be designed to incorporate choice, privacy, and understanding.

Early Adolescence. Nursing care plans must be oriented to the adolescent's age. Illness during early adolescence, approximately 10 to 13 years of age, is seen mainly as a threat to body image. There is a **narcissistic** concern about height, weight, and sexual development. Patients are aware of heightened body sensations and often have numerous physical complaints. Intense relationships with members of one's own sex are prevalent; they precede heterosexual involvement. Patients in this age group are anxious about how the illness will affect their physical appearance, functioning, and mobility; however, they are not usually overwhelmed by forced dependence. Self-portrait drawings are effective at this time. Maintaining privacy and same-sex room assignments are essential.

Middle Adolescence. During middle adolescence (approximately 14 to 16 years of age), adolescents are anxious about their ability to appeal to the opposite sex and to meet gender role expectations. Physical growth is practically complete. The peer group assumes greater importance in determining acceptability and behavior. During middle adolescence the struggle for emancipation from the family, although erratic, is at its peak. It is disturbing not only to the adolescent but also to parents, who must relinquish much of their control to hospital personnel. Incorporating choice, privacy, appropriate hair and cosmetic appearance, and the opportunity for peer visitors is important during hospitalization.

Late Adolescence. Late adolescents, approximately 17 to 21 years of age, are mainly concerned with the tasks of education, career, marriage, children, community, and lifestyle. The dating partner becomes the person of primary importance. Hospitalization may pose the threat of postponement of career and future plans. Contact with school personnel, counselors, and teachers is important to prevent long-term impact on the education and development of the adolescent.

Adjustment to Illness. The adolescent has many intellectual strengths, including the ability to think abstractly and to solve problems. Adolescents can understand the implications of their disease both in the present and in the future, and they are capable of participating in decisions related to treatment and care. The nurse who recognizes these skills and encourages their practice helps patients gain confidence in their intellectual abilities, thus increasing patients' sense of independence and self-esteem.

Roommate Selection. Roommate selection, although often overlooked, is extremely important for this age group. Adolescents usually do better with one or more roommates than in a single room. Because few community hospitals have adolescent wings, it is helpful when the patients participate in the decision regarding whether the adolescent is admitted to the pediatric or the adult unit. A few adjoining rooms at the ends of these units will suffice for adolescents. Placing the teenager next to a senile, dying, or severely debilitated patient in the adult unit or an infant in the pediatric unit should be avoided.

CONFIDENTIALITY AND LEGALITY

Respecting the confidentiality of children is important in establishing trust. In general, information should not be divulged or shared without consent. Many problems can be avoided if the confidentiality of the relationship is clearly defined during initial meetings. Patient records must be carefully monitored to prevent loss or observation by unauthorized personnel. The nurse must avoid giving to telephone callers or visitors any private information about a patient. Appointment books and computer screens in an office are concealed rather than kept open at the desk to view.

The term **emancipated minor** generally refers to an adolescent younger than 18 years of age who is no longer under the parent's authority. Married minors or minors in the military are automatically considered emancipated and may give consent for medical treatment for themselves and their children.

In some parts of the United States the young adolescent may receive medical assistance without parental awareness for certain conditions, such as sexually transmitted infections, contraception, pregnancy, abortion, and drug abuse. These laws are designed to afford the young person immediate medical help without fear of reprisal. However, some laws are being challenged in the courts. In a medical emergency a minor can be treated without the consent of parents if the situation is life threatening.

Because laws vary from state to state, nurses must keep abreast of policies and legislation within their practice. Such information is available from the local medical or state nursing licensing boards.

DISCHARGE PLANNING

Preparation for the patient's discharge ideally begins on admission, because the goal of hospitalization is to return a healthier and happier child to the parents. An approach directed only toward good physical care of the patient's disease is not sufficient. The nurse must also consider the emotional growth of the child and the education of the patient and family. This will provide a positive learning experience for all involved.

If a patient requires specific home treatment, such as hyperalimentation, colostomy care, crutches, special diet, or insulin therapy, instructions are given to the parents gradually throughout their child's hospitalization. The instructions are written so they can be referred to as needed. If the older child is to administer any self-treatment, careful explanations and supervision are required until both patient and parents are confident they can carry out the procedure safely at home. This may require the participation of home health services.

Parents also must be prepared for behavioral problems that may arise after hospitalization. Severe stress may be obvious during the patient's stay. The services of a children's counselor are helpful if nightmares and regression occur. Guidance includes the following suggestions:

- Anticipate behaviors such as clinging, regression in bowel and bladder control, aggression, manipulation, and nightmares.
- Allow the child to become a participating family member as soon as possible.
- Take the focus off the illness; praise accomplishments unrelated to it.
- Be kind, firm, and consistent regarding misbehavior.
- Build trust by being truthful.
- Provide suitable materials for play such as clay, paints, and doctor and nurse kits.
- Allow time for free play.
- Listen to and clarify misconceptions about the illness.
- Prevent long periods of separation until a sense of security is regained.

- Allow the child to visit hospital staff during routine clinic visits if desired.

Whenever possible, parents are provided at least 1 days' notice of their child's discharge from the hospital so they can make the necessary arrangements. This is particularly important if both parents work, or if transportation is a problem. The physician writes the discharge order. The approximate hour of dismissal is relayed to the parents. The child is weighed and dressed, and all personal belongings are collected. Parents are given a written return clinic appointment card when indicated.

Parents sign a release form and visit the hospital business office according to hospital procedure. The nurse may accompany the child and parents to the hospital exit to say good-bye. According to condition, the child is placed in a hospital wagon, wheelchair, or stretcher for transport. The nurse supervises the use of a car seat or seatbelt to secure the child safely into the vehicle. Documentation includes when and with whom the child departed, patient's behavior (smiling, alert, crying, and so on), method of transportation from the facility, patient's weight at the time of discharge, and any instructions or medications given to the child or the parents.

⚖ Legal & Ethical Considerations

Discharge Documentation

Discharge documentation should include who accompanied the child (and identification given), time of discharge, behavior and condition of the child, method of transportation, vital signs and weight, medications, and instructions given to parents or caregiver.

HOME CARE

Many children with acute and chronic conditions are cared for in the home. Home health care and other community agencies work together to provide holistic care (Jackson et al, 2009). **Respite care** provides trained workers who come into the home for brief periods to relieve parents of the responsibility of caring for the child. This enables the parents to shop, do business transactions, or simply take time for much needed self-care. The school system also shares in the responsibility for care, which is crucial if a family is to be successful in home care. The health care worker assisting in the home should do the following:

- Observe how the parents interact with the child.
- Observe facial expressions and body language.
- Post signs above the bed denoting special considerations, such as "Never position on left side" and "Do not feed with plastic spoon."
- Listen to the parents and observe how they attend to the physical needs of the youngster.
- Ask questions or discuss apprehensions the parents may have about their ability to care for the child.
- Be attuned to the needs of other children in the home.
- Be creative in exploring avenues for socialization, because these children may not often be invited to slumber parties or community activities.
- Explore community facilities or support groups that might benefit the family.

Get Ready for the NCLEX® Examination!

Key Points

- The care of sick children can take place in a variety of settings.
- Play is an important part of a nursing care plan for children.
- Nursing care plans for hospitalized children should include measures to minimize negative impact on growth and development.
- There are various pain scales available to help the nurse determine the pain level in a nonverbal child.
- Pain is the fifth vital sign and should be assessed and treated in infants and children.
- Three major causes of stress for children of all ages are separation, pain, and fear of bodily harm.
- Separation anxiety is most pronounced in the toddler.
- The three stages of separation anxiety are protest, despair, and detachment.
- When a school-age child requires hospitalization, a school, home, or hospital teacher can be requested by the nurse to prevent loss of grade status.
- Nurses caring for children must maintain a high level of suspicion for pain, because children are often unable to verbalize discomfort.

- Techniques such as drawing, distraction, imagery, and relaxation; cognitive strategies; and analgesia provide relief from pain.
- A culturally sensitive attitude toward families with hospitalized children decreases anxiety.
- Treatments should not be performed in the playroom.
- The surgical patient should be shown the part of the body where the operation will be performed. Children are assured that this is the only area of the body that will be involved.
- Respecting the confidentiality of the adolescent is important to establishing trust.
- The pediatric nursing care plan is a product of the nursing process as applied to the child.
- Clinical pathways are a multidisciplinary plan of care with outcome goals that involve timelines.
- The developmental level of the child influences specific needs during the hospitalization experience.
- The child's age, sex, developmental level, and diagnosis are factors that influence placement on a unit.
- Discharge planning begins on the day of admission.

Additional Learning Resources

SG Go to your Study Guide for additional learning activities to help you master this chapter content.

evolve Go to your Evolve website (http://evolve.elsevier.com/Leifer) for the following learning resources:
- Animations
- Answer Guidelines for Critical Thinking Questions
- Answers and Rationales for Review Questions for the NCLEX® Examination
- Glossary with English and Spanish pronunciations
- Interactive Review Questions for the NCLEX® Examination
- Patient Teaching Plans in English and Spanish
- Skills Performance Checklists
- Video clips and more!

 Online Resource
- City of Hope Pain & Palliative Care Resource Center—City of Hope: http://prc.coh.org

Review Questions for the NCLEX® Examination

1. What are the stages of separation anxiety in the toddler?
    1. Protest, despair, and denial
    2. Denial, dependence, and submission
    3. Protest, sadness, and despair
    4. Despair, anxiety, and regression

2. Assessment of pain is considered a fifth vital sign to be documented by the nurse. The nurse understands that pain in infants:
    1. cannot be reliably assessed.
    2. will not be remembered by the infant.
    3. can be assessed by observation of behavior.
    4. is usually caused by fear and anxiety.

3. The best way to minimize separation anxiety in a hospitalized infant is to:
    1. explain routines carefully.
    2. encourage parent to room-in.
    3. provide age-appropriate roommates.
    4. provide an age-appropriate toy.

4. Which statement by the parent of a hospitalized 4-year-old child indicates an understanding of the child's needs?
    1. "I am going to buy him a box of new toys to keep him busy while in the hospital."
    2. "I am going to bring some of his favorite toys from home for him to play with while in the hospital."
    3. "I'm glad there is a television in the room for him to watch all day."
    4. "I will stay every day until he falls asleep and then I will go home."

5. A 4-year-old hospitalized child wets his bed. The parents tell the nurse that the child was completely toilet trained. What should the nurse understand?
    1. The parents are denying a problem exists.
    2. The child may be developmentally delayed.
    3. The child may be experiencing regression.
    4. The child is probably "punishing" the parents.

Critical Thinking Question

1. A 5-year-old child has been hospitalized for 2 days. She is watching the television mounted above her bed. She is expressionless but does not cry or appear to be in distress. Her mother calls on the telephone and states that because her child seems to be adjusted, she may not come in today to visit because she does not want to "upset her." How should the nurse interpret the child's behavior? How should the nurse respond to the mother?

Objectives

1. Define each key term listed.
2. List five safety measures applicable to the care of the hospitalized child.
3. Illustrate techniques of transporting infants and children.
4. Plan the basic daily data collection for hospitalized infants and children.
5. Identify the normal vital signs of infants and children at various ages.
6. Devise a nursing care plan for a child with a fever.
7. Discuss the techniques of obtaining urine and stool specimens from infants.
8. Position an infant for a lumbar puncture.
9. Calculate the dosage of a medicine that is in liquid form.
10. Demonstrate techniques for administering oral, eye, and ear medications to infants and children.
11. Compare the preferred sites for intramuscular injection for infants and children.
12. Discuss two nursing responsibilities necessary when a child is receiving parenteral fluids and the rationale for each.
13. Demonstrate the appropriate technique for gastrostomy tube feeding.
14. Summarize the care of a child receiving supplemental oxygen.
15. Recall the principles of tracheostomy care.
16. List the adaptations necessary when preparing a pediatric patient for surgery.

Key Terms

auscultation (ăw-skŭl-TĀ-shŭn, p. 491)
body surface area (BSA) (p. 507)
dimensional analysis (p. 509)
fever (p. 493)
gastrostomy (găs-TRŎS-tŏ-mē, p. 513)
hyperthermia (p. 493)
informed consent (ĭn-FŎRMD kŏn-SĔNT, p. 486)
intramuscular (IM) injection (ĭn-tră-MŬS-kyū-lăr ĭn-JĔK-shŭn, p. 503)
low-flow oxygen (p. 519)
lumbar puncture (LŬM-băhr PŬNK-chŭr, p. 498)
mist tent (p. 518)

mummy restraint (p. 488)
nomogram (NŎM-ŏ-grăm, p. 507)
parenteral (pă-RĔN-tŭr-ŭl, p. 506)
phototoxicity (fō-tō-tŏk-SĬS-ĭ-tē, p. 513)
saline lock (SĀ-lēn LŎK, p. 506)
subcutaneous (SQ or SC) injection (sŭb-kyū-TĀ-nē-ŭs ĭn-JĔK-shŭn, p. 503)
total parenteral nutrition (TPN) (TŌT-ŭl pă-RĔN-tŭr-ŭl nū-TRĬ-shŭn, p. 506)
tracheostomy (trā-kē-ŎS-tŏ-mē, p. 516)
tympanic thermometer (tĭm-PĂN-ĭk thŭr-MŎM-ă-tŭr, p. 495)

ADMISSION TO THE PEDIATRIC UNIT

Specific pediatric skills can be found in the chapters that discuss related diagnoses or conditions.

INFORMED CONSENT

When the child is admitted to the pediatric unit, a written informed consent is obtained for treatments that are provided. An **informed consent** implies that the parent or legal guardian is capable of understanding information given to him or her, including the purpose and risks of the procedure, and the parent or guardian voluntarily agrees to that procedure. The parent, the health care provider who provides the information, and a witness must sign the consent. The nurse acts as a patient advocate by ensuring that the proper consent has been signed *before* a procedure and that the child is also given age-appropriate information concerning the procedure and its possible outcomes.

IDENTIFICATION

Every child admitted to the pediatric unit must have an identification (ID) bracelet applied. The ID bracelet of the patient should be checked before medications are administered or treatments are administered. If a bracelet applied on admission is taken off by the child or if it falls off, identification should be verified and a new bracelet applied (Figure 22-1). The bracelet should be snug enough to prevent voluntary removal by the child. Many hospitals attach a security chip to the identification band that will activate an alarm if the child leaves the unit. Documentation that the security chip is

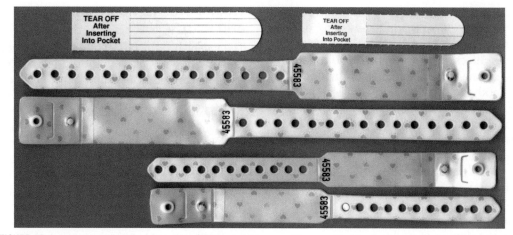

FIGURE 22-1 Identification (ID) bracelet. All hospitalized children must have an identification bracelet that is checked before the nurse administers medications or provides care. Some ID bracelets may have a computer chip sensor attached to alert the staff if the child leaves the unit. (Courtesy Prosec Protection Systems Inc., Lakewood, N.J.)

secured on the child should be reviewed at the time of patient hand-off/shift report.

ESSENTIAL SAFETY MEASURES IN THE HOSPITAL SETTING

The nurse must be especially conscious of safety measures in the children's unit of the hospital. Accidents are a major cause of death among infants and children. By demonstrating concern about safety regulations, the nurse not only reduces unnecessary accidents but also sets a good example for parents. Although personnel cannot alter the physical layout of each institution, many simple safety measures can be performed by the entire hospital team. The following lists of positive (Do's) and negative (Do Not's) measures are applicable to the children's unit:

DO's

- Keep crib sides up and locked in place at all times when the child is unattended in bed (Figure 22-2).
- Identify a child by ID bracelet, not room number.

- Use a bubble-top or plastic-top crib for infants and children capable of climbing over the crib rails (Figure 22-3).
- Place cribs so that children cannot reach sockets and appliances.
- Inspect toys for sharp edges and removable parts.
- Keep medications and solutions out of reach of the child.
- Identify the child properly before giving medications.
- Document the infant/child's weight in kilograms in a prominent place on the medical record and review during each hand-off report.

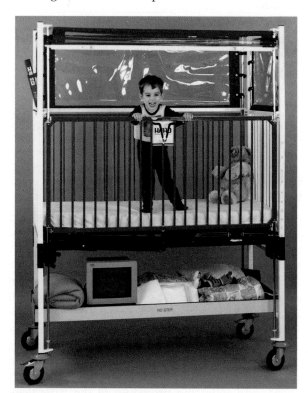

FIGURE 22-3 A hard plastic "bubble top" or a soft plastic crib extender must be in place on the crib if the child is capable of climbing over the side rails. The extender stays in place when the side rails are lowered. (Courtesy Hard Manufacturing Co., Buffalo, N.Y.)

FIGURE 22-2 The nurse should maintain hand contact if it is necessary to turn away from the infant or toddler. The side of the crib should be raised before leaving the infant or child to retrieve equipment that is out of reach or to fulfill any other purpose. (Courtesy Pat Spier, RN-C.)

- Keep items such as powder, lotions, tissues, baby wipes, disposable diapers, and safety pins out of the infant's reach.
- Prevent cross-infection. Diapers, toys, and materials that belong in one patient's unit should not be borrowed for another patient's use.
- Remain with the child who uses the bathtub or shower.
- Apply a safety belt to the child in a high chair.
- Take proper precautions when oxygen is in use.
- Locate fire exits and extinguishers on your unit and learn how to use them properly.
- Become familiar with your hospital's fire procedure.

DO NOT's

- Do not prop nursing bottles or force-feed small children. There is a danger of choking.
- Do not allow ambulatory patients to use wheelchairs or stretchers as toys.
- Do not leave an active child in a baby swing, feeding table, or high chair unattended.
- Do not leave a small child unattended when out of the crib.
- Do not leave medications at the bedside.

Many other safety measures must be implemented as the nurse becomes more familiar with the hazards of individual units. Nurses must use their eyes to scrutinize, not just to look at, and then must take the necessary precautions.

 Safety Alert!

Crib Safety

- The mattress must fit securely into the crib.
- Blankets should not be tucked in.
- Soft or contour pillows should not be placed in cribs.
- The distance between crib slats should be no more than 6 cm (2⅜ inches).
- Decorative extensions on the corners of cribs can become caught on clothing and strangle the child.
- A bubble top or extension should be in place if the child is capable of climbing over the crib side.

PREPARATION STEPS FOR PERFORMING PROCEDURES

Nurses must take specific steps to prepare for performing any procedure on any patient. A simple explanation and discussion with the parent or an age-appropriate explanation to the child should precede any nursing intervention. The parent can be allowed to assist whenever possible, and the child should be familiarized with the equipment to be used or even allowed to assist in the simple aspects of the procedure when appropriate. Common nursing actions before the actual skill is performed include checking the written order of the health care provider, gathering equipment, identifying the patient, explaining the procedure to the parent and the child, providing privacy, performing hand hygiene, and using standard precautions or transmissions-based precautions as needed. These preparatory steps appear as icons within each skill as appropriate.

TRANSPORTING, POSITIONING, AND RESTRAINING

The means by which the child is transported within the unit and to other parts of the hospital depends on age, level of consciousness, and how far the child must travel. Older children are transported in the same way as adults. Younger children are often transported in their cribs, in a wagon or wheelchair, or on a stretcher. The side rails on a stretcher are raised during transport. The nurse ensures that the child's ID band is secured before leaving the unit. A notation is made describing where the child is being taken, for what purpose, and who is accompanying the child.

Figure 22-4 depicts four safe methods for holding an infant. Head and back support are necessary for young infants. The movements of small children are often random and uncoordinated; therefore the children must be held securely. The *football hold* is useful when one hand needs to be free, such as for bathing the infant's head. The **mummy restraint** is a short-term restraint that might be necessary for examination or treatments such as a venipuncture or placement of a nasogastric tube. This restraint effectively controls the child's movements and can be modified to expose an arm, a leg, or the chest as needed. *Swaddling* of the newborn infant is accomplished by the same technique. Many young infants respond positively to snug wrapping with a light baby blanket. Skill 22-1 describes the application of a mummy restraint (swaddling) for infants and children.

Restraints may be used for infants and children to facilitate examinations or treatments and to maintain safety. The reason for the restraint must be explained to the parents and the child. Restraints are used only when necessary. They are not a substitute for close observation, and should involve the fewest joints possible in order to enable free movement, which is necessary for growth and development. Excessive restraints can result in the infant or child fighting the restraint, thereby wasting energy and increasing oxygen consumption needs. Parents should be taught the importance of fastening safety straps on infants who are in high chairs, shopping carts, and infant seats. The *colic carry* (Figure 22-4, *D*) is a position that can be used for infants when they are irritable, because the carry typically confers a calming effect.

ASSESSMENT AND BASIC DATA COLLECTION

Children are different from adults both anatomically and physiologically. Basic data collection is done to determine the level of wellness, the response to medication or treatment, and any need for referral.

ORGANIZING THE INFANT ASSESSMENT

To obtain accurate results, the organization of the infant assessment is important:

1. Select an area or room that is warm and not stimulating for the infant.
2. To prevent heat loss, expose only those areas of the body to be examined.

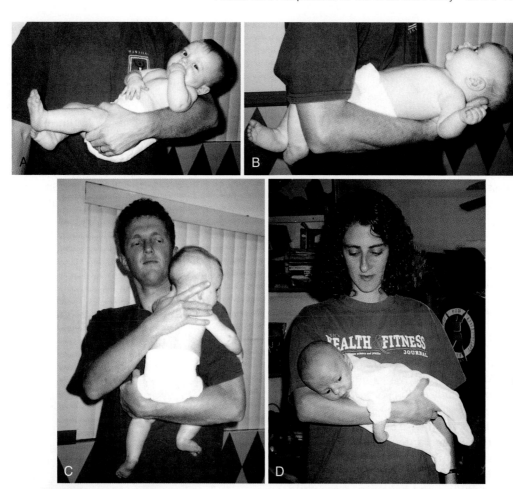

FIGURE 22-4 A, The cradle position. **B,** The football position. **C,** The upright position. **D,** The colic carry.

The Mummy Restraint (Swaddling)

PURPOSE

To promote comfort or confine movements for procedure

STEPS

1. Place a small, light blanket flat on the bed with the top at the infant's shoulders.
2. Fold the blanket over the body and under the arm at the opposite side, tucking in the excess under the infant.
3. Place the other arm at the side and fold the blanket over the body, tucking the excess under the infant. The weight of the infant holds the restraint in place.
4. Separate the bottom of the blanket and fold upward toward the shoulder, tucking the sides under the infant's body.
5. The arms should be in anatomical position. This restraint provides a feeling of snug security for the infant. It may be used for jugular venipunctures, nasogastric tube insertion, and other procedures.

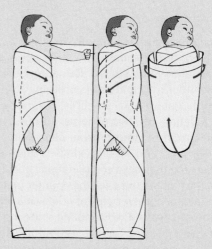

(From Leifer G: *Principles and techniques in pediatric nursing*, ed 4, Philadelphia, 1982, Saunders.)

3. Without touching the infant, observe the following:
   - Position
   - Attitude
   - Flexion
   - Color
   - Respiratory rate
   - Ability to focus
4. Using minimal touch:
   - Auscultate lung sounds
   - Auscultate heart sounds
   - Auscultate bowel sounds
   - Measure head, chest, abdomen, and length
5. Using invasive touch last:
   - Assess reflexes and blood pressure
6. Talk softly.
7. Use pacifier to comfort infant.
8. Swaddle and hold after assessment is complete.
9. Use parent-teaching opportunities.
10. Document findings.

BASIC DATA COLLECTION

Basic data collection involves casual observation without touching. The child's general appearance will indicate if his or her condition is serious or within normal limits. In general, serious illness may be suspected if the child is not alert and responsive to the environment. If the child is lethargic, prompt intervention by a health care provider is essential. Applying knowledge of basic growth and development will enable the nurse to determine whether the activities and behavior of the child are age appropriate. A child who has not mastered age-appropriate milestones should be referred for follow-up care. The presence of bruises on the body of the child that may be in different stages of healing, the lack of body cleanliness or appropriate dress, and the interaction or lack of interaction between parent and child are also areas that may require prompt referral for follow-up care. Is the child tipping his head or rubbing the ears? Is the child maintaining a rigid body position to breathe? If stridor or grunting sounds are heard during respiration, prompt referral should be made.

THE HISTORY SURVEY

The *personal history survey* affords the nurse the opportunity to teach parents about the child's needs and prevention of injury and illness. The admission history should include information concerning the child's usual health habits and practices regarding eating, sleeping, toileting, activity patterns, and use of special words or gestures. Information concerning coping patterns, siblings, and family values is helpful. Questions concerning the use of complementary and alternative medicine (CAM) and over-the-counter medications should be included in every history data collection. This information can be used to formulate a nursing diagnosis in the plan of care for the individual child. The immunization record should be reviewed and plans for future immunizations discussed. Encouraging safe environments that include the use of car seats and protective gear for sports activities should be part of every teaching plan.

THE PHYSICAL SURVEY

The physical survey includes a head-to-toe review that should be completed, at minimum, once each shift or once each clinic visit, even if the clinic visit is for a specific problem. The nurse may assist with an ear examination by properly restraining the child in a position that will enable safe and quick assessment by the health care provider (Figure 22-5). Obtaining vital signs is a priority. Often the first sign of shock or body stress in infants or children is tachycardia (a rapid heartbeat). However, a drop in blood pressure may be a late sign of shock in children because of a compensatory mechanism that is activated early. Therefore hypotension in an infant or child is considered an acute emergency. Extreme irritability or pupils that are unequal in response to light should be reported immediately. The anterior fontanelle, which is usually open until

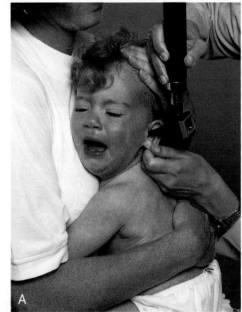

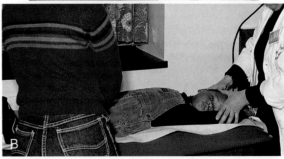

FIGURE 22-5 Positioning the child for an ear examination. **A,** The parent or nurse can hold the infant close with one hand immobilizing the head. **B,** The nurse holds the arms above the child's head and prevents movement of the head with the thumbs. The parent or assistant can hold the hips or thighs. (**A** from Hockenberry M, Wilson D: *Wong's nursing care of infants and children,* ed 9, St Louis, 2011, Mosby; **B** from Zitelli B et al: *Atlas of pediatric physical diagnosis,* ed 6, St Louis, 2012, Saunders.)

Table 22-1	Average Pulse Rates at Rest			
AGE	**AVERAGE (BEATS/MIN, AWAKE)**		**UPPER LIMITS OF NORMAL (BEATS/MIN)**	
Newborn	125		160	
1-11 months	120		160	
2 years	110		130	
4 years	100		120	
6 years	100		115	
8 years	90		110	
10 years	90		110	
	GIRLS	**BOYS**	**GIRLS**	**BOYS**
12 years	90	85	110	105
14 years	85	80	105	100
16 years	80	75	100	95
18 years	75	70	95	90

Data from Kliegman R et al: *Nelson's textbook of pediatrics*, ed 19, St Louis, 2011, Saunders.

Table 22-2	Normal Respiratory and Blood Pressure Ranges for Children	
AGE	**BLOOD PRESSURE**	**RESPIRATORY RATE**
Birth-1 month	65-85/45-55	30-60
1 month-1 year	80-100/55-65	26-40
1-3 years	90-100/55-70	20-30
3-6 years	95-100/55-75	20-25
6-10 years	100-115/60-75	16-22
Adolescent	110-120/65-75	14-18

Data from Kliegman R et al: *Nelson's textbook of pediatrics*, ed 19, St Louis, 2011, Saunders.

age 18 months, should be palpated. A sunken fontanelle may indicate dehydration, whereas a bulging fontanelle indicates increased intracranial pressure (ICP). A fontanelle that feels flat to the contour of the head is normal. Increased ICP in the older child and adult is manifested by an increase in systolic blood pressure and a widening pulse pressure, irregular respirations, and bradycardia. In the infant, however, the open fontanelles allow brain swelling to occur without these classic signs, and a decreased level of consciousness may be the only manifestation of increased ICP.

Bradycardia (a slow heartbeat) is always treated as a medical emergency in infants and young children. Unlike adults, infants and children cannot increase the stroke volume of their heart for a more effective cardiac output when the heart slows; instead, they must rely on increased heart rate alone to increase output. Therefore fatigue and heart failure may result. Mottling of the skin of the extremities may be normal in young infants because of their immature temperature control mechanisms. Maintaining warmth during observation is essential for infants. Because of their large body surface area and high metabolic rate, they are prone to fluid loss and hypothermia as well as to cold stress.

An accurate kilogram weight should be recorded (see Figure 12-11) because the dosage of medications for infants and children is based on milligrams per kilogram of body weight (AAP, 2013). The weight should be updated each day for infants and at least twice a week for children. The temperature of infants may be taken via the axilla or in the ear or appropriate electronic thermometer (see Skill 22-3). The lungs should be clear to auscultation, and the chest should move symmetrically. Bowel sounds should be active in all four quadrants, and the abdomen should not be distended or tender to palpation. The skin should be observed for rashes or lesions.

Pulse and Respirations

The nurse counts a pulse rate by placing the finger pads over the site and feeling the wave of blood as it is forced through the artery. The pulse rate varies considerably in different children of the same age and size. The pulse rate and respiratory rate of the newborn are high (Tables 22-1 and 22-2). Both pulse rate and respiratory rate gradually decelerate with age until adult values are reached.

The pulse of the older child is taken just like that of an adult. Apical pulses are advised for children younger than 5 years of age (see Figure 12-10). The apical pulse is heard through a stethoscope at the apex of the heart. The nurse counts the rate for 1 full minute. Another common site is the radial pulse (at the thumb side of the wrist just above the radial artery). Actually, the pulse may be assessed in any area where a large artery lies close to the skin, especially if the artery runs across a bone and has little soft tissue around it. The following are the most common sites: radial, temporal (just in front of the ear), mandibular (on the lower jawbone), femoral (in the groin), and carotid (on each side of the front of the neck). The carotid pulse may not be appropriate to use in infants with chubby necks.

The child's respirations are counted in the same way as for an adult. The nurse notes the number of times the chest or abdomen rises and falls for 1 minute. The rate and character of respirations are important in determining the patient's general condition. The relationship of the pulse rate to the temperature and the respiratory rate should be assessed; the pulse rate will increase as the temperature increases because of the increased cardiac output and increased oxygen consumption needs that occur with an elevated temperature. When taking the vital signs in infants, the respirations are often taken first because they are the least invasive, and after the infant cries, it is difficult to obtain an accurate respiratory rate.

Blood Pressure

Blood pressure is defined as the pressure of the blood on the walls of the arteries. It is an index of elasticity of arterial walls, peripheral vascular resistance, efficiency of the heart as a pump, and blood volume. Common sites for measuring blood pressure in children are the brachial artery, popliteal artery, and posterior tibial artery. The 50th percentile is the midpoint of the normal range of blood pressure for children. Blood pressure readings in the 90th percentile are defined as prehypertension. Readings in the 90th percentile are considered stage 1 hypertension, and those in the 99th percentile are considered stage 2 hypertension (see Appendix J).

All children should have their blood pressure checked and recorded using an appropriately sized blood pressure cuff.

Auscultation. **Auscultation** of blood pressure is done the same way as for an adult but with a pediatric stethoscope and blood pressure cuff. The cuff should be long enough to encircle the extremity. The width of the cuff should cover two thirds of the upper arm. The following sizes are suggested: birth to 1 year, 3.8 cm (1½ inches); 2 to 8 years, 7.6 cm (3 inches); and 8 to 12 years, 11.4 cm (4½ inches). Pressure is normally slightly higher in the lower extremities. The American Heart Association designates the muffled tone as the most accurate index of diastolic pressure but recommends recording both that and the final distinct sound as the complete record; thus 120/80/78 mm Hg. Nurses should clarify this with the physician or institution to ensure uniformity. To determine *pulse pressure,* the diastolic reading is subtracted from the systolic reading. This usually varies from 20 to 50 mm Hg. Widening pulse pressure may be a sign of increased ICP. The American Medical Association has recommended that mercury manometers not be used when taking the blood pressure of patients. Digital manometers are environmentally safer (Skill 22-2).

Palpation. Palpation is one of the oldest methods of measuring blood pressure. The cuff is applied and inflated above the expected pressure. The fingers are placed over the brachial or radial artery. The systolic pressure is recorded at the point when the pulse reappears. Diastolic pressure is unobtainable. This method is useful in newborns.

Electronic or Ultrasonographic Measurement. This is a noninvasive type of blood pressure monitoring that ultrasonically detects motion of the arterial wall. A transducer with an attached cuff is secured over an artery in the arm or leg. The cuff is inflated above systolic pressure and is then gradually deflated. The transducer transmits vascular sounds, and the measurement appears on a digital readout. Both systolic and diastolic pressures are recorded. Electronic blood pressure machines do not require auscultation with a stethoscope. A cuff is applied, the machine is turned on, and a digital reading is obtained, usually in less than 1 minute.

The nurse should explain what is about to happen; for example, "This will hug your arm and feel tight for a few seconds." The child is allowed to examine the sphygmomanometer and cuff.

Blood pressure is lower in children than in adults. If a patient needs blood pressure measurements throughout hospitalization, the nurse observes the previous readings before charting the current one. Many factors account for variations in blood pressure measurements, including time of day, sex, age, exercise, pain, and emotion. A blood pressure reading taken when a child is frightened or crying is not accurate. If a significant change is observed, the blood pressure should be rechecked. Abnormal readings are charted and reported to the nurse in charge. See Appendix J for blood pressure readings in infants and children.

Temperature
Pathogenesis of Fever and the Use of Antipyretics

An infection from bacteria or other toxins stimulates immune substances to work along with prostaglandins in the body to stimulate the hypothalamus to raise the body temperature. This triggers a body response of vasoconstriction, shivering, and decreased peripheral perfusion that decreases body heat loss while maintaining homeostasis, and therefore the body temperature rises. Antipyretic medications such as ibuprofen or acetaminophen inhibit prostaglandin production, thereby preventing shivering, vasoconstriction, and alteration in perfusion, resulting in heat loss and lowering of body temperature.

Fever differs from hyperthermia. **Hyperthermia** is an increase in core body temperature occurring with central nervous system impairment. Prostaglandins are not involved, and the homeostasis mechanism is bypassed. Hyperthermia can result from a drug reaction, trauma, or environmental overheating, such as when a baby is bundled and left in a hot automobile. Treatment of hyperthermia involves vigorous cooling measures such as cold blankets and intravenous (IV) fluids.

Fever results in an increased metabolic demand on the heart and lungs, and children with cardiopulmonary disease require antipyretics to minimize the increase in oxygen consumption that causes an increased demand

Blood Pressure Measurement in Children

Common sites for measuring blood pressure in children are the radial artery, brachial artery, popliteal artery, and posterior tibial artery. Blood pressure may be taken with a manometer and stethoscope or by an electronic machine using a cuff with a sensor that provides a digital readout of the blood pressure. A stethoscope is not necessary when this method is used.

PURPOSE

To assess blood pressure

STEPS

Radial Artery

1. Position limb at level of heart.
2. Place cuff above wrist.
3. Auscultate radial artery.

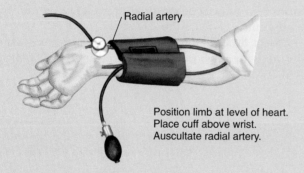

Radial artery

Position limb at level of heart.
Place cuff above wrist.
Auscultate radial artery.

Brachial Artery

1. Position limb at level of heart.
2. Place cuff on upper arm.
3. Auscultate brachial artery.

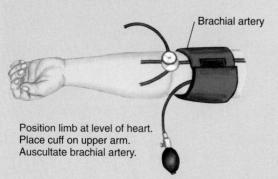

Brachial artery

Position limb at level of heart.
Place cuff on upper arm.
Auscultate brachial artery.

Posterior Tibial Artery

1. Place cuff above malleoli or at midcalf.
2. Auscultate either the posterior tibial artery or the dorsal pedal artery.

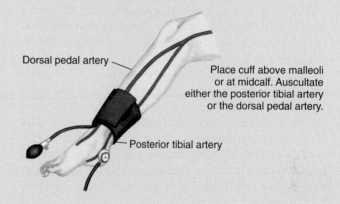

Dorsal pedal artery

Place cuff above malleoli or at midcalf. Auscultate either the posterior tibial artery or the dorsal pedal artery.

Posterior tibial artery

Popliteal Artery

1. Place cuff above knee.
2. Auscultate the popliteal artery.

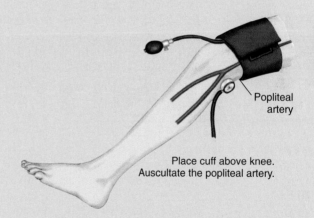

Popliteal artery

Place cuff above knee.
Auscultate the popliteal artery.

Figures from McKinney ES, James SR, Murray SS, & Ashwill JW: *Maternal-child nursing*, ed 2, Philadelphia, 2005, Saunders.

on the heart. Antipyretics also provide comfort and may aid in enabling the child to consume fluids, lessening the risk of dehydration. Antipyretics may also be recommended for children with a history of febrile seizures to prevent a second seizure. Excessive use of antipyretics should be avoided, because these drugs can burden the kidneys and liver. Fever is thought to be a protective mechanism that aids in the recovery from infection.

Temperature Measurement. Fever is most often defined as a rectal temperature at or above 38° C (100.4° F), a tympanic temperature at or above 38° C (100.4° F), an oral temperature at or above 37.8° C (100° F), or an axillary temperature above 37.2° C (99° F) (Crocetti and Serwirt, 2005).

When evaluating the degree of illness in a febrile child, the response of the child to cuddling, alertness, hydration, sociability, and quality of cry should be assessed and recorded. A quiet, lethargic child who does not respond readily to the environment may be acutely ill. Because dehydration is a common problem in infants and children, skin turgor should be assessed (see Figure 12-13). Measures to reduce fever may promote comfort for the child.

There are several types of thermometers available to measure body temperature. The American Medical Association has recommended that thermometers containing mercury not be used. Temperatures are most often measured using the axillary technique. An oral temperature technique may be used in children more than 5 years of age if the child can keep his or her mouth closed and has not ingested hot or cold fluids before measurement. Rectal temperatures are not recommended for pediatric patients. The electronic thermometer, the plastic strip thermometer, and the tympanic membrane sensor are commonly used in the pediatric unit. The electronic thermometer works quickly and is ideal because the plastic sheath is replaceable. The disposable plastic strip changes color according to sensed temperature changes. Tympanic thermometers have a blunt tip that is covered with a disposable cover and can be inserted into the ear. They record temperature from the tympanic membrane (eardrum) by an infrared emission. This site is of importance because the hypothalamus (temperature-regulating center) and the eardrum are perfused by the same circulation. Table 22-3 shows normal temperature ranges. The documentation of the patient's temperature should indicate the method used, such as "O" for oral; "Ax" for axillary; or "T" for tympanic.

Oral temperature. The procedure is the same as for adults and may be appropriate for older children or adolescents.

Axillary temperature. Axillary temperatures are usually taken for newborns and/or according to unit policy (Skill 22-3).

Axillary Temperature Technique

PURPOSE
To assess body temperature

STEPS
1. Hold the thermometer in the axilla with the infant's arm pressed against the side.
2. Use a paper thermometer, digital thermometer, or long-term sensor to measure the axillary temperature.
3. Perform hand hygiene.
4. Document the temperature and route used in the medical record.

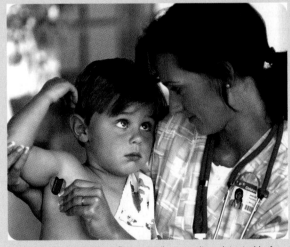

A skin sensor thermometer adheres to the armpit on intact skin for up to 48 hours. Raising the arm will facilitate reading the temperature level. The last dot to turn black indicates the correct temperature. The sensor is intended for single use and is disposable. The temperature range of this continuous-reading thermometer is 35.0° to 40.0° C (95.0° to 104.0° F). (Courtesy Medical Indicators, Carlsbad, CA).

METHOD	RANGE
Table 22-3 Normal Temperature Ranges for Children	
Oral	36.4°-37.4° C (97.6°-99.3° F)
Rectal	37.0°-37.7° C (98.6°-100.0° F)
Axillary	35.8°-36.6° C (96.6°-98.0° F)
Tympanic	36.9°-37.5° C (98.4°-99.5° F)

Temporal artery temperature. The temporal artery thermometer measures infrared emissions over the temporal artery by rolling the transducer over the child's forehead.

Tympanic temperature. The **tympanic thermometer** measures core body temperature by detecting the infrared energy emitted from the tympanic membrane. (Core body temperature is the estimated temperature of the internal body organs.) The tympanic technique is accurate for all ages. However, some brands of tympanic thermometers have ear probes that do not fit well into the auditory canal of infants younger than age 3 months. These thermometers should be used only for infants greater than 3 months of age (Skill 22-4).

The accuracy of the tympanic temperature is not affected by illness such as otitis media. A table of Celsius and Fahrenheit temperature equivalents appears in Appendix H. Nursing Care Plan 22-1 reviews the care of a child with a fever. The use of acetaminophen or NSAID in the treatment of fever in infants and children and the risk for poisoning is discussed in Chapter 28.

Pain

Pain is a fifth vital sign that must be addressed in the plan of care. See Chapter 12 for pain in the newborn and Chapter 21 for pain in the child or adolescent.

Weight

Weight must be accurately recorded in *kilograms* on admission (see Figure 12-11). The weight of a patient provides a means of determining progress and is necessary for determining the dosage of medications. The way in which the nurse weighs the child depends on the child's age.

The infant is weighed completely naked in a warm room. A fresh absorbent pad or scale paper is placed on the scale. This prevents cross-contamination (the spread of germs from one infant to another). The scale is balanced to compensate for the weight of the pad. The infant is placed gently on the scale. The nurse's hand is held slightly above the infant to prevent falling. After the exact weight appears on the digital readout, the infant is removed from the scale, wrapped in a blanket, and soothed. The weight is immediately recorded. The scale paper is disposed of in the proper receptacle.

The older child is weighed in the same manner as an adult. A paper towel is placed on the scale for the patient to stand on. The patient is generally weighed in a hospital gown. The shoes are removed. If the child is unable to stand on the scales, it may be necessary for the nurse to hold the child and read the combined weights. The nurse is then weighed and that number subtracted from the combined weight to obtain the

Tympanic Temperature Technique

PURPOSE

To assess body temperature

STEPS

1. Gently pull the pinna (earlobe) down and back in infants less than 3 years of age and pull the auricle slightly up and back in children more than 3 years of age to straighten the auditory canal and provide an accurate temperature reading.
2. Aim the probe of the thermometer at the opposite eyebrow.
3. Perform hand hygiene.
4. Document the temperature and route used in the medical record.

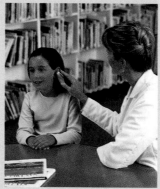

This tympanic thermometer captures the temperature within 3–7 s. It signals stable probe positioning to ensure accuracy, so the infrared ray will reach the tympanic membrane. (Braun ThermoScan® PRO 4000. Courtesy Welch Allyn, Inc.)

⭐ Nursing Care Plan 22-1 | The Child with a Fever

PATIENT DATA A 6-year-old child is admitted with a diagnosis of dehydration and a fever of 39.6° C (103.3° F) and is unable to retain food because of nausea and vomiting

Selected Nursing Diagnosis: Deficient fluid volume, potential for dehydration because of increased metabolic rate

Goals	Nursing Interventions	Rationales
The child will not become dehydrated as evidenced by good skin turgor, moist mucous membranes, and no weight loss.	Increase fluid intake; offer juice, water, popsicles, and yogurt, as age appropriate.	Body's metabolic rate increases with fever. Children have a higher proportion of body water; therefore more water can be lost rapidly. Body systems such as the kidneys are immature at some ages.
Child's temperature will be between 36.1° and 37.4° C (97.0° and 99.3° F).	Administer tepid sponge bath for fever of 40.0° C (104.0° F).	Tepid baths help to reduce fever and may make the child more comfortable.
	Determine vital signs before a sponge bath.	Provides baseline data.
	Retake vital signs 30 minutes after procedure.	Comparison of vital signs will show whether fever is decreasing.
	Expose skin to air after procedure; prevent shivering.	Promotes evaporation and cooling of skin.
	Administer antipyretic medications according to physician's instructions.	Frequently, child with a fever also has a headache and painful joints; antipyretic medications will relieve these discomforts and reduce fever.
Injury during treatments will be prevented.	Keep side rails raised.	Side rails provide safety from falls.
	Observe child frequently.	Frequent observation will allow subtle changes to be detected and possibly reduce complications.
	Remain with child if tub bath is given.	Threat of drowning is always present with small children and water.
	Explain nature of fever (not always bad); control that is too vigorous may mask signs of illness.	Potential benefits of fever have been cited; it is thought to enhance the body's defense mechanisms and to increase antibody activity.
Parent will understand and verbalize nature and treatment of fever.	Emphasize removal of clothes when child has fever.	Removal of clothing cools child.
	Call physician if child looks sick or acts in a way different from normal.	Degree of fever does not always reflect the severity of disease.
Parent will verbalize understanding of how to read a thermometer.	Demonstrate how to read a thermometer.	This gives parents a sense of control; accuracy of fever detection will be ensured on discharge.
Parent will verbalize understanding of potential for convulsion.	Discuss with parent potential for convulsion.	Only a small number of children convulse with fever; however, discussion is advisable.
Parent will understand how to give appropriate care during a convulsion.	Review management of a convulsion.	Knowledge allays anxiety.
	Discourage use of alcohol sponge baths, which may cause toxicity and skin irritation.	Alcohol sponge baths may still be suggested by older relatives.
	Discourage use of cold water.	Cold water may cause shivering and raise body temperature.

Critical Thinking Question
1. A mother states that her child has developed a fever after receiving an immunization, and she requests antibiotic treatment. What data collection and parent teaching are indicated?

patient's weight. Occasionally a child is weighed while wearing a cast. The nurse records this; for example, "weight 34 lb (15.4 kg) with cast on right arm." It is often desirable to record the weight in pounds as well as kilograms. Some parents find pounds a more familiar term. Kilograms are necessary to calculate safe dosages of medications.

Height
The child's height is measured along with weight. The infant's height must be measured while the infant is lying on a flat surface alongside a metal tape measure or yardstick. The knees should be pressed flat on the table. The measurement is taken from the top of the head to the heels and recorded (see Skill 15-1).

Head Circumference

Head circumference increases rapidly during infancy as a result of brain growth. It is generally measured on infants and toddlers and on all children with neurological defects. The tape measure is placed around the head slightly above the eyebrows and ears and around the occipital prominence of the skull (see Skill 12-1). The measurement is recorded.

SPECIMEN COLLECTION

Urine Specimens

A urine specimen is usually obtained from the newly admitted patient. There are certain general principles of collecting specimens:

- Explain the procedure to the child (as age appropriate).
- Use a clean container or urine collection device.
- Check frequently for results.
- Label all specimens clearly and attach the proper laboratory slip.
- Send specimen to laboratory according to hospital policy.
- Record in nurses' notes and on intake and output (I&O) sheet.

The procedure for collecting a urine specimen from an infant is described in Skill 22-5.

Urine collected directly from ultraabsorbent disposable diapers may yield inaccurate protein, pH, and specific gravity measurements because of the chemicals in the diaper.

Obtaining a Clean-Catch Specimen. Special sterile containers are available for clean-catch specimens; the manufacturer's directions should be followed. The procedure necessitates cleansing of the perineum with an antiseptic. Rinsing and drying the perineum are important to prevent contamination of urine from the antiseptic. Wiping is done from front to back. After the urine stream has started, the midstream specimen is caught in the sterile container. The nurse's participation is either direct or supervisory depending on the child's age or the availability of a parent. Adolescents, who may be embarrassed by carrying a urine specimen through the halls, may be given a bag or other suitable camouflage. The specimen should be sent to the laboratory promptly.

Obtaining a 24-Hour Specimen. At times a 24-hour urine specimen may be requested to determine the rate of urine production and measure the excretion of specific chemicals from the body. The nurses on each shift must closely supervise this test to maintain its accuracy, because lost specimens necessitate restarting the test. Problems can arise if the collection device does not adhere to the skin properly; therefore the nurse must be alert for this occurrence. Diversions suitable to the child's age are used. A sign is attached to the infant's crib to alert personnel of a 24-hour urine collection. The average daily amount of urine excreted, by age, is shown in Table 22-4.

Testing for Albumin. The nurse working in a physician's office or clinic may also be requested to test urine for albumin (protein). Normally, little or no albumin is found in the urine of a healthy child. Reagent strips especially intended for this purpose are available. The nurse dips the end of the strip into urine and compares the strip with a special color chart. Specific instructions accompany test materials.

Stool Specimens

Stool specimens are obtained from older children in the same manner as from adults. This is embarrassing for most children, who are "turned off" by the suggestion. The ambulatory child can use a bedpan or "hat" placed beneath a toilet seat. It is difficult for a child to tell the nurse that the sample has been collected. The nurse can acknowledge these feelings by giving the child permission to express them without being critical; for example, the nurse could say, "I know this must be embarrassing for you. It is for grown-ups, too, but we need this specimen." An infant's stool specimen can be obtained from the infant by scraping the specimen from the diaper with a tongue depressor and placing it in the specimen container. Some specimen containers contain a portion of liquid. The label indicates a "fill line." The amount of infant stool needed for a specimen is the amount which, when placed into the container, results in the fluid level rising to the fill line.

Some specimens must be sent to the laboratory while they are warm. The specimen container is labeled properly and placed in a plastic bag, and the laboratory slip is attached. The nurse charts the time; color, amount, and consistency of the stool; the purpose for which it was collected (e.g., blood, ova, parasites, or bacteria); and any related information.

Blood Specimens

Positioning the Child. Positioning the child for drawing blood is extremely important. The nurse is often asked to assist in these procedures. Figure 22-6 depicts how to position the patient for a femoral venipuncture. Both the jugular and the femoral veins are large; therefore the patient is frequently checked to ensure that there is no bleeding afterward. These sites are used mainly when other areas have been exhausted. Therefore the infant is soothed, because crying and thrashing may precipitate oozing. Distraction and simple pain relief techniques should be used during any painful procedure and the infant soothed after. The nurse charts the site used, the name of the blood test, and any untoward developments.

Collecting a Urine Specimen in Infants

PURPOSE

To obtain a specimen for clinical laboratory assessment

STEPS

1. Clean and dry the infant's skin, avoiding use of oil, baby powder, or lotion soap, which may leave a residue on the skin and interfere with the ability of the adhesive to stick.

2. Begin by applying the urine collector to the tiny area of skin between the anus and the perineum. The narrow "bridge" on the adhesive patch keeps feces from contaminating the specimen and helps to position the collector correctly. After applying the adhesive section between the anus and perineum, the remainder of the urine collector is fitted to the rest of the genital area.

3. Recover the specimen. Drain the urine bag collector into a clean beaker or specimen bottle by removing the tab in the lower corner, or seal the specimen inside the collector itself by folding the sticky adhesive sides together.

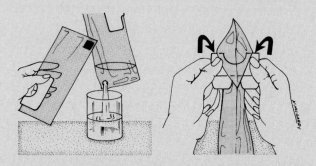

4. Place the collector with specimen into a plastic bag.
5. With small infants a cotton ball may be placed at the opening of the collector. When the infant voids into the cotton ball, aspirating the cotton ball with a syringe can retrieve even a small volume of urine.
6. Replace infant's clean diaper, position in crib, and raise side rails.
7. Remove gloves and perform hand hygiene.
8. Label specimen container for transport to laboratory according to hospital protocol.
9. Document in medical record amount of urine collected and time sent to laboratory.

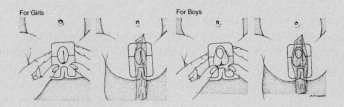

For Girls   For Boys

Permission to reproduce this copyrighted material has been granted by the owner, Hollister, Inc., Libertyville, IL.

Lumbar Puncture

The nurse often assists the physician with a **lumbar puncture**, which is also referred to as a *spinal tap*. It is done to obtain spinal fluid for examination or to reduce pressure within the brain in conditions such as hydrocephalus or meningitis. Disposable lumbar puncture sets are used.

Normal spinal fluid is clear like water. The opening pressure ranges from 60 to 180 mm Hg. It is somewhat lower in infants. The procedure for children is essentially the same as that for adults. The main difference lies in the patient's ability to cooperate with positioning. The nurse explains that the child must lie quietly, and the child will be helped to do this. Sensations

Table 22-4	Average Daily Excretion of Urine	
AGE	**FLUID OUNCES**	**MILLILITERS (mL)**
Days 1-2	1-2	30-60
Days 3-10	3-10	100-300
Day 10-2 months	9-15	250-450
2 months-1 year	14-17	400-500
1-3 years	17-20	500-600
3-5 years	20-24	600-700
5-8 years	22-34	650-1000
8-14 years	27-47	800-1400

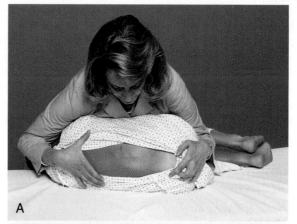

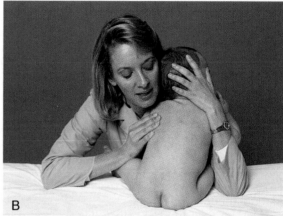

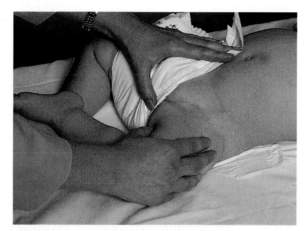

FIGURE 22-6 An infant positioned for femoral venipuncture. This position exposes the groin area. (From Hockenberry M, Wilson D: *Wong's nursing care of infants and children,* ed 9, St Louis, 2011, Mosby.)

FIGURE 22-7 A child positioned for a lumbar puncture. **A,** An older child may be placed in a side-lying fetal position and held firmly by the nurse. **B,** Placing an infant in a sitting position allows for flexion of the lumbar spine. The nurse hugs the child for support and security. (From Hockenberry M, Wilson D: *Wong's nursing care of infants and children,* ed 9, St Louis, 2011, Mosby.)

during a lumbar puncture include a cool feeling when the skin is cleansed and a feeling of pressure when the needle is inserted. The way in which the child is held can directly affect the success of the procedure.

The child lies on the side with the back parallel to the side of the treatment table. The knees are flexed, and the head is brought down close to the flexed knees. The nurse can keep the child in this position by placing the child's head in the crook of one arm and the knees in the crook of the other arm. The nurse's hands are then clasped together or placed as shown in Figure 22-7. The nurse leans forward, gently placing the chest against the patient.

After the infant is positioned, the physician prepares the lower back using sterile technique. A vial of local anesthetic may be necessary unless this is provided in the sterile setup. The top of the vial is cleansed according to hospital protocol. After the area has been locally anesthetized, the physician inserts a special hollow needle into the patient's lower back and collects the spinal fluid in two or three test tubes. Pain relief techniques, such as allowing the infant to suck on a sucrose-sweetened nipple, or distraction techniques should be used during any painful procedure. When the procedure is completed, a sterile bandage is placed over

the injection site, and the child is comforted. Specimens are labeled and taken to the laboratory with the appropriate requisition form.

The adolescent may avoid post–lumbar puncture headache by lying flat for some time. The nurse charts the date and time of the lumbar puncture and the name of the attending physician. Also charted are the amount of fluid obtained and its character (e.g., cloudy or bloody), whether or not specimens were sent to the laboratory, and the patient's reaction to the procedure.

PHYSIOLOGICAL RESPONSES TO MEDICATIONS IN INFANTS AND CHILDREN

Medication administration is a primary responsibility of the nurse. It is important for the nurse to understand that the responses of infants differ from those of children and that the responses of infants and children differ from those of adults. These concepts must also be communicated to the parents, who often administer over-the-counter medications to their growing child. The most common over-the-counter medication administered by parents to infants and children is acetaminophen (Tylenol). The toxic effects of Tylenol overdose are discussed in Chapter 28.

Understanding the differences in drug absorption, distribution, metabolism, and excretion between children and adults is essential to provide safe pediatric medication administration. Age is the most important variable in predicting response to any drug therapy. The functions of various organs in the body mature as the child grows and develops.

ABSORPTION OF MEDICATIONS IN INFANTS AND CHILDREN

Gastric Influences

In the neonate there is an absence of free hydrochloric acid in the stomach. The acid content of the stomach reaches adult levels by age 2 years. Therefore medications that require an acid medium in the stomach for absorption may not be completely absorbed if the child is less than 2 years of age. The administration of such medications near the time of formula feedings will further decrease the acid content of the stomach. After 2 years of age, the ingestion of orange juice increases gastric acidity, causing more effective absorption of medication that requires an acid medium to absorb.

Intestinal Influences

Children less than 5 years of age have a more rapid intestinal transit time than adults. Medication may move out of the small intestines before it is completely absorbed. Therefore delayed or timed-release oral medication may not be fully absorbed by children younger than 5 years of age. There may be a low amount of pancreatic enzymes for infants less than 1 year of age. Some medications depend on pancreatic enzymes to help absorb the drug.

Topical Medications (Ointments)

Pediatric patients have a thin stratum corneum that allows topical medications to be absorbed. The larger skin surface area also increases the amount of absorption of topical medication as compared to adults. The use of a plastic diaper can also cause increased absorption of a topically applied medication in the diaper area of the skin. Hydrocortisone and hexachlorophene may produce adverse systemic responses when applied to the buttocks and covered with a plastic diaper or dressing.

Parenteral Medications

Poor peripheral perfusion in the young infant will slow intramuscular (IM) drug absorption. IM drugs administered to infants and children less than 4 years of age should be water soluble to prevent precipitation. In neonates, medication may pass through the blood–brain barrier more easily than in older children and adults. Therefore medications that depress respiration may have a more powerful effect on neonates than in adults.

METABOLISM OF MEDICATIONS IN INFANTS AND CHILDREN

Most medications are metabolized in the liver. Because the liver and its enzymes do not function at a mature level until 2 to 4 years of age, drugs generally metabolize more slowly in the infant and young child compared to the adult. Medications given at frequent intervals to infants and children may result in toxic levels and responses.

EXCRETION OF MEDICATIONS IN INFANTS AND CHILDREN

Many medications such as penicillin and digoxin depend on the kidneys for excretion. The immature kidney function prevents effective excretion of drugs from the body in infants less than 1 year of age.

The combination of slow stomach emptying (delays medication from being absorbed), rapid intestinal transit time (may prevent the full amount of medication from being absorbed), unpredictable liver function (may impair metabolism of the drug), and inability to excrete medications effectively via the kidney can result in altered responses to medication and a high risk for toxicity.

NURSING RESPONSIBILITIES IN ADMINISTERING MEDICATIONS TO INFANTS AND CHILDREN

It is a legal and ethical responsibility of the nurse to understand that children who are growing differ in their ability to respond to medications. Nurses must observe for toxic symptoms whenever medications are administered and must document positive and negative responses. Close attention must be paid to pediatric dose calculations. Every medication administered should have the safety of the prescribed dose calculated and confirmed by the nurse before administration. The manufacturer's pocket insert, the *Physician's Desk Reference (PDR)*, or other current drug reference books, or www.drugguide.com or www.PDR.net provide official sources for safe dosage levels for various age groups.

PARENT TEACHING

Parent teaching is essential to ensure compliance when the child is sent home. Instructions should cover the following six areas:

1. The importance of administering the medicine.
2. The importance of completing the prescribed course of treatment.
3. Techniques for measuring the amount of medication to administer in each dose. The use of the teaspoon in the home is not advisable when administering medication to infants and children. Inexpensive and accurate measuring devices are available in pharmacies.
4. Techniques for administering medications to the infant or child:
   • Using a dropper, a syringe, or a measured cup
   • Not mixing medication with formula, food, or water

- Shaking medication before administering
- Refrigerating unused portions of medication if indicated

5. Techniques of encouraging child compliance:
   - Allowing toddlers and young children autonomy of assisting with taking their own medication by squirting the contents into their own mouth or drinking it from the cup
   - Providing praise for cooperation and perhaps a chart of stars or stickers for compliance
   - Providing a good-tasting liquid or an ice-pop following administration of a medication that has a bad taste

6. The importance of writing a schedule and documenting the administration to avoid forgetting or double dosing.

ADMINISTERING ORAL MEDICATIONS

The administration of medication by mouth is preferred in children but is not always possible because of vomiting, malabsorption, or refusal. Children younger than 5 years of age cannot safely swallow tablets or capsules. Most pediatric medications are available in liquid, suspension, or chewable tablets. Only scored tablets should be divided. Extended release tablets should not be chewed or crushed. Gel tablets should not be cut or dissolved. Suspensions must be fully shaken before use.

Medications should not be diluted in formula or water, because medications should be given in the smallest amount possible to assure the complete dose is consumed. If the medication is placed in the formula bottle and the infant does not finish all of the formula in the bottle, the complete dose of the medication will not have been administered. The use of important sources of nutrients, foods, or liquids (e.g., orange juice) for disguising the taste of the medication is discouraged because the child may develop distaste for these foods. The medication is never referred to as "candy." Medication is administered slowly, especially if the child is crying. The child's head and shoulders are elevated to prevent aspiration. Toddlers may attempt to push away the medicine cup. In anticipation of this response, the nurse holds the child in a "hug" position in the nurse's lap in a semisitting position (Skill 22-6).

If a nasogastric tube is in place, the nurse tests for proper placement of the tube *before* pouring medication into the funnel. A small amount of water is administered afterward to flush (cleanse) the tube. The procedure is recorded on the intake and output (I&O) sheet.

For infants, an oral syringe is an excellent device for measuring small quantities. It is easily transported, and

Administering Oral Medications

PURPOSE

To safely administer oral medications

STEPS

1. Verify medication orders and assemble supplies.
2. Place the infant's legs between your knees to maintain control of them.
3. Place one of the infant's arms behind your back and restrain the other arm by "hugging" the child (this helps to prevent the child from tipping the medication cup).
4. Give the medication slowly by cup or syringe to allow the child time to swallow. An older child may be given the choice to self-administer the medication by cup or syringe.
5. Provide "chasers" of water, fruit juice, or frozen ice-pops to help lessen the residual taste of the medicine. The patient's age and diet prescription are considered when choosing a chaser.
6. Remove gloves and perform hand hygiene.
7. Document in the medication administration record (MAR) the medication, route, time, and dose given.

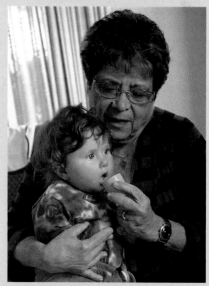

The syringe or cup method of administering oral medications to infants or children. Note that one of the infant's arms is behind the nurse's back while the nurse restrains the other. The legs of the infant can be held firmly between the knees of the nurse for better control during medication administration.

medication can be provided directly from the syringe. The syringe is placed midway back at the side of the mouth. The medication can also be administered via the syringe while the infant is sucking on a pacifier. A Medibottle, a device that consists of a syringe attached to a nipple, can be used for infants who will suck the medication from the nipple while the plunger of the syringe is slowly depressed (Figure 22-8).

A plastic medicine dropper is useful, and the drug manufacturer may provide one with the medication. It is used only for the medication specified; it is not intended for measuring other liquids. A drug ordered in teaspoons should be measured in milliliters to ensure accuracy (5 mL, 1 teaspoon). The nurse administering

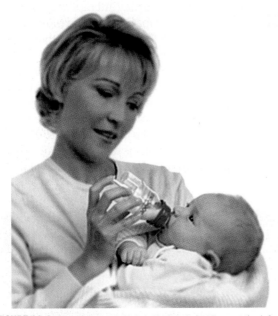

FIGURE 22-8 The Medibottle is attached to the syringe so the infant can suck on the nipple to consume the medication. The nurse controls the flow with gentle pressure on the syringe barrel. (Courtesy The Medicine Bottle Co., Inc.)

medications on the pediatric unit must keep the medicine tray or cart in sight at all times. This prevents other patients from upsetting or ingesting the contents.

ADMINISTERING PARENTERAL MEDICATIONS
Nose Drops, Ear Drops, and Eyedrops

Except for a few differences, the principles for administering nose drops, ear drops, and eyedrops to children are essentially the same as for adults. Infants and small children may need to be restrained in a mummy restraint (see Skill 22-1).

Nose Drops. The procedure for administering nose drops to a small child is detailed in Skill 22-7.

Ear Drops. The health care provider may prescribe a drug to be instilled into the ear to relieve pain. If the drops were refrigerated, they are allowed to warm to room temperature before administration (Skill 22-8).

Eyedrops and Creams. Ophthalmic medication is administered to a child in the same manner as for the adult. The child is informed of the need for the medication. The patient is identified, and the orders and the label on the bottle are checked for correct medication and concentration. The nurse ascertains which eye requires treatment. Hand hygiene is performed before and after the procedure, and clean gloves are worn. With the thumb and index finger, gentle pressure is applied in opposite directions to open the eye. The older child is instructed to "look up." Supporting the hand on the patient's forehead, the medication is instilled into the center of the lower lid (conjunctival sac) (see Skill 6-6 and accompanying illustration). The child is instructed to close the eye but not to squeeze it, because this could expel some of the solution.

Ointment is applied to the same conjunctival sac as eyedrops. The mummy restraint is applied when only

---

Administering Nose Drops

PURPOSE
To administer medication by nasal route

STEPS
1. Immobilize the infant with a mummy restraint.
2. Wipe excess mucus from nose with a tissue.
3. Place the infant on his or her back, with the head over the side of the mattress or the neck extended over a pillow.
4. Encircle the infant's cheeks and chin with the left arm and hand to steady.
5. Instill drops with the right hand.
6. Keep infant in this position for 30 seconds to 1 minute to allow the drops to reach the proper area.
7. Remove restraints. Make the infant comfortable.
8. Remove gloves and perform hand hygiene.
9. Chart the following: time, name of nose drops, strength, and number of drops instilled, how the patient tolerated the procedure, and untoward reactions.

Administering Ear Drops

PURPOSE
To administer medications into the ear canal

STEPS
1. Place child in supine position with unaffected ear down.
2. Instill the ordered number of drops:
   a. In children less than 3 years of age, pull the pinna (earlobe) of the affected ear down and back to straighten the canal.
   b. In older children, pull the upper pinna (auricle) up and back to straighten the canal.
3. Gently massage the area in front of the ear to facilitate entry of the drops.
4. Keep the patient in a supine position for a few minutes to permit the fluid to be absorbed.
5. Remove gloves and perform hand hygiene.
6. Document the time, name of drug, number of drops administered, area (right or left ear), untoward reactions, and whether or not the patient obtained relief.

---

one nurse is available and the patient is an infant. Occasionally children refuse to open their eyes. The nurse must use ingenuity to coax reluctant children. It may help to involve the parents.

Rectal Medications

Some drugs, such as sedatives and antiemetics, come in the form of suppositories. Children's suppositories are long and thin in comparison with the cone-shaped types administered to adults. Wearing a latex glove or finger cot, the nurse inserts the lubricated suppository well beyond the anal sphincter about half as far as the forefinger will reach. The nurse applies pressure to the anus by gently holding the buttocks together until the child's desire to expel the suppository subsides.

Subcutaneous and Intramuscular Injections

Most medications are given to infants and children by the oral or intravenous (IV) route. However, some medications must be given by the subcutaneous (SC/SQ) route, such as insulin for diabetic children. Some medications must be administered via the intramuscular route (IM), such as immunizations or vitamin K to newborn infants. The site and technique of injection can affect the absorption rate and the effect of the drug on the child. Needles should not be recapped, and the syringe must be disposed of in the appropriate container after use.

The Subcutaneous Route. In **subcutaneous (SC/SQ) injections**, absorption occurs by slow diffusion into the capillaries. If a medication such as epinephrine is given IM instead of SC/SQ, a life-threatening cardiac dysrhythmia could occur. If the extremity in which the SC/SQ medication was given is exercised immediately before or after a SC/SQ injection, the absorption rate is increased. (If insulin is the drug injected, hypoglycemia could occur because of the rapid absorption.)

Sites should be rotated. Irritating solutions should not be injected SC/SQ.

The Intramuscular Route. An **intramuscular (IM) injection** places medication into the skeletal muscle below the subcutaneous tissue. The medication spreads among the muscle's elastic fibers and absorbs rapidly. Aspirating the plunger after insertion and observing for a flashback of blood serves to prolong a painful procedure and is not necessary when the needle is inserted appropriately at a 45 or 90 degree angle according to the World Health Organization (WHO), the American Academy of Pediatrics (AAP), and the American Academy of Family Physicians (AAFP) (Crawford, 2012). Because there are no large vessels in the recommended injection sites for infants and children, aspiration is not necessary (Immunization Coalition, 2012; Hensel, 2013).

 Medication Safety Alert!

Maximum volume for IM administration in infants is 0.5 mL; in the toddler 1 mL; in the school-aged or adolescent, in the deltoid 1 mL, and in the *vastus lateralis* 2 mL.

Intramuscular Sites. IM injections are administered into the thickest part of the *vastus lateralis* muscle of the anterolateral thigh in all infants (Figure 22-9). The site is free of major nerves and blood vessels, but small nerve endings can cause the injection to be painful. The *ventrogluteal* site places the medication into the gluteus medius and gluteus minimus muscles, which are free of major nerves and blood vessels. This site is usually used for adolescents and adults.

The *dorsogluteal* site involves a high risk for sciatic nerve injury or piercing of a major blood vessel. ***This site is small and poorly developed in infants and***

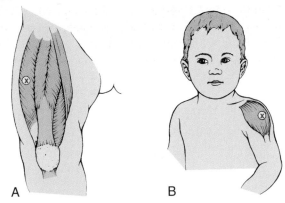

FIGURE 22-9 Appropriate sites for intramuscular (IM) injection in children. **A,** The thigh. **B,** Deltoid. The thigh is preferred in children less than 3 years of age.

children and is not used for IM injections. The *deltoid* site in the upper arm has a small muscle mass that limits the amount of medication that can be injected at one time. Immunizations are often administered via the deltoid site.

Reducing the Pain of Injections. Nurses can take the time to reduce the discomfort associated with injections. *Positioning* the patient properly can minimize muscle tenseness and ease the procedure. The infant or child can be held in the "hug" position on the lap of the parent or co-worker. Administering an injection while the infant is restrained and lying down on a bed or a table is a traumatic experience for the infant or child (Hensel, 2013). Infants should be given a sucrose-sweetened nipple to suck on or should breastfeed during or after the procedure. The older child should be distracted. For an injection into the deltoid area, the child can be held in the "hug" position with the elbow flexed and the arm supported and restrained. A *topical anesthetic* such as a eutectic mixture of local anesthetics (EMLA) (see Figure 21-3) can be used when the time of injection can be planned in advance. Storing alcohol sponges in the refrigerator or rubbing the site with an ice cube before injection will numb the site. The current design of many syringes minimizes accidental needle punctures to the caregiver that can spread infections and increase risk of blood-borne pathogen exposure. The needle should be inserted rapidly. The medication is injected rapidly unless the package insert states that slow injection is preferred (Hensel, 2013). Rapid removal of the needle and mild massage or exercise of the extremity will increase absorption and comfort. Distraction and other pain management techniques should be used.

The sizes of the syringe and needle vary with the size of the child, the volume of medication prescribed, the amount and general condition of the muscle tissue, the frequency of injections, and the viscosity (thickness) of the drug. A small needle, such as 25-gauge with a length of 1.3 to 2.5 cm (½ to 1 inch), is commonly

used for infants. As a general rule, 1 mL is the maximum volume to be given in one site to infants and small children. Small or premature infants may tolerate even less. For volumes less than 1 mL, a tuberculin syringe or low-dose syringe is preferred. Some syringes are designed automatically to retract the needle into the syringe after injections, and some have a plastic sleeve (Figure 22-10) to push over the needle after use. This eliminates the practice of recapping the needles and reduces the risk of an accidental needle stick. Although a change of needle may be recommended after drawing up a medication from a glass ampule before injecting the infant, a change of needle is not necessary when drawing up medication from a vial (Hensel, 2013).

The nurse should anticipate some protest from children about injections. The child's first injection is particularly important because it establishes the pattern for future reactions (Figure 22-11). The school-age child may assist in selecting the site, if possible. This helps to increase feelings of mastery and control. Injections are more of a threat to toddlers and preschool children, who are too young to understand their necessity. The nurse should be careful not to shame the uncooperative child. Fortunately, the necessity for administering IM injections to children is decreasing, because most medications can now be administered orally, rectally, or intravenously. The skill/technique of administering intramuscular injections is reviewed in Chapter 6, Skill 6-7.

Intravenous Medications

An IV injection places the drug directly into the bloodstream in a faster, more predictable time frame.

Medications provided by the IV route are being administered routinely in pediatric patients. In some

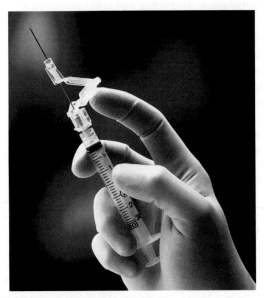

FIGURE 22-10 This syringe has a plastic sleeve that covers the needle after medication is administered. This helps to protect the nurse from an accidental needle stick. (Courtesy Becton, Dickinson & Co., Franklin Lakes, NJ.)

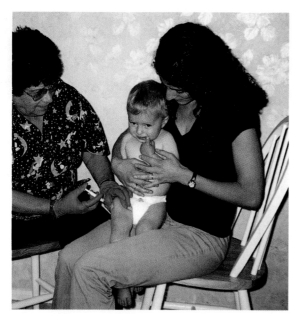

FIGURE 22-11 The "hug" restraining position for administration of intramuscular injections. Note that the mother restrains the arms, and that the child's legs are restrained between the mother's knees. The mother comforts the child during the procedure and may breastfeed after the procedure. The site for intramuscular injections in infants is the thigh, and the nurse wears a protective glove.

cases this prevents repeated IM injections. Other drugs are effective only if given by this method. The medication is also absorbed more rapidly, which is of value. The nurse monitors the IV site carefully for patency, infiltration, and inflammation.

IV medications can cause phlebitis, and the nurse must observe the child's IV site hourly for reddened areas or signs of inflammation. Infiltration is a risk for children who are active, and the site should be observed hourly, because infants cannot communicate the burning or pain that may accompany infiltration. Leakage at the IV site, a tense tissue turgor, and cool, blanched skin around the IV site may indicate infiltration; the registered nurse (RN) should be notified. Because the medication reaches the heart and brain within seconds, adverse reactions can occur quickly. The nurse must be aware of the side effects associated with each drug administered. A rapid rate of flow of IV solution can cause fluid overload (manifested by increased pulse rate or blood pressure, distended neck veins, and puffy eyes), or a slow rate of infusion can result in clot formation that obstructs the patency of the IV line. The nurse should monitor the rate of the IV flow, observe condition of the IV site hourly, identify the responses of the child, and document findings. IV pumps are usually set to alarm hourly so that the nurse will be reminded to observe the IV site and the responses of the infant or child and to document findings.

Sites for IV infusion in children are illustrated in Figure 22-12. A pediatric arm board is used (Figure 22-13) to restrain the extremity used for IV access, and the insertion site is secured and covered to prevent tampering by the child or parents. The child

with an IV in the extremity or in the scalp will benefit from being held and rocked. Infusion pumps and syringe pumps are used in pediatrics to control the administration of small volumes of fluid and to prevent

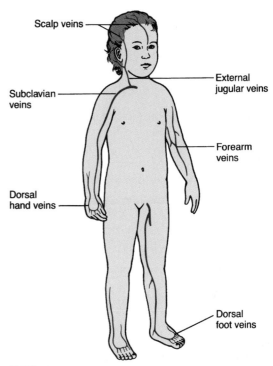

FIGURE 22-12 Sites for intravenous (IV) infusion in children.

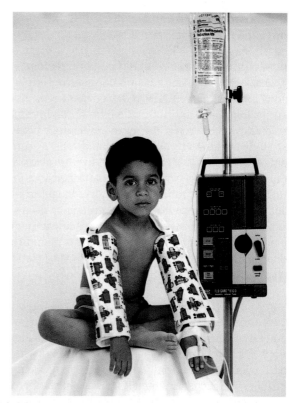

FIGURE 22-13 The arm board immobilizes the arm during intravenous (IV) therapy and permits movement. (Courtesy the Medi-Kids Co., Post Office Box 5398, Hemet, Calif., 92544, 888-463-3543, www.medi-kid.com.)

Removal of a Peripheral Intravenous Catheter

PURPOSE

To safely remove the peripheral intravenous (IV) catheter

STEPS

1. Turn off the infusion pump and clamp the IV tubing.
2. Perform hand hygiene and don clean gloves.
3. Remove the tape:
   a. To remove the Tegaderm or Opsite, pull the opposing edges parallel to the skin to loosen the bond.
   b. To remove sticky adhesive, use an adhesive removal pad and wash the skin afterward.
4. When all tape is removed and the catheter is movable and free, pull the catheter out of the vessel (in the opposite direction to that of insertion), keeping a straight line and not pulling upward or downward.
5. Exert firm pressure at the site with a dry sterile gauze.
6. Apply dry dressing or adhesive bandage at the insertion site.
7. Inspect catheter tip to ensure it is intact.
8. Remove gloves and perform hand hygiene.
9. Document on chart.

NOTE: Encourage the child's participation when appropriate (for example, when removing the tape).

changes in rate resulting from changes in position or activity in the infant or child. A pacifier should be provided for infants who are given nothing by mouth (NPO status) to fulfill their developmental need for sucking. When the health care provider orders IV access discontinued before discharge from the hospital, the licensed practical or vocational nurse (LPN/LVN) can remove the IV catheter (Skill 22-9).

Long-Term Peripheral Venous Access Devices

Saline lock. A **saline lock** is a long-term peripheral venous access device (VAD), a device that keeps a vein open for long-term intermittent medication administration. It allows children to be more ambulatory because they are freed from IV tubing. Repeated "sticks" can be avoided when a patient has a saline lock in place. The apparatus consists of an IV catheter attached to an 8.3-cm (3 1/4-inch) plastic tube plugged by a resealable rubber insert. This rubber top allows the insertion of a needle so that blood can be drawn or medications administered. The original catheter remains in place and is periodically flushed with sterile saline solution to prevent clotting. Each catheter flushing should be documented.

Central Venous Access Devices (CVAD).
A peripherally inserted central catheter (PICC) is a type of central venous access device that is inserted for moderate-length therapy. The tip of the catheter usually terminates in the superior vena cava. Specially trained RNs may insert the PICC line. Dressings are changed per established protocol, the insertion site is assessed, and care is taken to prevent dislodgement during this procedure.

Total parenteral nutrition. Total parenteral nutrition (TPN) is also known as *hyperalimentation* and provides the total nutritional needs for infants and children who cannot use the gastrointestinal tract for nourishment for a prolonged period. It allows highly concentrated solutions of proteins, glucose, and other nutrients to infuse directly into a large vessel such as the superior vena cava via a CVAD. In general, these concentrated solutions are not administered through peripheral veins. The nursing responsibilities are similar to those for other IV infusions. The solution is prepared by the pharmacist and is sterile. Monitoring vital signs, recording I&O, and tracking laboratory reports are essential nursing responsibilities.

Hypoglycemia, hyperglycemia, and electrolyte imbalances can occur. Before discontinuing TPN therapy, the rate is *gradually* decreased, and the child is monitored for adverse responses. Parents may need extensive teaching and return demonstrations if they are expected to care for their child who is to receive TPN treatment at home. Community agencies should be contacted to aid and support the family.

Nursing Care of a Child Receiving Parenteral Fluids.
Parenteral (*para,* "beside or apart from," and *enteron,* "intestine") fluids are those given by some route other than the digestive tract. They are necessary when vomiting or loss of consciousness accompanies sickness, or when the gastrointestinal system requires rest. The extremity in which the IV catheter is inserted is restrained on an arm board, and the insertion site is secured and covered. If the infant is on NPO status, a pacifier should be offered. Diversional therapy will prevent the child from focusing on the IV tubing and using it as a toy. The infant should be picked up, rocked, and played with.

IV pumps prevent a change in IV infusion rate when position or activity changes. The IV pump allows the administration of microdrops of IV solution so that a slow rate of infusion can be maintained. Adult IV sets administer 15 drops per 1 mL. Pediatric IV sets administer 60 drops per 1 mL. The infusion pump sounds an alarm every hour to alert the staff that the IV site must be assessed and the response of the infant can be documented. The nurse observes the child hourly for the following:

- Low volume in the bag
- The rate of flow of the solution
- Pain, redness, or swelling at the catheter insertion site
- Moisture at or around the catheter insertion site

An accurate I&O record is kept for all children receiving IV fluids. Nursing guidelines for IV therapy at various stages of development are described in Table 22-5.

PREVENTING MEDICATION ERRORS

Adhering to the six rights of medication administration used for any patient, adult or pediatric, is not always a guarantee of error-proofing medication administration to children.

 Medication Safety Alert!

The fact that the medication dose is ordered by the health care provider is not in itself a guarantee of safety, and the nurse has a responsibility to double-check the medication dosage with the recommended dosage published in a current recognized drug source.

Prescribing medication in a tense emergency setting increases the challenge of maintaining safety of the dosage prescribed for the small infant or young child.

Medication Safety Alert!

There are six rights of adult and pediatric medications administration:

1. Right patient
2. Right drug
3. Right dose
4. Right time
5. Right route
6. Right documentation

There have been many efforts to reduce the number of medication errors by the design of charts and the use of color-coding systems, and nurses must be familiar with those used at their hospital or clinic. Broselow pediatric emergency tape is used to determine the length of the child and serves as a guide in the administering of emergency medications by correlating dosage calculation and equipment sizes for emergency use. Based on the successful use of Broselow tape for many years, a system of color-coded ID bracelets for each child admitted to a hospital unit, based on the child's weight, correlates to reference guides for each weight group and provides an extra check point for the nurse to monitor the safety of the dose for that individual child before administering (Broselow et al, 2008).

The PEDI Slide Chart from A.C.T.N.T. Healthcare Services is another product used to help decrease the number of medication errors; it was developed in 2007 and is used in many hospitals. Also a length-based tool (as is the Broselow tape), it serves to determine accurate weight in kilograms of a child by using Centers for Disease Control (CDC) weight-to-height growth charts. The PEDI Slide system uses a disposable tape to measure from the top of the head to the heel of the foot of the fully extended leg. The body type is also estimated to determine if the child is average weight (50th percentile), at risk for overweight (75th percentile), or overweight (95th percentile). When the PEDI Slide is aligned with the appropriate length and body type, the estimated weight and correlated dosages of commonly used drugs will appear on the slide. The nurse should be familiar with the use of these systems as tools to reduce medication errors in pediatric patients (Figure 22-14).

Medication Safety Alert!

For each pediatric patient, the right dose involves calculating the recommended dose in mg/kg, comparing with the dose ordered, and checking with the pharmacist or health care provider if there is any question or discrepancy. A second licensed nurse must check insulins, hypoglycemics, narcotics, digoxin, inotropic drugs, anticoagulants, potassium, and calcium salts before being administered.

Selected tips for providing medication to children of various ages are offered in Box 22-1.

Calculating Pediatric Drug Dosages

Body Surface Area. Most pediatric medications are prescribed in milligrams per kilogram of body weight per 24 hours. A hospital drug reference is usually available on the unit to enable the nurse to determine the safety of a particular dose. If there is any question, one should consult the charge nurse, the physician who wrote the order, or the hospital pharmacist. The nurse should not be interrupted when preparing medications.

The physician calculates a particular dosage of a medication for each child. One method, calculation by **body surface area (BSA)**, is considered to be the most accurate. In this method, a **nomogram** is used (Figure 22-15).

On the nomogram, the child's height is located on the left scale and the weight on the right scale. A line is drawn between the two points. The point at which the line transects the surface area (SA) shows the BSA of the individual child. If the patient's size is roughly average, the SA can also be estimated from the weight alone by using the shaded area of Figure 22-15.

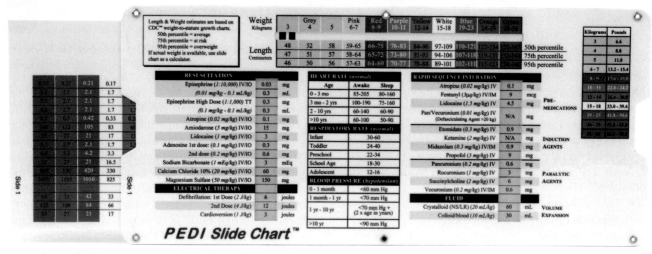

FIGURE 22-14 The *PEDI Slide Chart* is a tool for determining the correct dosage of medication and equipment sizes for the pediatric patient based on the patient's length, and it is most useful in emergency situations in which the child cannot be weighed. The PEDI Slide comes with disposable tape measures to measure head-to-toe length. This system also takes into consideration the body type—whether 50th, 75th, or 95th percentile—to refine further the dosage accuracy. (Courtesy A.C.T.N.T. Healthcare Services, Mineral Wells, Tex.)

Box 22-1 Selected Age-Appropriate Techniques for Giving Medications to Children

INFANT
Support and elevate head and shoulders.

Plastic disposable oral syringe is accurate and safe for administering oral medications.

Depress chin with thumb to open mouth.

Slowly insert medication along the side of the infant's mouth; this helps to prevent gagging.

Allow time for swallowing. The syringe may be placed at the corner of the mouth while the infant is sucking on the pacifier.

The recommended site for intramuscular (IM) injections is the vastus lateralis muscle.

The buttocks are never used for IM injections, because the gluteal muscles are undeveloped in infants and there is danger of injury to the sciatic nerve.

As a rule of thumb, provide no more than 1 mL of solution in a single site; if in doubt, confer with the charge nurse or physician.

Soothe infant after procedure is completed.

TODDLER
Place the child in the "hug position" for secure restraint.

Let child explore an empty medicine cup.

Explain reasons for the medication.

Crush tablets if they are not chewable. *Do NOT crush enteric-coated tablets.*

If child is cooperative, he or she may hold the medicine cup.

Allow the child to drink at his or her own pace.

When administering IM medications, perform the injection quickly and gently.

Be prepared to find that resistive behavior is at its peak, particularly kicking, crying, and thrashing about.

Be prepared to be surprised, because some toddlers are very cooperative.

PRESCHOOL
Chewable tablets and liquids are preferred.

Regression in pill taking may be seen.

Watch for loose teeth that may be swallowed.

Avoid prolonged reasoning.

Involve parents whenever possible.

Have child make choices when appropriate.

Whenever possible, follow bad tasting medicine with good tasting fluid.

Provide puppet play to help child express frustrations concerning injections.

Praise child after procedure.

SCHOOL AGE
Child can take pills and capsules; instruct child to place pill near the back of the tongue and immediately swallow water.

Emphasize swallowing of fluid to distract the child when swallowing the pill.

Some children continue to have a difficult time swallowing pills, and other forms of the medication should be explored (many come in suspensions); never ridicule the child.

Child can be unpredictable from day to day regarding cooperation; allow more time for giving pediatric medication.

Allow child to make realistic choices before, during, and after procedures. Child can choose if he wants to self-administer liquid medication via syringe or cup.

Whenever possible follow bad tasting medicine with good tasting fluid.

Always ascertain that the child is fully awake (particularly after nap time and during the night shift).

Always inform the child of what you are about to do.

Remain with the fearful child after the procedure until he or she regains composure.

ADOLESCENT
Adolescent needs more time to process information and needs to know the results of blood studies and other tests.

Prepare the adolescent with explanations suitable to his or her level of understanding.

Always ensure privacy.

Teach the adolescent what side effects to report.

Identify adolescents on contraceptives to prevent drug interactions (may have been too embarrassed to provide information during history or may be attempting to keep secret from significant others).

Remain with patient until medication is consumed (especially if patient has a behavior disorder).

Anticipate mood swings affecting compliance.

Consider possibility of adolescent addiction (e.g., drugs, alcohol) even though this may not be a presenting problem; metabolism of many medications is altered by such conditions.

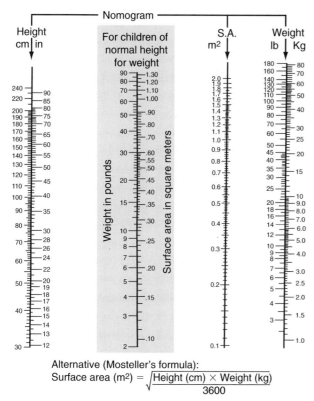

Alternative (Mosteller's formula):

$$\text{Surface area (m}^2) = \sqrt{\frac{\text{Height (cm)} \times \text{Weight (kg)}}{3600}}$$

FIGURE 22-15 Nomogram for estimating surface area. The body surface area of the child is at the point where the height and weight levels intersect the surface area column. If the patient is of average size, the surface area can be deduced based on weight alone (see *shaded* box).

The results are inserted into a formula, as follows (note that the average adult BSA is approximately 1.7 m²):

$$\frac{\text{BSA (child)}}{\text{BSA (adult)}} \times \text{Average adult dose} = \text{Child's dose}$$

Calculating the Safe Drug Dose

Milligrams per Kilogram (mg/kg). For adults, most medications have an "average dose." There is no average dose in pediatrics, because the weight of the child can vary from 1 kg (2.2 lb) to 68 kg (150 lb), and at different ages the ability to metabolize and excrete drugs may be limited. Therefore it is necessary for the nurse to calculate whether the ordered dose is safe. The nurse can use the mg/kg protocol when calculating safe doses for an infant or child. For example, the physician orders 25 mg of a medication to be administered. The nurse checks the *PDR* or other current drug reference books or resources and finds that the safe dose for that medication is 2 to 4 mg/kg. This child weighs 7 kg. Using the highest safe dose, the nurse inserts the actual weight of the child in kilograms (kg) into the formula so that the formula now reads as follows: the safe dose of *this* medication for *this* child is 4 mg × 7 kg, or 28 mg. The physician's order does not exceed 28 mg, and therefore the dose ordered is safe to give. If the physician's order had exceeded the computed safe dose, the nurse calls a supervisor or the physician.

Formula for Dimensional Analysis

$$\frac{\text{Unit}}{\text{Dosage on hand}} \times \frac{\text{Dosage wanted}}{\text{Unit to give}}$$

Dimensional Analysis. **Dimensional analysis** is one method of calculating dosages using basic arithmetic and algebra (Box 22-2). Some examples are provided in this section.

Example: A physician orders 0.025 g of a drug. Each tablet is 12.5 mg. How many tablets will you give?

You know that 1000 mg = 1 g. Therefore:

$$\left(\frac{\text{Unit}}{\text{Dosage on hand}} \times \frac{\text{Dosage wanted}}{\text{Unit to give}} \right.$$
$$\left. \frac{1000 \text{ mg}}{1 \text{ g}} \times \frac{0.025 \text{ g}}{?\text{mg}} = 1000 \times 0.025 = 25 \text{ mg} \right)$$

You will give 25 mg. Remember that each tablet is 12.5 mg:

What you have : What you want to give :

$$\frac{1 \text{ tablet}}{12.5 \text{ mg}} \times \frac{25 \text{ mg}}{?\text{tablets}} = 2 \text{ tablets}$$

You would give 2 tablets.

Example: A physician orders 5 mg of a drug. The label reads 10 mg/2 mL. How many mL do you administer?

$$\frac{\text{Unit}}{\text{Dose}} = \frac{2 \text{ mL}}{10 \text{ mg}} \times \frac{5 \text{ mg}}{?\text{mL}} = \frac{10}{10} = 1 \text{ mL}$$

You will give 1 mL.

Determining Whether a Dose Is Safe for an Infant. A physician orders 200 mg q6h. The *PDR* states that a 40-mg/kg dose is a safe dose for infants. This infant weighs 12 lb.

Dose ordered		Convert pounds to kg		Weight of child		What child is receiving
$\frac{200 \text{ mg}}{\text{Dose}}$	×	$\frac{2.2 \text{ lb}}{1 \text{ kg}}$	×	$\frac{1 \text{ infant}}{12 \text{ lb}}$	=	36.6 mg/kg/dose

Because 36.6 mg/kg does not exceed the stated safe dose of 40 mg/kg, the dose ordered is safe for this child.

In addition to knowing the correct amount and route of a drug, the nurse must also be aware of the toxic side effects that might occur. The absorption, distribution, metabolism, and excretion of drugs differ substantially in children, who also react more quickly and violently to medication. Drug reactions are therefore not as predictable as they are in adult patients. The drug's

Table 22-5 Nursing Guidelines for Pediatric Intravenous (IV) Lines at Various Stages of Development

DEVELOPMENTAL CHARACTERISTICS	IV PLACEMENT (IDEAL SITES)	PREPARATION OF CHILD	FAMILY INVOLVEMENT	RELATED NURSING ACTIONS	PROTECTION OF IV SITE	MOBILITY CONSIDERATIONS	SAFETY NEEDS
Infant (First Year)							
Infant is dependent on others for all needs. Needs to feel physically safe through close relationship with one caregiving person (usually mother). Trust develops through needs being met consistently. Mistrust and anxiety develop when needs are met inconsistently. Stranger anxiety begins at approximately 6-8 months.	Scalp vein; foot, hand, forearm	It is best not to feed infant immediately before IV insertion (vomiting and aspiration possible).	Prepare family about need for IV therapy, insertion procedure, appearance of infant with IV, and fluid needs. Encourage family to continue providing infant with tactile and verbal stimulation and tender, loving care. Demonstrate safe ways to hold an infant with IV.* Encourage questions and clarify misconceptions.	Restrain infant during insertion. Comfort and cuddle during and after insertion. Observe carefully during insertion for problems such as vomiting and aspiration. Firmly restrain extremity with IV (see next column). Use of pacifier diminishes stress, especially for infants who are on nothing-by-mouth (NPO) status.	IV may be secured with tape and is wrapped. Extremity may be restrained by using small arm board.	Allow for motion. Use minimal restraint such as elbow restraint or arm board. Mitten hands with cotton and stockinette to prohibit infant from grasping IV. Restraining all extremities is rarely necessary. Remember infant's need for sensory stimulation.	Maintain strict intake and output (I&O) record. Secure IV tubing out of range of kicking legs and flailing arms. Check restraints frequently for effectiveness and presence of adequate circulation. Check IV pump pressure settings and administration rate.
Toddler (Age 1-3 Years)							
Discovers and explores self and surrounding world. Enjoys new mobility skills. Develops egocentric thinking and need for parallel play. Tolerates short separations from mother. Transitional objects (security blanket, special toy) provide some comfort. Oppositional syndrome ("no" stage).	Hand, arm, foot Important: for this age group and older, the less dominant extremity should be used for IV whenever possible. Determine handedness before IV insertion	Prepare child immediately before procedure (child has limited attention span and is likely to become more anxious if prepared sooner). Give very simple explanation in concrete terms. Show equipment to be used. Do not offer choice. See discussion of preparation for preschool age and assess ability of each child to understand.†	Prepare family about need for IV therapy, insertion procedure, and appearance of child with IV. Whether parents remain with child during procedure varies. If they stay with child, their role is to comfort rather than to assist with restraining. Demonstrate to parents how to handle child with IV safely.	Restraining toddler for an IV usually requires more than one person. Reassure child through verbal and tactile stimulation during procedure. Provide toys such as pegs to hammer for therapeutic and distraction techniques. Many hospitals have child-life specialists who help provide atraumatic care.	See Infant (above). A securely anchored IV is essential for normally active toddler. Even the best site protection will not remain effective unless it is coupled with close nursing supervision and distracting activities for child.	Toddlers cope with world and learn about it through action. Therefore minimal restraints should be used. Parental presence during waking hours permits child to be constantly supervised. Appropriate play and distraction can be effective.	Child is unaware of danger at this age and will not know that movement of IV causes pain. Constant supervision is needed when child is out of bed. Frequently remind child not to touch IV, but do not expect compliance. Distracting activities accomplish much more than does a scolding. Tape securely.

Preschool (Age 4-6 Years)

Magical thinking, based on what child would like to believe. Cannot always distinguish fantasy from reality. Fears intrusive procedures. Castration fears common. Develops conscience (guilt), while asserting independence and mastering new skills. Learning to share.	Hand, forearm (less dominant)	Prepare child just before procedure. Using small bottle, tubing, and doll or stuffed animal, explain in literal terms the need for IV and insertion procedure. Allow child to see and touch equipment. Explain how child can help with procedure by cleaning site, opening packages, and taping, for example. Allow child some control in situation. State that you will help child to hold still and that it is OK to cry.	As with toddlers, parents may or may not stay with child during procedure. If they stay, they should provide comfort and support, but they should not be asked to restrain child for IV insertion. Reinforce child's need for honest, simple explanations. Reassure parents that child can still play and be active, even with IV.	Tell child purpose of IV in simple terms. Never bribe or threaten with IVs (e.g., "Drink, or you'll get another IV"). Praise for cooperation or any efforts in that direction. Maintain patient privacy. Do not start an IV in the sight of other patients, visitors, or staff. Child needs support to cope with intrusiveness of this procedure. Show understanding.	See Infant (earlier in this table). As with toddlers, securely anchored IVs are essential but inadequate unless coupled with close supervision and age-appropriate activities.	Preschoolers need maximum mobility to master surroundings. Provide a range of out-of-bed activities whenever possible.	Child will be curious about IV. Child is capable of understanding instructions not to touch it but needs frequent reminders and distraction. IV clamps should be out of reach or taped over. Constant supervision is needed when child is out of bed. Child is likely to take off running down hall, heedless of the IV bag, for example. Short attention span limits duration of cooperation with instructions.

School-Age Child (Age 7-11 Years)

Struggles between mastery of new skills and failure. Enjoys school, learning skills, and games with rules. Needs to succeed. Fears body mutilation. May feel need to be brave. Can understand hospital rules. World now expanding beyond family. Peer group becomes important. Competitiveness.	Hand, forearm (less dominant)	Prepare child ahead of time but on same day of insertion. Carefully explain and demonstrate equipment and reasons for IV therapy, letting patient watch or help set up equipment. Ask child for questions about need for IV and procedure. Give child choices and let child help in procedure whenever possible. Tell child	Whenever possible, family and child should be prepared together so that family can reinforce what child has been told. Stress to family the child's need for some independence in activities of daily living, even with an IV. Parental presence or participation in IV insertion may be appropriate, but child's preference should be	Approach child expecting cooperation (this age group likes to please adults), but expect that child will need help remaining still. Allow child to clean site with alcohol swab and to cut tape before insertion. Praise cooperative efforts. Give child step-by-step explanation of procedure as it progresses. Child may like to take	Child will need less protection than younger children owing to interest in making IV work correctly. May naturally protect extremity with IV. Some children appreciate a warning sign, "Hands Off," on a piece of tape over IV as a reminder. Use child's natural curiosity and interest in learning. Tell child the rules of safe IV handling.	Show patient and family how to manipulate IV safely for out-of-bed activities (e.g., walking in hall with IV bag, keeping tubing out of wheelchair wheels).	Remind patient periodically about necessary caution with IV. Show patient clamps and caution against handling them. Teach patient signs of IV problems. Enlist child's help in interest of good compliance, but do not entirely depend on it. Tape tubing connections. Child may forget about IV.

Continued

Table 22-5 Nursing Guidelines for Pediatric Intravenous (IV) Lines at Various Stages of Development—cont'd

DEVELOPMENTAL CHARACTERISTICS	IV PLACEMENT (IDEAL SITES)	PREPARATION OF CHILD	FAMILY INVOLVEMENT	RELATED NURSING ACTIONS	PROTECTION OF IV SITE	MOBILITY CONSIDERATIONS	SAFETY NEEDS
School-Age Child (Age 7-11 Years), cont'd							
		crying is OK because needles hurt; child can help by remaining still.	considered primary.	some responsibility in keeping I&O record.			Emphasize need for caution in some activities, especially if play includes other children.
Adolescent (Age 12-18 Years)							
Vacillates between needs for independence and dependence. Adult cognitive abilities, deductive reasoning. Coping mechanisms: rationalization, intellectualization. Peer acceptance is very important. Egocentric, rebellious at times, especially against parents and authority figures. Very concerned with body image, body changes, sexuality, and role. Searching for "who I am."	Hand, forearm (less dominant)	Prepare patient several hours to a day before procedure, if possible. Needs time between preparation and insertion to absorb explanations and ask questions. For most adolescents, approach discussions on an adult level. Explain need for IV therapy and expected duration, and show equipment. May need much support for acceptance of therapy.	Explain therapy needs and duration as with patient. Decision regarding parental presence during procedure should be patient's, not parents'. Stress that patient's participation in decisions affecting care is important.	Be aware of IV adding to patient's dependency status and need for some control. Encourage child to keep own I&O sheet and to help in counting drip rate, for example.	See School-Age Child (earlier in this table). If patient is very active, will need well-protected, well-anchored IV, because movements may be more forceful and strength may be greater than those of younger patients.	See School-Age Child (earlier in this table). Encourage mobility as much as possible as a means of independence for adolescent.	Be aware of possibility of adolescent rebellion showing itself by lack of cooperation with therapy. These patients may rebel if feeling threatened and may be very manipulative in testing behaviors. Consistent limits, clearly communicated to patient, parents, and staff, are needed. Instruct patient about signs of infiltration and phlebitis, for example.

Modified from Guhlow LJ, Kolb J (1979). Pediatric IVs: special measures you should take. RN, 42, 40. Published in RN, the full-service nursing journal. Copyright 1979 Medical Economics Co. Inc., Oradell, NJ. Reprinted by permission.
*No child should be restricted to bed simply because he or she has an IV!
†Each stage builds on the earlier ones, and during hospitalization many children regress to behaviors appropriate to earlier levels of development. Age-appropriate pain relief measures should be implemented for every infant or child. Appropriate distraction will enhance pain relief measures.

Table 22-6   Selected Drug–Environment Interactions

DRUGS	INTERACTS WITH	RESULT OF INTERACTION
Imipramine (Tofranil), phenothiazines, griseofulvin, tetracyclines, chlorothiazide (Diuril)	Sun	Skin rash when child is exposed to sun
Vitamin C	Air	Decomposes when exposed to air

impact on normal growth and development must be considered. Drug inserts must be read carefully to determine the suitability of a particular drug for children. **Drugs should be administered only by the route indicated.**

Double-checking with another nurse is required in most hospitals when administering drugs such as digoxin (Lanoxin), insulin, or heparin. Two identifiers on the hospital ID band should be used to correctly identify the child. The child's assigned nurse must always know what medications the patient is receiving, whether or not the nurse personally administers them. See Box 22-1 for further age-appropriate techniques of administering pediatric medications.

Preventing Drug Interactions

Selected Drug–Environment Interactions. Some medications can cause skin reactions when the child is exposed to the sun (**phototoxicity**). Parents should be advised to keep their child protected from the sun while he or she is taking these medications. Drugs that decompose when exposed to the air or light are dispensed in darkened bottles. These drugs should not be purchased in the large economy size because some tablets may deteriorate before all are used. Table 22-6 lists some examples of drug–environment interactions.

Selected Drug–Drug Interactions. The nurse should be alert to possible interactions between drugs prescribed and between prescription drugs and drugs that parents may purchase without a prescription. Table 22-7 includes a partial list of some common drug–drug interactions.

Selected Drug–Food Interactions. The nurse should be aware that food and nutrients can influence the absorption, metabolism, and excretion of certain drugs. Foods that influence gastrointestinal motility or the pH of gastric secretions can affect absorption, thus lessening the drug's therapeutic value. Table 22-8 lists some drug–food interactions.

SELECTED PROCEDURES AND THEIR ADAPTATION TO CHILDREN

NUTRITION, DIGESTION, AND ELIMINATION

Gavage Feedings

A gavage feeding may be ordered when an infant cannot take food or fluids by mouth but the gastrointestinal tract is functioning. A gavage feeding places nutrients directly into the stomach so that natural digestion can occur. This can be accomplished by placing a nasogastric tube into the stomach via the nose, securing it in place with tape or by using the oral route, and reinserting a new tube with each feeding. When long-term feeding is required, a gastrostomy may be performed and a tube inserted directly into the stomach (see Skill 22-10).

Gastrostomy

A **gastrostomy** (*gastro,* "stomach," and *stoma,* "opening") is designed to introduce food directly into the stomach through the abdominal wall by means of a surgically placed tube or button (Skill 22-10). It is used in infants or children who cannot have food by mouth because of anomalies or strictures of the esophagus or who are severely debilitated or in a coma. Cleansing of the skin around the tube prevents irritation from formula or gastric secretions. The nurse observes and reports vomiting or abdominal distention. Brown or green drainage may indicate that the tube has slipped through the pylorus into the duodenum. This could cause an obstruction and is reported immediately.

 Nursing Tip

One way of determining fluid loss in infants is to weigh a wet diaper and then weigh a dry diaper of the same type and size and to mark the weight on the outside of the dry diaper. Subtract the weight of the dry diaper from the weight of the wet diaper, and record results on the I&O record. Include both urine and liquid stools (1 g = 1 mL of output).

Enema

Administering an enema to a child is essentially the same as for adults; however, the type, the amount, and the distance for inserting the tube require modifications. In addition, a child's bowel is more easily perforated under pressure. An isotonic solution (saline) is used in children. Tap water enemas are contraindicated, because plain tap water is hypotonic to the blood and could cause rapid fluid shift and overload if absorbed through the intestinal wall. The type of solution intended is always confirmed. The amount of fluid varies somewhat in procedure recommendations. The smaller the child, the less solution is used. The exact amount for infants should be prescribed by the health care provider's order. Guidelines range from a low of 50 mL (1.7 oz) for infants to a high of 500 to 750 mL (16.9 to 25.4 oz) for the adolescent. The nurse consults the procedure manual for the institution's guidelines.

Table 22-7   Selected Drug–Drug Interactions

DRUG	INTERACTS WITH	RESULT OF INTERACTION
Antacids	Steroids	Decreased absorption
	Digoxin	Decreased absorption
	NSAIDs	Decreased absorption
	Tetracycline	Decreased absorption
	Theophylline	Increased toxicity
Barbiturates	Oral contraceptives	Decreased protection
	Steroids	Decreased steroid effectiveness
	Influenza vaccine	Barbiturate toxicity
	Theophylline	Decreased theophylline effect
Bleomycin	Oxygen	Increased lung toxicity
Erythromycin	Phenytoin	Decreased phenytoin effect
	Theophylline	Increased theophylline toxicity
Isoniazid	Antacid	Decreased absorption
	Phenytoin	Increased phenytoin toxicity
	Valproate	Hepatic and central nervous system toxicity
Phenytoin	Alcohol	Acute toxicity
	Antacid	Decreased phenytoin effect
	Antidepressants (tricyclic)	Increased phenytoin toxicity
	Contraceptives	Decreased protection
	Steroids	Decreased steroid effectiveness
	Digoxin	Decreased digoxin effect
	Folic acid	Decreased phenytoin effect
	Isoniazid	Increased phenytoin toxicity
	Theophylline	Decreased effect of both medications
	Valproate	Increased phenytoin toxicity

NSAIDs, Nonsteroidal antiinflammatory drugs.

Table 22-8   Selected Drug–Food Interactions

DRUG	INTERACTS WITH	RESULT OF INTERACTION
Aminoglycosides Gentamicin Penicillin Tetracycline	Any food	Decreased absorption rate
Theophylline	High-protein foods Low-carbohydrate diet	Decreased time of drug activity in body
Monoamine oxidase (MAO) inhibitors (phenelzine [Nardil], tranylcypromine [Parnate], isocarboxazid [Marplan])	Tyramine-containing foods such as yogurt, processed meats, beer	Possible hypertensive crises
Iron supplements	Starch, egg yolks	Decreased iron absorption
Antihypertensives	Licorice or natural licorice extract	Can counteract effect of antihypertensive drugs
Vitamin C	Foods high in vitamin B_{12}	Decreased absorption of vitamin B_{12} if both vitamins are taken together

Gastrostomy Tube Feeding

PURPOSE

To introduce nutrition directly into the stomach

STEPS

1. Verify order for type and amount of feeding.
2. Position child comfortably either flat or with head slightly elevated if not contraindicated. Provide pacifier to relax infant. Place absorbent pad under gastrostomy tube extender to protect bed linens.
3. Check residual stomach contents by attaching syringe to gastrostomy tube and aspirating. If amount of residual is large (10 to 25 mL for newborns, more than 50 mL for older children), replace residual and decrease present formula by equal amount, or delay feeding for a short time. (This may vary according to the pediatrician's protocol.) Overloading the stomach can cause reflux and increases the danger of aspiration. If residual continues or increases, report this to the physician. If no residual is obtained, inject 2 to 5 mL of water into the tubing to clear tubing and test residual again. (Verification of tube placement is usually obtained via x-ray after initial insertion and when any question of placement occurs.)
4. Attach the syringe barrel (if not already present for continuous infusion) to the gastrostomy tube. If the tube has more than one lumen, be sure to use the port labeled for *food or formula*. Fill with formula. Remove clamp. This prevents air from entering the stomach and causing distention. (Note: When administering medication via gastric tube, first flush the tubing so medication will not mix with the milk or formula and flush between each medication administered. Flushing after giving a medication assures all the medication has entered the body and none is left in the tubing.)
5. Elevate the receptacle. Allow the formula to flow slowly by gravity—force should not be used. (Note: Medications and feedings should flow by gravity and be followed with enough fluid as a flush to ensure the medication or feeding is in the stomach and does not remain in the tubing.)
6. Continue to add formula to the syringe before it empties completely (to prevent excess air from entering the tubing).
7. Clamp the tube as the final formula or water is passing through the lower part of the syringe. The gastrostomy tube extender may remain in place and be clamped or it may be removed from the gastrostomy button and the button closed and locked. (Note: With infants, some physicians may prefer that the gastrostomy tube remain open at all times to produce a safety valve in the event that the infant vomits. In such cases, the tube is elevated above the patient's body.)
8. Whenever possible, hold the patient quietly after feeding. Reposition in Fowler's position or on right side to promote gastric emptying.
9. Remove gloves and perform hand hygiene.
10. Record in the medical record the type (gastrostomy feeding), the amount given, the amount and characteristics of residual, and how the child tolerated the procedure.
11. Record the intake on the Intake and Output record.
12. An increase in gastric residual, abdominal distention, vomiting, or bradycardia should be reported to the health care provider promptly.

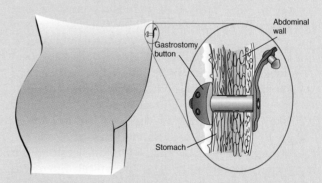

The gastrostomy button allows feedings to be administered directly into the stomach through the abdominal wall. (From Hockenberry M, Wilson D, et al: *Wong's nursing care of infants and children*, ed 7, St Louis, 2003, Mosby.)

The tube is inserted from 0.4 to 1.6 cm (1 to 4 inches) according to the size and age of the child. Infants and small children may be unable to retain the solution; therefore it may be necessary to hold the buttocks together for a short time. Commercial enemas specific for the child may be used; however, some are not recommended for infants and children. The Fleet Enema contains sodium biphosphate and sodium phosphate and has an osmotic action that can result in metabolic acidosis. Other commercially prepared enemas can cause complications in a dehydrated child. An oral polyethylene-glycol lavage solution, GoLytely or NuLytely, can be used to cleanse the bowel, as can a solution of magnesium citrate, without causing a risk for an electrolyte imbalance.

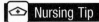 **Nursing Tip**

Saline enemas may be made by combining 1 teaspoon of table salt with 500 mL of tap water.

RESPIRATION

Tracheostomy Care

A **tracheostomy** is a surgical procedure in which an opening is made in the trachea to enable the patient to breathe. This artificial airway may be necessary in emergency situations, may be an elective procedure, or may be combined with mechanical ventilation. Some of the childhood conditions that may require tracheostomy are acute epiglottitis, head injury, and burns. Nursing care is indispensable to the survival of the child, because blockage of the tube by mucus or other secretions can lead to suffocation. In many hospitals the child is placed in the intensive care unit immediately after surgery because this is a critical period that requires frequent suctioning and close observation. The child is placed on heart and respiratory monitors. When the child's condition stabilizes, the child is usually transferred to a general unit.

The child is placed in an area of high visibility. This is important, because small children communicate their needs by crying and the tracheostomy prohibits vocalization. Whenever possible, one person is assigned to the child and to work with the parents. The nurse reinforces preoperative teaching and explains what happened; for example, "You were having a lot of trouble breathing. This operation is called a tracheostomy and helps you to breathe more easily. A small opening has been made in your neck. A hollow tube was inserted to keep the area open. It is frightening not to be able to speak. When you are better, the hole will close by itself and your voice will return." An explanation of suction might be, "We have to keep the area in your neck open. This tube goes into the throat and clears it." The use of suction can be shown with a glass of water. The child is then prepared for the unfamiliar sound. "You might feel like gagging, but afterward you will feel better. I know this is difficult for you and I'm sorry."

The nursing care of the child with a tracheostomy is a significant responsibility. The anatomical differences between children and adults and the small child's inability to communicate through writing increase the need for close observation. In addition, toddlers often have short, stubby necks that become easily irritated. It may be helpful to place a reminder on the intercom at the clerk's desk or in other suitable areas indicating that this patient cannot cry or speak. The nurse's touch and quiet voice and the presence of significant others help to make the child feel secure. Repeating familiar stories incorporates calming routines. A favorite article, such as a blanket or toy, is kept nearby. A supply of teaching aids and of dramatic play material is made available. Puppets are particularly valuable.

Tracheostomy Tube. Maintaining patency of the tracheostomy tube is of utmost importance. Plastic or Silastic tubes are generally used because they are flexible and reduce crust formation. They are lightweight and disposable, and most do not have inner cannulas. Cuffed tubes are not usually necessary in infants and small children, because their air passages are smaller and the tracheostomy tube provides a sufficient seal. The surgeon chooses a tracheostomy tube that is appropriate for the patient's neck size and condition. Administering oxygen by manual resuscitator ("bagging") before or after the procedure helps to prevent hypoxia.

Suctioning. Selection of a suction catheter is important. The nurse chooses one that does not block the tube during suctioning. The diameter should be about half the size of the tracheostomy tube. Hands are washed before proceeding. The nurse uses sterile gloves for the procedure, and all equipment used in the care of a tracheostomy should be sterile. Suction is applied as the catheter is *withdrawn.* The tube is rotated to allow the removal of secretions on all sides. With Y-tube technique, suction is achieved by closing the port with the thumb. A drop of saline solution may be inserted before suctioning to aid in loosening secretions. Because variations in this procedure exist and modifications are often required, the nurse must understand what is intended for the particular patient and must ask for clarification of specific procedures of the institution.

Suctioning is done periodically and when necessary. Indications for suctioning include noisy breathing, bubbling of mucus, and moist cough or respirations. Patients can rapidly become hypoxic during suctioning, and therefore it is limited to no more than 15 seconds. Two or three breaths for reoxygenation are allowed between suctioning. The depth of suctioning is important. In general, suctioning is limited to the length of the tracheostomy tube or slightly beyond to stimulate coughing. The catheter is cleared with sterile water between insertions. Unnecessary suctioning is avoided. The suction catheter is discarded after use. Disposing of water after suctioning prevents the growth of opportunistic organisms.

Tracheal Stoma. The tracheal stoma is treated as a surgical wound. The area is kept free of secretions and exudate to minimize the risk of infection. Cotton-tipped applicators dipped in half-strength hydrogen peroxide and saline solution can be used to remove crusted mucus. Tapes around the child's neck should be loose enough to allow one finger to be easily inserted between tape and neck. The knot is placed to the side of the neck (Figure 22-16). The condition of the skin beneath the tape is assessed. The tape is changed as necessary. Two people are used for this procedure—one to hold the outer cannula and the other to change the tape. When feeding the infant, the nurse covers the tracheostomy with a bib or a moist piece of gauze to prevent aspiration of food particles.

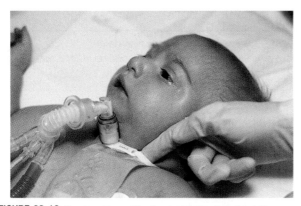

FIGURE 22-16 Tracheostomy. The tracheostomy ties should be snug but should allow one finger to be inserted between ties and neck to ensure that it is not too tight. (From Hockenberry M, Wilson D: *Wong's nursing care of infants and children*, ed 9, St Louis, 2011, Mosby.)

Observing for Complications. The nurse observes the patient for symptoms such as restlessness, rising pulse rate, fatigue, apathy, dyspnea, sternal retractions, pallor, cyanosis, and inflammation or drainage around the incision. Possible complications include tracheoesophageal fistula, stenosis, tracheal ischemia, infection, atelectasis, cannula occlusion, and accidental extubation. Baseline monitoring of the patient is done on each shift and before suctioning. The patient's mental status, respirations, pulse rate and rhythm, and chest sounds are of particular importance. Accurate recording of observations is essential to evaluation. The time and frequency of suctioning, the character of secretions, the relief afforded the patient, the behavior of the patient, the appearance of the wound, and other pertinent data are recorded.

A sterile hemostat is kept at the bedside for emergency use. Accidental *extubation,* or expulsion of the tube, is uncommon but can occur as a result of severe coughing if the tapes are too loose. Patency of the airway is maintained by spreading the edges of the wound with the sterile clamp until a duplicate sterile tube is inserted. An extra tracheostomy tube and the equipment needed for its replacement are always kept in a visible, easily reached area at the bedside for use in such emergencies. As the child's condition improves, he or she is weaned from the tube. The opening gradually closes by granulation. Children whose tubes must remain in place for a longer time may require periodic tube changes.

Additional Nursing Measures. Additional nursing measures include frequent changes of position, use of elbow restraints, oral feedings (unless contraindicated), and careful bathing to prevent water from entering the tube. Range-of-motion exercises are a must for long-term patients, and in acute cases arm restraints are removed one at a time to allow for passive exercises. The health care provider orders the diet. Although patients may initially have nothing by mouth, they progress to a soft or normal diet as the condition improves. The Fowler's position is preferred during feedings. The older child can cooperate by holding the head flexed with the chin down. This decreases swallowing difficulties, because the esophagus opens and the airway narrows.

Discharge. Certain patients are discharged with a tracheostomy. This is anticipated, and instruction and demonstration for the parents begin early. Parents who are comfortable with the procedure during hospitalization will feel more secure when the child returns home. Information about parent support groups, visiting home nurses, and other referrals is provided before discharge.

Oxygen Therapy

Box 22-3 shows a review of selected considerations for the child receiving oxygen. See Chapter 13 for care of a child in an incubator.

Safety Considerations. All equipment used for oxygen therapy must be inspected periodically. Combustible materials and potential sources of fire are kept away from oxygen equipment. These materials are essentially the same as for adults; for the child, however, friction toys are also to be avoided, because the sparks the toys can create could ignite the oxygen. Nylon or wool blankets are not to be used. One should know where the nearest fire extinguisher is located. Parents are alerted to the precautions and to the presence of "no smoking" signs.

Infection prevention and control are extremely important. It is imperative that cross infection via unclean equipment be prevented. Humidifiers and nebulizers, which are warm and moist, serve as an excellent medium for the growth of disease-producing organisms. Although most masks, tents, and cannulas that come into direct contact with the child are disposable, other pieces of mechanical equipment cannot be discarded. They require periodic cleansing if therapy is extended and terminal cleansing according to product direction. The respiratory therapy department should be contacted as necessary.

Prolonged exposure to high oxygen concentrations can be toxic to some body tissues (e.g., the retina in preterm infants and the lungs in the general population) but particularly in children with pulmonary diseases such as asthma or cystic fibrosis. The amount of oxygen administered depends on the child's arterial oxygen concentration. Blood gas determinations (oxygen and carbon dioxide pressures, or Po_2 and Pco_2, respectively) ensure safe and accurate therapy. Noninvasive pulse oximeters that measure blood oxygen saturation via the skin are used whenever oxygen is administered to patients (see Skill 13-1). Saturation rates displayed on the pulse oximeter should be frequently documented on the medical record.

Oxygen is a dry gas and requires the addition of moisture to prevent irritation of the respiratory tract. High-humidity concentrations may be achieved by the use of jet humidifiers on several oxygen units. Compressed air rather than oxygen may also be used for this purpose.

Box 22-3   Selected Considerations for the Child Receiving Oxygen

GENERAL CONSIDERATIONS

Signs of respiratory distress include an increase in pulse rate and respirations, restlessness, flaring nares, intercostal and substernal retractions, and cyanosis. In addition, children with dyspnea often vomit, which increases the danger of aspiration. Maintain a clear airway by suctioning if needed.

Organize nursing care so that interruptions are kept at a minimum.

Observe children carefully, because vision may be obstructed by mist, and young children are unable to verbalize their needs.

NEWBORN

Oxygen may be provided via hood, which may be used in the warming unit.

Oxygen may be provided via Isolette; keep sleeves closed to decrease oxygen loss.

Oxygen must be warmed to prevent neonatal stress from cold.

Analyze oxygen concentration carefully.

Parents are the primary focus of preparations; help to develop good parenting skills and self-confidence in their ability to care for the newborn who is ill.

INFANT

Nose may need to be suctioned by bulb syringe to remove mucus.

Infant may benefit from use of infant seat; secure seat to bed frame; watch for slumping in seat.

Make sure crib sides are up; a canopy often gives the illusion of safety.

Avoid the use of baby oil, A+D ointment, petroleum jelly (Vaseline), or other oil-based or alcohol-based substances around nares.

Anticipate stranger anxiety at around 6 to 8 months of age; infant clings to parents and turns away from nurse.

An extremely irritable infant may benefit from comforting in parent's lap followed by sleeping in tent; clarify at report time.

Nasal catheters often are well tolerated and allow in-bed activity of infant.

TODDLER

Anticipate that a toddler will be distressed by a tent. A nasal catheter is tolerated best.

Anticipate regression.

When toddlers are restless and fussy, they may pull tent and covers apart.

Toddler cannot tell nurse if tent is too hot or too cold.

Change clothing and bed linen when damp.

Toddler may be comforted by a transitional object, such as a blanket.

Parents may have suggestions as to how to keep toddler happy in the tent if one is necessary.

PRESCHOOL

Tent plastic distorts view. Nasal catheters are better tolerated.

Because thought processes are immature in preschool children, reality and fantasy are inseparable.

To decrease fear, prepare child for all procedures.

Anticipate that child will feel lonely and isolated.

Child will enjoy stories, puppets, and dramatic play.

If extremely restless and anxious, child may benefit from holding parent's hand through small opening in zippers.

Do not allow child to play with toys that spark.

SCHOOL AGE

The tent usually frightens school children less; fears center around body mutilation and loss of control. Nasal catheters are tolerated best.

Preparatory information continues to focus on what the child will see, hear, feel, and be expected to do.

Child may benefit from writing a story about the experience; nurse reviews story with child and clarifies misconceptions; posting story on unit affirms child's self-esteem and mastery (always ask permission to post).

Allow child to make realistic choices before, during, and after procedures.

Encourage child to draw "what it feels like to be in a tent" and discuss.

ADOLESCENT

Nurse remains available to the patient to answer questions as they arise.

Trust is extremely important as the adolescent attempts to move beyond the nuclear family.

Anticipate problems of being restricted by apparatus. Nasal catheter is tolerated best.

May feel weird when visited by peers; wavers between feeling self-confident and feeling ineffective.

Reiterate no smoking and other safety precautions with patient and peers.

Include patient in therapy; he or she may be able to manage own oxygen needs.

For comfort and survival, review safe use of oxygen in the home if required.

Oxygen therapy is terminated gradually. This allows the patient to adjust to *ambient* (environmental) oxygen. The nurse slowly reduces liter flow, opens air vents in Isolette incubators, or opens zippers in croup tents. The child's response is closely monitored via a pulse oximeter. An increase in restlessness and in pulse rate and respirations indicates that the child is not tolerating withdrawal from the oxygen-enriched environment.

Methods of Administration. Oxygen is administered to children as appropriate for age via Isolette, nasal cannula, mask, hood, tent, or tracheostomy. Regardless of the method used, the child is observed frequently to determine the effectiveness of the oxygen therapy. The desired goals include decreased restlessness and improved breathing, vital signs, and color. High concentrations of oxygen can be delivered by way of a plastic hood (see Figure 13-4). Warmed, humidified oxygen is delivered directly over the child's head. It may be used in a radiant warmer.

Mist tent. A **mist tent** provides an atmosphere of fine particles of water suspended in a cool air or oxygen environment. The zippered openings in the clear plastic canopy facilitate easy access and observation of the

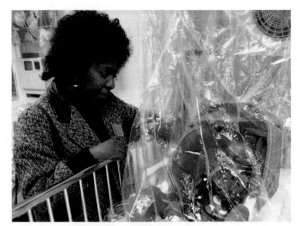

FIGURE 22-17 This infant is in an infant seat to maintain Fowler's position while in a mist tent. This method of oxygen administration allows the parent and the child to see each other. (From Hockenberry M, Wilson D, et al: *Wong's nursing care of infants and children*, ed 7, St Louis, 2003, Mosby.)

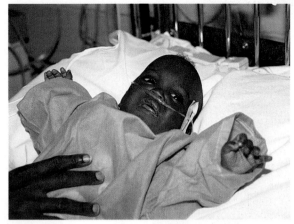

FIGURE 22-18 Child receiving blow-by oxygen therapy via nasal catheter. The prongs may be placed below (blow-by) or in the nares, and the loop is slipped over the ears to stabilize the position. The cannula can be taped to the side of the child's face to prevent slippage. (From James SR, Nelson K, Ashwill JW: *Nursing care of children: principles and practice*, ed 4, Philadelphia, 2012, Saunders.)

child (Figure 22-17). A nebulizer can be attached to provide medicated inhalation therapy. The child should be dressed warmly when inside the tent to prevent hypothermia. The oxygen concentration should be checked periodically, and a pulse oximeter assessment of oxygen saturation should be monitored.

A physician's order often reads, "Keep O₂ saturation at 93%." This means that if the O₂ saturation on the pulse oximeter reads above 93%, the oxygen liter flow can be lowered and the child carefully monitored. If the O₂ saturation level reads below 93%, the liter flow can be gradually increased and the child closely monitored until the reading reaches 93% (see Chapter 13 for discussion of pulse oximeters). A parent at the bedside stroking the infant through the zippered opening in the canopy can have a calming effect. Keeping a child dry in a high-humidity tent can be a challenge. Frequent linen and clothing changes are essential. Often, high humidity oxygen can be administered via nasal catheter rather than by a tent.

> ### ⊙ Safety Alert!
>
> The nurse should inspect all toys when a child is undergoing oxygen therapy. Stuffed toys absorb moisture from the humidity in the oxygen tent, and mechanical or battery toys can create a spark that can be dangerous in high-oxygen environments. Neither toy is acceptable for a child receiving oxygen therapy.

Low-flow oxygen. **Low-flow oxygen** is a method of oxygen delivery used for children with chronic lung disease (e.g., cystic fibrosis) who are oxygen dependent for prolonged periods. These children react poorly to high oxygen concentrations. Approximately 1 or 2 L/min of oxygen is administered via nasal cannula or a "blow-by" catheter that is placed on the upper lip just below the nostrils (Figure 22-18). Because this type of oxygen delivery is used for prolonged periods, parent teaching concerning home management is a nursing responsibility.

Management of Airway Obstruction

Emergency abdominal thrusts and back blows are recommended to dislodge food or foreign bodies from the airway. These techniques work on the principle that forcing the diaphragm upward causes residual air in the lung to be forcefully expelled, resulting in popping the obstruction out of the airway.

Older Child Standing or Sitting. The nurse stands behind the standing or sitting victim and wraps the arms around the victim's waist, with one hand made into a fist (Figure 22-19, C). The thumb side rests against the victim's abdomen, slightly above the navel and well below the tip of the sternum (xiphoid process). The fist is grasped with the other hand and is pressed into the victim's abdomen with a quick upward thrust. From 6 to 10 thrusts may be necessary to dislodge the object. Each thrust should be a separate and distinct movement. The child may be placed in a side-lying position for the recovery phase.

Older Child Lying Down (Conscious or Unconscious). The child is positioned on his or her back. The nurse kneels at the child's feet if the child is on the floor or stands at the child's feet if the child is on a table. The heel of one hand is placed on the child's abdomen in the midline, slightly above the navel and well below the rib cage. The fist is grasped with the other hand and pressed into the victim's abdomen with a quick upward thrust. The 6 to 10 thrusts are repeated as needed. Thrusts are directed upward into the midline and not to either side of the abdomen. The smaller the child, the gentler the procedure.

Infant. The nurse should determine airway obstruction. If the object is visualized, it is removed, trying not to push the object deeper into the throat. If this approach is unsuccessful, the infant is positioned prone with the

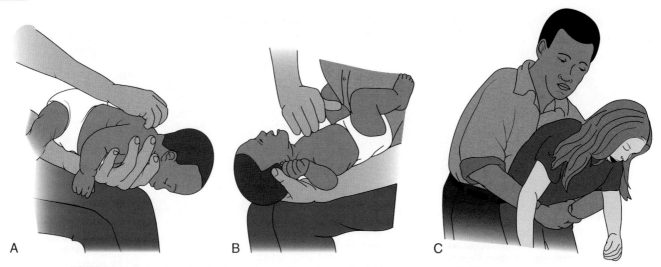

A   B   C

FIGURE 22-19 Procedures for clearing an airway obstruction. **A,** Back blow on an infant. **B,** Chest thrust on an infant. **C,** Abdominal thrust on a child. (From Hockenberry MJ, Wilson D: *Wong's essentials of pediatric nursing,* ed 9, St Louis, 2013, Mosby.)

head lower than the trunk. Support the head and neck with one hand and straddle the infant face down over the forearm, which is supported on the nurse's thigh (see Figure 22-19, *A*). Resting the infant on the thigh, the nurse performs five forceful back blows between the shoulder blades with the heel of one hand. After delivering the back blows, the free hand is placed on the infant's back so that he or she is sandwiched between the two hands; the infant is then turned on his or her back, with the head still lower than the trunk. Five thrusts are delivered in the midsternal region in the same manner as for external chest compressions, but at a slower rate (3 to 5 seconds) (Figure 22-19, *C*). This is repeated until the foreign body is expelled. The nurse should not perform abdominal thrusts, because this may cause injury to the infant's abdominal organs. Conventional cardiopulmonary resuscitation (CPR) can be initiated when the airway is cleared. Because all student nurses are required to have basic CPR certification, the technique is not reviewed in the context of this chapter.

 Safety Alert!

Blind finger sweeps in the mouths of infants and children should be avoided, as foreign bodies may be pushed further into the throat and aspirated.

PREOPERATIVE AND POSTOPERATIVE CARE

Children are particularly fearful of surgery and require both physical and psychological preparation at the child's level of understanding. Listening to the child is especially valuable to clarify misunderstandings. The child is asked to point to the operative site on a body outline. "Show me what they are going to fix." Anesthesia is explained, and the child is allowed to play with a mask (Figure 22-20). Children and adults need reassurance.

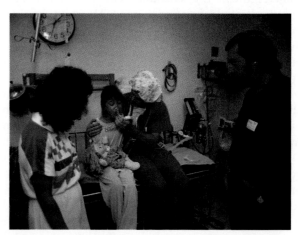

FIGURE 22-20 Preparing the child for the sights and sounds of surgery. The parents may be present during early induction of anesthesia to relieve anxiety during the preoperative period. (From Hockenberry M, Wilson D, et al: *Wong's nursing care of infants and children,* ed 7, St Louis, 2003, Mosby.)

Nursing interventions after surgery are aimed at assisting the child to master a threatening situation and minimizing physical and psychological complications. Tables 22-9 and 22-10 summarize preparation for surgery and postoperative care. Parents are included in all aspects of preoperative and postoperative care.

When adults are prepared for surgery, they are usually kept on NPO status from midnight before the scheduled surgery date. The surgery may be done in the morning or afternoon. Infants should not be maintained on NPO status for longer than 4 to 6 hours because of the high risk for dehydration. It is a nursing responsibility to check that the test procedure or surgery is scheduled as early as possible in the morning to avoid a prolonged wait. Pacifiers should be provided to infants who are on NPO status to meet their developmental need for sucking.

Table 22-9 Comparative Summary of Surgery Preparation of the Adult and Child

PROCEDURE	ADULT	CHILD	MODIFICATION
Consent	Yes	Yes	Parent or legal guardian
Blood work	Yes	Yes	Age-appropriate restraint
Urinalysis	Yes	Yes	Age-appropriate collection (U-bag) Assist school child Age-appropriate instructions
Evaluate for respiratory infection, nutritional status	Yes	Yes	Use more objective observations in infants and toddlers because of child's limited verbal skills
Allergies	Yes	Yes	Indicate clearly on chart
Nothing by mouth (NPO)	Yes	Yes	Increase fluids before NPO Length of time may vary with age and type of surgery (4-12 hours) If surgery is late, place appropriate notice on child: "Do not feed me" Remove "goodies" from bedside stand No gum or hard candy Supervise hungry ambulatory patients carefully
Vital signs	Yes	Yes	Approach child carefully, explain, demonstrate Allow more time
Void before surgery	Yes	Preferred	Not always possible in infants and toddlers
Clothing	Yes	Yes	Hospital gown; may wear underwear or pajama bottoms depending on age, type of surgery
Identification	Yes	Yes	ID bracelet
Teeth	Yes	Yes	Check for loose teeth, orthodontic appliance
Skin preparation	Yes	Possible	May be done in operating room
Nails	Yes	Yes	Trim, remove nail polish
Glasses or contact lenses	Yes	Yes	Have children and adolescents remove glasses or contact lenses
Enemas	Possible	Possible	Not routine
Transportation	Yes	Yes	Crib or stretcher Parents may accompany to operating room door
Emotional preparation	Yes	Yes	Preoperative tour Group and individual puppet play Body drawings of parts involved Play selected by child as mode of expression Support parents during surgery
Sedation	Yes	Yes	Usually 20 minutes before surgery
Record all pertinent data	Yes	Yes	Essentially the same with pediatric modifications as indicated previously

Table 22-10 Comparative Summary of Postoperative Care of the Adult and Child

PROCEDURE	ADULT	CHILD	MODIFICATION
Return from recovery room	Yes	Yes	Notify parents Smaller patients generally in crib Age-appropriate safety precautions
Note general condition, alertness	Yes	Yes	Infant and toddler cannot verbalize fear or pain
Vital signs	Yes	Yes	Every 15-30 minutes until stable Blood pressure is sometimes omitted for infant
Evaluate for shock	Yes	Yes	Essentially the same
Assess operative site for bleeding, condition of dressing	Yes	Yes	Essentially the same Elevate casted extremities Circle drainage on dressing

Continued

| Table 22-10 | Comparative Summary of Postoperative Care of the Adult and Child—cont'd |||

PROCEDURE	ADULT	CHILD	MODIFICATION
Restraints	Possible	Probable	May be necessary to protect intravenous line (IV) such as joint restraints Remove periodically for range of motion
Connect dependent drainage (urinary catheter, nasogastric tubes)	Yes	Yes	Prepare child for sight and noises of equipment; draw pictures to clarify purpose
Position patient	Yes	Yes	Prop on side unless contraindicated, no pillow
Intravenous line (IV)	Yes	Yes	Should have pediatric adapting device and infusion pump with appropriate pressure Monitor rate meticulously, because infants and small children respond quickly to fluid shifts Measure and record intake and output
Assess elimination	Yes	Yes	Bowel and bladder
Relief of pain	Yes	Yes	Hold, comfort small children unless contraindicated Be sensitive to behavioral changes such as increase in irritability, crying, regression, nail biting, passivity, withdrawal Administer pain relievers Involve parents in care Provide transitional object such as blanket, favorite toy, pacifier Be aware of transcultural considerations that provide familiarity and comfort
Nothing by mouth (NPO)	Yes	Yes	Until fully awake Infants are started on clear fluids by bottle unless contraindicated Avoid brown or red liquids, which may be confused with old or fresh blood Monitor bowel sounds
Consider diet	Yes	Yes	Advance from clear to full liquids to soft to regular diet
Observe for complications	Yes	Yes	Turn, cough, deep breathe; dangle feet; ambulate early; less of a problem in children Hold operative site with hands as a splint when child coughs

Surgery and Body Piercing, Body Jewelry, and Tattoos

Body piercing jewelry and tattoos are very common today among teens at every socioeconomic level. Most body jewelry is designed to stay in place and can be covered with an occlusive dressing during surgery without being removed as long as it is not in the operative area (DeBoer, 2008). If removed, the teen should supply a flexible plastic retainer to preserve the opening. Although nipple rings need to be removed before mammography, most body jewelry is made of titanium, niobium, or stainless steel and is not ferromagnetic and therefore can safely remain in place during magnetic resonance imaging (MRI) (DeBoer et al, 2008a). Patients with tattoos or permanent cosmetics are at risk for developing edema or burning during MRI. Tattoo pigments can interfere with the quality of the MRI results; therefore, the radiologist should be made aware of the tattoo through accurate documentation. Appropriate equipment such as ring-opening pliers should be used to remove body jewelry when necessary to avoid skin trauma. The nurse needs to know policies and best practices when the teen with body art is hospitalized (Armstrong, 2009).

Get Ready for the NCLEX® Examination!

Key Points

- The nurse must be especially conscious of safety measures on the children's unit, particularly the following: keeping crib sides up when the child is unattended, careful application of restraints, safe transport, and proper identification of the child.
- The parents are included in both planning and implementing care. Children are prepared for and encouraged to express their feelings about treatments.
- Weight measurements must be accurately recorded in kilograms because medication is calculated according to the child's weight as mg/kg per day or per dose.
- The child's weight in kilograms is part of the mandatory nursing assessment and must be prominently recorded on the medical record and reviewed on each shift hand-off report.

- The correctly sized blood pressure cuff must be used for children to obtain an accurate reading. It should cover two thirds of the upper arm.
- Special urine collection bags are used for newborns and infants.
- Proper positioning of the child for jugular and femoral puncture is important. Because these are large veins, the infant is frequently checked for bleeding after these procedures.
- Medications for children must be adapted to size, age, and body surface. The absorption, distribution, metabolism, and excretion of drugs differ substantially in children. Their reactions to drugs are less predictable than those of adults.
- The nurse should be familiar with tools and techniques that decrease medication errors in pediatric patients.
- The recommended IM injection site for children is the vastus lateralis.
- Careful observation of the child receiving IV fluids is necessary because overload of fluids in an infant can lead to cardiac failure. IV pumps are used to ensure accurate rate and safe administration of intravenous fluid. Intake and output sheets must be accurate.
- The nurse must monitor the rate of the IV flow, observe the condition of the IV site, and document hourly the response of the child.
- When administering ear drops to children younger than 3 years old, the pinna of the ear is pulled down and back to straighten the ear canal. In the older child, the pinna of the ear is pulled up and back.
- A pacifier should be offered to infants whose status is NPO (nothing by mouth).
- Weighing a wet diaper and subtracting the dry weight of a similar diaper is one method of recording the output of infants.
- Preoperative and postoperative care assists the child to master threatening situations and minimize physical and psychological complications.
- Most body jewelry made of titanium or surgical stainless steel is not ferromagnetic and may not need to be removed before MRI or surgery.

Additional Learning Resources

SG Go to your Study Guide for additional learning activities to help you master this chapter content.

evolve Go to your Evolve website (http://evolve.elsevier.com/Leifer) for the following learning resources:
- Animations
- Answer Guidelines for Critical Thinking Questions
- Answers and Rationales for Review Questions for the NCLEX® Examination
- Glossary with English and Spanish pronunciations
- Interactive Review Questions for the NCLEX® Examination
- Patient Teaching Plans in English and Spanish
- Skills Performance Checklists
- Video clips and more!

 Online Resources
- Children's blood pressure measurements: www.scribd.com/doc/8791142/Pediatrics-Hypertension-2008
- Electronic medical library: www.statref.com
- Pediatric information: www.drgreene.com
- Trauma information: www.trauma.org
- Ask the Experts General Vaccine Questions: www.immunize.org/askexperts/experts_general.asp

Review Questions for the NCLEX® Examination

1. Which approach is best when administering an oral medication to a young child?
   1. "Would you please take your medicine now, David?"
   2. "Look how good Johnny took his medication. Can you do that too, David?"
   3. "You must take your medicine now if you want to get better."
   4. "It's time for your medication, David. Would you like water or juice after it?"

2. The preferred site for an intramuscular injection in small infants is:
   1. dorsogluteal.
   2. ventrogluteal.
   3. vastus lateralis.
   4. deltoid.

3. The physician orders 10 mg of Demerol for an infant after surgery. If the label reads 50 mg/mL, the nurse would administer:
   1. 2.0 mL.
   2. 0.8 mL.
   3. 0.5 mL.
   4. 0.2 mL.

4. Which of the following medications can be crushed when administered to a pediatric patient?
   1. Potassium chloride (Slo-K) capsule
   2. Colace gel tablet (Docusate)
   3. Ditropan XL tablet (oxybutynin)
   4. Simethicone tablet

5. The mother and grandmother of a child are at the bedside, rubbing the skin of the child. When the nurse enters the room, the visitors are startled and drop the item they were using to rub the child's skin. The nurse picks up the item and recognizes it as a penny. The best response of the nurse is to:
   1. ask, "What on earth are you doing to that child with this penny?"
   2. give the penny back to the mother and leave the room to give them their privacy.
   3. tell them they could hurt the child with the penny and there are many germs on coins.
   4. return the penny to the mother and open a dialogue about the practice they are using.

Objectives

1. Define each key term listed.
2. Discuss the prevention and treatment of ear infections.
3. Outline the nursing approach to serving the hearing-impaired child.
4. Discuss the cause and treatment of amblyopia.
5. Compare the treatment of paralytic and nonparalytic strabismus.
6. Review the prevention of eyestrain in children.
7. Discuss the functions of the 12 cranial nerves and nursing interventions for dysfunction.
8. Outline the prevention, treatment, and nursing care for the child with Reye's syndrome.
9. Describe the symptoms of meningitis in a child.
10. Discuss the various types of seizures and the relevant nursing responsibilities.

11. Formulate a nursing care plan for the child with a decreased level of consciousness.
12. Describe four types of cerebral palsy and the nursing goals involved in care.
13. Prepare a plan for success in the care of an intellectually or developmentally disabled child.
14. Describe signs of increased intracranial pressure in a child.
15. Describe three types of posturing that may indicate brain damage.
16. Describe the components of a "neurological check."
17. Discuss neurological monitoring of infants and children.
18. State a method of determining level of consciousness in an infant.
19. Identify the priority goals in the care of a child who experienced near drowning.

Key Terms

amblyopia (ăm-blē-Ō-pē-ă, p. 530)
athetosis (ăth-ě-TŌ-sĭs, p. 544)
aura (ĂW-ră, p. 539)
barotrauma (p. 529)
clonic movement (p. 539)
cognitive impairment (p. 546)
concussion (p. 548)
conjunctivitis (p. 532)
dyslexia (p. 530)
encephalopathy (ĕn-sĕf-ă-LŎP-ă-thē, p. 533)
enucleation (ē-nū-klē-Ā-shŭn, p. 533)
epicanthal folds (p. 530)
extensor posturing (p. 550)
flexor posturing (p. 550)
generalized seizures (p. 539)
grand mal (p. 539)
hyperopia (hī-pŭr-Ō-pē-ă, p. 530)
idiopathic (íd-ē-ō-PĂTH-ĭk, p. 539)
intracranial pressure (ICP) (p. 533)

intellectual impairment (p. 546)
ketogenic diet (p. 541)
myringotomy (mĭr-ĭng-GŎT-ŏ-mē, p. 527)
neurological check (p. 533)
nystagmus (nĭs-TĂG-mŭs, p. 538)
opisthotonos (ō-pĭs-THŎT-ō-nŏs, p. 536)
papilledema (păp-ĭl-ă-DĔ-mă, p. 538)
paroxysmal (păr-ŏk-SĬZ-mŭl, p. 539)
partial seizures (p. 541)
petit mal (p. 541)
postictal lethargy (pōst-ĬK-tăl lethargy, p. 541)
posturing (p. 550)
sepsis (SĔP-sĭs, p. 535)
shaken baby syndrome (p. 550)
sign language (p. 528)
status epilepticus (p. 543)
strabismus (stră-BĬZ-mŭs, p. 530)
tonic movement (p. 539)

THE EARS

The ear, which can be considered a part of the nervous system, contains the receptors of the eighth cranial (acoustic) nerve. The fetus can hear at 20 weeks gestation and the auditory nerve function is mature by 5 months of age. The ear performs two main functions: hearing and balance. Figure 23-1 summarizes ear, eye, and neurological differences between children

EARS

- The eustachian tube in infants is shorter, wider, and straighter than in older children and adults, and this may contribute to infections.
- In newborns and young infants, the walls of the ear canal are pliable because of underdeveloped cartilage and bony structures.

EYES

- Infants' eyes may occasionally cross until about 6 weeks of life.
- Tears are scant or absent for the first 2 to 4 weeks of life.

NERVOUS SYSTEM

- Brain and nerve cell growth and specialization are most rapid from birth until about 4 years of age.
- The suture lines and fontanelles of the infant allow for molding during birth and also help compensate for increases in intracranial pressure.
- By the end of the first year, the brain has increased in weight about 2½ times. Brain growth is almost complete by 2 years of age. Measuring head circumference in infants helps determine neurological growth.
- Myelinization of nerve tracts in the central nervous system accelerates after birth and follows the cephalocaudal and proximodistal sequence. This allows for progressively more complex neurological and motor functions.

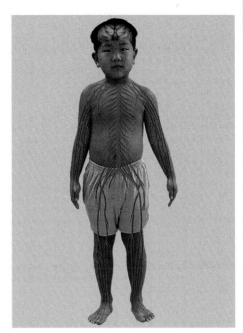

FIGURE 23-1 Summary of the ear, eye, and neurological differences between the child and adult. (Art overlay courtesy Observatory Group, Cincinnati, Ohio.)

and adults. The three divisions of the ear are the external ear, the middle ear, and the inner ear (Figure 23-2). In the newborn, the tympanic membrane is almost horizontal and is more vascular than in the adult. It has a dull and opaque appearance and an inconsistent light reflex. The eustachian tube is shorter and straighter in the infant than in the adult. Three functions of the eustachian tube are *ventilation* of the middle ear, *protection* from nasopharyngeal secretions and sound pressure, and *drainage*. Middle-ear infections are common during early childhood.

When nurses examine the ear, they observe both the exterior and the interior. Ear alignment is observed. The top of the ear should cross an imaginary line drawn from the outer canthus of the eye to the occiput (see Figure 12-6). Low-set ears may be associated with kidney disorders and intellectual or developmental disabilities. The outer ear and the area around it are inspected for cleanliness and drainage. The inner ear is examined with an otoscope. One method of restraint used when assisting with the examination of the inner ear is to lay the child on a table with the arms held alongside the head, which is turned to the side. Another method of positioning a child for an ear examination is to place the child in the lap of the adult (see Figure 22-5).

🏠 Nursing Tip

Before instilling ear drops in *infants*, gently pull the pinna of the ear *down and back*. In *children*, gently pull the pinna of the ear *up and back* to straighten the external auditory canal.

DISORDERS AND DYSFUNCTION OF THE EAR

Otitis Externa

An acute infection of the external ear canal is called *otitis externa* and is often referred to as *swimmer's ear*, because prolonged exposure to moisture is often the precipitating factor. Pain and tenderness on manipulating the pinna or tragus of the ear are specific signs of this type of infection. The ear canal may be erythematous, but the tympanic membrane is normal. A foreign body, cellulitis, diabetes mellitus, and herpes zoster should be ruled out. Irrigation and topical antibiotics or antivirals are the treatments of choice. The health care provider may insert a loose cotton gauze (wick) into the outer third of the ear canal. The wick is kept moist with frequent drops of the appropriate medicated solution.

Acute Otitis Media

Pathophysiology. Otitis media (*ot*, "ear," *itis*, "inflammation of," and *media*, "middle") is an inflammation of the middle ear. The middle ear is a tiny cavity in the temporal bone. Its entrance is guarded by the sensitive tympanic membrane, or eardrum, which transmits sound waves through the "oval window" to the inner ear, which contains the organs of hearing and balance. The middle ear opens into air spaces, or *sinuses*, in the mastoid process of the temporal bone. It is also connected to the throat by a channel called the *eustachian tube*. These structures—the mastoid sinuses, the middle ear, and the eustachian tube—are lined by mucous membranes. As a result, an infection of the throat can

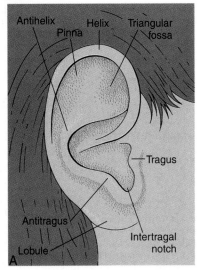
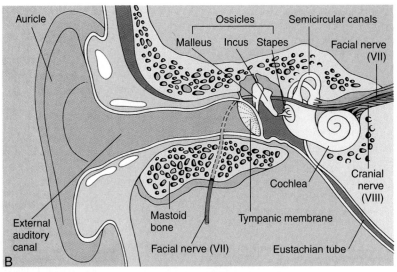

FIGURE 23-2 Anatomy of the ear. **A,** The normal external ear—the auricle (pinna) and tragus—is shown with common landmarks labeled. **B,** There are three divisions of the ear: outer ear, middle ear, and inner ear. In the newborn the mastoid process and the bony part of the external canal are not fully developed, leaving the tympanic membrane vulnerable to injury. Newborns can hear as soon as amniotic fluid is drained by the first sneeze. The eustachian tube connects the middle ear and the pharynx, and it serves to vent the middle ear. In infants the eustachian tube is shorter, wider, and straighter than in adults. Pooling of fluids such as milk in the throat of an infant who falls asleep with a bottle of milk can contribute to ear infections. The external auditory canal is more angulated (curved) in infants, and therefore pulling the pinna (auricle) is required to straighten the canal for an accurate tympanic temperature. (From Zitelli BJ, Davis HW, editors: *Atlas of pediatric physical diagnosis,* ed 4, St Louis, 2002, Mosby.)

easily spread to the middle ear and can lead to mastoiditis. The eustachian tube also protects the middle ear from nasopharyngeal secretions, provides drainage of middle ear secretions into the nasopharynx, and equalizes air pressure between the middle ear and the outside atmosphere. These protective functions are diminished when the tubes are blocked. Unequalized air pressure within the ear creates a negative pressure that allows organisms to be swept up into the eustachian tube.

Otitis media (OM) occurs most often after an upper respiratory tract infection and usually affects children between 6 and 24 months of age and in early childhood. It is caused by various organisms, of which *Streptococcus pneumoniae* and *Haemophilus influenzae* are the most common. Polyvalent pneumococcal polysaccharide vaccines have reduced the incidence of pneumococcal otitis media, but these vaccines are not effective in children less than 2 years of age, because they are not capable of producing an antibody response.

Infants are more prone to middle ear infections than older children and adults because their eustachian tubes are shorter, wider, and straighter. When infants lie flat for long periods, microorganisms have easy access from the eustachian tube to the middle ear. Feeding methods may have a bearing on middle ear infection; for instance, the pooling of fluids such as milk in the throat of an infant who falls asleep with a bottle of milk provides a source for growth of organisms. The infant's *humoral* (*humor,* "body fluid") defense mechanisms are immature. Children in passive smoking environments have more respiratory infections

because of the effect of secondary smoke on the protective cilia that line the nose. Day care attendance can contribute to the risk of upper respiratory infections and OM because of increased exposure to ill children. Upper respiratory infections are discussed in detail in Chapter 25.

> **Nursing Tip**
>
> Signs and symptoms of ear infection can include the following:
> - Rubbing or pulling at the ear
> - Rolling the head from side to side
> - Hearing loss
> - Loud speech
> - Inattentive behavior
> - Articulation problems
> - Speech development problems

Manifestations. The symptoms of OM are pain in the ear, which is often very severe, irritability, and diminished hearing. Fever, which may be as high as 40° C (104° F), headache, vomiting, diarrhea, and febrile seizures may also occur. Earaches in infants may be manifested by general irritability, frequent rubbing or pulling at the ear, and rolling of the head from side to side. The older child can point to the place that is tender. Visualization of the tympanic membrane via otoscope shows a reddened and bulging membrane.

If an abscess forms, a rupture of the eardrum may result, and drainage from the ear may be evident. When this happens, the pressure is relieved and the child is more comfortable. Some amount of hearing loss may result from the rupture. OM is considered chronic if the condition persists for more than 3 months. Recurrent attacks can lead to serious complications. Chronic OM can lead to cholesteatoma (*chole*, "bile," *steato*, "fat," and *oma*, "tumor"), a cyst-like sac filled with keratin debris. This may occlude the middle ear and erode adjacent ossicle bones, causing hearing loss. This condition is best treated by an otolaryngologist. Complications of repeated attacks of acute OM can include the development of chronic OM with effusion (fluid accumulation). Hearing loss can result. Treatment may be indicated because hearing loss may impair cognitive and language development that can hamper the education and communication abilities in developing children.

Treatment. When an infection is evident, treatment is directed toward finding the causative organism and relieving the symptoms. A throat culture may be taken to determine the specific organism. Broad-spectrum antibiotics may be administered orally and should be continued until the prescribed amount of medication has been taken. Analgesics are provided to relieve pain. Antihistamines and decongestants are not effective in treating acute OM.

🖂 Nursing Tip

Instruct caregivers that the child's condition may improve dramatically after antibiotics are taken for a few days. To prevent recurrence, caregivers must continue to administer the medication until the prescribed amount has been completed.

Surgical Treatment. Surgical intervention may be necessary when medical treatment is unsuccessful. The physician may incise the tympanic membrane to relieve pressure and to prevent a tear by spontaneous rupture. This is called a **myringotomy** (*myringa*, "eardrum," and *otomy*, "incision of"). A *tympanic membrane* (TM) button or tympanostomy ventilating tube (pressure equalizer [PE]) may be inserted if the condition becomes chronic, lasts more than 3 months, or causes hearing difficulties that impair school performance. The PE tube may fall out spontaneously within 6 to 12 months. In some children, the tubes may have to be reinserted to continue ventilation. Care no longer needs to be taken to avoid getting water in the ears while bathing or showering, and use of earplugs is no longer required when PE tubes are in place (Rosenfeld, 2013). All children should be followed up to make sure that the condition is resolved and to evaluate any hearing loss that may have occurred.

Comfort Measures. Antipyretics may be given to reduce fever, and a warm compress may be applied locally for comfort. If the eardrum has ruptured, the child is placed on the affected side. Cold may also be beneficial. An ice pack may be prescribed to reduce edema and pressure. The skin around the ears must be kept clean and protected from any drainage to prevent tissue breakdown. Parents are instructed not to insert cotton swabs into the ears.

Hearing Impairment

Pathophysiology. Approximately 1 in 1000 newborns is born with some type of hearing impairment. This number may increase to 5 in 1000 for hearing loss occurring during childhood. Hearing-impaired children present special challenges to the health care team. Hearing loss can affect speech, language, social and emotional development, and behavior, as well as academic achievement. The nurse should have a basic understanding of how to approach and work with a hearing-impaired child.

The inner ear is fully formed during the early months of prenatal life. If an expectant mother contracts German measles or other viral infection during this period, the child may be born with a hearing loss; this is termed *congenital deafness*. Deafness can also be *acquired*. Infectious diseases such as measles, mumps, chickenpox, or meningitis can result in various degrees of hearing loss. The common cold, some medications, exposure to loud noise levels, certain allergies, and ear infections may also be responsible. Hearing problems can also be temporary if they are caused by cerumen (wax) accumulation. Some rattles and squeaky toys can emit sounds as loud as 110 decibels. (Sounds above 80 decibels can cause damage.) These types of toys should not be held close to the infant's ear.

Early diagnosis and treatment of hearing-impaired children are important to prevent adverse physical and mental complications from developing. Members of the health care team concerned with the child who is hearing impaired include the physician, otologist (ear specialist), audiologist, speech therapist, specially trained teacher, social worker, psychologist, school nurse, and members of the child's family.

The various degrees of hearing loss range from a complete bilateral loss (which affects both ears) to a loss so mild that the problem is never recognized. Hearing loss can result from defects in the transmission of sound to the middle ear, from damage to the auditory nerve or ear structures, or from a mixed hearing loss that involves both a defect in nerve pathways and interference with sound transmission. If hearing loss is complete, the child misses all the pleasures of sound and has difficulty in communication (children learn to talk by imitating what they hear). Behavior problems may arise because these children do not understand verbal directions. They may become aggressive with other children in their attempt to communicate. If playmates ridicule them, personality development will be affected. Unless these children are helped early in life, they may become socially isolated.

Partial bilateral deafness may be responsible for behavior problems and poor progress in school. It is most commonly caused by chronic ear infections, such as OM, or by blockage of the eustachian tube. Children who have hearing losses in one ear are less affected if hearing in the other ear is normal.

Nursing Tip

When addressing a hearing-impaired child, the nurse should do the following:

- Be at eye level with the child.
- Be face-to-face with the child.
- Establish eye contact.
- Talk in short sentences.
- Avoid using exaggerated lip or face movement.

Diagnosis and Treatment. The American Academy of Pediatrics recommends a goal of universal detection of hearing impairment in infants before 3 months of age, with interventions started no later than 6 months of age to minimize problems with growth and development (Wolff et al, 2010). The evoked otoacoustic emissions (OAE) test is a preferred method for neonatal testing. The brainstem auditory evoked response (BAER) test records brain wave responses generated by the auditory system. These tests are easily administered to the newborn infant, and many hospitals routinely screen newborns for hearing ability before discharge. Lack of response by the infant to sounds or music or lack of the startle reflex in infants less than 4 months of age are the first signs that may alert the parents or nurse to the possibility of hearing impairment. Early diagnosis and prompt treatment are primary requisites, regardless of the child's age. Complete bilateral deafness is usually discovered during infancy. Partial deafness may be unrecognized until the child begins school. The school nurse, who administers standard hearing tests, detects many hearing problems.

Tympanometry measures ear pressure but is difficult to perform adequately on an active infant or small child. A tuning fork is used to evaluate for air conduction (Rinne test) or bone conduction (Weber test). These types of tests require the child to be cooperative and able to communicate what is heard or felt. Diagnosis of hearing loss can be confirmed by visual reinforcement audiometry (VRA), which identifies sensitivity to sounds in young infants.

Many hearing defects are amenable to medical or surgical treatment. Hearing aids can amplify sound waves. Surgically placed cochlear implants are used for some children with nerve damage. Children who suffer a severe loss of hearing need more extensive help from personnel at an auditory training center. These children must begin treatment as soon as the hearing loss is discovered.

Nursing Care. Various methods are used to bring the child into the world of sound. Lip reading, sign language, writing, visual aids, and amplified sound are but a few examples. The parents are instructed in means of communication that correspond with those used by the teachers.

The nurse must be aware of the symptoms of deafness in the child. Newborns are observed for their responses to auditory stimuli. The Brazelton Neonatal Behavioral Assessment Scale evaluates the infant's orientation response to the sound of a voice. The persistence of the Moro reflex beyond 4 months of age may also be an indication of deafness. The infant who makes no verbal attempts by 18 months of age should undergo a complete physical examination. Indifference to sound, behavior problems, or poor school performance may also be signs of deafness. The nurse inquires into the facilities that are available in the community for such a child.

The hearing-impaired child in the hospital needs the same opportunities to communicate as the child who does not have this disability. The nurse smiles when approaching the child. Body language communicates a lot, especially if there is a severe communication problem. The nurse faces the child when speaking and is positioned at eye level with the child. The nurse must ensure that the child sees him or her before touching to avoid startling the child. **Sign language** is the use of hand signals that correspond to words and assist in communication with a deaf child. Previously developed speech patterns may regress during hospitalization. Visual aids, writing, or drawing can be used to enhance communication.

If a hearing aid is indicated, the child is equipped with one and is taught how to use it. Regular checkups ensure that the hearing aid is working properly. A hearing aid is expensive and invaluable to the child. It is put in a safe place when not in use. When the child goes to surgery, it is given to the parents or placed in the hospital safe. The pockets of hospital gowns are checked before the gowns are placed in the laundry.

The National Hearing Center provides information about hearing aids. Hearing aids are designed to fit in the ear, behind the ear, on eyeglass frames, or on the body with wires to the ear. The nurse should check ear hygiene and be sure hairs are not caught on the end of the hearing aid to ensure a proper fit and to minimize noise and whistling problems. Teaching safe battery handling and storage and promoting self-care are important nursing responsibilities.

Home care of the hearing-impaired child should include speech therapy. Flashing lights should be installed in the home to alert the child to doorbells and other sound-based devices.

Telecommunication devices for the deaf (TDD) are available to enable telephone communication. Closed captioning devices for television are available to the child who can read.

The school nurse can help the family nurture socialization skills. Some hearing-impaired children attend special schools for the deaf, and some are mainstreamed into the general school population. The multidisciplinary health care team should follow each hearing-impaired child and each family unit.

Barotrauma

Barotrauma occurs when there is a change in the atmospheric pressure between the internal body systems and the surrounding environment. An example of barotrauma would be the painful obstruction of auditory tubes when in a pressurized cabin of an airplane. Today many children travel with their families via airplanes and may react to a change in altitude and barometric pressure. During airplane descent, children should be encouraged to yawn or chew on gum to promote swallowing. Infants should be bottle-fed juice or water to promote swallowing, which produces autoinflation and relief of symptoms. Systemic decongestants can be taken before air travel and timed so that their peak effectiveness occurs during airplane descent.

Adolescents may participate in recreational underwater diving that can cause barometric pressure stress to the ear and result in severe earaches and other serious problems. Underwater diving should be slow during the descent phase to minimize negative pressure buildup. Sensory hearing loss and vertigo with nausea and vomiting may be early signs of decompression sickness when it occurs during the ascent phase of diving. The diver should be referred for medical care. Upper respiratory infections or tympanic membrane perforation are contraindications to diving, because vertigo, nausea, vomiting, and disorientation can occur, with dangerous results.

THE EYES

The eye is the organ of vision. The anatomy of the eyeball is depicted in Figure 23-3. The eyes begin to develop as an outgrowth of the forebrain in the 4-week-old embryo. The retinal vessels vascularize (develop) at 40 weeks of gestation, and therefore infants born prematurely often have vision problems throughout their lives. At birth, the eye is 65% of adult size. The newborn's sight is not mature, but the newborn can see. Visual acuity is estimated to be in the range of 20/400. This improves rapidly and may reach 20/40 to 20/30 by 2 or 3 years of age and 20/20 by 6 or 7 years of age. The shape of the newborn's eye is less spherical than the adult's eye. Newborns keep their eyes closed most of the day, can focus and fixate on objects 12 to 30 cm (8 to 12 inches) away for only a few seconds at a time, and cannot coordinate or follow without turning their heads. By 2 to 4 months infants can move their eyes to follow people or objects that may be 6 feet away. By 4 to 5 months their eyes are open most of the day and the tears, when crying, overflow on to the face (visible tears). Eye–hand coordination develops. The nurse should document this, because the ability to transfer objects from one hand to another is partially dependent on the ability to see the object. The development of the ability to crawl is also partially dependent on the ability to see an object at a distance and attempt to reach it. Depth perception is not developed until 9 months of age. When the child walks or runs, visual depth perception influences the child's ability to run without falling.

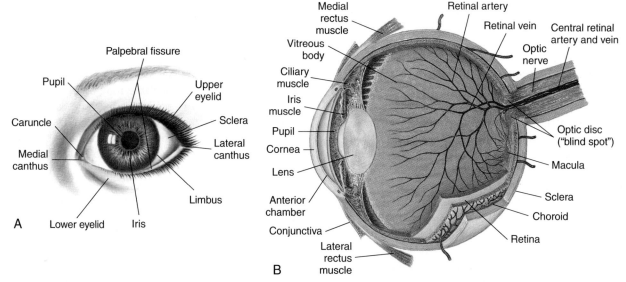

FIGURE 23-3 The normal eye. **A,** External view. **B,** Internal view showing relationship of the optic nerve, eye muscles, and chambers of the eye. (**A** from Hockenberry M, Wilson D: *Wong's nursing care of infants and children,* ed 9, St Louis, 2011, Mosby. **B** from Seidel HM, Ball JW, Dains JE, Benedict GW: *Mosby's guide to physical examination,* ed 5, St Louis, 2003, Mosby.)

The American Academy of Pediatrics (AAP) recommends that all children undergo preschool visual screening during well-child visits between 2 and 3 years of age (Kuhn, 2009).

> **Nursing Tip**
>
> At birth, the quiet, alert infant will respond to visual stimuli by ceasing to move. Visual responsiveness to the mother during feeding is noted. The infant's ability to focus and follow objects in the first months of life should be documented. Coordination of eye movements should be achieved by 3 to 6 months of age.

On physical examination the nurse observes the eyes to see if they are symmetrical and are an equal distance from the nose. **Epicanthal folds** (*epi*, "upon," and *canthus*, "angle") are folds of skin that extend on either side of the bridge of the nose and cover the inner eye canthus. Some folds are broad and cover a large portion of the inner eye, causing the eye to appear crossed. Large epicanthal folds occur as part of some chromosomal anomalies. Pupils are observed for size, shape, and movement. Shining a penlight into the eye, and then quickly removing it allows observation of the eyes' reaction to light. The healthy pupil constricts (gets smaller) as the light approaches and dilates (gets larger) as it disappears (see Figure 23-14). Older children are given explanations concerning the examination. The nurse should assess and document the general appearance of the child as well as achievement of developmental milestones. This includes observing for symmetry of the eye orbit and eyelids, excessive tearing, squeezing of the eyelids, and strabismus (crossed eyes).

> **Nursing Tip**
>
> The achievement of developmental milestones such as transferring objects from hand to hand is partially dependent on seeing the object. Therefore, assessment of visual ability is part of assessment of growth and development.

VISUAL ACUITY TESTS

The ability of an infant to fixate and focus on an object can be demonstrated by 6 weeks of age. The object should not emit a sound so it is certain the infant is turning toward a sight stimulus rather than a sound stimulus.

There are a variety of visual acuity charts (Figure 23-4, *A*). The Snellen alphabet chart and the Snellen E version for preschoolers who have not learned the alphabet are commonly used to assess the ability to see near and far objects. Picture cards are also useful for children who do not know letters. Visual acuity can be tested by 2½ to 3 years of age (Figure 23-4, *B*).

The Titmus machine is often used for school-age children and adolescents. Directions for testing are standardized and must be carefully adhered to for proper results. Computerized tests, such as the random-dot stereogram, are also useful in the visual screening of children. Visual acuity is important in the learning process. Retinopathy of prematurity (ROP) is discussed in Chapter 13.

DISORDERS AND DYSFUNCTION OF THE EYE

Dyslexia

Dyslexia (*dys*, "difficult," and *lexis*, "diction") is a reading disability that involves a defect in the cortex of the brain that processes graphic symbols. Although an eye evaluation is recommended when a child has mirror vision or word reversal, the problem does not involve any local eye defect. Correcting vision problems will aid in optimal visual function, but treatment for dyslexia involves remedial instruction.

Amblyopia

Pathophysiology. **Amblyopia** (lazy eye) is a reduction in or loss of vision that usually occurs in children who strongly favor one eye. If both retinas do not receive a clearly defined image, bilateral amblyopia may result. However, it is more common for one eye to be affected. When abnormal binocular interaction occurs (such as crossed eyes or strabismus), the prognosis depends on how long the eye has been affected and on the age of the child when treatment begins. The earlier the treatment is given, the better the results. One commonly accepted diagnostic sign is that vision in the normal eye is at least two Snellen lines (E charts) better than that in the affected eye. There are various types of amblyopia. Strabismus is the most common; however, dissimilar refractory errors can also result in this condition. Because amblyopia occurs as a result of sensory deprivation of the affected eye, children are at risk for developing the problem until visual stability occurs, usually by 9 years of age.

Treatment and Nursing Care. Early detection and prompt treatment are essential. The goal of treatment is to obtain normal and equal vision in each eye. Treatment consists of eyeglasses for significant refractive errors such as **hyperopia** (farsightedness) or myopia (nearsightedness) and patching (occlusion) of the *good eye*. The good eye is patched to force the use of the affected eye. Daytime patching may be tried first, since part-time occlusion is sufficient in some cases. Occlusion therapy is often difficult to maintain. The nurse can help by explaining the importance of the procedure and by offering support, but the child is often subjected to teasing by peers. Providing a safe place to express feelings is important to promoting a healthy self-image. In most cases an opaque contact lens or a contact lens of sufficiently high power to blur the vision in the better eye is used (Kliegman et al, 2011).

Strabismus

Pathophysiology. **Strabismus** (cross-eye), also known as *squint*, is a condition in which the child is not able to direct both eyes toward the same object. There is a lack of coordination between the eye muscles that direct movement

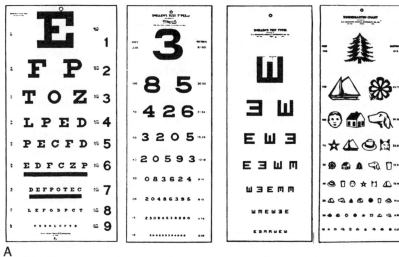

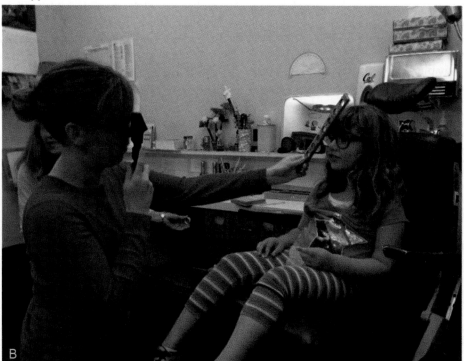

FIGURE 23-4 **A,** Various types of visual acuity charts. The "E" chart is often used for young children who can "show which way the fingers of the *E* are pointing." **B,** A 4-year-old child responds to a detailed vision assessment. (**A** from Behrman RE, Kliegman RM: *Nelson textbook of pediatrics,* ed 14, Philadelphia, 1992, Saunders.)

of the eye. When the eyes cannot coordinate sight together, the brain will disable one eye to provide a clear image. The disabled eye can develop permanent visual impairment because of sensory deprivation (amblyopia). Normal binocular vision is the goal and must be accomplished by intervening early before the eye matures.

There are several types of strabismus. *Nonparalytic strabismus* (concomitant) involves a constant deviation in the gaze related to faulty insertion of the eye muscle. One eye always looks crossed. The extraocular muscles are normal. *Paralytic strabismus* (nonconcomitant) involves a paralysis or weakness in the extraocular muscle. Double vision is experienced. Deviation of the gaze occurs with movement, when the eye attempts to focus. To prevent double vision (*diplopia*) the child

will tilt his or her head or squint when focusing on an object. Strabismus may be present at birth or may manifest after a disease or injury. This type of strabismus can occur after head trauma or a neurological disease. It is important to note that epicanthal folds can provide a false impression of strabismus.

Nursing Tip

Symptoms of strabismus include the following:
- Eye "squinting" or frowning to focus
- Reaching for objects and missing them
- Covering one eye to see
- Tilting the head to see
- Dizziness and/or headache

Treatment. In nonparalytic strabismus, the refractory error is usually corrected with eyeglasses. When paralytic strabismus is seen during early infancy, the physician may recommend that a patch cover the unaffected eye until the infant is old enough to wear glasses. The affected eye may improve through use and often becomes normal. Eye exercises and glasses are effective ways of treating the condition medically. If they do not help, surgery should be considered. It is generally performed when the child is 3 or 4 years of age. Early correction is necessary to prevent amblyopia. If strabismus is left untreated, blindness in the affected eye may result, because the brain tends to obliterate the confusing double image by disabling the eye.

Nursing Care. The child undergoing surgery for strabismus might be hospitalized for only a brief period. The surgery involves structures outside the eyeball; therefore the child is allowed to be up and about postoperatively. Eye dressings are kept at a minimum, and elbow restraints may be sufficient to keep the child from touching the dressings.

Prevention of Eyestrain. Children, who are beginning to read, need books with large type in which the letters are spaced far apart. The lighting must be adequate and without glare. Chairs and desks must be of the proper height.

Symptoms that may indicate eyestrain include inflammation, aching or burning of the eyes, squinting, a short attention span, frequent headaches, difficulties with schoolwork, or an inability to see the blackboard. It is important for the nurse to *observe* the child for eyestrain, to *teach* proper eye care, to *prevent* complications of eyestrain or strabismus, to *refer* as needed for follow-up care, and to assist in *rehabilitation.*

Conjunctivitis

Conjunctivitis (*conjungere,* "to join together," and *itis,* "inflammation") is an inflammation of the conjunctiva, which is the mucous membrane that lines the eyelids (Figure 23-5). A wide range of bacterial and viral agents, allergens, irritants, toxins, and systemic diseases can cause conjunctivitis. Conjunctivitis that

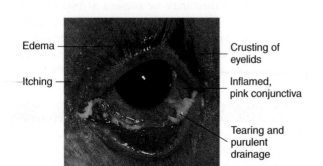

Edema

Itching

Crusting of eyelids

Inflamed, pink conjunctiva

Tearing and purulent drainage

FIGURE 23-5 Acute bacterial conjunctivitis. Signs of conjunctivitis are evident in this highly contagious infection. (From Newell FW: *Ophthalmology: principles and concepts,* ed 7, St Louis, 1992, Mosby.)

occurs with viral exanthems such as measles is usually self-limiting. It is common in childhood and may be infectious or noninfectious. The acute, infectious form is commonly referred to as *pinkeye.* Pinkeye is considered no longer contagious after 24 hours of appropriate antimicrobial therapy. Conjunctivitis can also result from an obstruction of the lacrimal duct. In general, the common forms of conjunctivitis respond to warm compresses and topical antibiotic eye drops or eye ointments. Ointments blur vision and are not generally used during daytime hours in the ambulatory child.

The nurse instructs parents to administer the eye medication for the prescribed time to prevent recurrence. Parents and older children are taught to wipe secretions from the **inner canthus downward and away from the opposite eye.** Because conjunctivitis spreads easily, affected children should use separate towels and be instructed to wash their hands frequently. *Ophthalmia neonatorum,* an acute conjunctivitis in the newborn, is discussed in Chapter 6. Allergic conjunctivitis is often associated with allergic rhinitis (*rhin,* "nose," and *itis,* "inflammation") in children with hay fever. Symptoms include itching, tearing of one or both eyes, and edema of the eyelids and periorbital tissues. The child may appear distracted and irritable.

Periorbital Cellulitis

An infection of the eyelid and tissues surrounding the eye sometimes occurs in school-age children as a complication of bacterial sinusitis (inflammation of the sinus). Pain and swelling around the eye are common symptoms of periorbital cellulitis. Intravenous antibiotics may be required to prevent spread of the infection to the brain.

Hyphema

Hyphema, the presence of blood in the anterior chamber of the eye, is one of the most common ocular injuries. It can occur from either a blunt or a perforating injury. Blows from flying objects (e.g., baseballs, snowballs) and forceful coughing or sneezing can cause this condition. These accidents are common among active school-age children. Hyphema appears as a bright red or dark red spot in front of the lower portion of the iris.

Treatment includes bed rest and topical medication. The head of the bed is elevated 30 to 45 degrees to decrease intraocular pressure and decrease intracranial pressure if there is an associated head injury. The condition generally resolves itself without residual problems.

Retinoblastoma

Pathophysiology. *Retinoblastoma* is a malignant tumor of the retina of the eye. There are hereditary and spontaneous forms. The average ages at diagnosis are 12 months for bilateral tumors and 21 months for unilateral tumors (Kliegman et al, 2011). Gene-mapping techniques have shown chromosome 13 to be affected in hereditary forms. Chromosome 13 is also known to cause other congenital defects.

Manifestations. A yellowish white reflex is seen in the pupil because of a tumor behind the lens. This is called the *cat's eye reflex* or *leukokoria* (*leuk*, "white," and *kore*, "pupil"). This may be accompanied by loss of vision, strabismus, hyphema, and, in advanced tumors, pain. Metastasis to the unaffected eye is common in unilateral tumors. When retinoblastoma is suspected in children, an examination is performed using an anesthetic so the pediatric ophthalmologist may carefully examine the fundus of the eye.

Treatment and Nursing Care. The standard treatment for unilateral disease is **enucleation** (removal) of the eye if there is no possibility of saving the vision. Small tumors are treated with laser photocoagulation to destroy the blood vessels supplying the tumor. Larger tumors can be treated with chemotherapy or external beam irradiation.

On return from enucleation surgery, the child has a large pressure dressing on the eye. Elbow restraints may be necessary to prevent removal of the dressing. The bandage is observed for bleeding, and the vital signs are assessed. After a few days the surgeon removes the dressing and applies an eye patch. Other structures of the eye, such as the lids, lashes, and tear glands, are not affected. An eye prosthesis is fitted when the socket has healed. Instructions for care of the prosthesis are provided at the time of final fitting. Providing education and emotional support for the child and family and referral to the multidisciplinary health care team are essential.

THE NERVOUS SYSTEM

The nervous system is the body's communication center; it receives and transmits messages to all parts of the body. It also records experiences (memorization) and integrates certain stimuli (learning). The anatomy of the nervous system is depicted in Figure 23-6. Neural tube development occurs during the third to fourth week of fetal life. This eventually becomes the central nervous system (CNS). The fusing process of the neural tube is critical. Its failure to fuse may lead to congenital conditions such as spina bifida (see Chapter 14). Most neurological disabilities in childhood result from congenital malformation (birth defects), brain injury, or infection. The 12 cranial nerves and their functions are shown in Figure 23-7.

Skull x-ray films, electroencephalography (EEG), computed tomography (CT), magnetic resonance imaging (MRI), electromyography, and other methods, including a **neurological check** may detect central nervous system dysfunction (see Box 23-6 and Table 23-6). The reflexes of the newborn are good indicators of neurological health. A decreased level of consciousness in the ill child may be an indication of a neurological problem. Box 23-1

describes the causes of altered levels of consciousness. In the finger–nose test (used to determine coordination), the child is asked to extend the arm and then to touch his or her nose with the index finger. This is done with the eyes opened and closed. The inability to balance on one foot in a school-age child necessitates further follow-up. The 12 cranial nerves, selected forms of dysfunction, and nursing interventions are described in Table 23-1.

> **! Safety Alert!**
>
> The sudden appearance of a fixed and dilated pupil is a neurologic emergency.

DISORDERS AND DYSFUNCTION OF THE NERVOUS SYSTEM

Reye's Syndrome

Pathophysiology. **Reye's syndrome** is an acute noninflammatory **encephalopathy** (pathology of the brain) and *hepatopathy* (pathology of the liver) that follows a viral infection in children. There may be a relationship between the use of aspirin (acetylsalicylic acid) during a viral flu or illness such as chickenpox (varicella) and the development of Reye's syndrome. For this reason, aspirin use is generally contraindicated for the pediatric population. Some studies show that a genetic metabolic defect triggers Reye's syndrome.

> **! Medication Safety Alert!**
>
> Discourage the use of aspirin and other medications that contain salicylates in children with flulike symptoms. Advise parents to read medication labels carefully to determine their ingredients.

Manifestations. Liver cell pathology causes an accumulation of ammonia in the blood. Toxic levels of ammonia cause cerebral manifestations (e.g., cerebral edema, increased **intracranial pressure [ICP]**), which results in neurological changes such as altered behavior, altered level of consciousness, seizures, and coma.

In children, the sudden onset of effortless vomiting and altered behavior (e.g., lethargy, combativeness) or altered level of consciousness after a viral illness is characteristic of Reye's syndrome. The results of blood tests assessing liver function will be abnormal. In infants, diarrhea, hypoglycemia, tachypnea with apneic episodes, and seizures may occur approximately 1 week after a respiratory illness.

Prevention. The education of the public concerning the dangers of using salicylate-containing medications during viral illnesses such as varicella in children may have contributed to the decline in the occurrence of Reye's syndrome. The availability of the varicella vaccine may also have an impact on the reduced incidence of Reye's syndrome.

Treatment. Early treatment can result in recovery with some neuropsychological deficits. However, progression to the acute stage is often rapid and unpredictable. The goals of treatment include reducing ICP and maintaining a patent airway, cerebral oxygenation, and fluid and electrolyte balance.

Frequent assessment of vital signs and a careful assessment of neurological status are essential.

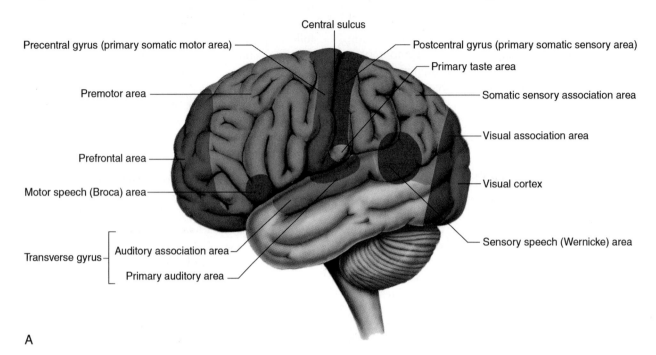

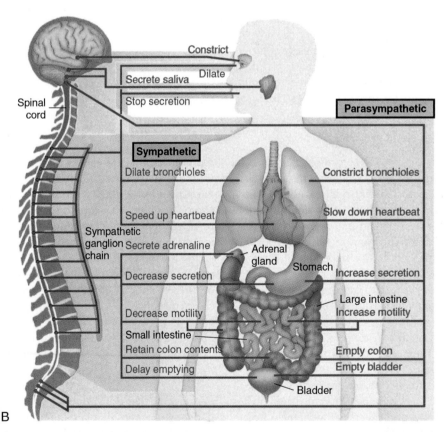

FIGURE 23-6 A, Functional areas of the brain. Each area of the brain has a specific function. Damage to the local area can cause loss of that function. **B,** The nervous system, and the innervation of target organs by the autonomic nervous system. The sympathetic pathways are shown in orange, and the parasympathetic pathways are shown in green. (**A** from Patton KT, Thibodeau GA: *Anatomy & physiology,* ed 9, St Louis, 2013, Mosby. **B** from Thibodeau GA, Patton KT: *Structure and function of the body,* ed 13, St Louis, 2008, Mosby.)

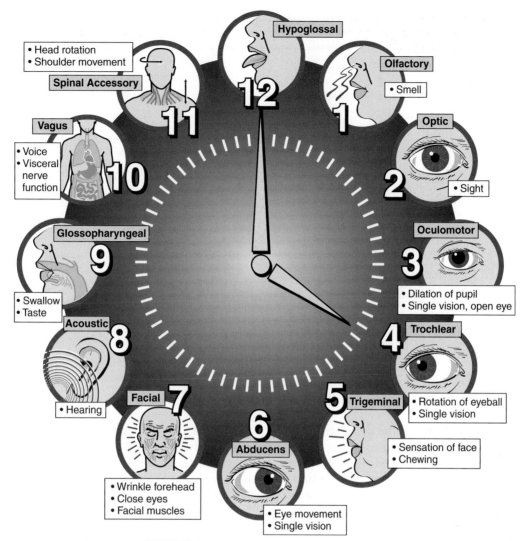

FIGURE 23-7 The 12 cranial nerves and their functions.

Box **23-1** | **Causes of Altered Level of Consciousness (LOC)**

- A fall to 60 mm Hg or below of Pao_2
- A rise above 45 mm Hg of $Paco_2$
- Low blood pressure causing cerebral hypoxia
- Fever (1° F rise in fever increases oxygen need by 10%)
- Drugs (sedatives, antiepileptics)
- Seizures (postictal state)
- Increased intracranial pressure (ICP)

Observation for signs of bleeding is important because liver dysfunction causes blood-clotting abnormalities. Parental education and support are necessary. Encouraging parents to participate in their child's care helps to reduce the parents' and child's levels of anxiety.

Sepsis

Sepsis is the systemic response to infection with bacteria and can also result from viral and fungal infections. Sepsis causes a systemic inflammatory response syndrome (SIRS) because of the endotoxin of the bacteria that causes tissue damage. Untreated sepsis results in septic shock, multiorgan dysfunction syndrome (MODS), and death. Children who are immune-compromised, who have neutropenia, or who are in intensive care receiving invasive therapy are at increased risk for developing sepsis.

Manifestations. Manifestations of sepsis include fever, chills, tachypnea, tachycardia, and neurological signs such as lethargy. Septic shock is not diagnosed by a decrease in blood pressure, because the infant's body initially compensates for the poor circulation and tissue perfusion by increasing the heart rate and vasoconstriction of peripheral blood vessels. Hypotension is an ominous sign that may indicate that the body is unable to compensate adequately and cardiorespiratory arrest is about to occur. Laboratory test results may include positive blood cultures, reduced fibrinogen and thrombocyte levels, and the presence of immature white blood cells. Neutropenia (neutrophil count below $1000/mm^3$) is an ominous sign. The nursing responsibilities include monitoring neurological status and vital

Table 23-1   **The 12 Cranial Nerves: Selected Dysfunctions and Nursing Interventions**

CRANIAL NERVE		DYSFUNCTION	NURSING INTERVENTIONS
I	Olfactory	Inability to smell	Appetite may be suppressed; present food attractively.
II	Optic	Inability to control pupil reflex	Protect eyes from glaring lights.
III	Oculomotor	Double vision	Cover eyes.
IV	Trochlear	Inability to move eyes	When communicating, remain in child's view.
V	Trigeminal	Difficulty in chewing	Provide soft foods.
VI	Abducens	Inability to control corneal reflex	Have eye ointment or eye patch on hand to protect cornea.
VII	Facial	Inability to close eye	Protect eyes with moist dressing.
VIII	Acoustic	Inability to hear	Maintain body language for communication.
IX	Glossopharyngeal	Inability to taste or to control gag and cough reflexes	Provide visually attractive food. Keep tracheotomy tray and suction at bedside.
X	Vagus	Difficulty in talking or swallowing; visceral malfunction	Provide means of communication. Assess for aspiration. Assess body system functions and vital signs.
XI	Spinal accessory	Controls head, turns, and shrugs shoulders	Provide position change and support.
XII	Hypoglossal	Controls tongue movement, thick speech	Have suction ready; observe ability to chew and swallow. Provide method of communication.

signs; observing for shock; and maintaining strict standard and expanded precautions (see Appendix A). Intravenous antibiotics are prescribed. To prevent sepsis, immunization against *H. influenzae* type B (Hib) and administration of pneumococcal conjugate vaccine (PCV) that are recommended for all children between 2 months and 4 years of age may prevent some cases of sepsis, however sepsis may be the result of other bacterial sources.

Meningitis

Pathophysiology. **Meningitis** is an inflammation of the meninges (the covering of the brain and spinal cord). Various organisms can cause bacterial meningitis. Organisms may invade the meninges indirectly by way of the bloodstream (sepsis) from centers of infection such as the teeth, sinuses, tonsils, and lungs, or directly through the ear (otitis media), or from a fracture of the skull.

Bacterial meningitis is often referred to as *purulent,* that is, pus forming, because a thick exudate surrounds the meninges and adjacent structures. This can lead to certain sequelae such as subdural effusion and, less frequently, hydrocephalus. The peak incidence for bacterial meningitis is between 6 and 12 months of age. Meningococcal meningitis is readily transmitted to others. Meningitis is less common in children older than 4 years of age. *H. influenzae* is the most common causative agent. *H. influenzae* type B vaccine and PCV have decreased the incidence of bacterial meningitis. The approaches to nursing care for all types of meningitis are similar.

Manifestations. The symptoms of purulent meningitis result mainly from intracranial irritation. They may be preceded by an upper respiratory infection and several days of gastrointestinal symptoms such as poor feeding. Severe headache, drowsiness, delirium, irritability, restlessness, fever, vomiting, and stiffness of the neck (nuchal rigidity) are other significant symptoms. A characteristic high-pitched cry is noted in infants. Seizures are common. Coma may occur fairly early in the older child. In severe cases, involuntary arching of the back caused by muscle contractions is seen (Figure 23-8). This condition is called **opisthotonos**

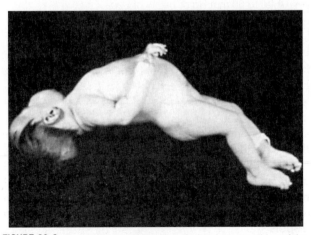

FIGURE 23-8 The opisthotonos position. An involuntary arching of the back and extension of the neck are seen in children with brain injury or meningeal irritation. Note that the back is arched so that the head is on an even level with the heels. (From Behrman R, Kliegman R, Jenson HB: *Nelson textbook of pediatrics,* ed 17, Philadelphia, 2004, Saunders.)

(*opistho*, "backward," and *tonos*, "tension"). The presence of *petechiae* (small hemorrhages beneath the skin) suggests meningococcal infection. Diagnosis is confirmed by examination of the cerebrospinal fluid (CSF).

 Safety Alert!

The acutely ill and lethargic child who develops a rash with petechiae must be referred for immediate follow-up care.

Treatment. At the first indication of meningitis, the physician performs a spinal tap (lumbar puncture, see Chapter 22) to obtain a specimen of CSF for laboratory testing. The spinal fluid may be clear in the early stages of the illness, but it rapidly becomes cloudy. The CSF pressure is increased, and further laboratory analysis indicates a high white cell count, an increase in protein, and a decrease in glucose.

The child is placed in isolation until 24 hours after antibiotic therapy has been initiated. An intravenous (IV) line is established for the administration of antibiotics and to restore fluid and electrolyte balance. Antibiotics are selected on the basis of culture and sensitivity laboratory results. Antibiotics are usually administered for a minimum of 10 to 14 days. A sedative may be provided to reduce the child's restlessness. An anticonvulsant such as phenytoin (Dilantin) may also be required to decrease the risk of seizure activity. Dexamethasone reduces complications of bacterial meningitis but is not used in nonbacterial meningitis.

Nursing Care. The single room is prepared in accordance with hospital protocol (see Appendix A for transmission-based precautions). Nursing responsibilities include performing frequent neurological checks and maintaining an accurate recording of the child's vital signs and intake and output. The nurse should also organize care so that the child is disturbed as little as possible.

The child with meningitis may be overly sensitive to stimuli; therefore the room should be dimly lit and the noise kept to a minimum. The nurse carefully raises and lowers the sides of the crib to avoid jarring the bed. The nurse avoids startling the child and so uses a soft voice and gentle touch. These precautions are also explained to the parents.

Frequent monitoring of the child's vital signs is necessary. A slowed pulse rate, irregular respirations, and increased blood pressure are reported immediately, because they could indicate increased ICP. Antipyretics, sponge baths, or a hypothermia (cooling) mattress may control fever. The nurse observes the child for additional or subtle signs of increased ICP, especially a change in alertness or muscles twitching. The joints are also observed for swelling, pain, and immobility. Oxygen is given as ordered.

The child's intake and output are carefully observed and recorded. Careful attention is given to maintaining the IV line. Good oral hygiene is essential during this stage when the child is receiving nothing by mouth. As the child's condition improves, the diet progresses from clear fluids to an age-appropriate diet. A special formula may be given when nasogastric feedings are necessary. During the convalescent period, oral fluids are encouraged unless contraindicated. The nurse promptly reports a decrease in output of urine (oliguria), which could signal urinary retention. Bowel movements are recorded each day to detect constipation and prevent *fecal impaction* (an accumulation of feces in the rectum). The nurse continues to monitor neurological status and to record and report findings such as weakness of the limbs, speech difficulties, mental confusion, and behavior problems. The child should be assessed for developmental deficiencies. When recovery is uneventful, the child may be discharged home. The parents are taught the principles of intermittent IV therapy that can be accomplished in the home setting with visits from a home health agency nurse.

Nursing Tip

When a spinal tap is planned, the infant can be sedated and EMLA cream applied to the area to reduce discomfort during needle insertion.

 Safety Alert!

A child diagnosed with meningitis remains on transmission-based droplet precautions until 24 hours after appropriate antimicrobial therapy has been started.

Encephalitis

Pathophysiology. *Encephalitis* (*encephalo*, "brain," and *itis*, "inflammation") is an inflammation of the brain. The condition is known as *encephalomyelitis* (*myelo*, "spinal cord") when the spinal cord is also infected. "Togaviruses" (ribonucleic acid [RNA] viruses) and herpesvirus types 1 and 2 can cause this disorder; it can be the aftermath of disorders such as upper respiratory tract infections, German measles (rubella), or measles (rubeola), or, rarely, an untoward reaction to vaccinations such as diphtheria, tetanus, and pertussis (DTaP); and it may also result from lead poisoning. Other causative agents include bacteria, spirochetes, and fungi.

Nursing Tip

Encephalitis may occur as a complication of childhood diseases such as measles, mumps, or chicken pox. It is crucial that children receive the immunizations available for the diseases that are preventable.

Manifestations. The symptoms of encephalitis result from the CNS response to irritation. Characteristically, the history is that of a headache followed by drowsiness that may proceed to coma. Because coma is sometimes prolonged, encephalitis is sometimes referred to as "sleeping sickness." Seizures are seen, particularly in infants. Fever, cramps, abdominal pain, vomiting, stiff neck (nuchal rigidity), delirium, muscle twitching, and abnormal eye movements are other manifestations of the disease.

Treatment and Nursing Care. The treatment is supportive and aimed at providing relief from specific symptoms. Sedatives and antipyretics may be prescribed. Seizure precautions are taken. Adequate nutrition and hydration are maintained. The nurse provides a quiet environment, good oral hygiene, skin care, and frequent changes of position. Oxygen is administered as ordered, and the mouth and nose are kept free of mucus by gentle aspiration. Bowel movements are recorded daily, because the child may be constipated from the lack of activity. Preventing the secondary effects of immobilization is paramount.

The nurse closely observes the child for neurological changes. Fatality rates and residual effects are higher among infants than among older children. Speech, mental processes, and motor abilities may be slowed, and permanent brain damage and intellectual or developmental disabilities can result. Growth and development and hearing evaluations should be monitored. Parents are encouraged to help with the care of the child as soon as the condition is stable. They are instructed about the nursing procedures for home care and any required follow-up care.

Brain Tumors

Pathophysiology. **Brain tumors** are the second most common type of neoplasm in children (the first is leukemia). The majority of childhood tumors occur in the lower part of the brain (cerebellum or brainstem).

The etiology of these tumors is unknown. They occur most commonly in school-age children.

Manifestations. The signs and symptoms are directly related to the location and size of the tumor. Most tumors create increased ICP with the hallmark symptoms of headache, vomiting, drowsiness, and seizures (Figure 23-9). **Nystagmus** (constant jerky movements of the eyeball), strabismus, and decreased vision may be evident. **Papilledema** (edema of the optic nerve) may occur. Other symptoms include ataxia, head tilt, behavioral changes, and cerebral enlargement, particularly in infants. Deviations in vital signs are noticeable when the tumor presses on the brainstem.

Treatment and Nursing Care. Clinical manifestations, laboratory tests, CT, MRI, and EEG confirm the diagnosis. Angiography is used to assist in the surgical approach by identifying the tumor's blood supply. Radiotherapy, chemotherapy, or surgery may be indicated.

Preoperative emphasis is placed on carefully explaining various procedures and on familiarizing the child and family with the recovery room, intensive care unit (ICU), and hospital personnel. The nurse explains that the child will have part or all of his or her head shaved. The size of the postoperative dressing is carefully explained. Applying a similar dressing to a doll may be helpful to the child. Trendelenburg position is avoided, because it increases ICP.

Postoperative care is usually provided in the ICU. Adjuncts to care may include using a hypothermia (cooling) blanket or a mechanical respirator. Parents must be prepared for the appearance of the child after surgery. Empathic family support and appropriate referral are offered.

Radiation treatment may be prescribed. The radiologist outlines the areas to be treated on the child's head.

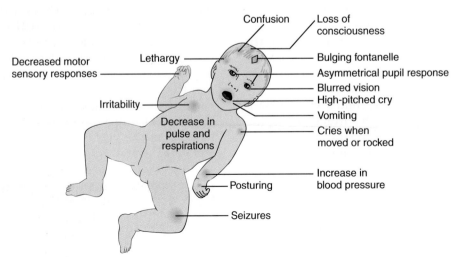

FIGURE 23-9 Signs of increased intracranial pressure (ICP) in infants and children.

These marks are not to be washed off. Small doses of radiation are provided throughout a period of weeks. Chemotherapy may follow irradiation.

Nursing Tip

The timing of providing information is important when preparing the child for various procedures.

Safety Alert!

Sluggish, dilated or unequal pupils may indicate increased ICP and must be reported promptly.

Seizure disorders

Seizures are the most commonly observed neurological dysfunction in children. The etiology varies (Box 23-2). Seizures are sudden, intermittent episodes of altered consciousness that last seconds to minutes and may include involuntary tonic and clonic movements. A **tonic movement** is a stiffening (contraction) of muscles. A **clonic movement** is an alternating contraction and relaxation of muscles. It may include changes in perception, behavior, sensations, and posture.

Febrile Seizures. Febrile seizures are a transient condition common in children between 6 months and 5 years of age. There may be a genetic predisposition explaining why children in the same family have this problem. The seizure occurs in response to a rapid rise in temperature—often above a level of 38.8° C (102° F). Because the seizure lasts a short time and is no longer present when the child reaches a hospital, causes other than fever may have to be ruled out. Simple febrile

Box 23-2 Causes of Seizures in Children

INTRACRANIAL
Epilepsy
Congenital anomaly
Birth injury
Infection
Trauma
Degenerative diseases
Vascular disorder

EXTRACRANIAL
Fever
Heart disease
Metabolic disorders
Hypocalcemia
Hypoglycemia
Dehydration and malnutrition

TOXIC
Anesthetics
Drugs
Poisons

seizures are treated by teaching the parent to control the fever by appropriate use of antipyretics (e.g., acetaminophen) and cooling measures (e.g., removing heavy blankets and clothing). Parents should be reassured that the condition is self-limiting. The use of phenobarbital is not effective and may decrease cognitive function. Valproic acid (Depakene) produces side effects. These drugs are not recommended for first-time treatment. Rectal or oral diazepam (Valium) for the duration of a febrile illness may be prescribed if febrile seizures recur. Side effects such as lethargy, irritability, or ataxia (lack of muscular coordination) should be reported. Febrile seizures rarely develop into epilepsy, and the affected child has an excellent prognosis without residual problems.

Epilepsy

Pathophysiology. The term *epilepsy* (chronic recurrent seizures) derives from the Greek *epilepsia*, which means "seizure." In the past, words such as fit, spell, and blackout were commonly used to describe this entity. These terms are nonspecific, and they tend to create confusion.

Epilepsy is a disorder manifested by a variety of symptom complexes. It is characterized by recurrent **paroxysmal** (sudden, periodic) attacks of unconsciousness *or* impaired consciousness that may be followed by contraction (tonic movements) and relaxation (clonic movements) resulting in alternating tonic and clonic movements of the muscles *or* abnormal behavior. It is a disorder of the CNS in which the neurons or nerve cells discharge in an abnormal way. These discharges may be focal or diffuse. The site of general discharge can sometimes be ascertained by observing the child's symptoms during the attack. It may be caused by a head injury or meningitis. When the cause is unknown, the term **idiopathic** epilepsy is used.

The nurse observes and records the following: the child's activity immediately before the seizure; body movements; changes in color, respiration, or muscle tone; any incontinence; and the parts of the body involved. When possible, the seizure is timed. The child's appearance, behavior, and level of consciousness after the seizure are also documented. Table 23-2 describes the first aid response and nursing responsibilities during a seizure.

Types of epilepsy. Childhood epilepsy is classified into partial seizures and generalized seizures.

Grand mal

Generalized seizures. **Generalized seizures** involve a loss of consciousness. The most common generalized seizure is the *tonic-clonic* or **grand mal**. A grand mal epilepsy has three distinct phases:

1. An *aura* (subjective sensation)
2. A *tonic-clonic seizure*
3. **Postictal lethargy**—a short period of sleep after a generalized seizure

Table 23-2   Seizure Recognition and First Aid Response

SEIZURE TYPE	WHAT IT LOOKS LIKE	OFTEN MISTAKEN FOR	WHAT TO DO	WHAT NOT TO DO
1. General: generalized tonic-clonic (also called *grand mal*)	Sudden cry (or *aura*), fall, rigidity, followed by *muscle jerking;* shallow, irregular breathing; possible loss of bladder or bowel control; usually lasts seconds to minutes, followed by some confusion, a period of sleep (*postictal lethargy*), and then return to full consciousness	Heart attack, stroke	Look for medical identification. Protect from nearby hazards. Observe and record stages and manifestations. Following seizure, maintain patent airway, turn on side, loosen clothing, reassure person. If multiple seizures, or if one seizure lasts longer than 5 minutes, call ambulance (911). If person is pregnant, injured, or diabetic, call for aid at once.	Do not put any hard implement in the mouth. Do not try to hold tongue; it cannot be swallowed. Do not try to give liquids during or just after seizure. Do not restrain person.
2. Absence (also called *petit mal*)	A blank stare, beginning and ending abruptly, lasting only a few seconds; most common in children; may be accompanied by rapid blinking, some chewing movements of the mouth; person is unaware of what is going on during the seizure but quickly returns to full awareness after it has stopped; may result in learning difficulties if not recognized and treated	Daydreaming, lack of attention, deliberate ignoring of adult instructions	No first aid necessary, but if this is first observation of seizure(s), medical evaluation should be recommended. Can be triggered by flashing lights or hyperventilation.	
3. Partial A. Simple partial (also called *Jacksonian*)	Jerking may begin in one area of body such as arm, leg, or face; cannot be stopped, but person stays awake and aware; jerking may proceed from one area of the body to another and sometimes spreads to become a generalized seizure	Acting-out, bizarre behavior, hysteria, mental illness, psychosomatic illness, parapsychological or mystical experience, tics	No first aid necessary unless seizure becomes generalized, then first aid as indicated. No immediate action needed other than reassurance and emotional support. Medical evaluation should be recommended.	
B. Complex partial (also called *psychomotor* or *temporal lobe*)	Usually starts with blank stare, followed by chewing, followed by random activity; person appears unaware of surroundings, may seem dazed and may mumble; is unresponsive; actions are clumsy, not directed; may pick at clothing, pick up objects, try to take off clothes; may run, appear afraid; may struggle or flail at restraint; after pattern established, same set of actions usually occurs with each seizure; can last 1 to 2 minutes; no memory of actions or behavior	Disorderly conduct	Speak calmly and reassuringly to person and others. Guide person gently away from obvious hazards. Stay with person until completely aware of environment. Offer to help getting home.	Do not grab hold unless sudden danger threatens (such as a cliff edge or an approaching car). Do not try to restrain person. Do not shout. Do not expect verbal instructions to be obeyed.
4. Atonic seizures (also called *drop attacks* or *myoclonic* or *infantile spasms*)	More frequent occurrence in the morning with jerking motions on awakening; suddenly collapses; after 10 seconds to 1 minute, person recovers and can stand and walk again	Clumsiness, normal childhood stage; lack of good walking skills; drunkenness	No first aid needed (unless hurt during fall), but the person should be given a thorough medical evaluation.	

Petit mal, or *absence,* seizures often are recognized when an intelligent child is referred for medical evaluation because of unexplained failure to achieve in school. The reason for school failure is found to be absence seizures, which cause a temporary loss of awareness that results in a lack of continuity in the learning environment.

Other types of general seizures include *myoclonic spasms,* where repetitive muscle contractions occur, and *infantile spasms,* which occur in infants less than 1 year of age and are manifested by a jackknife posture for frequent but brief periods.

Partial seizures. **Partial seizures** account for 40% of childhood seizures. Consciousness may be intact or slightly impaired. *Simple partial seizures* (Jacksonian) are often mistaken for alterations in behavior or "tics," which usually involve only the face or shoulders. *Complex partial seizures* can be manifested by motor activities, sensory signs, or psychomotor (behavioral) activity.

Treatment. Initially, treatment is aimed at determining the type, site, or cause of the disorder. Diagnostic measures include a complete history and physical and neurological examinations. Skull radiography and CT or MRI scans are used to establish the presence or absence of tumors, skull abnormalities, hematomas, and intracranial calcifications. The EEG is also a valuable tool in diagnosing seizures. It is especially helpful in differentiating between an absence seizure and a complex partial seizure. Prolonged EEG monitoring (24 hours) is another diagnostic technique.

Laboratory studies such as complete blood count (CBC), determinations of serum calcium and blood urea nitrogen (BUN), and tests to rule out lead poisoning or other metabolic disorders are performed. Anticonvulsant medications are prescribed when epilepsy is the diagnosis (Table 23-3). The drug of choice depends on the type of seizure, and the goal is the use of only one drug that will control the seizures with the fewest side effects.

The duration of therapy is based on the individual child. Initially, the physician prescribes the lowest dose of anticonvulsant medication likely to control the seizures. The goal is to control the seizures and minimize the toxic effects of the medication. Drowsiness, a common side effect of many anticonvulsants, may interfere with the child's activities. Careful recording of seizure activity and compliance with the drug regimen are of particular importance in determining a suitable program. The medication is administered at the **same time each day,** generally with meals or at bedtime.

If it is necessary for the child to take medication during school hours, the parents sign a consent form so that the school nurse can monitor the administration. The responses of the nurse and teacher, particularly during and after a seizure, will have a significant effect on the attitude of classmates toward the child.

Abrupt withdrawal of anticonvulsant medications is the most common cause of status epilepticus (prolonged seizures). In the hospital, the nurse clarifies with the physician whether anticonvulsants are to be withheld if the child is to be given nothing by mouth (NPO). When children are old enough, they can assume responsibility for their own medications. They should wear a medical identification bracelet. During puberty and adolescence, the dosages may have to be adjusted to meet growth needs. Anticonvulsant drugs should not be taken during pregnancy, because birth defects can occur. Premenstrual fluid retention in girls can sometimes trigger seizures. Surgery is being performed on children who are unresponsive to anticonvulsants and who have a well-defined focus of seizure activity in the brain.

> **! Medication Safety Alert!**
>
> Children taking phenobarbital or phenytoin (Dilantin) should receive vitamin D and folic acid supplementation. Phenytoin should not be given with milk.

The **ketogenic diet** is sometimes prescribed for children who do not respond well to anticonvulsant therapy. The diet is high in fats and low in carbohydrates, with adequate protein. This diet produces ketoacidosis in the body, which appears to reduce convulsive episodes. A reduction of fluid intake tends to increase the ketogenic effect. The use of this diet is limited, because it is boring and requires strict adherence to intake, and compliance tends to be a problem. Long-term effects of this type of diet, such as hyperlipidemia, are unknown but may lead to heart attack or stroke if used long-term (Epilepsy Foundation, 2010).

Rebellion against medical routine is not uncommon during adolescence. Some states do not allow controlled epileptics to obtain a driver's license, which is disheartening to the child. Other states have stipulations regarding the amount of seizure-free time required before licensing. Excess intake of fluids, particularly alcoholic beverages, can trigger a seizure. Parents can obtain valuable information and support from the Epilepsy Foundation of America. Other major resources include the Department of Vocational Rehabilitation, the Department of Public Health, the Department of Social Services, and other community agencies.

The greatest untapped resource for persons with epilepsy is often within themselves. A fundamental principle of comprehensive epilepsy management is that the child must become an active member of the health care team. In a comprehensive multidisciplinary treatment approach, team members help the child to mobilize his or her inner resources to handle the lifelong treatment and to lead a fully

Table 23-3   Properties of Selected Anticonvulsant Drugs

DRUG	SIDE EFFECTS	COMMENTS
Carbamazepine (Tegretol)	Grapefruit juice may increase levels Causes photosensitivity Interacts with erythromycin	Few side effects, fewer sedative properties; used for general and partial seizures Give with food.
Phenobarbital (Luminal)	Drowsiness, irritability, hyperactivity	Altered sleep patterns, often combined with other drugs
Phenytoin (Dilantin)	Ataxia, insomnia, nystagmus, gum overgrowth, hirsutism (hairiness), rash, nausea, vitamin D and folic acid deficiencies	Generally effective and safe; may cause cognitive impairment; regular massaging of gums decreases hyperplasia; used in combination with phenobarbital. Intravenous (IV) doses should not be mixed with glucose solutions.
Valproic acid (Depakene)	Gastrointestinal upset, liver toxicity, amenorrhea, weight gain	Take with food. Do not chew; potentiates action of phenobarbital and other drugs. Do not administer with carbonated beverages. Should not be taken during pregnancy. Monitor platelets.
Primidone (Mysoline)	Personality changes, anorexia, fatigue, dermatitis	May be used alone or in combination; side effects minimized by starting with small amounts. Provide folic acid supplements.
Ethosuximide (Zarontin)	Anorexia, gastrointestinal upset	Often used for absence seizures Give with food.
Felbamate (Felbatol)	Monitor liver and blood reports	Used in partial seizures Can be used as only antiseizure medication
Topiramate (Topamax)	Slow cognition, fatigue May cause psychomotor slowing	Used for complex partial seizures Increase fluid intake.
Gabapentin (Neurontin)	Weight gain and somnolence	Used in poorly controlled seizures. Do not take with antacid. Monitor vision and concentration.
Lamotrigine (Lamictal)	Ataxia, rash, photosensitivity, and drowsiness	Do not give with valproic acid.
Keppra (Levetiracetam)	Sleepiness, incoordination, behavior changes	Used with other medications for partial seizures. Monitor coordination.

Note: The physician determines the child's medication by the type of seizure and other factors. The goal is to achieve the best control with the minimum dosage and the least number of side effects. An important aspect of nursing intervention includes reinforcing the need for drug supervision and compliance.
Data from David R: *Pediatric neurology*, New York, 2010, Demos Medical Publishing; Ferril C: Rufinamide: an antiepileptic drug for Lennox-Gastaut syndrome, *Exp Rev Neurotherapeutics* 19(6):857-860, 2010; Wilson B, Shannon M, Shield K: *Nurses drug guide*, Upper Saddle River, N.J, 2011, Pearson-Prentice-Hall.

productive, normal life. With a few safety guidelines, this is possible.

Restriction of physical activity is not necessary, but adult supervision during swimming or bathing is advisable. A family assessment is helpful in establishing rapport and setting realistic short- and long-term goals. Too much attention to seizures by well-meaning adults can make control difficult. The child may learn to use the threat of a seizure to manipulate caregivers. Teaching should include first aid treatment for seizures (see Table 23-2), the importance of compliance with long-term medication regimens, and general reassurance that the child can lead a normal life. Medications used in the treatment of epilepsy are outlined in Table 23-3. The gum hypertrophy (Figure 23-10) that occurs as a side effect of phenytoin (Dilantin) will require meticulous oral hygiene and special care, especially if orthodontic treatment is necessary. Death or serious injury rarely occurs from a seizure, and it does not cause mental deterioration. The Individuals with Disabilities Education Act (IDEA) guarantees children with disabilities the right to publicly financed educational programs in the least restrictive environment possible.

Safety Alert!

The nurse is responsible for maintaining seizure precautions for a child diagnosed with a seizure disorder.

In the hospital:
- Keep side rails up.
- Pad all sharp or hard objects around the bed.

In the community:
- Make sure child wears a medical ID bracelet.
- Provide supervision during potentially hazardous play, such as swimming.
- Avoid triggering factors.
- Teach the importance of compliance with the medication regimen.

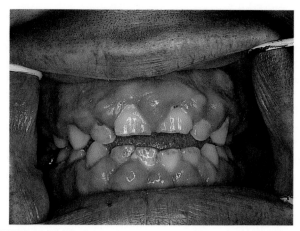

FIGURE 23-10 Phenytoin-induced gum hyperplasia. (From Callen JP, Greer KE, Paller AS, Swinyer LJ: *Color atlas of dermatology*, ed 2, Philadelphia, 2000, Saunders.)

Status epilepticus. A prolonged seizure that does not respond to treatment for 30 minutes or more is called **status epilepticus**; it can result in brain hypoxia. A common cause is sudden stopping of epilepsy medication or generalized infection. Treatment includes managing the airway, providing oxygen, observing and documenting details of the seizure, and providing IV therapy. Diazepam, lorazepam, phenytoin, or a pentobarbital drug may be given intravenously. Rectal diazepam or intranasal midazolam are safe and effective approaches for treating status epilepticus. The child may need to be supported on a mechanical ventilator until seizures are controlled.

Nursing Tip

Common triggering factors for seizures include the following:
- Flashing of dark/light patterns
- Startling movements
- Overhydration
- Photosensitivity

Other Conditions Causing Decreased Level of Consciousness

Several conditions are mistaken for epilepsy because they involve paroxysmal altered levels of consciousness. These conditions do not respond to antiepileptic drugs.

Benign Paroxysmal Vertigo. This condition occurs in children less than 3 years of age, who often develop ataxia and fall. Nausea, vomiting, and complaints of motion sickness and migraine headache follow. The condition responds to dimenhydrinate (Dramamine) medication.

Night Terrors. Night terrors occur in children between 5 and 7 years of age. The child may sleepwalk, thrash, scream, and be unaware of his or her surroundings. A period of sleep follows. Brief treatment with diazepam (Valium) or imipramine (Tofranil) may be helpful, but family dysfunction should be investigated.

Breath-Holding Spells. Breath holding can result in cyanosis or extreme pallor. Episodes of breath holding are most common between 2 and 5 years of age. The child loses consciousness, and the parents are frightened. Counseling parents to avoid reinforcing the behavior by refusing to play with or hold the child after the episode is helpful.

Cough Syncope. Cough syncopes are paroxysmal coughing spells, usually at night, that result in a diminished cardiac output, cerebral hypoxia, and loss of consciousness. The condition usually occurs in asthmatic children. Prevention involves avoidance of bronchoconstriction.

Prolonged QT Syndrome. One type of sudden loss of consciousness is associated with vigorous exercise. It can be caused by a heart problem and reflected as a prolonged QT segment on the ECG, and it can result in loss of consciousness and death. It usually occurs during adolescence and arises from a defect in chromosome 11. Beta-blockers may be lifesaving. Knowledge of cardiopulmonary resuscitation (CPR) and exercise restriction are essential.

Rage Attacks, or Episodic Dyscontrol Syndrome. Rage attacks are sudden recurrent attacks of violent physical behavior. These attacks appear out of control and are followed by fatigue, remorse, and amnesia. The EEG is usually normal. This condition is often mistaken for complex partial seizure epilepsy.

Cerebral Palsy
Pathophysiology. **Cerebral palsy** (CP) is a term used to describe a group of motor disorders caused by dysfunction of various motor centers in the brain. A definition proposed in 2007 suggests that CP "is a group of permanent disorders of the development of movement and posture, causing activity limitations that are attributed to nonprogressive disturbances occurring in the developing fetal or infant brain" (Rosenbaum, 2007). It also involves problems with sensation and communication secondary to the musculoskeletal problems. It is now believed that CP results most often from existing prenatal brain abnormalities, exposure to maternal chorioamnionitis in utero, prematurity, or severe hypoglycemia. CP can be acquired as a result of shaken baby syndrome, meningitis, or encephalitis. Some 15% to 60% of children with CP also develop epilepsy. CP is not fatal in itself, but currently there is no cure. It is one of the most common disabling conditions seen in children and occurs in as many as 2 per 1000 live births (Kliegman, 2011).

Manifestations. The symptoms of CP vary with each child and may range from mild to severe. Many children with CP have normal intelligence. The disease is suspected during infancy if there are feeding problems,

Table 23-4   Types of Cerebral Palsy

TYPE	CHARACTERISTICS
Spastic	Involves damage to the cortex of the brain Spasms occur with movement Related to cerebral asphyxia
Athetoid (dyskinetic)	Involves damage to the basal nuclei ganglion Continuous involuntary writhing movements Often associated with hyperbilirubinemia
Ataxic	Uncoordinated movements and ataxia from a lesion in the cerebellum
Mixed	Usually a combination of spastic and athetoid

seizures not associated with high fever, and developmental delays. Developmental milestones are not achieved at the expected age levels. Persistence of primitive reflexes such as the Moro and tonic neck reflexes may be seen. Diagnostic tests may include metabolic and genetic testing and MRI. Early recognition is important for appropriate referrals.

There are four types of CP (Table 23-4). Two of the more common are those marked by spasticity and athetosis (Figure 23-11). These conditions occur in about 75% of the cases. *Spasticity* is characterized by tension in certain muscle groups. The stretch reflex

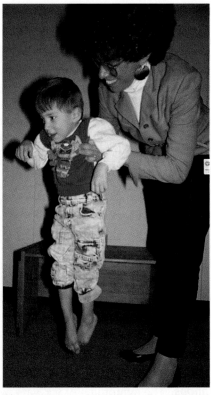

FIGURE 23-11 A child with spastic cerebral palsy. Note the legs crossing in a scissorlike pattern when the child is supported in vertical suspension. (From Zitelli BJ, Davis HW, editors: *Atlas of pediatric physical diagnosis,* ed 4, St Louis, 2002, Mosby.)

is present in the involved muscles. When the child tries to move the voluntary muscles, jerky motions result. Eating, walking, and other coordinated movements are difficult to accomplish. The lower extremities are usually involved. The legs cross and the toes point inward. The arms and trunk may also be affected. In **athetosis** the child has involuntary, purposeless movements that interfere with normal motion. Speech, sight, and hearing defects or seizures may be complications. The success in preventing kernicterus in the newborn by effective treatment of hyperbilirubinemia has reduced the incidence of the athetoid type of CP.

Treatment and Nursing Care. The goal of treatment of children with CP is to assist them in making the most of their assets and to guide them in becoming well-adjusted adults, performing at their maximum ability. Both short- and long-term goals must be realistic. Parents need help in accepting the child and should not be deceived into expecting miraculous cures from treatment. Early diagnosis can result in fewer physical and emotional problems. Botulinum toxin has been used successfully to manage spasticity problems, and levodopa has helped control some athetoid symptoms. An implanted pump that delivers baclofen directly into the intrathecal space around the spinal cord can reduce spasticity. This type of medication delivery produces less acute side effects than oral baclofen. Antiepileptic drugs such as carbamazepine (Tegretol) and valproic acid (Depakote) may be prescribed if seizures are present. Pain management and medication for gastroesophageal reflux may be prescribed. Dental hygiene is important because phenytoin, often prescribed for seizures, causes gum hyperplasia. Computerized toys that are customized to the child aid in developing hand–eye coordination. Voice-activated computer technology can also aid the child to communicate needs and manage wheelchairs. Physical therapy is essential to prevent contractures and deformities. Approximately 30% to 50% of children with CP are mentally handicapped, but many children with severe, spastic quadriplegia have normal intelligence. Gastrostomy tube feedings may be required to augment nutritional intake (see Skill 22-10).

Parents must be informed of community resources available to them. The family's religious affiliation should not be overlooked, because it can be a source of support and help during times of stress. The long course of this disability can place a financial burden on the family. Caregivers need respite care from time to time to enhance their coping skills.

The specific treatment is highly individualized and depends on the severity of the disability. It is not uncommon for the parents of children with CP to become the experts in caring for their children. Therefore the parent should be an integral part of the health care team.

Good skin care is essential for the child with CP. The nurse observes the skin for redness and other evidence of pressure sores. All precautions are taken to prevent the formation of *contractures* (degeneration or shortening of the muscles because of lack of use), which could result in permanent loss of function of the part involved (e.g., leg, arm, or finger). The nurse encourages these children to do as much as they can for themselves. When they bathe, they are encouraged to put their muscles and joints through the normal range of motion. The nurse must use judgment in assessing their capabilities and assist only in those areas where they are lacking.

Other measures necessary to prevent contractures include frequent changes of position, the use of splints, and the performance of passive, range-of-motion, and stretching exercises. The nurse must also ensure that the child maintains good posture while in bed. This is done through the use of footboards and the proper positioning of pillows and other comfort devices.

Braces are often used to treat contractures. A brace is a mechanical aid that supports weakened muscles or limbs. All braces are routinely checked for correct alignment, loose or missing parts, and the condition of straps and buckles. The child needs assistance to adjust to this unfamiliar device. Wheelchairs and crutches are designed to fit the child.

Orthopedic surgery may be indicated and may be followed by an extensive period of rehabilitation. The nurse must remember that the child is in a continuous state of psychological and physical growth during this period. Maintaining interest and efforts in achieving developmental milestones whenever possible may have a decided effect on the personality of the child in later years.

Feeding problems can lead to nutritional deficiencies. Vitamin, mineral, or protein supplements may be indicated for some children. Swallowing and sucking may be difficult. Vomiting is common because the gag reflex is overactive. The entire body may become tense. The nurse must be especially careful to feed the child slowly to prevent aspiration. It is difficult for these infants to adjust to solid foods, and it takes a great deal of patience on the part of parents and nurses to help the child to adapt to this new experience (Skill 23-1 and Figure 23-12). As the children grow, they can be taught to manage special feeding equipment so they are able to eat independently. They are also taught such activities as dressing and combing their hair. Dental care is discussed in Chapter 15.

The physically challenged child needs opportunities to play alone and with other children. Games suited to ability, such as finger painting, are fun and allow freedom of expression. Activities that require fine muscular movements of the hand cause frustration in the child whose arms and hands are affected by the disease. The nurse can learn a great deal from the parents about the types of play the child enjoys. Children with CP tire easily but find it difficult to relax. They use a great deal of energy to accomplish the simplest of tasks, and they do not respond well to being hurried or overly stimulated.

Educational opportunities geared to the child's abilities are essential. Public Law 94-142 mandates that public schools provide education for disabled children.

General Modifications and Precautions in Pediatric Feeding Techniques for Children with Cerebral Palsy

PURPOSE

To facilitate safe feeding and prevent aspiration

STEPS

1. Ensure proper positioning and support of the head and back before feeding solid foods.
2. Place small amounts of food on a spoon to prevent choking.
3. Avoid tilting the head back during feeding of solid foods, because this will place the swallowing mechanisms out of alignment.
4. Do not touch the tip of the child's tongue with the spoon, because this can activate the tongue extrusion reflex.
5. Use rubber-coated spoons for children with hyperactive bite reflex to protect the teeth from injury.
6. Gently stroke the angle of the jaw below the ears to relax the bite of a child who has clamped down on a spoon.
7. Gently stroke the area under the chin in a circular motion to stimulate chewing when food is held in the mouth.
8. Gently press upward under the chin to stimulate swallowing when fluid is held in the mouth.
9. To help a disabled child drink from a cup, cut the top portion of the paper or plastic cup away to provide space for the nose. This will enable the cup to be tilted without the child's head being tilted back.
10. Avoid excessive pressure on the back of the head when positioning a disabled child for feeding to prevent reflex responses in the body or torso position.

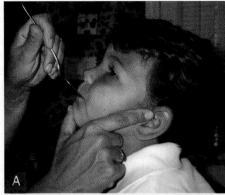

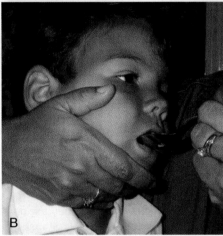

FIGURE 23-12 Feeding the disabled child. **A,** Manual jaw control is supplied anteriorly. **B,** Manual jaw control is provided from the side. (From Hockenberry M, Wilson D: *Wong's nursing care of infants and children*, ed 9, St Louis, 2011, Mosby.)

The child's mental capacity is determined not just in the light of the intelligence quotient (IQ) itself but also by the demonstrated potential of the individual.

Preschools and summer camps for exceptional children are available. These programs vary in quality and extent of services. Parents are also referred to the United Cerebral Palsy Association, a national organization that provides education and support services. The expanding role of nurses in the home and schools may further assist in mainstreaming these children into educational and social situations (Box 23-3).

Successful experiences help to improve a child's self-concept; repeated failures are demoralizing and may lower self-esteem. The health care team works to bring satisfaction to these children by making it possible for

---

Box 23-3 **Treatment Protocol for Cerebral Palsy**

1. Establish communication.
2. Establish locomotion.
3. Use and optimize existing motor functions.
4. Provide intellectual stimulation.
5. Promote socialization.
6. Provide technology to encourage self-care and promote growth and development.
7. Provide multidisciplinary approach to care.

---

them to succeed. The amount of confidence and self-respect that a disabled child has depends a great deal on a supportive environment.

Mental Health Needs of the Physically Challenged Child. The requirements for good mental health in the physically challenged child do not differ from those of other children. They need to have their basic human requirements satisfied and they need people who are genuinely interested in them. The disabled child must participate to the fullest extent in family, school, and community activities. Friendships with other disabled and nondisabled peers are encouraged. Extended family and the community are important resources. Educational programs are integrating the disabled more fully into the community. Barrier-free buildings and modifications that improve accessibility contribute positively to these efforts.

Cognitive Impairment

Cognitive impairment or **intellectual impairment** is a term that encompasses any type of mental deficiency or mental disability.

Intellectual Impairment. Intellectual impairment and disability are terms that replace "mental retardation," which was often used to describe a type of developmental disability characterized by mental and physical impairment. Intellectual impairment or disability have been defined as below-average mental functioning (IQ below 70) and a deficit in adaptive behavior, conceptual skills, or social skills manifested during the developmental period (before 18 years of age) (Box 23-4). Since 1992, the American Association of Intellectual and Developmental Disabilities (AAID) refocused the definition of mental retardation and the emphasis was shifted away from IQ alone and onto a relationship-oriented concept of the cognitively impaired person functioning within an environment (American Association on Mental Retardation [AAMR], 2010; AAID, 2013). That classification involved four levels of support systems needed for activities of daily living (ADLs): the

---

Box 23-4 **Identifying Adaptive Behavior Deficits**

Intellectual functioning below IQ of 75
Limitations in at least two of the following 10 areas of adaptive behaviors:

1. Communication
2. Self-care
3. Home living
4. Social skills
5. Community use
6. Self-direction
7. Health and safety
8. Functional academics
9. Leisure
10. Work

need for intermittent support, limited support, extensive support, or pervasive (total) support. Intellectual disability had many descriptive labels. The specific terminology most often used in the medical field in the past, was mental retardation, whereas the education system most often used mentally handicapped, mentally deficient, mentally disabled, mentally impaired, or mentally challenged. The education system uses various criteria for classroom placement and eligibility for available resources. For educational purposes, cognitively impaired children may be classified as educable, educable-mildly impaired, or trainable moderately impaired. U.S. federal law provides for services from birth to 21 years of age. Public law requires providing the least restrictive environment possible for learning, and mainstreaming with nonimpaired students whenever possible.

The *DSM-5 2013* clearly identifies the use of the term *intellectual impairment*. The American Psychological Association published the *DSM-5* in 2013 in an attempt to help clinicians identify and diagnose mental disorders. The *DSM-5* standardizes criteria in agreement with the WHO International Classification of Diseases. The *DSM-5* also identifies symptom severity for individual disorders and is compatible with disabilities resulting from the disorders as described in the International Classification of Functioning Disabilities and Health (ICF). The term *intellectual disability* or *intellectual developmental disorder* currently replaces the term "mental retardation" that involves impairment of general mental abilities that affect functioning related to everyday tasks and includes language, reading, math, reasoning, memory, social skills, judgment, communication skills, and self-management abilities.

When a child is diagnosed as intellectually impaired, it is important to correlate growth and development with mental functioning. For example, abstract thinking does not begin to appear before 12 years of age. A child classified as intellectually impaired is not necessarily impaired in all areas of mental functioning (Box 23-5). There are numerous tests to measure intelligence. One test that is often given to children and adolescents is the Stanford-Binet.

Intelligence in children is difficult to evaluate and is best tested on an individual basis. Personality tests such as picture story tests, ink blot tests, drawing tests, and sentence completion tests may also be administered. All such tests have their limitations, and of course their accuracy is subject to the abilities of the person interpreting them. Nonetheless, the tests are of value when used in conjunction with a thorough study of the child's physical, mental, emotional, and social development.

There are many causes of intellectual impairment. Some conditions that can be detected during the neonatal period are phenylketonuria, hypothyroidism, fetal alcohol syndrome, Down syndrome, malformations of the brain (e.g., microcephaly, hydrocephalus, craniosynostosis), and maternal infections such as cytomegalovirus (CMV). Birth injuries or anoxia during or shortly after delivery may also cause intellectual impairment. Conditions such as meningitis, lead poisoning, neoplasms, and encephalitis can cause intellectual impairment in a child or adult of any age. Heredity is a factor in intellectual impairment. It is also possible that living in a physically and emotionally deprived environment causes the child to be intellectually impaired. A diagnosis of intellectual disability is determined after a thorough study is made. The American Psychiatric Association (2013) provides diagnostic criteria for intellectual impairment in the *DSM-5*.

Autism spectrum disorders, eating disorders, PTSD, specific learning disorders involving academic skills, substance abuse, and disruptive mood regulation disorders are defined. Disruptive mood regulation disorders replace bipolar disorder in children and are characterized by disruptive irritability with outbursts more than three times a week for more than 1 year (*DSM-5, 2013*). Conditions such as epilepsy, CP, severe malnutrition, emotional disturbances, blindness, deafness, and speech disorders must be ruled out. In certain cases, early recognition and intervention can lessen or prevent intellectual impairment. The child may be classified as having a developmental delay before a diagnosis of cognitive impairment is made.

Other symptoms of intellectual impairment are associated with milestones of the growth process. Children who do not achieve milestones at the expected age may be cognitively impaired. Unusual clumsiness and failure to respond to stimuli are also early indications. Sometimes this disorder is not discovered until the child enters school. There are many tests for assessing adaptive behaviors including the Vineland Social Maturity Scale and the Adaptive Behavior Scale. Each case must be frequently reevaluated according to the child's individual progress. The goal of care is to normalize the child and family as much as possible.

Specific behavioral disorders are discussed in Chapter 33.

Box 23-5	**Elements Involved in Mental Functioning**

LEVEL OF CONSCIOUSNESS
Attention
Short- and long-term memory
Perceptions

THOUGHT PROCESSES
Insight
Judgment
Affect
Mood

EXPRESSIVE LANGUAGE
Vocabulary
Abstract thinking
Intelligence

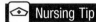 **Nursing Tip**

Cognitively or intellectually impaired children have the same psychosocial needs as all other children, but they cannot express themselves or respond as other children do.

The importance of success in the approach to the intellectually impaired child. We cannot all run at the same speed, sing with the same ability, dance as gracefully or draw as skillfully as some of our peers. Yet most of us get by. However, problems can develop if one is not good in something such as reading, writing, and communicating (which, in our culture, are very important). The problems usually relate to the consequences of chronic failure. Computers can assist with spelling deficiencies, and calculators can assist with math deficiencies.

The pediatric nurse must assist the parents to understand that providing experiences in which the child can be successful, and concentrating on his or her strengths rather than weaknesses, are the keys to helping a child who is developmentally different. A child who experiences consistent failure becomes angry. The anger causes behavior difficulties that can cloud the problem and the therapy.

 Nursing Tip

The intellectually impaired child needs to develop a sense of accomplishment. Do not "take over" projects because of your own need to assist or speed up the process.

Management and nursing goals. An individualized plan of care with goals and objectives is vital to managing intellectually impaired children and helping their families. The initial step is to present the findings to the family and to provide the emotional support necessary to cope with a disabled child. The child's competence and adaptive behaviors should be discussed along with the deficiencies. Introduction to the multidisciplinary team for long-term management is important. Play therapy should be prescribed to nurture growth and development. The Special Olympics introduce healthy competition to the cognitively and physically impaired child. Receptive and expressive communication skills are developed with professional help.

Nurses must be familiar with the resources of the community so that they can direct the family to them. The local chapter of the AAMR may provide information and support. Summer camps, such as those run by the Easter Seals Society, provide stimulation and opportunities for socialization to children with intellectual and developmental disabilities. The child guidance clinic or the psychological services of a nearby college or hospital may be used. Arrangements for proper dental care must be made because some children may be unable to cooperate with the necessary procedures.

The nurse caring for the intellectually impaired child in the hospital must know the child's stage of

maturation and ability. A detailed history, including a habit and care sheet, is completed. Self-help activities are documented. Home routines are to be followed as closely as possible to avoid the reversal of gains already made. Good communication between the parents and the nurse can help to make the transition from home to hospital as smooth as possible for the child. A positive approach is recommended when obtaining information about the child from the parents. A request such as "Tell me about Carla's eating habits" is preferable to "Does she feed herself?" and the former is likely to yield more helpful information.

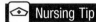 **Nursing Tip**

Nursing responsibilities for disabled children include the following:

- Emphasizing the *strengths* present.
- Maintaining communication with the family.
- Avoiding labels.
- Using simple terms.
- Contacting the school nurse and planning for school needs.
- Providing daily experiences in which the child can succeed.
- Referring family to local, state, and national support groups.

Prevention. The outlook is good for continued success in the prevention of intellectual impairment. Nurses can contribute to this by promoting genetic counseling, immunizations, newborn screening, and good prenatal care (Table 23-5). Comprehensive programs for early assessment and treatment of children with intellectual impairment must also be promoted. The nurse can serve as an advocate for the child and/or adolescent to help ensure that his or her rights are upheld.

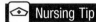 **Nursing Tip**

Many intellectually impaired children have a normal facial appearance, and many children with unusual faces are not intellectually impaired.

Head Injuries

Head injuries are the major cause of death and permanent injury in children older than 1 year of age. More physical force is needed to produce brain trauma when the head is in a fixed position than when it is freely moving—a fact that supports the use of infant car seats. The incidence of head injury among children is high. Children have poorly developed neck muscles and participation in collision sports increases the risk of concussion and a second injury before the first one heals, resulting in prolonged cognitive changes. A **concussion** is a temporary disturbance of the brain that is usually followed by a period of unconsciousness. It jars the brainstem and is often accompanied by a loss of memory for events that occurred immediately before

Table 23-5	Interventions Currently Available to Prevent Intellectual and Developmental Disabilities
FACTOR	**INTERVENTION**
Nearly Total Elimination	
Congenital rubella	Early immunization, antibody screening
Phenylketonuria, galactosemia, congenital hypothyroidism	Newborn screening, dietary management, replacement therapy
Kernicterus	Reduction of sensitization (RH negative/ABO incompatibility)
Major Reduction	
Tay-Sachs disease	Carrier screening, prenatal diagnosis in high-risk persons
Morbidity from prematurity	Newborn intensive care nurseries
Measles encephalitis	Early vaccination
Significant Reduction	
Neural tube defects	Prenatal folic acid supplements
Lead intoxication	Early screening for lead levels, improvement in environment, chelation when necessary
Fetal alcohol syndrome	Public education
Morbidity from head injury	Automobile child restraints, safety helmets and equipment; education
Child neglect and abuse	Parenting classes and family life education through the schools
Special Assistance and Relief	
Multiple disabilities, hearing, speech, Down syndrome	Early identification, support for families, genetic counseling of special risks

Modified from Carey W, Crocker A, Elias E, Coleman W: *Developmental-behavioral pediatrics,* ed 3, Philadelphia, 2009, Saunders.

(retrograde amnesia), during, and after the accident. A skull fracture indicates that the skull bone is broken or depressed. Bleeding may occur, resulting in pressure being exerted on the brain.

The response of the child to a head injury may differ from that of the adult. Loss of consciousness may not be evident, but changes in behavior, sleep, cognition, and balance may occur (McGuire, 2011). For example, the child may find it difficult to stand on one foot with the eyes closed. The location and type of skull fracture may not correlate with clinical findings. Careful clinical assessment is essential to determine the extent of brain injury. The surface area of a child's scalp is large and very vascular. Significant blood loss can result from scalp lacerations.

⚠ Safety Alert!

A concussion with resulting amnesia and confusion can be more serious than the presence of a fractured skull with no clinical symptoms.

Pathophysiology. A skull fracture, brain concussion, contusion, or intracranial hemorrhage may occur at the time of injury. Brain injury may occur at the point of impact, or on the opposite side of the brain *(coup-contre-coup).* Therefore, a blow to the occiput can result in an injury to the temporal area as the brain hits the bony skull. Children are more susceptible to the effects of a concussion than adults because children have muscles that are not fully developed framing the

central nervous system (CNS). The myelin sheath development is not yet mature so that conduction of impulses from the CNS to the rest of the body are not completely developed, making the signs and symptoms of concussion difficult to recognize by the untrained eye. Cognitive skills such as focusing, processing information, and recall are often the functions of the brain that are affected by a concussion. Concussion is not limited to a direct head injury and can be the result of a biomechanical impulsive force transmitted from a blow to another site of the body transmitted to the brain (Norton, 2013). Hypoxia, increased ICP, cerebral edema, and infection can occur within a few days. Hypoxia causes the brain to need increased energy, which results in increased cerebral blood flow. This increased blood flow (hyperemia) increases cerebral edema. If the ICP rises too high, cerebral perfusion diminishes, and brain damage or death results. If the fontanelles are open, the tolerance for increased ICP is higher in infants. Older children and adults do not have this advantage.

A child who sustains a mild bump to the head, retains consciousness, and does not vomit may have a covered ice pack applied to the site. During the first night after a bump on the head, parents are advised to be sure that they can arouse the child at least once, because intracranial bleeding occasionally occurs from a minor injury. They should be advised to contact a physician if the child appears confused, has trouble seeing or speaking, or walks unsteadily. Confusion and amnesia after any head injury may indicate a concussion even if consciousness is not lost.

Roughly shaking an infant can cause the brain to strike the inside of the skull (**shaken baby syndrome**). This can cause tearing of the nerve fibers within the brain, which can result in retinal, subarachnoid, and subdural hemorrhages as well as high-level cervical spine injuries and permanent disability or death. Teaching coping techniques to parents of children who cry inconsolably can prevent this type of injury. Infants suspected of shaken baby syndrome must be reported to local authorities. This type of pathologic condition can also result from an infant being held by a person who is repeatedly jumping high on a trampoline.

A child who has suffered a blow to the head is often brought to the hospital for overnight observation to rule out or confirm the extent of injury. The child may experience all or some of the following symptoms:
- Headache (manifested by fussiness in the toddler)
- Drowsiness
- Blurred vision
- Vomiting
- Dyspnea

In severe cases, the child may be completely unconscious. Decerebrate posturing (**extensor posturing**) or decorticate posturing (**flexor posturing**) may be evident (Figure 23-13). In decerebrate (extensor) rigidity, all four limbs are extended and the hands are pronated. This may indicate brainstem injury. In decorticate (flexor) rigidity, the arms, wrists, and fingers are flexed. Plantar flexion occurs in the feet. This may indicate damage to the cortex of the brain. These pathological postures (**posturing**) are seen with severe brain injury.

A careful history is obtained to determine any preexisting conditions and to ascertain the exact circumstances of the accident. Of particular importance is the child's state of consciousness immediately after the accident.

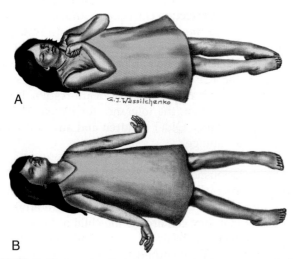

FIGURE 23-13 Posturing. Pathological posturing that may occur in the children with severe brain damage. **A,** Decorticate (flexor) posturing. **B,** Decerebrate (extensor) posturing. (From Hockenberry M, Wilson D: *Wong's nursing care of infants and children*, ed 9, St Louis, 2011, Mosby.)

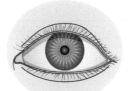 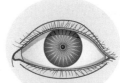

A In room light   **B** After flashlight beam

FIGURE 23-14 The response of the pupil of the eye to a flashlight beam. **A,** The pupil of the eye is a *3* in room light. **B,** The pupil of the eye is a *1* after a flashlight beam is directed at the eye. The letters *B*, *S*, and *N* may be used to denote brisk movement, slow movement, or nonmovement of the pupil response. This illustration would be recorded "3/1 B." The other eye should respond symmetrically. Sluggish movement, nonmovement, or asymmetrical response should be reported immediately.

The nurse observes the child for signs of increasing ICP. There are four components of a cranial or neurological check:
1. Level of consciousness
2. Pupil and eye movement (Figure 23-14)
3. Vital signs
4. Motor activity (Box 23-6)

Children are handled gently and are inspected for injuries to other areas. They are placed in a crib or bed in accordance with their age. Side rails are raised, because seizures are not uncommon. The head of the bed is slightly elevated to decrease cerebral edema.

Nursing Tip

Nurses should stress to parents the dangers of shaking infants roughly, including jumping on a trampoline with an infant in their arms.

Safety Alert!

After a head injury, the presence of asymmetrical pupils is a medical emergency.

Level of Consciousness. Changes in level of consciousness are particularly meaningful and necessitate immediate medical attention. Consciousness implies awareness or the ability to respond to stimuli. It also includes cognitive power, which is the ability to produce verbal and motor responses. The child's alertness on admission is recorded for use as baseline data. The response should be correlated with the child's developmental age. Parents can be helpful in providing information about the child's usual capabilities. In general, children should be oriented to person, time, and place (according to developmental capabilities). The nurse asks, "What is your name?" and "Where are you?" Older children may know the day of the week. The child should recognize parents. The nurse points to the mother and asks, "Who is this?" The child should be able to follow simple commands, such as "Turn over."

| Box 23-6 | **Neurological Monitoring of Infants and Children** |

Many subtle clues to a change in neurological status in infants and children can be missed unless the nurse performs aggressive assessment in looking for them. The lack of the child's ability to communicate and cooperate poses challenges in the neurological assessment of infants, but a knowledge of normal growth and development aids the nurse in evaluating the status of his or her little patient. For example, we know that an infant should turn his or her head toward the spoken word by age 6 months. However, assessing after a full feeding may cause a delayed response that may not be pathological.

PAIN STIMULI

There are two types of pain stimuli: *central,* a response of the brain; and *peripheral,* a response of the spinal cord. The pain stimulus should continue for 30 seconds to determine the optimal function response.

Central pain stimulus:

Trapezius muscle: Firmly pinch large muscle mass at the angle where the neck and shoulder meet.

Suborbital pressure: Exert firm pressure on the "notch" that can be located under the center of the eyebrow.

LEVEL OF CONSCIOUSNESS

In children and adolescents we can determine the difference between arousal, awareness, orientation, and memory. In infants, the Glasgow Coma Scale is used (see Table 23-6).

AROUSAL AWARENESS

Child responds to his or her name, which is indicative of basic cerebral function.

Child can interact with environment, indicating cerebral cortex functioning.

Orientation: Determine awareness of person, place, or time. Use open-ended or multiple-choice questions rather than questions that can be answered by "yes" or "no."

Attention span: Although attention span can differ with the age of child, the child would not normally fall off to sleep in the middle of a response requiring re-arousal stimuli. This should be recorded if it occurs.

Language: Understanding the level of language development is essential in determining if the language pattern is normal or abnormal. Speaking clearly and recognizing familiar objects is a skill that is age related in the pediatric setting.

Irritability, lethargy, and vomiting: These are clinical symptoms of increased intracranial pressure (ICP) in infants, in addition to signs such as a bulging fontanelle.

Memory: A child's ability to recognize family members or repeat what he or she had for breakfast is a valid observation for memory.

CRANIAL NERVE RESPONSES

Cranial nerve responses are valuable in determining priority of need related to survival and safety.

Olfactory (I): A strong-smelling substance under the nose of an alert infant will elicit a grimace or a startle response.

Optic (II): Infant is able to fix eyes on object and follow a short distance. Pupils react equally to light.

Oculomotor (III): Pupils respond to light. In "doll's-eye test," eyes move away from direction head is rotated; infant is able to open eyes.

Trochlear (IV): Infant is able to move eyes and follow object.

Trigeminal (V): Infant turns head in response to stroking cheek.

Abducens (VI): Corneal reflex is present; eyes follow past midline.

Facial (VII): Wrinkles brow; facial movements symmetrical; closes eyes when crying.

Auditory (VIII): Tested via auditory screening machine; infant turns head toward sound source.

Glossopharyngeal (IX): Elicits a positive gag reflex, moves tongue in mouth.

Vagus (X): Infant has ability to swallow and a lusty cry and cough.

Accessory (XI): Turn infant's head to one side, and infant will return head to midline.

Hypoglossal (XII): Infant able to suck and swallow; tongue protrusion is present.

MOTOR RESPONSE

Symmetrical spontaneous body movements are an important observation to record. Asking the child to follow a simple motor request is more accurate than a hand grasp, because in some age groups a hand grasp is a reflex rather than a voluntary response. A purposeful voluntary motor response is a more valuable observation than a reflex response to remove irritants such as an attempt to pull out a nasogastric tube.

Glasgow Scale motor responses may be recorded as follows: 5—obeys; 4—withdraws; 3—flexion; 2—extension; 1—none.

POSTURING

In children and adolescents, posturing can indicate a change in neurological status that necessitates immediate notification to the physician.

Decorticate (flexor): Flexion of the arms to center of body and flexing of wrists indicate partial brain function (indicates injury to the cerebral cortex of the brain) (see Figure 23-13, *A*).

Decerebrate (extensor): Arms are extended along the side of the body and the hands are pronated. This indicates brainstem function only (see Figure 23-13, *B*).

Opisthotonos position: Hyperextension of the neck and arching of the spine is a position assumed by infants with pathologic cerebral disturbance (see Figure 23-8).

EYES

The pupils of the eyes should be observed for size, equality, and response to light (see Figure 23-14). It may be best to evaluate the eye in a slightly darkened room so the pupils may be somewhat dilated and the response to sudden light from a flashlight can be readily assessed.

Pupils that remain *pinpoint* can indicate damage to the pons or part of the brainstem or can indicate drug toxicity.

Bilateral dilated pupils can be indicative of hypoxia or intoxication with atropine-like drugs.

Pupils that are *unequal* in size can signal brain herniation; *immediate action is required.*

Pupillary response to light can be brisk, sluggish, or absent. Recording should indicate the size of the pupil in normal light (e.g., 3), size of pupil after flashlight intervention (e.g., 1), and how fast the change occurred (*B*, brisk; *S*, sluggish or slow; *A*, absent). A normal recording for pupillary response would be as follows: R 3/1 B; L 3/1 B.

Keep in mind that infants and children who are blind will not have a meaningful light response test.

Continued

| Box 23-6 | Neurological Monitoring of Infants and Children—cont'd |

When the pupil constricts in response to light, be sure that constriction is maintained and that the eye does not dilate again before light is removed.
Glasgow Scale eye opening responses may be recorded as follows: 4—spontaneous; 3—to sound; 2—to pain; 1—none.

FONTANELLE
A bulging anterior fontanelle is indicative of increased ICP.

SCALP VEIN DISTENTION
Scalp veins distend because of the obstruction of flow from the bridging veins of the scalp to the sagittal sinus.

ATAXIA: SPASTICITY OF LOWER EXTREMITIES
These occur with damage to the corticospinal pathways.

REFLEXES: MORO OR TONIC NECK WITH WITHDRAWAL
In infants, an absence of these reflexes can occur with increased ICP.

When the child does not respond to verbal stimuli, the upper arm is gently pinched and the response is observed. The presence or absence of crying or speech is noted. It is not unusual for children to fall asleep, but he or she should be easily aroused. The nurse records changes in sleeping posture, movements of extremities, and any signs of tremors or restlessness. The bladder is observed for distention, which can contribute to irritability. Incontinence in the child who is toilet-trained is significant. The child's behavior is described in the nurse's notes. The *Glasgow Coma Scale* is valuable in standardizing the description and interpretation of various levels of consciousness. It includes eye opening and motor and verbal responses. The lower the score, the deeper the level of unconsciousness or coma. A score of less than 15 requires a CT scan and less than 8 usually necessitates immediate medical intervention (Horeczko, 2012) Table 23-6 shows a scale modified for infants.

Vital Signs. An increase in blood pressure and a decrease in pulse and respiration are evidence of increased ICP. Temperature elevations may result from inflammation, systemic infection, or damage to the hypothalamus, which regulates body temperature. Mild elevations caused by trauma are not uncommon during the first 2 days after a head injury.

Motor Activity. Because nerves energize the muscle tissue, any damage to the nervous system affects body movement. The quality and strength of muscle tone are observed in all four extremities. The child should be able to move the legs and push against the nurse's hands with both feet. The face should be symmetrical. The child can smile and frown. Drooping of the eyes (*ptosis*), inability to close the eyes tightly, and drooping of the corner of the mouth are considered pathological. The child should be able to raise the arms and extend the palms upward and downward. Abnormal posturing is described and recorded.

Nursing Care. Nursing care includes examination of wound swelling if a laceration of the head is present. The type and amount of drainage from the ears and nose are recorded. The nurse checks for *nuchal* (neck) rigidity, which might indicate infection such as meningitis. Occipital-frontal circumference of the head is monitored in infants, as are tension of the fontanelles and the presence of a high-pitched cry. Fluids are carefully monitored to control *cerebral edema*. Feeding difficulties should be noted as the child's diet is increased. The child is observed for signs of shock, which can also occur. Children whose condition has remained stable are discharged. Parents are instructed about any additional observations and follow-up care. Most children are advised to decrease cognitive activities after a concussion, including texting, cellphone use, TV, loud music, and computer use, with a gradual return to full activity. Signs of postconcussion syndrome include headache, fatigue, photophobia, and disturbed thinking (Norton, 2013). Nurses should teach parents and children the importance of using appropriate protective equipment when engaging in sports activities.

Nursing Tip

A positive glucose (Dextrostix) test can determine if watery nasal discharge is CSF or a concurrent cold (rhinorrhea).

Following even a slight head injury, the child should be assessed before continuing in sports activities. Mild traumatic brain injury (MTBI) can occur even without loss of consciousness and long-term effects can result. Complications of concussion can include postconcussion syndrome that involves cognitive and emotional problems and chronic traumatic encephalopathy caused by repeated head injuries and may be associated with the development of early Alzheimer's disease (Mcguire, 2011). Coaches are not qualified to assess head injuries (Norton, 2013) and a baseline function should be established before entering into contact sports activities. The Sports Concussion Assessment Tool (SCAT), and the Standardized Assessment of Concussion (SAC) are tools that are available. A decline of one point or more from baseline is important. The American Academy of Clinical Neuropsychology (AACN) and the National Academy of Neuropsychology (NAN) have endorsed practice guidelines for the use of Computerized neuropsychological testing devices.

Legislation is pending concerning education, prevention, and management of head injuries in sports.

Table 23-6   The Glasgow Coma Scale Modified for Infants

AGE IN MONTHS	RESPONSE
1	1. None 2. Crying to stimuli 3. Crying spontaneously 4. Blinks when eyelashes are touched 5. Throaty noises
2	1. None 2. Crying to stimuli 3. Shuts eyes to light 4. Smiles when caressed 5. Babbles—single vowel sounds
3	1. None 2. Crying to stimuli (moans) 3. Stares to response and looks at environment 4. Smiles to sound stimulation 5. Coos, chuckles, pronounces *vowels* in a prolonged way
4	1. None 2. Crying to stimuli (moans) 3. Turns head to sound 4. Smiles spontaneously or when stimulated, laughs when socially stimulated 5. Modulating voice and perfect vocalization of vowels
5 and 6	1. None 2. Crying to stimuli (moans) 3. Localizes general direction of sound 4. Discriminates family members 5. Babbles to people, toys
7 and 8	1. None 2. Crying to stimuli (moans) 3. Recognizes familiar voices and family 4. Babbles 5. "Ba," "Ma," "Da"
9 and 10	1. None 2. Crying to stimuli (moans) 3. Recognizes (smiles or laughs) 4. Babbles 5. "Mama," "Dada"
11 and 12	1. None 2. Crying to stimuli (moans) 3. Recognizes—smiles 4. Babbles

Motor Responses	Eye Opening
5 Obeys	
4 Withdraws	4 Spontaneous
3 Flexion	3 To sound
2 Extension	2 To pain
1 None	1 None
In the older child, the best verbal, motor, and eye-opening responses are scored and recorded.	

Modified from Kliegman RM, Marcdante K, Jenson HB, Behrman RE: *Nelson's essentials of pediatrics,* ed 5, Philadelphia, 2005, Saunders; Kliegman, R, Stanton B, St Geme III J, Schor N, Behrman R: *Nelson's textbook of pediatrics,* ed 19, Philadelphia, 2011, Saunders.

Near Drowning

Accidental drowning or near drowning is the fourth leading cause of death for U.S. children less than 19 years of age. Near drowning is defined as survival beyond 24 hours after submersion. Proper supervision and environmental safety precautions are the best measures to prevent drowning. In adolescents, the use of illicit drugs and alcohol during recreational swimming contributes to drowning incidents. The priorities include the immediate treatment of hypoxia, aspiration, and hypothermia.

Cardiorespiratory survival has increased with advances in emergency medical treatment by paramedics on site and with the technology available in intensive care units in the hospital. However, CNS injury remains the major cause of death or long-term disability.

Submersion for more than 10 minutes with failure to regain consciousness at the scene or within 24 hours is an ominous sign and is predictive of severe neurological deficits if the child survives. Respiratory and cardiovascular support, controlled rewarming, and maintenance of adequate cerebral oxygenation are priorities of care (Nursing Care Plan 23-1). The parents need to be offered support, explanations of the therapy, and referral to social services, religious organizations, or community agencies for follow-up. Adult supervision, and water safety and survival training can prevent most drownings, and nurses can advocate for these in schools and communities.

 Safety Alert!

All children who experience near drowning should be admitted for a 24-hour observation period of close monitoring for the development of cerebral edema, which may be evidenced by an altered level of consciousness.

★ Nursing Care Plan 23-1 | The Child with Altered Level of Consciousness

PATIENT DATA A 4-year-old child fell into a pool while playing, hitting his head on the pool deck. Cardiopulmonary resuscitation reestablished a heartbeat and spontaneous respirations. The child is admitted with signs of increased intracranial pressure, including a decreased level of consciousness and an absence of the gag reflex.

Selected Nursing Diagnosis: Ineffective airway clearance/ineffective breathing pattern related to decreased level of consciousness

Goals	Nursing Interventions	Rationales
Child will demonstrate effective airway clearance and breathing pattern as evidenced by patent airway, age-appropriate respiratory rate (RR), lungs clear to auscultation, and ability to breathe on his or her own without mechanical assistance.	Observe airway for patency. Observe for presence/absence of gag/swallow reflex, RR, rhythm, and effort; note any irregularities. Auscultate breath sounds, noting and reporting any adventitious breath sounds. Provide meticulous pulmonary toilet to prevent respiratory compromise.	Diminished oxygenation can lead to cerebral anoxia and/or death. Inability to protect the airway can lead to aspiration pneumonia. A marked increase or decrease in respiratory pattern can be a sign of impending respiratory failure. Adventitious breath sounds are indicative of accumulated respiratory secretions, thereby increasing the risk for pneumonia or atelectasis. Good oral hygiene, suctioning of oral secretions, cleaning of buccal cavity, and turning child every 2 hours will help prevent respiratory problems.

Selected Nursing Diagnosis: Risk for impaired skin integrity, related to physical immobility

Goals	Nursing Interventions	Rationales
Child will maintain intact skin without signs or symptoms of tissue breakdown or decubitus ulcer formation.	Inspect all skin surfaces, noting areas of erythema, blanching, or edema. Pay particular attention to all bony prominences and areas in direct contact with the bed. Reposition every 2 hours. Place child in prone position periodically (unless contraindicated by medical condition). Bathe child daily and keep bedding free of wrinkles and crumbs.	Lying in one position for extended periods increases the risk of tissue breakdown and decubitus ulcer formation. Repositioning helps to improve circulation and relieves pressure areas. Bathing increases circulation because of the massaging of the skin with the washcloth. Having a bed free of wrinkles and crumbs prevents additional areas of potential skin breakdown and decubitus ulcer formation.

Selected Nursing Diagnosis: Compromised family coping related to loss of well-being of child

Goals	Nursing Interventions	Rationales
Parent and/or family will demonstrate effective coping skills as evidenced by expressing a realistic understanding of child's illness and active participation in child's care.	Assess level of anxiety or concern of parent(s) and/or family members. Provide opportunities for instruction on how to care for the ill child. Reinforce and/or clarify medical explanation of child's condition and prognosis. Identify community agencies and support services within the community available to the family.	Provides data to determine type of assistance or support that is needed. Enhances feelings of control and involvement in the health care of the child. Ensures parent and family have a clear understanding of information received. Provides family with sources of emotional and spiritual support in time of crises.

Get Ready for the NCLEX® Examination!

Key Points

- Infants are more prone to ear infections than older children because their eustachian tubes are shorter, wider, and straighter.
- When instilling ear drops in infants, gently pull the pinna **down** and back. In children, the pinna is gently pulled **up** and back.
- In paralytic strabismus the **unaffected** eye is patched.
- Level of consciousness is the most important indicator of neurological health.
- Nursing care of the unconscious child includes assessing the child for increased intracranial pressure (ICP), maintaining an open airway, providing adequate nutrition and fluids, positioning, maintaining flexibility of joints, and preventing injury.
- A high-pitched cry may be indicative of increased ICP.
- Do not give aspirin or other salicylates to children with symptoms of influenza or chickenpox, because the drug is linked to Reye's syndrome, a serious and life-threatening illness.
- Meningitis is an inflammation of the meninges that cover the brain and spinal cord.
- A seizure is a symptom of an underlying pathological condition.
- Grand mal seizures involve an *aura, tonic and clonic* phases, and *postictal lethargy*.
- Decerebrate, decorticate, or opisthotonos posturing indicates brain damage.
- The response of the pupils to light and ascertaining level of consciousness are essential assessments to determine brain injury.
- The Glasgow Coma Scale is used to determine level of consciousness in infants and children.
- "Shaken baby syndrome" can result in subdural hematoma and death.
- Confusion and amnesia after a head injury may indicate concussion even if consciousness is not lost.
- The four types of cerebral palsy are *spastic, athetoid, ataxic,* and *mixed.*
- Many children with spastic quadriplegia have normal intelligence.
- Computer technology can help the physically impaired child communicate and achieve mobility.
- Intellectual disability involves three components: intelligence, adaptive behavior, and failure to meet developmental milestones with onset before 18 years of age.
- The priority of care for a child who has experienced near drowning is to prevent hypoxia, aspiration, and hypothermia.

Additional Learning Resources

SG Go to your Study Guide for additional learning activities to help you master this chapter content.

evolve Go to your Evolve website (http://evolve.elsevier.com/Leifer) for the following learning resources:

- Animations
- Answer Guidelines for Critical Thinking Questions
- Answers and Rationales for Review Questions for the NCLEX® Examination
- Glossary with English and Spanish pronunciations
- Interactive Review Questions for the NCLEX® Examination
- Patient Teaching Plans in English and Spanish
- Skills Performance Checklists
- Video clips and more!

 Online Resources
- Epilepsy Foundation: www.epilepsyfoundation.org/
- Hydrocephalus Foundation: www.hydroassoc.org
- National Hearing Center: http://nationalhearingcenter.com/
- Pediatric head injuries: www.brainline.org
- Sight and Hearing Association: www.sightandhearing.org

Review Questions for the NCLEX® Examination

1. Symptoms of an earache in an infant include:
   1. external drainage, pain, and decrease in temperature.
   2. tugging at the ear and rolling head from side to side.
   3. crying and pointing to affected ear.
   4. redness of the cheeks and cyanosis of the ear.

2. Signs of increased intracranial pressure in a 3-year-old child include:
   1. headache, lethargy.
   2. high pitched cry, bulging fontanelles.
   3. apnea, crossed eyes.
   4. painful head movement, anorexia.

3. An important nursing intervention when administering Dilantin (phenytoin) to a patient diagnosed with epilepsy includes:
   1. recording blood pressure.
   2. providing detailed oral hygiene.
   3. encouraging bed rest.
   4. administering it with milk.

4. A practice that has been helpful in preventing intellectual disability is:
   1. administering the Stanford-Binet test.
   2. a blood test at birth.
   3. careful preschool developmental screening.
   4. a urine test at age 6 months.

5. Distinct phases of a grand-mal epileptic seizure include (select all that apply):
   1. aura.
   2. agitation.
   3. tonic/clonic movements.
   4. postictal lethargy.

Critical Thinking Question

1. After resuscitation in the emergency department, the child has regained consciousness, is interacting with the mother, and has stable vital signs. The mother states, "Now that my child is OK I want to take him home." What is the best response of the nurse?

The Child with a Musculoskeletal Condition

Objectives

1. Define each key term listed.
2. Discuss the musculoskeletal differences between the child and adult and how it influences orthopedic treatment and nursing care.
3. Demonstrate an understanding of age-specific changes that occur in the musculoskeletal system during growth and development.
4. Describe the management of soft tissue injuries.
5. Discuss the types of fractures commonly seen in children and their effect on growth and development.
6. Differentiate between Buck's extension and Russell traction.
7. Compile a nursing care plan for the child who is immobilized by traction.
8. Describe a neurovascular check.
9. Discuss the nursing care of a child in a cast.
10. List two symptoms of Duchenne's muscular dystrophy.
11. Describe the symptoms, treatment, and nursing care for the child with Legg-Calvé-Perthes disease.
12. Describe two topics of discussion applicable at discharge for the child with juvenile rheumatoid arthritis.
13. Describe three nursing care measures required to maintain skin integrity for an adolescent child in a cast for scoliosis.
14. Describe three types of child abuse.
15. Identify symptoms of abuse and neglect in children.
16. State two cultural or medical practices that may be misinterpreted as child abuse.

Key Terms

arthroscopy (p. 558)
Bryant's traction (p. 560)
Buck's extension (p. 560)
compartment syndrome (p. 563)
compound fracture (p. 559)
contusion (kŏn-TŪ-zhŭn, p. 558)
epiphysis (ĕ-PĬF-ă-sĭs, p. 560)
gait (p. 557)
genu valgum (JĒ-nū VĂL-găm, p. 557)
genu varum (JĒ-nū VĂR-ăm, p. 557)
greenstick fracture (p. 559)

hematoma (hē-mă-TŌ-mă, p. 558)
Legg-Calvé-Perthes disease (p. 568)
Milwaukee brace (p. 570)
neurovascular checks (p. 563)
osteomyelitis (p. 566)
Russell traction (p. 560)
slipped femoral capital epiphysis (p. 567)
spiral fracture (p. 560)
sprain (p. 558)
strain (p. 558)

The musculoskeletal system supports the body and provides for movement. The muscular and skeletal systems work together to enable a person to sit, stand, walk, and remain upright. In addition, muscles move air into and out of the lungs, blood through vessels, and food through the digestive tract. They also produce heat, which aids in numerous body chemical reactions. Bones act as levers and provide support. Red blood cells are produced in the bone marrow, and minerals such as calcium and phosphorus are also stored there.

The musculoskeletal system arises from the mesoderm in the embryo. A great portion of skeletal growth occurs between the fourth and eighth weeks of fetal life. As the limbs elongate before birth, muscle masses form in the extremities. The Ballard scoring system (see Figure 13-2) is one measure of assessing neuromuscular maturity at birth. Testing various reflexes is another.

Locomotion develops gradually and in an orderly manner in the growing child. A marked deceleration of growth is always a signal for investigation.

MUSCULOSKELETAL SYSTEM: DIFFERENCES BETWEEN THE CHILD AND THE ADULT

The pediatric skeletal system differs from the adult skeletal system in that bone is not completely ossified, epiphyses are present, and the periosteum is thicker and produces callus more rapidly than in the adult. The lower mineral content of the child's bone and its greater porosity increase the bone's strength. However,

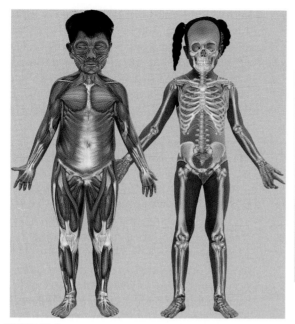

MUSCULOSKELETAL SYSTEM

- Skeletal growth is most rapid during infancy and adolescence. Assessing growth and development is an integral part of the physical examination for children.
- The bones of children are more resilient, tend to bend, and may deform before breaking.
- The blood supply to bone in children is rich; therefore healing occurs more quickly. Their periosteum is thick, and osteogenic activity is high.
- Epiphyseal plate fractures in children can disrupt the growth of bones.
- Musculoskeletal problems may be growth related.
- Rapid growth of the skeletal frame of children can cause deformities to become more severe.

FIGURE 24-1 Some musculoskeletal system differences between the child and the adult. The muscular system consists of the large skeletal muscles that enable movement as well as the cardiac muscle of the heart and the smooth muscle of the internal organs. The skeletal system consists of bones and cartilage. This system helps to support and protect the body. (Art overlay courtesy Observatory Group, Cincinnati, Ohio.)

rotational or angular forces can stress ligaments that insert at the epiphyseal area of the bone, and injury to the epiphysis can affect bone growth. Because of the presence of the epiphysis and hyperemia caused by the trauma, bone overgrowth is common in healing fractures of children less than 10 years of age. At birth, the thoracic and sacral areas of the child's spine are convex curves. When the child sits and stands these curves must change to be concave or kyphosis or lordosis will result. Figure 24-1 describes some differences between the child's and the adult's skeletal and muscular systems.

OBSERVATION AND ASSESSMENT OF THE MUSCULOSKELETAL SYSTEM IN THE GROWING CHILD

To assess the musculoskeletal system of the growing child and to identify deviations, the nurse must have a basic understanding of the effect of growth, neurological development, and motor milestones at various ages. The newborn hip has limited internal rotation range of motion (ROM). The legs are maintained in a flexed position, and the lower leg has an internal rotation (internal tibial torsion) caused by the effects of uterine positioning; this can last 4 to 6 months. The general curvature of the newborn spine is a C shape from the thoracic to the pelvic level; it changes with the mastery of motor skills to a double S curve in childhood (see Figure 17-1). The newborn's feet normally turn inward *(varus)* or outward *(valgus),* but the turning-in self-corrects when the sole of the foot is stroked. The toddler's feet appear flat because of the presence of a fat

pad at the arch. Any delay in neurological development can cause a delay in the mastery of motor skills, which can result in altered skeletal growth.

Assessment of the musculoskeletal system includes observation, palpation, ROM, and gait assessment in children who can walk. Children who do not walk independently by 18 months of age have a serious delay and should be referred to a health care provider for follow-up.

OBSERVATION OF GAIT

A **gait** is a characteristic manner of walking. The toddler who begins to walk has a wide, unstable *gait*. The arms do not swing with the walking motion. By 18 months of age the wide base narrows and the walk is more stable. By 4 years of age the child can hop on one foot, and arm swings occur with walking. By 6 years of age the gait resembles the adult walk with equal stride lengths and associated arm swing. The trunk is centered over the legs, and movement is symmetrical. When a child favors one side, pain may be present. Toe walking after 3 years of age can indicate a muscle problem.

In most cases, excessive in-toeing, or pointing of the toe inward, will resolve by 4 years of age. These children trip and fall easily. Teaching proper sitting and body mechanics is the treatment of choice. Participation in ballet classes and in-line skating will enhance hip flexibility. If the problem does not resolve, a brace may be prescribed. Failure to treat can result in hip, knee, or back problems in adulthood.

Young children appear bowlegged (**genu varum**) or knock-kneed (**genu valgum**), with the knees turned inward until 5 years of age. Bowing is seldom pathological.

The ligaments that support the arch are not mature before 6 years of age, and therefore the child may appear to have flat feet. If the condition interferes with walking, an orthotic appliance can be prescribed for the child to wear inside the shoes. When the flat foot is painful, a referral for follow-up examination should be initiated. The role of the nurse is to reassure parents that unless there is associated pain or a problem with motor or nerve functions, many minor abnormal-appearing alignments will spontaneously resolve with activity.

OBSERVATION OF MUSCLE TONE

The nurse should assess symmetry of movement and the strength and contour of the body and extremities. Having the child push away the examiner's hand with his or her foot or hand can test the strength of the extremities.

NEUROLOGICAL EXAMINATION

A neurological assessment is a vital part of a comprehensive musculoskeletal examination. An assessment of reflexes, a sensory assessment, and the presence or absence of spasms should be noted.

DIAGNOSTIC TESTS AND TREATMENTS

Radiographic Studies

Radiographs (x-ray films) are taken to confirm a suspected pathological condition, and the affected area is compared with the unaffected area.

Bone Scans. Bone scans are helpful in identifying pathological conditions that may not clearly be seen on a routine x-ray study, such as septic arthritis or tumors.

Computed Tomography. Computed tomography (CT) provides a cross-sectional picture of the bone and its relationship to other structures within the area of examination.

Magnetic Resonance Imaging. Magnetic resonance imaging (MRI) does not involve harmful radiation. MRIs produce detailed pictures of the brain, spinal cord, and soft tissue lesions, including a slipped femoral epiphysis.

Ultrasound. Ultrasound does not involve harmful radiation. It is used to rule out foreign bodies in soft tissues, joint effusions, and developmental dysplasia of the hip.

LABORATORY TESTS AND TREATMENTS

A complete blood count (CBC) and erythrocyte sedimentation rate (ESR) may rule out septic arthritis or osteomyelitis. Human leukocyte antigen (HLA) B-27 may help diagnose rheumatological disorders.

A thorough history is necessary to determine the basis for musculoskeletal problems, which are often insidious. The nurse determines the history of the injury; the location of pain; when symptoms started; any weakness, numbness, or loss of function in an extremity; and whether the problem is affecting the daily activities of the child. An **arthroscopy** is commonly performed on adolescents with sports injuries. The physician is able to look inside the joint (usually the knee or shoulder) to determine the extent of injury. The area is inspected, foreign particles are removed, or repairs are made to the torn menisci. A bone biopsy may show a malignancy. Muscle biopsy may detect muscular dystrophy.

Traction, casting, and splints are used in accordance with the patient's needs. Three types of skin traction are often used for the lower extremities of children: *Bryant's traction, Buck's extension,* and *Russell traction.* Children with musculoskeletal disorders may require lengthy hospitalization. Immobility causes a deceleration in body metabolism. Nursing interventions focus on maintaining body functions. ROM exercises and the use of a trapeze prevent muscle atrophy. Foods high in roughage stimulate the digestive tract and prevent constipation. Respiratory exercises prevent pneumonia. These and other measures can prevent complications that can lengthen hospitalization for the child. (Clubfoot, congenital hip dysplasia, and spica casts are discussed in Chapter 14. Rickets is discussed in Chapter 28.)

PEDIATRIC TRAUMA

SOFT TISSUE INJURIES

Soft tissue injuries usually accompany traumatic fractures in the child at play or the adolescent involved in sports activities and include the following:

- ***Contusion***: A tearing of subcutaneous tissue resulting in hemorrhage, edema, and pain. The escape of blood into the soft tissue is referred to as a **hematoma**, or a "black and blue mark."
- ***Sprain***: When the ligament is torn or stretched away from the bone at the point of trauma, there may be resulting damage to blood vessels, muscles, and nerves. Swelling, disability, and pain are major signs of a sprain.
- ***Strain***: A microscopic tear to the muscle or tendon that occurs over time and results in edema and pain.

Treatment of Soft Tissue Injuries

Soft tissue injuries should be treated immediately to limit damage from edema and bleeding. A cold pack and elastic wrap will reduce edema and bleeding and relieve pain, and should be applied at **alternating 30-minute intervals**. (After a 30-minute period, ischemia can occur and impede the tissue perfusion.) Elevating the extremity above heart level reduces edema. When an elastic bandage is used for compression, a priority nursing responsibility is to perform frequent neurovascular checks to ensure adequate tissue perfusion.

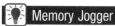
Memory Jogger

Principles of managing soft tissue injuries include the following:

Rest
Ice
Compression
Elevation

PREVENTION OF PEDIATRIC TRAUMA

Accidents are common in childhood, but much can be done to prevent morbidity and mortality. Parents are responsible for maintaining a safe environment for their children. Nurses are responsible for educating parents and schoolteachers about how to prevent accidental injury and maintain a safe environment.

The proper use of pedestrian safety practices, car seat restraints, bicycle helmets and other athletic protective gear, pool fences, window bars, deadbolt locks, and locks on cabinets can prevent many injuries to children. Pediatric trauma can cause permanent disability or premature death. Nursing assessment and interventions can assist the injured child toward recovery. The nurse also has a community responsibility to support legislation that would maintain safe environments for children.

TRAUMATIC FRACTURES

Pathophysiology. A fracture is a break in a bone and is usually caused by accidents. It is characterized by pain, tenderness on movement, and swelling. Discoloration, limited movement, and numbness may also occur. In a *simple fracture*, the bone is broken, but the skin over the area is not. In a **compound fracture** a wound in the skin accompanies the broken bone, and there is an added danger of infection. A **greenstick fracture** is an incomplete fracture in which one side of the bone is broken and the other is bent. This type of fracture is common in children because their bones are soft, flexible, and more likely to splinter. In a complete fracture the bone is entirely broken across its width. Figure 24-2 illustrates

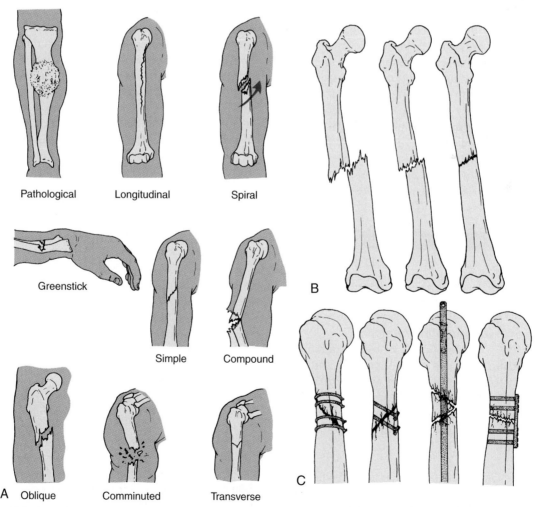

FIGURE 24-2 A, Types of fractures. **B,** Reduction of a fractured bone. A gradual pull is exerted on the distal (lower) fragment of the bone until it is in alignment with the proximal fragment. **C,** Various methods of internal fixations, using plates, pins, nails, and screws to hold fragments of bone in place. (Redrawn from deWit SC: *Keane's essentials of medical-surgical nursing,* ed 3, Philadelphia, 1992, Saunders.)

various types of fractures. When an x-ray film shows multiple fractures at various stages of healing, child abuse should be suspected.

A fracture heals more rapidly in a child than it does in an adult. The child's periosteum is stronger and thicker, and there is less stiffness on mobilization. Injury to the cartilaginous **epiphysis**, the growth plate which is found at the ends of the long bones, is serious if it happens during childhood because it may interfere with longitudinal growth. A fat embolism can occur within a few hours after fractures of the long bones or multiple fractures, when fat particles escape from the site into the circulation and lodge in the lung. Although it is more common in adults than children, the nurse must be observant for signs of hypoxia following traumatic fractures. Care of a child in a cast is discussed in Chapter 14. Casts may be made of plaster or fiberglass.

Fractures of the Femur in Early Childhood. The femur (thigh bone) is the largest and strongest bone of the body. It is one of the most prevalent serious breaks that occur during early childhood. A forceful twisting motion of the femur causes a **spiral fracture**. When the history of an injury does not correlate with x-ray findings, child abuse should be suspected, because spiral fractures can be the result of manual twisting of the extremity. The child complains of pain and tenderness when the leg is moved and he or she cannot bear weight on it. Clothes are gently removed, starting at the uninjured side and proceeding to the injured side. It may be necessary to cut the clothes; x-ray films confirm the diagnosis. Skin traction is used to reduce the fracture and keep the bones in proper alignment. A spica cast may be applied. See Chapter 14 for care of the child in a spica cast.

> **⚠ Safety Alert!**
>
> A spiral femur fracture in a young child may indicate child abuse and must be referred to an assessment team.

Treatment of Fractures with Traction

Traction in the Younger Child. **Bryant's traction** is used for treating fractures of the femur in children less than 2 years of age or lighter than 20 to 30 lb. Weights and pulleys extend the limb as in the Buck's extension; however, the legs are suspended vertically (Figure 24-3). The weight of the child supplies the countertraction.

Traction in the Older Child. Traction is used when the cast cannot maintain alignment of the two bone fragments. Skeletal muscles act as a splint for the fracture. Traction aligns the injured bone by the use of weights and countertraction. Immobilization is maintained until the bones fuse.

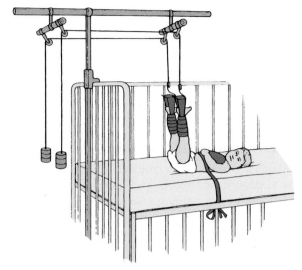

FIGURE 24-3 Bryant's traction is used for the young child who has a fractured femur. Note that the buttocks are slightly off the bed to facilitate countertraction. Active infants may require a jacket restraint to maintain body alignment.

Buck skin traction (**Buck's extension**) is a type of skin traction used in fractures of the femur and in hip and knee contractures. It pulls the hip and leg into extension. The child's body supplies countertraction; therefore it is essential that the child does not slip down in bed and that the bed is not placed in high-Fowler's position. Buck's extension is sometimes used preoperatively, either unilaterally or bilaterally, to reduce pain and muscle spasm associated with a slipped capital femoral epiphysis. **Russell traction** is similar to Buck's extension. In Russell traction, however, a sling is positioned under the knee, which suspends the distal thigh above the bed (Figure 24-4). Skin traction is applied to the lower extremity. Pull is in two directions, vertically from the knee sling and longitudinally from the footplate (Figure 24-5). This prevents posterior subluxation of the tibia on the femur, which can occur in children who are in traction. Split Russell traction uses two sets

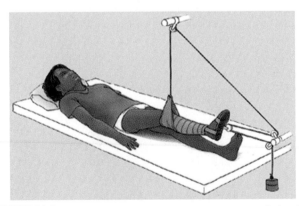

FIGURE 24-4 Russell skin traction. A skin traction system applied to the lower extremity using a footplate and a knee sling. When there are separate weights attached to both the footplate and the knee sling, it is known as a *split Russell traction.* (From Bowden VR, Dickey SB, Greenberg SC: *Children and their families: the continuum of care,* Philadelphia, 1998, Saunders.)

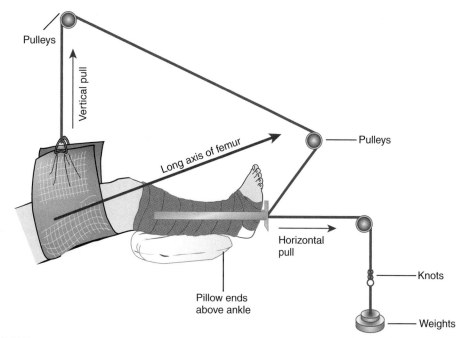

FIGURE 24-5 Forces involved in traction. The placement of pulleys and the angle of the joints determine the line of pull. In this case the combined vertical and horizontal pull results in a pull on the long axis of the femur to reduce fracture displacement.

of weights, one suspending the thigh and the other exerting a pull on the leg, with weights at the head and foot of the bed. Balanced suspension using the *Thomas splint* and *Pearson attachments* is used to treat diseases of the hip as well as fractures in older children and adolescents. It may be used both before and after surgery.

In *skeletal traction,* a Steinmann pin or Kirschner wire is inserted into the bone, and traction is applied to the pin. Daily cleansing of the pin site is essential. "Ninety-ninety" (or ninety degree–ninety degree) traction with a boot cast or sling on the lower leg may be used (Figure 24-6). Crutchfield, or Barton, tongs may be used in the skull to provide cervical traction (Figure 24-7). Skeletal traction carries the added risk of infection from skin bacteria that may cause osteomyelitis. The child in traction experiences certain effects as a result of immobilization (Figure 24-8). Visitors are important to the

child in traction, and a school tutor should be contacted so that the child will be able to return to class after healing occurs.

> **Nursing Tip**
>
> Checklist for a traction apparatus:
> - Weights hanging freely
> - Weights out of reach of the child
> - Ropes on the pulleys
> - Knots not resting against pulleys
> - Bed linens not on traction ropes
> - Countertraction in place
> - Apparatus does not touch foot of bed

> **Safety Alert!**
>
> The nurse should never lift or remove weights from the traction apparatus during the delivery of patient care.

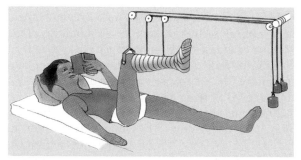

FIGURE 24-6 Ninety degree–ninety degree skeletal traction. A wire pin is inserted into the distal segment of the femur. The lower leg may be placed in a boot cast or is supported by a sling. (From Bowden VR, Dickey SB, Greenberg SC: *Children and their families: the continuum of care,* Philadelphia, 1998, Saunders.)

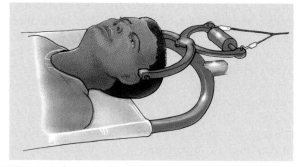

FIGURE 24-7 Cervical traction. A special bed may be used to turn a patient who is in cervical traction. (From Bowden VR, Dickey SB, Greenberg SC: *Children and their families: the continuum of care,* Philadelphia, 1998, Saunders.)

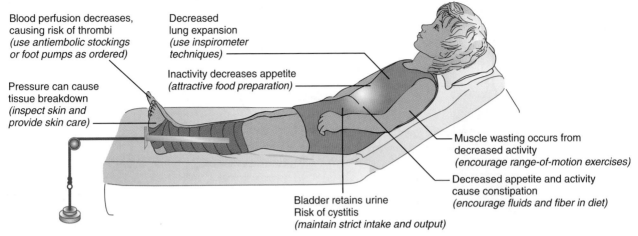

Prolonged treatment requires absence from school
(request home tutor, maintain written or e-mail
contact with friends)

Blood perfusion decreases,
causing risk of thrombi
(use antiembolic stockings
or foot pumps as ordered)

Decreased
lung expansion
(use inspirometer
techniques)

Pressure can cause
tissue breakdown
(inspect skin and
provide skin care)

Inactivity decreases appetite
(attractive food preparation)

Muscle wasting occurs from
decreased activity
(encourage range-of-motion exercises)

Decreased appetite and activity
cause constipation
(encourage fluids and fiber in diet)

Bladder retains urine
Risk of cystitis
(maintain strict intake and output)

FIGURE 24-8 Overcoming the effects of traction on a child.

Nursing Responsibilities for Traction. The nurse observes the traction ropes to be sure they are intact and in the wheel grooves of the pulleys and that the child's body is in good position. In Bryant's traction, the legs should be at right angles to the body, with the buttocks raised sufficiently to clear the bed. In all types of traction, elastic bandages should be neither too loose nor too tight. A jacket restraint may be used to prevent the child from turning from side to side. The weights are not removed after they are applied. **Continuous traction is necessary.** The weights must hang free, and room furnishings, such as a chair, must not obstruct the pull of the weights. The weights are *not* lifted or supported when the bed is moved.

The nurse performs frequent neurovascular checks to the toes to see that they are warm and that their color is good (Figure 24-9). Observations of conditions such as cyanosis, numbness, or irritation from attachments; tight bandages; severe pain; hypoxia or the absence of pulse rates in the extremities are reported immediately to the nurse in charge. A specific and serious complication of any traction is *Volkmann's ischemia* (*ischein,* "to hold back," and *haima,* "blood"), which occurs when the circulation is obstructed. When the legs are elevated overhead, as in Bryant's traction, there is gravitational vascular drainage. Arterial occlusion can cause anoxia of the muscles and reflex vasospasm, which when unnoticed could result in contractures and paralysis.

The child is bathed, and back and buttock care are given. Sheepskin padding may also be used. The sheets are pulled taut and are kept free of crumbs. The jacket restraint is changed when it is soiled. The child is encouraged to drink plenty of fluids and to eat foods that are high in roughage to prevent constipation caused by a lack of exercise. Because the child in traction is unable to sit upright when eating, special precautions to prevent choking and aspiration during mealtime are a priority nursing responsibility. Stool softeners may be

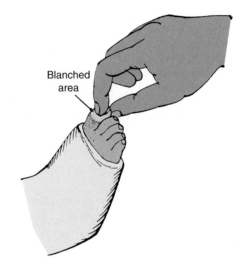

Blanched area

FIGURE 24-9 Checking circulation to the toes or fingers. To check circulation (capillary refill), squeeze or press a toe or finger to blanch the skin. If the circulation is adequate, the color should return in less than 3 seconds when the pressure is released. (1) If the toes do not blanch, congestion may be present and should be reported to the physician. (2) If the blanching persists after pressure is released, the circulation is impaired. The physician must be notified. (3) Report to the physician if extreme pain results from touching or moving the toes. (From Leifer G: *Principles and techniques in pediatric nursing,* Philadelphia, 1982, Saunders.)

necessary. A fracture pan is used for bowel movements, and a careful record is kept of eliminations. Deep-breathing exercises are encouraged to prevent the collection of fluid in the lungs caused by the child's immobility. These exercises may be done by blowing bubbles or by blowing a pinwheel.

Diversional therapy is important because hospitalization may be lengthy. Toys may be securely suspended over the child's head so they are within easy reach. The child's crib is taken to the playroom when possible so the child can experience the excitement of the activities there.

DVDs, CDs, MP3 players, video games, stories, and other forms of entertainment are important aspects of a total nursing care plan. Pain control is essential. Parents are encouraged to visit the child as often as possible. With proper treatment the prognosis for the child with this condition is good.

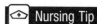 **Nursing Tip**

Checklist for the patient in traction:
- Body in alignment
- Head of bed no higher than 20 degrees (for countertraction)
- Heels of feet elevated from bed
- ROM of unaffected parts checked at regular intervals
- Antiembolism stockings or foot pumps in place as ordered
- Neurovascular checks performed regularly
- Skin integrity monitored regularly
- Pain and its relief by medication recorded
- Measures to prevent constipation
- Use of trapeze for change of position encouraged

Neurovascular checks. A priority nursing responsibility in the care of a child with a fracture who is in traction or who has a cast or Ace bandage in place is to perform neurovascular assessments or **neurovascular checks** at regular intervals (Skill 24-1). Any abnormalities should be reported promptly so that early intervention can prevent complications from developing (Figure 24-10).

! **Safety Alert!**

The "neurovascular check" for tissue perfusion is performed on the toes or fingers distal to an injury or cast and includes the following:
- Peripheral pulse rate and quality
- Color
- Capillary refill time
- Warmth
- Movement and sensation

Nursing Care Plan 24-1 describes interventions for the child in traction.

Assessing for compartment syndrome. Compartment syndrome is a progressive loss of tissue perfusion caused by an increase in pressure resulting from edema or swelling that presses on the vessels and tissues. Circulation is compromised, and the neurovascular check is abnormal.

Compartment syndrome can be caused by a cast that is too tight and compromises circulation or by excessive edema that causes ischemia. Often, surgical intervention (fasciotomy) is required to relieve pressure and to restore circulation. An important nursing responsibility is to provide frequent neurovascular checks on the distal fingers or toes of any injured limb to enable early intervention.

Neurovascular Checks

PURPOSE

To determine if tissue perfusion is adequate

STEPS

1. *Pain:* Assess and record the location and quality of pain. Initiate pain control strategies and medication as soon as possible. Pain at the trauma site that does not respond to medication may indicate a serious complication called *compartment syndrome.* Compartment syndrome is a term used to describe *ischemia* to an extremity caused by pressure on the tissues as a result of excessive edema. A surgical procedure called a fasciotomy (a cutting into the tissue) may be needed to reduce the pressure and increase tissue perfusion.

2. *Pulse:* Compare the quality of the pulse on the affected extremity to that on the unaffected extremity. A strong pulse indicates good blood flow necessary for healing.

3. *Sensation:* Reduced sensation to touch (numbness or tingling) at a site distal to the fracture may indicate poor tissue perfusion and should be reported.

4. *Color:* Pallor at the site distal to the fracture can indicate arterial insufficiency, whereas cyanosis of the site distal to the fracture can indicate venous stasis. Adequate blood supply and vascular drainage are essential for optimal healing.

5. *Capillary refill:* A compressed nail bed should return to its original color in *less than 3 seconds.* The findings should be compared with the unaffected extremity and the results recorded frequently (see Figure 24-9). Any delay in capillary refill time should be reported promptly.

6. *Movement:* Test the toes and fingers distal to the fracture site for movement. Because nerve injury can occur as a complication of skeletal fractures, the movement associated with specific nerve supply should also be tested (see Figure 24-10).

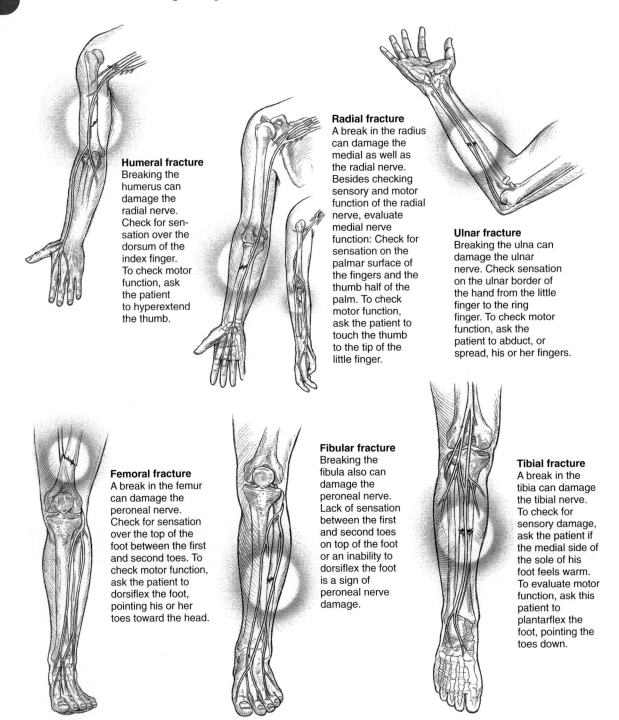

Humeral fracture
Breaking the humerus can damage the radial nerve. Check for sensation over the dorsum of the index finger. To check motor function, ask the patient to hyperextend the thumb.

Radial fracture
A break in the radius can damage the medial as well as the radial nerve. Besides checking sensory and motor function of the radial nerve, evaluate medial nerve function: Check for sensation on the palmar surface of the fingers and the thumb half of the palm. To check motor function, ask the patient to touch the thumb to the tip of the little finger.

Ulnar fracture
Breaking the ulna can damage the ulnar nerve. Check sensation on the ulnar border of the hand from the little finger to the ring finger. To check motor function, ask the patient to abduct, or spread, his or her fingers.

Femoral fracture
A break in the femur can damage the peroneal nerve. Check for sensation over the top of the foot between the first and second toes. To check motor function, ask the patient to dorsiflex the foot, pointing his or her toes toward the head.

Fibular fracture
Breaking the fibula also can damage the peroneal nerve. Lack of sensation between the first and second toes on top of the foot or an inability to dorsiflex the foot is a sign of peroneal nerve damage.

Tibial fracture
A break in the tibia can damage the tibial nerve. To check for sensory damage, ask the patient if the medial side of the sole of his foot feels warm. To evaluate motor function, ask this patient to plantarflex the foot, pointing the toes down.

FIGURE 24-10 Checking for nerve damage. Nerve damage can result from trauma, and the motor sensory status of the extremity should be assessed and recorded frequently. (Courtesy Bert Oppenheim.)

Treatment of Fractures with Casts
Nursing Care of a Child in a Cast. A cast is a device used to immobilize a fracture site, usually including the joints above and below the fracture. Casts are constructed of plaster of Paris or a synthetic material such as fiberglass. Fiberglass casts are lighter than plaster casts and come in various bright colors but cannot be written on as easily as plaster casts can. If the proper lining is used under the fiberglass cast, the cast is water resistant and can be washed and dried, whereas the plaster cast will deteriorate if it becomes wet. When applied, the fiberglass cast dries within half an hour compared to the plaster cast that takes 10 to 72 hours to dry and must be handled carefully with *open palms* and *extended fingers* to prevent indents that can create pressure areas on the skin during this drying time.

Nursing responsibilities include elevating the affected extremity on a pillow and performing frequent neurovascular checks on the distal digits (see Skill 24-1). Before discharge, the nurse teaches the child and

★ Nursing Care Plan 24-1 | The Child in Traction

PATIENT DATA A 6-year-old child is admitted with a fractured femur after falling from a tree while playing. His leg is placed in Steinmann pin traction.

Selected Nursing Diagnosis: Impaired physical mobility related to fixation devices

Goals	Nursing Interventions	Rationales
Child will demonstrate how to obtain help via call light.	Draw picture of fracture for child and explain traction apparatus.	An understanding of condition and of the type of traction used reduces anxiety and promotes compliance with treatment protocol.
	Place call light within easy reach of child.	It is frightening to be immobilized; a call light provides reassurance that help is at hand.
	Change position as traction allows every 2 hours.	Position changes every 2 hours help to prevent skin breakdown.
	Encourage exercise through play by doing pull-ups on trapeze apparatus.	Exercise will help to prevent atrophy, joint contractures, and muscle weakness.
	Institute range-of-motion (ROM) exercises on unaffected extremities.	Unaffected limbs need exercise to prevent stiffness, muscle atrophy, and deformities.
	Encourage self-care.	Self-care promotes self-directed wellness.
	Encourage deep breathing with incentive spirometer or a toy.	Deep-breathing exercises help to prevent pneumonia and atelectasis.
Child will not develop complications of immobility as evidenced by intact skin and absence of respiratory and urinary tract infections.	Observe for urinary tract infection.	Kidney filtration slows with immobilization; immobility causes minerals (e.g., calcium) to leave bones and pool in renal pelvis; stasis of urine is likely to occur, causing renal calculi.
Child will have a bowel movement on a regular basis.	Provide high-fiber diet and stool softeners.	Bulk improves stool consistency and prevents constipation. Stool softeners prevent straining during defecation.
	Provide adequate fluids; monitor intake and output.	Increased fluids are necessary to hydrate body, and they decrease the risk of urine stasis and constipation.

Selected Nursing Diagnosis: Acute pain, related to tissue trauma

Goals	Nursing Interventions	Rationales
Child will be comfortable as evidenced by a decrease in irritability, crying, body posturing, and anorexia.	Administer pain medication before activity and before pain escalates.	Child may be unable to verbalize pain. Premedication for pain allows for muscle relaxation and participation in activities.
Older child verbalizes relief of pain.	Allow choice in method of pain relief, if possible.	Allowing some choice, if there is one, promotes self-control.
	Encourage child to hold favorite possession; provide pacifier for toddler.	Favorite possessions and a pacifier are comforting, particularly to a small child.
	Distract child with music box or tapes as age appropriate.	Distraction from a problem reduces stress and tension.
	Listen and communicate with child.	Listening to child gives nurse clues about amount of pain; nonverbal cues are important in infants and toddlers.
	Use touch as a comfort measure.	Touch is particularly important in infants and toddlers but is comforting for all ages; proceed with caution if there is reason to suspect abuse.
	Involve family in supporting child's ability to cope with pain.	Child trusts family; family members may be able to suggest favorite types of comfort for child.
	Consider cultural background in relation to pain expression.	In some cultures, showing pain is considered cowardly.
	Monitor vital signs.	A change in vital signs can indicate pain, infection, or poor tissue perfusion.
	Provide support and education to family members.	Family members who understand and participate in care can help the child to develop effective coping skills.

Continued

★ Nursing Care Plan 24-1   The Child in Traction—cont'd

Selected Nursing Diagnosis: Risk for impaired skin integrity, related to immobility, traction, poor circulation

Goals	Nursing Interventions	Rationales
Skin will remain intact with no evidence of breakdown.	Inspect skin regularly.	Provides for early assessment of developing skin problems.
Circulation of affected extremity will be adequate as evidenced by normal capillary refill, equal and strong peripheral pulses, and sensation and motion in extremity.	Check capillary refill of nail beds in affected extremity.	Impaired tissue perfusion will result in an increased capillary refill time.
	Have child wiggle toes or fingers of affected extremity to determine sensation and motion.	Wiggling toes and fingers demonstrates extent of mobility and sensation.
	Inspect restraining devices and elastic bandages for wrinkles or looseness.	Excessive tightness or wrinkles in bandages can cause swelling and irritation of underlying tissue.
	Use sheepskin underneath hips and back.	Sheepskin may protect susceptible areas, such as bony prominences on sacrum.
	Monitor traction device, including ropes, pulleys, and weights.	To maintain effective traction, weights must be hanging freely, ropes must be securely on pulleys, and the traction device must be free of friction.
	Maintain body alignment.	Proper body alignment maintains a pull on the long axis of the bone.
	Inspect pin sites for redness, swelling, or discharge; provide pin care according to protocol.	Early intervention can prevent infection; pin care removes debris that can lead to infection or osteomyelitis.

Selected Nursing Diagnosis: Delayed growth and development, related to separation from family and friends

Goals	Nursing Interventions	Rationales
Child's developmental level will be maintained.	Allow child to choose age-appropriate games.	Allowing child to choose activities increases active participation.
	Encourage peer contact.	Children, particularly those of school age and adolescents, must remain in contact with their peers to prevent feelings of isolation.
	Involve child-life specialist or schoolteacher to provide appropriate learning activities.	Maintaining age-appropriate studies will allow the child to rejoin peers in school.

parents how to care for the cast and how to support the cast to prevent the extremity from assuming a dependent position that could compromise circulation. The child is taught safe transfer from bed to wheelchair and safe crutch-walking techniques (e.g., being sure to keep the body weight on the hands and not the axillae). Parents are also taught how to check whether the cast is too loose or too tight and when to return to the clinic or health care provider.

⊘ Safety Alert!

Pain unrelieved by medication, swelling, cyanosis or pallor of digits, or decreased pulse and skin temperature should be immediately reported because they may be signs of compartment syndrome.

The child should be prepared for the experience of cast removal because the cast cutter can appear and sound threatening. After cast removal, the skin can be expected to be dry and caked. Lotion and soothing baths are advised. Care of a child in a spica cast is discussed in Chapter 14.

DISORDERS AND DYSFUNCTION OF THE MUSCULOSKELETAL SYSTEM

OSTEOMYELITIS

Pathophysiology. **Osteomyelitis** is an infection of the bone that generally occurs in children younger than 1 year of age and in those between 5 and 14 years of age. Long bones contain few phagocytic cells (white blood cells [WBCs]) to fight bacteria that may come to the bone from another part of the body. The inflammation produces an exudate that collects under the marrow and cortex of the bone.

Staphylococcus aureus is the organism responsible for osteomyelitis in 75% to 80% of cases in children more than 5 years of age, and *Haemophilus influenzae* is the most common cause in younger children. This incidence may be reduced by the widening practice of routine infant immunization against this organism. Other causative organisms include group A streptococci and pneumococci. *Salmonella* and *Pseudomonas* are organisms often found in adolescents who are intravenous (IV) drug users. Osteomyelitis may be preceded by a local injury to the bone, such as an open fracture, burn, or contamination during surgery. It may also follow a furuncle, impetigo, and abscessed teeth. In neonates a heel puncture or scalp vein monitor can be the predisposing site of infection. Infective emboli may travel to the small arteries of the bone, setting up local destruction and abscess. For this reason, a careful search for infection in other bones and soft tissues is necessary.

The vessels in the affected area are compressed, and thrombosis occurs, producing ischemia and pain. The collection of pus under the periosteum of the bone can elevate the periosteum, which can result in necrosis of that part of the bone. If the pus reaches the epiphysis of the bone in infants, infection can travel to the joint space, causing septic arthritis of that joint.

Local inflammation and increased pressure from the distended periosteum can cause pain. Older children can localize the pain and may limp. Younger children and infants will show decreased voluntary movement of that extremity. Associated muscle spasms can cause limited active ROM. The child may refuse to stand or walk. Signs of local inflammation may be present. A detailed history may show possible sources of primary infection. Blood cultures to identify the organism may be valuable if the child has not been given antibiotics for the primary infection. A urine test for the presence of bacterial antigens and a tissue biopsy may be helpful to establish the diagnosis.

Diagnosis. There is an elevation in WBC count and sedimentation rate. X-ray examination may initially fail to reveal the infection. A microbiology culture of aspirated drainage or a bone scan may be diagnostic.

Treatment and Nursing Care. Prompt and vigorous treatment is essential to ensure a favorable prognosis. Intravenous antibiotics are prescribed for a 4- to 6-week period. The high doses required indicate a nursing responsibility to monitor the infant or child for toxic responses and to ensure long-term compliance. The joint may be drained of pus arthroscopically or surgically to reduce pressure and to prevent bone necrosis. A complication should be suspected if fever lasts beyond 5 days. The use of appropriate pain-relieving medications and gentle handling to minimize pain are essential. The child should be positioned comfortably with the limb supported by pillows or blanket rolls.

Bed rest is followed by wheelchair access, but weight bearing should be avoided. Diversional therapy, physical therapy, and tutorial assistance for school-age children should be provided so that they can return to their classes and classmates after discharge. Close interaction with home care providers is indicated.

DUCHENNE'S MUSCULAR DYSTROPHY

Pathophysiology. The **muscular dystrophies** are a group of disorders in which progressive muscle degeneration occurs. The childhood form (Duchenne's

muscular dystrophy) is the most common type. It has an incidence of about 1 in 3600 live born male infants of all races and ethnic groups. It is a sex-linked inherited disorder that occurs only in boys. Dystrophin, a protein in skeletal muscle, is absent. Becker's pseudohypertrophic muscular dystrophy occurs later in childhood, progresses more slowly and is not as common as Duchenne's muscular dystrophy.

Manifestations. The onset is generally between 2 and 6 years of age; however, a history of delayed motor development during infancy may be evidenced. The calf muscles in particular become hypertrophied. The term *pseudohypertrophic* (*pseudo,* "false," and *hypertrophy,* "enlargement") refers to this characteristic. Other signs include progressive weakness as evidenced by frequent falling, clumsiness, contractures of the ankles and hips, and Gowers' maneuver (a characteristic way of rising from the floor).

Laboratory findings show marked increases in serum creatine phosphokinase. Muscle biopsy shows a degeneration of muscle fibers and their replacement by fat and connective tissue. A myelogram (a graphic record of muscle contraction as a result of electrical stimulation) shows decreases in the amplitude and duration of motor unit potentials. A serum blood polymerase chain reaction (PCR) for the gene mutation is diagnostic for this condition (Sarnat, 2007). The disease becomes progressively worse, and wheelchair confinement may be necessary. Death usually results from cardiac failure or respiratory tract infection. Mental retardation is not uncommon.

Treatment and Nursing Care. The use of prednisone has shown some promise. Studies are in place concerning the use of glutamine and creatine for muscle weakness, the enzyme transferase to block muscle wasting, and urotrophin to replace the missing dystrophin. Treatment at this time is mainly supportive to prevent contractures and to maintain the quality of life. Cardiac and respiratory complications are common. A multidisciplinary team should provide psychological support, nutritional support, physiotherapy, social and financial assistance, and, when necessary, respite and hospice care.

Compared with other children with disabilities, some children with muscular dystrophy may appear passive and withdrawn. Early on, depression may be seen because the child cannot compete with peers. Social and emotional pressures on the child and family are great.

SLIPPED FEMORAL CAPITAL EPIPHYSIS (SCFE)

Pathophysiology. A **slipped femoral capital epiphysis,** also known as *coxa vara,* is the spontaneous displacement of the epiphysis of the femur. It most often occurs during rapid growth of the preadolescent and is not related to trauma. More than 80% of children with SCFE are obese (Chen, 2009). Increased rates of obesity have correlated with increased rates of the occurrence of SCFE. The epiphysis of the femur widens, and then the femoral head and epiphysis remain in the acetabulum. The head of the femur then rotates and displaces. Symptoms include thigh pain and a limp or the inability to bear weight on the involved leg. An x-ray study confirms diagnosis.

Treatment. The child is placed in traction to minimize further slippage, and then surgery is scheduled to insert a screw to stabilize the bone. Serious complications may include disturbance of circulation to the epiphysis, resulting in necrosis of the head of the femur.

Nursing Care. The general principles of caring for a child in traction and preoperative and postoperative care are used (see Chapters 14 and 22). The nurse assists in performing orders regarding range-of-motion activities, guides gradual resumption of weight bearing with the help of crutches, and encourages referrals to maintain school studies. Education concerning management of weight is important postoperatively.

LEGG-CALVÉ-PERTHES DISEASE (COXA PLANA)

Pathophysiology. **Legg-Calvé-Perthes disease** is one of a group of disorders called the osteochondroses (*osteo,* "bone," *chondros,* "cartilage," and *osis,* "disease") in which the blood supply to the epiphysis, or end of the bone, is disrupted. The tissue death that results from the inadequate blood supply is termed *avascular necrosis* (*a,* "without," *vasculum,* "vessels," and *nekros,* "death"). Legg-Calvé-Perthes disease affects the development of the head of the femur. The incidence is approximately 1:1250 (Perry, 2011). The disease is seen most commonly in boys between 5 and 12 years of age. It is more common in Caucasians. This disease is unilateral in about 85% of cases. Healing occurs spontaneously during 2 to 4 years; however, marked distortion of the head of the femur may lead to an imperfect joint or degenerative arthritis of the hip in later life. Symptoms include a painless limp and limitation of motion. X-ray films and bone scans confirm the diagnosis.

Treatment. Legg-Calvé-Perthes disease is a self-limiting disorder that heals spontaneously, but slowly, throughout the course of 2 to 4 years. The treatment involves keeping the femoral head deep in the hip socket while it heals and preventing weight bearing. This is accomplished through the use of ambulation-abduction casts or braces that prevent subluxation (*sub,* "beneath," and *luxatio,* "dislocation") and enable the acetabulum to mold the healing head in such a way that it does not become deformed. Bed rest and traction may precede this treatment. The prognosis in Legg-Calvé-Perthes disease is fair. Some affected people may require hip joint replacement procedures as adults.

Nursing Care. Nursing considerations depend on the age of the patient and the type of treatment. The general principles of traction, cast, and brace care are used when immobilization of the child is necessary. Teaching and counseling are directed toward a holistic understanding of and interest in the individual child and family. Total immobility or partial mobility is particularly trying for children. The natural inclination to compete physically is thwarted. In some cases surgical immobilization is required. Preoperative and postoperative care and care of a patient in a cast are discussed in Chapters 14 and 22.

OSTEOSARCOMA

Pathophysiology. **Osteosarcoma** (*osteo,* "bone," *sarx,* "flesh," and *oma,* "tumor") is a primary malignant tumor of the long bones. The two most common types of bone tumors in children are osteosarcoma and Ewing's sarcoma. The mean age of onset of osteosarcoma is between 10 and 15 years of age. Children who have had radiation therapy for other types of cancer and children with retinoblastoma have a higher incidence of this disease. Metastasis occurs quickly because of the high vascularity of bone tissue. The lungs are the primary site of metastasis; the brain and other bone tissue are also sites of metastasis.

Manifestations. The patient experiences pain and swelling at the site. In adolescents this is often attributed to injury or "growing pains." Flexing the extremity may lessen the pain. Later a pathological fracture may occur. Diagnosis is confirmed by biopsy. A complete physical examination, including CT and a bone scan, is performed. Radiological studies help to confirm the diagnosis.

Treatment and Nursing Care. Treatment of the patient with osteosarcoma consists of radical resection or amputation surgery. Internal prostheses are available for most sites. Long-term survival is possible with early diagnosis and treatment.

The nursing care is similar to that for other types of cancer. Problems of body image are particularly important to the self-conscious adolescent. If amputation is necessary, the family and patient will need much support. The nurse anticipates anger, fear, and grief. Immediately after surgery the stump dressing is observed frequently for signs of bleeding. Vital signs are monitored. The child is positioned as ordered by the surgeon.

Phantom limb pain is likely to be experienced. This is the continued sensation of pain in the limb even though the limb is no longer there. It occurs because nerve tracts continue to report pain. This pain is very real, and an analgesic may be necessary. Rehabilitation measures follow surgical recovery.

EWING'S SARCOMA

Pathophysiology. Dr. James Ewing first described **Ewing's sarcoma** in 1921. It is a malignant growth that occurs in the marrow of the long bones. It occurs mainly in older school-age children and early adolescents. When metastasis is present on diagnosis, the prognosis is poor. Without metastasis there is a 60% survival rate. The primary sites for metastasis are the lungs and long bones.

Treatment and Nursing Care. Amputation is not generally recommended for Ewing's sarcoma because the tumor is sensitive to radiation therapy and chemotherapy. This is a relief to the child and family. The child is warned against vigorous weight bearing on the involved bone during therapy to help prevent pathological fractures. Patients must be prepared for the effects of radiation therapy and chemotherapy. The nurse supports the family members in their efforts to gain equilibrium after such a crisis.

JUVENILE IDIOPATHIC ARTHRITIS (JUVENILE RHEUMATOID ARTHRITIS)

Pathophysiology. **Juvenile rheumatoid arthritis** (JRA) is now referred to as juvenile idiopathic arthritis (JIA) and is the most common arthritic condition of childhood. It is a systemic autoimmune disease that involves the joints, connective tissues, and viscera, and it differs somewhat from adult rheumatoid arthritis. It is not a rare disease. Approximately 1 of 1000 children in the United States has JIA (Stanley, 2011). The exact cause is unknown, but an autoimmune response is believed to be the cause.

Manifestations and Types. JIA has several distinct classifications.
1. *Oligo Arthritis* involves 4 or fewer joints, and uveitis (inflammation of the eye) is common in about 30% of the children.
2. *Polyarthritis* involves 5 or more joints, and uveitis occurs in about 10% of the children.
3. *Systemic arthritis* is characterized by fever, rash, and joint inflammation. Uveitis occurs in about 10% of these children (Nistala, 2009). The *systemic* form is manifested by intermittent spiking fever above 39.5° C (103° F) persisting for more than 10 days, a nonpruritic macular rash, abdominal pain, an elevated ESR, C-reactive protein in laboratory tests, presence of antinuclear antibodies, and possibly an enlarged liver and spleen. It occurs most often in children ages 1 to 3 years and 8 to 10 years. Joint symptoms may be absent at onset, but usually arthritis develops in most patients.

Treatment. The goals of therapy are to accomplish the following:
- Reduce joint pain and swelling
- Promote mobility and preserve joint function
- Promote growth and development
- Promote independent functioning
- Help the child and family to adjust to living with a chronic disease

Medications such as nonsteroidal antiinflammatory drugs (NSAIDs) and methotrexate may also be provided. The child should undergo frequent CBC tests to monitor closely for side effects. Steroids may be administered for incapacitating arthritis, uveitis, or life-threatening complications. Etanercept (Enbrel) is a tumor necrosis factor–inhibitor used in children unresponsive to methotrexate. It is administered subcutaneously, weekly, and may have serious side effects. Slow-acting antirheumatic drugs (SAARDs) such as sulfasalazine, hydroxychloroquine, gold, and d-penicillamine can be used with NSAIDs but are not as popular today as in the past.

Nursing Care. The nurse functions as a member of a multidisciplinary health care team that includes the pediatrician, rheumatologist, social worker, physical therapist, occupational therapist, psychologist, ophthalmologist, and school and community nurses. Physical and occupational therapy preserve joint function and mobility. Occupational therapy helps with activities of daily living. Resting in a bed with a supportive, flat mattress is helpful. Resting splints during sleep can prevent flexion contractures from developing. Moist heat and exercise are advised, and whirlpool baths and hot packs relieve pain and stiffness. Therapeutic play facilitates compliance with exercise regimens. Pool exercise, kick ball, and biking can help maintain joint mobility. Sleep, rest, and general health measures are important. The school nurse can be contacted to help promote normal growth and development in school-related activities. Homeschooling, if needed, is available in most school districts. Unnecessary restrictions should be avoided because they can lead to rebellion and noncompliance. JIA inhibits the child's social interactions and can interfere with development of a positive self-concept. The Arthritis Foundation provides services to parents and nurses involved in patient care.

This long-term disease is characterized by periods of remission and exacerbations. Nurses can serve as advocates for the child; that is, they can help alleviate stress by recognizing the impact of the disease and by openly communicating with the child, the family, and other members of the health care team. Nurses support the child and family members and instill hope.

TORTICOLLIS (WRY NECK)

Pathophysiology. **Torticollis** (*tortus,* "twisted," and *collium,* "neck") is a condition in which neck motion is limited and the cervical spine is rotated because of shortening of the sternocleidomastoid muscle. It can be either congenital or acquired and can also be either acute or chronic. The most common type is a congenital anomaly in which the sternocleidomastoid muscle is injured during birth. It is associated with breech and forceps delivery and may be seen in conjunction with other birth defects, such as congenital hip dysplasia.

Manifestations. In congenital torticollis the symptoms are present at birth. The infant holds the head to the side of the muscle involved. The chin is tilted in the opposite direction. There is a hard, palpable mass of dense fibrotic tissue (fibroma). This is not fixed to the skin and resolves by 2 to 6 months of age. Passive stretching and ROM exercises and physical therapy may be indicated. Feeding and playing with the infant can encourage turning to the desired side for correction. Surgical correction is indicated if the condition persists beyond 2 years of age.

Acquired torticollis is seen in older children. It may be associated with injury, inflammation, neurological disorders, and other causes. Nursing intervention is primarily that of detection. Infants who have limited head movement require further investigation.

SCOLIOSIS

Pathophysiology. The most prevalent of the three skeletal abnormalities shown in Figure 24-11 is *scoliosis.* Scoliosis refers to an S-shaped curvature of the spine. During adolescence, scoliosis is more common in girls. Many curvatures are not progressive and may necessitate only periodic evaluation. Untreated progressive scoliosis may lead to back pain, fatigue, disability, and heart and lung complications. Skeletal deterioration does not stop with maturity and may be aggravated by pregnancy.

Causes. There are two types of scoliosis: functional and structural. *Functional* scoliosis is usually caused by poor posture, not by spinal disease. The curve is flexible

and easily correctable. *Structural* or fixed scoliosis is caused by changes in the shape of the vertebrae or thorax. It is usually accompanied by rotation of the spine. The hips and shoulders may appear uneven. The patient cannot correct the condition by standing in a straighter posture.

There are many causes of structural scoliosis. Some are congenital and develop in utero. These are noticeable at birth or during periods of rapid growth. Neuromuscular scoliosis is the result of muscle weakness or imbalance. It is seen in children with cerebral palsy, muscular dystrophy, and other conditions. The cause of idiopathic scoliosis is unknown; there may be a hereditary link.

Signs and Symptoms. Symptoms develop slowly and are not painful so that detection is usually via an incidental screening at school by the school nurse. The shoulders are different heights with one higher than the other, and a one-sided rib hump and a prominent scapula are seen. This asymmetry is seen from the back when the child leans forward. Diagnosis is made by moiré photography that highlights the asymmetry, and by a spinal x-ray study.

Treatment. Treatment is aimed at correcting the curvature and preventing more severe scoliosis. Curves up to 20 degrees do not necessitate treatment but are carefully followed with exercise to increase muscle tone and posture. Curves between 20 and 40 degrees require the use of a **Milwaukee brace** (Figure 24-12). This apparatus exerts pressure on the chin, pelvis, and convex (arched) side of the spine. It is worn approximately 23 hours a day and is worn *over* a T-shirt to protect the skin. An underarm modification of the brace (the Boston brace) is proving effective for patients with low curvatures. It is less cumbersome and is more acceptable to the self-conscious young person. Transcutaneous electrical muscle stimulation (TENS) and exercise have also proven effective in the treatment of scoliosis (Kliegman, 2011).

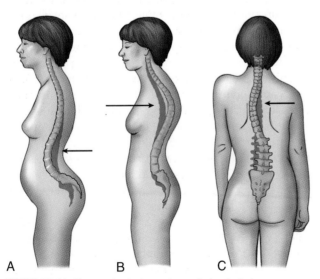

FIGURE 24-11 Abnormal spinal curvatures. **A,** *Lordosis,* known as "sway back," is commonly seen during pregnancy. **B,** *Kyphosis,* known as "hunchback," is an increased roundness in the thoracic curve commonly found in the elderly. **C,** *Scoliosis,* an abnormal side-to-side curvature of the spine, is commonly found in adolescents. (From Patton KT, Thibodeau GA: *Anatomy & physiology,* ed 8, St Louis, 2013, Mosby.)

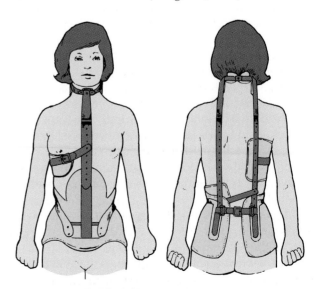

FIGURE 24-12 The Milwaukee brace.

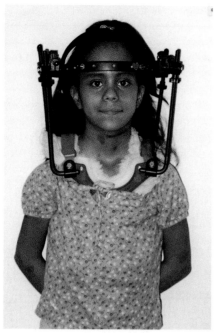

FIGURE 24-13 Halo traction. This halo jacket and apparatus is used for cervical fractures and spinal disorders. (Courtesy Pat Spier, RN-C.)

Severe scoliosis necessitates surgery to fuse the bones. A Harrington rod, Dwyer instrument, or Luque wires may be inserted for immobilization during the time required for the fusion to become solid. Halo traction may be used when there is associated weakness or paralysis of the neck and trunk muscles (Figure 24-13); this traction is also used in treating cervical fractures and fusions. An anterior/posterior plastic shell or orthotic may be worn for several months until the spine is stable. Helping the teen cope with a body brace and maintain a positive self-image is an important aspect of care.

Nursing Tip

Insertion of a Harrington rod or other metal device may delay a patient at an airport or other security scanner because the metal could activate the alarm.

Nursing Care

Community nursing. The management of scoliosis begins with screening. This is undertaken before middle school. It should be a part of every yearly physical examination for prepubescent youngsters. Camp nurses also need to be aware of symptoms. Early recognition is of utmost importance in detecting mild cases amenable to nonsurgical treatment.

The adolescent is prepared by explaining the purpose of the procedure and by being reassured that it merely entails observing the back while standing and bending forward. Adolescents must know that it is simple, quick, and painless and that privacy will be afforded. They are instructed to wear clothing that is easy to remove, such as a pullover top. Boys disrobe to the waist, girls generally to the bra. No slip or undershirt should be worn.

The procedure consists of the nurse examining the spine from the front, side, and back while the adolescent stands erect and then observing the back as the adolescent bends forward. One looks initially for general body alignment and *asymmetry* (lack of proportion). In scoliosis, one shoulder may be higher than the other, a scapula may be prominent, the arm-to-body spaces may be unequal, or a hip may protrude; one arm may appear longer than the other when the person bends forward. Referrals are made as indicated to those who must obtain further treatment.

The nurse's knowledge of preadolescent and adolescent developmental tasks is imperative, because therapy often conflicts with these tasks.

Routine preoperative nursing care of the adolescent is necessary for spinal fusion. This includes instructing the adolescent and family about the purpose and extent of the cast or brace that may be prescribed. It is important for the nurse to evaluate and document the adolescent's neuromuscular status at this time so that it may be used as a basis for comparison after the procedure is completed.

Much postoperative nursing care is directly related to combating the physical results of immobilization (see Figure 24-8). The body systems become sluggish because of inactivity. This is evidenced in the gastrointestinal tract by anorexia, irregularity, and constipation. Allowing the adolescent to select foods with the aid of the dietitian is helpful in improving appetite. Increasing fluid intake reduces constipation. The adolescent and parents are introduced to the multidisciplinary health care team. Postoperative exercise, physical therapy, and promotion of adolescent school and developmental tasks are essential aspects of nursing care.

SPORTS INJURIES

A high percentage of adolescent males and females participate in athletic activities. The American Academy of Pediatrics (AAP) recommends that a complete physical examination be given at least every other year during adolescence and that sports-specific examinations be provided for those involved in strenuous activity on entry into middle school or senior high school. Such examinations should be updated by an annual questionnaire. The family history and an orthopedic screening are important in identifying risk factors.

Prevention. Several factors help to prevent sports injuries. Some of these are adequate warm-up and cool-down periods; year-round conditioning; careful selection of activity according to physical maturity, size, and skill necessary; proper supervision by adults; safe, well-fitting equipment; and avoidance of participation when in pain or injured. Proper diet and fluids are also necessary. A few of the more common injuries are listed in Table 24-1. The nurse has a major role in educating and directing parents to sources of accurate information to ensure that the physical, emotional, and maturational levels of the adolescent are appropriate for the activity (see Health Promotion box). Parents

Table 24-1	Common Sports Injuries
TYPE	**DESCRIPTION**
Concussion	Any blow to the head followed by alterations in mental functioning should be treated as a possible concussion; observe carefully for sequelae
"Stingers" or "burners"	A common neck injury when a player hits another in the head in such sports as football or soccer; caused by brachial plexus trauma; feels like an electrical jolt; usually mild and disappears suddenly; restrict sports activity until symptoms disappear; reassess protective gear
Injured knee	Usually a result of stress on the knee ligaments; potentially serious; should be evaluated by an experienced trainer or physician; may necessitate arthroscopic surgery
Sprain or strained ankle	May injure growth plate; x-ray films important in adolescent
Muscle cramps	Caused by injury, alterations in blood flow, or electrolyte deficiencies; important to warm up before activity; ensure fluid intake is adequate
Shin splints	Pain and discomfort in lower leg caused by repeated running on a hard surface such as concrete; avoid such activity; use well-fitting shoes; decrease inflammation by rest

are encouraged to inquire about the capabilities of personnel and the availability of emergency services before the beginning of the competition.

FAMILY VIOLENCE

Violence has become a problem that affects children of all social classes across the nation. Family violence includes spousal abuse and child abuse, neglect, and maltreatment. Community violence is seen in neighborhoods where even non–gang-related adolescents arm themselves with guns and knives for protection. Preschoolers who are repeatedly allowed to watch violent programs on television or play aggressive computer games may be learning antisocial coping skills they will use as they grow and mature. Parents should control the time spent watching television and the content of the programs, so that television exposure results in the acquisition of knowledge, skills, and information that will motivate learning. In homes where spousal and/or child abuse occurs, children learn the behaviors they will likely practice when they become adults, and the abuse cycle continues. Parents who are abusive are not usually psychotic or criminal. They

---

⛹ Health Promotion

Selected Recreational Activities and Their Risks

ACTIVITY	RISK
Gymnastics	Common problems associated with children engaging in gymnastics are delayed menstruation and eating disorders. Trauma and overuse injuries of the large joints and spine are common. Prevention includes muscle strengthening exercises, flexibility exercises, and wrist braces. Nutritional planning and education are essential.
Ballet	Common problems associated with ballet include delayed menarche and eating disorders. There is a high risk for stress fractures, strains, shin splints, and spinal deviations. Prevention includes skilled coaching and nutrition planning and education.
Wrestling	Placement in a wrestling match is based on weight. A bingeing and purging behavior is commonly found in athletes participating in wrestling. Concussions, neck strains, and spinal injuries are common. Skin dermatitis and infection occur from contact with floor mats. Skilled coaching and nutrition education and planning are important.
Football	Improvements in techniques, protective equipment, and game exercises have decreased serious injuries in children participating on football teams.
Hockey	Injuries can occur from both collisions with other athletes and collisions with pucks or sticks. Proper protective equipment and sporting rules decrease the seriousness of injuries.
Basketball, volleyball	These are jumping sports that involve injury risk to ankles, knees, and fingers. Ankle sprain, tendonitis, stress fractures, and blisters are common complications of these sports.
Running	Involves repeated, poorly absorbed foot impact. Muscle fatigue, environmental temperature, and running surface contribute to injuries. Engaging in proper exercises before running, using good impact-absorbing shoes, cross-training, and adequate rest are essential. *Shin splints* involve pain over the anterior tibia and result from tearing the collagenous fibers that connect muscle to bone. Shoe orthotics, running on a soft surface, cross-training, and rest are the priorities of management.
Skiing, snowboarding	Injuries are usually related to falls. Better equipment, controlled slope conditions, and separation of skiers by skill level contribute to a decreased rate of injury.
Cheerleading	Includes acrobatics, pyramid climbing, and tossing. Falls related to injuries such as sprains, fractures, dislocations, and head injuries. Safety instruction is important, and a certified coach should be present.

may have a knowledge deficit about child care needs and child growth and development. Abusive parents are often without a support system and are perhaps alone, angry, or in crisis, or have unrealistic expectations.

CHILD ABUSE

Kempe (1962) coined the term *battered child syndrome* in his landmark article in the *Journal of the American Medical Association*. It refers to "a clinical condition in young children who have received serious physical abuse, generally from a parent or foster parent." The impact of Kempe's research was considerable and focused the attention of physicians on unexplained fractures and signs of physical abuse. Today, most authorities consider Kempe's definition narrow and have broadened it to include neglect and maltreatment.

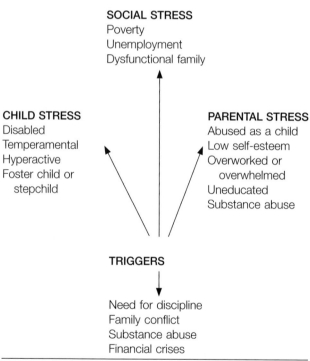

Health Promotion

Factors That May Contribute to or Trigger Child Abuse

SOCIAL STRESS
Poverty
Unemployment
Dysfunctional family

CHILD STRESS
Disabled
Temperamental
Hyperactive
Foster child or
    stepchild

PARENTAL STRESS
Abused as a child
Low self-esteem
Overworked or
    overwhelmed
Uneducated
Substance abuse

TRIGGERS

Need for discipline
Family conflict
Substance abuse
Financial crises

NOTE: Abusive parents may love their children but respond to stress and triggers that provoke abusive behavior.

According to the National Center on Child Abuse and Neglect (Nooner et al, 2010), the incidence of the following aspects of child abuse has been increasing:

- *Emotional abuse:* Intentional verbal acts that result in a destruction of self-esteem in the child; can include rejection or threatening the child
- *Emotional neglect:* An intentional omission of verbal or behavioral actions that are necessary for development of a healthy self-esteem; can include social or emotional isolation of a child

- *Sexual abuse:* Involves an act that is performed on a child for the sexual gratification of the adult
- *Physical neglect:* The failure to provide for the basic physical needs of the child, including food, clothing, shelter, and basic cleanliness
- *Physical abuse:* The deliberate infliction of injury on a child; suspected when an injury is not consistent with the history or developmental level of the child

The temperament of the child and the parent can be a causal factor in child abuse. Children who are different from others in any way are at particular risk. This includes preterm infants, sick or disabled children, and merely unattractive children. Unwanted or illegitimate infants and stepchildren are especially vulnerable. It has been noted that people are often reluctant to report occurrences in middle- and upper-income families or when the incident involves friends or relatives.

FEDERAL LAWS AND AGENCIES

By 1963 the U.S. Children's Bureau drafted a model mandatory state reporting law that has been adopted in some form in all states (see Legal & Ethical Considerations box). This law aids in establishing statistics and is based on the need to provide therapeutic help to both child and family. Immunity from liability is provided for persons reporting suspected cases. Most states have penalties for failure to report suspected child abuse. Referrals usually are made to the local child protective services, and a caseworker is assigned.

Legal & Ethical Considerations

Reporting Suspected Abuse or Neglect

A citizen can report suspected child abuse or neglect by contacting the child protective services using the Internet or in the yellow pages of the telephone directory under "Social Service Organizations." This can be done anonymously. After obtaining the facts, the agency informs the parents that a report is being filed and checks the condition of the child. A visit must be initiated within 72 hours. In most cases, this is accomplished within 48 hours or earlier if the situation is life threatening. All persons who report suspected abuse or neglect are given immunity from criminal prosecution and civil liability if the report is made in good faith. Many professionals, such as physicians, nurses, and social workers, must report child abuse.

NURSING CARE AND INTERVENTIONS

Nursing intervention for high-risk children is of utmost importance (Box 24-1). One approach currently taken is to identify high-risk infants and parents during the prenatal and perinatal periods. Predictive questionnaires are being used as screening tools in some clinics. Many hospitals also provide closer follow-up of mothers and newborns. Maternal–infant bonding and its significance to later parent–child relationships has been explored.

Nurses in obstetrical clinics have the opportunity to observe parents and their abilities to cope. The history of the parent(s), desirability of the pregnancy, number of children already in the family, financial and personal

| Box 24-1 | Nursing Interventions for Abused and Neglected Children and Adolescents |

TEACH CHILD ANXIETY-REDUCING TECHNIQUES
Teach child gradual relaxation.
Teach child relaxation to music.
Teach child visual imagery.
Teach child how to use exercise to reduce anxiety.
Teach child to talk to safe, appropriate people about feelings.
Teach child to choose, build, and maintain positive support systems.
Teach child to ensure personal safety.
Teach child to set boundaries.
Teach child to establish a safe, supportive relationship.
Teach child to clarify expectations and rules.
Teach child self-soothing techniques.

ASSIST CHILD IN MANAGING HIS OR HER FEELINGS
Teach child to identify feelings.
Teach child to express feelings appropriately.
Teach child to modulate and control feelings.
Teach child to identify events that elicit strong positive and negative feelings.
Teach child to express feelings verbally instead of physically.
Teach child to normalize feelings resulting from abuse.
Teach child to share feelings appropriately with peer group.
Teach child to find commonality and support within group for feelings resulting from abuse.

TEACH CHILD ASSERTIVENESS SKILLS
Teach child to identify differences between assertiveness, passivity, and aggression.
Teach child to practice assertiveness skills.
Teach child to identify boundaries.
Teach child to understand when someone violates boundaries.
Teach child to practice responses when someone violates boundaries.

ASSIST CHILD IN DEVELOPING PROBLEM-SOLVING SKILLS
Provide simple problem-solving model.
Increase awareness of child's control and decision making.
Teach child to generate a list of possible solutions to problem situations.
Help child look at consequences of each solution.
Help child make best choice.
Help child give positive and gentle negative feedback to self.
Coach problem solving with actual situations as much as possible.
Teach about good touch and bad touch.
Teach refusal skills.
Teach age-appropriate sexual expression.
Teach the effects of substance abuse.

ASSIST CHILD IN VALUE BUILDING AND CLARIFICATION
Define values.
Identify role of values.
Assist child in identifying and verbalizing values.
Help link child's values to child's actions.
Assist child in development of values.
Help child practice value-based decision-making.

ASSIST CHILD IN ENHANCING HIS OR HER COPING MECHANISMS
Teach child to practice positive self-talk.
Help child set realistic expectations for self.
Assist child in learning to nurture self.
Teach child to practice relaxation.
Teach child to practice assertiveness and appropriate expression of feelings.
Assist child in learning to accept defeat and failure.
Help child identify and build skills and hobbies.
Encourage child to identify and focus on strengths.
Help child set and accomplish goals.
Assist child in developing organizational skills.

Data from: Bowden VR, Dickey SB, Greenberg CS: *Children and their families: the continuum of care*, Philadelphia, 1998, Saunders; Santrock J: *Child development*, ed 13, Philadelphia, 2011, McGraw-Hill; DiMarco M, Melnyk B: The mental health needs of children and adolescents, *Arch Psychiatr Nurs* 23:334-336, 2009; Storch E, Elder J: Introduction to special series on child and adolescent mental health, *Pediatr Nurs* 24:1-2, 2009.

stability of the family, types of support systems, and other factors may have a bearing on how the parents accept the new offspring. Pertinent observations include a description of parent–newborn interaction. Both verbal and nonverbal communications are important, as is the level of body and eye contact. Lack of interest, indifference, or negative comments about the sex, looks, or temperament of the infant could be significant.

In other areas, a cooperative team approach is necessary. This may include services such as family planning, protective services, day care centers, homemakers, parenting classes, self-help groups, family counseling, child advocates, and a continued effort to reduce the incidence of preterm birth. Other related areas include financial assistance, employment services, transportation, emotional support and encouragement, and long-term follow-up care.

Individual nurses can help to detect child abuse by maintaining a vigilant approach in their work settings. Record keeping should be *factual* and *objective*. The pediatric nurse should make a point of reviewing old records of their patients, which may show repeated hospitalizations, x-ray films of multiple fractures, persistent feeding problems, a history of failure to thrive, and a history of chronic absenteeism from school. Neglect or delay in seeking medical attention for a child or failure to obtain immunization and well-child care can be significant findings. Children who seem overly upset about being discharged must be brought to the attention of the health care provider. Runaway teenagers are often victims of abuse.

The abused child is approached quietly, and preparation for any treatment is carefully explained in advance. The number of caretakers should be kept to a minimum. The child may be able to express some hostility and fear through play or drawing. It is not unusual for these children to be unresponsive or openly hostile or to show affection indiscriminately. Direct questioning is kept to a minimum. Praise is used when appropriate. Activities that promote physical and sensory development are encouraged. The nurse avoids speaking to the child about the parents in a negative manner. Other professionals are consulted about setting limits for poor behavior.

The nurse must acknowledge that there are always two victims in cases of child abuse: the child *and* the abuser. Because of personal problems, the abuser often leads an isolated life. Some have themselves been battered or neglected as children. Many have unrealistic expectations about the child's intelligence and capabilities. There may be a role reversal in which the child becomes the comforter. Although removing the child from the home is one answer, many authorities believe this can be more detrimental in the long run.

Being open to parents during this type of crisis is difficult but essential if the nurse wishes to be part of the solution rather than part of the problem. When placement in a foster home is necessary, parents experience grief, loss, and remorse. The child also mourns the loss of the family, even though there has been abuse. The nurse should be aware of the child's needs and facilitate the expression of feelings of loss. The nurse who recognizes the potential for violence within all of us is better able to respond to this complex problem.

! Safety Alert!

Bruises heal in various stages that are indicated according to color:

- 1 to 2 days: **swollen, tender**
- 2 to 5 days: **red or purple**
- 5 to 7 days: **green**
- 7 to 10 days: **yellow**
- 10 to 14 days: **brown**
- 14 to 28 days: **clear**

It is important to ask yourself, "Does the bruise match the caregiver's explanation of what happened and when?"

CULTURAL AND MEDICAL ISSUES

Multiple factors should be considered when evaluating the child. A culturally sensitive history is essential. The nurse should be aware that what appears to be a cigarette burn could be a single lesion of impetigo. Mongolian spots can be mistaken for bruises. A severe diaper rash caused by a fungal infection can look like a scald burn. In some cases, loving parents can injure infants when shaking them to wake or feed them. They are not aware of the danger of "shaken baby syndrome."

Some cultural practices can be interpreted as physical abuse if the nurse is not culturally aware of folk healing and ethnic practices. For example, "coining" of the body by the Vietnamese to allay disease can cause welts on the body (see Chapter 34). Burning small areas of the skin to treat enuresis is practiced by some Asian cultures. Forced kneeling is a common Caribbean discipline technique. Yemenite Jews treat infections by placing garlic preparations on the wrists, which can result in blisters. The Telugu people of Southern India touch the penis of a child to show respect.

The nurse should document all signs of abuse and interaction as well as verbal comments between the child and parents (Figure 24-14). Child protective services should oversee any investigation that is warranted. Providing support to parents and child, including an opportunity to talk in privacy, and planning for follow-up care are basic nursing responsibilities. Parent education concerning growth and development is valuable.

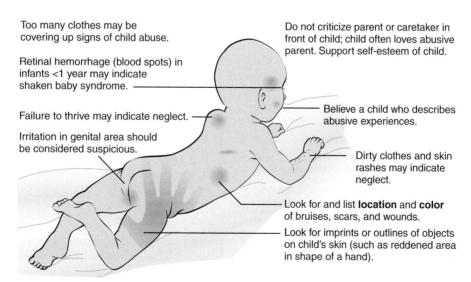

Too many clothes may be covering up signs of child abuse.

Retinal hemorrhage (blood spots) in infants <1 year may indicate shaken baby syndrome.

Failure to thrive may indicate neglect.

Irritation in genital area should be considered suspicious.

Do not criticize parent or caretaker in front of child; child often loves abusive parent. Support self-esteem of child.

Believe a child who describes abusive experiences.

Dirty clothes and skin rashes may indicate neglect.

Look for and list **location** and **color** of bruises, scars, and wounds.

Look for imprints or outlines of objects on child's skin (such as reddened area in shape of a hand).

Divide the body into four planes: front, back, right side, and left side.
Injuries occurring in >1 plane should be considered suspicious.

FIGURE 24-14 Assessing for child abuse. The nurse should be alert for inconsistent statements about injuries, bruises at various stages of healing, delay in seeking care, and a history that is not compatible with injury or development.

Get Ready for the NCLEX® Examination!

Key Points

- The age, neurological development, and motor milestones achieved will influence the nursing assessment of the musculoskeletal system in a growing child.
- The normal gait of a toddler is wide and unstable. By 6 years of age, the gait resembles an adult walk.
- Immobility causes a deceleration of body metabolism.
- Injury to the epiphyseal plate at the ends of long bones is serious during childhood because it may interfere with longitudinal growth.
- In a compound fracture a wound in the skin accompanies the broken bone, and there is added danger of infection.
- Any delay in neurological development can cause a delay in mastery of motor skills, which can result in altered skeletal growth.
- Children who do not walk by 18 months of age should be referred for follow-up care.
- Rest, ice, compression, and elevation are the principles of managing soft tissue injuries.
- Pain over a muscle area that does not respond to medication may indicate a complication known as *compartment syndrome*.
- A neurovascular check includes color, warmth, capillary refill time, movement, pulse, sensation, and pain.
- Frequent neurovascular checks should be performed on the distal digits of a patient with a cast to determine adequate tissue perfusion.
- Tutorial assistance should be provided to school-age children who are hospitalized or immobilized for long periods of time.
- A complication of any traction is an arterial occlusion termed Volkmann's ischemia.
- Legg-Calvé-Perthes disease affects the blood supply to the head of the femur.
- Juvenile idiopathic arthritis is the most common arthritic condition of childhood.
- Juvenile idiopathic arthritis can inhibit social interaction and the development of a positive self-image.
- Treatment of scoliosis includes bracing, exercise, and surgery (spinal fusion).
- Adolescents who participate in sports are subject to injuries such as concussions and ligament injuries. Activities must be selected carefully according to physical maturity, size, and skill required.
- A spiral fracture of the femur or humerus may be a sign of child abuse.
- Child abuse may be physical, emotional, or sexual, or may involve neglect.

Additional Learning Resources

SG Go to your Study Guide for additional learning activities to help you master this chapter content.

evolve Go to your Evolve website (http://evolve.elsevier.com/Leifer) for the following learning resources:
- Animations
- Answer Guidelines for Critical Thinking Questions

- Answers and Rationales for Review Questions for the NCLEX® Examination
- Glossary with English and Spanish pronunciations
- Interactive Review Questions for the NCLEX® Examination
- Patient Teaching Plans in English and Spanish
- Skills Performance Checklists
- Video clips and more!

 Online Resources
- Arthritis Foundation: www.arthritis.org
- Scoliosis: www.kidshealth.org/kid/health_problems/bone/scolio.html

Review Questions for the NCLEX® Examination

1. A type of fracture in a young child that may be indicative of child abuse is:
   1. greenstick fracture of the tibia.
   2. spiral fracture of the femur.
   3. pathological fracture of the fibula.
   4. aligned fracture of the wrist.

2. A teenager who had a cast applied after a tibia fracture complains that his pain medication is not working and his pain is still a 9 or 10. The nurse notices some edema of the toes and a capillary refill of 6 seconds. The priority action of the nurse would be:
   1. call the health care provider immediately.
   2. check if there is an order for a stronger pain medication.
   3. try nonpharmacological techniques of pain relief.
   4. explain to the teen that a new fracture is expected to be painful the first day.

3. A "neurovascular check" for tissue perfusion includes which of the following observations (select all that apply)?
   1. Pulse
   2. Color and capillary refill
   3. Movement and sensation
   4. Equal pupil size of eyes

4. An abnormal S-shaped curvature of the spine seen in school-age children is:
   1. sclerosis.
   2. sciatica.
   3. scabies.
   4. scoliosis.

5. A yellow bruise is approximately:
   1. 2 days old.
   2. 5 to 7 days old.
   3. 7 to 10 days old.
   4. 10 to 14 days old.

Critical Thinking Question

1. The nurse enters the room of a child who is in skeletal traction for a fractured femur. He is sitting in a high-Fowler's position watching television and eating snacks. What nursing observations relating to the traction would the nurse make, and what interventions are necessary?

The Child with a Respiratory Disorder

Objectives

1. Define each key term listed.
2. Distinguish the differences between the respiratory tract of the infant and that of the adult.
3. Compare bed rest for a toddler with bed rest for an adult.
4. Discuss how sinusitis in children is different from that in adults.
5. Discuss the nursing care of a child with croup, pneumonia, or respiratory syncytial virus.
6. Recognize the precautions involved in the care of a child diagnosed with epiglottitis.
7. Describe smoke inhalation injury as it relates to delivery of nursing care.
8. Discuss the postoperative care of a 5-year-old who has had a tonsillectomy.
9. Recall the characteristic manifestations of allergic rhinitis.
10. Assess the control of environmental exposure to allergens in the home of a child with asthma.
11. Interpret the role of sports and physical exercise for the asthmatic child.
12. Express five goals of asthma therapy.
13. Recall four nursing goals in the care of a child with cystic fibrosis.
14. Devise a nursing care plan for the child with cystic fibrosis, including family interventions.
15. Review the signs and symptoms of respiratory distress in infants and children.
16. Review the prevention of bronchopulmonary dysplasia.
17. Examine the prevention of sudden infant death syndrome.

Key Terms

alveoli (ăl-VĒ-ō-lī, p. 584)
atelectasis (ă-tĕ-LĔK-tă-sĭs, p. 596)
carbon dioxide narcosis (p. 578)
clubbing of the fingers (p. 596)
coryza (kō-RĪ-ză, p. 578)
dysphagia (dĭs-FĀ-jhă, p. 580)
laryngeal spasm (p. 582)
meconium ileus (p. 597)

orthopnea (ŏr-thŏp-NĒ-ă, p. 581)
pursed-lip breathing (p. 599)
reactive airway disease (RAD) (p. 584)
stridor (STRĪ-dŏr, p. 581)
surfactant (sŭr-FĂK-tănt, p. 577)
tachypnea (tăk-ĭp-NĒ-ă, p. 584)
ventilation (p. 578)

THE RESPIRATORY SYSTEM

DEVELOPMENT OF THE RESPIRATORY TRACT

Pulmonary structures differentiate in an orderly fashion during fetal life. This makes it possible to determine at what point a particular defect may have occurred. The laryngotracheal groove appears at 2 to 4 weeks of gestation. The trachea and the esophagus originate as one hollow tube; gradually, by 4 weeks of gestation, a septum forms to completely separate them. If the septum fails to form completely, a tracheoesophageal fistula occurs (see Chapter 28). By the seventh week of fetal life the diaphragm forms and separates the chest from the abdominal cavity. If the diaphragm fails to close completely, a *diaphragmatic hernia* allows the abdominal contents (intestines, spleen, and stomach) to enter the chest cavity and prevents the lungs from expanding fully. Alveoli and capillaries, which are necessary for gas exchange in the human body, are formed between 24 and 28 weeks of gestation.

At the twenty-fourth week, the formed alveolar cells begin to produce surfactant. **Surfactant** is composed of lecithin and sphingomyelin and prevents the alveoli from collapsing during respirations after birth. A premature birth is accompanied by problems with respiratory gas exchange. During fetal life the lungs are filled with a fluid that has a low surface tension and viscosity; this is rapidly absorbed after birth. Spontaneous respiratory movements occur in the fetus, although gas exchange occurs via placental circulation. When surfactant is present in the lungs, the respiratory movements force some of the surfactant into the amniotic fluid. At about 35 weeks of gestation, the lecithin component is twice that of the sphingomyelin component. The analysis of the lecithin/sphingomyelin ratio (L/S ratio) by amniocentesis (see Table 5-1) is one method of

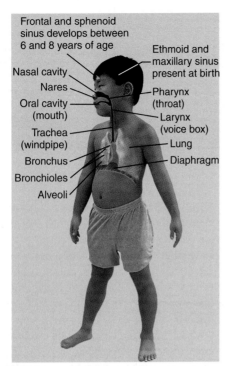

Frontal and sphenoid sinus develops between 6 and 8 years of age

Ethmoid and maxillary sinus present at birth

Nasal cavity

Nares

Oral cavity (mouth)

Trachea (windpipe)

Bronchus

Bronchioles

Alveoli

Pharynx (throat)

Larynx (voice box)

Lung

Diaphragm

RESPIRATORY SYSTEM

- Respiratory rates are higher in children. Diaphragmatic abdominal breathing is common in infants.
- Oxygen consumption is high in children in proportion to body size; metabolic rate is higher than in adults.
- Airway diameter is smaller in children, which increases the potential for obstruction.
- Mucous membranes of airways are highly vascular and are susceptible to trauma, edema, and spasm.
- Surfactant is lacking in preterm infants, which contributes to respiratory distress syndrome.
- Accessory muscles of respiration are not as strong in children, particularly in infants.
- Chest wall retractions are common in infants with respiratory problems because the chest wall is supple.

FIGURE 25-1 Summary of respiratory tract in children. The ribs and the diaphragm allow for inspiration of air. Air enters the body through the *nares,* or nostrils. The mucous membranes and cilia that line the respiratory tract warm, moisten, and filter the air as it passes to the *pharynx.* The pharynx contains the tonsils, which assist in infection control. The *larynx* at the upper end of the trachea contains the epiglottis, the glottis, and the vocal cords, which prevent food and fluids from entering the trachea and allow voice sounds. The *trachea* is encircled by smooth muscle and cartilage to maintain patency and carries the air to the bronchi and then to the smaller bronchioles. The bronchioles continue to divide and lead to small, thin air sacs *(alveoli)* that are kept open on inspiration by the air contained in them. During expiration when the air sacs collapse, *surfactant* prevents the walls from sticking together, allowing for reinflation. Gas exchange occurs in the alveoli by diffusion to the bloodstream. The volume of air inhaled with each breath is related to body size. (Art overlay courtesy Observatory Group, Cincinnati, OH.)

determining fetal maturity and the ability of the fetus to survive outside the uterus.

NORMAL RESPIRATION

The process of normal respiration is described in Figure 25-1.

Ventilation

Ventilation, the process of breathing air into and out of the lungs, is affected by several elements and their interaction with each other:

- *Intercostal muscles, diaphragm, ribs:* These allow chest expansion and contraction. Expansion of the chest lowers pressure in the chest cavity, and air flows from the higher pressure of the atmosphere into the lower pressure of the chest cavity. The opposite occurs during expiration.
- *Brain:* The vagus nerve and the respiratory centers in the medulla of the brain regulate rhythmic respiratory movements. Signals sent to the respiratory center will increase or decrease respiratory rates.
- *Chemoreceptors:* These sensors respond to changes in the oxygen saturation of the blood by sending a signal to the pons in the brainstem, which is stimulated to increase respirations when the oxygen (O_2) saturation is low.

Note that a high carbon dioxide (CO_2) level in the blood and a low O_2 saturation stimulate the brain to increase the respiratory rate. In chronic lung disease, however, the receptors become tolerant to the high CO_2 and low O_2 concentration in the blood. Administration of supplemental oxygen increases the O_2 saturation level and may result in a decreased respiratory effort (**carbon dioxide narcosis**), leading to respiratory failure. The differences between the respiratory tracts of the growing infant and the adult are shown in Table 25-1.

Procedures that may be performed on the child with a respiratory condition include throat and nasopharyngeal cultures, bronchoscopy, lung biopsy, arterial blood gas (Pao_2, $Paco_2$) and pH analysis, pulse oximetry, and various pulmonary function tests (PFTs). Chest x-ray films, computed tomography, radioisotope scan, bronchogram, and angiography may prove useful, depending on symptoms. The inspection, percussion, and auscultation procedures performed by the nurse are of utmost value in data collection.

DISORDERS AND DYSFUNCTION OF THE RESPIRATORY SYSTEM

Nasopharyngitis

Pathophysiology. A cold, also known as acute **coryza,** is the most common infection of the respiratory tract. It can be caused by a number of viruses, principally

Table 25-1   **Differences in the Respiratory Tracts of the Growing Infant and the Adult**

DIFFERENCE	SIGNIFICANCE
The infant relies primarily on the abdominal muscles and the diaphragm for breathing. The intercostal muscles only stabilize the chest wall.	Assessment of respiration is best accomplished by monitoring the rise and fall of the abdomen until 3 years of age, when thoracic breathing begins. Adult types of breathing patterns are typically developed by 7 years of age. Substernal retraction is a sign of respiratory distress in infants.
In infants, the diaphragm is attached higher than in the adult and is stretched longer, limiting its ability to contract forcefully.	Abdominal distention from formula or gas can interfere with movement of the diaphragm.
The infant depends on the accessory muscles for respiratory efforts.	Muscle fatigue can result in respiratory arrest.
Infants are nose breathers and do not breathe through the mouth unless crying.	Swelling of the nasal mucosa will interfere with sucking and will cause irritability.
In infants, the tissue below the vocal cords is not firm, and portions of the larynx are very narrow.	Any edema or swelling can cause respiratory obstruction.
In infants, the cartilage that maintains the patency of the airway is soft, not firm.	Vagal nerve stimulation or muscle constriction can cause collapse of the airway and respiratory obstruction.
The larynx and trachea are higher in the chest in infancy and descend slowly as the child grows.	Positioning the infant or child for airway clearance and resuscitation is different than for adults. Excess flexion or extension of the neck can cause respiratory obstruction.
Alveoli in the lung divide and thin as the child grows and develops, resulting in increased surface area for gas exchange. The number of alveoli present at puberty is nine times that found in the infant.	Less surface area in the alveoli is available for gas exchange, which predisposes infants and young children to respiratory distress.
Lung growth is inhibited by phenobarbital and excess insulin.	Drugs and disease can inhibit lung development.
Infants and young children have a small airway diameter.	Edema or muscle spasm can rapidly cause respiratory obstruction.
Newborns and infants produce less respiratory mucus (which serves as a cleansing agent).	Infants and children are more susceptible to respiratory infections.
Infants have a smaller amount of developed smooth muscle lining the airway than do older children and adults.	Bronchospasm may not occur in infants, and therefore wheezing may not be a presenting sign of a narrowed airway.
In infants, the respiratory rate is higher and the breathing pattern is irregular.	Meaningful assessment of respiration must be related to the age of the child. Irregular respirations with short periods of apnea is a normal pattern for a young infant but abnormal for an adult.

the rhinoviruses, which are spread from one child to another by sneezing, coughing, or direct contact. The age, state of nutrition, and general health of the child contribute to the susceptibility level.

The rhinovirus is spread by contact with contaminated fingers that touch the conjunctiva of the eyes or the mucous membranes of the mouth. Routine hand-washing practices, especially before rubbing the nose or sucking the fingers, can prevent the spread of the common cold.

The common cold differs from allergic rhinitis in that a child who has allergic rhinitis has no fever, no purulent nasal discharge, and no reddened mucous membranes. Sneezing, watery eyes, and itching of the skin are the primary manifestations of *allergic rhinitis*. In the older child or adolescent, persistent naso-pharyngitis may be related to inhaled cocaine or other drug abuse.

Manifestations. The symptoms of a cold in an infant or small child are different from those in an adult. Children's air passages are smaller and more easily obstructed. The virus causes inflammation and edema of the membranes of the upper respiratory tract, which damage cilia and prevent the drainage of mucus. Fever as high as 40° C (104° F) is not uncommon in children younger than 3 years of age. Nasal discharge, irritability, sore throat, cough, and general discomfort are present, and there may be vomiting and diarrhea. The diagnosis is complicated by the fact that many infectious diseases resemble the common cold during their onset. Complications of a cold include bronchitis, pneumonitis, and ear infections.

Treatment and Nursing Care. There is no cure for the common cold. Treatment should begin early, when a cold is suspected. The following treatment is designed to relieve symptoms:

- *Rest:* Fatigue should be prevented. Confinement to bed for a child does not always result in physical rest. In pediatrics, "bed rest" means providing play therapy that promotes minimal activity. The nurse should consider the age and developmental level of the child and the activity level involved in the play when designing appropriate activities and guiding parents in the home care of their child.

- *Clear airways:* Congested nasal passages cause discomfort and impede nursing or sucking of formula. Because fluid consumption is essential to prevent fever and dehydration, the airways must be cleared before feeding and before bedtime to provide a restful sleep. The nurse can teach the parents that instilling a few drops of saline solution into the nose and then suctioning with a bulb syringe (Skill 12-2) is the best way to clear the nostrils. Medicated nose drops can be irritating to the mucosa of a young child's nasal passages. Use of nose drops with an oily base should be avoided because they are readily aspirated and can cause respiratory problems. Rebound congestion can be avoided by limiting the use of medicated nose drops to no more than 3 days. Use of over-the-counter combination cold remedies should be avoided. Contents on the label should be checked for safe dosage.
- *Adequate fluid intake:* Anorexia is common in children with nasopharyngitis. Intake of fluids should be encouraged to prevent dehydration. Cool, bland liquids are usually tolerated well in a child who has a sore throat.
- *Prevention of fever:* Ibuprofen (Motrin) or acetaminophen (Tylenol) can be administered when a high fever accompanies a cold.
- *Skin care:* A petroleum-based ointment can be applied to the nares and upper lip to prevent skin irritation from a nasal discharge.

! Medication Safety Alert!

Parents should be cautioned to check the label of any medication for appropriate dosages and to use the measuring devices that are supplied with the medication.

Moist air soothes the inflamed nose and throat. An electric cold-air humidifier is safe and convenient. It must be cleaned and disinfected daily. If a great deal of moisture is indicated (as in croup), the infant may be taken to a small room, such as the bathroom, and the hot water faucets or shower can be turned on to produce sufficient steam to help soothe the infant.

The older child is taught the proper way to remove nasal secretions from the nose. The mouth is opened slightly, and secretions are gently blown out through both nostrils at the same time. This method prevents the infection from being forced into the eustachian tubes. Children must be taught to cover the mouth and nose when sneezing and to wash their hands afterward. Tissues must be properly discarded. Antibiotics are not effective against the common cold because it is viral in origin.

Otitis media is an inflammation of the middle ear. The middle ear is connected to the throat by the eustachian tube, which provides drainage of middle ear secretions into the nasopharynx and equalizes pressure between the middle ear and the outside atmosphere. When the lining of the eustachian tube becomes infected as a complication of nasopharyngitis, otitis media often develops, usually following an upper respiratory infection. Infants are more prone to middle ear infections because their eustachian tubes are shorter, straighter, and wider than those of older children or adults. For a detailed discussion of otitis media, see Chapter 23.

Nursing Tip

Children and parents should be taught to wash their hands frequently and use hand sanitizers to prevent the spread of infection.

Acute Pharyngitis

Pathophysiology. Acute pharyngitis is an inflammation of the structures in the throat. This infection is common among children between 5 and 10 years of age. In 80% of cases the causative organism is a virus. Group A beta-hemolytic streptococcus (strep throat) occurs in about 37% of the cases. The bacterium *Haemophilus influenzae* is common in children younger than 3 years of age.

Manifestations, Treatment, and Nursing Care. Symptoms include fever, malaise, **dysphagia** (*dys,* "difficult," and *phagia,* "swallowing"), and anorexia. It is difficult to distinguish viral from bacterial types by symptoms only. Conjunctivitis, rhinitis, cough, and hoarseness with a gradual onset and persisting no longer than 5 days are characteristic of viral pharyngitis. In a child more than 2 years of age, streptococcal pharyngitis characteristically includes high fever (40° C [104° F]) and difficulty in swallowing, and it may last longer than 1 week. A strep throat is determined by throat culture. When the culture is positive, antimicrobial therapy such as penicillin is administered orally for 10 days. Compliance may be a problem; therefore the nurse carefully explains to parents the need for the child to finish all of the medication. Erythromycin may be prescribed if the child is allergic to penicillin. Acetaminophen may be taken to relieve soreness of the throat. If the child is old enough to gargle, a solution of warm water and salt may be used.

Prompt treatment of strep throat is important to prevent serious complications such as rheumatic fever, glomerulonephritis, peritonsillar abscess, otitis media, mastoiditis, meningitis, osteomyelitis, or pneumonia. The persistence of a positive streptococcal culture after careful follow-up and therapy may indicate that the child is a group A beta-hemolytic streptococcus carrier. However, it may also mean that the child did not complete the 10-day course of medication or that a drug-resistant organism has evolved. The child with strep throat is no longer infectious to others after drug therapy has begun and fever has decreased.

Sinusitis in Children

The frontal sinuses are present at 8 years of age but may not be fully developed until age 18. Some ethmoid sinus cells are present at birth. The sphenoid sinus is present by 3 years of age and is fully developed by age 12. The maxillary sinuses are present at birth and develop as long as teeth are erupting. The proximity of this sinus to the tooth roots often results in tooth pain when the sinus is infected. The maxillary and ethmoid sinuses are most often involved in childhood sinusitis. Therefore the signs and symptoms of sinusitis in children are different from those in adults, depending on the age of the child and which sinus is fully developed. An acute sinusitis is suspected when an upper respiratory infection lasts longer than 10 days, with a daytime cough. Halitosis is often present. Untreated sinusitis can lead to periorbital cellulitis, because the infection spreads from the ethmoid sinus to the subperiosteal space around the eye. Treatment involves a 10- to 14-day course of antibiotic therapy.

Croup Syndromes

Pathophysiology. *Croup* is a general term applied to a number of conditions whose chief symptom is a "barking" (croupy) cough and varying degrees of inspiratory **stridor** (a harsh, high-pitched sound). When the larynx is involved, the clinical picture becomes more intense because of possible alterations in respiratory status, such as airway obstruction, acute respiratory failure, and hypoxia (Figure 25-2). Acute viral spasmodic laryngitis is the milder form of the syndrome. Acute laryngotracheobronchitis is the most common. It is also referred to as subglottic croup. The area below the glottis is firm cartilage and therefore cannot expand outward when edema occurs, as other regions of the respiratory tract can. For that reason, subglottic edema that occurs with epiglottitis or bacterial tracheitis results in acute respiratory obstruction (Sobol, 2008). Croup can be benign or acute. Benign croup is frightening but rarely life threatening. Acute croup can develop into a respiratory emergency.

Benign Crouplike Conditions

Congenital laryngeal stridor (laryngomalacia). Some infants are born with a weakness of the airway walls and a floppy epiglottis that causes a stridor on inspiration. There may be inspiratory retractions. The symptoms lessen when the infant is placed prone or propped in the side-lying position. Respiratory infection and crying may cause the symptoms to become frightening to the parents. The condition usually clears spontaneously as the child grows and the muscles strengthen. The nurse should provide reassurance and suggest slow, small feedings and a prone or side-lying position for the infant.

Spasmodic laryngitis (spasmodic croup). Spasmodic croup usually occurs in children between 1 to 3 years of age and can be caused by a virus, allergy, or psychological trigger. Very often, gastroesophageal reflux (GER) will trigger an attack. Spasmodic croup has a sudden onset, usually at night, and is characterized by a barking, brassy cough and respiratory distress. The child appears anxious, and the parents become frightened. The attack lasts a few hours, and by morning the child appears normal and is in no distress. Increasing humidity and providing fluids are helpful treatment measures.

Acute Croup

Laryngotracheobronchitis. The viral condition laryngotracheobronchitis is manifested by edema, destruction of respiratory cilia, and exudate, resulting in respiratory obstruction. A mild upper respiratory infection usually precedes the development of a characteristic barking or brassy cough. Stridor develops, and classic symptoms of respiratory distress follow (see Figure 25-2). The infant prefers to be held upright or sit up in bed (**orthopnea**). Crying and agitation worsen the symptoms. Hypoxia can develop and can be accompanied by tachycardia and diminished breath sounds.

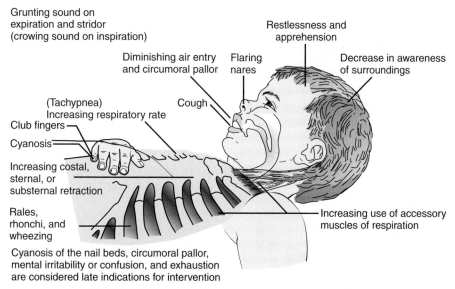

Grunting sound on expiration and stridor (crowing sound on inspiration)

Restlessness and apprehension

Diminishing air entry and circumoral pallor

Flaring nares

Decrease in awareness of surroundings

Cough

(Tachypnea) Increasing respiratory rate

Club fingers

Cyanosis

Increasing costal, sternal, or substernal retraction

Rales, rhonchi, and wheezing

Increasing use of accessory muscles of respiration

Cyanosis of the nail beds, circumoral pallor, mental irritability or confusion, and exhaustion are considered late indications for intervention

FIGURE 25-2 Signs of respiratory distress in infants and children.

Treatment and nursing care. When the child is treated at home, parents are often instructed to increase humidity levels around the child. This can be accomplished by using an electric cold-water humidifier. The humidifier must be emptied, washed, and disinfected each day to prevent the growth of microorganisms that occur in stagnant tap water. The child can also be taken into the bathroom, where the hot water in the shower is turned on to increase humidity. The child inhales the moist air, which usually relieves the respiratory distress and **laryngeal spasm** (constriction of laryngeal muscles).

When continuing symptoms of respiratory distress necessitate hospitalization, the child may be given nebulizer therapy or placed in a mist tent, or *croupette* (see Figure 22-17). The cool air, well saturated with microdroplets that can enter the small airway of a child, causes mucosal cooling and vasoconstriction and relieves the respiratory obstruction and distress. However, the value of mist tent therapy in the acutely ill child is unproven. Intravenous (IV) fluids are prescribed to prevent dehydration and to decrease the risk of vomiting and aspiration that can occur after a coughing episode. Organization of care is essential to enable the child to have long periods of rest. The child is placed on a cardiorespiratory monitor (CRM), and the vital signs are observed closely. Oxygen is provided to reduce hypoxia (see Chapter 22). Oxygen saturation is monitored, and saturation levels are maintained above 90% (see Skill 13-1 for pulse oximeter sensor application).

Opiates are contraindicated because they depress respiration. Sedatives are contraindicated because increased restlessness is a primary sign of increased respiratory obstruction, and sedatives can mask signs of restlessness. Nebulized epinephrine may be used to relieve the symptoms of respiratory obstruction (Figure 25-3). Corticosteroids are often prescribed to reduce the edema caused by inflammation and to prevent further destruction of ciliated epithelium in children hospitalized with croup, providing there is no history of recent exposure to varicella (chicken pox) (Lenney, 2009).

 Safety Alert!

Respiratory illness is always potentially more serious in children than in adults.

Epiglottitis

Pathophysiology. Epiglottitis is a swelling of the tissues above the vocal cords, that is, supraglottic swelling. This results in narrowing of the *airway inlet,* with the possibility of total obstruction. It is caused by *H. influenzae* type B and most often occurs in children 3 to 6 years of age. It can occur in any season. The course is rapid and progressive. Blood gasses fluctuate and there is leukocytosis. **Epiglottitis is a life-threatening medical emergency!**

Manifestations. The onset of epiglottitis is abrupt, and the child presents with classic symptoms. The child insists on sitting up, leans forward with the mouth open, and drools saliva because of the difficulty in swallowing. The child appears wide-eyed, anxious, and restless, and he or she may emit a froglike croaking sound on inspiration. Cough is absent. Inspection of the throat shows an enlarged, reddened edematous epiglottis, much like a "beefy-red thumb." However, the examining tongue blade may trigger a laryngospasm and result in sudden respiratory arrest.

 Safety Alert!

It is a primary nursing responsibility to be sure there is a tracheotomy set at the bedside before any examination of the throat is attempted.

Treatment. The treatment of choice is immediate tracheotomy or endotracheal intubation and oxygen to prevent hypoxia, brain damage, and sudden death caused by respiratory arrest. Parenteral antibiotic therapy usually results in a dramatic improvement within a few days.

Prevention. The AAP recommends that *H. influenzae* type B conjugate vaccines be administered beginning at 2 months of age as part of a regular immunization program for all children. This type of program has decreased the incidence of acute epiglottitis in children (D'Augustino, 2010).

Bronchitis

Pathophysiology. A study of the respiratory system shows that the air tubes leading to the lungs resemble an upside-down tree. The trachea is the main trunk, with the bronchi, bronchioles, and alveoli as branches. These passages proceed from large to small and are lined with a continuous membrane. If there is an

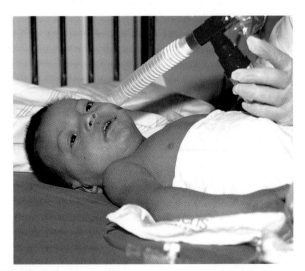

FIGURE 25-3 A child receiving aerosol therapy (medicated nebulizer treatments). (From McKinney ES, James SR, Murray SS, Ashwill JW: *Maternal-child nursing,* ed 2, Philadelphia, 2005, Saunders.)

infection of the bronchial tree, it is seldom confined to one area but more often involves other structures.

Acute bronchitis is an infection of the bronchi. It seldom occurs as a primary infection but is usually secondary to a cold or other communicable disease. It is caused by a variety of organisms. Poor nutrition, allergy, and chronic infection of the respiratory tract may precipitate this condition. Most patients are younger than 4 years of age.

Manifestations. The gradual onset of an unproductive "hacking" cough is preceded by an upper respiratory infection, or cold. The cough may become productive with purulent sputum. Children less than 7 years of age cannot voluntarily cough and usually swallow their sputum.

Treatment. The use of cough suppressants before bedtime may be helpful in promoting restful sleep. Antihistamines, expectorants, and antibiotics are usually not helpful. Most children recover uneventfully with symptomatic care at home.

Bronchiolitis

Pathophysiology. Acute bronchiolitis is a viral infection of the small airways (bronchioles) in the lower respiratory tract. It occurs in infants and children 6 months to 2 years of age, with a peak at 6 months of age. The small diameters of the bronchioles in the infant are susceptible to obstruction when inflammation results in edema and excess mucus. The obstruction often leads to atelectasis. The gas exchange in the lungs becomes impaired, and hypoxia can occur.

Manifestations. An upper respiratory infection or cold with a mild fever, and serous (clear) nasal discharge, is followed by the development of a wheezing cough and signs of respiratory distress. The increase in respiratory rate interferes with successful feeding, and the infant becomes irritable and dehydrated. The respiratory syncytial virus (RSV) is the causative organism in 50% of cases in infants. An apneic episode is usually the cause of hospitalization. Infants who have bronchiolitis may develop a hyperreactive airway or asthma later in life.

Treatment and Nursing Care. The treatment of an infant with bronchiolitis is symptomatic and similar to that of the child with croup. A semi-Fowler's position with a slightly hyperextended neck facilitates respirations. Oral feedings are often supplemented by IV fluids. Intake and output are recorded. Bronchodilating aerosol therapy and high-humidity tents are prescribed. Frequent assessment of vital signs and monitoring of oxygen saturation levels are essential.

Respiratory Syncytial Virus

Respiratory syncytial virus (RSV) is responsible for 50% of cases of bronchiolitis in infants and young children and is the most common cause of viral pneumonia.

RSV is the single most important respiratory pathogen in infancy. RSV occurs worldwide and causes annual epidemics during the winter months. Most children who are infected with RSV experience it before their second birthday, and reinfection is common, especially in children attending day care centers. Infants between 2 and 7 months of age can become seriously ill with this condition because their airways are so small and prone to obstruction by the thick mucus produced. Older children and adults are not as seriously ill and continue to go to work or school, becoming carriers and spreading the infection. Children with RSV bronchiolitis have an increased risk for developing asthma later in life (Sorce, 2009).

Transmission. RSV is spread by direct contact with respiratory secretions, usually by contaminated hands to the mucous membranes (eyes, mouth, nose). RSV survives for more than 6 hours on countertops, tissues, and soap bars. RSV is not spread via the airborne route. The incubation period is approximately 2 to 8 days. Reinfection is common, as infection does not result in immunity (AAP, 2012).

Hospital-acquired infection can be a major problem because caregivers may be carrying the organism. For this reason, an infant diagnosed with RSV infection is placed on transmission-based *contact isolation* precautions to prevent the spread of RSV to other sick children.

RSV immunoglobulin may be used for preterm newborns with bronchopulmonary dysplasia who are at risk for infection.

Diagnosis. An examination of nasopharyngeal washings for RSV antigens can be performed while the child waits in the admitting unit so that the diagnosis is established before the infant is admitted to the pediatric unit.

Prevention. Prevention of RSV is available via a monoclonal antibody, palivizumab (Synagis), given in monthly intramuscular injections. This medication is started at the onset of RSV season and is terminated at the end of the season (the season usually lasts from November through March). The AAP practice guidelines state that candidates for preventive therapy include infants with bronchopulmonary dysplasia, severe immunodeficiencies, or significant congenital heart disease and those on continuous mechanical respiratory support (Meissner and Bocchini, 2009). The powder form of palivizumab should be administered within 6 hours of reconstitution because it is preservative free.

Treatment and Nursing Care. The care of infants with RSV infection should be assigned to personnel who are not caring for other patients that may be at high risk for adverse response to RSV. Infection prevention and control techniques (see Appendix A) are used to prevent the spread of infection to others on the unit.

Contact isolation precautions are used to prevent fomite spread. Frequent hand washing is essential. Liquid soap dispensers should be available at the sink, because the organism survives for a long time on a dry bar of soap.

Support of the Infant and Family. Effective communication skills are necessary to provide support for parents of the infant who is seriously ill. The parent can be familiarized with the mist tent and encouraged to participate in the care and feeding of the infant. Adults who have RSV can shed the virus for 1 week after the infection, and precautions should be taken if that adult is caring for infants (see Appendix A for infection prevention and control precautions).

Symptomatic Care. An ineffective breathing pattern is the priority nursing diagnosis for an infant hospitalized with RSV infection. Reporting **tachypnea** (increased respiration) and *tachycardia* (increased heart rate) is essential, because these vital sign changes may be indicative of hypoxemia. It is also important to auscultate breath sounds and to report wheezing, rales, or rhonchi. A child who has been wheezing and suddenly has a "quiet chest" on auscultation may be at risk for respiratory arrest. The higher-pitched the wheeze, the more constricted the airway. Signs of respiratory distress should be assessed and reported. Oxygen saturation levels are monitored, and oxygen is administered at levels needed to maintain a minimum of 90% to 95% saturation. Suctioning of mucus may be necessary to maintain a patent airway. Monitoring IV fluids and recording intake and output are essential to prevent dehydration. Urine output should be a minimum of 1 to 2 mL/kg/hr for infants and children. Pedialyte or Ricelyte are examples of clear liquid electrolyte formulas prescribed for infants at risk of dehydration. The child should be weighed daily to detect early signs of dehydration. Inhaled bronchodilators or steroids are not helpful in relation to RSV infections.

Antiviral Medication. Antiviral medication such as ribavirin (Virazole) may be prescribed for use with severely ill infants or infants who have heart or lung problems that place them at high risk for serious complications. The medication has been found effective in the treatment of RSV infection but is rarely used prophylactically because of its serious side effects. The medication is administered by fine-droplet aerosol mist while the infant is in a mist tent. It is administered 18 to 24 hours a day for a minimum of 3 days. If the infant is on a ventilator, the nurse must monitor the ventilator tubes, which may be warped by ribavirin. Caregivers and visitors who are of childbearing age, pregnant, or breastfeeding should not care for infants receiving ribavirin, because teratogenic effects have been reported. The ribavirin mist can cause precipitation on the surface of plastics, and caregivers with contact lenses may develop conjunctivitis because of the lens changes that this mist causes. When providing care to an infant receiving ribavirin therapy, the nurse should turn off the nebulizer and allow the mist to settle before opening the mist tent and providing care. Linen removed from the bed should be slowly rolled and then carefully folded to avoid releasing droplets of ribavirin into the air.

An IV immune globulin (RespiGam) may be prescribed for high-risk infants to prevent complications from RSV disease. RespiGam is administered intravenously and necessitates close observation for fluid volume overload. Routine immunizations may have to be postponed for 9 months if antiviral medication for RSV is prescribed. Intramuscular palivizumab (Synagis) can also be given to high-risk infants every month for 5 months, and this does not interfere with mumps-measles-rubella (MMR) or varicella vaccines (AAP, 2012).

> **!** | **Medication Safety Alert!**
>
> Caregivers who are pregnant or who wear contact lenses should not give direct care to infants who are receiving ribavirin aerosol therapy.

Complications. Infants who have a small airway size and are severely ill and hospitalized with RSV infection may be at risk for wheezing and **reactive airway disease (RAD)** later in life. Some studies (Kliegman, 2011) have shown that the inflammation caused by RSV injures the respiratory epithelial cells, resulting in exposed sensory nerve fibers that respond easily to environmental irritants.

Pneumonia
Pathophysiology. Pneumonia or pneumonitis is an inflammation of the lungs in which the **alveoli** (air sacs) become filled with exudate and surfactant may be reduced. The affected portion of the lung does not receive enough air. Breathing is shallow. As a result, the bloodstream is denied sufficient oxygen.

Pneumonia may occur as the initial or primary disease, or it may complicate another illness, in which case it is termed *secondary pneumonia*. There are many types of pneumonia. Classification may be by causative organism (i.e., bacterial or viral) or by the part of the respiratory system involved (i.e., lobar or bronchial). Group B streptococci are the most common cause of pneumonia in newborns, whereas *Chlamydia* is the most common cause of pneumonia in infants 3 weeks to 3 months of age. The incidence of *H. influenzae* type B infection has been decreasing with current immunization programs. RSV, rhinovirus, adenovirus, and pneumococcus are other organisms that are responsible for pneumonia in infants and children. Immunocompromised children may develop pneumonia caused by a gram-negative organism or a fungus such as *Pneumocystis jiroveci* (formerly known as *Pneumocystis carinii*).

Toddlers often aspirate small objects such as peanuts or popcorn and develop pneumonia as a result; therefore such foods are to be discouraged for this age group. *Lipoid pneumonia* occurs when the infant inhales an oil-based substance into the airways. It is less common today because children are seldom given cod liver oil or castor oil routinely, as they were in the past. Nose drops with an oil base must not be used for children because the oil can be aspirated and can cause lipoid pneumonia. A toddler who drinks kerosene may also develop a type of pneumonia. *Hypostatic pneumonia* may occur in patients who have poor circulation in their lungs and remain in one position too long. The child recovering from anesthesia must be turned frequently to stimulate circulation through the lungs. Early ambulation also accomplishes this.

Severe acute respiratory syndrome (SARS) is a severe type of pneumonia caused by the coronavirus (SARS-CoV). Symptoms are similar to pneumonia, but often the severity of the respiratory distress necessitates assisted ventilation and treatment in the intensive care unit (ICU). Nursing care and treatment involve supportive care. Airborne infection isolation precautions are recommended in the care and treatment of these patients (see Appendix A).

Manifestations. The symptoms of pneumonia vary with the patient's age and the causative organism. They may develop suddenly or may be preceded by an upper respiratory tract infection. The cough is dry at first, but it gradually becomes productive. Fever rises as high as 39.5° to 40° C (103° to 104° F) and may fluctuate widely during a 24-hour period. The respiratory rate may increase (tachypnea) to 40 to 80 breaths/min in infants and to 30 to 50 breaths/min in older children. Respirations are shallow as the child attempts to reduce the amount of chest pain. The chest pain may be caused by a pleural irritation or a musculoskeletal irritation from frequent coughing. Sternal retractions may be seen when the accessory muscles of respiration are used. The nostrils may flare. The child is listless, has a poor appetite, and tends to lie on the affected side. X-ray films confirm the diagnosis and determine whether there are complications such as atelectasis. A differential white blood cell count is routinely performed. Blood specimens show a marked increase in the number of white blood cells (16,000 to 40,000/mm^3). Culture specimens may be obtained from the nose, the throat, or sputum.

Treatment. Treatment depends on the causative organism. Antipyretics are given to reduce fever. Oxygen is administered for dyspnea or cyanosis. When this treatment is begun early, the child is less restless and does not require as many sedatives or drugs to relieve pain. Because drug therapy has become so effective, many uncomplicated cases can be treated at home. Fluid intake should be increased, particularly clear fluids and "flattened" soft drinks. Pediazole, (a combination of erythromycin ethylsuccinate and sulfisoxazole acetyl) may be prescribed for infants younger than 6 months of age, but amoxicillin is the drug of choice for children up to 5 years of age.

Rest, fluids, and a cough suppressant before bedtime are the basics of home care. Parent education concerning the need to complete all medication prescribed is essential. Tobacco use in the environment should be avoided, and the need for *H. influenzae* type B (Hib) immunizations is stressed. The proper use and disposal of tissues, covering the mouth during a cough, and the modeling of proper handwashing techniques are preventive measures the nurse should teach the family.

Nursing Care. Nursing care for all types of pneumonia is basically the same. The age of the patient determines the nurse's approach and the type of equipment used. (The newborn receives oxygen in the Isolette, whereas the older child requires a croupette or a larger tent.) Rest is an important part of the treatment. The nurse must organize care so that the child is not disturbed unnecessarily. Planned, quiet activities for the child are recommended (Pictorial Pathway 25-1).

The nurse checks the vital signs at regular intervals. When a child is flushed with fever, heavy clothing and blankets should be removed. The nurse encourages the child to take fluids, flavored ice pops, or small sips of water frequently. If vomiting persists, parenteral fluids are given.

Smoke Inhalation Injury

Smoke inhalation injury may cause carbon monoxide poisoning. Poisonous substances inhaled from burning material may also cause pathological disturbance. There are three stages of inhalation injury:

1. Pulmonary insufficiency in the first 6 hours
2. Pulmonary edema from 6 to 72 hours
3. Bronchopneumonia after 72 hours, which may cause atelectasis

When the child is injured by fire and burns are evident around the face or mouth, heat injury to the upper airway should be suspected. Burned materials can be carried deep into the respiratory tract in the form of insoluble gases and may cause chemical injury. Smoke from burning synthetic materials and plastic are especially toxic to the airways. Severe exposure to these chemicals can inhibit secretion of surfactant and cause a hyaline membrane to form, resulting in acute respiratory distress syndrome also known as Adult

Respiratory Distress Syndrome (ARDS). Carbon monoxide is not toxic to the lungs, but, by combining with hemoglobin to form carboxyhemoglobin (COHb), it prevents oxygen from binding to hemoglobin and thus inhibits cellular respiration.

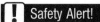

! Safety Alert!

Pulse oximetry readings are of little value in carbon monoxide poisoning because pulse oximetry does not detect COHb and readings may appear normal.

Pictorial Pathway 25-1   Care of a Child with Pneumonia

Nursing diagnoses
- Ineffective breathing pattern as evidenced by rapid respiration rate, retractions, and nasal flaring
- Deficient knowledge related to home care as evidenced by unfamiliarity with suction, metered-dose inhaler (MDI), and medication

NIC: Airway management
NOC: Ventilation

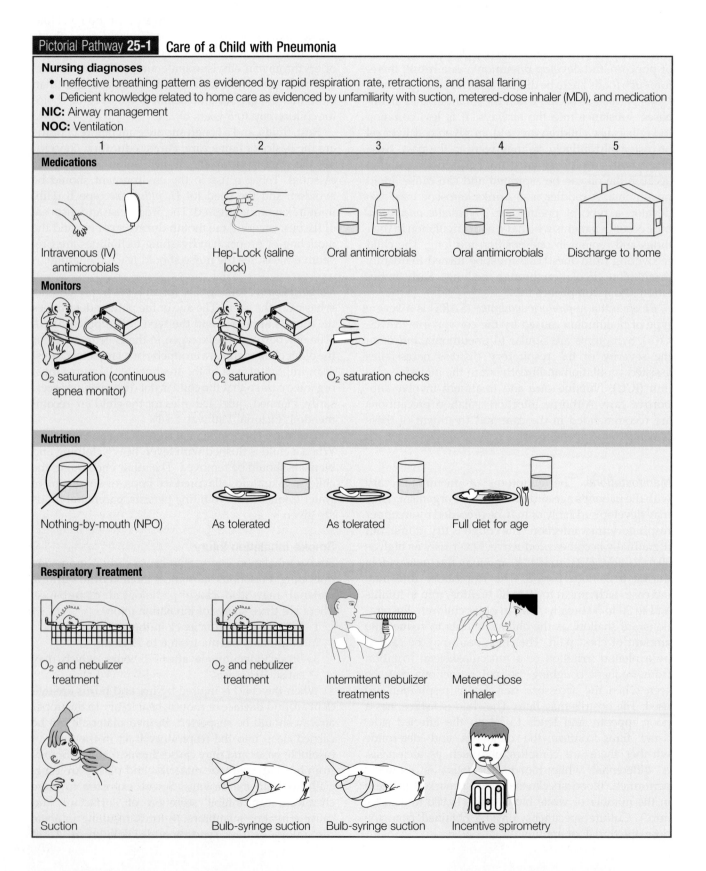

	1	2	3	4	5
Medications	Intravenous (IV) antimicrobials	Hep-Lock (saline lock)	Oral antimicrobials	Oral antimicrobials	Discharge to home
Monitors	O₂ saturation (continuous apnea monitor)	O₂ saturation	O₂ saturation checks		
Nutrition	Nothing-by-mouth (NPO)	As tolerated	As tolerated	Full diet for age	
Respiratory Treatment	O₂ and nebulizer treatment	O₂ and nebulizer treatment	Intermittent nebulizer treatments	Metered-dose inhaler	
	Suction	Bulb-syringe suction	Bulb-syringe suction	Incentive spirometry	

Pictorial Pathway 25-1   Care of a Child with Pneumonia—cont'd

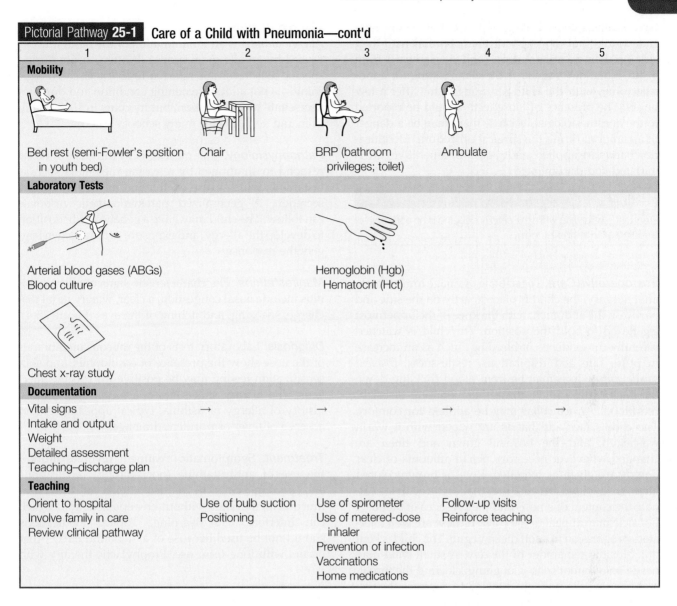

	1	2	3	4	5
Mobility	Bed rest (semi-Fowler's position in youth bed)	Chair	BRP (bathroom privileges; toilet)	Ambulate	
Laboratory Tests	Arterial blood gases (ABGs) Blood culture, Chest x-ray study		Hemoglobin (Hgb) Hematocrit (Hct)		
Documentation	Vital signs Intake and output Weight Detailed assessment Teaching–discharge plan	→	→	→	→
Teaching	Orient to hospital Involve family in care Review clinical pathway	Use of bulb suction Positioning	Use of spirometer Use of metered-dose inhaler Prevention of infection Vaccinations Home medications	Follow-up visits Reinforce teaching	

Treatment is often symptomatic and includes oxygen administration, careful monitoring of intake and output, and frequent assessments of arterial blood gas reports. In severe carbon monoxide poisoning hyperbaric oxygenation (see Chapter 34) may be the treatment of choice. See Chapter 32 for agents used in bioterrorism attacks.

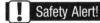 **Safety Alert!**

Respiratory arrest can occur suddenly in children who have smoke inhalation injuries. An intubation tray should be readily available.

Tonsillitis and Adenoiditis

Pathophysiology. The tonsils and adenoids, located in the pharynx (throat), are made of lymph tissue and are part of the body's defense mechanism against infection. The symptoms of tonsillitis include difficulty in swallowing and breathing. Enlarged adenoids block the nasal passage, resulting in mouth breathing. Other symptoms are similar to those of nasopharyngitis. Nursing care involves providing a cool mist vaporizer to keep the mucous membranes moist; salt water gargles; throat lozenges (if age-appropriate); a cool, liquid diet; and acetaminophen to promote comfort. Antibiotics are not usually prescribed unless a throat culture is positive for the streptococcal organism.

Treatment. The removal of the tonsils and adenoids, referred to as a "T&A," is usually not recommended for children less than 3 years of age. It is thought that the condition may correct itself if surgery is postponed, because the tissues become smaller as the child grows. A *tonsillectomy* (removal of the palatine tonsils) is indicated only if persistent airway obstruction, repeated infections, or difficulty in breathing occurs. The surgery is not performed during an acute infectious episode because inflamed tissue responds poorly to surgery.

Age-appropriate explanations are provided to children to prepare them for the surgery. Wording should be carefully selected, because young children may associate being "put to sleep" for the operation with their sick pet being "put to sleep" and never heard from again. Same-day surgery is the usual setting for a tonsillectomy, with the child returning home after a few hours. The presence of loose teeth should be reported to the anesthesiologist, because there may be a danger of aspiration during the surgical procedure. Identification bands are applied, and routine preoperative care is initiated and documented.

> ### 🔲 Nursing Tip
>
> Frequent swallowing while the child is sleeping is an early sign of bleeding after a tonsillectomy.

Postoperative Care. To facilitate drainage immediately after surgery, the child is placed partly on the side and partly on the abdomen, with the knee of the uppermost leg flexed to hold the position. The child is watched carefully for evidence of bleeding, such as an increase in pulse rate and respirations, restlessness, *frequent swallowing* (which may be from blood trickling down the back of the child's throat), or vomiting of bright red blood. An ice collar may be applied for comfort. The child's face and hands are wiped with a warm washcloth, and the hospital gown and linen are changed whenever necessary. Small amounts of clear liquids are given as tolerated. Red- or brown-colored juices are avoided, because they make it difficult to evaluate the content of emesis and the presence of blood. A Popsicle may appeal to the child. If these are well tolerated, progression to a soft diet is begun. The child is kept quiet for the remainder of the day. A small child may nestle on a parent's lap. Coughing, clearing the throat, and blowing the nose are avoided to decrease the risk of precipitating bleeding at the operative site. Appropriate pain relief is important and will help to minimize crying, which may further irritate the throat. Hemorrhage is the most common postoperative complication. The nurse should not assume that because the surgery is minor it does not involve certain risks.

Written instructions are given to the parents when the child is discharged. The child should be kept quiet for a few days and should receive nourishing fluids and soft foods. After this, the child may continue to take a nap or to have a rest period so that he or she has sufficient convalescent time. Acetaminophen may be administered to reduce throat discomfort. The child must be protected from exposure to infections. Gargling and highly seasoned food should be avoided during the first postoperative week.

> ### 🔲 Nursing Tip
>
> After a tonsillectomy, milk and milk products may coat the throat and cause the child to "clear" the throat, further irritating the operative site.

Allergic Rhinitis

Allergic rhinitis is an inflammation of the nasal mucosa caused by an allergic response. It often occurs during specific seasons and is referred to as *hay fever*. Allergic rhinitis is not a life-threatening condition and does not necessitate hospitalization, but it occurs in 10% of children and accounts for many school absences.

Pathophysiology. The mast cells in the nasal mucosa respond to an antigen by releasing mediators such as histamine, which cause edema and increased mucous secretion. A generalized parasympathetic response can follow. The child may have a genetic predisposition to develop the allergy, and exposure to the allergen triggers the response.

Manifestations. The characteristic signs of allergic rhinitis include nasal congestion, a clear, watery nasal discharge, sneezing, and itching of the eyes (Figure 25-4).

Diagnosis. Laboratory tests of the mucous membranes of the nose show the presence of eosinophils, and skin sensitization testing may be positive for specific allergens. The history shows seasonal occurrence, family history of allergy or asthma, typical appearance, and absence of fever or purulent drainage.

Treatment. Symptomatic treatment revolves around the use of antihistamine (nonsedating) medications and decongestants to reduce edema of the nasal mucous membranes without creating sedation, which can interfere with learning. Topical medications should not be used because of a "rebound effect" that occurs with long-term use. Prophylactic therapy with

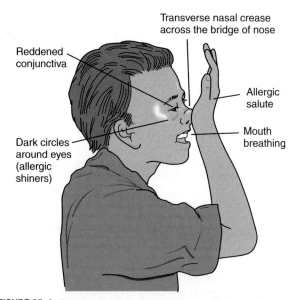

FIGURE 25-4 The allergic salute. Signs of allergic rhinitis include a typical rubbing of the nose in response to nasal discharge *(allergic salute)*, darkened circles under the eyes *(allergic shiners)* caused by an obstruction of lymphatic and vein flow, and a *transverse crease* across the bridge of the nose resulting from the allergic salutes.

cromolyn inhalants or glucocorticoid nasal sprays may be prescribed if antihistamines are not effective, but this type of medication requires daily administration and parent and child compliance. Immunotherapy for identified allergens may be prescribed. A drug, carbinoxamine maleate (KarbinalER), was recently approved by the FDA as the first liquid sustained release histamine H-1 receptor blocker indicated for the relief of allergic rhinitis in children more than 2 years of age. It may be mildly sedating and is prescribed for a q12h dosage schedule.

The main goals of the nurse are to help the parent identify the difference between the allergy and a cold and to provide a referral for medical care and support during the long-term allergy testing and immunotherapy process. Teaching the family about controlling the environmental exposure to allergens is very important. Dust control, prevention of contact with animal dander, the use of air-conditioners and high-efficiency particulate air (HEPA) filters in the home, and the planning of vacation locales that do not present pollen challenges are some of the vital issues to discuss with the family. Leukotriene antagonist drugs have also been effective in the treatment of allergic rhinitis (Kliegman, 2011).

Asthma

Pathophysiology. Asthma is a syndrome caused by increased responsiveness of the tracheobronchial tree to various stimuli that results in reversible, *paroxysmal* (intermittent) constriction of the airways (Figure 25-5). The term *asthma* is a Greek word for *panting* or *breathlessness*. Asthma is the principal cause of chronic illness in children. It is the leading cause of school absenteeism, emergency department visits, and hospitalization. Although it may occur at any age, about 80% of asthma sufferers have their first symptoms before 5 years of age. Before puberty, about twice as many boys as girls are affected; thereafter the gender incidence is equal.

Asthma is a recurrent and reversible obstruction of the airways in which bronchospasm, mucosal edema, and secretion of and plugging by mucus contribute to

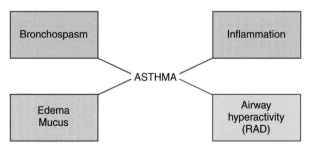

FIGURE 25-5 There are four main components of asthma, and the medication prescribed by the physician is specifically designed to manage the component manifested by the individual child. Inhaled corticosteroids may be prescribed for children with reactive airway disease (RAD), whereas an inhaled bronchodilator is the treatment of choice for bronchospasm. A child with asthma can manifest one or more of the components of the asthma syndrome.

significant narrowing of the airways and subsequently impaired gas exchange (Figure 25-6). Both large and small airways may be involved. The onset of asthma may be triggered by house dust, animal dander, wool, feathers, pollen, mold, passive smoking, strong odors, (as from wet paint, wood stoves, or fireplaces), and certain foods. Vigorous physical activity (especially in cold weather) and rapid changes in temperature and humidity may precipitate an attack. Viral infections are also responsible. Emotional upsets, which affect smooth muscle and vasomotor tone (*vas*, "vessel," and *motor*, "mover"), are closely intertwined with the condition. Environmental factors such as smoking combined with a genetic disposition may trigger the onset of asthma (Caliskan, 2013). Whatever the precipitating cause, the response of the airways is similar. As the attack worsens, arterial blood gases change. $Paco_2$ rises and the blood pH falls, increasing respiratory acidosis and producing a strain on the heart. Children who are prone to allergies often develop asthma. Some children who suffer from infantile eczema (see Chapter 30) develop asthma as they grow older. A family history of allergies is often seen.

Diagnosis. A history, physical examination, and response to bronchodilator therapy are the first diagnostic tools. An elevated level of eosinophils in the blood is typical. Eosinophils in the sputum are also diagnostic. Allergy skin testing and a radioallergosorbent test (RAST) are measures that can identify a sensitivity to allergens. Exercise testing and pulmonary function tests help to diagnose asthma and assess the progress of the syndrome.

Asthma is rarely diagnosed in infancy; the increased susceptibility of infants to respiratory obstruction and dyspnea in response to many different illnesses has many causes:

- Decreased smooth muscle of an infant's airway
- Presence of increased mucous glands in the bronchi
- Normally narrow lumen of the normal airway
- Lack of muscle elasticity in the airway
- Fatigue-prone and overworked diaphragmatic muscle on which infant respiration depends

The symptom of wheezing in infancy can be caused by gastroesophageal reflux, cystic fibrosis, or the chronic aspiration often seen in developmentally delayed infants, or it may be a manifestation of a milk or food allergy.

Manifestations. The symptoms of asthma may begin slowly or abruptly. They may be mild, moderate, or severe. Obstruction is most severe during expiration because the airways become smaller during this phase of respiration. The trapped air in the lung causes hyperinflation and results in an increase in the effort needed for breathing. This increased work of breathing can eventually put a strain on the heart. The hypoxia and

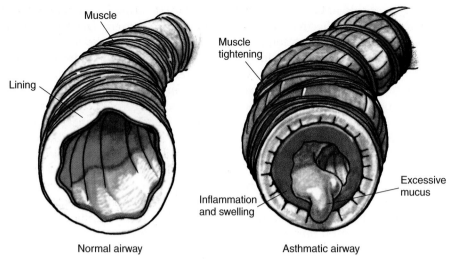

FIGURE 25-6 An asthmatic airway compared to a normal airway. (From Bowden VR, Dickey SB, Greenberg SC: *Children and their families: The continuum of care.* Philadelphia, 1998, Saunders.)

resulting acidosis can then cause general pulmonary vasoconstriction that damages alveoli, decreases surfactant, and causes a chronic respiratory problem.

In acute episodes the patient coughs, wheezes, and has difficulty breathing, particularly during expiration. The child may complain that his or her chin, neck, or chest itches. Signs of air hunger, such as flaring of the nostrils, and the use of the accessory muscles of respiration (chest and abdominal muscles) may be evident. Orthopnea appears. The child is restless, perspires, and sometimes complains of abdominal pain; participation in activities decreases. Pulse and respirations are increased, and rales (abnormal respiratory sounds) may be heard in the chest. Inflammation of the nose and sinuses may accompany asthma.

Asthma attacks often happen during the night and are frightening for both the child and the parents. Repeated attacks over a long period may lead to emphysema. Chronic asthma is manifested by discoloration beneath the eyes (allergic shiners), slight eyelid eczema, and mouth breathing.

Laboratory studies may show eosinophilia (increased blood eosinophils). Pulmonary function tests assess the degree of respiratory obstruction. Exercise testing may reveal bronchoconstriction with prolonged physical exercise.

> **! Safety Alert!**
>
> Shortness of breath accompanied by restricted breath sounds and a rising respiratory rate may indicate imminent respiratory failure and should be reported promptly to the health care provider.

Treatment and Long-Term Management. The main goals of asthma therapy are as follows (Figure 25-7):
- Maintain a near-normal pulmonary function.
- Maintain a near-normal activity level.
- Prevent chronic signs and symptoms.
- Prevent exacerbations that necessitate hospital treatment.
- Prevent adverse responses to medication.
- Promote self-care and monitoring consistent with developmental level.

Medications. Medications used for outpatient treatment of asthma are for quick relief ("rescue") in case of the return of acute symptoms and for long-term control (Table 25-2). An asthma specialist is usually responsible for the follow-up care of the child with asthma.

The nurse should teach the family how to use the inhalation devises and the precautions concerning frequency of dosages. The nurse should also instruct the family concerning drug–drug interactions (Table 25-3).

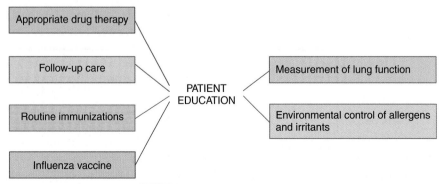

FIGURE 25-7 Management of asthma.

Slow inhalation of an inhaled drug enables the drug to reach the lower airway. Rapid inhalation causes some of the dose to be lost by being deposited on the sides of the pharynx. The respiratory therapist in the hospital administers nebulized inhalation therapy (often referred to as *med-nebs*), and home care units are also available.

Nursing Care. The necessary general control of the environment is explained to the child and family. Avoiding pet dander, mold, smoking, and dust is essential. Stuffed toys are not desirable. Humidity in living areas of the house should be controlled to between 25% and 50%, because excess humidity (above 50%) promotes mold growth. Dust collectors such as carpets, upholstery, or drapes should not be in the bedroom of an asthmatic child. Mattress covers, foam rubber pillows, and cotton blankets are preferred. Wool, down, and feather-stuffed items should be avoided. Upholstery, drapes, and carpets can be sprayed every 3 months with benzyl benzoate (Acarosan) to kill dust mites, followed by cleaning and vacuuming. The use of HEPA air-filtering devices in the bedroom and HEPA filters in the vacuum is advisable. Children can be taught to monitor their own lung function with the use of a peak flow meter at home (Skill 25-1). Involvement in self-care aids in compliance, and it results in better control of asthmatic symptoms.

Very often the parents and teachers exclude the child from physical activity in school because of the fear of

Table 25-2   Medications Commonly Used to Treat Asthma

DRUG	ACTIONS	NURSING CONSIDERATIONS
Short Acting Beta₂ Agonists (SABA)		
Albuterol (nebulizer or metered-dose inhaler [MDI])	Bronchodilator acts in 5-10 minutes	Child should hold breath 5-10 seconds after inhaling or use spacer. Rinse mouth after administration. Observe for tachycardia, headache and nervousness.
Corticosteroids		
Prednisone; prednisolone (oral)	Decreases signs of inflammation Enhances bronchodilation	Give with food to reduce gastric irritation. Administer in early AM when normal hormones peak. Prolonged therapy/high doses may cause immunosuppression.
Anticholinergic		
Ipratropium (Atrovent) (MDI or nebulizer)	Bronchodilation and decreases mucus within 30-90 minutes	Rinse mouth to relieve bitter taste. Observe for dry mouth, tachycardia. Assess for peanut allergy.
Daily Medications		
Long Acting Beta₂ Agonists (LABA)		
Salmeterol; Formoterol (dry powder inhaler)	Bronchodilator used for exercise-induced asthma	Not used during acute episodes. Take 30-60 minutes before exercise Observe for tachycardia, tremor.
Inhaled Steroids		
Beclomethasone (MDI or nebulizer)	Antiinflammatory; reduces mucus in airway	Administer with spacer. Clean inhaler between uses. Rinse mouth after dose. Observe for GI distress.
Methylxanthenes		
Theophylline (oral)	Bronchodilator	Do not crush or chew tablet. Give same time each day. Monitor blood levels. Watch for dysrhythmia and tremors.
Mast Call Inhibitors		
Cromolyn sodium Nedocromil (MDI or nebulizer)	Antiinflammatory; inhibits response to allergens and exercise-induced asthma	Do not use during acute episode. Must use several times a day on a regular basis to prevent attacks. Observe for nasal congestion; throat irritation.
Leukotriene Receptor Agonists (LTRA)		
Montelukast (Singulair) Zafirlukast (oral)	Antiinflammatory; improves lung function	Administer in evening. Mix granules in applesauce or ice cream (not liquids) or chew tablet. Administer between meals. Do not give with theophylline or warfarin.
Immunotherapy		
Omalizumab (Xolair) (Sub Q)	An antibody that blocks allergic reactions	Used for child older than 12 years. Injections given every 2 weeks, based on IgE levels.

Data from Wilson B, Shannon M, Shields K: *Nurses drug guide,* Upper Saddle River, N.J., 2011, Pearson, Prentice-Hall; Banasiah N: Childhood asthma: management update, *J Pediatr Health Care* 21(3):184-191, 2007; Robinson P, Van Asperen P: Asthma in childhood, *Pediatr Clin North Am* 56:191-226, 2009; Fong E, Lewin R: Inhaled corticosteroids for asthma, *Pediatr Rev* 28(6):30-35, 2007; Zagara M: Inhalant agents for asthma, bronchospasm and COPD: focus on delivery, devises, and technique, *Am J Nurse Pract* 14(3):21-25, 2010; McKinney E, James SR, Murray SS, Nelson S, Ashwill J: *Maternal-child nursing,* ed 4, St Louis, 2013, Saunders.

Table 25-3   Asthma Drug Interactions

ASTHMA DRUG	INTERACTING SUBSTANCE	EFFECT
Ephedrine	Antihypertensive drugs	Decrease antihypertensive effects
	Antidepressants—monoamine oxidase inhibitors (MAOIs) such as isocarboxazid (Marplan), phenelzine (Nardil), tranylcypromine (Parnate)	Can cause a rise in blood pressure
	Antacids	Increase serum level of ephedrine
	Ammonium chloride expectorants	Reduce effectiveness of ephedrine
	Steroids	Lessen steroid effectiveness
Epinephrine	Antidepressants—tricyclics (e.g., imipramine [Tofranil], amitriptyline [Elavil]) and MAOIs)	Can cause tachycardia, high blood pressure, and cardiac dysrhythmia
	Beta-adrenergic blockers, such as propranolol (Inderal)	Can cause high blood pressure
	Digitalis	Can cause cardiac dysrhythmia
Theophylline	Allopurinol (Zyloprim)	Can cause tachycardia and allopurinol toxicity
	Antibiotics (erythromycin)	Can cause theophylline toxicity
	Antibacterials (ciprofloxacin [Cipro])	May increase theophylline levels significantly
	Rifampin	Decreases effectiveness of theophylline
	Cimetidine (Tagamet)	Can cause theophylline toxicity
	Phenytoin (Dilantin)	Can decrease effect of both drugs
	Phenobarbital	Decreases effect of theophylline
	Ephedrine	Can cause dysrhythmia and nervousness
	Beta-adrenergic blockers, such as propranolol (Inderal)	Decrease effect of theophylline
	Oral contraceptives	Can increase theophylline blood levels
	High-fat foods	Increase absorption of theophylline

Using the Peak Flow Meter

PURPOSE

To monitor lung function

STEPS

1. Be sure the arrow points to 0 or is at the bottom of the numbered scale.
2. Instruct the child to close his or her mouth over the mouthpiece.
3. Instruct the child to take a deep breath and blow as hard as possible into the peak flow meter.
4. Observe and record the score or measurement on the peak flow meter.
5. Repeat three times and report the highest of the three readings.
6. Compare the score with previous scores and correlate with the plan of care.
7. Document for future reference.

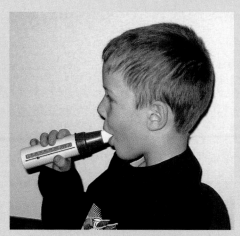

Using the peak flow meter. Assessments should be done daily at home. The reading in the morning should be within 20% of the evening reading. (Courtesy KW-Med Inc.)

triggering an asthmatic attack. The school nurse must teach school personnel the types of activities that are best tolerated by the asthmatic child. Swimming is best tolerated, probably because of the high humidity in the air inhaled, and the exhaling of air underwater is similar to "pursed-lip" exhaling. Sports such as baseball, short sprints, and gymnastics are well tolerated, because the activity is intense but short. Individuals with asthma are less able to tolerate prolonged intense activity such as jogging, lap running, race running, or basketball. Preexercise puffs of a prescribed inhaler and a warm-up before vigorous exercise can enable the child to participate more fully in age-appropriate school physical exercise. Many Olympic athletes have successfully managed their asthma symptoms. The promotion of normal growth and development is a basic goal in asthma care, and participation with peers is important.

The child is hospitalized for more severe asthma attacks. The nurse limits conversation with the child during the emergency period to questions that can be answered "yes" or "no." Oxygen reduces hypoxia and improves the patient's color. Nasal prongs, hood, or facial mask can be used to administer the oxygen.

If the child is in respiratory distress on admission, oxygen is administered per the physician's protocol, and the child is positioned comfortably. One method is to place a pillow on the overbed table and have the child extend the arms over it, elbows bent. This is comfortable and allows maximum use of the accessory muscles of breathing. Lung sounds are assessed for rhonchi, wheezing, or rales. Arterial blood gases and vital signs are monitored. The child is evaluated for clinical improvement (quieter, slower respirations, relaxed facial expressions, cessation of retractions). Oral fluids are encouraged because they help to liquefy secretions and are needed to compensate for fluid loss from dyspnea and diaphoresis. Carbonated beverages, such as ginger ale and colas, are avoided when the child is wheezing. Beverages are served at room temperature because cold liquids can trigger reflex bronchospasm. Milk products are avoided because they tend to increase the production of mucus. Intake and output should be recorded. The patient is observed for cracked lips, the absence of tears, poor skin turgor, and a decrease in urine output, all of which signal dehydration.

A well-balanced diet and adequate fluids are necessary for general health. Ample time is allowed for meals, because respiratory distress may interfere with eating. The nurse organizes tasks so that the child obtains sufficient rest. The child is assisted with the use of the nebulizer.

! Medication Safety Alert!

Oxygen is a drug, and administration should be correlated with monitoring of oxygen saturation levels. Too little oxygen can result in hypoxia; too much oxygen can result in lung damage.

Self-care. The child is gradually taught self-care. The importance of exercise to strengthen vulnerable lungs is emphasized. *Pursed-lip breathing* (blowing out as if blowing a kiss) and biofeedback are also helpful. The child is taught to observe "personal triggers" that are forewarnings of an attack. He or she is taught how to use the peak flow meter. Other aspects of care include how to administer MDIs and understanding medications and their possible side effects. Specific information about how often and when to use inhalers is paramount. The child is encouraged to discuss daily school routines. The health care provider is seen regularly to evaluate progress and to readjust the medications as needed. The nurse reviews the signs of respiratory infection with the child and where, when, and whom to call for help. Early attention to symptoms may prevent escalation of the disease.

Nursing Tip

Health promotion outcome: The goal of treatment is to maintain long-term asthma control, using the least amount of medication to avoid adverse events, and to maintain a normal developmental lifestyle with no more than one acute episode a year (Vanhoose, 2009).

Metered-dose inhalers (MDIs). Routine monitoring of airway obstruction should be part of comprehensive asthma management. A child 6 years of age can self-test with adult supervision. A diary of peak flow readings (PFRs) should be brought to the physician at each follow-up visit (Figure 25-8). The nurse should be alert to the fact that compliance may be a problem with older children and adolescents, who may cause false results by manipulating the unit.

An MDI consists of a pump that is a mouthpiece and an actuator (or holder) into which a medicine canister is inserted. The child breathes *out* and then places the mouth around the mouthpiece and inhales slowly as a puff is released by pushing down on the actuator. Pushing down on the actuator releases a dose of medication (puff), which is inhaled through the mouthpiece. This delivers the medicine directly to the lungs without systemic side effects. The use of a spacer slows the movement of the medicine, allowing more time to inhale the medicine. Some spacers reduce the need for hand-press-breath coordination during inhalation. Aerochambers with masks are available for infants. Practice to acquaint the infant to the treatment is helpful, because crying reduces delivery of medication to the lungs. Parents should be taught to use distractions such as books, music, or toys to minimize crying. Dry powder inhalers are popular because more medications are coming in powder form and often the dose administered does not need to be coordinated with inhalation. The child should be taught to rinse the mouth after steroid inhalation to prevent the development of candidiasis. Activators should be cleaned regularly.

SAMPLE DIARY:

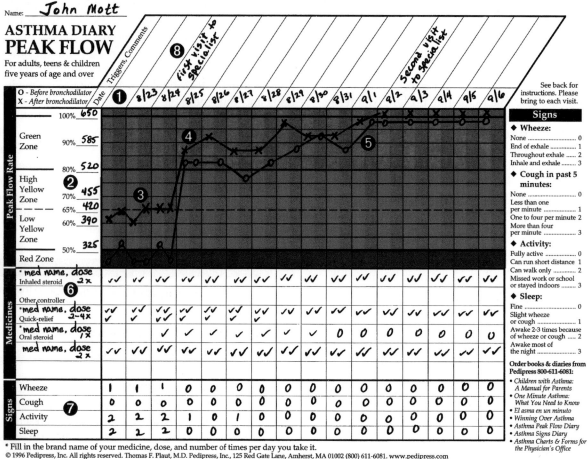

Name: **John Mott**

ASTHMA DIARY
PEAK FLOW
For adults, teens & children
five years of age and over

See back for instructions. Please bring to each visit.

O - Before bronchodilator
X - After bronchodilator

Signs

◆ **Wheeze:**
None 0
End of exhale 1
Throughout exhale 2
Inhale and exhale 3

◆ **Cough in past 5 minutes:**
None 0
Less than one per minute 1
One to four per minute 2
More than four per minute 3

◆ **Activity:**
Fully active 0
Can run short distance 1
Can walk only 2
Missed work or school or stayed indoors 3

◆ **Sleep:**
Fine 0
Slight wheeze or cough 1
Awake 2-3 times because of wheeze or cough 2
Awake most of the night 3

Order books & diaries from Pedipress 800-611-6081:
• *Children with Asthma: A Manual for Parents*
• *One Minute Asthma: What You Need to Know*
• *El asma en un minuto*
• *Winning Over Asthma*
• *Asthma Peak Flow Diary*
• *Asthma Signs Diary*
• *Asthma Charts & Forms for the Physician's Office*

* Fill in the brand name of your medicine, dose, and number of times per day you take it.
© 1996 Pedipress, Inc. All rights reserved. Thomas F. Plaut, M.D. Pedipress, Inc., 125 Red Gate Lane, Amherst, MA 01002 (800) 611-6081. www.pedipress.com

This asthma diary can help you learn about asthma and asthma medicines. With this information, you and your doctor can work out a written plan that will help you care for your (child's) asthma at home.

❶ **DATE:** Fill in date above the grid.

❷ **ASTHMA CARE ZONES:**
• *Green Zone:* Your current treatment plan is effective.
• *High Yellow Zone:* Avoid triggers and change your medication routine.
• *Low Yellow Zone:* Intensify treatment if your peak flow score does not increase into the high yellow zone within 10 minutes after inhaling a quick-relief medicine, or if it falls back into the low yellow zone within four hours.
• *Red Zone:* Take emergency medicine and see your doctor or go to the Emergency Room if your peak flow score does not increase into the low yellow zone within 10 minutes after inhaling a quick-relief medicine, or if it falls back into the red zone within four hours.

Put your (child's) personal best peak flow score here: _____.
This is the top of the *Green Zone.* Find your (child's) personal best score on the table below. List it and the numbers below it on the front of this sheet.

If your (child's) personal best peak flow score has not yet been determined, use the average peak flow score for your (child's) height from a standard chart, e.g., *Children with Asthma,* page 100.

If your (child's) personal best peak flow score reaches a higher level on two separate days, start a new section by drawing a thick

vertical line to indicate the change. Enter the new numbers from the chart below.

❸ **DAY/NIGHT COLUMNS:** Use the clear column for daytime scores (7 AM-7 PM) and the shaded column for nighttime scores (7 PM-7 AM).

❹ **PLOT PEAK FLOW SCORE:** Use an *"O"* to plot scores blown before taking an inhaled bronchodilator and an *"X"* to plot scores blown after taking an inhaled bronchodilator. Estimate placement of mark between zone lines.

❺ **PEAK FLOW TREND:** Connect the *O's* with a line to illustrate a trend. Do the same thing for the *X's.*

❻ **MEDICINES:** Enter the name, dose, and number of doses per day for each medicine. Put one check mark (✔) in the box for each dose given.

❼ **SIGNS:** Sign scores are listed on the right side of diary. Enter each score by time of day. Cough is assessed during a five minute period.

❽ **COMMENTS:** Enter comments above the date such as *"Exposed to cigarette smoke," "Had cold," "Rabbit in school"* and *"Painting bedroom."*

◆ **RELATIONSHIPS:** Try to see connections between triggers, medicines and signs. For example, did peak flow drop after contact with a cat or a rabbit? Does peak flow always change with a cold? If not, why not? Any time there is a change in peak flow, you should look for a trigger.

◆ **ILLNESS:** If you (or your child) are sick, and you want to record peak flow more often, use several sections to record each day.

FIGURE 25-8 The asthma diary. The clear column is for daytime peak flow reading (PFR) score, and the shaded column is for nighttime peak flow scores. An *X* indicates PFR following inhaler therapy. An *O* indicates PFR without inhaler therapy. A check mark indicates medication taken. Asthma triggers and comments are recorded. The diary is brought to each follow-up clinic visit.

Using a Metered-Dose Inhaler

PURPOSE

To promote home self-care

STEPS

1. Insert the metered-dose inhaler (MDI) canister into the holder.
2. Shake the MDI vigorously.
3. Instruct the child to exhale a normal breath.
4. Instruct the child to close mouth around the mouthpiece (or hold 2 to 4 cm [0.8 to 1.6 inches] from the open mouth).
5. Push down on the canister for one puff.
6. Instruct the child to inhale deeply and slowly for 3 to 5 seconds.
7. Instruct the child to hold the breath for 10 seconds.
8. Remove MDI from mouth.
9. Instruct the child to exhale slowly from the nose.

Most near-empty inhaler canisters will float in a bowl of water. Some canisters have an alert system to notify user of remaining doses available in the canister. Knowing the canister content level enables the child to request a refill and avoid missing medication doses. Inhalers are designed for use with an open-mouth technique or a closed-mouth technique (Skill 25-2). A nebulizer machine can be used in the home when inhalers are not appropriate for the individual child.

The nurse should help the child see connections between triggers, medicines, and signs of respiratory distress. For example, did the peak flow drop after contact with a cat or rabbit? Does the peak flow always change with a cold? Any time there is a change in peak flow, the child should know to look for a cause that triggered it.

During every clinic visit, the nurse should have the child demonstrate the use of the inhaler or spacer and reinforce the principles involved.

> **Medication Safety Alert!**
>
> Medicated inhalers should be used as prescribed. Overuse can be dangerous.

Status Asthmaticus

Status asthmaticus is continued severe respiratory distress that is not responsive to drugs, including epinephrine and aminophylline. **This is a medical emergency.** The child requires immediate admission to the ICU. Oxygen is administered via nasal cannula because mist in a mist tent can cause coughing or wheezing. Vital signs and the flow of IV medications are carefully monitored. Complying with the prescribed medical regimen, promptly seeking medical care when indicated, minimizing exposure to known allergens, wearing medical identification bracelets, and having a written plan for crisis management can minimize the life-threatening occurrence of status asthmaticus.

> **Nursing Tip**
>
> The principles of asthma treatment are as follows:
> - Daily monitoring
> - Symptom diary
> - Treatment plan with active participation of the child
> - Identification and avoidance of triggers

Cystic Fibrosis

Pathophysiology. Cystic fibrosis (CF) is a major worldwide cause of serious chronic lung disease in children. It occurs in approximately 1 in 2500 live births of Caucasian infants and 1 in 13,000 births of African American infants in the United States. Approximately 1 in 31 healthy people in the United States are carriers (Gott, 2010). It is an inherited recessive trait, with both parents carrying a gene for the disease. There is a defect in chromosome number 7 that is thought to have developed many years ago as a protective response of the human body against cholera. As the chromosomes mutated to develop the body's resistance to cholera, the change in the gene resulted in another defect that caused CF. Newborn screening for cystic fibrosis is performed in all states in the United States and the District of Columbia (Cystic Fibrosis Foundation, 2011c). A sweat chloride test is considered diagnostic.

The basic defect in CF is an exocrine gland dysfunction that includes (1) increased viscosity (thickness) of mucous gland secretions, and (2) a loss of electrolytes in sweat because of an abnormal chloride movement. CF is considered a *multisystem* disease because of the following effects of the thick, viscid secretions:

- *Respiratory system:* Small and large airways are obstructed by the thick secretions, resulting in difficulty breathing. The accumulation and stasis of the thick secretions create a medium for growth of organisms that cause repeated respiratory infections. The thick secretions in the lungs and

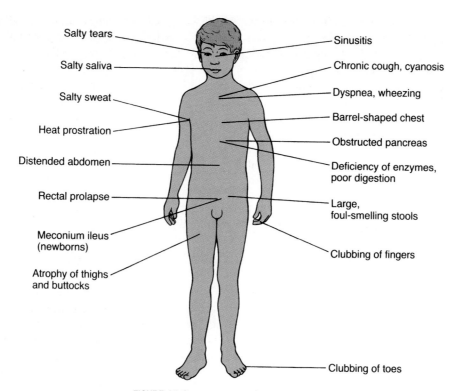

Salty tears

Salty saliva

Salty sweat

Heat prostration

Distended abdomen

Rectal prolapse

Meconium ileus
(newborns)

Atrophy of thighs
and buttocks

Sinusitis

Chronic cough, cyanosis

Dyspnea, wheezing

Barrel-shaped chest

Obstructed pancreas

Deficiency of enzymes,
poor digestion

Large,
foul-smelling stools

Clubbing of fingers

Clubbing of toes

FIGURE 25-9 Manifestations of cystic fibrosis.

response of tissues to infections cause hypoxia that can result in heart failure. Emphysema, wheezes, and respiratory distress are common.

- *Digestive system:* The thickened secretions prevent the digestive enzymes from flowing to the gastrointestinal tract, resulting in poor absorption of food and general growth failure. Bulky, foul-smelling stools that are frothy because of the undigested fat content are characteristic. Thick, impacted feces can cause rectal prolapse. Pancreatic, liver, and biliary obstruction occur.
- *Skin:* Loss of electrolytes (sodium and chloride) in the sweat causes a "salty" skin surface. Loss of electrolytes via the skin predisposes the child to electrolyte imbalances during hot weather.
- *Reproductive system:* Thick secretions can decrease sperm motility. Thick cervical mucus can inhibit sperm from reaching the fallopian tubes.

Manifestations. The manifestations of CF are illustrated in Figure 25-9.

Lung Involvement. The air passages of the lungs become clogged with mucus. There is widespread obstruction of the bronchioles. It is difficult for the child to breathe; expiration is especially difficult. More and more air becomes trapped in the lungs (*obstructive emphysema*), and small areas of collapse (**atelectasis**) may occur. Eventually the chest assumes a barrel shape, with increased diameter across the front and back. The right ventricle of the heart, which supplies the lungs, may become strained and enlarged. **Clubbing of the fingers**

and toes (Figure 25-10), a compensatory response indicating a chronic lack of oxygen, may be present. *Staphylococcus* and *Pseudomonas* infections can easily occur in the lungs, which provide a suitable medium for the organism's growth. This causes more thickening of the abnormal secretions, irritates and damages lung tissues, and further increases lung obstruction.

Dyspnea, wheezing, and cyanosis may occur. The child is irritable and tires easily. There is a gradual change in physical appearance. Evidence of obstructive emphysema, atelectasis, and fibrosis of lung tissue may also be present. The prognosis for survival depends on the extent of lung damage. However, this is only part of the picture, because CF also affects the pancreas and sweat glands.

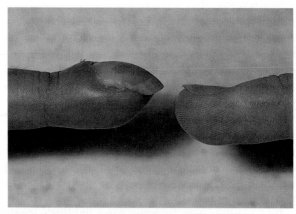

FIGURE 25-10 Clubbing of the fingers, a sign of chronic hypoxia. (From Swartz MH: *Textbook of physical diagnosis: History and examination,* ed 7, Philadelphia, 2014, Saunders.)

Pancreatic Involvement. The pancreas lies behind the stomach. Some of its cells secrete pancreatic enzymes that drain from the pancreatic duct into the duodenum in the same area in which bile enters. Changes occurring in the pancreas result from obstruction by thickened secretions that block the flow of pancreatic digestive enzymes. As a result, foodstuffs, particularly fats and proteins, are not properly digested and used by the body.

The stools in infants may be loose. Because of impaired digestion and food absorption, the feces of the child become large, fatty, and foul smelling. They are usually light in color. The child does not gain weight despite a good appetite, and he or she may look undernourished. The abdomen becomes distended, and the buttocks and thighs *atrophy* (waste away) as fat disappears from the main deposit sites.

A condition known as **meconium ileus** exists when the intestine of the newborn becomes obstructed with abnormally thick meconium while in utero. This condition is caused by the absence of pancreatic enzymes that normally digest proteins in the meconium. The abnormal, puttylike stool sticks to the walls of the intestine, causing blockage. The presenting symptoms develop within hours after birth. The absence of stools and the presence of vomiting and of abdominal distention lead to suspicion of intestinal obstruction. X-ray films confirm the diagnosis.

Sweat Glands. The sweat, tears, and saliva of the patient with CF become abnormally salty because of an increase in sodium chloride levels. Up to about 20 years of age, more than 60 mEq/L of sodium chloride in sweat is diagnostic of CF. Levels of 40 to 60 mEq/L are highly suggestive. The analysis of sweat is a major aid in diagnosing the condition. The *sweat test* is the best diagnostic study. Because these children lose large amounts of salt through perspiration, they must be watched for heat prostration. Liberal amounts of salt should be included with food, and extra fluids and salt should be provided during hot weather.

Complications. CF is often responsible for rectal prolapse in infants and children partly because of poor muscle tone in the rectal area and because of the excessive leanness of the buttocks of the patient.

As the disease progresses, the liver may become hard, nodular, and enlarged. *Cor pulmonale* (*cor*, "heart," and *pulmon*, "lung"), which is heart strain caused by improper lung function, is often a cause of death. There is a deficiency of vitamin A because the child is unable to absorb fats from which this vitamin is obtained. Sexual development may be delayed in these patients. Males are generally sterile, but sexual function is unimpaired. Adolescent girls may experience secondary amenorrhea during exacerbations.

Treatment and Nursing Care

Respiratory relief. See Chapter 22 for a discussion of oxygen therapy. Antimicrobials may be administered as a preventive measure against respiratory infection; however, this treatment is controversial. Nursing Care Plan 25-1 summarizes interventions for the CF patient. Intermittent aerosol therapy is administered to provide

---

⭐ **Nursing Care Plan 25-1   The Pediatric Patient with Cystic Fibrosis**

PATIENT DATA A 5-year-old child diagnosed with cystic fibrosis is admitted to the unit. The child has loose, foul-smelling stools, a persistent cough with some nasal flaring, and chest retractions.

Selected Nursing Diagnosis: Ineffective airway clearance related to inability to clear mucus from respiratory tract secondary to cystic fibrosis as evidenced by thick mucus production, unproductive or minimal cough, and adventitious breath sounds (wheezes, crackles, dyspnea, tachypnea, cyanosis)

Goals	Nursing Interventions	Rationales
Child will have an effective airway as demonstrated by effective cough, thin respiratory secretions, age-appropriate respiratory rate and effort, and O$_2$ saturation >92% on room air.	Observe respiratory status (rate, depth, effort, breath sounds, oxygen saturation, and skin color) *at least* every 4 hours.	Allows for early detection of and intervention for changes in child's respiratory status.
	Administer humidified O$_2$ as ordered by physician; monitor O$_2$ saturation frequently.	Humidification helps to thin and loosen secretions. In chronic obstructive respiratory diseases, the respiratory center in the brain becomes tolerant of low O$_2$ saturation in the blood. Administering high concentrations of O$_2$ to a child with chronic lung disease can lead to carbon dioxide narcosis.
	Administer bronchodilators and expectorants as ordered by physician.	These medications help the thinning, loosening, and expectoration of respiratory mucus.
	Encourage age-appropriate oral intake of fluids.	Helps to decrease the viscosity (thickness) of secretions.

Continued

Goals	Nursing Interventions	Rationales
	Perform chest physiotherapy treatments (CPT) and postural drainage (PD) every 4 hours or as needed. Perform CPT/PD 1 hour before or 2 hours after meals.	CPT and PD help to mobilize secretions and to increase oxygenation. Performing 1 hour before or 2 hours after meals lessens the risk of vomiting and/or aspiration.
	Teach the child how to do coughing and deep-breathing exercises. Use play therapy whenever possible. For example, using an inspirometer, "blow up" the fingers of a clean glove.	Children younger than age 7 years cannot voluntarily produce an effective cough. Coughing and deep-breathing exercises help expand the lungs and mobilize secretions.
	Teach parents and caregivers *not* to give over-the-counter (OTC) medications, especially cough suppressants, to the child with cystic fibrosis.	Cough suppressant medication inhibits the cough reflex, leading to secretions being retained and the possibility of respiratory infection.

Selected Nursing Diagnosis: Imbalanced nutrition: less than body requirements related to decrease in the availability of pancreatic enzymes; poor intestinal absorption of nutritional intake; anorexia secondary to cystic fibrosis as evidenced by decreased oral intake, weight loss or failure to thrive, diarrhea, steatorrhea, or constipation

Goals	Nursing Interventions	Rationales
Child will be able to ingest age-appropriate nutrition and maintain weight or gain height and weight according to the normal growth and development charts. Stools will be of normal color, consistency, and amount for age.	Determine child's normal feeding patterns, dietary likes and dislikes, and activity level.	Knowing the child's preferences and activity level will aid in the plan of care with regard to feeding the child.
	Administer pancreatic replacement enzymes and fat-soluble vitamin supplements as directed by the physician before meals and snacks.	Digestive and nutritional therapy consists of replacement of pancreatic enzymes and dietary adjustments. Administering supplemental fat-soluble vitamins is necessary because of the inability of the body to absorb fats.
	Teach the child (and parents) *not* to chew the capsules or "beads" but to swallow the medication whole; if using powder form, to sprinkle over a nonfat, nonprotein food, such as applesauce. Do not mix enzymes with hot (heated) foods, high-starch, or high-acid–containing foods. Wipe any powder from oral mucosa or lips.	Pancreatic enzymes are inactivated by heat, and acids are known to degrade the enzymes. Wipe the excess powder off mucosa to prevent excoriation or breakdown of mucosal membranes.
	Note color, consistency, amount, and frequency of stools. Notify the physician of any changes (e.g., diarrhea, constipation, or steatorrhea).	Pancreatic enzymes are known to cause constipation if taken in high doses, or they can cause steatorrhea from malabsorption of fats and proteins or because of low intake of the enzymes.

Selected Nursing Diagnosis: Interrupted family processes related to chronicity of disease, need for outside support, the risk of life-threatening complications as evidenced by frequent physician office visits or hospitalizations, a diminished focus on other siblings in home, and the need for therapeutic interventions and compliance with home care routines

Goals	Nursing Interventions	Rationales
Family members will verbalize their feelings about the impact cystic fibrosis has on them; will be able to comply with the therapeutic treatment plan; and will use available resources within their community to assist in the care and treatment of their child.	Determine the educational level and amount of knowledge each family member has on cystic fibrosis *before* planning any family interventions or teaching sessions.	Educational level will help to determine the type of teaching methods to be used (i.e., written, visual, hands-on, auditory). Having this information in advance helps the nurse to map out the plan of care and teaching. It also prevents the repetition of the same information or guides the nurse as to the amount of teaching/information required or needed by the family.
	Determine the level of impact that the disease has had on the family.	Guides the nurse in selecting appropriate referrals to community or support agencies needed by the family.
	Teach and/or review with family the skills required in the daily care of the child with cystic fibrosis: for example, assessing respiratory rate and status, CPT and PD methods, monitoring stools, caring for skin, and medication administration.	Return demonstration enables the nurse to evaluate the ability of the family to provide effective home care.

medication to the lower respiratory tract and to promote the evacuation of secretions. An inhaler that acts as a mucus clearance device can be used in the home care of these children. Bronchodilators are used to increase the width of the bronchi, allowing free passage of air into the lungs. Recombinant human deoxyribonuclease dornase alfa (Pulmozyme) in a single daily aerosol dose is effective in decreasing thickness of secretions, thereby improving pulmonary function.

Postural drainage and chest-clapping therapy are also of value (Figure 25-11). The physical or respiratory therapist performs these procedures during hospitalization. When postural drainage and chest clapping are done properly, the secretions in the chest are moved up and out. This should be explained to the parents so they will continue this valuable procedure when the child returns home. Instructions may need to be repeated frequently to encourage full cooperation of the parents and child. These procedures are done after nebulization and at least 2 hours after eating. General exercise is good for the patient because it stimulates coughing. Play activities such as somersaults and headstands within the child's endurance limits are therapeutic.

Breathing exercises may also be recommended for the older child. **Pursed-lip breathing** is one technique that is simple and effective. The patient is instructed to inhale through the nose, then to exhale through the mouth with the lips pursed as if whistling. Exhalation should be at least twice as long as inhalation. (If it takes 3 seconds to breathe in, 6 seconds are taken to allow all the air to escape.) The child is taught not to force the air out but to let it escape naturally.

Prevention of respiratory infections is essential. The child is isolated from patients and personnel who may harbor infections. The period of hospitalization is kept brief, if possible, to avoid cross infection. The necessary immunizations against childhood diseases must be given to this child (see Chapter 32).

An oral pancreatic preparation, such as pancrelipase (Pancreaze), is given to the child with each meal and snack to replace the pancreatic enzymes that the child's body cannot produce. This medication is considered specific for the disease because it helps the child to digest and absorb food, thus improving the condition of the stools. If the child is ill and not eating, the medication is withheld. When meals are erratic, such as during vacations, medication is given when the largest amount of food will be consumed. High doses have been associated with the development of gastrointestinal strictures, and the child should be monitored. Vitamins A, D, E, and K, iron, and zinc supplements are also prescribed.

> **Nursing Tip**
>
> Chest physiotherapy should be performed *between* meals.

Diet. The maintenance of adequate nutrition is essential. The diet should be high in protein and calories. Supplemental enzymes are provided with the food to aid in digestion, and fat-soluble vitamins may be prescribed. The child should be weighed daily. Intake and output are recorded. Children should have free access to salt, although a regimented salt supplementation is no longer recommended. Infants can breastfeed with added enzyme intake. Formula-fed infants do best with a higher calorie-per-ounce formula, such as Pregestimil or Alimentum. Parenteral alimentation (total parenteral nutrition [TPN]) may be indicated in some cases.

> **Nursing Tip**
>
> Pancreatic enzyme powder should be given with applesauce or other nonstarch, nonfat, nonprotein food.

General hygiene. The nurse must pay special attention to the skin of the child with CF. The diaper area is cleansed after each bowel movement. An ointment to protect the skin is advisable because the character of the stool subjects the diaper area to irritation. The buttocks are exposed to air when a rash occurs. Because the child has little fat and muscle, the position must be changed frequently, especially if the child is weak and cannot get out of bed. Frequent changes of position also prevent the development of pneumonia.

The child wears light clothing to avoid becoming overheated; it should be loose to allow freedom of movement. Good oral hygiene is necessary, because the teeth may be in poor condition because of dietary deficiencies. Mouth care is given after postural drainage because foul mucus may be raised, leaving an unpleasant taste in the patient's mouth.

Long-term care. The goals of care include minimizing pulmonary complications, ensuring adequate nutrition, promoting growth and development, and assisting the family to adjust to the chronic care required at home. This is extremely taxing financially, physically, and emotionally. The parents must distribute their time and energy within the family yet give careful attention to their sick child or, sometimes, children. How do they keep from spoiling the child? Do they limit the normal activities of the remaining children to spare the sick one? What about birthday parties, camping, scouts, pets, and epidemics at school? What does a trip to the shore or mountains entail? When do the parents find time for themselves? Coping techniques must be developed and used.

Parents need explicit instructions regarding diet, medication, postural drainage, prevention of infection, rest, and continued medical supervision. Many families require the assistance of a social worker to secure funds for equipment and drugs. Genetic counseling is also advised.

Emotional support. The child who is chronically ill finds it hard to accept restricted activity. The amount and types of diversion required vary in CF because

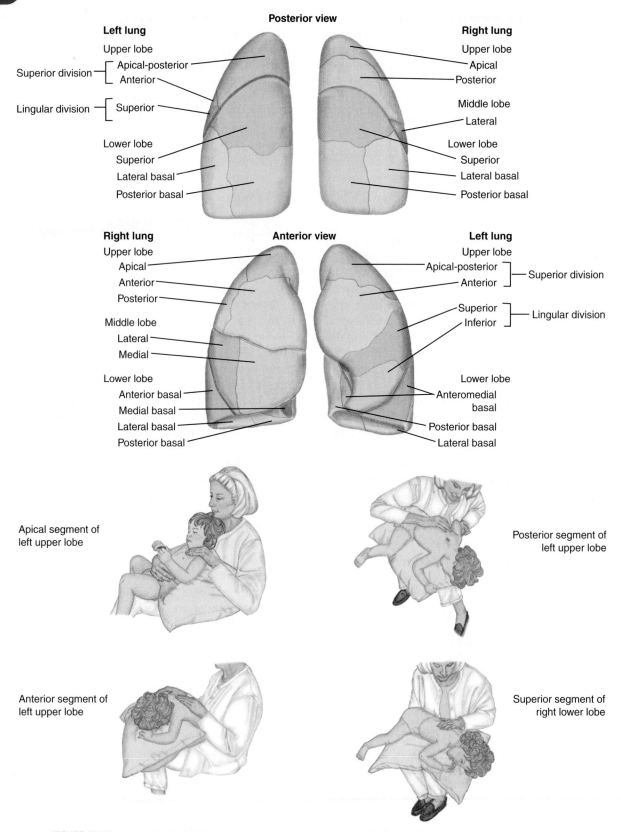

FIGURE 25-11 Postural drainage. The positions for postural drainage are correlated with the segment being drained. (From McKinney ES, James SR, Murray SS, Ashwill JW: *Maternal-child nursing*, ed 2, Philadelphia, 2005, Saunders.)

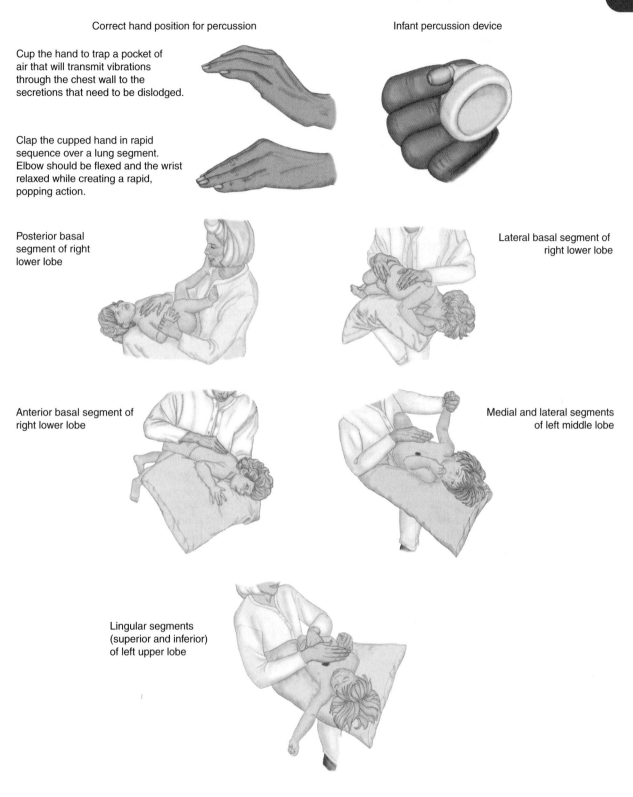

Correct hand position for percussion

Cup the hand to trap a pocket of air that will transmit vibrations through the chest wall to the secretions that need to be dislodged.

Clap the cupped hand in rapid sequence over a lung segment. Elbow should be flexed and the wrist relaxed while creating a rapid, popping action.

Infant percussion device

Posterior basal segment of right lower lobe

Lateral basal segment of right lower lobe

Anterior basal segment of right lower lobe

Medial and lateral segments of left middle lobe

Lingular segments (superior and inferior) of left upper lobe

FIGURE 25-11, cont'd Postural drainage.

the disease affects children of all ages and varies in severity.

It is thought that children benefit from simple, straightforward answers to questions about their illnesses. An uncomplicated diagram might be helpful. They should know why they must take medications with each meal, use the nebulizer, and have postural drainage. They should see and handle the unfamiliar equipment necessary for care.

The young child finds it more difficult to be separated from parents during hospitalization. Even when the prognosis is grave, a child's courage is sustained if parents are there. Rooming-in is encouraged whenever possible. Close contact by mail, telephone, or e-mail with school, church, and clubs is important for the school-age child. It is helpful for patients to develop an activity that they enjoy, such as piano or art. This increases feelings of worth and provides outlets for feelings. Consideration must be given to ways of fostering love, acceptance, trust, fair play, security, freedom of choice, creativity, and maintenance of self-identity.

Bronchopulmonary Dysplasia

Pathophysiology. Bronchopulmonary dysplasia (BPD) is a fibrosis, or thickening, of the alveolar walls and the bronchiolar epithelium. It occurs in premature infants (less than 32 weeks) who have abnormal or arrested lung development and who receive ventilation and oxygen for more than 28 days to survive (Gott, 2010). Swelling of the tissues causes edema, and the respiratory cilia are paralyzed by the high oxygen concentrations and lose their ability to clear mucus from the airways. Respiratory obstruction, mucus plugs, and atelectasis follow.

Prevention. Respiratory distress in the newborn is the major reason that oxygen and ventilators are used for prolonged periods. The main cause of respiratory distress in the newborn is prematurity. Therefore the prevention of preterm births is the best way to prevent BPD. The goal of treatment for respiratory distress in the newborn should be to administer only the amount of oxygen required to prevent hypoxia, at the minimum necessary ventilator pressures, so as to prevent tissue trauma. The use of antenatal steroids to hasten lung development during preterm labor and the administration of surfactant within 15 minutes after delivery in a very premature infant may prevent respiratory distress that would necessitate oxygen and prolonged ventilation treatment.

Symptoms. Symptoms of chronic respiratory distress include the following:

- Wheezing
- Retractions
- Cyanosis on exertion
- Use of accessory respiratory muscles
- Clubbing of the fingers
- Failure to thrive
- Irritability caused by hypoxia

Treatment. After BPD has developed, the goal of therapy is to reduce inflammation of the airway and to wean the infant from the mechanical ventilator. The infant may become oxygen dependent and develop reactive airway bronchoconstriction. Noninvasive ventilation techniques have been developed, such as synchronous intermittent mandatory ventilation (SIMV) via nasal cannula prongs, continuous positive airway pressure (CPAP), high-flow blended nasal cannulas, and high-flow humidified oxygen, which are safer and may minimize the development of BPD. Right-sided heart failure may also develop. Fluid restriction, bronchodilators, and diuretics may be prescribed. A tracheostomy may

also be needed. Nasogastric tube feedings may be required to conserve energy while maintaining adequate nutrition. Infants with BPD often develop respiratory stridor and retractions with even minor respiratory infections, which result in repeated hospitalizations. Ongoing home care is required, and respiratory problems persist through adulthood. Maintaining optimum growth and development is a challenge. Education and support of the family for a technology-dependent child at home are essential, and a multidisciplinary health care team approach is essential.

 Safety Alert!

When oxygen is used in the home, the family should be taught safety precautions to prevent fire and injury.

Sudden Infant Death Syndrome

Sudden infant death syndrome (SIDS) is clinically defined as the sudden, unexpected death of an apparently healthy infant between 2 weeks and 1 year of age, for which a routine autopsy fails to identify the cause. It is also referred to as "crib death" or sudden unexplained infant death (SUID). The peak incidence is between 2 and 4 months of age. The clinical features of the disease remain constant:

- Death occurs during sleep.
- The infant does not cry or make other sounds of distress.

It has occurred even when the parents were sleeping in the same room. The occurrence of SIDS accounted for 15% of all infant deaths in 2010 and has decreased by 38% since 1992 when the "back to sleep" program was first implemented. SIDS is thought to be caused by a brainstem abnormality of cardiorespiratory control. Overheating, irregular respiratory patterns, and decreased arousal responses are contributing factors. Increased risk factors for SIDS may include maternal smoking or cocaine use that causes hypoxia of the fetus, preterm birth, and poor postnatal care. A facedown sleeping position may cause rebreathing of expired air or airway occlusion. Wrapping the infant who is placed face down may increase the risk for SIDS by preventing the infant from lifting and turning the face to the side.

Prevention. Infants should be placed on a firm mattress with no loose bedding surrounding the infant. The use of a pacifier may be protective (Moon, 2011). For high-risk infants, home apnea monitors have been used to warn parents of an impending problem and enable them to try to resuscitate the infant manually. All parents should have cardiopulmonary resuscitation education. However, frustrations with frequent alarm malfunctions and noncompliance have made this intervention less effective. The AAP recommends that all healthy infants be placed in the supine (back-lying) position on firm mattresses to prevent SIDS. The use of soft pillows or fluffy blankets for the infant to lie on and sharing a bed with parents are discouraged because these practices can prevent the infant from raising and turning his or her head. A national educational media campaign for this recommended positioning of infants has decreased the occurrence of SIDS. The SUID/SIDS Resource Center offers "safe to sleep campaign" educational materials (www.sidscenter.org).

When infants are in car seats, care should be taken to avoid flexion of the infant's head so that the chin rests on the chest, as this can cause oxygen desaturation and hypoxia. Car seats should not be used as a prolonged sleeping arrangement (Moon, 2011). When an infant is placed in a "sling carrier" care should be taken that the infant's face is above the fabric and the nose and mouth are unobstructed.

 Safety Alert!

The AAP recommends that all healthy infants be placed on their backs for sleep to help prevent the occurrence of SIDS.

Nursing Care. In talking with grieving parents after the death of their infant, the nurse must convey some important facts: that the infant died of a disease entity called sudden infant death syndrome, that currently the disease cannot be predicted or prevented, and that they are *not* responsible for the child's death. Grieving parents need time to say good-bye to their child. They are encouraged to hold and rock the infant, shed tears, and assist in burial preparations. This process is conducive to the resolution of grief.

Parents experience much guilt and are catapulted into a totally unexpected bereavement that creates the need for numerous explanations to relatives and friends. Often needless blame has been placed on one parent by the other or by relatives. The family babysitter and physician may also be targets of attack. Emergency department personnel must be especially sensitive and supportive during this crisis. There have been crib deaths for which parents have been mistakenly charged with child abuse.

Get Ready for the NCLEX® Examination!

Key Points

- Routine handwashing practices can prevent the spread of the common cold.
- Quiet play may be more restful than confinement to bed for toddlers and young children.
- Use of nose drops with an oil base should be avoided.
- Laryngomalacia and acute spasmodic laryngitis are benign forms of croup.
- Laryngotracheobronchitis and epiglottitis are acute types of croup.
- A croupette, or mist tent, provides moist air supersaturated with microdroplets that can enter the small airway of a child and relieve respiratory distress.
- A tongue blade examination of the throat can cause sudden respiratory arrest in a child with epiglottitis.
- Frequent swallowing while the child is sleeping is an early sign of bleeding immediately after a tonsillectomy.
- Coughing, clearing the throat, and blowing the nose should be avoided in the immediate postoperative period after a tonsillectomy.
- Swimming and sports activities that involve intermittent activity are well tolerated by asthmatic children.
- Cystic fibrosis is a multisystem disease characterized by an increased viscosity of mucous gland secretions.
- Bulky, frothy, foul-smelling stools are characteristic of cystic fibrosis.
- The maxillary and ethmoid sinuses are most often involved in childhood sinusitis.
- Periorbital cellulitis is a complication of childhood sinusitis.

- Pulse oximetry readings are of little value in carbon monoxide poisoning.
- An intubation tray should be readily available at the bedside for infants with carbon monoxide poisoning.
- An infant should be positioned for sleep on the back, on a firm mattress without pillows or fluffy blankets. A car seat should not be used as a prolonged sleeping arrangement for infants.

Additional Learning Resources

 SG Go to your Study Guide for additional learning activities to help you master this chapter content.

evolve Go to your Evolve website (http://evolve.elsevier.com/Leifer) for the following learning resources:

- Animations
- Answer Guidelines for Critical Thinking Questions
- Answers and Rationales for Review Questions for the NCLEX® Examination
- Glossary with English and Spanish pronunciations
- Interactive Review Questions for the NCLEX® Examination
- Patient Teaching Plans in English and Spanish
- Skills Performance Checklists
- Video clips and more!

Online Resources

- Guidelines for the Diagnosis and Management of Asthma: www.nhlbi.nih.gov/guidelines/asthma/asthgdln.pdf
- National Asthma Control Initiative (NACI): http://rover.nhlbi.nih.gov/health/prof/lung/asthma/naci
- Respiratory syncytial virus: www.cdc.gov/rsv

Review Questions for the NCLEX® Examination

1. Which is a priority nursing diagnosis in a child admitted with acute asthma?

   1. Risk for infection
   2. Imbalanced nutrition
   3. Ineffective breathing pattern
   4. Disturbed body image

2. Which sign or symptom observed in a sleeping 2-year-old child immediately after a tonsillectomy necessitates reporting and follow-up care?

   1. A pulse of 110 beats/min
   2. A blood pressure of 96/64 mm Hg
   3. Nausea
   4. Frequent swallowing

3. The nurse is reinforcing teaching concerning the use of a cromolyn sodium inhaler for a 10-year-old with asthma. Which would be an accurate concept to emphasize?

   1. You should use the inhaler whenever you feel some difficulty in breathing.
   2. You should use the inhaler between meals.
   3. You should use the inhaler regularly every day even if you are symptom free.
   4. You can discontinue using the inhaler when you are feeling stronger.

4. A health care provider is preparing to examine the throat of a child diagnosed with acute epiglottitis. A priority nursing responsibility would be to:

   1. have a tracheotomy set at the bedside.
   2. immobilize the child's head.
   3. restrain the child's arms.
   4. have oxygen available.

5. An infant is admitted with a diagnosis of respiratory syncytial virus (RSV) infection. The type of transmission-based isolation precaution the nurse would set up would be (select all that apply):

   1. standard precautions.
   2. droplet precautions.
   3. contact precautions.
   4. airborne infection isolation precautions.

Critical Thinking Question

1. The father of a child diagnosed with cystic fibrosis visits his child in the hospital. He states that he thinks the hospital food does not agree with his child because he notices the child has a loose stool with a very bad odor. None of his other children have that type of stool. He brought some loperamide (Imodium) pills from the drugstore to give to the child. What is the best response of the nurse?

Objectives

1. Define each key term listed.
2. Distinguish the differences between the cardiovascular system of the infant and that of the adult.
3. List the general signs and symptoms of congenital heart disease.
4. Differentiate between patent ductus arteriosus, coarctation of the aorta, atrial septal defect, ventricular septal defect, and tetralogy of Fallot.
5. Discuss six nursing goals relevant to the child with acquired heart disease.
6. List the symptoms of rheumatic fever.
7. Discuss the prevention of rheumatic fever.
8. Discuss hypertension in childhood.
9. Differentiate between primary and secondary hypertension.
10. Identify factors that can prevent hypertension.
11. Describe heart-healthy guidelines for children older than 2 years.
12. Recognize the manifestation of Kawasaki disease and the related nursing care.

Key Terms

carditis (kăhr-DĪ-tĭs, p. 614)
chorea (kŏ-RĒ-ă, p. 614)
hemodynamics (hē-mō-dī-NĂM-ĭks, p. 606)
hypothermia (hī-pō-THŬR-mē-ă, p. 606)
Jones criteria (p. 614)
polyarthritis (p. 614)
polycythemia (pŏl-ē-sī-THĒ-mē-ă, p. 609)

pulse pressure (p. 609)
shunt (p. 606)
stenosis (p. 609)
stroke volume (p. 612)
tachycardia (p. 612)
"tet" spells (p. 610)
thoracotomy (thŏ-ră-KŎT-ō-mē, p. 606)

THE CARDIOVASCULAR SYSTEM

The cardiovascular system consists of the heart, the blood, and the blood vessels. See Figure 3-7 for changes that occur in cardiovascular circulation at birth. As the heart beats, blood, oxygen, and nutrients are transported to all tissues of the body, and waste products are removed. Because of anatomical and physiological immaturity, the cardiovascular system of the child differs from that of the adult. Figure 26-1 summarizes some of these differences.

The cardiovascular system develops between the third and the eighth week of gestation. It is the first system to function in intrauterine life. When cardiovascular development is incomplete, heart defects occur. Fetal circulation is designed to serve the metabolic needs during intrauterine life and also to permit safe transition to life outside the womb.

Congenital heart defects can occur as an isolated defect or they can be part of a genetic syndrome with other defects present.

SIGNS RELATED TO SUSPECTED CARDIAC PATHOLOGY

Although signs and symptoms of specific congenital heart defects relate to the specific pathology involved, several signs and symptoms are common to most infants with congenital cardiac problems. When the nurse assesses the child, the following observations should be reported:

- Failure to thrive and/or poor weight gain
- Cyanosis, pallor
- Visually observed pulsations in the neck veins
- Tachypnea, dyspnea
- Irregular pulse rate
- Clubbing of fingers
- Fatigue during feeding or activity
- Excessive perspiration, especially over forehead

🔷 Nursing Tip

Bradycardia may be a sign that cardiovascular arrest is imminent in children with hypoxia (Zidemar, 2008).

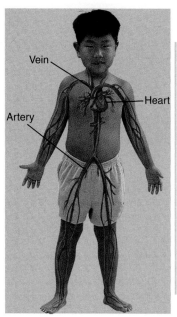

CARDIOVASCULAR SYSTEM

- Pulse, respiration, blood pressure, and hematological values vary with the age of the child.
- Chest walls are thin in infants and young children because of the relative lack of subcutaneous and muscle tissue compared with older children. "Innocent" murmurs can be heard in structurally normal hearts.
- The newborn's circulation differs from fetal circulation; if adaptations do not take place, congenital heart problems may arise.
- Capillary function is immature in newborns. It takes several weeks for the small capillaries to expand and contract in response to external temperatures.
- The heart rate is higher in newborns and infants than in adults.
- Children have limited ability to increase stroke volume in response to decreased cardiac output.
- Most heart conditions in children result from defects in embryonic structure.

FIGURE 26-1 Summary of some cardiovascular system differences between the child and the adult. The cardiovascular system consists of the heart, blood, and blood vessels. As the heart beats, blood, oxygen, and nutrients are transported to all the tissues of the body, and waste products are removed. (Art overlay courtesy Observatory Group, Cincinnati, Ohio.)

CONGENITAL HEART DEFECTS

Congenital heart defects may be caused by genetic or maternal factors (e.g., drug intake or rubella illness) or environmental factors. Fetal echocardiography can detect cardiac malformations in high-risk cases. Acquired heart disease occurs *after* birth, as a result of a defect or illness.

Pathophysiology. Congenital heart defects are not a problem for the fetus because the fetal–maternal circulation compensates for all fetal oxygen needs. At birth, however, the infant's circulatory system must take over and provide for the child's own oxygen needs. Any heart defect or patent (open) fetal pathways in the cardiovascular system after birth produce signs and symptoms that indicate an anatomical heart defect. Congenital heart disease occurs in approximately 8 of 1000 births, and 50% of these infants evidence signs and symptoms before the first year of life. Some defects, such as mitral valve prolapse, may not be manifested until later in life.

Of the congenital anomalies, heart defects are the principal cause of death during the first year of life. Therefore nurses must stress the need for good prenatal care and impress on parents the value of regular checkups at well-baby clinics. Many organic heart murmurs have been detected early in infancy at periodic checkups.

Diagnosis and Treatment. The appearance of clinical symptoms and the results of diagnostic tests aid in the diagnosis of congenital heart disease (Table 26-1). The treatment of most cardiac defects is surgical. A **thoracotomy** (chest incision) is performed, and the use

of a cardiopulmonary bypass machine and hypothermia during the procedure minimize blood loss and enhance patient response. **Hypothermia** (*hypo,* "under," and *thermal,* "heat") reduces the temperature of body tissues, resulting in a decreased need for oxygen. The cardiopulmonary bypass machine provides oxygenation of the body tissues while the surgeon stops the heart to perform surgery. Heart transplants may be the treatment of choice in cases such as a three-chambered heart. Interventional cardiac catheterization can correct some heart defects without open heart surgery.

Classification. Congenital heart defects can be divided into two categories: cyanotic and acyanotic. A more accurate classification is based on the effect of the defect on blood circulation. The study of blood circulation is termed **hemodynamics** (*hemo,* "blood," and *dynamics,* "power"). Blood always flows from an area of high pressure to an area of low pressure and takes the path of least resistance. Physiologically, defects can be organized into (1) lesions that increase pulmonary blood flow, (2) lesions that restrict blood flow, and (3) lesions that decrease pulmonary blood flow. There are also lesions that result in mixed oxygenated and non-oxygenated blood. A **shunt** refers to the flow of blood through an abnormal opening between two vessels of the heart. Figure 26-2 compares the normal heart and the heart with various congenital defects.

Defects That Increase Pulmonary Blood Flow

Congenital heart defects that cause the blood to return to the right ventricle and recirculate through the lungs before exiting the left ventricle through the aorta are known as defects that increase pulmonary blood flow.

Table 26-1   Diagnostic Tests Used in Congenital Heart Defects

TEST	DEFINITION	VALUE
Angiocardiography (selective)	Serial x-ray films of the heart and great vessels after injection of an opaque substance; a radiopaque catheter is moved into the heart chambers, and contrast medium is injected in specific areas	Abnormal communications in the heart can be observed; the course of the blood through the heart and great vessels can be traced
Aortography	X-ray films of the aorta after the injection of an opaque material	Useful in showing patent ductus arteriosus
Radionuclide angiocardiography	Noninvasive nuclear procedure that permits visualization of the course of blood through the heart	May be used as a precardiac catheterization screening study; provides assessment of congenital and acquired cardiovascular lesions and monitors the effects of therapy; an intravenous (IV) device is necessary to permit injection of the radionuclide
Barium swallow	Barium given by mouth	Shows indentation of the esophagus by the aorta or other vessels
Cardiac catheterization	A radiopaque catheter is passed through the femoral artery directly into the heart and large vessels	Shows blood pressure within the heart; physician can examine the heart closely with the tip of the catheter to detect abnormalities; blood samples can be obtained to determine oxygen content
Chest x-ray film	A radiographic image of a body structure	Provides a permanent record; shows abnormalities in the shape and position of heart
Cineangiocardiography	Motion pictures of images recorded by fluoroscopy	Useful recording and monitoring device
Echocardiography	The use of ultrasound to produce an image of sound waves of the heart; transducer placed directly on chest; sounds are analyzed	Noninvasive procedure; localizes murmurs; determines if heart is structurally normal
Electrocardiogram	Tracing of heart action by electrocardiography	Detects variations in heart action and shows the condition of the heart muscle; may also be used as a monitoring device during cardiac catheterization
Magnetic resonance imaging (three-dimensional [3-D] imaging)	Noninvasive imaging technique that uses low-energy radio waves in combination with a magnetic field to generate signals that produce tomographic images	Very useful in diagnosing coarctation of the aorta

For example, the defect in the atrial septum in the fetus allows blood to flow from the right atrium through the defect into the left atrium, providing a bypass of the lungs. After birth, the pressure is higher in the left atrium; if the atrial opening persists, the blood flows back into the right atrium (*left-to-right shunt*) and then recirculates to the lungs, causing *increased pulmonary flow*. Some defects that increase pulmonary flow are atrial septal defect, ventricular septal defect, and patent ductus arteriosus (see Figure 26-2). In heart defects that result in increased pulmonary flow because of a left-to-right shunt, the oxygenated blood recirculates to the lungs, and cyanosis is rare.

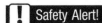 **Safety Alert!**

In congenital heart disease, cyanosis is *not always* a clinical sign.

Atrial Septal Defect. Atrial septal defect (ASD) involves an abnormal opening between the right and left atria. Blood that already contains oxygen is forced from the left atrium back to the right atrium. Most patients do not have symptoms. The defect may be recognized when a murmur is heard during a routine health examination. Cardiac catheterization, electrocardiogram, and echocardiography may be performed to help to confirm the diagnosis. The surgical repair involves application of a surgical Dacron patch or repair with open cardiac surgery or robotic surgery using a portion of the pericardium to secure a patch. Nonsurgical closure during cardiac catheterization can sometimes be accomplished. Continued cardiology follow-up is necessary. Low-dose aspirin therapy is usually prescribed for 6 months after repair. Prognosis is excellent.

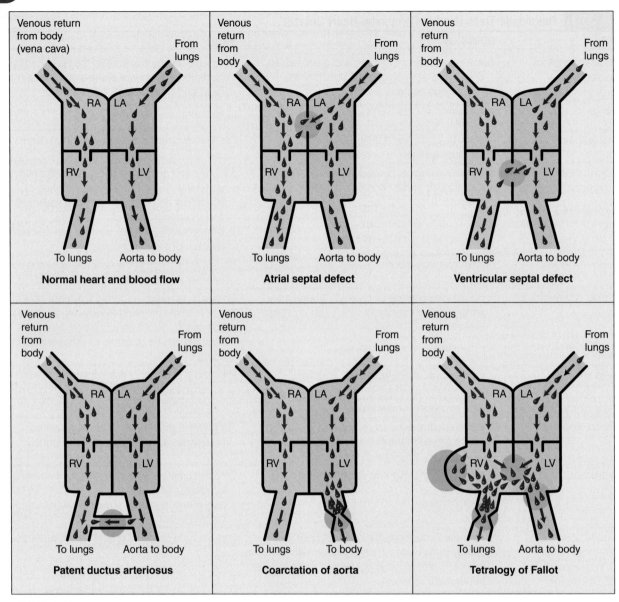

FIGURE 26-2 The normal heart and various congenital heart defects. *LA*, Left atrium; *LV*, left ventricle; *RA*, right atrium; *RV*, right ventricle.

Ventricular Septal Defect. Ventricular septal defect (VSD) is the most common heart anomaly. As the name suggests, there is an opening between the right and left ventricles of the heart. Increased pressure within the left ventricle forces blood back into the right ventricle (left-to-right shunt). A loud, harsh murmur combined with a systolic thrill is characteristic of this defect. The condition may be mild or severe. It is often associated with other defects. Many children with small defects may experience spontaneous closure during the first year of life as a result of growth. Small defects may be closed during cardiac catheterization (Kliegman, 2011).

Early surgical intervention has a low risk for most infants, and the prognosis is excellent. Normal growth and development are usually achieved within 1 or 2 years after surgery.

Open heart surgery is performed under hypothermia. With the use of the heart-lung bypass machine the condition can be corrected in a fairly dry or bloodless field. The hole is ligated (closed) with sutures or a synthetic patch.

Patent Ductus Arteriosus. The circulation of the fetus differs from that of the newborn in that most of the fetal blood bypasses the lungs. The ductus arteriosus is the passageway (shunt) through which the blood crosses from the pulmonary artery to the aorta and avoids the deflated lungs. This vessel closes shortly after birth; when it does not close, blood continues to pass from the aorta, where the pressure is higher, into the pulmonary artery. This causes oxygenated blood to recycle through the lungs, overburdening the pulmonary circulation and making the heart pump harder.

The symptoms of patent ductus arteriosus (PDA) may go unnoticed during infancy. As the child grows, dyspnea is experienced, the radial pulse becomes full and bounding on exertion, and there is an unusually wide range between systolic and diastolic blood pressures. This is referred to as the **pulse pressure**. A characteristic machinery type of murmur may be heard. A two-dimensional echocardiogram is useful in visualizing and determining blood flow across the PDA.

PDA is one of the more common cardiac anomalies. It occurs twice as frequently in girls as in boys. Premature infants with hypoxia often respond to indomethacin drug therapy that results in closure of the PDA. Heart surgery is performed on all full-term newborns diagnosed with PDA to prevent congestive heart failure (CHF), embolus formation, and other complications. The ductus may be ligated via thoracotomy (incision into the chest) or via the visually assisted thoracoscopic surgery (VATS) technique that eliminates the need for a large chest incision. Nonsurgical options include the insertion of coils to occlude the PDA, which is done in a cardiac catheterization lab. Prostaglandin E_1 may be administered to maintain patency of the ductus arteriosus until surgery can be performed when an anomaly such as hypoplastic heart is diagnosed in the newborn. The prognosis is excellent.

Defects That Restrict Ventricular Blood Flow

Some congenital cardiac defects can restrict blood flow from the ventricles because of a **stenosis** (narrowing) of a vessel.

Coarctation of the Aorta. The word *coarctation* means "a tightening." In coarctation of the aorta, there is a constriction or narrowing of the aortic arch or of the descending aorta (i.e., the blood meets an obstruction) (see Figure 26-2). Hemodynamics consist of increased pressure proximal to the defect and decreased pressure distally. The characteristic symptoms are a marked difference in the blood pressure and pulses of the upper and lower extremities. The patient may not develop symptoms until late in childhood. X-ray examination may show cardiac enlargement and "notching" of the ribs caused by vessels developed as collateral circulation. Pulses and blood pressure will differ in the upper and lower extremities. Two-dimensional echocardiography can aid in the diagnosis. If the condition is untreated, hypertension, CHF, and infective endocarditis may develop. Treatment depends on the type and severity of the defect. Infants who have associated CHF are treated medically until the optimal time for surgery.

Percutaneous balloon angioplasty is the treatment of choice for older children, and stents can be inserted to maintain patency. The surgeon resects the narrowed portion of the aorta and joins its ends. The joining is called an anastomosis. If the section removed is large, an end-to-end graft using tubes of synthetic polyester (Dacron) or similar material may be necessary. Some children complain of leg pain after exercise. As in PDA, closed heart surgery is performed because the structures are outside the heart. The prognosis is good if there are no other defects and the child's physical condition is favorable at the time of surgery. If restenosis occurs after surgery for coarctation, a balloon angioplasty can relieve the obstruction. The nurse should observe the child after coarctation surgery for the development of hypertension and abdominal pain associated with nausea and vomiting, leukocytosis, and gastrointestinal bleeding or obstruction. Antihypertensive drugs, steroids, and nasogastric tube decompression are the priority treatments for these postsurgical complications.

ⓘ Safety Alert!

A significant difference in the blood pressure between the upper extremities and the lower extremities is a characteristic sign of coarctation of the aorta.

Defects That Decrease Pulmonary Blood Flow

A **decrease** in pulmonary blood flow occurs when a congenital heart anomaly allows blood that has not passed through the lungs (unoxygenated blood) to enter the aorta and the general circulation. Cyanosis caused by the presence of unoxygenated blood in the circulation is a characteristic feature of this type of congenital heart anomaly.

Tetralogy of Fallot. *Tetra* means "four." In *tetralogy of Fallot* there are four defects:
1. Stenosis or narrowing of the pulmonary artery, which decreases the blood flow to the lungs
2. Hypertrophy of the right ventricle, which enlarges because it must work harder to pump blood through the narrow pulmonary artery
3. Dextroposition (*dextro*, "right," and *position*) of the aorta, in which the aorta is displaced to the right and blood from both ventricles enters it
4. VSD (see Figure 26-2)

When venous blood enters the aorta, the infant displays symptoms of cardiac problems. Cyanosis increases with age, and clubbing of the fingers and toes is seen (see Figure 25-10). The child rests in a "squatting" position to breathe more easily. This position alters systemic venous return. Feeding problems, growth retardation, frequent respiratory infections, and severe dyspnea on exertion are prevalent. The red blood cells (RBCs) of the body increase, causing **polycythemia** (*poly*, "many," *cyt*, "cells," and *hema*, "blood") to compensate for the lack of oxygen.

Narrowing of the pulmonary artery causes CHF as a result of the increased muscular force necessary to propel blood through the narrowed orifice. When unoxygenated blood enters the general circulation, *hypoxia* occurs and may be manifested by cyanosis.

The increased oxygen consumption and decreased energy and ability to eat, result in failure to thrive. Multiple hospitalizations, cyanotic skin, and limited energy can impede growth and development both physically and socially.

Paroxysmal hypercyanotic episodes, or **"tet" spells**, occur during the first 2 years of life. Spontaneous cyanosis, respiratory distress, weakness, and syncope occur. They can last a few minutes to a few hours and are followed by lethargy and sleep. Parents and day care personnel must be instructed to place the child in a knee-chest position when a tet spell occurs (Figure 26-3). Often the child will pause and voluntarily squat in position until the attack abates. Recovery from the tet spell is usually rapid.

Diagnosis of tetralogy of Fallot is confirmed by a chest x-ray study that shows a typical boot-shaped heart. An electrocardiogram, three-dimensional echocardiography, and cardiac catheterization aid in confirming the diagnosis.

Complications such as cerebral thrombosis caused by polycythemia (thickened blood as a result of increased RBCs) are a problem, especially if dehydration occurs. Iron deficiency anemia develops because of decreased appetite and increased energy required to suck or eat. Bacterial endocarditis can occur and is prevented with prophylactic antibiotic therapy.

Treatment is designed to increase pulmonary blood flow to relieve hypoxia. A Blalock-Taussig surgical procedure (temporary shunt) can be performed successfully on newborns or premature infants. Open heart surgery using cardiopulmonary bypass provides total correction of all defects and is usually performed, with excellent results, on the older, stable child. The nurse should be observant for signs of congestive heart failure and an irregular heartbeat postoperatively.

> **Nursing Tip**
>
> There are four defects in tetralogy of Fallot:
> 1. Pulmonary artery stenosis
> 2. Hypertrophy of the right ventricle
> 3. Dextroposition of aorta
> 4. VSD

Defects That Cause Mixed Pathology

Hypoplastic Left Heart Syndrome. In hypoplastic left heart syndrome there is an underdevelopment of the left side of the heart, usually resulting in an absent or nonfunctional left ventricle and hypoplasia of the ascending aorta. This condition can be diagnosed before birth and the infant placed on a transplant list early so surgery can be performed soon after birth. The initial survival of the infant depends on a patent foramen ovale and ductus arteriosus to provide a pathway for oxygenated blood to the general body system. Prostaglandin E_1 may be administered to maintain patency of the ductus arteriosus. Other serious congenital anomalies may be present, and the infant should be carefully assessed.

Symptoms include a grayish blue color of the skin and mucous membranes and signs of CHF, including dyspnea, weak pulses, and a cardiac murmur. Survival beyond the first few months of life without intervention is rare. A multistage shunting procedure can be done as a temporary holding measure until a new heart is available. With the advent of successful heart transplants, however, the prognosis for these infants is much brighter, and emphasis is placed on maintaining life and hope until an appropriate heart is available for transplant. After a transplant, immunosuppressive therapy to prevent organ rejection is required.

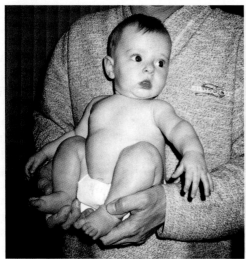
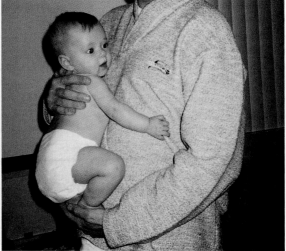

FIGURE 26-3 Tet position. Infants and children with tetralogy of Fallot can have paroxysmal hypercyanosis or "tet" spells. Placing the child in the tet position (a knee-chest position) will relieve these symptoms. Older children will spontaneously squat when a tet spell occurs.

General Treatment and Nursing Care of Children with Congenital Heart Defects

Recent technological advances have enabled therapeutic catheterization procedures for valvuloplasty, angioplasty, and other corrections of pediatric heart pathologies as alternatives to open heart surgery. After the procedure the nursing care involves monitoring vital signs, observing for thrombosis formation, and performing neurovascular checks of the limb (see Figure 24-9), including pedal pulses. Emotional support of the family and education concerning what to do and expect during and after therapy is a nursing responsibility. In most cases, hospitalization after cardiac catheterization is limited to 2 or 3 days. Parents must be guided to understand that the child should not be overprotected or restricted from normal activities related to optimum growth and development. Fear and anxiety can be transferred from the parents to the child. Education concerning general health, hygiene, dental care, balanced diet, and routine immunizations should be emphasized. Immunizations after cardiac transplantation must be placed on hold.

Immunizations are not recommended before cardiac surgery, because immune-suppressants are used to prevent rejection of the transplanted heart, and the child's ability to manufacture antibodies in response to routine immunizations will be impaired. Dental health care in children with heart disease is important to prevent bacteremia, which can cause bacterial endocarditis. Antibiotics are usually required before dental care. Competitive sports are avoided for children with congenital heart disease, because the pressure for a team win can interfere with the child's need to stop activity if specific symptoms arise. Some children benefit from being transported to school so that energy can be consumed *during* school activities rather than by walking to and from school.

Nutritional guidance is aimed at preventing anemia and promoting optimal growth and development. Parents should be instructed in the techniques of preventing dehydration in children with polycythemia. Family trips or vacations during the hot summer months require attention to the child's fluid needs to replace fluid lost from sweating. Vacations to high altitudes or very cold environments may cause adverse responses in a child who is already hypoxic or who has cardiac problems.

Cardiac surgery—if needed to repair a defect that causes heart failure—is generally performed at a regional medical center where the necessary costly equipment is available. Chest tubes may be used postoperatively to remove secretions and air from the pleural cavity and to allow reexpansion of the lungs. These are attached to underwater-seal drainage systems or to a commercially manufactured disposable system such as Pleur-evac. Units for infants and older children are available. This system must be *airtight* to prevent collapse of the lung. Drainage systems are always kept below the level of the chest to prevent the backflow of secretions. This is especially important during transportation. **Two padded Kelly clamps must be available at all times** for emergency clamping of tubes. These are applied to the tubes as close as possible to the child's chest if a break in the system occurs.

Cardiac transplants are a treatment option when other treatments fail. The 1-year survival rate is 80% and the 5-year survival rate is 68% (Conway, 2010). Infection, hyperlipidemia, and rejection of the new tissue are some causes of deaths.

Postoperative cardiac care usually takes place in an intensive care unit (ICU), where high-technology monitoring minimizes complications. The licensed vocational nurse will have contact with the child who is returning for postoperative checkups or is on a home care program after discharge. Providing routine supportive care, encouraging appropriate medical follow-up, and designing activities that promote optimal growth and development are primary goals of care.

> **⚠ Medication Safety Alert!**
>
> CAM therapy with ginkgo, ginseng, and St. John's Wort may interact with drugs used for congenital heart disease and should not be used (Holcomb, 2009).

ACQUIRED HEART DISEASES

Acquired heart disease is a cardiac problem that occurs *after* birth. It may be a complication of a congenital heart disease or a response to respiratory infection, sepsis, hypertension, or severe anemia. *Heart failure* is defined as cardiac output inadequate to meet the metabolic needs of the body.

Congestive Heart Failure

Manifestations. Manifestations of congestive heart failure (CHF) depend on the side of the heart affected. The *right side* of the heart moves unoxygenated blood to the pulmonary circulation. A failure results in the backup of blood in the systemic venous system. The *left side* of the heart moves oxygenated blood from the pulmonary circulation to the systemic circulation. A failure results in backup into the lung. When the body tries to compensate for the problems, peripheral vasoconstriction occurs and results in cold and/or blue hands and feet, tachycardia, and tachypnea. Although heart failure may start as a right- or left-sided failure, eventually *both* sides become involved.

Signs and symptoms may differ somewhat and are more subtle in infants. Some of these signs are cyanosis, pallor, rapid respiration, rapid pulse, feeding difficulties, fatigue, a weak cry, excessive perspiration (especially on the forehead), failure to gain weight, edema, and frequent respiratory infections.

Safety Alert!

Early signs of CHF in infants that should be reported:
- Tachycardia at rest
- Fatigue during feeding
- Sweating around scalp and forehead
- Dyspnea
- Sudden weight gain

Cyanosis. When observing color, the nurse notes whether the cyanosis is general or localized. If it is localized, the exact location is recorded in the nurse's notes, for example, hands, feet, lips, or around the mouth. Is the cyanosis deep or light? Is it constant or transient? Sometimes color improves during crying, and sometimes it gets worse; this is significant. If overt cyanosis is not apparent in the African American infant, the palms of the hands and bottoms of the feet are observed. Clubbing of the fingers and toes (see Figure 25-10) may be evident as a result of blood pooling in the capillaries of the extremities in children with chronic hypoxia. The skin may be very pale or mottled. Sweating, particularly of the head, may be seen.

Rapid respiration. Rapid respiration is called *tachypnea*. A rate of more than 60 breaths/min in a newborn at rest indicates distress. The amount of dyspnea, or shortness of breath, varies. In more acute cases, dyspnea is accompanied by flaring of the nostrils, mouth breathing, grunting, and sternal retractions. The infant has more trouble breathing when flat in bed than when held upright. Air hunger is evidenced if the child is irritable and restless. The cry is weak and hoarse.

Rapid pulse. A rapid pulse is termed **tachycardia**. An increase in pulse rate is one of the first signs of CHF. The heart is pumping harder in an effort to increase its output and to provide sufficient oxygen to all the tissues of the body. Cardiac output can be increased by one of two mechanisms: tachycardia or increased **stroke volume**. Stroke volume is the amount of blood ejected during one contraction. Because infants and small children have a limited ability to increase stroke volume, their heart rate must increase to meet the demand.

Feeding difficulties. When the nurse feeds these infants, they tire easily and may stop sucking after a few ounces. When placed in the crib, they cry and appear hungry. They may choke and gag during feedings; the pleasure of sucking is spoiled by their inability to breathe.

Poor weight gain. The child fails to gain weight. A sudden increase in weight may indicate edema and the beginning of heart failure.

Edema. Blood flow to the kidneys is decreased, and the glomerular filtration rate slows. This causes both fluid and sodium to be retained. The nurse watches for puffiness about the eyes and, occasionally, in the legs, feet, and abdomen. Urine output may decrease.

Frequent respiratory tract infections. Resistance is very low. Slight infections can be highly dangerous because the heart and lungs are already compromised.

Immunizations are reviewed and updated as needed. The nurse prevents exposure to other children who have upper respiratory tract infections and other illnesses.

Treatment and Nursing Care. The nursing goals significant to the care of children with heart failure are the following:
- Reduce the work of the heart
- Improve respiration
- Maintain proper nutrition
- Prevent infection
- Reduce the anxiety of the patient
- Support and instruct the parents

The nurse must organize care so that the infant is not unnecessarily disturbed. A complete bath and linen change for an infant with a serious heart defect may not be a priority. The infant is fed early if crying and late if asleep. The physician orders the position in which the infant is placed. In some cases the knee-chest position facilitates breathing; in other cases, a position with the head elevated (Fowler's position) may be helpful. Older infants may be placed in infant seats.

Feedings are small and frequent. A soft nipple with holes large enough to prevent the infant from tiring is provided. Often, formulas with increased caloric density are used. In some cases, nasogastric tube feedings are advantageous because they are less tiring for the child. Oxygen is administered to relieve dyspnea. As breathing becomes easier, the infant begins to relax. A soft voice and gentle care are soothing. Whenever possible, the infant is held and comforted during feedings.

Digitoxin and digoxin (Lanoxin) are common oral digitalis preparations. In pediatric patients, Lanoxin is preferred because of its rapid action and shorter half-life. These agents slow and strengthen the heartbeat. The nurse counts the patient's pulse for 1 full minute before administering them. A resting apical pulse is most accurate. As a rule, if the pulse rate of an infant or child is below 100 beats/min the medication is withheld and the physician is notified. In older children the pulse rate should be more than 70 beats/min. Because the pulse rate varies with the age of the child, it is ideal for the physician to specify in the written drug order at what heart rate the nurse should withhold the drug. When this is not done, the nurse obtains clarification. The physician is notified when the drug is withheld.

The physician is contacted if the patient vomits. Digitalis administration is not repeated until the physician confirms that it is safe to do so. Tachycardia and irregularities in the rhythm of the pulse are significant and should be reported. Symptoms of toxicity include nausea, vomiting, anorexia, irregularity in rate and rhythm of the pulse, and a sudden change in pulse. If the infant is discharged while still receiving medication, the parents are taught how to take the pulse and what signs to be alert for when administering the drug.

A group of drugs called angiotensin converting enzyme inhibitors (ACE-Is) may be prescribed. Captopril, enalapril, and lisinopril are examples of these drugs. The nurse should observe for signs of hypotension, cough, renal dysfunction, and hyperkalemia. Serum potassium should be carefully monitored.

> **! Medication Safety Alert!**
>
> Two nurses should check dosage of drugs such as digoxin. A single dose larger than 0.05 mg, or 50 mcg, should be reconfirmed with the health care provider.

Diuretics such as furosemide (Lasix) or chlorothiazide (Diuril) are useful in reducing edema. Careful monitoring of serum electrolyte levels prevents electrolyte imbalance, particularly potassium depletion. Parents of older patients are taught to recognize foods high in potassium, such as bananas, oranges, milk, potatoes, and prune juice. Diapers are weighed to determine urine output. Daily weighing of the infant also helps the physician to determine the effectiveness of the diuresis.

An accurate record of intake and output is essential. Signs of dehydration such as thirst, fever, poor skin turgor, apathy, sunken eyes or fontanelle, dry skin, dry tongue, dry mucous membranes, and decreased urination should be brought to the immediate attention of the nurse in charge. Pneumonia can occur rapidly. Fever, irritability, and an increase in respiratory distress may indicate this condition. The child's position is changed regularly to help prevent hypostatic pneumonia.

The nurse working in a cardiac unit assesses the child frequently for complications of cardiac and respiratory failure and should be competent in cardiopulmonary resuscitation techniques and the necessary modifications required for pediatric patients (Pediatric Advanced Life Support [PALS] certification).

The parents of the child need support and understanding throughout a long period. Because the heart is the body's major vital organ, this type of diagnosis causes much apprehension. The physician must reassure the parents without minimizing the danger involved.

The patterns formed during infancy can build the framework of a healthy personality for the patient. Children who have heart conditions but who are well integrated into family life have a decided advantage over children who are made to think they are invalids. Routine naps and early bedtimes provide adequate rest for most children.

As children grow, they usually set their own limits on the amount of activity they can handle. Prompt treatment of infections is important. A suitable diet with adequate fluids is necessary. Eating iron-rich foods is encouraged. Dental care should be regular. All-day attendance in school may be too tiring for the child; therefore special arrangements may be necessary. The child needs careful evaluation before any type of minor surgery is performed.

Detailed discharge planning and coordination of community services are of value to the family.

Rheumatic Fever

Pathophysiology. **Rheumatic fever (RF)** is a systemic disease involving the joints, heart, central nervous system (CNS), skin, and subcutaneous tissues. It belongs to a group of disorders known as *collagen diseases.* Their common feature is the destruction of connective tissue. RF is particularly detrimental to the heart, causing scarring of the mitral valves. Its peak incidence is between 5 and 15 years of age. RF is common worldwide in lower-income groups and where overcrowded conditions exist. It is more prevalent during winter and spring, and carrier rates among school-age children are believed to be higher during these seasons. Genetic factors have implicated an abnormal immune response.

RF is an autoimmune disease that occurs as a complication of untreated group A beta-hemolytic streptococcus infection of the throat. The disease almost disappeared during the 1960s and 1970s; since the late 1980s, however, a resurgence has occurred in the United States. This has highlighted the need for more aggressive diagnosis and treatment of streptococcal pharyngitis.

Manifestations. Symptoms of RF range from mild to severe and may not occur for 1 to 6 weeks after a strep throat infection (Figure 26-4). The classic symptoms are *migratory polyarthritis* (wandering joint pains), skin eruptions, chorea (a nervous disorder), and inflammation of the heart. Subcutaneous nodules may appear

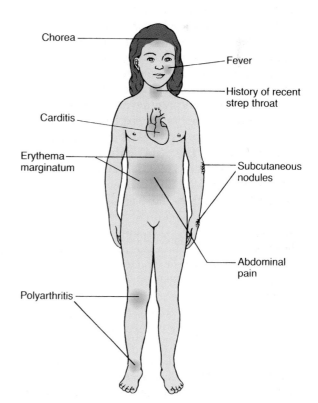

FIGURE 26-4 Manifestations of rheumatic fever.

beneath the skin but are less common in children. Abdominal pain, often mistaken for appendicitis, sometimes occurs. Fever varies from slight to very high. Pallor, fatigue, anorexia, and unexplained nosebleeds may be seen. An elevated antistreptolysin O titer (ASO) is a standard diagnostic test for RF. Rheumatic fever tends to *recur*, and each attack carries the threat of further damage to the heart. The recurrences are most frequent during the first 5 years after the initial attack, and they decline rapidly thereafter.

Migratory polyarthritis. The **polyarthritis** (*poly*, "many," *arthr*, "joint," and *itis*, "inflammation of") seen in RF is distinctive in that it does not result in permanent deformity to the joint. It involves mainly the larger joints: knees, elbows, ankles, wrists, and shoulders. The joints become painful and tender and are difficult to move. The symptoms last for a few days, disappear without treatment, and frequently return in another joint. This pattern may continue for a few weeks. The symptoms tend to be more severe in older children. The joint may be visibly swollen and inflamed. On diagnosis, salicylates are administered to relieve the pain.

Skin eruptions. *Erythema marginatum*, the rash seen in RF, consists of small red circles with red-colored margins, a pale center, and wavy lines appearing on the trunk and abdomen. They appear and disappear rapidly and are significant in diagnosing the disease.

Sydenham's chorea. **Chorea** is a disorder of the CNS characterized by involuntary, purposeless movements of the muscles. It may occur as an acute rheumatic involvement of the brain. Sydenham's chorea is primarily seen in prepubertal girls.

Attacks of chorea, which begin slowly, may be preceded by increased tension and behavioral problems. The child becomes "clumsy," may stumble and spill things, and may have difficulty buttoning clothes and writing. When the facial muscles are involved, grimaces occur. The child may laugh and cry inappropriately. In severe cases the patient may become completely incapacitated, and deterioration in speech may be noticeable. Treatment of Sydenham's chorea is directed toward the relief of symptoms. The condition usually disappears spontaneously within weeks to months. Medication may also be required. The presence of Sydenham's chorea alone can support the diagnosis of RF.

Rheumatic carditis. **Carditis**, an inflammation of the heart, is a manifestation of RF that can be fatal. It occurs more often in the young child. The tissues that cover the heart and the heart valves are affected. The heart muscle (myocardium) may be involved, as may the pericardium and the endocardium. The *mitral valve*, which is located between the left atrium and the left ventricle, is often involved. Vegetations form, which interfere with the proper closing of the valve and disturb its normal function. When this valve becomes narrowed, the condition is called *mitral stenosis*. Myocardial lesions called *Aschoff's bodies* are also characteristic of the disease. The burden on the heart is great, because it must pump harder to circulate the blood. As a result, it may become enlarged. Symptoms of poor circulation and heart failure may appear.

The child has an irregular, low-grade fever; is pale and listless; and has a poor appetite. Moderate anemia and weight loss are apparent. The child may experience dyspnea on exertion. The pulse and respiration rates are out of proportion to the body temperature. The physician may detect a soft murmur over the apex of the heart.

Diagnosis. The diagnosis of RF is difficult to make, and for this reason the **Jones criteria** have been developed and modified throughout the years (Box 26-1). The presence of two major criteria or one major and two minor criteria supported by evidence of recent streptococcal infection, indicates a high probability of rheumatic fever. A careful physical examination is performed, and a complete history of the patient is obtained. Certain blood tests are helpful. The erythrocyte sedimentation rate (ESR) is elevated. Abnormal proteins, such as C-reactive protein, may also be evident in the blood serum. Leukocytosis may occur but is not regularly present. Antibodies against the streptococci (measured by ASO titer) may also be detected. Additional studies may include chest x-rays, throat culture, and pulmonary function tests. The electrocardiogram, a graphic record of the electrical changes caused by the beating of the heart, is very useful. Changes in conductivity, particularly a prolonged P-R interval (indicating a first-degree heart block), may reflect carditis. These tests are repeated throughout the course of the disease so that the physician may determine when the active stage has subsided.

Box 26-1	Modified Jones Criteria

A positive diagnosis of rheumatic fever cannot be made without the presence of two major criteria, or one major and two minor criteria, plus a history of streptococcal infection.

MAJOR CRITERIA	**MINOR CRITERIA**
Carditis	Fever
Polyarthritis	Arthralgia
Erythema marginatum	Previous history of rheumatic heart disease
Chorea	Elevated erythrocyte sedimentation rate
Subcutaneous nodules	Leukocytosis
	Abnormal electrocardiogram (altered P-R interval)
	Positive test for C-reactive protein

A useful mnemonic for remembering the Jones criteria is:

MAJOR CRITERIA	MINOR CRITERIA
Joint (arthritis)	**P**-R interval
Obvious carditis	**E**SR elevated
Nodules subcutaneous	**A**rthralgia
Erythema marginatum	**C**RP elevated
Sydenham's chorea	**E**levated temperature (fever)

Treatment and Nursing Care. Treatment is aimed at preventing permanent damage to the heart. This is accomplished by antibacterial therapy, physical and mental rest, relief of pain and fever, and management of cardiac failure should it occur. Initial antibacterial therapy is directed toward eliminating the streptococcal infection. Penicillin is the drug of choice (given for a 10-day period) unless the patient is sensitive to it, in which case erythromycin is substituted.

Elimination of infection through medication is followed by long-term *chemoprophylaxis* (prevention of disease by drugs); intramuscular benzathine penicillin G is administered monthly to children with a history of RF or evidence of rheumatic heart disease for a minimum of a 5-year period or until an age of 18 years is attained. Oral administration is considered for patients with minimal involvement whose reliability about taking medications can be confirmed. Erythromycin is recommended for long-term therapy for children who cannot tolerate penicillin. Financial assistance may be available to patients and their families. Local heart associations, rehabilitation services, and state and municipal health departments are sources of such aid.

Antiinflammatory drugs are used to decrease fever and pain. Aspirin is the drug of choice for joint disease without evidence of carditis. The use of steroids is reserved for severe cardiac symptoms or when aspirin does not relieve cardiac pain. Concerns during therapy include aspirin toxicity and the effects of aspirin on blood clotting. Mild signs of Cushing's disease, such as moon face, acne, and hirsutism (increased hairiness), should be anticipated with the use of steroids. More severe reactions such as gastric ulcer, hypertension, overwhelming infection, and toxic psychosis may occur. Phenobarbital is effective in reducing chorea. Padded side rails are used to protect the patient who experiences spasms. If CHF occurs, symptomatic treatment is provided.

Bed rest during the initial attack is recommended until the ESR returns to normal levels. The amount of work the heart must do must be limited by resting the entire body. In this way the circulation of the heart is slower, and the heart does not need to work as fast or as hard as when a child is active. The nurse should teach parents and children about the need for rest and the types of play activity appropriate during home care.

Nursing activities should be organized to ensure as few interruptions as possible to prevent tiring the patient. A bed cradle can be used to prevent pressure on painful extremities. Care includes special attention to the skin, especially over bony prominences; back care; good oral hygiene; and small, frequent feedings of nourishing foods. Maintaining healthy teeth and preventing cavities is of special importance. The pa tient with RF is particularly susceptible to *subacute bacterial endocarditis,* which can occur as a complication of dental or other procedures likely to cause bleeding or infection. Prophylactic antibiotic treatment is required before any dental procedure. Nutrition consists of small servings from the basic food groups. These are increased as the child's appetite improves. A record of fluid intake and output is kept, because overhydration may tax the heart. All efforts are made to provide emotional support for the child and family. Provision should be made for the child to continue school studies.

Prevention. Prevention of infection and prompt treatment of group A beta-hemolytic streptococcal infections can prevent the occurrence of RF. All throat infections should be cultured. After a diagnosis of strep throat is established, the nurse stresses the need to complete antibiotic therapy even if symptoms disappear and the child "feels better." Close medical supervision and follow-up care are essential. The prognosis is favorable.

The nurse should teach parents about the need for prophylactic antibiotic therapy before any dental procedure.

Systemic Hypertension

Pathophysiology. Hypertension, or high blood pressure, is being seen more often during childhood and adolescence. Blood pressure is a product of peripheral vascular resistance and cardiac output. An increase in cardiac output or peripheral resistance results in an increase in blood pressure. Systemic blood pressure increases with age and is correlated with height and weight throughout childhood and adolescence. (See Appendixes H and I for blood pressure measurements in infants and children.) Significant hypertension is considered when measurements are persistently at or above the 95th percentile for the patient's age and sex (Gill, 2012). Hypertension is referred to as secondary when a disease process can explain the increased pressure. Renal, congenital, vascular, and endocrine disorders represent the majority of illnesses that account for secondary hypertension. Primary, or essential, hypertension implies that no known underlying disease is present. Nevertheless, heredity, obesity, stress, and a poor diet and exercise pattern can contribute to any type of hypertension.

There is increasing evidence that essential hypertension, although not generally seen until adolescence or adulthood, may have its roots in childhood. Prevention is thus significant in reducing the incidence of stroke or myocardial infarction as a person ages. The assessment of blood pressure levels should be part of every physical examination during childhood. Hypertension is more prevalent in children whose parents have high blood pressure. High blood pressure in children is usually discovered during a routine physical examination. Measuring blood pressure in young children requires careful attention to cuff size (see Chapter 22).

> **Nursing Tip**
>
> The blood pressure cuff should encircle two thirds of the length of the upper arm for an accurate blood pressure assessment.

Treatment and Nursing Care. Treatment and nursing care involve nutritional counseling, weight reduction, and an age-appropriate program of aerobic exercise. Adolescents should be counseled concerning the adverse effects of drugs, alcohol, and tobacco on blood pressure. Drug therapy to reduce high blood pressure may not be effective in adolescents, who often are noncompliant with long-term regimens. The focus of treatment for secondary hypertension is the underlying disease causing the high blood pressure.

Prevention. The main focus of a hypertensive prevention program is patient education. The nurse can work with school personnel to promote awareness of the problem at parent–teacher association (PTA) meetings. Community health fairs should offer opportunities for blood pressure screening. Blood pressure measurement must be part of every routine physical examination. Risk factors such as obesity, elevated serum cholesterol levels, sedentary lifestyle, and drug, alcohol, or tobacco use should be discussed.

> **Health Promotion**
>
> **Nonpharmacological Methods for Preventing and Treating High Blood Pressure**
>
> - Aerobic exercise
> - Reduction of sedentary activities such as computer, TV, and video games
> - Weight reduction
> - Dietary management with fresh vegetables and low-fat foods
> - Adequate intake of potassium and calcium
> - Avoidance of smoking and those who smoke

Hyperlipidemia

Hyperlipidemia refers to excessive lipids (fat and fatlike substances) in the blood. Lipoproteins contain lipids and proteins and include the following:

- *Low-density lipoproteins (LDL),* which contain a low amount of triglycerides, high level of cholesterol, and some protein. LDL carries cholesterol to the cells, which aids in cellular metabolism and steroid production.
- *High-density lipoproteins (HDL)* contain low amounts of triglycerides, little cholesterol, and high levels of protein. HDL carries cholesterol to the liver for excretion.

Children with a parental history of cholesterol levels exceeding 240 mg/dL or a family history of early cardiac death (less than 55 years of age) should have their cholesterol levels tested because genetics can play a role in hypercholesterolemia (Gidding, 2012a). However, screening only those children who are identified as high risk may not identify all children who need follow-up care. Because there is evidence that the factors responsible for degenerative vascular disease may begin in childhood and may be somewhat controllable, considerable interest has developed in screening children for risk factors and in attempting to change these risks (Table 26-2).

According to the 2011 National Heart, Lung and Blood Institute (NHLBI), statins are not the treatment choice for children with increased lipids associated with obesity and a sedentary lifestyle (Gidding, 2012a). The guidelines endorsed by the National Lipid Association (NLA) and American Academy of Pediatrics (AAP) recommend universal screening for cholesterol in children 9 to 11 years of age to identify the genetic form of inherited familial hypercholesterolemia. Lipid screening of younger children may be recommended if there is an established diagnosis of diabetes mellitus, hypertension, tobacco use, obesity, or a positive family history. A borderline blood lipid level should be interpreted as a signal for family education and lifestyle change rather than a need for treatment (Gidding, 2012b). For elevated cholesterol, a fat intake reduction of 25% to 35% of total calories with less than 7% saturated fat and less than 200 mg cholesterol per day is advised. Most children with high triglycerides are obese and therefore reduction of calories, increase of fiber, and regular exercise should be stressed in their education. Drug therapy is only for children between 8 to 10 years of age with very high risk factors (Gidding, 2012b). There are 6 statin

Table 26-2	Average Lipid Profile Levels in Childhood			
	CHOLESTEROL (mg/dL)	**TRIGLYCERIDES (mg/dL)**	**LDL (mg/dL)**	**HDL (mg/dL)**
Newborn	68	35	29	35
1-9 years	155-165	55-65	93-100	53-56
10-14 years	160	62-72	97	52-55
15-19 years	150-160	73-78	94-96	46-52

drugs approved for children: Lovastatin, pravastatin, atorvastatin, simvastatin, fluvastatin, and rosuvastatin. Regular follow-up of liver function tests and lipid levels is important. If liver enzymes are 3 times normal, statin therapy should be discontinued (Gidding, 2012b).

An active prevention program for all children and adolescents is essential. Lifelong healthy eating habits should be nurtured early and practiced by the entire family. The Step I dietary program advocated by the National Cholesterol Education Program embraces the aforementioned guidelines. Children less than 2 years of age should not have a fat-restricted diet, because calories and fats are necessary for CNS growth and development. The American Academy of Pediatrics (AAP) recommendations for heart-healthy guidelines are presented in the Health Promotion box.

 Health Promotion

Heart-Healthy Guidelines for Children

INFANTS

Provide breast milk or formula for 1 year.
Provide rice or other single-grain cereal for 4 to 6 months.
Provide a balanced mixture of cereal, vegetables, fruits, and meats for the second 6 months of life.
Baby foods are labeled regarding calories and nutrient composition; avoid foods with added sugar or salt. Most baby foods, with the exception of combined foods and desserts, do not have these additives.
Infants do not need desserts to grow; infant fruits are more nutritious.
Fats do not have to be restricted in healthy infants.

TODDLERS AND PRESCHOOLERS

Avoid excessive fats, salt, and refined sugars.
Avoid salty snacks and sweet desserts.
Offer heart-healthy snacks of vegetables, fruits, and finger foods.
Offer a variety of foods from the basic food groups.
Discourage the consumption of large amounts of milk, which can lead to nutritional imbalances.

SCHOOL-AGE CHILDREN

Provide heart-healthy school lunches. Limit juice intake.
Role-model good daily exercise.
Screen children with family history of congenital heart disease (cholesterol, triglycerides, blood pressure).
Avoid obesity. Use recommended portion sizes.
Discourage smoking.

ADOLESCENTS

Emphasize the importance of heart-healthy foods to improve endurance and good body image.
Avoid a sedentary lifestyle.
Discourage the excessive intake of dietary saturated fat, sodium, sugar, and excess calories.
Be a nonsmoking parent as a model for the adolescent.
Assess stress management capabilities; counsel accordingly.
Screen periodically for serum cholesterol elevations and blood pressure measurements.
Provide serial monitoring of adolescents deemed to be at high risk (sustained high blood pressure readings on at least three separate occasions).

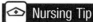 **Nursing Tip**

Contact in the clinic or during hospitalization provides an excellent opportunity for the nurse to review heart-healthy information. Reviews of family history, lifestyle, and eating patterns are suitable interventions, even in the absence of high risks.

Kawasaki Disease

Kawasaki disease (KD) (mucocutaneous lymph node syndrome) occurs worldwide and is the leading cause of acquired cardiovascular disease in the United States. It usually affects children less than 5 years of age. Studies have shown that no known microbe is associated with KD, although it may be a response to a mild asymptomatic viral infection in children with a genetic predisposition (Rowley, 2012). KD is not spread from person to person. Clinical signs and symptoms make the diagnosis because specific laboratory findings are not diagnostic. KD causes inflammation of the vessels in the cardiovascular system. The inflammation weakens the walls of the vessels and often results in an *aneurysm* (an abnormal dilation of the wall of a blood vessel). Aneurysms can cause thrombi (blood clots) to form, resulting in serious complications. Approximately 40% of untreated children develop aneurysms of the coronary vessels, which can be life threatening. For this reason, it is essential that a diagnosis of KD be made as early as possible.

Manifestations. The onset is abrupt with a sustained fever, sometimes above 40° C (104° F), that does not respond to antipyretics or antibiotics. The fever lasts for more than 5 days. Conjunctivitis without discharge, fissured lips, a "strawberry tongue" (enlarged reddened papilla on the tongue), inflamed mouth and pharyngeal membranes, and enlarged nontender lymph nodes are seen. An erythematous skin rash develops, with swollen hands and desquamation (peeling) of the palms and soles (Figure 26-5). The child is very irritable and may develop signs of cardiac problems. Abnormalities in an echocardiogram can be detected by the tenth day and this observation is an important diagnostic tool

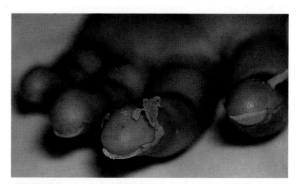

FIGURE 26-5 Peeling of the fingertips. The appearance of fingertip or toe tip peeling is characteristic of the subacute phase of Kawasaki disease. (From Zitelli BJ et al: *Zitelli and Davis' atlas of pediatric physical diagnosis,* ed 6, Philadelphia, 2012, Saunders.)

(Rowley, 2012). Lab results may show an elevated C-reactive protein, ESR, and white blood count.

Treatment and Nursing Care. Intravenous immune globulin (IVIG) administered early in the illness can prevent the development of coronary artery pathology. Salicylate therapy (aspirin) is prescribed for its antithrombus properties. If the child does not respond to IVIG therapy and aspirin, a second dose of IVIG may be prescribed or cyclosporine may be added to the treatment. Prednisolone may be used but its effectiveness has not been proven (Rowley, 2012).

Nursing care is symptomatic and supportive. Parent teaching should be reinforced concerning the need to postpone active routine immunizations for 11 months after the administration of immune globulin, which is an immunosuppressant.

Long-term, low-dose aspirin therapy may be prescribed to prevent clot formation. Compliance may be a problem for any long-term regimen in which medication must be taken when the child feels "well." The nurse should reinforce parent teaching concerning the recognition of cardiac problems and updating their CPR skills.

Get Ready for the NCLEX® Examination!

Key Points

- Signs and symptoms of congenital heart abnormalities in infants include dyspnea, difficulty with feedings, choking spells, recurrent respiratory infections, cyanosis, poor weight gain, clubbing of the fingers and toes, and heart murmurs.
- The nursing goals significant to the care of children with heart failure are to (1) reduce the work of the heart, (2) improve respiration, (3) maintain proper nutrition, (4) prevent infection, (5) reduce the anxiety of the parent, and (6) support growth and development.
- Congenital heart defects may be caused by genetic factors, maternal factors such as drug use or illness, or environmental factors. Acquired heart disease occurs after birth as a response to a defect or illness.
- Congenital heart defects that result in a recirculation of blood to the lungs do not usually produce cyanosis as a clinical sign.
- A congenital heart defect can cause an increase in pulmonary blood flow, a decrease in pulmonary blood flow, or an obstruction of blood flow.
- A difference in the blood pressure between the arms and the legs is characteristic of coarctation of the aorta.
- The defects in tetralogy of Fallot include pulmonary artery stenosis, hypertrophy of the right ventricle, dextroposition of the aorta, and a ventricular septal defect.
- Hypercyanotic "tet" spells are relieved by placing the child in a knee-chest position.
- Signs of congestive heart failure in infants include tachycardia, at-rest fatigue during feedings, and perspiration around the forehead.
- Two nurses should check the dose of digoxin before administration. A dose exceeding 0.05 mg should be reconfirmed with the health care provider.
- The major Jones criteria diagnostic of rheumatic fever include polyarthritis, erythema marginatum, Sydenham's chorea, and rheumatic carditis.
- Chest tube drainage systems must always be kept below the level of the chest.

- Young infants should *not* have a fat-restricted diet because fat is needed for CNS growth and development.

Additional Learning Resources

SG Go to your Study Guide for additional learning activities to help you master this chapter content.

evolve Go to your Evolve website (http://evolve.elsevier.com/Leifer) for the following learning resources:
- Animations
- Answer Guidelines for Critical Thinking Questions
- Answers and Rationales for Review Questions for the NCLEX® Examination
- Glossary with English and Spanish pronunciations
- Interactive Review Questions for the NCLEX® Examination
- Patient Teaching Plans in English and Spanish
- Skills Performance Checklists
- Video clips and more!

  Online Resources
- American Heart Association: www.americanheart.org/presenter.jhtml?identifier=4498
- Kawasaki disease: www.mayoclinic.com/health/kawasaki-disease/DS00576
- Tetralogy of Fallot: www.nhlbi.nih.gov/health/dci/Diseases/tof/tof_what.html; www.Cincinnatichildrens.org/health/heart/

Review Questions for the NCLEX® Examination

1. When administering digoxin (Lanoxin) to an infant, the medication should be withheld and the physician notified if the:

    1. pulse rate is below 60 beats/min.
    2. infant is dyspneic.
    3. pulse rate is below 100 beats/min.
    4. respiratory rate is above 40 breaths/min.

2. An infant with tetralogy of Fallot is experiencing a tet spell involving cyanosis and dyspnea. In which position should the infant be placed?

   1. Fowler's
   2. Knee-chest
   3. Trendelenburg's
   4. Prone

3. Prevention of rheumatic fever can best be accomplished by:

   1. keeping children with fever home.
   2. sending children with sore throats home from school.
   3. having sore throats cultured as soon as possible.
   4. treating all colds with antibiotics.

4. The nurse is assessing a child admitted with possible Kawasaki disease. A characteristic sign or symptom that the nurse should observe and document would be:

   1. cardiac dysrhythmia.
   2. decreased urine output.
   3. peeling skin on fingers.
   4. decreased level of consciousness.

5. A child who has had heart surgery returns to the pediatric unit with a chest tube and drainage bottles in place. What is a priority nursing responsibility when caring for a child with chest tubes?

   1. Empty the chest tube drainage bottles each shift.
   2. Clamp the chest tubes when turning the patient.
   3. Place the drainage bottles on the bed when moving the bed.
   4. Keep the drainage bottles below the chest level at all times.

Critical Thinking Questions

1. A child who was diagnosed with Kawasaki disease is discharged home with directions to take a low-dose aspirin tablet once a day. The parent states that she heard that aspirin is contraindicated for use in children and asks if she can substitute Tylenol instead. What is the best response of the nurse?

2. A parent states that her 4-month-old infant is scheduled for heart transplant surgery in 2 weeks. She states that the infant is now due for her second immunization series and asks if the child will be better protected if she has the immunizations now before she has the surgery. What is the best response of the nurse?

Objectives

1. Define each key term listed.
2. Summarize the components of blood.
3. List two laboratory procedures commonly performed on children with blood disorders.
4. List the symptoms, prevention, and treatment of iron-deficiency anemia.
5. Review the effects of severe anemia on the heart.
6. Recommend four food sources of iron for a child with iron-deficiency anemia.
7. Examine the pathophysiology and the signs and symptoms of sickle cell disease.
8. Describe four types of sickle cell crises.
9. Devise a nursing care plan for a child with sickle cell disease.
10. Recognize the effects on the bone marrow of increased red blood cell production caused by thalassemia.
11. Recall the pathophysiology and the signs and symptoms of hemophilia A and hemophilia B.
12. Identify the nursing interventions necessary to prevent hemarthrosis in a child with hemophilia.
13. Compare and contrast four manifestations of bleeding into the skin.
14. Recall normal blood values of infants and children.
15. Plan the nursing care of a child with leukemia.
16. Review the nursing care of a child receiving a blood transfusion.
17. Discuss the effects of chronic illness on the growth and development of children.
18. Formulate techniques the nurse can use to facilitate the grieving process.
19. Contrast age-appropriate responses to a sibling's death and the nursing interventions required.
20. Recall the stages of dying.
21. Discuss the nurse's role in helping families to handle the death of a child.

Key Terms

alopecia (ăl-ō-PĒ-shă, p. 631)
anemia (p. 622)
Christmas disease (p. 628)
ecchymosis (ĕk-ĭ-MŌ-sĭs, p. 629)
erythropoietin (ĕ-rĭth-rō-POI-ă-tĭn, p. 620)
hemarthrosis (hē-măhr-THRŌ-sĭs, p. 628)
hematoma (hē-mă-TŌ-mă, p. 629)
hematopoiesis (hē-mă-tō-poi-Ē-sĭs, p. 620)
hemosiderosis (hē-mō-sĭd-ŭr-Ō-sĭs, p. 626)

lymphadenopathy (lĭm-făd-ĕn-ŎP-ă-thē, p. 621)
oncologists (p. 630)
petechiae (pĕ-TĒ-kē-ă, p. 621)
purpura (PŬR-pyŭ-ră, p. 621)
respite care (RĔS-pĭt kār, p. 636)
sickle cell crises (p. 624)
Sickledex (p. 624)
splenomegaly (splĕ-nō-MĔG-ă-lē, p. 621)

The blood and blood-forming organs make up the hematological system. Blood is vital to all body functions. *Blood dyscrasias* or disorders occur when blood components fail to form correctly or when blood values exceed or fail to meet normal standards.

Plasma and blood cells are formed at about the second week of gestation, primarily in the yolk sac. Later, blood forms in the spleen, liver, thymus, lymph system, and bone marrow. In the fetus, blood is formed primarily in the liver until the last trimester of pregnancy. During childhood, the red blood cells (RBCs) are formed in the marrow of the long bones (such as the tibia and femur); by adolescence, **hematopoiesis** (blood formation) takes place in the marrow of the ribs, sternum, vertebrae, pelvis, skull, clavicle, and scapulae. The rate of RBC production

is regulated by **erythropoietin**. The liver of the fetus produces this substance, but at birth the kidneys take over erythropoietin production. The blood volume of a newborn is approximately 85 mL/kg weight (London, 2011). The newborn has a high hemoglobin and red blood cell count at birth because of the high erythropoietin level, placental shift of blood to the vascular system at birth, and a low extracellular fluid volume. A high white blood cell (WBC) level is evident at birth but decreases by 1 week to a stable level. The vitamin K level is low in the newborn and is required for the development of several blood clotting factors, therefore vitamin K is administered immediately after birth (Greenbaum, 2011).

The lymphatic system includes lymphocytes, lymphatic vessels, lymph nodes, the spleen, the tonsils,

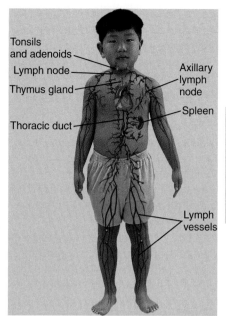

LYMPHATIC SYSTEM

- The increased size of tonsils and adenoids is normal in preschool and school-age children and is one of the body's defense mechanisms.
- The thymus gland is important in the development of the immune response in newborns.
- Preterm and term infants are at greater risk for viral and bacterial infections because of immature T-cell activity.

FIGURE 27-1 Summary of lymphatic system differences between the child and the adult. The lymphatic system is a subsystem of the circulatory system. It returns excess tissue fluid to the blood and defends the body against disease. (Art overlay courtesy Observatory Group, Cincinnati, Ohio.)

the adenoids, and the thymus gland. The lymphatic system drains regions of the body to lymph nodes, where infectious organisms are destroyed and antibody production is stimulated. Lymph nodes are not palpable in the newborn, but the cervical, auxiliary, and inguinal nodes may be palpable by childhood. **Lymphadenopathy** is an enlargement of lymph nodes that is indicative of infection or disease. Figure 27-1 summarizes some of the differences between the child's and the adult's lymphatic systems.

Figure 27-2 depicts the main types of blood cells in the circulating blood. Circulating blood consists of two portions: plasma and formed elements. The formed elements are erythrocytes (red blood cells), leukocytes (WBCs), and thrombocytes (platelets). Erythrocytes primarily transport oxygen and carbon dioxide to and from the lungs and tissues. Leukocytes act as the body's defense against infections. Thrombocytes, along with portions of blood plasma, are involved with blood coagulation. In the young child, every available space in the bone marrow is involved with blood formation.

Lymphocytes, unlike other WBCs, are produced in the lymphoid tissues of the body. They travel in the circulation but are more commonly found in the lymph tissue. They are released into the body to fight infection and to provide immunity. Their numbers greatly increase in chronic inflammatory conditions. The spleen is the largest organ of the lymphatic system. One of the main functions of the spleen is to bring blood into contact with lymphocytes. Aside from trauma and rupture, the most commonly seen pathological condition of the spleen is enlargement. This is termed **splenomegaly**. The spleen enlarges during infections, congenital and acquired hemolytic anemias, and liver malfunction.

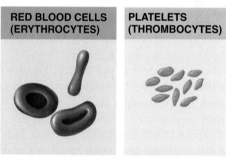

RED BLOOD CELLS (ERYTHROCYTES)

PLATELETS (THROMBOCYTES)

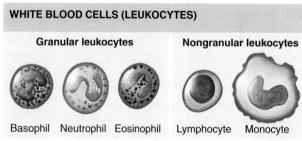

WHITE BLOOD CELLS (LEUKOCYTES)

Granular leukocytes

Nongranular leukocytes

Basophil   Neutrophil   Eosinophil

Lymphocyte   Monocyte

FIGURE 27-2 The formed elements of the blood. Red blood cells (RBCs; erythrocytes), white blood cells (WBCs; leukocytes), and platelets (thrombocytes) constitute the formed elements of the blood. (From Patton KT, Thibodeau GA: *Anatomy & physiology*, ed 8, St Louis, 2013, Mosby.)

Bone marrow aspiration is a procedure helpful in determining disorders of the blood. Numerous types of blood counts are used as well. Many are specific to a particular disease. The skin is sometimes an indicator of certain conditions of the blood. **Petechiae** (pinpoint hemorrhagic spots) and **purpura** (large petechiae) are often seen and these conditions should alert the nurse to the possibility of blood dyscrasias. The physician examines the liver and spleen by palpation and percussion to determine whether they are enlarged.

ANEMIAS

Anemia can result from many different underlying causes. A reduction in the amount of circulating hemoglobin reduces the oxygen-carrying ability of the blood. A hemoglobin level below 8 g/dL results in an increased cardiac output and a shunting of blood from the periphery of the body to the vital organs. Pallor, weakness, tachypnea, shortness of breath, and congestive heart failure can result.

IRON-DEFICIENCY ANEMIA

Pathophysiology. The most common nutritional deficiency of children in the United States today is anemia caused by insufficient amounts of iron in the body. The incidence is highest during infancy and adolescence—two rapid growth periods. Anemia (*an*, "without," and *emia*, "blood") is a condition in which there is a reduction in the amount and size of the RBCs, or in the amount of hemoglobin, or both. Iron-deficiency anemia may be caused by severe hemorrhage, the child's inability to absorb the iron received, excessive growth requirements, or an inadequate diet. Researchers have also found that feeding whole cow's milk to infants can precipitate gastrointestinal bleeding, resulting in anemia.

Prevention of iron-deficiency anemia begins with good prenatal care to ensure that the mother has a suitable intake of iron during pregnancy. During the first few months after birth, the newborn relies on iron that was stored in the system during fetal life. Preterm infants may be deprived of a sufficient supply, because iron is obtained late in the prenatal period. In addition, the iron stores of low-birth-weight infants and infants from multiple births are relatively small.

The highest incidence of iron-deficiency anemia occurs from the ninth to the twenty-fourth month. During this rapid growth period, the infant outgrows the limited iron reserve that was in the body; in addition, iron-fortified formula and infant cereals may have been eliminated from the diet. Poorly planned meals or feeding problems also contribute to this deficiency. The mother may sometimes rely too heavily on bottle feedings to avoid conflict at meals. Unfortunately, milk contains very little iron. Instead, the amounts of solid food should be increased and the amount of milk decreased. Boiled egg yolk, liver, leafy green vegetables, Cream of Wheat, dried fruits (apricots, peaches, prunes, raisins), dry beans, crushed nuts, and whole-grain bread are good sources of iron. Iron-fortified cereals eaten out of the box provide a nutritious snack. Unfortunately, the body does not absorb all the iron found in a food source. The bioavailability of iron in vegetables is less than that in meat.

Manifestations. The symptoms of iron-deficiency anemia are pallor, irritability, anorexia, and a decrease in activity. Many infants are overweight because of excessive consumption of milk (so-called "milk babies"). Blood tests for anemia may include RBC count, hemoglobin and hematocrit levels, and determination of morphological cell changes and iron concentration. The stool may be tested for occult blood. A dietary history is also obtained. Sometimes a slight heart murmur is heard. The spleen may be enlarged.

Untreated iron-deficiency anemias progress slowly, and in severe cases the heart muscle becomes too weak to function. If this happens, heart failure follows. Children with long-standing anemia may also show growth retardation and cognitive changes. Screening procedures are suggested at 9 and 24 months for full-term infants and earlier for low-birth-weight infants.

Treatment. Iron-deficiency anemia responds well to treatment. Iron, usually ferrous sulfate, is administered orally two or three times daily between meals. Vitamin C aids in the absorption of iron; therefore providing juice when administering iron is suggested. Liquid preparations are taken through a straw to prevent temporary discoloration of the teeth. (Some iron preparations without this disadvantage are available.) The toddler needs solid foods that are rich sources of iron. An iron-dextran mixture (Imferon) given intramuscularly is also highly effective. It must be injected deep in a large muscle using the Z-track technique to minimize staining and tissue irritation.

> ### Nursing Tip
>
> Oral iron supplements should not be ingested with milk or milk products because milk interferes with iron absorption.

Parent Education. Parents need explicit instructions on proper foods for the infant. The nurse stresses the importance of breastfeeding for the first 6 months and the use of iron-fortified formula throughout the first year of life (the absorption of iron from human milk is much better than from cow's milk). The amount of milk consumed during the day and night is determined. Solid food intake is reviewed, and specific iron-enriched nutrients are suggested. The nurse considers financial, ethnic, and family preferences in teaching plans. Behavior concerns at mealtime may also have to be addressed.

The stools of infants who are taking oral iron supplements are tarry green. An absence of this finding may indicate poor parental compliance with therapy. Oral iron preparations are not to be provided with milk, which interferes with absorption. To increase absorption, these preparations should be given between meals, when digestive acid concentration is highest. It is important to emphasize that both dietary changes and supplemental iron therapy are necessary to eradicate iron-deficiency anemia. Good dietary practices must be lifelong to maintain good health. Parents are encouraged to return for periodic evaluation of the child's blood status. Nursing Care Plan 27-1 specifies interventions for the child with iron-deficiency anemia.

⭐ Nursing Care Plan 27-1   The Child with Iron-Deficiency Anemia

PATIENT DATA: A parent brings a 10-month-old boy to the clinic. The child is pale and listless. Laboratory results show iron-deficiency anemia. The parent states that the child loves to drink milk.

Selected Nursing Diagnosis: Deficient parental knowledge related to cause and treatment of anemia

Goals	Nursing Interventions	Rationales
Parents will verbalize an understanding of the importance of dietary factors and iron supplements in the prevention and treatment of this condition.	Encourage breastfeeding.	Absorption of iron from human milk is much better than that from cow's milk.
Infant will ingest iron-rich formula plus two servings of iron-fortified cereal and iron supplement, if prescribed.	Encourage iron-rich formula for full first year.	Cow's milk contains little iron.
	Dispel the myth that milk is a perfect food.	Parents often rely too heavily on milk because it is easier than preparing solid foods, which the infant may initially dislike; ingestion of large amounts of milk may interfere with absorption of iron supplements.
	Between meals, give iron supplement with juice.	Vitamin C aids in the absorption of iron.

Selected Nursing Diagnosis: Imbalanced nutrition: less than body requirements, related to iron-poor diet

Goals	Nursing Interventions	Rationales
Patient's hemoglobin level will improve with therapy; there will be no recurrence of anemia.	Review 24-hour dietary history.	Nurse can determine what foods are missing and quantities of food ingested; this information can be used as a baseline for teaching.
	Review height and weight chart.	Determines child's status in relation to norms; compares patient's present measurements with former rate of growth and progress.
	Review solid food intake and suggest iron-rich foods as age appropriate.	Solid foods high in iron must be increased as age appropriate (egg yolk, liver, leafy green vegetables, Cream of Wheat, dried fruits, whole-grain bread, iron-fortified cereal).
	Educate parents in administration of the iron supplement.	Usually administered orally two or three times a day between meals. Supplements are easily forgotten because evidence of improvement is slow and signs of disease may not be noticeable. Poisoning can result from overdose.
	Stress the importance of compliance with the dietary regimen to prevent recurrence.	Dietary changes must be lifelong to maintain good health.

Critical Thinking Question

1. The mother of a child diagnosed with anemia comes to the clinic and states she is worried about the pallor and lack of energy her child continues to show. She states she works outside the home but has her child in "good day care" that provides good meals. What further questions would be appropriate for the nurse to ask in this interview?

 Medication Safety Alert!

Prevent iron poisoning in children by keeping preparations well out of reach. Educate parents about this hazard.

SICKLE CELL DISEASE

Pathophysiology. Sickle cell disease is an inherited defect in the formation of hemoglobin. It occurs mainly in people of African descent, but it is also carried by some persons of Mediterranean descent, such as some Arabs, Greeks, Maltese, Sicilians, as well as those originating from other Mediterranean areas. Many researchers believe that the gene for sickle cell disease developed in these populations as protection against malaria. Sickling (clumping) caused by decreased blood oxygen levels may be triggered by dehydration, infection, physical or emotional stress, or exposure to cold. Laboratory examination of the affected child's blood shows that the RBC has changed its shape to resemble that of a sickle blade, from which the name of the disorder is derived (Figure 27-3).

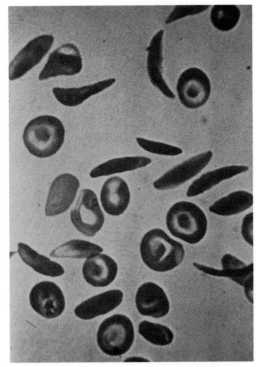

FIGURE 27-3 Scanning electron micrograph of erythrocytes. Note that the normal red blood cell is round. The sickle-shaped cell can clump as it flows through the circulation, causing a vasoocclusive sickle cell crisis. (From Zitelli BJ et al: *Zitelli and Davis' atlas of pediatric physical diagnosis*, ed 6, Philadelphia, 2012, Saunders.)

Sickle cells contain an abnormal form of hemoglobin termed *hemoglobin S* (the sickling type). The membranes of these cells are fragile and easily destroyed. Their crescent shape makes it difficult for them to pass through the capillaries, causing a pileup of cells in the small vessels. This clumping may lead to a thrombosis (clot) and cause an obstruction. Infarcts, or areas of dead tissue, may result when the tissue is denied proper blood supply. These generally develop in the spleen but may also be seen in other areas of the body, such as the brain, heart, lungs, gastrointestinal tract, kidneys, and bones. The patient feels acute pain in the affected area.

There are two types of sickle cell disease: an asymptomatic (*a*, "without," and *symptoma*, "symptom") version (sickle cell trait) and much more severe forms that necessitate intermittent hospitalization (sickle cell anemia).

Sickle cell trait. This form of the disease occurs in about 1 of 12 of the African American population in the United States (American Sickle Cell Anemia Association, 2010). The blood of the patient contains a mixture of normal (hemoglobin A) and sickle (hemoglobin S) hemoglobins. The proportions of hemoglobin S are low because the disease is inherited from only one parent. The physician can distinguish sickle cell trait from the more severe disease by electrophoresis study of the patient's RBCs and hemoglobin. Sickling is more rapid and extreme with sickle cell disease. In sickle cell trait the hemoglobin and RBC counts are normal.

Sickle cell trait does not develop into sickle cell disease. Although there is no need to treat the patient with sickle cell trait, the patient is a carrier, and genetic counseling is important.

Sickle cell anemia. This severe form of sickle cell disease results when the abnormality is inherited from both parents (Figure 27-4). Each offspring has a one in four chance of inheriting the disease (which is not the same as one in four children inheriting it). In general, the clinical symptoms do not appear until the last part of the first year of life. There may be an unusual swelling of the fingers and toes. The specific symptoms of sickle cell disease are caused by the enlarged bone marrow sites that develop to produce more red blood cells and the abnormal sickle cell shape that causes clumping and obstruction in the vessels and ischemia to the organ.

There is chronic anemia. The hemoglobin level ranges from 6 to 9 g/dL or lower. The child is pale, tires easily, and has little appetite. These manifestations of anemia are complicated by characteristic episodes called **sickle cell crises**, which are painful and can be fatal. Specific types of crises have been identified. They differ in their pathological causes and manifestations and may necessitate somewhat different treatments (Table 27-1). Unfortunately, in some cases the sickle cell crisis is the first obvious manifestation of the condition. The patient appears acutely ill. There is severe abdominal pain. Muscle spasms, leg pain, or painful swollen joints may be seen. Fever, vomiting, hematuria, convulsions, stiff neck, coma, or paralysis can result, depending on the organs involved. Children with sickle cell disease have a risk for stroke as a complication of a vasoocclusive sickle cell crisis.

The sickle cell crises recur periodically throughout childhood; however, they tend to decrease with age. Patients should be kept in good health between episodes. Immunizations of these children are particularly important, including those for *Haemophilus influenzae*, hepatitis A, and hepatitis B as well as the pneumococcal vaccine. Patients should refrain from becoming overly tired. They also should avoid situations such as flying in an unpressurized airplane or exercising at a high altitude, because oxygen concentrations in their blood are already reduced. Extra stress and exposure to cold may lower resistance, causing additional problems. Overheating, which can lead to dehydration, is also to be avoided. Oral intake of iron is of no value.

📖 Nursing Tip

During sickle cell crises, anticipate the child's need for tissue oxygenation, hydration, rest, protection from infection, pain control, blood transfusion, and emotional support for this life-threatening illness.

Diagnosis. Sickle cell disease can be detected before birth by chorionic villi sampling. Early diagnosis by mandatory screening of all newborns in the United States allows early detection before symptoms occur. The sickling test (**Sickledex**) is commonly used for screening. Hemoglobin electrophoresis ("fingerprinting") is used when the result

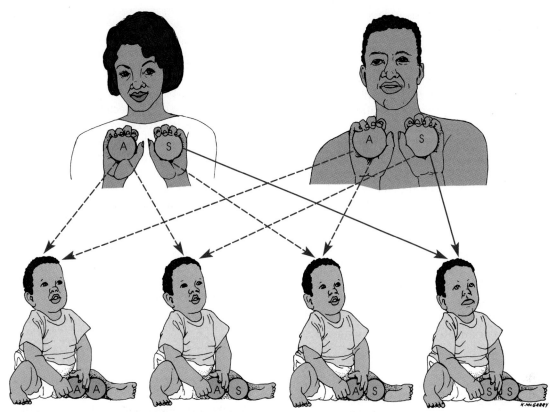

FIGURE 27-4 Transmission of sickle cell disease from parents to children. Parents who are carriers of the sickle cell trait do not show symptoms of the disease because hemoglobin A (the normal form of hemoglobin) in their red blood cells protects them from hemoglobin S (the sickling form). When two carriers become parents, however, the possibilities are as follows: One child in four will inherit all normal hemoglobin and thus be free of the disease (AA); two children in four will inherit both hemoglobin A and hemoglobin S and thus become carriers (AS) of the trait (similar to their parents); and one child in four will inherit all sickling hemoglobin and thus be affected by sickle cell disease (SS).

Table 27-1	Types of Sickle Cell Crises
TYPE	**COMMENT**
Vasoocclusive (painful crises)	Most common type; there is an obstruction of blood flow by cells, infarctions, and some degree of vasospasm. Dactylitis, painful joints and extremities, abdominal pain (infarction or bleeding within liver, spleen, abdominal lymph node), central nervous system strokes, pulmonary disease, and/or priapism may be present. Morphine, codeine or Vicodin are commonly prescribed with intravenous hydration.
Splenic sequestration	Large amounts of blood pool in liver and spleen. Spleen becomes massive. Abdominal pain Circulatory collapse and shock are present. Children between 8 months and 5 years of age are particularly susceptible. Death may occur within hours of appearance of symptoms. Minor episodes may resolve spontaneously. Splenectomy may be indicated for children who have one or more severe crises.
Aplastic crises	Bone marrow stops producing red blood cells (RBCs); a number of infections may precipitate this (usually viral). Decreased reticulocyte count may be present. Child may be transfused with fresh packed RBCs if severe anemia occurs.
Hyperhemolytic	Rapid rate of hemolysis is superimposed on an already severe process; rare condition. Functional hyposplenism and overwhelming infection occur. Progressive fibrosis of spleen reduces its function; patient becomes more susceptible to infection.

Data from Jackson-Allen P, Vessey J, Shapiro N: *Primary care of the child with a chronic condition,* ed 5, Philadelphia, 2010, Saunders; Kliegman R, Stanton B, St Geme III J, Schor N, Behrman R: *Nelson textbook of pediatrics,* ed 19, Philadelphia, 2011, Saunders.

is positive. This procedure separates and records the various peptide patterns of the blood. It distinguishes between patients with the trait and those with the disease.

Treatment and Nursing Care. When the infant or child is hospitalized during a crisis, the treatment is supportive and symptomatic. The patient is confined to bed. Analgesics are provided to relieve pain. Children in severe pain may need a continuous intravenous (IV) infusion containing a narcotic. Meperidine (Demerol) is not recommended for children with sickle cell disease because of the risk of normeperidine-induced seizures (Ellison, 2012). A patient-controlled analgesia (PCA) pump enables children older than 7 years to maintain control and participate in care. Every effort is made to combat dehydration and acidosis. Small blood transfusions may be administered to increase the hemoglobin count, but the results are only temporary. Packed RBCs are often given for this purpose. An accurate record of intake and output is kept. The patient's body position is changed frequently but gently. Hemopoietic stem cell transplantation may provide a cure in the near future.

Sickle cell disease may take a wide variety of courses. As always, the individual patient's progress is followed. Sometimes it is difficult to distinguish between abdominal pain caused by a sickle cell crisis and abdominal pain caused by appendicitis. The nurse must remember that pain experienced by a child with sickle cell disease may also be caused by an unrelated condition.

Prevention of infection and prevention of dehydration are very important goals in the care of a child with sickle cell disease. Infants and children with sickle cell disease often have impaired immune function, and bacteremia (sepsis) is a leading cause of death in this group. Pneumococcal and meningococcal vaccinations and annual influenza vaccination are recommended. Oral penicillin prophylaxis before any invasive treatment, including dental care, is also advised (Kliegman, 2011). Multiple transfusions of packed cells may be required to maintain adequate hemoglobin levels. The nurse should observe the child for reactions to the blood transfusion. **Hemosiderosis** (the deposit of iron into organs and tissues in the body) is a complication of this type of hemolytic disease. The drug deferoxamine mesylate (Desferal) binds with iron and allows its excretion via the kidney. An oral form is also available. An exchange transfusion may reduce the number of circulating sickle cells and prevent complications such as thrombus formation and stroke. High-dose IV methylprednisolone may be used to decrease severe pain (Rees, 2010).

The main goals of therapy are to prevent sickling, dehydration, hypoxia, and infection, which can cause a sickle cell crisis. Erythropoietin and some chemotherapy regimens can increase the production of fetal hemoglobin and reduce complications. Bone marrow transplantation and gene replacement therapy may hold a promising cure.

> **⚠ Medication Safety Alert!**
>
> Meperidine (Demerol) should not be used for pain control in children with sickle cell disease due to risk of seizures.

Surgery. The use of splenectomy in children with sickle cell disease has been conservative. A recurrence of acute splenic sequestration becomes less likely after 5 years of age. Routine splenectomy is not recommended because the spleen generally atrophies on its own because of fibrotic changes that take place in patients with sickle cell disease. Hematopoietic stem cell transplantation can cure sickle cell disease, but this therapy is currently available only to those with a human leukocyte antigen (HLA) compatible sibling (Rees, 2010).

> **👁 Nursing Tip**
>
> It is essential to teach parents the signs and symptoms of dehydration, hypoxia, and infection to prevent the occurrence of sickle cell crisis.

> **⚠ Safety Tip**
>
> Cold or hot compresses should not be used to relieve pain in a child with sickle cell anemia, because cold promotes sickling and ischemia, and ischemic tissues have reduced sensation and therefore burns can occur.

THALASSEMIA

Pathophysiology. The thalassemias are a group of hereditary blood disorders in which the patient's body cannot produce sufficient adult hemoglobin. The RBCs are abnormal in size and shape and are rapidly destroyed. This abnormality results in chronic anemia. The body attempts to compensate by producing large amounts of fetal hemoglobin. Thalassemias are caused by a deficiency in the normal synthesis of hemoglobin polypeptide chains. They are categorized according to the Greek letters designating the polypeptide chain affected but α- and β- thalassemia are the most common.

The thalassemia that involves impaired production of beta chains is known as *β-thalassemia*. This variety consists of two forms: thalassemia minor and thalassemia major. Thalassemia major is also called *Cooley's anemia*. Thalassemia occurs mainly in persons of Mediterranean origin, such as Greeks, Syrians, and Italians, and their descendants elsewhere. The term is derived from the Greek *thalassa*, which means "sea." Thalassemia can also occur from spontaneous mutations.

Thalassemia minor. Thalassemia minor, which is also termed *β-thalassemia trait*, occurs when the child inherits a thalassemia gene from only one parent (heterozygous inheritance). It is associated with mild anemia. Hemoglobin concentration averages 2 to 3 g/dL, which are lower than normal age-related values. These patients are often misdiagnosed as having an iron-deficiency anemia. Symptoms are minimal. The patient is pale, and the spleen may be enlarged. The patient may lead a normal life, with the illness going undetected. This condition is of genetic importance, particularly if both parents are carriers of the trait. Prenatal blood samples can detect thalassemia major in such cases.

Thalassemia major (Cooley's anemia). When two thalassemia genes are inherited (homozygous inheritance), the child is born with a more serious form of the disease. A progressive, severe anemia becomes evident within the second 6 months of life.

The child is pale and hypoxic, has a poor appetite, and may have a fever. Jaundice, which at first is mild, progresses to a muddy bronze color resulting from *hemosiderosis*, a deposit of iron (released by blood cell destruction) into the tissues. The liver enlarges, and the spleen grows enormously as defective red blood cells are destroyed. Abdominal distention is great, which causes pressure on the organs of the chest. Cardiac failure caused by the profound anemia is a constant threat. Bone marrow space enlarges to compensate for an increased production of blood cells. *Hematopoietic (hema,* "blood," and *poiesis,* "to make") defects and a massive expansion of the bone marrow in the face and skull result in changes in the facial contour that give the child a characteristic appearance (Figure 27-5). The teeth protrude because of an overgrowth of the upper jawbone; the bone becomes thin and is subject to pathological fracture.

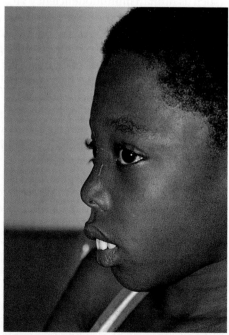

FIGURE 27-5 Appearance of child with thalassemia major (Cooley's anemia). Note the overgrowth of the upper jawbone (maxillary hyperplasia). (From Zitelli BJ, Davis HW, editors: *Atlas of pediatric physical diagnosis,* ed 4, St Louis, 2002, Mosby.)

Diagnosis is aided by a family history of thalassemia, radiographic bone growth studies, and blood tests. Hemoglobin electrophoresis is helpful in diagnosing the type and severity of the various thalassemias. Prenatal screening and diagnosis are available, and genetic counseling is advised.

Treatment and Nursing Care. The goals of care for children with thalassemia are to: (1) maintain hemoglobin levels at 9.5 g/dL to prevent overgrowth of bone marrow and resultant deformities, and (2) provide for growth and development and normal physical activity. Prevention or early treatment of infection is important. Some patients require splenectomy. A hematopoietic stem cell transplantation can provide a cure if an HLA matched donor is available (Muncie, 2009).

The mainstay of treatment for thalassemia major is frequent blood transfusions to maintain the hemoglobin level above 9.5 g/dL. As a result of repeated blood transfusions, excessive deposits of iron may be stored in the tissues. This is termed *hemosiderosis* and is seen especially in the spleen, liver, heart, pancreas, and lymph glands. Deferoxamine mesylate (Desferal), an iron-chelating agent, is provided to counteract hemosiderosis. This drug causes red discoloration of the urine. Blurred vision should be reported. Severe splenomegaly may occur in some children. Splenectomy may make the patient more comfortable, increase the ability to move about, and allow for more normal growth. After surgery, these children are given prophylactic antibiotics to prevent infection.

Nursing measures adhere to the principles of long-term care. The observation of the patient during a blood transfusion is discussed on p. 632. Monitoring of vital signs is necessary to detect irregularities of the heart. Whenever possible, to provide security and trust, the same nurse cares for the patient during transfusions, blood tests, and other unpleasant procedures. Children are taught to regulate their activities according to their own tolerance.

The emotional health of the child and parents calls for special consideration by the nurse. Every attempt to ease the strain of this prolonged illness must be made. Home care arrangements can be provided through community agencies. The family can be referred to the Cooley's Anemia Foundation for support and education. Older children need special support to accept changes in their body image caused by the disease. Suggestions applicable to the care of the chronically ill child are discussed throughout the text. Care of the dying child is discussed later in this chapter.

BLEEDING DISORDERS

HEMOPHILIA

Pathophysiology. Hemophilia is one of the oldest hereditary diseases known to humanity. In this disorder, the blood does not clot normally, and even the slightest injury can cause severe bleeding. It has been called the disease of kings because it has occurred in the children of several royal families in Russia and Europe. This congenital disorder is confined almost exclusively to males but is transmitted by symptom-free females.

Hemophilia is inherited as a sex-linked recessive trait. It is termed sex-linked because the defective gene is located on the X, or female, chromosome. Different combinations of genes account for the fact that some children inherit the disease, some become carriers, and others neither inherit nor carry the trait. New mutations do occur, and the reason for this is unclear. The sex of the fetus can be determined by amniocentesis. Fetal blood sampling detects hemophilia. Some carrier women can also be identified.

There are several types of hemophilia. More than 10 identified factors in blood are involved in the clotting mechanism. A deficiency in any one of the factors will interfere with normal blood clotting. The two most common types of hemophilia are *hemophilia B,* or **Christmas disease** (a factor IX deficiency), and *hemophilia A* (a deficiency in factor VIII). This discussion is limited to classic hemophilia, or hemophilia A, which accounts for approximately 85% of cases (Scott, 2011).

Hemophilia A is caused by a deficiency of coagulation factor VIII, or antihemophilic globulin (AHG). The severity of the disease depends on the level of factor VIII in the plasma of the patient's blood. Some patients' lives are endangered by minor injury, whereas a child with a mild case of hemophilia might just bruise a little more easily than the normal person. The degree of severity tends to remain constant within a given family. The aim of therapy is to increase the level of factor VIII high enough to ensure clotting. It is possible to determine the level of factor VIII in the blood by means of a test called the *partial thromboplastin time (PTT),* which can help to diagnose and assess the child's condition. Prenatal diagnosis by amniocentesis is possible.

🔲 Nursing Tip

A classic symptom of hemophilia is bleeding into the joints (hemarthrosis).

Manifestations. Hemophilia can be diagnosed at birth because maternal factor VIII cannot cross the placenta and be transferred to the fetus. However, it is usually not apparent in the newborn unless abnormal bleeding occurs at the umbilical cord or after circumcision. As the child grows older and becomes more subject to injury, the slightest bruise or cut can induce extensive bleeding. Normal blood clots in about 3 to 6 minutes. In a patient with severe hemophilia, however, the time required for clotting may be 1 hour or longer.

Anemia, leukocytosis, and a moderate increase in the number of platelets may be seen in the hemorrhaging

child. There may also be signs of shock. Spontaneous hematuria is seen. Death can result from excessive bleeding anywhere in the body, but particularly when hemorrhage into the brain or neck occurs. Severe headache, vomiting, and disorientation may reflect cranial bleeding. Bleeding into the neck can cause airway obstruction. Bleeding into the ears and eyes can affect hearing and vision. Bleeding into the spinal column can lead to paralysis.

The circumstances leading to diagnosis may be the inability of a parent to stop a child's bleeding from a cut around the mouth or gums. A deciduous tooth loss may precipitate problems in a child who has a bleeding disorder. *Hematomas* may develop after immunizations. An injured knee, elbow, or ankle presents particular problems. Hemorrhage into the joint cavity, or **hemarthrosis** (*hema,* "blood," *arthron,* "joint," and *osis,* "condition of"), is considered a classic symptom of hemophilia. The effusion (*ex,* "out," and *fundere,* "to pour") into the joint is very painful because of the pressure buildup. Repeated hemorrhages may cause permanent deformities that could incapacitate the child. This deformity is sometimes referred to as an ankylosis (*ankyle,* "stiff joint," and *osis,* "condition of").

Treatment and Nursing Care. In a newborn with a family history of hemophilia, circumcision, heel sticks, and intramuscular injections are delayed to prevent bleeding and tissue injury. The principal therapy for hemophilia is to prevent bleeding by replacing the missing factor. The development of recombinant antihemophilic factor, a synthetic product, has eliminated the need for repeated blood transfusions and its accompanying dangers (such as human immunodeficiency virus [HIV] and hepatitis infection). After the parents and child are taught how to administer the medication, treatment is handled in the home. Diagnosed infants may receive prophylactic factor replacements at regular intervals to prevent hemarthrosis. Desmopressin acetate (DDAVP) is a nasal spray that increases factor VIII in the blood, which leads to decreased bleeding. It may be the treatment of choice for mild cases of hemophilia. Aminocaproic acid (Amicar) is an antifibrinolytic agent that can control bleeding that might occur because of dental care or other oral bleeding.

Prophylactic factor VIII concentrate replacement combined with specific treatment before planned invasive procedures, such as dental extraction or minor surgery, and also education concerning the prevention of injuries that can cause bleeding enable the hemophiliac child to live a normal life. Because young children often fall while playing, padding their play outfits can protect the joints of knees, hips, and elbows. Appropriate sports activities should be selected to prevent undue injury and the risk of bleeding into joints. When bleeding does occur, the traditional approach to care includes **r**est, **i**ce, **c**ompression, and **e**levation (RICE). A medical alert identification band should be worn at all times. In addition to factor VIII concentrate to treat hemophilia A and von Willebrand disease, and factor IX concentrate to treat hemophilia B, a recombinant antihemophilic factor, *Kyntha,* and a version of factor VIII, Kogenate *FS,* are currently approved for use to reduce joint damage in hemophilia (Foster, 2008). Gene therapy offers hope in the near future (Matrai, 2010). The FDA approved "Rixubis," a recombinant coagulation factor IX for routine use in children who are older than 16 years and are diagnosed with hemophilia B to prevent bleeding episodes and for perioperative management. It is administered twice a week intravenously. Research concerning the use of gene therapy for hemophilia is underway and may be available in the near future (Nordquist, 2013).

Home care programs are the treatment of choice. These greatly reduce the cost of treatment and decrease the risk of psychological trauma. Using a multidisciplinary approach to care assists families to develop healthy coping strategies to manage a child who has a chronic illness. The multidisciplinary approach to care is supported by the National Hemophilia Foundation.

It is difficult for parents not to be overly protective. The struggle to protect these children and still foster independence and a sense of autonomy may seem monumental to parents who work away from home. Allowing children to participate in decision-making about their care and focusing on their strengths are helpful.

Parent groups and professional counseling may provide support to enable children and parents to develop a healthy attitude toward the child's medical condition.

 Medication Safety Alert!

Drugs that contain salicylates are contraindicated for use in children with hemophilia.

PLATELET DISORDERS

The reduction or destruction of platelets in the body interferes with the clotting mechanism. Skin lesions that are common to these disorders include petechiae, a bluish, nonblanching, pinpoint-sized lesion; purpura, groups of adjoining petechiae; **ecchymosis,** an isolated bluish lesion larger than a petechia; and **hematoma,** a raised ecchymosis.

Idiopathic (Immunological) Thrombocytopenia Purpura

Pathophysiology. Idiopathic (immunological) thrombocytopenic purpura (ITP) is an acquired platelet disorder that occurs in childhood. It is the most common of the purpuras, which is a group of disorders affecting the numbers of platelets or their function. The cause is unknown, but it is thought to be an autoimmune system reaction to a virus. Platelets become coated with antiplatelet antibody, are "perceived" as foreign material, and are eventually destroyed by the spleen. ITP occurs in all age groups, with the main incidence between 2 and 4 years of age.

Manifestations. The classic symptom of ITP is slowed blood clotting and easy bruising, which result in petechiae (pinpoint hemorrhagic spots beneath the skin) and purpura (hemorrhage into the skin). Approximately 30% of patients also have nosebleeds. There may have been a recent history of rubella, rubeola, or viral respiratory infection. The interval between exposure and onset is about 2 weeks. The platelet count is below $20,000/mm^3$ (normal range is between $150,000/mm^3$ and $400,000/mm^3$). Diagnosis is confirmed by bone marrow aspiration to rule out leukemia.

 Nursing Tip

The bruises of idiopathic (immunological) thrombocytopenic purpura (ITP) must be distinguished from those of child abuse.

Treatment and Nursing Care. When platelet counts are low, the greatest danger is spontaneous intracranial bleeding. Neurological assessments are therefore a priority of care. Treatment is not indicated in most cases of ITP. Spontaneous remission occurs in about 6 weeks to 4 months. A few children progress to chronic ITP. Drugs that interfere with platelet function should be avoided to prevent bleeding. These include aspirin, phenylbutazone (Butazolidin), and phenacetin, acetylsalicylic acid, and caffeine (APC). Activity is limited during the acute stage to prevent bruises from falls and trauma. Nursing considerations for the more acutely ill child focus on observing the patient for signs of bleeding. The child should use soft toothbrushes for oral hygiene to minimize tissue trauma. Packed RBCs may be administered when there has been a large amount of blood loss. Platelets are usually not provided because the disease process destroys them. Corticosteroids such as prednisone may be prescribed. IV gamma globulin may be used to elevate platelet counts. In some patients, infusion with anti-D antibody may be an effective treatment when there is no active bleeding present. A splenectomy may be indicated for cases of chronic ITP. Complications of ITP include bleeding from the gastrointestinal tract, hemarthrosis, and intracranial hemorrhage. Mortality in childhood ITP is less than 1%. All children must keep recommended immunizations against the viral diseases of childhood current to prevent this complication from occurring.

 Medication Safety Alert!

After administration of anti-D antibody the child should be observed for 1 hour for fever, chills, headache, or alteration in vital signs.

DISORDERS OF WHITE BLOOD CELLS

LEUKEMIA

Leukemia refers to a group of malignant diseases of the bone marrow and lymphatic system. There are many types and classifications, each with its own therapy and prognosis. The two most common forms are acute lymphoid leukemia (ALL) and acute nonlymphoid (myelogenous) leukemia (AMLL or AML). Cytochemical markers, chromosome studies, and immunological markers differentiate the types of leukemia. The discussion in this test refers to ALL, the most common type of childhood leukemia.

Pediatric **oncologists** (physicians who specialize in the treatment of tumors) are challenged with the treatment of cancer in children because irradiation, surgery, and chemotherapy often have adverse effects on growth and development. Most children with cancer are treated in large medical centers to maximize the availability of high technology and newer treatment methods.

Survival rates for children diagnosed with leukemia have greatly improved. However, close monitoring of late side effects of leukemia therapy is essential, and long-term follow-up care should be monitored.

Pathophysiology. Leukemia (*leuko,* "white," and *emia,* "blood") is a malignant disease of the blood-forming organs of the body that results in an uncontrolled growth of immature WBCs. The immature cells are termed *blasts,* or *stem cells.* This term comes from the Greek *blastos,* meaning "germ" or "formative cell." The nurse may see references to the terms *lymphoblasts* or *myeloblasts* in descriptive histories. Leukemia is the most common form of childhood cancer. It was considered fatal in the past, but the prognosis has improved greatly with modern treatments and medication. Approximately 2000 new cases of childhood leukemia are diagnosed in the United States every year. About 4 children per 100,000 less than 15 years of age are affected annually, with the typical onset occurring between 2 and 5 years of age. Chromosomal abnormalities can be identified in 80% of cases of acute lymphocytic leukemia (Tubergen, 2011).

The leukemias involve a disruption of bone marrow function caused by the overproduction of immature WBCs in the marrow. Although the WBC count can be as high as $50,000/mm^3$ to $100,000/mm^3$, the cells are immature and do not function as healthy WBCs to fight infection; increased susceptibility to infection results. The WBCs take over the centers that are designed to form RBCs, and anemia results. When the WBCs infiltrate and take over the marrow centers that form platelets, the reduced platelet counts cause bleeding tendencies. The invasion of the bone marrow causes weakening of the bone, and pathological fractures can occur.

Leukemia cells can infiltrate the spleen, liver, and lymph glands, resulting in fibrosis and diminished function. The cancerous cells invade the central nervous system and other organs, draining these organs of their nutrients and finally causing metabolic starvation of the body.

Manifestations. The most common symptoms during the initial phase of leukemia are low-grade fever, pallor, bruising tendency, leg and joint pain, listlessness,

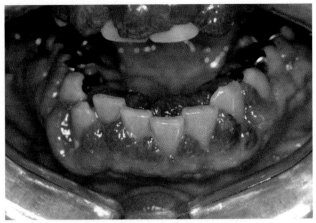

FIGURE 27-6 The mouth lesions of leukemia. (From Regezi JA, Sciubba JJ, Jordan RCK: *Oral pathology: clinical pathologic correlations,* ed 6, St Louis, 2012, Saunders.)

abdominal pain, and enlargement of lymph nodes. These symptoms may develop gradually or may be sudden in onset. As the disease progresses, the liver and spleen become enlarged. The skin may have an unusual lemon yellow color. *Petechiae* and *purpura* may be early objective symptoms. Anorexia, vomiting, weight loss, and dyspnea are also common. The kidneys and testicles may enlarge, and the patient may develop hematuria.

Because the WBCs are not functioning normally, bacteria easily invade the body. Ulcerations develop around the mucous membranes of the mouth and anal regions and have a tendency to bleed (Figure 27-6). Anemia becomes severe despite transfusions. The child may die as a direct result of the disease or from secondary infection. The symptoms are the same regardless of the type of WBC affected, but they vary widely with each patient depending on the parts of the body involved.

Diagnosis. The diagnosis of leukemia is based on the history and symptoms of the patient and the results of extensive blood tests that demonstrate the presence of leukemic blast cells in the blood, bone marrow, or other tissues. Because many WBCs and RBCs are formed in the bone marrow, a bone marrow aspiration is commonly performed. A piece of bone marrow is aspirated from the sternum or, more often in children, from the iliac crest. A special needle is used to obtain the sample, and the marrow is studied in the laboratory (Figure 27-7). X-ray films of the long bones show changes. After the diagnosis has been confirmed, a spinal tap determines central nervous system involvement. Kidney and liver function studies are also performed because normal functioning of these organs is absolutely necessary for chemotherapy to be safely used in treating the disease.

Treatment and Nursing Care. Long-term care is provided on an outpatient basis whenever possible. The treatment of a child with cancer involves the

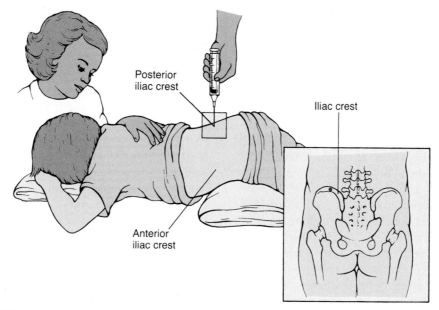

FIGURE 27-7 Bone marrow aspiration. Because many white blood cells and red blood cells are formed in the bone marrow, a bone marrow aspiration can determine the type and quantity of cells present and help to rule out or to confirm a serious disease.

multidisciplinary health care team (pediatrician, pathologist, oncologist, nurse, radiotherapist, nutritionist, psychologist, and school personnel). As with any diagnosis of cancer, the child with leukemia is usually referred to a specialized center where facilities for required care are available. Chemotherapy is performed in specialized units with specially trained and certified personnel.

Although chemotherapy may be effective in reducing leukemic cells, the side effects as well as the long-term effects of treatments must be addressed. In chemotherapy, bone marrow suppression makes it essential for the family to be taught about infection prevention. Neutropenia may require protective isolation precautions. Adequate hydration should be emphasized to minimize kidney damage. Active routine immunizations must be delayed while the child is receiving immunosuppressive drugs, because the body will not be able to manufacture antigens as expected. Parents should report any exposure to infections such as chicken pox so that immunoglobulin can be administered. Chickenpox can be life threatening to a child who is immunosuppressed. Nausea and vomiting are common complications of chemotherapy and result in decreased appetite, weight loss, and generalized weakness. Presenting the child's favorite foods in an attractive manner may help stimulate the appetite. Total parenteral nutrition (TPN) may be indicated to support nutritional needs. An intake and output record is maintained, and meticulous oral hygiene is provided.

The nurse should refer parents to available support groups. The Ronald McDonald house and hospice programs help parents and families cope with this illness. Because hair loss (**alopecia**) is a side effect of chemotherapy, the child can be offered a hat or a wig to help preserve a positive body image. School tutoring and counseling should be continuous in the hospital setting and in the home during home care to provide optimal growth and development.

Nursing Tip

Four priority challenges in the care of leukemic children are: (1) the complications of anemia from decreased red blood cell (RBC) infection, (2) infection from neutropenia, (3) bleeding from decreased platelets, and (4) fractures resulting from the involvement of the bone marrow.

Radiation and chemotherapy target specific cells (Rabin, 2011). Chemotherapy includes the following components:

- An induction period
- Central nervous system prophylaxis for high-risk patients
- Maintenance
- Reinduction therapy (if relapse occurs)
- Extramedullary disease therapy

The list of medications for treatment of this disease is growing. A combination of drugs used to induce remissions includes prednisone, vincristine sulfate, and daunorubicin or l-asparaginase. They work within 4 to 6 weeks in about 95% of children with ALL. The therapeutic effects of these drugs are of short duration, and therefore it is necessary to use additional drugs that help to maintain the remissions. The steroid prednisone has the side effects of masking the symptoms of infection, increasing fluid retention, inducing personality changes, and causing the child's face to take on a moon-shaped appearance. Methotrexate and 6-mercaptopurine are useful in maintaining remissions because they act against chemicals vital to the life of the WBC. These powerful medications produce side effects of varying degrees, such as nausea, diarrhea, rash, hair loss (alopecia), fever, anuria, anemia, and bone marrow depression. Peripheral neuropathy may be signaled by severe constipation caused by decreased nerve sensations to the bowel. The nurse should consult a pharmacology text for information about the particular drugs used for the patient to anticipate potential problems.

A bone marrow transplant may be useful. An autologous transplant uses the child's own bone marrow that has been purged of malignant cells. An allogeneic bone marrow transplant is taken from a donor who matches the child. Transplanted marrow rejection is a risk. When the child is hospitalized, protective environmental precautions and transmission-based precautions may prevent health care-associated infections (see Appendix A). Hemopoietic stem cell transplantation (HSCT) has been used successfully in children with AML and children with ALL who do not respond to chemotherapy. Prevention of infection is the challenge for the health care team after transplant. HSCT is a risky procedure because the immune system of the child must first be destroyed before the transplant procedure starts. However, approximately 80% of children with leukemia are cured (Tubergen, 2011).

Children's anxiety often centers on their symptoms. They fear that the treatments necessary to correct their problems may be painful, as indeed some are, such as venipunctures, bone marrow aspirations, and blood transfusions. Their trust in others is in a precarious balance. Nurses must inform children of what they are about to do and why it is necessary. The explanation is given in terms the child will understand.

The child may ask the nurse the inevitable question, "Am I going to die?" One suggestion is to reply with a question, such as "Why do you ask that? Do you feel sick today?" This may encourage the child to verbalize feelings. The pediatric nurse who encourages patients to discuss their concerns will find opportunities to clear up misconceptions and to decrease children's feelings of isolation.

The patient is frequently observed for signs of infection. Particular attention is paid to potential sites of infection, such as the patient's mucous membranes and puncture breaks in the skin from laboratory or therapeutic procedures. Pierced ears or other pierced body parts are observed for inflammation. Vital signs are observed for subtle variances, because steroid therapy may mask these indicators. The patient is turned often and is observed for skin breakdown, particularly in the perianal area. Nutritious meals and supplemental feedings that are high in protein and calories are offered. Parents and children are taught what they should look for and report.

Thrombocytopenic bleeding is a common complication of leukemia. The nurse observes the patient's skin for petechiae and ecchymosis. Nosebleeds are common and are treated by the application of cold and pressure.

The mouth is inspected daily for ulcerations and bleeding from the gums. It may be rinsed with a prescribed solution of one part hydrogen peroxide to four parts saline solution. Commercial mouthwashes are used with caution because they may alter normal flora and may cause fungal overgrowth. A water pick is helpful in massaging and toughening the gums. If the child is comatose, mouth care supplies are kept at the bedside. A soft tooth sponge is helpful. The nurse may also clean food particles from the patient's teeth with a piece of gauze wrapped around the finger. Lip balm is applied to dry, cracked lips.

🔊 Nursing Tip

Bleeding from the nose or mouth may be evidenced by a soiled pillowcase or sheet.

Care of a child receiving a transfusion. Platelets and packed RBCs may be given to the child. Hemolytic reactions caused by mismatched blood are rare. Nevertheless, the registered nurse should positively identify donor and recipient blood types and groups on labels and the patient's chart together with another licensed professional. Blood is infused through a blood filter to exclude impurities. Medications are *never* added to blood. Blood is administered *slowly*. The IV site is frequently checked for infiltration. The patient is observed for *signs of transfusion reaction*, which include *chills, itching, rash, fever, headache,* and *pain* in the back. If such a reaction or reactions occur, the tubing should be clamped off immediately, the line kept open with normal saline solution, and the nurse in charge notified.

Transfusions with piggyback setups are common. A stopcock connects blood, normal saline, or other suitable IV solutions. When a blood transfusion must be stopped, tube patency can be maintained by opening the saline line. Necessary emergency medications can thus be administered and the site preserved for future infusions.

Circulatory overload is always a danger with children. An infusion pump is routinely used to regulate blood flow. Dyspnea, precordial pain, rales, cyanosis, dry cough, and distended neck veins are indicative of circulatory overload. Apprehension can also be a warning signal of air emboli or electrolyte disturbance. The nurse must maintain a high level of alertness for such signs, particularly in children whose conditions warrant repeated transfusions. If a reaction occurs, the blood bag and tubing are saved and returned to the blood bank. Most transfusion reactions occur within the first 10 minutes of administration; nevertheless, the patient is carefully monitored throughout this treatment. Diphenhydramine (Benadryl) may be ordered for allergic reactions. Aminophylline may be ordered for wheezing. Oxygen may be necessary to relieve dyspnea and cyanosis. To prevent cardiac dysrhythmias, a blood warmer must warm blood transfusions that are administered through central lines. Baseline data (temperature, pulse, respiration, and blood pressure) are established before transfusion, and the nurse monitors for changes. It is helpful if the parents remain with the child during this time. Suitable diversions minimize boredom.

> **Nursing Tip**
>
> If a blood transfusion reaction occurs, stop the infusion, keep the vein open with normal saline solution, and notify the charge nurse. Take the patient's vital signs and observe closely.

> **Safety Tip**
>
> Medications are never added to blood transfusions and the drip rate should be slow.

HODGKIN'S DISEASE

Pathophysiology. Also known as *Hodgkin's lymphoma,* Hodgkin's disease is a malignancy of the lymph system that primarily involves the lymph nodes. It may metastasize to the spleen, liver, bone marrow, lungs, or other parts of the body. The presence of giant multinucleated cells called *Reed-Sternberg cells* is diagnostic of the disease. Hodgkin's disease is rarely seen before 5 years of age, with the incidence increasing during adolescence and early adulthood. It is twice as common in boys as in girls. It may have a genetic origin or may be linked to a virus infection (Waxman, 2011).

Manifestations. The presenting symptom of Hodgkin's disease is generally a painless lump along the neck. Characteristically, there are few other manifestations. In general, the patient or parents first note the swelling. In more advanced cases, there may be unexplained low-grade fever, anorexia, unexplained weight loss, night sweats, general malaise, rash, and itching. Diagnosis is confirmed by x-ray films, blood tests, PET bone scans, and a biopsy of the node. The stages of Hodgkin's disease are defined in Table 27-2.

Treatment. Well-established treatment regimens are now being used to combat this illness. Both radiation therapy and chemotherapy are used in accordance with the clinical stage of the disease. The combination of cyclophosphamide and vincristine (Oncovin), procarbazine hydrochloride, and prednisone is a common protocol. It is referred to as the COPP regimen. Long-term prognosis is excellent, but long-term effects of

Table 27-2	**Criteria for Staging Hodgkin's Disease**
STAGE	**CRITERIA**
I	Restricted to single site or localized in a group of lymph nodes; asymptomatic
II	Involves two or more lymph nodes in area or on same side of diaphragm
III	Involves lymph node regions on both sides of diaphragm; involves adjacent organ or spleen
IV	Is diffuse disease; least favorable prognosis

therapy have to be monitored. Autologous or allogenic stem cell transplant is a treatment option.

Nursing Care. Nursing care is mainly directed toward symptomatic relief of the side effects of radiation therapy and chemotherapy. Education of the patient and family is paramount because most patients are cared for in the home. The nurse should explain the myriad diagnostic tests to be performed and prepare the child for the typical procedures and their aftereffects. After a lymphangiogram, for example, the skin and urine may take on a bluish color.

Children and parents should be prepared to handle the impact on self-image. The school nurse should be contacted to implement a schedule that will promote growth and development while preventing overfatigue. A common side effect of irradiation is malaise. The adolescent tires easily and may be irritable and anorectic. The skin in the treated area may be sensitive and must be protected against exposure to sunlight and irritation. After treatment, a sun-blocking agent containing para-aminobenzoic acid (PABA) should be used to prevent burning. The attending physician may prescribe an ointment to relieve itching. Nothing should be applied to the treatment area without the recommendation of the physician. There may be diarrhea after abdominal irradiation. The patient does *not* become radioactive during or after therapy.

Emotional support of the adolescent is age appropriate. Nurses must be particularly prepared for periods of anger, which may be directed at them. Suitable outlets, such as the use of a punching bag, allow for the safe direction of anger. Routine use helps to prevent a buildup of tension. The patient generally regulates his own activity. The physician advises the patient if special precautions are necessary.

The appearance of secondary sexual characteristics and menstruation may be delayed in pubescent patients. Sterility is often a side effect of the treatment. This can be a source of anxiety. Adolescents may be interested in sperm banking before immunosuppressive therapy is initiated. The nurse respects the patient concerns and can be most effective by listening empathically (Nursing Care Plan 27-2).

⭐ Nursing Care Plan 27-2   The Adolescent Receiving Cancer Chemotherapy

PATIENT DATA An adolescent is admitted for initiation of chemotherapy. She appears thin, anxious, and fearful. She asks if she is going to die.

Selected Nursing Diagnosis: Deficient knowledge related to prevention of infection that is a result of myelosuppression

Goals	Nursing Interventions	Rationales
Patient will remain free of infection as evidenced by temperature of 37.1° to 37.6° C (98.7° to 99.6° F); skin and mucous membranes will show no signs of irritation or inflammation. Patient's hemoglobin level will improve with therapy; there will be no recurrence of anemia.	Instruct patient about the body's immune system and immunotherapy as age appropriate; use visual aids. Monitor white blood cell (WBC) count and interpret blood values at patient's level of understanding. Place the patient in a private room, avoid crowds, and practice proper handwashing and good personal hygiene; monitor temperature.	A malignant process depresses the immune system at the onset of disease; chemotherapy further suppresses it and causes some physical changes that increase chances of infection. Leukopenia (decreased WBCs), which predisposes patient to infection, and thrombocytopenia (decreased platelets), which predisposes patient to bruising and bleeding, are the most serious side effects. Anemia caused by decreased erythrocyte count is also a side effect but is more easily treated. Bone marrow suppression as a side effect of chemotherapy or radiation predisposes the child to anemia, infection, and bleeding. In addition to treatment effects, patients with leukemia are particularly vulnerable because their bone marrow is depressed as a result of disease; neutropenia may result. Infection can be life threatening.
	Observe the mouth and perianal area for infection and bleeding.	Ulcerations of mouth and anus are common; meticulous rectal care will prevent natural microbial flora (*Escherichia coli*) from being introduced by a break in the mucosa. Enemas and rectal temperatures are avoided because of this. Stomatitis is a common side effect of chemotherapy.
	Use a soft toothbrush, Waterpik, and soothing mouthwashes.	Protecting membranes decreases the likelihood of capillary damage and of mucous membrane breakdown.
	Limit exposure to direct sunlight.	Photosensitivity is a side effect of some chemotherapeutic drugs.

Selected Nursing Diagnosis: Risk for impaired tissue integrity related to platelet deficit from bone marrow suppression

Goals	Nursing Interventions	Rationales
Patient shows no signs of bleeding, as evidenced by stable vital signs and absence of hematuria, petechiae, and ecchymosis.	Observe for hematuria, hematemesis, melena, epistaxis, petechiae, and ecchymosis. Increase fluid intake. Use local measures if necessary to control bleeding. Monitor platelet counts and assist the patient in types of safe activity when the count is low.	Bleeding from these sites can occur because of myelosuppression. Patient may be febrile; a liberal fluid intake also prevents hemorrhagic cystitis. Vomiting from chemotherapy may deplete fluid volume, and the patient may become dehydrated. Direct pressure reduces small hemorrhages. Avoid creating puncture wounds whenever possible; bandages and old blood are promptly removed because they provide media for infection. Children with low platelet counts are advised to avoid activities temporarily that might cause bleeding or injury (e.g., skateboarding, contact sports); aspirin is avoided because it destroys platelets.

Selected Nursing Diagnosis: Imbalanced nutrition caused by stomatitis, nausea, and vomiting

Goals	Nursing Interventions	Rationales
Patient is able to eat frequent small meals; caloric intake is adequate for age. Nausea and vomiting will decrease; patient's weight will stabilize.	Inspect mouth daily for ulcerations. Serve bland, moist, soft diet. Apply local anesthetics to ulcerated areas before meals. Monitor weight.	Mouth lesions may lead to anorexia; early treatment is necessary. Prevents trauma to mouth and lesions of the esophagus. Protects lesions and makes eating easier. Malnutrition may be present; weight loss is common owing to nature of treatments and side effects of medication, such as nausea and vomiting.

Nursing Care Plan 27-2 — The Adolescent Receiving Cancer Chemotherapy—cont'd

Alert patient to expected reactions to treatment protocol.	Preparing patient in advance reduces anxiety.
Give antiemetic before onset of nausea and vomiting.	Regularly scheduled antiemetics reduce discomfort of nausea and vomiting.
Suggest appropriate relaxation techniques.	Symptoms can be controlled or lessened by relaxation techniques.

Selected Nursing Diagnosis: Disturbed body image related to moon face, hair loss

Goals	Nursing Interventions	Rationales
Patient will verbalize some satisfaction with appearance.	Allow the adolescent to vent feelings about his or her body.	Allowing the adolescent to vent shows acceptance.
Patient will participate in self-care.	Provide continuity of care.	Adolescents need persons they can trust; continuity of care provides this.
Patient will remain in contact with peers.	Use wigs, scarves, eyebrow pencil, false eyelashes. Stress that hair loss is temporary. Suggest clothing that minimizes body changes and enhances appearance.	Looking and feeling attractive are morale boosters.
	Have the patient draw "How it feels to be sick," "How it feels to be well"; discuss.	Indirect communication is helpful for the self-conscious adolescent; drawing provides an outlet for the expression of feelings.
	Involve the patient in decision-making.	Control is important to a teen.
	Provide an opportunity for groups.	Group identity is a task of adolescence.

Selected Nursing Diagnosis: Fear of death related to treatment or nature of disease

Goals	Nursing Interventions	Rationales
Patient will express concerns regarding life expectancy.	Convey empathic understanding of patient's and family's worries, fears, and doubts.	Fear of death is like the elephant in the living room: by pretending it does not exist and refusing to discuss it, the family can also pretend that it will not happen. Because no feelings are shared, each member suffers in isolation; sharing a threat lessens the burden and brings members closer; nevertheless, sharing cannot be forced on persons who are not ready for it.
	Determine the patient's perception of diagnosis, for example, "What are your concerns?" and "How can I help?"	Misconceptions abound in life-threatening illness because the patient is in crisis and less able to absorb information.
Patient will express hope, although this may be changed from "hope" of cure to prolonged life.	Support "hope" by clarifying and by educating patient about the disease and side effects.	Hope is important to the patient and family members; it may be hope of celebrating a birthday or seeing a special friend; it may be hope that suffering will end.
	Avoid discounting the patient's experience by making statements such as "I know exactly how you feel" or "You shouldn't feel that way" or by changing the subject.	Discounting shuts down the patient's self-expression, and expression of feelings is the basis for identifying effective coping methods.
	Have patient draw and discuss "the strongest feeling I've had today."	The patient can distance himself or herself from feelings through drawings. This makes the feelings less threatening.

Critical Thinking Question

1. An adolescent receiving cancer chemotherapy has withdrawn from contact with her peers and states she is not interested in attending school. What is the best response of the nurse?

Table 27-3	The Effects of Chronic Illness on Growth and Development*	
AGE	**FEATURE**	**EFFECT**
Infancy	Trust	A visible defect can delay bonding. Prolonged illness may separate child from family.
		Irritability promotes parental negativity.
Toddler	Autonomy	Physical restrictions impede development of motor and language skills. Toilet training may be delayed. Fear may erode self-confidence. Separation anxiety occurs.
Preschooler	Initiative	Impaired ability to experience world outside of family impedes social skills. Overprotective parents delay teaching self-discipline. Child may develop negative body image. Child develops sense of guilt at his or her inability to master tasks.
School age	Industry	Loss of grade level in school because of illness and inability to participate or compete can lead to sense of inferiority. Sense of independence and accomplishment can be lost. Being different from peers may impede child's sense of belonging.
Adolescent	Identity	Adolescent feels loss of control and inability to conform to peers. The developing self-concept may become negative. Adolescent may grieve for a lost ability. Enforced dependence may impair plans for future goals. Rebellion results in decreased compliance.

*Chronic illness can impede growth and development. The nurse should reinforce teaching concerning the developmental needs of chronically ill children at different age levels to promote self-acceptance and positive self-esteem.

NURSING CARE OF THE CHRONICALLY ILL CHILD

CHRONIC ILLNESS

Chronic illness during childhood often affects growth and development (Table 27-3). Specific programs that foster feelings of security and independence within the limits of the situation are essential. Behavior problems are lessened when patients can verbalize specific concerns with persons sensitive to their problems. To be in school, and to be considered one of the group, is very important to children. If they feel rejected by and different from their peers, they may be prone to depression. Hospital school programs provide familiarity and enable patients to keep pace with their classmates. The recreational therapist may also be helpful in combating boredom and providing outlets for tension.

Nurses must help patients to accept their body with all its strengths and imperfections. They must develop an awareness of the adolescent's particular fears of forced dependence, body invasion, mutilation, rejection, and loss of face, especially within peer groups. The nurse anticipates a certain amount of reluctance to adhere to hospital regulations, which reflects the adolescent's need for self-determination. Recognizing this as an asset rather than a liability enables the nurse to respond creatively.

DEVELOPMENTAL DISABILITIES

Children who have a developmental disability that affects their intellect or ability to cope face some unique difficulties. They may often be overprotected, unable to break away from supervision, and deprived of necessary peer relationships. The pubertal process with its emerging sexuality is a concern to parents and may precipitate a family crisis.

HOME CARE

Most children with acute and chronic conditions are cared for in the home. Home health care and other community agencies work together to provide holistic care. **Respite care** provides trained workers who come into the home for brief periods to relieve parents of the responsibility of caring for the child. This enables the parents to shop, take care of business transactions, or simply take a much-needed vacation. The school systems also share in the responsibility of care, which is crucial if a family is to be successful in home care. One mother, whose 13-year-old daughter has a severe developmental disability (cerebral palsy, blindness, scoliosis, mental retardation), offered the following suggestions for the health care worker assisting in the home:

- Observe how the parents interact with the child.
- Do not wait for the child to cry out for attention, because the youngster may be unable to communicate in this way.
- Watch for facial expressions and body language.
- Post signs above the bed denoting special considerations, such as "Never position on left side" and "Do not feed with plastic spoon."
- Listen to the parents and observe how they attend to the physical needs of the youngster.
- Do not be afraid to ask questions or discuss apprehensions you may feel about your ability to care for the child.
- Be attuned to the needs of other children in the home.
- Be creative in exploring avenues for socialization, because these adolescents are seldom invited to birthday or slumber parties.
- Explore community facilities or support groups that might benefit the family.

The Chronically Ill Child as Family Member

The chronically ill child must be a contributing member to the family unit. Faced with having to choose, the child and parent will often discard the health care practice when health care activities inhibit development and prevent peer socialization opportunities. The child must be treated normally and overprotection and excessive restriction avoided. Focusing on what the child can do and providing successful experiences are more effective than focusing on the disability.

Involvement of the entire family with the care of the chronically ill child aids in normal family interaction. Respite care is needed to provide parents with the opportunity for a normal spousal relationship. The child should be integrated into, rather than isolated from, the community and society. Nurses can assist the child and the family to develop strategies to cope with chronic illness and to promote optimal growth and development. The wellness of the child should be the center of the child's life, rather than the disability.

> **Nursing Tip**
>
> When caring for a child who has a chronic illness, explain to the child what to expect, include the child in decisions and treatment, and allow the child some control whenever possible. Promote normality of routines.

NURSING CARE OF THE DYING CHILD

FACING DEATH

Facing death is often a difficult personal issue for the nurse. The nurse must understand the grieving process, personal and cultural views concerning that process, the views of a parent losing a child, and the perceptions of the child facing death. Integrating these understandings and helping all involved to cope successfully involve a multidisciplinary approach. The response to a child's death is influenced by whether there was a long period of uncertainty before the death or whether it was a sudden, unexpected event. The nurse must show compassion but function in a clinically competent, professional manner. Demonstrating a nonjudgmental approach when the personal or cultural practices of the family conflict with the nurse's own values presents a challenge. Sensitive, effective care can be provided only if the nurse is aware of these needs of the family. The nurse can facilitate the grief process by anticipating psychological and somatic responses and maintaining open communication. The family's efforts to cope, to adapt, and to grieve must be supported.

The response of the family to the death of the child may initially be manifested by somatic distress such as weakness, anguish, or shortness of breath. A family member may feel detached from the world and have a sense of unreality or disbelief. A sense of guilt and blame may follow ("I should have" or "I could have"). Hostility is a normal response and may drive away those who do not understand its normality in the acute grieving process. A restlessness and general irritability or inability to function may follow. Assistance in the care of other children or household responsibilities may be necessary. Nursing priorities include being a patient advocate and family advocate, providing support, and facilitating the grieving process.

SELF-EXPLORATION

One important, if not the most important, task to prepare for in working with the dying patient is self-exploration. Our own attitudes about life and death affect our nursing practice. Emotions buried deep within can form barriers to effective communication unless they are recognized and released. How nurses have or have not handled their own losses affects present lives and the ability to relate to patients. Nurses must recognize that **coping is an active and ongoing process.** At times, nurses need compassionate detachment from patients and their families to become revitalized. We must find constructive outlets, such as exercise and music, to maintain equilibrium. An active support system consisting of nonjudgmental people who are not threatened by natural expressions of feelings is crucial. Proper channeling of these emotions can be a valuable part of the empathetic response to others. It is vital that nurses support one another in the work environment.

THE CHILD'S REACTION TO DEATH

Each child, like each adult, approaches death in an individual way, drawing on limited experience. Nurses must become well acquainted with patients and view them within the context of the family and social culture. Their anxiety often centers on symptoms. They fear that treatments may be painful. Nurses must be honest and inform patients about the upcoming procedures in terms the child will understand. Expressing feelings is encouraged: "You seem angry." Sufficient time should be given for a response. Children should be allowed to have as much control as possible regarding what happens to them; including them in decisions concerning their welfare fosters this control. However, the child should not be offered a choice when there is none. Children often communicate symbolically. The nurse listens to what they say to adults, to their toys, and to other children. Crayons and paper are provided for self-expression.

Although age is a factor, the child's level of cognitive development, rather than chronological age, affects the response to death. Children younger than 5 years of age are mainly concerned with separation from their parents and abandonment. (Even adults are threatened by thoughts of dying alone.) Preschool children respond to questions about death by relying on their experience and by turning to fantasy. They may believe death is reversible or that they are in some way responsible. Children do not develop a realistic concept of death as a permanent biological process until 9 or 10 years of age.

Health Promotion

A Child's Response to a Sibling's Death

AGE	RESPONSE OR UNDERSTANDING	PARENTAL GUIDANCE
Infant	Does not understand concept of death; reacts on emotional level to anxiety of parents	Maintain normal routine. Use a support network to assist in care.
Preschooler	Thinks death is temporary; may blame self for sibling's death	Use accurate terms and simple explanations. Reassure child, and *listen.*
School age	Realizes death is final; may be interested in details of death; may fear parents will die; may try to "take care of" parents	Respond to child's need for reassurance and security. Refer to death using accurate terms. Allow child to participate in funeral and feel useful.
Adolescent	Can understand abstract concept of death but has feelings of own immortality; may express anger at death of sibling	Accept adolescent's behavior. Encourage communication and discussion.

Dying adolescents face conflicts between their treatment regimens and their need to establish independence from their parents and conformity with their peers. This leads to anger and resentment, which are often displaced onto hospital staff members. An atmosphere of acceptance and nonjudgmental listening allows adolescents freedom to vent their hostility in a nonthreatening environment. Nursing Care Plan 27-3 specifies nursing interventions for the dying child.

Nursing Tip

Brothers and sisters often feel neglected and lonely. They are frustrated because they are unable to comfort their parents and loved ones. They need to be included in the plan of care.

THE CHILD'S AWARENESS OF HIS OR HER CONDITION

Surprising as it may seem, many investigators have shown that terminally ill children are generally aware of their condition, even when it is carefully concealed. This is reflected in their drawings and play, and can be detected through psychological testing. Failure to be honest with children leaves them to suffer alone, unable to express their fears and sadness or even to say good-bye. The family should be referred as needed for support and social services.

PHYSICAL CHANGES OF IMPENDING DEATH

The physical changes that occur with impending death include cool, mottled, cyanotic skin and the slowing of all body processes. There may be a loss of consciousness, but hearing is intact. Rales in the chest may be heard, which result from increased secretions pooling in the lungs. Movement and neurological signs lessen. If thrashing or groaning occurs, the patient is assessed for pain, and pain relief should be provided.

STAGES OF DYING

The stages of dying as detailed by Kübler-Ross (1975)—*denial, anger, bargaining, depression, acceptance,* and reaching out to help others—can be applied to parents and siblings as well as to the sick child. (Nurses may also respond with similar feelings.) It is important to accept and support each participant at whatever stage has been reached and to refrain from directing progress. Nurses should be available and should make their availability known (Box 27-1).

Parents are encouraged to assist in the care of their child; hospice care and the movement toward supervised home care facilitate this assistance. It is therapeutic for children to be in their own surroundings whenever possible. Siblings involved in patient care feel less neglected, and the sacrifices they must make become more meaningful. Discussions before death allow them to make amends for their hostilities toward the sick child. The family's religious and spiritual philosophy can be a source of strength and support, as can caring neighbors and friends.

Statistics show a high correlation between the death of a child and divorce. Nurses must observe signs of tension between parents so that suitable intervention may be implemented. Each parent grieves in an individual time and way, often making it difficult for spouses to be supportive of each other. The suppression of strong feelings of guilt, helplessness, and outrage can be devastating. Feelings left unexpressed can cause depression and/or physical illness.

Kübler-Ross (1969) reminds us that dying is the easy part. Helping patients to live until they die is the real challenge. She discusses this beautifully in *A Letter to a Child with Cancer,* which she wrote in response to a child's question, "What is life, what is death, and why do little children have to die?" A library may be consulted to locate this classic book and other literature published especially to help children and parents with dying and grief. There are several hospices in the United States that limit their services to children. St. Mary's Hospice in Bay Side, New York, is credited as being the first of these.

Nursing Tip

Grandparents, teachers, and friends are also grieving. Be alert for the emotional responses of all of the significant others.

★ Nursing Care Plan 27-3 | The Dying Child

PATIENT DATA The parents of a terminally ill school-age child sit stoic and silent at the bedside of their child. The child appears cranky and withdrawn and states he wants to go home and see his friends.

Selected Nursing Diagnosis: Anxiety (family members), death, related to potential death of child

Goals	Nursing Interventions	Rationales
Parents will express anxieties to the nurse. Communications among parents, other children, patient, and nurse remain open.	Remain available to family as child grows weaker.	Nurse's presence provides support.
	Give parents permission to talk and grieve about the upcoming death and to think about funeral arrangements if they choose.	Helps to prepare family for the inevitable; sorts out and identifies actual sources of feelings.
	Involve siblings in plans and progress of brother or sister.	Siblings will feel less isolated.
	Provide permission for laughter, play, friends (make every day count).	Laughter and play reduce tension.
	Suggest that overprotection and inordinate attention, even when provided out of love, can be detrimental to the dying child.	Child will feel more in control if not overprotected.
	Encourage family to maintain as normal a lifestyle as possible, and encourage each member to take time for his or her own needs (e.g., continue to go to hairdresser or a movie—whatever was previously enjoyed).	When all members are taking care of themselves, they will have more energy to cope with crises.
	Facilitate honesty about child's imminent death among family members and the patient.	Information helps to relieve anxiety.
	Explain that family members often cannot support one another, because each grieves in his or her own way.	Explaining this to the family helps to relieve the guilt stemming from irritability or anger.
	Recognize that grief is often expressed as anger.	Anger is a natural emotion; it does not provoke fear in itself, although its expression may. Family has a right to all feelings.
	Provide for ventilation of guilt (e.g., "If only I had taken her to the physician sooner").	Prevents accumulation or repression of guilt.
	Suggest meditation, progressive relaxation, and/or guided imagery.	Helps to reduce stress.

Selected Nursing Diagnosis: Anxiety (dying child) related to pain, isolation, lack of information

Goals	Nursing Interventions	Rationales
Child will verbalize feelings of comfort; if nonverbal, child rests comfortably, with no crying.	Administer pain relievers as necessary.	Child may deny pain because of fear of treatment.
	Encourage parents to hold, cuddle, and touch their child as condition permits.	Reduces anxiety, thereby reducing pain.
Child is not isolated.	Encourage visits from friends and siblings as age appropriate.	Provides emotional support and distraction from the disease.
	Decorate hospital room with cards, pictures, mementos; provide telephone as age appropriate.	Attractive environment promotes mental health.
Child will verbalize understanding of treatment, procedures, and outcome as age appropriate.	Investigate possibility of home or hospice care.	Familiar and stable environment may facilitate child's emotional healing.
	Explain all procedures.	Information relieves anxiety.
	Determine child's knowledge about impending death.	Nurse can determine level of understanding as age appropriate; this aids in communication.
	Answer all questions about death honestly; use open-ended questions to assist patient in the expression of feelings.	Conveys that all feelings are acceptable.
	Listen to what child says in play.	Children work through many fears in play.
	Assist child in drawing "a wish," "yesterday, today, tomorrow."	Drawings promote the release of feelings and provide a means of communication.
	Allow the child to grieve (behavior may be sulky, cranky, withdrawn).	Therapeutic grieving prevents depression.

Continued

⭐ Nursing Care Plan 27-3 The Dying Child—cont'd

Selected Nursing Diagnosis: Grieving related to death of child

Goals	Nursing Interventions	Rationales
Family members will have an opportunity to say good-bye. Family members will express feelings of grief, fear, anger, loss, and guilt.	Provide time for family to be alone with the dead child as desired. Remain available; express your own loss and grief. Assist parents in making decisions. Offer a beverage. Determine spiritual need; refer to pastoral counseling if desired. Respect family's beliefs, worldview, and philosophy. Listen to expressions of grief.	Family needs to say good-bye. Parents derive comfort from knowing others loved their child. Even a simple decision such as when to telephone relatives becomes monumental at this stage. Denotes concern. A belief in God provides strength for many persons; pastoral counselors are effective. Many beliefs may be unconventional, but failure to be open shuts down the supportive relationship. Family needs to repeat story to work through grief.

Critical Thinking Question

1. The parents of a child dying from a terminal illness stay in the corner of the child's room, hugging each other and crying. What would be the best nursing intervention?

Box 27-1 The Nurse's Role in Helping the Family Cope with the Dying Child

Listen. Giving advice is a reflection of the nurse's need to "solve the problem."

Provide privacy. Family members need to express their emotions and comfort one another without being embarrassed.

Provide therapeutic intervention. Assess coping behaviors and work with clergy and social workers to meet immediate needs for patient comfort and family coping.

Provide information. Avoid the tenseness of waiting for test results. Be truthful to the child and family.

Use appropriate phrases and open-ended questions and concrete statements. When speaking with a sibling of a child who has died, avoid using phrases such as "he isn't hurting anymore," "he is living with God," or "he has passed away." These terms are confusing to children; explanations should be short, direct, and truthful.

Get Ready for the NCLEX® Examination!

Key Points

- Circulating blood consists of two portions: plasma and formed elements.
- Bone marrow aspiration is one procedure that is helpful in determining disorders of the blood.
- The most common nutritional deficiency of children in the United States is iron-deficiency anemia.
- Sickle cell disease is an inherited defect in the formation of hemoglobin. The cells become crescent shaped and clump together.
- Pain control with meperidine (Demerol) should not be used for children with sickle cell anemia.
- Massive expansion of the bone marrow in thalassemia causes changes in the contour of the child's skull and face.
- Hemophilia A results from a deficiency in coagulation factor VIII, and hemophilia B (Christmas disease) involves a deficiency of factor IX.
- Hemarthrosis (bleeding into the joints) is a characteristic sign of hemophilia A.

- Hemosiderosis (deposits of iron in the organs and tissues) is a complication of multiple transfusions in hemolytic blood disorders.
- Signs of transfusion reactions include chills, itching rash, fever, and headache.
- *Petechiae* are bluish pinpoint lesions on the skin. *Purpura*s are groups of adjoining petechiae, *ecchymosis* is an isolated bluish lesion larger than a petechiae, and a *hematoma* is a raised ecchymosis.
- Leukemia is the most common form of childhood cancer.
- Four priority challenges in the care of a child with leukemia are anemia, bleeding, infection, and fractures.
- Diagnostic procedures for patients with blood disorders are often invasive or painful. The nurse prepares and supports the patient and family during these procedures.
- Maintenance of schooling, adequate hydration and nutrition, prevention of infection, promotion of a positive self-image, and meticulous oral hygiene are essential components of nursing care for a child with leukemia.

- Reed-Sternberg cells are diagnostic for Hodgkin's disease.
- Children who are chronically ill must be aided in mastering developmental tasks.
- The stages of dying according to Kübler-Ross include denial, anger, bargaining, depression, acceptance, and reaching out to help others.
- The nurse can help the family of a dying child by listening and assessing their needs, reinforcing information, providing privacy, and using appropriate phrases and open-ended concrete questions and statements.

Additional Learning Resources

SG Go to your Study Guide for additional learning activities to help you master this chapter content.

evolve Go to your Evolve website (http://evolve.elsevier.com/Leifer) for the following learning resources:

- Animations
- Answer Guidelines for Critical Thinking Questions
- Answers and Rationales for Review Questions for the NCLEX® Examination
- Glossary with English and Spanish pronunciations
- Interactive Review Questions for the NCLEX® Examination
- Patient Teaching Plans in English and Spanish
- Skills Performance Checklists
- Video clips and more!

Online Resources

- Hodgkin's lymphoma and leukemia: www.lls.org
- Cooley's Anemia Foundation: www.thalassemia.org
- National Hemophilia Foundation. www.hemophilia.org
- Non-Hodgkin's lymphoma: www.oncologychannel.com/nonhodgkins

Review Questions for the NCLEX® Examination

1. When the patient experiences apprehension and urticaria while receiving a blood transfusion, the nurse:

   1. slows the transfusion and takes the patient's vital signs.
   2. observes the child for further transfusion reactions.
   3. stops the transfusion, allows normal saline solution to run slowly, and notifies the charge nurse.
   4. stops what he or she is doing and obtains the patient's history.

2. A child who is in a vasoocclusive crisis caused by sickle cell anemia is experiencing acute pain. The nurse understands that Demerol (meperidine) is not an appropriate pain medication to administer to this child because it:

   1. is very addictive.
   2. is not strong enough.
   3. may induce seizures.
   4. cannot be given by mouth.

3. Which principle should the nurse teach the parent concerning administering liquid iron preparations to the child with iron-deficiency anemia?

   1. Allow the preparation to mix with saliva and bathe the teeth before swallowing.
   2. Warm the medication before administering.
   3. Administer between meals.
   4. Administer in the bottle of formula.

4. Thalassemia major (Cooley's anemia) is treated primarily with:

   1. a diet high in iron.
   2. multiple blood transfusions.
   3. bed rest until the sedimentation rate is normal.
   4. oxygen therapy.

5. What is a characteristic manifestation of Hodgkin's disease?

   1. Petechiae
   2. Erythematous rash
   3. Enlarged lymph nodes
   4. Pallor

Objectives

1. Define each key term listed.
2. Discuss three common gastrointestinal anomalies in infants.
3. Discuss the postoperative nursing care of an infant with pyloric stenosis.
4. Discuss the dietary management of celiac disease.
5. Understand the symptoms, treatment, and nursing care of a child with Hirschsprung's disease.
6. Understand the treatment and nursing care of a child with intussusception.
7. Interpret the nursing management of an infant with gastroesophageal reflux.
8. Explain why infants and young children become dehydrated more easily than adults.
9. Differentiate between three types of dehydration.
10. Understand how nutritional deficiencies influence growth and development.
11. Review the prevention of the spread of thrush in infants and children.
12. Trace the route of the pinworm cycle and describe how reinfection takes place.
13. Prepare a teaching plan for the prevention of poisoning in children.
14. List two measures to reduce the effect of acetaminophen poisoning in children.
15. Indicate the primary source of lead poisoning.

Key Terms

anasarca (ăn-ă-SĂHR-kă, p. 658)
anthelmintics (ănt-hěl-MĬN-tĭkz, p. 662)
colitis (p. 650)
colonoscopy (p. 643)
currant jelly stools (p. 649)
encopresis (ĕn-kō-PRĒ-sĭs, p. 652)
endoscopy (p. 643)
enterocolitis (ĕn-tĕr-ō-kō-LĪ-tĭs, p. 648)
guarding (p. 661)
herniorrhaphy (hŭr-nē-ŎR-ă-fē, p. 650)
homeostasis (hō-mē-ō-STĀ-sĭs, p. 656)
hypertonic (hī-pŭr-TŎN-ĭk, p. 657)
hypotonic (hī-pō-TŎN-ĭk, p. 657)
incarcerated hernia (p. 649)

isotonic (ī-sō-TŎN-ĭk, p. 657)
McBurney's point (p. 661)
parenteral fluids (pă-RĔN-tŭr-ăl, p. 655)
pediatric capsule endoscopy (p. 667)
peritoneal dialysis (pĕ-rĭ-tŏ-NĒ-ăl dī-ĂL-ĭ-sĭs, p. 665)
pica (p. 666)
plumbism (p. 666)
polyhydramnios (pŏl-ē-hī-DRĂM-nē-ŏs, p. 644)
projectile vomiting (p. 645)
pruritus (p. 643)
pyloric stenosis (p. 645)
rebound tenderness (p. 661)
reflux (p. 651)
sigmoidoscopy (p. 643)

THE GASTROINTESTINAL TRACT

The gastrointestinal (GI) tract transports and metabolizes nutrients necessary for the life of the cell. It extends from the mouth to the anus. Nutrients are broken down into absorbable products by enzymes from various digestive organs. The anatomy of the digestive tract, with some of the differences between that of the child and that of the adult, is depicted in Figure 28-1. The primitive digestive tube is formed by the yolk sac and is divided into the foregut, the midgut, and the hindgut. The foregut evolves into the pharynx, the lower respiratory tract, the esophagus, the stomach, the duodenum, and the beginning of the common bile duct. The midgut elongates in the fifth fetal week to form the primary intestinal loop. The remainder of the large colon is derived from the primitive hindgut. The liver, pancreas, and biliary tree evolve from the foregut. The anal membrane ruptures at 8 weeks of gestation, forming the anal canal and anal opening.

As the child grows, the gastrointestinal capacity increases. A 1-week-old infant has the stomach capacity of 30 to 90 mL; a 1-month-old infant has the stomach capacity of 90 to 150 mL; a 1-year-old infant has the stomach capacity of 210 to 360 mL; and a 2-year-old has a stomach capacity of approximately 500 mL. The adult stomach has a 2000 to 3000 mL capacity

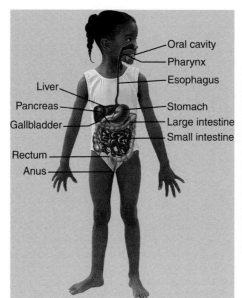

GASTROINTESTINAL SYSTEM

- At birth the resistance of the newborn's intestinal tract to bacterial and viral infection is incompletely developed.
- As children grow, they have higher nutritional, metabolic, and energy needs.
- Children with nausea and vomiting dehydrate more quickly than do adults with those symptoms.
- The infant's stomach is small and empties rapidly.
- Newborns produce little saliva until 3 months of age.
- Swallowing is a reflex for the first 3 months.
- Hepatic efficiency in the newborn is immature, sometimes causing jaundice.
- The infant's fat absorption is poor because of a decreased pool of bile acid.

FIGURE 28-1 Some of the gastrointestinal system differences between the child and adult. The digestive system consists of the digestive tract and the glands that secrete digestive juices into the digestive tract. This system mechanically and chemically breaks down food and eliminates wastes. (Art overlay courtesy Observatory Group, Cincinnati, OH.)

(Collopy, 2010). Many enzymes necessary for digestion are deficient until 4 to 6 months of age. Understanding the physiology of the pediatric digestive tract is the basis to the plan for introduction of new foods during the first year and avoidance of problems that can occur with overfeeding (AAP, 2011).

DISORDERS AND DYSFUNCTION OF THE GASTROINTESTINAL TRACT

A number of procedures are available to determine GI disorders. Laboratory work, such as a complete blood count (CBC) with differential, will show anemia, infections, and chronic illness. An elevated erythrocyte sedimentation rate (ESR) is indicative of inflammation. A comprehensive chemical panel will show electrolyte and chemical imbalances. Often-used x-ray studies include GI series, barium enema, and flat plates of the abdomen. **Endoscopy** allows direct visualization of the GI tract through a flexible lighted tube. Upper endoscopy permits visualization and biopsy of the esophagus, the stomach, and the duodenum. It is also valuable for use in removing foreign objects and cauterizing bleeding vessels. Visualization of the bile and pancreatic ducts is also possible through endoscopy. The lower colon is inspected by **sigmoidoscopy**. **Colonoscopy** provides visualization of the entire colon to the ileocecal valve. Stool cultures and rectal biopsy are also important diagnostic tools. Ultrasonography is a noninvasive procedure useful in visualizing intestinal organs and masses, particularly of the liver and pancreas. Some liver function blood tests include alanine aminotransferase (ALT), aspartate aminotransferase (AST), prothrombin time (PT), and partial thromboplastin time (PTT). Liver biopsy may also be indicated.

Overall malabsorption tests, such as the 72-hour fecal fat test and the Schilling test (which can determine the absorption capacity of the lower ileum) are also useful. For more detailed information concerning preparation for various tests, refer to a laboratory diagnostics textbook.

Symptoms of GI disorders may be manifested by systemic signs, such as *failure to thrive* (FTT; failure to develop according to established growth parameters such as height, weight, and head circumference) or jaundice. **Pruritus** (itching) in the absence of allergy may indicate liver dysfunction. Local manifestations of a GI disorder include pain, vomiting, diarrhea, constipation, rectal bleeding, and hematemesis.

Nursing intervention focuses on providing adequate nutrition and freedom from infection, which can result from malnutrition or depressed immune function. Developmental delays in children should be investigated to determine whether they are related to the GI system. Skin problems in these patients may be related to pruritus from liver disease, irritation from frequent bowel movements, or other disorders. Pain and discomfort may occur during acute episodes; however, they may also result from medication side effects, or they may be referred pain. Cleft lip and cleft palate are discussed in Chapter 14. Anorexia is discussed in Chapter 33, and necrotizing enterocolitis is discussed in Chapter 13. Oral care in health and in illness are discussed in Chapter 15.

CONGENITAL DISORDERS

Esophageal Atresia (Tracheoesophageal Fistula)

Pathophysiology. **Atresia of the esophagus** (tracheoesophageal fistula [TEF]) is caused by a failure of the tissues of the GI tract to separate properly from the

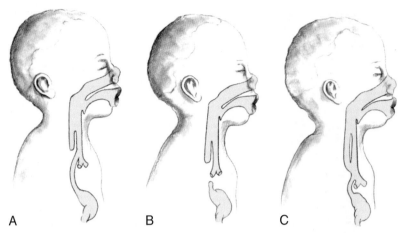

FIGURE 28-2 Esophageal atresia (failure of the esophagus to contact with the stomach), or tracheoesophageal fistula (TEF). The three most common types of TEF are **(A)** the upper esophagus ending in a blind pouch and the lower esophagus ending in the trachea; **(B)** the upper esophagus and the lower esophagus ending in a blind pouch (fetal swallowing is prevented, and the mother will develop polyhydramnios during pregnancy); and **(C)** both the upper and the lower esophagus end in the trachea. In TEF, the newborn will have excessive mucous secretions (drooling) and may choke or vomit if fed.

respiratory tract early in prenatal life. There are four types of TEF:

1. The upper esophagus and the lower esophagus (leading from the stomach) end in a blind pouch.
2. The upper esophagus ends in a blind pouch; the lower esophagus (leading from the stomach) connects to the trachea.
3. The upper esophagus is attached to the trachea; the lower esophagus (leading from the stomach) is also attached to the trachea.
4. The upper esophagus connects to the trachea; the lower esophagus (leading from the stomach) ends in a blind pouch.

The diagnosis of this condition is based on clinical manifestations and is confirmed by x-ray study (Figure 28-2). TEF occurs in approximately 1 in 4000 neonates (Khan, 2011).

Manifestations. The earliest sign of TEF occurs prenatally when the mother develops **polyhydramnios**. When the upper esophagus ends in a blind pouch, the fetus cannot swallow the amniotic fluid, resulting in an accumulation of fluid in the amniotic sac (polyhydramnios). At birth the infant will vomit and choke when the first feeding is introduced. Because the upper end of the esophagus ends in a blind pouch, the newborn cannot swallow accumulated secretions and will appear to be drooling. Although drooling after age 3 months is related to teething, drooling in a newborn is pathological and is related to atresia. If the upper esophagus enters the trachea, the first feeding will enter the trachea and result in coughing, choking, cyanosis, and apnea. If the lower end of the esophagus (from the stomach) enters the trachea, air will enter the stomach each time the infant breathes, causing abdominal distention.

Nursing Tip

Drooling in the newborn is pathological because the salivary glands do not develop for several months.

Treatment and Nursing Care. The nursing goals involve preventing pneumonia, choking, and apnea in the newborn. Assessment of every newborn during the first feeding is essential. The first feeding usually consists of clear water or colostrum (if breastfed) to minimize the seriousness of aspiration should it occur. If symptoms are noted, the infant is placed on NPO status (nothing by mouth), suctioned to clear the airway, and positioned to drain mucus from the nose and throat. Surgical repair is essential for survival.

Imperforate Anus

Pathophysiology. **Imperforate anus** occurs in about 1 of every 5000 live births. The lower GI tract and the anus arise from two different tissues. Early in fetal life the two tissues meet and join; the tissue separating them then perforates, allowing for a passageway between the lower GI tract and the anus. When this perforation does not occur, the lower end of the GI tract and the anus end in blind pouches. This is called *imperforate anus.* There are four types of imperforate anus, ranging from a stenosis to complete separation or failure of the anus to form.

Manifestations. A routine part of the newborn assessment is determining the patency of the anus. Often the first temperature of the newborn is taken rectally to ascertain patency. (All subsequent and routine temperature readings are usually taken via the axillary route.) Failure to pass meconium in the first 24 hours must be reported. Infants should not be discharged to the home before a meconium stool is passed.

ⓘ Safety Alert!

Newborn infants should not be discharged before a meconium stool is observed and recorded.

Treatment and Nursing Care. After a diagnosis of imperforate anus is established, the infant is given nothing by mouth and is prepared for surgery. Diagnosis is confirmed by x-ray study or magnetic resonance imaging (MRI). The initial surgical procedure may be a colostomy. Subsequent surgery can reestablish the patency of the anal canal.

Pyloric Stenosis

Pathophysiology. **Pyloric stenosis** (narrowing) is an obstruction at the lower end of the stomach (pylorus) caused by an overgrowth (hypertrophy) of the circular muscles of the pylorus or by spasms of the sphincter. This condition is commonly classified as a congenital anomaly; however, its symptoms do not appear until the infant is 2 or 3 weeks old. Pyloric stenosis is the most common surgical condition of the digestive tract in infancy (Figure 28-3). Its incidence is higher in boys than in girls, and although it may have a genetic predisposition, bottle-fed infants are at higher risk because it is thought that the bottle-fed infant consumes a larger amount with each suck, causing increased pressure against the pyloric muscle that requires forceful contractions resulting in the development of muscle hypertrophy. Breast milk has a lower osmolarity and contains hormones and peptides that relax the GI muscles and therefore *may* protect against the development of muscle hypertrophy (Krogh, 2012).

Manifestations. Vomiting is the outstanding symptom of this disorder. The force progresses until most of the food is ejected a considerable distance from the mouth. This is termed **projectile vomiting**, and it occurs immediately after feeding. The vomitus contains mucus and ingested milk. The infant is constantly hungry and will eat again immediately after vomiting. Dehydration as evidenced by a sunken fontanelle, inelastic skin, and

decreased urination, as well as malnutrition, can develop. An olive-shaped mass may be felt in the right upper quadrant of the abdomen. Ultrasonography or scintiscans are commonly used today for diagnostic purposes, because they are noninvasive and accurate. In severe cases the outline of the distended stomach and peristaltic waves are visible during feeding.

Treatment. The surgery performed for pyloric stenosis is called a *pyloromyotomy* (*pylorus, myo,* "muscle," and *tomy,* "incision of"). The surgeon incises the pyloric muscle to enlarge the opening so food may easily pass through it again. This is done as soon as possible if the infant is not dehydrated.

Nursing Care. The dehydrated infant is given intravenous (IV) fluids preoperatively to restore fluid and electrolyte balance. If this is not done, shock may occur during surgery. Thickened feedings may be provided until the time of operation with the hope that some nutrients will be retained. The physician prescribes the degree of thickness of the formula, which is given by teaspoon or through a nipple with a large hole. The infant is burped *before* as well as *during* feedings to remove any gas accumulated in the stomach. The feeding is done slowly, and the infant is handled gently and as little as possible. The infant is placed on the right side after feedings to facilitate drainage into the intestine. Fowler's position is preferred to aid gravity in passing milk through the stomach (see Fowler's sling, Figure 28-8). If vomiting occurs, the nurse may be instructed to *refeed* the infant. Charting of the feeding includes time, type, and amount offered, the amount taken and retained, and the type and amount of vomiting. The nurse also notes whether the infant appeared hungry after the feeding or if vomiting occurred again.

The nurse obtains and records a baseline weight and weighs the infant at about the same time each morning. Other factors to be charted include the type and number of stools and the color of urine and frequency of voiding (intake and output). Position is changed frequently, because the infant is weak and vulnerable to pneumonia. All procedures designed to protect from infection must be strictly performed.

The care of the infant after surgery includes a careful observation of vital signs and the administration of IV fluids. The wound site is inspected frequently (see Chapter 22 for postoperative care). The surgery involves cutting into the hypertrophied muscle but not through the mucous membrane of the bowel; therefore the infant will not need nasogastric decompression postoperatively and will be able to resume oral feedings shortly after recovering from anesthesia. The physician prescribes oral feedings of small amounts of glucose water that gradually increase until a regular formula can be taken and retained. Overfeeding is avoided, and the nurse reviews feeding techniques with parents. The diaper is placed low over the abdomen to prevent contamination of the wound site (Clinical Pathway 28-1).

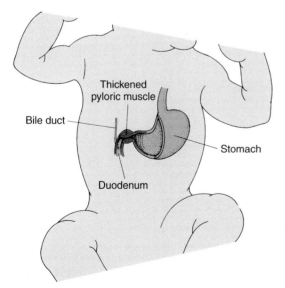

FIGURE 28-3 Pyloric stenosis. Hypertrophy or thickening of the pyloric sphincter blocks passage of the stomach contents, causing the infant to regurgitate forcefully. Serious electrolyte imbalances ultimately occur, and surgery is necessary to correct the condition. (From Betz C, Hunsburger M, Wright S: *Family-centered nursing care of children,* ed 2, Philadelphia, 1994, Saunders.)

Labels in figure: Thickened pyloric muscle; Bile duct; Stomach; Duodenum

Clinical Pathway 28-1 **An Interdisciplinary Plan of Care for the Infant with Pyloric Stenosis**

NURSING DIAGNOSIS	DAY: ADMISSION	DAY: POSTOP 1	DAY: POSTOP 2
Patient and Family Intermediate Outcomes			
Deficient fluid volume related to effects of persistent vomiting	Child shows improved fluid and electrolyte balance.	Child demonstrates normal fluid and electrolyte balance, as evidenced by normal urine output (1 mL/kg/hr), moist mucous membranes, good skin turgor, laboratory values within normal limits.	⟶
Imbalanced nutrition: less than body requirements related to persistent vomiting	Child stops vomiting.	Child ingests and retains small amounts of formula.	Child ingests and retains sufficient nutrients to meet dietary needs.
Acute pain related to incision, muscle cutting, and manipulation during surgery		Child has signs of pain recognized and interventions are promptly implemented. Child experiences minimal levels of pain.	⟶
Deficient knowledge related to treatments, surgery, postoperative care	Parents verbalize understanding of treatments and surgery.	Parents verbalize understanding of postoperative pain management, feeding, and incision care.	Parents verbalize understanding of home care and follow-up needs.
Care Intervention Categories			
Consults	Surgical consult		
Labs	CBC, electrolytes Repeat electrolytes prn to monitor Cl and CO_2 values.		
Medications and IVs	IV fluids: maintenance and replacement Provide acetaminophen with codeine or acetaminophen prn for pain.	Saline- or heparin-lock IV when tolerating PO fluids.	Discontinue IV if tolerating PO fluids.
Nutrition	NPO	Administer 10 mL oral electrolyte solution after recovery from anesthesia; start pyloric refeeding protocol (increasing feeding volumes from clear fluids to dilute to full-strength formula); repeat previous step if emesis x1, notify surgeon if emesis x2.	Provide full-strength formula at normal feeding volumes.
Pain management	Provide acetaminophen with codeine or plain (see "Medications and IVs" earlier in this table). Flex knees; position to avoid stretching abdominal muscles. Burp frequently to avoid abdominal distention.	⟶	⟶
Procedures	NG tube to gravity drainage	Discontinue NG tube before starting feedings.	
Radiology	Sonogram of abdomen and barium study as needed to confirm diagnosis		
Teaching and discharge planning	Teach parents about preoperative care routines. Teach parents about surgical routines; review postoperative care.	Teach parents methods of pain assessment and management; reintroduce feedings; provide incision care. Assess the supplies that will be needed at home (medications, dressings) and the ability of parents to obtain them.	Evaluate parent's ability to manage pain, feeding, and caring for incision; review techniques prn. Discharge child when full oral feedings are tolerated.

Continued

Clinical Pathway 28-1	An Interdisciplinary Plan of Care for the Infant with Pyloric Stenosis—cont'd		
NURSING DIAGNOSIS	**DAY: ADMISSION**	**DAY: POSTOP 1**	**DAY: POSTOP 2**
Care Intervention Categories			
Vital signs and baseline parameters	Vital signs with blood pressure on admission and q4h	⟶	⟶
	Daily weight	⟶	⟶
	Urine specific gravity each shift	⟶	⟶
	Intake and output	⟶	⟶

CBC, Complete blood count; *Cl*, chloride; *CO₂*, carbon dioxide; *IV*, intravenous route; *NG*, nasogastric; *NPO*, nothing by mouth; *PO*, by mouth; prn, as needed.
Modified from Bowden VR, Dickey SB, Greenberg CS: *Children and their families: the continuum of care*, Philadelphia, 1998, Saunders.

Celiac Disease

Pathophysiology. **Celiac disease** is also known as *gluten enteropathy* and *sprue* and is the leading malabsorption problem in children, affecting 1 in 266 people worldwide and 1% of the adult population in the United States (McCabe, 2012) (Figure 28-4). It is an autoimmune genetic illness that affects the small intestine because of gluten intolerance and resolves with removal of gluten from the diet.

Manifestations. Symptoms are not evident until 6 months to 2 years of age, when foods containing gluten are introduced to the infant. Gluten is found in *wheat, barley, oats,* and *rye*. Repeated exposure to gluten damages the villi in the mucous membranes of the intestine, resulting in malabsorption of food. The infant presents with failure to thrive. Stools are large, bulky, and frothy because of undigested contents. The infant is irritable. Diagnosis is confirmed by serum immunoglobulin A (IgA) test, other autoantibodies, and small bowel biopsy. The characteristic profile of a child with a malabsorption syndrome is abdominal distention with atrophy of the buttocks.

According to the National Institute of Health (Sapone, 2012), celiac disease is classified into 4 types:
1. *Classic celiac disease* involves atrophy of the villi of the small intestine and is characterized by malabsorption, diarrhea and abdominal pain.
2. *Atypical celiac disease* involves the duodenum and includes mild GI symptoms such as reflux and bloating. Malabsorption is manifested by anemia, fatigue, and peripheral nerve problems.
3. *Silent celiac disease* is diagnosed when the atrophy of the intestinal villi is discovered by endoscopy or biopsy that may be done for other reasons, or by a positive blood test.
4. *Latent celiac disease* may not have atrophy of the intestinal villi but may manifest a wheat sensitivity by a recurring rash.

> **! Safety Alert!**
> A bulky, frothy stool may indicate malabsorption.

Treatment and Nursing Care. The treatment for celiac disease involves a lifelong diet restricted in wheat, barley, and rye. Often, oats are avoided because they are routinely contaminated with wheat during the growing and processing (McCabe, 2012). It is a nursing challenge to teach the family the importance of dietary compliance, because tiny amounts of gluten can cause damage to the villi of the intestines. Maintaining a gluten-free diet is a challenge because gluten is often expressed on labels as a "malt," and it is in emulsifiers, stabilizers, meat substitutes, and thickening agents in many processed foods, soups, and candy. A professional nutritionist or dietitian can aid in identifying foods that are gluten free. Long-term bowel pathology can occur if dietary compliance is not lifelong.

Families may be referred to www.csaceliacs.org for information and resources.

Hirschsprung's Disease (Aganglionic Megacolon)

Pathophysiology. **Hirschsprung's disease,** or aganglionic megacolon, occurs when there is an absence of ganglionic innervation to the muscle of a segment of the bowel. This usually happens in the lower portion of the sigmoid colon. Because of the absence of nerve cells,

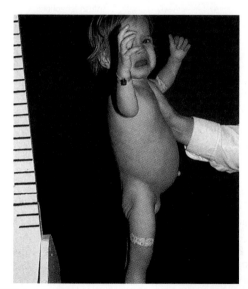

FIGURE 28-4 A child with celiac disease. Note that the classic profile of a child with a malabsorption syndrome is an enlarged abdomen with atrophy of the buttocks. (From Zitelli BJ et al: *Zitelli and Davis' atlas of pediatric physical diagnosis*, ed 6, Philadelphia, 2012, Saunders.)

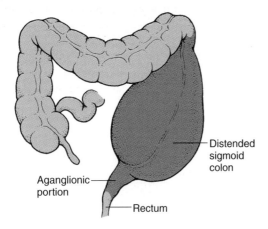

FIGURE 28-5 Hirschsprung's disease (megacolon). There is no ganglionic nerve innervation or peristalsis in the narrowed section. The adjacent bowel becomes enlarged, causing distention of the abdomen. (From Bowden VR, Dickey SB, Greenberg, SC: *Children and their families: The continuum of care*. Philadelphia, 1998, Saunders.)

there is a lack of normal peristalsis. This results in chronic constipation. Ribbonlike stools are seen as a result of feces passing through the narrow segment. The portion of the bowel nearest to the obstruction dilates, causing abdominal distention (Figure 28-5). It is seen more often in boys than girls, and it has familial tendencies. The incidence is approximately 1 in 5000 live births. There is a higher incidence in children with Down syndrome. The condition may be acute or chronic.

Manifestations. In the newborn, failure to pass meconium stools within 24 to 48 hours may be a symptom of Hirschsprung's disease. In the infant, constipation, ribbonlike stools, abdominal distention, anorexia, vomiting, and failure to thrive may be evident. Often the parent brings the young child to the clinic after trying several over-the-counter laxatives to treat the constipation without success. If the child is untreated, other signs of intestinal obstruction and shock might be seen. The development of **enterocolitis** (inflammation of the small bowel and colon) is a serious complication. A fever, explosive stools, and depletion of strength may signal enterocolitis. Diagnostic evaluation usually includes a barium enema and rectal biopsy, and it shows a lack of innervation. Anorectal manometry tests the strength of the internal rectal sphincter. In this procedure a balloon catheter is placed into the rectum, and the pressure exerted against it is measured.

Treatment and Nursing Care. Megacolon is treated by surgery. The impaired part of the colon is removed, and an anastomosis of the intestine is performed. In newborns a temporary colostomy may be necessary, and more extensive repair may follow at about 12 to 18 months of age. Closure of the colostomy follows in a few months.

Nursing care is age dependent. In the newborn, detection is a high priority. As the child grows older, careful attention to a history of constipation and

diarrhea is important. Signs of undernutrition, abdominal distention, and poor feedings are suspect.

Because the distended bowel in a child with megacolon provides a larger mucous membrane surface area that will come in contact with fluid inserted during an enema, an increased absorption of the fluid can be anticipated. For this reason, when a child is given an enema at home, normal saline solution, not tap water, is used. Tap water enemas in infants and small children can lead to water intoxication and death. Parents can obtain normal saline solution from the pharmacy without prescription, or they can make it at home by using one half of a teaspoon of noniodized salt in 1 cup of lukewarm tap water. The health care provider should determine the amount of fluid administered. The nurse stresses to parents the importance of using saline solution. Postoperative care of children is discussed in Chapter 22.

Intussusception

Pathophysiology. **Intussusception** (*intus*, "within," and *suscipere*, "to receive") is a slipping of one part of the intestine into another part just below it (Figure 28-6). It is often seen at the ileocecal valve, where the small intestine opens into the ascending colon. The mesentery, a double fan–shaped fold of peritoneum that covers most of the intestine and is filled with blood vessels and nerves, is also pulled along. Edema occurs. At first this telescoping of the bowel causes intestinal obstruction, but strangulation takes place as peristalsis forces the structures more tightly. This portion may burst, causing peritonitis.

Intussusception generally occurs in boys between 3 months and 6 years of age who are otherwise healthy. Its frequency decreases after age 36 months. Occasionally the condition corrects itself without treatment. This

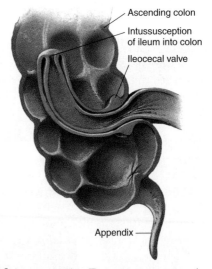

FIGURE 28-6 Intussusception. The most common type begins at or near the ileocecal valve, with this part of the intestines (bowel) pushing into the cecum and on to the colon. At first the obstruction is partial, but complete obstruction occurs as the bowel becomes inflamed and edematous. (From McKinney ES et al: *Nursing care of children: Principles and practice*, ed 2, Philadelphia, 2005, Saunders.)

is termed a spontaneous reduction. However, because the patient's life is in danger, the physician does not waste time waiting for this to occur. The prognosis is good when the patient is treated within 24 hours.

Manifestations. In typical cases the onset is sudden. The infant feels severe pain in the abdomen, as evidenced by loud cries, straining efforts, and kicking and drawing of the legs toward the abdomen. At first there is comfort between pains, but the intervals shorten and the condition becomes worse. The child vomits. The stomach contents are green or greenish yellow (this results from bile stain), and the contents are described as bilious. Bowel movements diminish, and little flatus is passed. Movements of blood and mucus that contain no feces are common about 12 hours after the onset of the obstruction; these are termed **currant jelly stools**. The child's fever may run as high as 41.1° C (106° F), and signs of shock, such as sweating, weak pulse, and shallow, grunting respirations are evident. The abdomen is rigid (DeLoach, 2013).

Treatment and Nursing Care. **Intussusception is an emergency,** and because of the severity of symptoms, most parents contact a physician promptly. The diagnosis is determined by the history and physical findings. The physician may feel a sausage-shaped mass in the right upper portion of the abdomen during bimanual rectal and abdominal palpation. Abdominal films also may indicate the mass. A barium enema is the treatment of choice, with surgery scheduled if reduction is not achieved. The recurrence rate after barium enema reduction is approximately 10%.

During the operation a small incision is made into the abdomen, and the wayward intestine is "milked" back into position. The intestine is inspected for gangrene; if all is well, the abdomen is sutured. Barring complications, recovery is straightforward. If the intestine cannot be reduced or if gangrene has set in, a bowel resection is performed and the affected area is removed. The cut end of the ileum is joined to the cut end of the colon; this is called an anastomosis. Routine preoperative and postoperative care is discussed in Chapter 22.

Meckel's Diverticulum
Pathophysiology. During fetal life the intestine is attached to the yolk sac by the vitelline duct. A small blind pouch may form if this duct fails to disappear completely. This condition is termed **Meckel's diverticulum**. It usually occurs near the ileocecal valve, and it may be connected to the umbilicus by a cord. A fistula may also form. This sac is subject to inflammation, much like the appendix. This disorder is the most common congenital malformation of the GI tract. It is seen more often in boys.

Manifestations. Symptoms may occur at any age but appear most often before 2 years of age. Painless bleeding from the rectum is the most common sign. Bright red or dark red blood is more usual than tarry stools. Abdominal pain may or may not be present. In some persons it may exist without causing symptoms. Barium enema and radionuclide scintigraphy are useful in diagnosing Meckel's diverticulum. X-ray films are not helpful, because the pouch is so small that it may not appear on the screen.

Treatment and Nursing Care. The diverticulum is removed by surgery. Nursing care is the same as for the patient undergoing exploration of the abdomen. Because this condition appears suddenly and bleeding causes parental anxiety, emotional support is of particular importance.

Hernias
Pathophysiology. An **inguinal hernia** is a protrusion of part of the abdominal contents through the inguinal canal in the groin. It is more common in boys than in girls. It is also commonly seen in preterm infants. An *umbilical* hernia is a protrusion of a portion of intestine through the umbilical ring (an opening in the muscular area of the abdomen through which the umbilical vessels pass, Figure 28-7). This type of hernia appears as a soft swelling covered by skin, which protrudes when the infant cries or strains. Hernias may be present at birth (congenital) or may be acquired, and they can vary in size. A hernia is called reducible if it can be put back into place by gentle pressure; if this cannot be done, it is called an *irreducible* or an **incarcerated hernia**. Incarceration (constriction) occurs more often in infants less than 10 months of age. Hernias may be bilateral.

Manifestations. The infant with a hernia may be relatively free of symptoms. Irritability, fretfulness, and constipation are sometimes evident. The diagnosis is made when physical examination shows a mass in the area that reappears from time to time, particularly when the child cries or strains. A *strangulated* hernia occurs when the intestine becomes caught in the passage and the blood supply is diminished. This happens

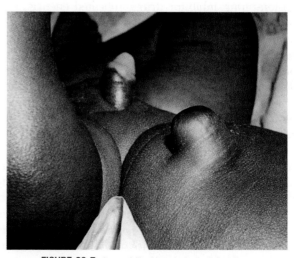

FIGURE 28-7 An umbilical hernia in an infant boy.

more often during the first 6 months of life. Vomiting and severe abdominal pain are present. Emergency surgery is necessary if strangulation occurs, and in some cases a bowel resection is performed.

Treatment and Nursing Care. Hernias are successfully repaired by the surgical operation called a **herniorrhaphy**. This is a relatively simple procedure and is well tolerated by the child. Most children are scheduled for procedures in same-day surgery units. The benefits of this method are both economic and psychological. Parents are instructed to bring the fasting child to the hospital about 1 hour before surgery. Parents remain with the child during the entire time except during the actual procedure. They are encouraged to assist in routine postoperative care.

Often no dressing is applied to the wound. Sometimes a waterproof collodion dressing, which looks like clear nail polish, is applied. Postoperative care is directed toward keeping the wound clean. Diapers are left open for this purpose. Wet diapers are changed frequently.

DISORDERS OF MOTILITY

Gastroenteritis

Pathophysiology. **Gastroenteritis** involves an inflammation of the stomach and the intestines; **colitis** involves an inflammation of the colon; enterocolitis involves an inflammation of the colon and the small intestine. The most common noninfectious causes of diarrhea involve food intolerance, overfeeding, improper formula preparation, or ingestion of high amounts of sorbitol (a substance found in sweetened "sugar-free" products). The priority problem in diarrhea is fluid and electrolyte imbalance and failure to thrive. *C. difficile* is a spore-forming, anaerobic grampositive bacillus and is the most common type of diarrhea associated with antimicrobial therapy and so is considered a health-care associated condition. Symptoms may include abdominal pain, fever, and bloody diarrhea. Risk factors for *C. difficile* diarrhea include contamination in the hospital environment, which is associated with the use of antimicrobial drugs, proton-pump inhibitor drugs, repeated enemas, prolonged nasogastric tube use, GI surgery, and impaired immunity. Diagnosis in children may be difficult because the *C. difficile* toxin tests are not reliable in children less than 3 years of age. The toxin can be shed in the stool for 4 weeks after treatment. Antidiarrheal drugs are not used because they hide the signs and symptoms. The child with *C. difficile* diarrhea should be placed on contact precautions (AAP, 2013).

Treatment and Nursing Care. Treatment of motility disorders is focused on identifying and eradicating the cause. *C. difficile* diarrhea is treated with metronidazole. The use of probiotics during broad-spectrum antibiotic treatment may prevent the development of *C. difficile* diarrhea (Johnston, 2012). Nursing

Table 28-1	Clarifying Food Labels
INGREDIENT LISTED	**MAY CONTAIN THIS:**
Binder	Egg
Bulking agent	Soy
Casein	Cow's milk (often in canned tuna)
Coagulant	Egg
Emulsifier	Egg
Protein extender	Soy

responsibilities include teaching parents and caregivers proper and age-appropriate diet and feeding techniques. The priority goal of care includes preventing fluid and electrolyte imbalance.

Oral rehydrating solutions (ORS) such as Pedialyte, Lytren, Ricelyte, and Resol are used for infants in small, frequent feedings. Although formula feeding is withheld, breastfeeding can accompany oral rehydration therapy (ORT) because of breast milk's osmolarity, antimicrobial properties, and enzyme content.

The nursing care of gastroenteritis includes maintaining intake and output records and providing skin care and frequent diaper changes to prevent excoriation from the frequent stools. Parents should be taught good handwashing techniques, proper food handling, and principles of cleanliness and infection prevention. The infant should be weighed daily, observed for dehydration or overhydration, and kept warm. Transmission-based contact precautions should be used to prevent the spread of infection (see Appendix A). Sometimes parents need help in interpreting food labels to avoid foods to which their child may be allergic. Table 28-1 lists some terms that often need clarification for the parents of a child who is food intolerant.

 Nursing Tip

Hand hygiene with soap and water rather than an alcohol-based hand sanitizer is recommended when caring for patients with *C. difficile* diarrhea. The environment should be cleaned with a bleach disinfectant by housekeeping staff.

Vomiting

Pathophysiology. **Vomiting,** a common symptom during infancy and childhood, results from sudden contractions of the diaphragm and the muscles of the stomach. It must be evaluated in relation to the child's overall health status. Persistent vomiting requires investigation because it results in dehydration and electrolyte imbalance. The continuous loss of hydrochloric acid and sodium chloride from the stomach can cause alkalosis. In this condition the acid-base balance of the body becomes disturbed because of a loss of chlorides and potassium. This can result in death if left untreated.

Manifestations. The child may vomit from various causes. Some causes stem from improper feeding techniques that should be assessed by the nurse. Sometimes the difficulty lies with formula intolerance. The introduction of foods of a different consistency may also precipitate this symptom.

Other causes of vomiting are systemic illness such as increased intracranial pressure or infection. Aspiration pneumonia is a serious complication of vomiting. In aspiration, vomitus is drawn into the air passages on inspiration, causing immediate death in extreme cases. Health professionals and laypersons should become familiar with lifesaving procedures such as cardiopulmonary resuscitation (CPR) for use in such emergencies.

Treatment and Nursing Care. To prevent vomiting the nurse must carefully feed and burp the infant. Treatments are avoided immediately after feedings. The infant is handled as little as possible after feedings. To prevent aspiration of vomitus the nurse places the infant on the right side following feedings. When an older child begins to vomit, the head is turned to one side, and an emesis basin and tissues are provided.

Factors to be charted include time, amount, color (e.g., bloody, bile-stained), consistency, force, frequency, and whether or not vomiting was preceded by nausea or by feedings. IV fluids may be given. Oral fluids are withheld for a short time to allow the stomach to rest. Gradually, sips of water are provided according to the infant's tolerance and condition. The infant's intake and output are carefully recorded so that the physician is able to compare the urine output with the total fluid intake.

Drugs such as trimethobenzamide (Tigan) or promethazine (Phenergan) may be prescribed when vomiting is persistent. They are available in rectal suppository form. The nurse lubricates the suppository and inserts it into the rectum, where it dissolves. Slight pressure is exerted over the anus for a short time to ensure that the suppository is not expelled. Charting includes the time administered and whether or not vomiting subsided.

Gastroesophageal Reflux (GER)

Pathophysiology. Gastroesophageal **reflux** (GER, or chalasia) results when the lower esophageal sphincter is relaxed or not competent, which allows stomach contents to be easily regurgitated into the esophagus.

The term *chalasia* is derived from the Greek word *chalasis*, which means "relaxation." Although many infants have this condition to a small degree, about 1 in 300 to 1 in 1000 has significant reflux and associated complications. The condition is associated with neuromuscular delay and is often seen in preterm infants and children with neuromuscular disorders, such as cerebral palsy and Down syndrome. In many infants the symptoms decrease at around age 12 months, when the child stands upright and eats more solid foods. Gastroesophageal reflux disease (GERD) implies inflammation of the esophagus, weight loss, abdominal pain, and back arching that accompanies the spitting-up or regurgitation.

Manifestations. Symptoms include vomiting, weight loss, and failure to thrive. The vomiting occurs within the first and second weeks of life. The infant is fussy and hungry. Respiratory problems can occur when vomiting stimulates the closure of the epiglottis and the infant presents with apnea. Aspiration of vomitus can also occur.

Treatment and Nursing Care. A careful history is taken. Of particular interest is when the vomiting started, type of formula, type of vomiting, feeding techniques, and the infant's eating in general. Tests used to determine the presence of GERD include scintigraphy, which involves the infant drinking a radioactively labeled formula and following the path of the fluid with imaging studies to determine the presence of reflux or poor swallowing coordination. Prolonged esophageal pH monitoring is one of the most definitive diagnostic tests, which helps to determine the acuity of the disease and the course of treatment to prevent esophagitis.

Therapy depends on the severity of symptoms. Most parents need only reassurance and education about feeding the infant. Teaching should include careful burping, avoiding overfeeding (which distends the stomach), and proper positioning. A general guide to determine optimum intake to prevent gastric distention is to feed the infant no more than the age in months plus 3, every 3 to 4 hours. For example, a 3-month-old infant should be fed a maximum of 6 oz in one feeding (Weill, 2008).

Medication and surgical intervention may be required for infants with more complicated GERD. Parents are instructed to burp the infant frequently. Feedings can be thickened with cereal (1 teaspoon to 1 tablespoon of cereal per ounce of formula). Adding cereal to the formula increases the caloric density from 20 calories per ounce to 27 calories per ounce. The formula Enfamil AR is a milk-based formula with added rice starch for thickness that provides 20 calories per ounce (see Table 16-3). However there may be an association between thickened formula and the development of necrotizing enterocolitis in preterm infants (Lightdale, 2013).

After being fed, the infant should be placed in an upright position or propped on the left side. The body is inclined about 30 to 40 degrees, and the infant is held in place by a Fowler's sling (Figure 28-8). Sitting upright in an infant seat or swing is not recommended because it increases intraabdominal pressure. The upright prone position has been recommended for the infant with GERD when awake and monitored. (The supine [back] sleep position is recommended for all healthy infants.) Medications that relax the pyloric sphincter, and promote stomach emptying may be used, such as histamine H_2-receptor antagonists Zantac (ranitidine), or Pepcid (famotidine); or proton pump

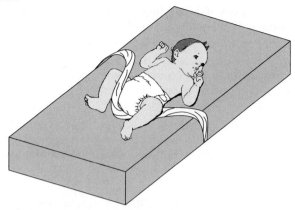

FIGURE 28-8 Fowler's sling. Fowler's sling is used to maintain Fowler's position and to prevent the infant from sliding down to the foot of the bed. The bed is in Fowler's position; the rolled blanket is tucked under the mattress on each side at armpit level; when the infant is in the side-lying position or prone, the legs straddle the sling to maintain positioning.

inhibitors such as Prilosec (Omeprazole). Chronic antacid therapy should be avoided (Lightdale, 2013). The medication must be administered before meals. Side effects such as drowsiness or restlessness can occur.

> ⬡ **Nursing Tip**
>
> A guide to prevent gastric distention is to feed infants no more than their age in months plus 3 every 3 to 4 hours.

Diarrhea

Pathophysiology. **Diarrhea** in the infant cannot be defined in the same way as diarrhea in the adult. The number of stools per day is not often significant in the infant. Diarrhea in infancy is a sudden increase in stools from the infant's normal pattern, with a fluid consistency and a color that is green or contains mucus or blood. *Acute sudden diarrhea* is most often caused by an inflammation, an infection, or as a response to a medication, food, or poisoning. *Chronic diarrhea* lasts for more than 2 weeks and may be indicative of a malabsorption problem, long-term inflammatory disease, or allergic responses. *Infectious diarrhea* is caused by viral, bacterial, or parasitic infection and usually involves gastroenteritis. The norovirus is the most common virus associated with diarrhea in infants (Payne, 2013).

> ⬡ **Nursing Tip**
>
> Green, watery stools may indicate diarrhea in infants.

Manifestations. The symptoms of diarrhea may be mild or extremely severe. The stools are watery and are expelled with force (explosive stools). They may be yellowish green. The infant becomes listless, refuses to eat, and loses weight. The temperature may be elevated, and the infant may vomit. Dehydration is evidenced by sunken eyes and fontanelle and by dry skin, tongue, and mucous membranes. Urination may

become less frequent. In severe cases the excessive loss of bicarbonate from the GI tract results in acidosis.

Infectious diarrhea in infants is commonly caused by the rotavirus that often occurs in day care centers; by *E. coli*, which is caused by lack of hygiene or by poorly cooked foods; by *Salmonella* from contaminated food or pet contact (especially turtles); by *Shigella*; and by other organisms. *C. difficile* infection often follows prolonged antibiotic therapy. *Giardia lamblia* is an intestinal protozoan that causes diarrhea. It is spread by contaminated water, unsanitary conditions, and fecal contamination by animals. Prevention is important and centers around teaching the basics of hygienic practices, handwashing, and the use of disinfectants.

Treatment and Nursing Care. Mild diarrhea in older children may be treated at home under a physician's direction, provided there is a suitable caregiver. Treatment is essentially the same. Reducing the intake of solid foods allows the intestine to rest. Oral rehydration (OR) solutions such as Pedialyte or Infalyte in liquid or frozen (ice pop) form are preferred, with the gradual introduction of a soft, bland diet. A regular intake is usually resumed within 2 to 3 days. Clear fluids, fruit juice without pulp, gelatin, and carbonated drinks have low electrolyte content and are avoided. Caffeinated sodas act as a diuretic and can worsen the dehydration. Chicken broth is often high in sodium and is not advisable. The BRAT diet (**b**ananas, **r**ice, **a**pplesauce, and **t**oast) is not nutritionally sound enough to support growth and development. Nursing Care Plan 28-1 provides nursing interventions for the care of a child with diarrhea.

> ⬡ **Nursing Tip**
>
> To prevent foodborne diarrhea, parents should be taught to keep perishable foods refrigerated, avoid thawing frozen food at room temperature for more than 2 hours, cook meat thoroughly, and wash hands, utensils, and work areas with soap and water.

Constipation

Pathophysiology. **Constipation** is defecation that is difficult or infrequent, with the passage of hard, dry fecal material. There may be associated symptoms, such as abdominal discomfort or blood-streaked stools.

Manifestations. The frequency of bowel movements varies widely in children. There may be periods of diarrhea or **encopresis** (constipation with fecal soiling). Constipation may be a symptom of other disorders, particularly obstructive conditions. Diet, culture, and social, psychological, and familial patterns may also influence its occurrence. The daily use of laxatives and enemas should be discouraged. Most children use the bathroom every day, but they may be hurried and have an incomplete bowel movement. Some children are embarrassed or even afraid to use school or public bathrooms.

★ Nursing Care Plan 28-1   The Child with Gastroenteritis (Diarrhea and Vomiting)

PATIENT DATA An 11-month-old infant is admitted with a history of diarrhea for several days and vomiting related to food ingestion. A diaper rash is evident, and skin tissue turgor is poor.

Selected Nursing Diagnosis: Deficient fluid volume related to diarrhea and/or vomiting as evidenced by weight loss, output greater than intake, emesis, liquid stools, decreased urine output, abdominal distention/rebound tenderness, excoriation of perianal mucosa, hypotension, increased pulse rate, change in skin turgor, lethargy, irritability

Goals	Nursing Interventions	Rationales
Infant's or child's weight will be within 5% of normal baseline.	Weigh infant or child daily.	Daily *accurate* weights are necessary to ascertain the amount of fluids lost through liquid stools and/or vomiting.
Bowel movements will be reduced in number within 24 hours of nursing intervention.	Monitor vital signs (e.g., temperature, pulse rate, respirations, blood pressure, and skin turgor).	Helps determine if the infant or child is responding appropriately to medical and nursing interventions.
Urine output will be above 1 mL/kg/hr.	Record intake and output accurately, including ice chips, intravenous (IV) fluids, gelatins, or other food products that become watery at room temperature.	Accurate recording of intake and output is necessary to determine the amount of fluid replacement required.
Infant or child will be free from fluid and electrolyte imbalance.	Observe and monitor IV fluid administration.	Fluid depletion occurs very rapidly in infants and small children because they have different proportions of both body water and fat than an adult. IV fluids may be needed to prevent dehydration, electrolyte imbalance, shock, and death.
	Notify health care provider of decreased number of stools, ability to drink liquids without emesis; increased urine output, and improvement in vital signs and skin turgor.	
	Obtain fresh stool specimen, if ordered, and send to laboratory for analysis.	
	Resume oral liquids, and foods gradually, starting with ordered rehydration fluids.	Prevents overhydration of infant or child. A fresh sample is required to determine if there are any ova (eggs) or parasites in the stool that could be the cause of the gastroenteritis. Rehydration fluids help to decrease the mobility of the colon, rest the intestinal tract, and decrease the risk of water toxicity.

Selected Nursing Diagnosis: Risk for impaired skin integrity related to frequency of stools as evidenced by excoriation of skin and tissue in perianal area, erythema, pain with each stooling; complaint of burning or pain in perianal area

Goals	Nursing Interventions	Rationales
Infant or child will show improvement or resolution of erythema and exhibit tissue intact and free from secondary infection.	Change diapers or underwear as soon as a stooling occurs; cleanse perianal area with warm water using a soft cloth free of any alcohol.	Liquid stools generally contain high amounts of acids. The longer the stool is in contact with the infant's or child's skin, the greater the risk of excoriated tissue. Alcohol can be very painful on impaired tissue.
	Leave buttocks exposed to air whenever possible (usually *after* the diarrhea slows down or stops).	Air helps to keep the skin dry and free from any irritation such as from diapers or underwear rubbing on the skin.
	Apply soothing balm or ointment to affected area (*after* thorough cleansing) sparingly.	The balm or ointment is a protective barrier on the infant's or child's skin. If the ointment is placed on uncleansed skin, the infant or child is at increased risk of excoriation.
	If medicated powders are prescribed and/or used, teach the parent to put powder in the hand and then apply on the infant's or child's buttocks and to keep powder container away from the infant or child.	If powder is "sprayed" onto the buttocks, the infant or child is at risk to inhale the powder.

Continued

⭐ Nursing Care Plan 28-1 The Child with Gastroenteritis (Diarrhea and Vomiting)—cont'd

Selected Nursing Diagnosis: Deficient parental knowledge related to diarrhea in infants and children as evidenced by lack of previous experience

Goals	Nursing Interventions	Rationales
Parents will verbalize understanding of the dietary restrictions, potential complications, and method of treatment for gastroenteritis or diarrhea.	Instruct parents on proper methods of making, reconstituting, and storing formulas, oral fluid replacements, and foods.	Ensure that parents understand that improper handling or storing of food products can increase the risk of further gastroenteritis.
	Teach and/or reinforce proper handwashing techniques, especially after handling soiled diapers and clothing and before preparing and/or eating a meal.	Handwashing is the first line of defense in preventing the spread of infection.
	Explain that dehydration occurs rapidly in infants and small children. Because of this fact, the parents need to seek help from their health care provider early to prevent potential hospitalization and/or further complications.	Early detection and interventions prevent more severe complications from the dehydration that occurs with gastroenteritis.
	Teach parents that some over-the-counter remedies for vomiting and diarrhea can be harmful to infants and small children.	Absorbents such as kaolin and pectin may alter the consistency and appearance of stools, decreasing the frequency of evacuation; however, they may mask actual fluid loss.

Critical Thinking Question

1. An 11-month-old infant is brought to the clinic. The mother states that he has watery diarrhea, and you notice that his eyes are sunken and that his skin turgor is only fair. The mother tells you she wants to give an antidiarrheal medicine that she has at home and asks how much to give. What is the best response of the nurse?

Treatment and Nursing Care. Evaluation begins with a thorough history of dietary and bowel habits. Some infants respond to formula with a high iron content by developing constipation. Changing to a low-iron formula may be helpful. The frequency, color, and consistency of the stool are noted. The nurse inquires about any medication the child may be taking. The parents are asked to define what they mean by constipation. Parent teaching concerning the prevention of constipation is essential.

Dietary modifications include adding more roughage to the diet. Foods high in fiber include whole-grain breads and cereals, raw vegetables and fruits, bran, and popcorn for older children. Increasing fluid intake is also important. A stool softener such as docusate sodium (Colace) may be prescribed. The child is encouraged to try to move the bowels at the same time each day to establish a routine. The child should not be hurried. Increased exercise may help sedentary children. Constipation can be defined as fewer than seven bowel movements in a 2-week period; within that context, the use of rectal suppositories, laxatives, and stool softeners offer relief and can prevent a chronic constipation problem from occurring (Borowitz et al, 2005).

FLUID AND ELECTROLYTE IMBALANCE

Principles of Fluid Balance in Children

Infants and small children have different proportions of body water and body fat than adults do (Figure 28-9), and the water needs and water losses of the infant (per unit of body weight) are greater. In children less than 2 years of age, *surface area* is particularly important in fluid and electrolyte balance because more water is lost through the skin than through the kidneys. The surface area of the infant is from 2 to 3 times greater than that of the adult in proportion to body volume or body weight. *Metabolic rate* and *heat production* are also 2 to 3 times greater in infants per kilogram of body weight. This causes more waste products to be produced, which must be diluted to be excreted. It also stimulates respiration, which causes increased evaporation through the lungs. Compared with adults, a greater percentage of body water in children less than 2 years of age is contained in the extracellular compartment.

Fluid turnover is rapid, and dehydration occurs more quickly in infants than in adults (Table 28-2). The infant cannot survive as long as the adult in the presence of continued water depletion. A sick infant does not adapt as rapidly to shifts in intake and output because the kidneys lack maturity. They are less able to concentrate urine and require more water than an adult's kidneys to excrete a given amount of solute. Disturbances of the GI tract often lead to vomiting and diarrhea. Electrolyte balance depends on fluid balance and cardiovascular, renal, adrenal, pituitary, parathyroid, and pulmonary regulatory mechanisms. Many of these mechanisms are maturing in the developing child and are unable to react at full capacity under the stress of illness, such as diarrhea and vomiting. Signs of dehydration in a child may not be evident until

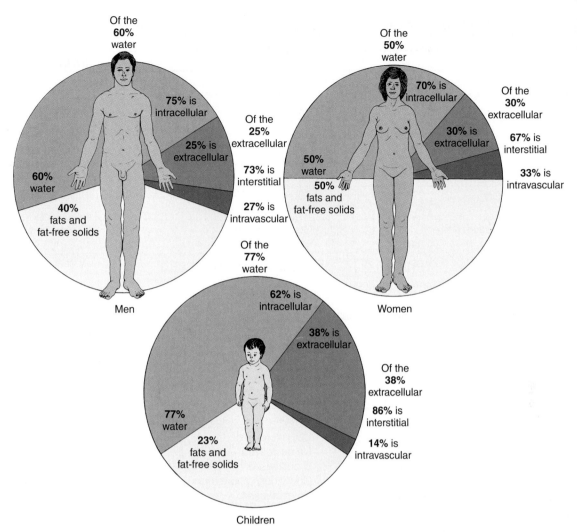

FIGURE 28-9 Relationship of body water and body solids to the body weight in the adult man and woman and in the child.

the fluid loss reaches 4%, and severe dehydration may not be evident until the fluid loss reaches 10% (Bender et al, 2005).

> **⚠ Safety Alert!**
>
> An accurate intake and output record must be kept for all children with vomiting or diarrhea.

Oral Fluids. Oral rehydrating solution (ORS) alternatives such as Pedialyte or Infalyte are preferred to IV therapy (Bender et al, 2005). Nurses must use their ingenuity to coax sick children to take enough fluids, because they may refuse food and water and do not understand their importance for recovery. Toddlers and infants are not capable of drinking by themselves. The busy nurse must find time to offer fluids and must be patient and gently persistent. Liquids are offered frequently and in small amounts. Brightly colored containers and drinking straws may help. ORS options are available in varied flavors and in frozen ice pop forms that are more acceptable to the young child.

The nurse keeps an accurate record of the patient's intake and output. General hygiene and principles of preventing diarrhea are discussed with the parents. In 2002, the World Health Organization (WHO) advised that the contents of an optimum oral rehydration solution should contain 75 mEq/L of sodium; 75 mEq/L of glucose; and a total osmolarity of 245 mOsm/L. In the United States, most commercial "lyte" solutions, such as Pedialyte, Oralyte, Infalyte, and others, meet these criteria with a more desirable lower sodium content. Fluids with a high glucose or sodium content, such as colas and juices, should not be used. Oral rehydration fluids are usually given as 1 milliliter of ORS for every gram of output. Replacement fluid needs are usually estimated as 10 mL/kg for each stool and 2 mL/kg for each emesis. In addition, a simple protein and starch feeding, such as rice, potato, yogurt, fruits, vegetables, cereal, or bread can lessen fluid loss (Bender et al, 2005).

Parenteral Fluids. **Parenteral fluids** (*para,* "beside or apart from," and *enteron,* "intestine") are those given by some route other than the digestive tract. They are

| Table 28-2 | Signs of Isotonic, Hypertonic, and Hypotonic Dehydration |

AREA OF ASSESSMENT	SIGNS OF DEHYDRATION		
	ISOTONIC	**HYPERTONIC**	**HYPOTONIC**
Weight loss	*Mild dehydration:* Up to 5% weight loss *Moderate dehydration:* 5% to 10% weight loss *Severe dehydration:* More than 10% weight loss		
Behavior	Irritable and lethargic	Irritable when disturbed; lethargic	Lethargic to delirious; coma
Skin turgor	Decreased elasticity	Good turgor; "foam rubber" feel	Very poor turgor; clammy
Mucous membranes	Dry	Parched	Clammy
Eyeballs and fontanelle	Sunken and soft	Sunken	Sunken and soft
Tearing and salivation	Absent or decreased	Absent or decreased	Absent or decreased
Thirst	Present	Marked	Present
Urine	Decreased output; serum globulin (SG) elevated	Normal to decreased output; SG elevated or decreased	Decreased output; SG elevated
Body temperature	Subnormal to elevated	Elevated	Subnormal
Respiration	Rapid	Rapid	Rapid
Blood pressure	Normal to low	Normal to low	Very low
Pulse	Rapid	Rapid	Rapid
Blood chemistry	BUN increased Na decreased K normal or increased Cl decreased pH usually decreased	BUN increased Na decreased K decreased Cl low during correction Ca decreased	BUN increased Na decreased K varies or increased Cl decreased

BUN, Blood urea nitrogen; *Ca,* calcium; *Cl,* chloride; *K,* potassium; *Na,* sodium.
Data from Bender B, Skoe C, Ozuah P: Oral rehydration therapy, *Contemp Pediatr* 22(4):72-76, 2005; Kliegman RM, Stanton BF, St Geme III JW, Schor NF, Behrman RE: *Nelson textbook of pediatrics,* ed 19, Philadelphia, 2011, Saunders.

necessary when vomiting or loss of consciousness accompanies sickness or when the GI system requires rest. Parenteral fluids are needed in severe cases of vomiting and diarrhea in which the loss of water and electrolytes will lead to death if untreated. It also provides a means for the safe and effective administration of prescribed parenteral medications. Solutions given parenterally must be sterile to prevent a general or local infection. The nurse must be aware of the importance of parenteral therapy and the assessments required.

The infant or child receiving parenteral fluids needs the nurse's warmth and affection. A pacifier should be used whenever infants are on NPO status. Parents should be encouraged to pick up and hold or rock their children who are receiving IV therapy. Arm boards prevent the child from pulling out the IV line and protect the tubing. Parenteral therapy is discussed in Chapter 22.

Dehydration
Pathophysiology. When a person is in good health, the intake and output of fluids are balanced and **homeostasis** (a uniform state) exists. This is accomplished by appropriate shifts of fluids and electrolytes across cellular membranes and by elimination of products of metabolism that are no longer needed or are in excess. The volume of blood plasma and interstitial and intracellular fluids remains relatively constant. Dehydration occurs whenever fluid output exceeds fluid intake, regardless of the cause.

Manifestations. Disorders of fluids and electrolytes—sodium (Na^+), potassium (K^+), calcium (Ca^{++}), and magnesium (Mg^{++})—are more complex in growing children. A newborn's total weight is comprised of approximately 77% water, compared with 60% in adults. This varies with the amount of fat. In addition, the daily turnover of water in infants is equal to almost 24% of total body water, compared with about 6% in adults. An infant's body surface in comparison with weight is 3 times that of the older child; therefore the infant is subject to greater evaporation of water from the skin. The younger the patient, the higher the metabolic rate and the more unstable the heat-regulating mechanisms. (Elevations in temperature also increase the rate of water loss.) Rapid respirations speed up this process;

when diarrhea is present, additional fluid is lost in the stools. Immaturity of the kidneys impairs the infant's ability to conserve water. The average urine output in infants and children is seen in Table 28-3. The average urine output in infants is 2 mL/kg/hr; the output for children is 0.5 mL/kg/hr; and the output for adolescents is 40 to 80 mL/hr. It is an important nursing responsibility to document the intake and output of hospitalized infants and children. Preterm and newborn infants are also more susceptible to dehydration from variations in room temperature and humidity. When this is coupled with higher fluid losses, life-threatening deficits can ensue within a few hours (Table 28-4).

Problems of fluid and electrolyte disturbance require evaluation of the type and severity of dehydration, clinical observation of the patient, and chemical analysis of the blood. The types of dehydration are classified according to the level of serum sodium, which depends on the relative losses of water and electrolytes. These types are usually termed **isotonic** (the patient has lost equal amounts of fluids and electrolytes), **hypotonic** (the child has lost more electrolytes than fluid), and **hypertonic** (more fluids are lost than electrolytes) (see Table 28-2). These classifications are important because each form of dehydration is associated with different relative losses from intracellular fluid (ICF) and extracellular fluid (ECF) compartments, and each requires certain modifications in treatment.

> **⚠ Safety Alert!**
>
> Life-threatening deficits can occur within a few hours of dehydration and fluid loss. Close assessment and reporting of signs and symptoms of dehydration are essential.

Treatment and Nursing Care. *Maintenance fluid therapy* replaces normal water and electrolyte losses, and *deficit therapy* restores preexisting body fluid and electrolyte deficiencies. The composition of IV fluids and the amount and rate of flow are important in preventing complications.

Shock (hypovolemia) is the greatest threat to life in isotonic dehydration. The electrolyte content of oral fluids is particularly significant in the care of infants and small children suffering from disorders of fluid balance and receiving infusions. Commercially prepared electrolyte solutions, or ORS, are available. Children with hypotonic dehydration (excess water with sodium electrolyte depletion) are at risk for water intoxication. This can also occur if tap water enemas are given to small children. Potassium is lost in almost all degrees of dehydration. Replacement potassium is administered only after normal urinary excretion is confirmed. Documentation must include accurate assessment of intake and output, vital signs, daily weight, skin and fontanelles, mucous membranes, and level of consciousness.

> **⌂ Nursing Tip**
>
> Intake and output records include information concerning oral and parenteral intake, suction, wound drainage, vomiting, urine and stool, and sweating. All must be documented accurately.

> **⚠ Safety Alert!**
>
> The nurse must document that at least one void has occurred before IV potassium is administered.

Table 28-3	Average Daily Excretion of Urine (Approximate)	
AGE	**FLUID OUNCES**	**MILLILITERS (mL)**
Days 1 and 2	1-2	30-60
Days 3-10	3-10	100-300
Day 10-2 months	9-15	250-450
2 months-1 year	14-17	400-500
1-3 years	17-20	500-600
3-5 years	20-24	600-700
5-8 years	22-34	650-1000
8-14 years	27-47	800-1400

Table 28-4 Estimation of Dehydration	DEGREE		
CLINICAL SIGN	**MILD**	**MODERATE**	**SEVERE**
Weight loss (%)	5	10	15
Behavior	Normal	Irritable	Hyperirritable to lethargic
Thirst	Slight	Moderate	Intense
Mucous membranes	May be normal	Dry	Parched
Tears	Present	Decreased	Absent
Anterior fontanelle	Flat	+/−	Sunken
Skin turgor	Normal	+/−	Decreased
Urinary output	Normal	Decreased	Minimal

Data from Kliegman RM, Stanton BF, St Geme III JW, Schor NF, Behrman RE: *Nelson textbook of pediatrics*, ed 19, Philadelphia, 2011, Saunders.

Overhydration

Pathophysiology. **Overhydration** results when the body receives more fluid than it can excrete. This can occur in patients with normal kidneys who receive IV fluids too rapidly. It also can occur in a patient receiving acceptable rates of fluid, especially when the patient's illness is related to disorders of fluid mechanism.

Manifestations. Edema is the presence of excess fluid in the interstitial (*interstitium*, "a thing standing between") spaces. Interstitial fluid is similar to plasma, but it contains little protein. In healthy persons, it responds well to shifts in fluid balance. Any factor causing sodium retention can cause edema. The flow of blood out of the interstitial compartments also depends on adequate circulation of blood and lymph. Low protein levels can also disturb osmotic cellular pressure, causing edema. This is seen in patients with nephrosis, in which large amounts of albumin are lost.

Trauma to or infections of the head can cause cerebral edema, which can be life threatening. Constrictive dressings may obstruct venous return, causing swelling, particularly in dependent areas. **Anasarca** (*ana*, "throughout," and *sarx*, "flesh") is a severe generalized edema.

Treatment and Nursing Care. Edema in infants may first be seen about the eyes and in the presacral, occipital, or genital areas. In pitting edema, the nurse notices an impression in the skin that lasts for several seconds after exerting gentle pressure with the finger.

Early detection and management of edema are essential. Taking an accurate weight daily is indispensable, as is close attention to body weight changes. Vital signs, physical appearance, and changes in urine character or output are noted.

Infants receiving IV therapy have their IV and oral intakes recorded. If the oral intake falls below prescribed rates, the IV rate is increased. If the oral intake exceeds prescribed levels, the IV rate is decreased or the IV is heparin- or saline-locked to maintain patency and prevent overhydration.

Electrolyte imbalance. The nurse must be able to assess the electrolyte needs of the child (Table 28-5). When fluid snacks or nourishment are ordered, the selection of fluid can influence the treatment given for dehydration. For example, if the child has a hypertonic type of dehydration (which means there is excess sodium), and the nurse offers the child tomato juice, the high sodium content of tomato juice will negatively affect the child's prescribed treatment. If the child has hypotonic dehydration (which

Table 28-5   Interpreting ABG Values

	ACID	NORMAL	ALKALINE
pH	>7.35	7.35-7.45	<7.45
$PaCO_2$ (Respiratory parameter)	>45	35-45	<35
HCO_3 (Metabolic parameter)	<22	22-26	>26

- The location where the patient's pH falls indicates acidosis or alkalosis.
- If the pH falls in the same column as the HCO_3, the problem is *metabolic*.
- If the pH falls in the same column as $PaCO_2$, the problem is *respiratory*.

Interpreting a Sample Patient's Laboratory Values: Case 1

	ACID	NORMAL	ALKALINE
pH	pH		
$PaCO_2$		$PaCO_2$	
HCO_3	HCO_3		

Interpretation
- Place the patient's laboratory values in the appropriate columns.
- The column in which the pH appears tells you that *acidosis* is the problem.
- The HCO_3 (the metabolic parameter) is in the same column as the pH; therefore the problem is *metabolic acidosis*.

Interpreting a Sample Patient's Laboratory Values: Case 2

	ACID	NORMAL	ALKALINE
pH			pH
$PaCO_2$			$PaCO_2$
HCO_3		HCO_3	

Interpretation
- Place the patient's laboratory values in the appropriate columns.
- The column in which the pH appears tells you *alkalosis* is the problem.
- The $PaCO_2$ (the respiratory parameter) is in the same column as the pH; therefore the problem is *respiratory alkalosis*.

Modified from Mays D: Turn ABGs into child's play, *RN* 58(1):37-38, 1995. Reprinted with permission. © 1995 Medical Economics.

means the child has deficient electrolytes), and the nurse offers plain water, this will also have a negative impact on the child's care. Therefore it is a nursing responsibility to correlate laboratory findings of the individual child with fluids and foods offered to the child.

NUTRITIONAL DEFICIENCIES

Because infancy is a period of rapid growth, poor nutrition is particularly dangerous at this time. Severe vitamin deficiencies are rare in prosperous countries; those that do occur are generally caused by poverty, ignorance, or neglect. Figure 28-10, *A* shows a child from the United States, with general, moderate malnutrition. Severe malnutrition is still rampant in many underdeveloped countries. Every person must be concerned with the plight of the starving child. Sometimes the infant's body is unable to use food even though the diet is adequate. An example of this is celiac disease, in which the intestines are unable to handle fats and starches. Severe malnutrition may also be seen in failure to thrive.

Failure to Thrive

Pathophysiology. **Failure to thrive** (FTT) describes infants and children who, without an obvious cause, fail to gain and often lose weight. This condition can be caused

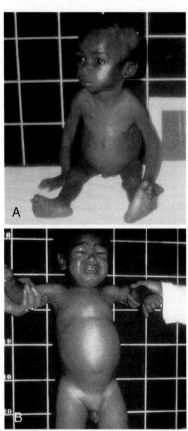

FIGURE 28-10 A, Failure to thrive is a general nutritional-calorie deficiency. Note the profound wasting found in malnutrition or starvation. **B,** Kwashiorkor, caused by a protein deficiency. The infant has generalized edema with a white streak in the hair. (From Zitelli BJ et al: *Zitelli and Davis' atlas of pediatric physical diagnosis*, ed 6, Philadelphia, 2012, Saunders.)

by physical (organic) pathological dysfunction (OFTT), such as congenital heart disease or malabsorption syndromes. It may be caused by a lack of parent–infant interaction that can result from environmental factors, neglect, or lack of information concerning the nutritional needs of infants, which is nonorganic failure to thrive (NFTT). FTT can be caused by environmental stresses.

Infants who fail to thrive are often admitted to the hospital for evaluation with presenting symptoms of weight loss or failure to gain, irritability, and disturbances of food intake such as anorexia or pica (abnormal consumption of nonfood materials). Vomiting, diarrhea, and general neuromuscular spasticity sometimes accompany the condition. These children fall below the third percentile (some authorities suggest the fifth) in weight and height on standard growth charts. Their development is delayed. Children who fail to thrive seem apathetic. Some have a "rag-doll limpness" (hypotonia), and they often appear wary of their caregivers. Others appear stiff and unresponsive to cuddling. The personality of the infant may not foster maternal attachment. FTT with malabsorption has been reported with frequency among autistic children and among institutionalized mentally retarded children. The child has a complete workup to identify organic reasons for FTT, and the cause is treated.

Manifestations. With NFTT, there may be a disturbance in the mother–child or caregiver–child relationship. The situation is complex and is often associated with marital discord, economic pressures, parental immaturity, low stress tolerance, and single parenthood. Alcohol and drug abuse can be present. Many mothers feel deprived and unloved and have conflicting needs. Infants suffer from the inability to establish a sense of trust in their caregivers. Their coping abilities are affected by a lack of nurturing. Obvious neglect and physical abuse are not uncommon.

Prevention of environmental FTT consists chiefly of social measures such as parenting classes, family planning, and early recognition of and support for families at risk. All children should receive routine health assessments. The pregnancy history may show circumstances that contribute to a lack of bonding, such as an unplanned pregnancy or desertion by the child's father. Planning interventions that will enhance parent–infant interaction is an important nursing responsibility.

Treatment and Nursing Care. Treatment involves a multidisciplinary approach in accordance with the circumstances; that is, the physician, the nurse, the social worker, the family agency, and the counselor may all participate. If no progress can be made, temporary or permanent placement of the child or children in a foster home may be required. During hospitalization, one nurse per shift is selected to increase nurturing and interaction with the infant and parent.

Treatment of the child who fails to thrive requires maturity on the part of the nurse. It is vital to support rather than to reject the mother. Listening and helping the mother to understand her feelings and frustrations, and helping her to explore her choices, can facilitate maternal attachment. The nurse encourages her to assist with the daily care of her child. The child's uniqueness and responses to the mother are stressed. The nurse points out developmental patterns and provides anticipatory guidance in this area. Often the mother's lack of interest stems from her own insecurities. Parents Anonymous and parent aides are other resources to help parents.

The prognosis of this condition is uncertain. Emotional starvation, particularly in the early years, can be psychologically traumatic. Inadequacies in intelligence, language, and social behavior have been documented in children who fail to thrive.

Kwashiorkor

Pathophysiology. **Kwashiorkor** is a protein deficiency. In many parts of the world, children still starve to death. There are no well-planned maternal and child health programs to elevate health standards in these localities. In some areas, superstition and ignorance prevent children from using nutritious foods found in their environments. In kwashiorkor, there is a severe deficiency of protein in the diet despite the fact that the number of calories consumed may be nearly adequate. It belongs to a class of disorders termed protein-energy malnutrition (see Figure 28-10, *B*).

Manifestations. Kwashiorkor occurs in children 1 to 4 years of age who have been weaned from the breast. *Kwashiorkor* means, in native dialect, "the disease of the deposed baby when the next one is born," indicating that the child no longer breastfeeds because a sibling is born and takes over the breast of the mother. Oral intake then is deficient in protein. The child fails to grow normally. The muscles become weak and wasted. There is edema of the abdomen that may become generalized. Diarrhea, skin infections, irritability, anorexia, and vomiting may be present. The hair becomes thin and dry. Because protein is the basis of melanin, which is a substance that provides color to hair, melanin becomes deficient. This is the reason that the earliest sign of this protein malnutrition is a white streak in the hair of the child (depigmentation). The child looks apathetic and weak.

Treatment and Nursing Care. Treatment for kwashiorkor is mainly preventive. Although hunger may never be completely eradicated in the world, many private, public, and world health agencies sponsor programs to alleviate such suffering. Simple protein powder sprinkled on the culturally prepared meal will help to alleviate the problem. Early dietary treatment in established cases may prevent more serious growth retardation later.

Rickets

Pathophysiology. **Rickets** is a disease of infancy and childhood caused by deficient amounts of vitamin D. Vitamin D and exposure to sunshine are necessary for the proper absorption and metabolism of calcium and phosphorus, which are needed for the normal growth of bones.

Manifestations. The classic symptoms of rickets are bowlegs; knock-knees; beading of the ribs, called the *rachitic rosary*; and improper formation of the teeth.

Treatment and Nursing Care. The widespread use of vitamin supplements and the fortification of foods have largely eliminated the problem of rickets in North America. The nurse should guide parents concerning the need for an optimal, well-balanced diet, exercise, and exposure to outdoor sunlight.

Scurvy

Scurvy is a disease caused by insufficient fruits and vegetables that contain vitamin C in the diet. The symptoms of scurvy include joint pains, bleeding gums, loose teeth, and lack of energy. Good sources of vitamin C are citrus fruits and raw, leafy vegetables. Vitamin C is easily destroyed by heat and exposure to air. Small amounts of water should be used for cooking vegetables to prevent vitamin C from being destroyed, because it is also water-soluble. It may be provided to infants in the form of orange juice, which should not be boiled. Vitamin supplements prescribed for infants and children contain vitamin C. The vitamin is not stored in the body, and daily intake from food sources is required.

INFECTIONS

Appendicitis

The most common reason for emergency abdominal surgery in childhood is appendicitis, with more than 70,000 cases occurring each year in the United States (Minkes, 2011). The average age of occurrence is 10 years old. The challenge in diagnosing appendicitis is that rupture or perforation of the appendix can occur with serious complications within 36 hours after the onset of abdominal pain. A delay in diagnosis often occurs because the child is unable to localize or express the symptoms experienced.

Pathophysiology and Manifestations. The appendix is a small appendage arising from the cecum; it is located on the right side of the abdomen. The lumen may become obstructed with fecal matter, with lymphoid tissue after a viral illness, or with parasites. There is stasis, increased swelling, edema, and growth of organisms. The initial pain perceived is usually periumbilical and increases within a 4-hour period. When the inflammation spreads to the peritoneum, the pain localizes in the right lower quadrant (RLQ) of the abdomen. The appendix may become gangrenous or rupture, causing peritonitis and septicemia. Vomiting may occur after periumbilical pain starts. (In children with gastroenteritis, vomiting precedes abdominal pain.) Infrequent mucus diarrhea may occur because of intestinal irritation caused by developing peritonitis. (Frequent watery stools are associated with gastroenteritis.) Fever is not a reliable sign of appendicitis in children. On examination, characteristic tenderness in the right lower quadrant, known as **McBurney's point**, will occur. Other diagnostic signs include the following:

- **Guarding**: There is a tightening of the abdominal muscles or rigidity of the abdomen on palpation.
- **Rebound tenderness**: Pressing the RLQ with rapid release of pressure causes severe pain.
- Pain on lifting the thigh while in the supine position is caused by muscle irritation.
- Pain in the RLQ when palpated and pain on rectal examination often occur.

Laboratory tests may be undertaken to confirm the diagnosis and to rule out other possible diagnoses. A urinalysis will rule out a urinary tract infection. C-reactive protein levels will be increased after 12 hours if any infection is present. An abdominal x-ray study (kidney, ureter, and bladder [KUB]) will show a right-sided curvature of the spine, a dilated cecum with an air or fluid level, and a decrease in bowel gas in the RLQ (if ruptured). An ultrasound will show a thickened appendix and a soft tissue mass in the RLQ, and it is used to rule out an ovarian cyst in females who may exhibit similar clinical signs. A computed tomography (CT) scan with rectal contrast (CTRC) is administered via the rectum to confirm the enlarged appendix. A culture of the stool may be performed to rule out gastroenteritis. A laboratory evaluation of the white blood cell (WBC) count will show an increased WBC count with neutrophils increased 75%, but this may not be helpful in diagnosing an unperforated appendix. Signs of ruptured appendix and peritonitis includes sudden relief of acute pain, rigid guarding of the abdomen, abdominal distention, tachycardia, chills, and irritability.

Treatment and Nursing Care. Observing the behavior of the child in relation to the developmental level and using pain perception scales can help assess the pain level. A warmed stethoscope should be used when auscultating the abdomen of a child; it is less frightening than the approaching fingers of the hand. The child and family are prepared for the diagnostic tests and possibility of surgery. An explanation of the reason for NPO status until the need for surgery is determined will help with compliance. The nurse should explain what to expect, discuss coping mechanisms, and provide referrals as necessary. Postoperative care is similar to that for any abdominal surgery. IV therapy is gradually replaced with fluids and food. A drain may be present at the wound site if perforation has occurred, and a frequent change of dressings may be necessary. Pain management, prevention of infection, and early ambulation are the primary goals.

Thrush (Oral Candidiasis)

Pathophysiology. **Thrush** is an infection of the mucous membranes of the mouth caused by the fungus *Candida*. This organism is normally present in the mother's vagina and is nonpathogenic. However, the altered conditions in the vagina produced by pregnancy may lead to the development of candidiasis vaginitis. The mucous membranes of the infant's mouth may become infected by direct contact with this infection during delivery or by contact with the mother's or nurse's contaminated hands. Cross infection of other newborns may result.

Manifestations. White patches that resemble milk curds appear on the tongue, inner lips, gums, and oral mucosa. They are painless but cannot be wiped away. Anorexia may be present. The systemic symptoms are mild if the infection remains in the mouth; however, it can pass along the mucous membranes into the GI tract, causing inflammation of the esophagus and the stomach. Pneumonitis may also develop. *Epstein's pearls,* which are small, white, epithelial cysts that appear along both sides of the midline of the hard palate, are sometimes mistaken for thrush. These are harmless and gradually disappear.

Treatment and Nursing Care. A thrush infection responds well to the local application of an antifungal suspension such as nystatin (Mycostatin). The mouth is swabbed 3 or 4 times a day between feedings with a sterile applicator moistened with the prescribed solution. With proper care, the condition disappears within a few days after its onset.

Newborns suspected of having thrush are cared for using isolation (standard) precautions. Individual feeding equipment is necessary, and the equipment should be sterile. Disposable bottles or prefilled formula bottles are used. Disposable nipples, pacifiers, and bottles are preferred.

Candida infection of the diaper area presents as a bright red, sharply demarcated diaper rash. Nystatin cream is often prescribed.

Nursing Tip

In the home, parents are taught to drop nystatin or other medication slowly into the **side of the infant's mouth**. Medication must remain in contact with "patches" as long as possible. Instruct parents to watch for dehydration (e.g., decrease in number of wet diapers) that can result from the infant's refusal to take fluids because of mouth discomfort.

Worms

The main nursing responsibility is the education of the patient and family concerning the prevention of worm infestation through general hygiene, food handling, and environmental controls.

Enterobiasis (Pinworms)

Pathophysiology. Of the several varieties of worms that affect humans, the most common is the pinworm, *Enterobius vermicularis* (*enteron*, "intestine," *bios*, "life," and *vermis*, "wormlike"). It is seen more often in toddlers but it can develop in older children and adults. The pinworm looks like a white thread about ⅓ of an inch long. It lives in the lower intestine but comes out of the anus to lay its eggs, generally during the night. These eggs become infective a few hours after they have been deposited. This type of parasite spreads from one person to another, particularly where large groups of children are in close contact with one another. The route of entry is the mouth; the child becomes infected by ingesting the eggs. Reinfection takes place by way of contact from the rectum to the fingers to the mouth or by way of the rectum to the clothing to the fingers to the mouth.

Manifestations. The nurse or parent may notice that the child scratches the anal area and may complain of itching. There may be associated irritability and restlessness. Weight loss, poor appetite, and fretfulness during the night can develop. The rectal area may become irritated from scratching. A special pinworm diagnostic tape or paddle, or a tongue blade covered with cellophane tape, sticky side out, may be placed against the anal region to obtain pinworm eggs (the "Scotch tape test"). This is done early in the morning, before the child has a bowel movement, bathes, or scratches the anal area with the fingers. The tape is put on a glass slide and is examined under a microscope. The eggs are typical of pinworms.

Treatment and nursing care. Several effective **anthelmintics** (*anti*, "against," and *helminth*, "worms") are available. Mebendazole (Vermox) is a single-dose, chewable tablet and is the drug of choice for children older than 2 years of age. Pyrantel pamoate (Antiminth) also controls the infestation. Pyrvinium pamoate (Povan) suspension, a one-dose treatment, is an alternative drug; nurses should advise parents that Povan stains and turns the stools red.

The child must be taught to wash the hands thoroughly after bowel movements. The child's fingernails are kept short. A soothing ointment is applied to the rectal area. The patient should wear clean underwear that fits snugly to prevent scratching the anus with the fingers.

All symptomatic members of the family should be treated for this condition to prevent reinfection. Pregnant women should not take Vermox and should consult a physician before taking any alternative drug. The toilet seats in the home are scrubbed daily. Cloth diapers and bed linens are washed in hot water.

Ascariasis (Roundworms). *Ascaris lumbricoides* is a roundworm, and infestation can be asymptomatic or can cause abdominal pain. The infestation is estimated to affect 1 billion persons worldwide. Roundworms thrive in warm climates and among the impoverished. In the United States, roundworms are seen more often in the Southern states and among immigrants and migratory workers living below poverty levels. The condition is caused by the unsanitary disposal of human feces and poor hygiene practices. An egg from an infected person can survive for weeks in the soil. The child ingests eggs from contaminated soil. The eggs develop into larvae in the intestine, penetrate the intestinal wall, and enter the liver, from which they circulate to the lungs and heart. The patient is generally without symptoms until the larvae reach the glottis, are coughed up, swallowed, and enter the small intestine. There they develop into adult male and female species. They survive on undigested food in the canal and produce eggs that are expelled in the child's feces. A chronic cough without fever is characteristic of this condition. Diagnosis is made by confirmation of the eggs in the patient's stool. The treatment of ascariasis is the medication albendazole, or a 3-day oral dose of nitazoxanide.

POISONING

Goals in the primary management of poisoning are the following:
- Remove access to the poison.
- Prevent further absorption.
- Call the poison control center.
- Provide supportive care—seek medical help.

Treatment of poisoning includes prevention of absorption, enhancement of excretion of the poison from the body, maintenance of fluid and electrolyte balance, and cardiopulmonary stabilization.

General Concepts

Volume of a Swallow. The volume of a swallow has been estimated at 0.21 mL/kg of body weight. Thus a child age 2 to 3 years who takes one swallow may have ingested about 3 mL of poison.

Principles of Care. Education of parents and children is the best way to prevent poisoning. The school and the clinic are the best resources to be used in an active accident prevention program.

Poison Control Centers. The telephone number of the poison control center is listed in the telephone directory and should be posted near the phone. Dialing 800-222-1222 anywhere in the United States will route the call to

Table 28-6	Detecting Poison by Specific Odor of Vomitus	
ODOR OF VOMITUS	**PROBABLE CONTENT**	
Sweet	Chloroform, acetone	
Bitter almond	Cyanide	
Pear	Chloral hydrate	
Garlic	Phosphorus, arsenic	
Shoe polish	Nitrobenzene	
Violet	Turpentine	

NOTE: The nurse should report and document the specific odor of vomitus, which can be helpful in determining the specific poison contained in the substance ingested.

the nearest poison control center that can identify the antidote or treatment needed for specific poisons.

Ipecac Syrup. Ipecac syrup is no longer sold in stores. Traditionally, syrup of ipecac was the treatment of choice to remove some types of poisons from a child's system, and parents were advised to keep a supply on hand in the home. However, the American Academy of Pediatrics (AAP) revised this policy in 2003 (Barclay and Nghiem, 2009). Parents are now advised to call the poison control center and bring the container of the substance ingested to the hospital emergency department as quickly as possible, because stomach lavage is rarely effective 1 hour or more after ingestion. Although ipecac syrup may be used in the hospital setting under the supervision of a health care provider, ipecac syrup should not be kept in the home. Uncontrolled vomiting can cause serious complications. Table 28-6 indicates how to assess the type of toxic substance ingested according to the smell of the vomitus.

Activated Charcoal. Activated charcoal will absorb poisons such as strychnine, atropine, malathion, arsenic compounds, phenobarbital, quinine, theophylline, salicylates, valproic acid, and phenytoin. When activated charcoal is given together with ipecac, however, they neutralize each other and render both ineffective in the treatment of poisoning. Activated charcoal may be given orally or by nasogastric tube. When administering oral activated charcoal it is first mixed with water to form a slurry, and then it is administered mixed with cola or chocolate milk or flavored with sorbitol via a straw to make it more palatable. The recommended dosage of activated charcoal is 1 to 2 g/kg of body weight. Charcoal or any gastric lavage may not be effective if administered more than 1 hour after ingestion and is therefore not routinely recommended.

Poisonous Plants

Many common plants used in home landscapes can be poisonous to the young child exploring in the backyard.

Health Promotion

Common Household Plants That Are Poisonous

PLANTS	CAUSE SYMPTOMS SIMILAR TO:
Azalea Buttercup Marigold	Aconite poisoning
Lantana Jimsonweed	Atropine poisoning
Sweet pea Black mountain laurel	Curare poisoning
Apricot pits Peach pits Elderberry	Cyanide poisoning
Camellia seeds Foxglove Oleander	Symptoms similar to digitalis poisoning
Goldenrod Nightshade Poinsettia	Nitrate poisoning
Laurel Water hemlock	Resin poisoning
Camellia Marigold Tulips Violets	Salicylate poisoning

NOTE: These plants should not be used to landscape the backyard of homes with young children who may place the leaves or flowers in their mouth.

Drugs

Drugs prescribed for family members and left within the reach of children are often the cause of accidental poisoning. Many over-the-counter medications are considered harmless by parents but can be deadly to toddlers, even in small doses (Table 28-7). Even a small amount of an oral hypoglycemic drug can lower blood sugar in a small child and can result in a coma. Herbal remedies can also be poisonous to small children (Hawke, 2005).

Acetaminophen Poisoning

Acetaminophen overdose is listed in Box 28-1 along with other poisons commonly encountered in pediatrics.

Pathophysiology. **Acetaminophen** (Tylenol) has now replaced aspirin as the most commonly ingested drug that causes toxicity. This is because it is so widely used and because aspirin, which has been associated with Reye's syndrome, is no longer recommended for fever in children with flulike symptoms. Because parents are often informed that acetaminophen is "safer" than aspirin, they may be more careless in storing it. Acetaminophen poisoning occurs most often from acute overdose rather than from the cumulative effects seen with aspirin. Acetaminophen is also found as an ingredient in multidrug medications, which, if taken with concentrated

Table 28-7 Selected Over-the-Counter Drugs That Are Deadly to Toddlers

GENERIC NAME	TRADE NAME	TOXICITY
Benzocaine	Orajel	Methemoglobinemia Seizures
Camphor	Vicks VapoRub Campho-Phenique	Central nervous system (CNS) depression Seizures
Diphenoxylate	Lomotil	CNS depression
Methyl salicylate	Oil of wintergreen Icy-Hot balm Arthritis ointments	Cardiovascular collapse
Tetrahydrozoline hydrochloride	Visine eye drops; Murine	Tachycardia; seizures

Data from Osterhardt K: The toxic toddler: drugs that can kill in small doses, *Contemp Pediatr* 17(3):73, 2000; Wong D, Perry S, Hockenberry M, Lowdermilk D, Wilson D: *Maternal-child nursing care*, ed 3, St Louis, 2012, Mosby; *Thomson physician's desk reference*, Montvale, N.J., 2015, Medical Economics; Isbistyer G, Kumar K: Indications for single dose activated charcoal administered in acute overdose, *Curr Opin Crit Care* 17(4):51-57, 2011; Frischknecht J: Setting the standard of treatment for acetaminophen toxicity, *Adv NPs PAs* 4(3):34-48, 2013.

Box 28-1 Poisons Commonly Encountered in Pediatrics

ACIDS
Toilet bowl cleaners
Swimming pool pH adjustment solutions
Concentrated acids in hardware and paint stores

ALKALINES
Clinitest tablets
Drain-cleaning crystals
Dishwasher soaps
Industrial cleaners (brought home in unlabeled containers)

MEDICATIONS
Diet pills
Sleeping pills
Sedatives
Cold remedies
Birth control pills
Vitamin supplements, iron supplements
Diarrhea remedies (Lomotil)
Menstrual pain relievers
Antipyretics (aspirin, acetaminophen)
Oil of wintergreen

CYANIDE
Pesticides
Metal polishes
Photographic solutions
Fumigating products

ETHANOL
Alcoholic beverages
Cold remedies
Perfumes
Mouthwashes
Aftershave lotions

PETROLEUM DISTILLATES
Heavy greases, oils
Turpentine
Furniture polishes
Gasoline, kerosene
Lighter fluid

Insecticides
Home gardening products
Recently sprayed lawns

CARBON MONOXIDE
Accidental administration
Suicidal administration

LEAD
Paint
Air
Food
Ant poison
Unglazed pottery
Colored newsprint
Curtain weights
Fishing sinkers
Lead water pipes
Acidic juices in leaded pottery

ARTHROPODS, INSECT STINGS
Spiders (brown recluse, black widow)
Certain scorpions
Insects (bees, wasps, hornets)

SNAKES
Rattlesnakes
Moccasins
Copperheads
Other snakes

POISONOUS PLANTS
Daffodil
Boston ivy
Split-leaf philodendron
Umbrella plant
Azalea
Foxglove
Mistletoe
Tulip
Others (see Health Promotion box on p. 663)

acetaminophen (Tylenol), can result in an overdose. Because acetaminophen is metabolized in the liver, overdose results in hepatic destruction. With early treatment, most children recover without complications.

Manifestations. Manifestations and treatment modalities that the nurse might anticipate in patients with acute poisoning are shown in Table 28-8.

Treatment and Nursing Care. Medical intervention is necessary if the ingested dose exceeds 200 mg/kg per day (Frischknecht, 2013). The stomach is emptied by lavage or induced emesis from syrup of ipecac. Activated charcoal can prevent the absorption of acetaminophen if it is administered a short time after acetaminophen ingestion (Isbister, 2011). Blood levels usually peak 4 to 6 hours after ingestion, and, depending on the serum acetaminophen level, this may be followed by the *N*-acetylcysteine (Mucomyst) antidote. In small children, it may be administered directly into the nasogastric tube after lavage. Otherwise it is generally given orally every 4 hours for 72 hours. This medicine has a bad smell and taste, and the patient needs coaxing and support to assist with compliance. The medicine may be mixed with a soft drink or juice.

Table 28-8	Anticipated Care for Poisoning
SYMPTOMS	**INTERVENTION**
Absorption	Lavage, activated charcoal
Central nervous system: restlessness, agitation, seizures, coma	Seizure precautions
Respiratory: airway obstruction, hypoventilation, hypoxia	Cardiopulmonary resuscitation, oxygen saturation monitoring, oxygen therapy, keep artificial airway handy
Cardiovascular: difficulties with electrolytes, blood urea nitrogen, creatinine, glucose	Monitor vital signs
Gastrointestinal: difficulty swallowing, abdominal pain	NPO status; possible gastrostomy
Kidney problems	Monitor intake and output; monitor IV lines
Need for increased elimination	Cathartic, forced diuresis, dialysis, hemoperfusion; monitor patient responses
Hypothermia or hyperthermia	Sponge baths, cooling blanket
Child: physical response or psychological trauma Parents: guilt, anger, family dysfunction	Crisis intervention Counseling, teaching, referral

IV, Intravenous; *NPO,* nothing by mouth.

Treatment within 8 hours of ingestion can reduce the risk of liver damage but a delay of more than 24 hours may increase the risk of liver damage. Levels of liver enzymes (ALT and AST) usually peak within 96 hours and are monitored along with prothrombin times. Prevention of overdose is of utmost importance. Even in uncomplicated cases the child is subjected to unpleasant, stressful procedures.

Salicylate Poisoning

Pathophysiology. **Aspirin** (acetylsalicylic acid) poisoning is seen less often than in the past because of safety packaging and the increased use of acetaminophen. Nevertheless, aspirin is often used in many homes and may be stored carelessly on bedside stands or in a mother's purse. Oil of wintergreen (methyl salicylate) is also extremely hazardous when mistakenly administered as cough medicine or swallowed by the curious child. It is sometimes used as a home remedy for arthritic pain. Even a dose as small as 1 teaspoon can cause a child's death.

Manifestations. Salicylate acts rapidly but is excreted slowly. Ingestion of 150 mg/kg of body weight causes symptoms. Although most cases of aspirin poisoning are emergencies, a child may unknowingly be poisoned by the cumulative effect of aspirin. The use of several aspirin-containing products at once, such as over-the-counter cold remedies combined with aspirin, can be hazardous. Time-release aspirin is especially dangerous because the symptoms of poisoning are delayed and aspiration of the stomach is of little value in these cases. Therefore it is wise to read labels carefully and to administer aspirin sparingly. It is even better to use it only under a physician's direction.

Treatment and Nursing Care. Vitamin K is administered to control bleeding. Hemodialysis may be indicated if blood levels exceed 100-120 mg/dL. Hemodialysis provides fluid and electrolyte stabilization as well as salicylate clearance. Oral activated charcoal removes salicylates from the circulation and enhances excretion from the gastrointestinal tract. Repeated doses of activated charcoal may be helpful if sustained release tablets were ingested. Whole bowel irrigation with doses of polyethylene glycol is most effective in reducing salicylate absorption. **Peritoneal dialysis** (*peritoneum* and *dialysis,* "passing of a solute through a membrane") is a therapeutic measure used in acute renal failure. The therapy uses the principles of osmosis and diffusion through the semipermeable peritoneal membrane, with the purpose of removing toxic substances from the blood.

The nurse must realize the danger of drug poisoning and must constantly practice and teach safety measures to prevent tragedies. Treatment rooms, utility rooms, and drug storage areas are scrutinized to ensure that nothing harmful is within the reach of ambulatory children.

Lead Poisoning (Plumbism)

Pathophysiology. **Lead poisoning** (plumbism) results when a child repeatedly ingests or absorbs substances containing lead. The lead levels in ½ million children in the United States in 2010 was high, with blood levels exceeding 5 mcg/dL (CDC, 2013). The primary source is paint from old, deteriorating buildings. The leading public health initiatives in the United States to prevent lead poisoning include the elimination of lead in gasoline; the banning of solder to seal food and beverage cans; and the limitation of lead used in household paint. In countries such as Nigeria, ore mining of gold disseminates lead containing dust, and most children in surrounding communities suffer from toxic lead ingestion. Lead poisoning is most common in children between 18 months and 3 years of age. Although the incidence is highest among the poor, lead poisoning is also found among suburban and middle-class children.

Children who chew on windowsills and stair rails may ingest flakes of paint, putty, or crumbled plaster. Eating nonfood items is called **pica**. Food, particularly fruit juices consumed from improperly glazed earthenware, is another source of poisoning. Lead poisoning among Mexican Americans may result from azarcon, a bright orange powder containing approximately 93.5% lead. Azarcon is used as a folk remedy to treat "empacho" and other digestive problems in infants. Lead poisoning among Hmong Laotian refugees may be caused by pay-loo-ah, a bright orange-red powder that may be used for fever or rash. Unwashed fresh fruit sprayed with insecticides, and dust from enclosed shooting galleries, are also culprits. Some alternative therapies such as ayurveda medicines contain lead (Cleveland et al, 2008). Another source is dust in homes near lead-processing plants. "Spitballs" made from the colored sections of newspaper comics or advertisements are also a source of lead poisoning. Older synthetic venetian or vertical blinds used as window coverings, brightly colored metal vases, and lead crystal are other common sources for lead poisoning in the home when a toddler handles the item and then places the hands in the mouth. Many toys and jewelry made in China have been recalled because of high lead content. Imported spices such as svanuri marili and saffron also contain lead (Karri, 2008).

Lead can have a lasting effect on the nervous system, especially the brain. Increased lead levels, even below 10 mcg/dL, can cause developmental delays and aberrant behaviors. Cognitive impairment may occur in severe cases. In much of the United States, lead poisoning is a reportable disease. The Agency for Toxic Substances and Diseases Registry (ATSDR) provides information on this condition.

Manifestations. The symptoms occur gradually and range from mild to severe. Because the infant's or young child's central nervous system is extremely vulnerable, acute symptoms of encephalitis may follow a relatively short period of exposure. The lead settles in the soft tissues and bones and is excreted in the urine. In the beginning, signs may be seen such as weakness, weight loss, anorexia, pallor, irritability, vomiting, abdominal pain, and constipation. In later stages, signs of anemia and nervous system involvement, such as muscular incoordination, neuritis, convulsions, and encephalitis, are seen. Being exposed to lead during pregnancy can lead to problems in the newborn.

Treatment and Nursing Care. Blood and urine tests are performed to determine the amount of lead in the system. Lead is especially toxic to the synthesis of heme in the blood; heme is necessary for hemoglobin formation and for the functioning of renal tubules. Blood lead levels are the primary screening test. X-ray films of the bones show further deposits of lead. The child's history may reveal *pica*, a condition in which the child has a distorted appetite and eats a variety of things that most persons consider unpalatable, such as sand, grass, wool, glass, plaster, coal, animal droppings, and paint from furniture.

Treatment is aimed at reducing the concentration of lead in the tissues and blood. Chelating agents that render the lead nontoxic and increase its excretion in the urine are administered in more severe cases. Calcium disodium edetate (calcium disodium versenate [CaEDTA]) and dimercaprol are commonly used. CaEDTA may be administered intravenously or as a deep intramuscular injection. Mild symptomatic lead poisoning may be treated with meso-2,3,-dimercaptosuccinic acid (DMSA). It can be given orally, has not been associated with serious side effects and, unlike CaEDTA, does not cause zinc depletion. British anti-Lewisite (BAL) is also used together with CaEDTA but may not be given to children who have a peanut butter allergy or who are taking supplemental iron. Complete deleading (chelation) takes several months, and retreatment may be necessary when the child has an acute infection or other metabolic disturbance.

 Safety Alert!

$CaNa_2EDTA$ is a chelating agent. Na_2EDTA is not interchangeable and should not be used.

The prognosis depends on the extent of poisoning. All children with elevated lead blood levels must be followed to evaluate developmental and intellectual milestone achievement. Providing an increased fluid intake and monitoring intake and output during therapy is an important nursing responsibility.

Prevention of this condition is of foremost importance. Lead paint should not be used on children's toys or furniture. Instead, one should use paint marked for indoor use. Inexpensive lead detection kits are available at most home improvement stores. The kit contains a "crayon" that can be rubbed on the vertical blind or other items in the home; it turns a different color if significant lead is present. Lead level screening of children by 12 months of age in high-risk areas is routine in many states.

 Nursing Tip

Documentation of adequate urine output is essential during chelation therapy.

FOREIGN BODY INGESTION

Approximately 80% of all foreign body ingestion occurs in children between 6 months and 3 years of age. About 80% of the foreign bodies ingested pass through the GI tract, but others require surgical removal (Uyemura, 2005). The high level of curiosity of the young child and the tendency to place objects in the mouth increase the susceptibility to accidental ingestion of a nonfood object. Unless the object is sharp or large, passage through the GI tract may be possible and can take up to 4 to 6 days. The child is cared for at home, and the nurse should emphasize the importance of cutting and examining each stool until the object is passed successfully.

The nurse should caution parents not to use laxatives and to maintain a normal diet to prevent the intestinal spasms that may precipitate an obstruction. Parents should be instructed to notify the physician if abdominal pain or vomiting occurs. Follow-up care and teaching concerning safety in the environment and the prevention of ingesting or inhaling foreign bodies are priority nursing responsibilities.

PEDIATRIC CAPSULE ENDOSCOPY

Pediatric capsule endoscopy involves the viewing of the internal GI tract without the use of an invasive endoscopic procedure that requires sedation and in-hospital care. A miniature camera that looks like a jellybean is swallowed like a pill and travels through the gastrointestinal tract, and it has been approved for pediatric use since 2009 (Cohen, 2012). The high-tech tiny capsule contains technology that provides color photos as it travels, propelled by natural peristalsis, through the intestines, and the images are wirelessly transmitted to an electrode contained in a small packet on the abdomen of the child and subsequently downloaded for viewing by the pediatric gastroenterologist. Preparation for the test includes a clear liquid diet and bowel preparation the day before ingestion of the capsule. The capsule is expelled within 72 hours and can be discarded in the normal trash (McCartney, 2013). Nursing responsibilities include assisting with the diet and bowel cleansing the day before and documenting the passage of the capsule. A website to explain the procedure to parents can be accessed at www.chp.edu/chp/capsule+endoscopy. Videos to help the nurse understand the procedure can be accessed at http://videos.NYP.org/videos/pediatriccapsule-endoscopy.

Get Ready for the NCLEX® Examination!

Key Points

- The newborn should be closely observed for signs of tracheoesophageal fistula (TEF), which include coughing, choking, cyanosis, and apnea during feedings.
- Drooling in the newborn may be a sign of an obstructed esophagus or TEF.
- The first stool of the newborn should be documented to record the patency of the anus.
- Pyloric stenosis is caused by hypertrophy of the pyloric muscles and is manifested by projectile vomiting.
- Nursing care for the child with pyloric stenosis involves frequent assessment, careful feeding, positioning on the right side after feedings, and education and support of the parents.
- Large, bulky, frothy stools are characteristic of malabsorption syndromes.
- Celiac disease is caused by a genetic sensitivity to gluten in the diet.
- To prevent the development of water intoxication, tap water should not be used for enemas in children with megacolon.
- Currant jelly stools characterize intussusception.
- Hirschsprung's disease occurs when there is an absence of ganglionic innervation of the muscle of a bowel segment.

- The treatment of gastroesophageal reflux includes thickened feedings, burping, and maintaining Fowler's position.
- A diarrheal stool in an infant is manifested by a watery consistency and a greenish color with the possible presence of mucus or blood. Frequency of bowel movements, by itself, is not an indication of diarrhea in infants.
- *C. difficile* is a health care–associated diarrhea that may occur with antimicrobial therapy.
- Hand hygiene with soap and water rather than an alcohol-based hand sanitizer is recommended when caring for patients with *C. difficile* diarrhea. Contact precautions are recommended, and the environment should be cleaned with a bleach disinfectant by housekeeping staff.
- Teaching parents basic hygienic practices, handwashing, and proper animal handling can prevent outbreaks of diarrhea.
- The functions of the gastrointestinal tract have a great influence on the fluid and electrolyte balance in infants and children.
- The higher daily exchange of water that occurs in infants leaves them less volume reserve when they are dehydrated.
- Oral rehydrating solutions are commercially prepared electrolyte solutions.

- Isotonic dehydration is the loss of equal amounts of water and electrolytes. Hypertonic dehydration is the loss of more water than electrolytes. Hypotonic dehydration is the loss of more electrolytes than water.
- Infants who are fed by the IV route should be picked up and held and allowed to suck on a pacifier.
- An intake and output record includes accurate documentation of information concerning oral and parenteral intake and suction, wound drainage, sweating, vomiting, urine, and stool output.
- Kwashiorkor is a protein deficiency characterized by a depigmented (white) streak of hair.
- Disposable nipples, pacifiers, and bottles should be used for infants with thrush.
- Pinworm is diagnosed by a "Scotch tape test." Preventing the child from scratching the anal area is an essential part of breaking the cycle of worm reinfestation.
- A chronic productive cough without fever is part of the roundworm life cycle in children.
- The nurse should teach parents not to store poisonous substances in food containers.
- Prevention of accidental poisoning should be part of every plan for teaching parents.
- Pica, the eating of nonfood items, is characteristic of children with lead poisoning.
- Lead poisoning (plumbism) can cause neurological damage.

Additional Learning Resources

SG Go to your Study Guide for additional learning activities to help you master this chapter content.

evolve Go to your Evolve website (http://evolve.elsevier.com/Leifer) for the following learning resources:
- Animations
- Answer Guidelines for Critical Thinking Questions
- Answers and Rationales for Review Questions for the NCLEX® Examination
- Glossary with English and Spanish pronunciations
- Interactive Review Questions for the NCLEX® Examination
- Patient Teaching Plans in English and Spanish
- Skills Performance Checklists
- Video clips and more!

 Online Resources
- Gastrointestinal conditions: http://digestive.niddk.nih.gov/ddiseases/ a-z.asp
- Poisoning: www.healthychild.net/articles/sf391ipecac.html

- Pyloric stenosis: http://kidshealth.org/parent/medical/digestive/ pyloric_stenosis.html
- Celiac Sprue Association: www.csaceliac.org/
- www.glutenfreediet.ca
- www.glutenfreedrugs.com/
- Celiac awareness: www.celiaccentral.com/
- Gluten-free restaurants and grocers: www.glutenfreeregistry.com/

Review Questions for the NCLEX® Examination

1. The pathologic disturbance of pyloric stenosis results from:
   1. edema of the pyloric muscle.
   2. ischemia of the pyloric muscle.
   3. hypertrophy of the pyloric muscle.
   4. neoplastic obstruction.

2. Which menu selections are best for a child diagnosed with celiac disease?
   1. Pizza and chocolate cake
   2. Spaghetti and blueberry muffin
   3. Chicken sandwich on whole-wheat bread
   4. Corn tortilla and fresh fruit

3. After surgery for pyloric stenosis, the nurse could anticipate that the infant will:
   1. have nasogastric suction for 24 hours.
   2. be fed clear liquids within 6 hours.
   3. remain NPO for 24 to 48 hours.
   4. be fed formula within 4 hours.

4. How are pinworms diagnosed?
   1. Seeing the worm in the stool
   2. A blood antigen level
   3. A "Scotch tape test" in the early morning
   4. A stool laboratory examination obtained at the hour of sleep

5. Priority teaching for a parent of a child who ingested a foreign body includes:
   1. encouraging the use of mild laxatives every night.
   2. slicing each stool passed to observe for the foreign body.
   3. encouraging a daily enema until the foreign body is passed.
   4. keeping the child NPO until the foreign body is passed.

The Child with a Genitourinary Condition

Objectives

1. Define each key term listed.
2. Name the functional unit of the kidney.
3. Recognize normal urine output for pediatric patients of various ages.
4. List four urological diagnostic procedures.
5. Recognize urinary tract anomalies in infants.
6. Discuss the cause and prevention of urinary tract infections in children.
7. Discuss the skin care pertinent to the child with nephrosis.
8. Explain any alterations in diet applicable to the child with nephrosis.
9. Differentiate between nephrosis and acute glomerulonephritis.
10. Outline the nursing care for a child who is diagnosed as having Wilms' tumor.
11. Discuss the impact of undescended testes on fertility.
12. Discuss the impact of genitourinary surgery on the growth and development of children at various ages.

Key Terms

chordee (KŎR-dē, p. 672)
cryptorchidism (krĭp-TŎR-kĭ-dĭz-ŭm, p. 681)
cystometrogram (sĭs-tō-MĔT-rō-grăm, p. 671)
dysuria (dĭs-YŪ-rē-ă, p. 672)
encopresis (ĕn-kō-PRĒ-sĭs, p. 671)
enuresis (ĕn-yū-RĒ-sĭs, p. 672)
epispadias (ĕp-ĭ-SPĀ-dē-ŭs, p. 672)
frequency (p. 672)
glomeruli (glō-MĔR-yū-lī, p. 675)
hydrocele (HĪ-drō-sēl, p. 680)
hydronephrosis (hī-drō-nĕ-FRŌ-sĭs, p. 673)
hyperkalemia (hī-pŭr-kă-LĒ-mē-ă, p. 678)
hypoalbuminemia (hī-pō-ăl-byū-mĭn-Ē-mē-ă, p. 675)
hypospadias (hī-pō-SPĀ-dē-ŭs, p. 672)
micturition (mĭk-tū-RĬSH-ŭn, p. 671)

nephron (NĔF-rŏn, p. 669)
neutropenia (nū-trō-PĒ-nē-ă, p. 677)
nocturia (nŏk-TŪ-rē-ă, p. 672)
oliguria (ŏl-ĭ-GŪ-rē-ă, p. 672)
orchiopexy (ŏr-kē-ō-PĔK-sē, p. 681)
paraphimosis (păr-ă-fī-MŌ-sĭs, p. 672)
phimosis (fī-MŌ-sĭs, p. 672)
polyuria (pŏl-ē-YŪ-rē-ă, p. 672)
pyelonephritis (pī-ĕ-lō-nĕ-FRĪ-tĭs, p. 674)
testicular torsion (tĕs-TĬK-yū-lăr TŎR-shŭn, p. 681)
ureteritis (yū-rĕ-tŭr-Ī-tĭs, p. 674)
urethritis (yū-rĕ-THRĪ-tĭs, p. 674)
urgency (p. 672)
vesicoureteral reflux (vĕs-ĭ-kō-yū-RĒ-tŭr-ăl RĒ-flŭks, p. 674)

DEVELOPMENT OF THE URINARY TRACT

The urinary system consists of two kidneys, two ureters, the urinary bladder, and the urethra. Figure 29-1 depicts these structures and illustrates how they differ in the developing child and in the adult. The function of the kidneys is to rid the body of waste products and to maintain body fluid homeostasis (Figure 29-2). The kidneys also produce substances that stimulate red blood cell formation in the bone marrow (e.g., erythropoietin-stimulating factor [ESF]), as well as renin, which regulates blood pressure. Microscopically, the functional unit of the kidneys is the **nephron**. Each kidney contains more than 1 million nephrons. Although the newborn's kidneys are immature, they function quite effectively. Nevertheless, the functional limitations must be considered carefully when the newborn is premature or ill. This applies especially to the administration of medications, formula, and parenteral fluids. The expected urine output for infants is 2 mL/kg/hr, and for children it is 0.5 to 1 mL/kg/hr.

Soon after implantation, the embryonic mass differentiates into three distinct layers of cells: the *ectoderm, mesoderm,* and *endoderm*. The urinary and reproductive organs originate from the mesoderm. At approximately the third month of gestation the fetal kidney begins to secrete urine. The amount gradually increases as the fetus matures and comprises a portion of the amniotic fluid volume. An absence or small amount of amniotic fluid (oligohydramnios) may indicate genitourinary difficulties.

The bladder capacity increases from 50 mL at birth to approximately 700 mL in adulthood. Adding 2 to the

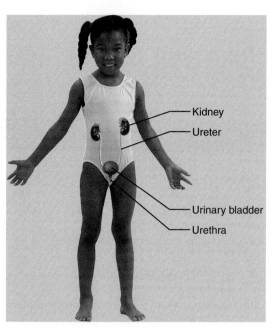

URINARY SYSTEM

- Fluid is of greater importance to the body chemistry of infants and small children, because it constitutes a larger fraction of their total body weight.
- Glomerular filtration and absorption are relatively low until 1 to 2 years of age. Infants are more prone to fluid volume excess and dehydration.
- Kidneys are more susceptible to trauma in children, because they usually do not have as much fat padding.
- Kidney function is immature until after 2 years of age.

Labels: Kidney, Ureter, Urinary bladder, Urethra

FIGURE 29-1 Summary of some urinary system differences between the child and the adult. The urinary system is the main excretory system. The kidneys remove wastes and excess materials from the blood and produce urine. This system helps to regulate blood chemistry. (Art overlay courtesy Observatory Group, Cincinnati, Ohio.)

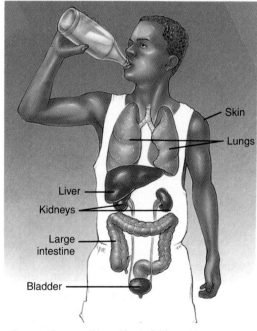

System	Organ	Excretion
Urinary	Kidney	Nitrogen compounds Toxins Water Electrolytes
Integumentary	Skin—sweat glands	Nitrogen compounds Water Electrolytes
Respiratory	Lung	Carbon dioxide Water
Digestive	Intestine	Digestive wastes Bile pigments Salts of heavy metals

Labels: Skin, Lungs, Liver, Kidneys, Large intestine, Bladder

FIGURE 29-2 The urinary system's chief function is to regulate the volume and composition of body fluids and to excrete unwanted materials, but it is not the only system in the body that is able to excrete unneeded substances. The table in this figure compares the excretory functions of several systems. Although all of these systems contribute to the body's effort to remove wastes, only the urinary system can finely adjust the water and electrolyte balance to the degree required for normal homeostasis of body fluids. (From Thibodeau GA, Patton KT: *Anatomy & physiology,* ed 6, St Louis, 2006, Mosby.)

age in years can provide an age-specific estimation of the bladder capacity in ounces, so that, for example, an 8-year-old child has a bladder capacity of 10 ounces.

There is an unexplained relationship between low-set ears in the newborn and urinary tract anomalies. When assessing the newborn, an imaginary line should be drawn between the outer canthus of the eye and the ear. The line should cross the tip of the auricle. If the tip of the auricle falls below this line, the assessment should be recorded and reported (see Figure 12-6). Because the kidney and the ear develop at about the same time in fetal life, an abnormality of the ear can be a signal that an abnormality of the urinary tract may also be present. Therefore, low-set ears may be a "red flag" to indicate that further assessment would be warranted.

DEVELOPMENT OF THE REPRODUCTIVE SYSTEMS

Figure 29-3 shows the female and male reproductive systems and lists some of the differences between children and adults. The reproductive system provides for perpetuation of the species. Members of each gender are equipped with gonads (which provide reproductive cells) and a set of accessory organs. The gonads (ovaries in the female and testes in the male) produce sex cells and hormones that affect the reproductive organs and other body systems.

Sex is genetically determined at the time of fertilization. The presence of a Y chromosome is essential for the development of the testes and their hormones. Sex differentiation in the embryo occurs early. The organs specific to the male or female child develop. Before this, the embryo has neither male nor female characteristics. The development of the ovaries occurs later than that of the testes. By the twelfth week the external genitalia of the fetus are recognizably male or female.

Several tests are helpful in diagnosing conditions of the reproductive tract. These include a Papanicolaou (Pap) smear, serological blood tests, cultures, ultrasound procedures, pregnancy tests, and routine blood and urine tests. Sexual abuse in children may be manifested by behaviors such as urinary frequency, excessive masturbation, **encopresis** (fecal soiling beyond 4 years of age), severe nightmares, bedwetting, irritation or pain in the genital area, and a decrease in physical or emotional development. Suggestive posturing by young children or an explicit knowledge of sex acts shown by children younger than 8 years of age calls for further investigation. Menstrual disorders and premenstrual syndrome are discussed in Chapter 11. Sexually transmitted infections are discussed in Chapters 11 and 32.

 Nursing Tip

Most newborns urinate within the first 24 hours of life. Recording and reporting the presence or absence of urination is very important.

ASSESSMENT OF URINARY FUNCTION

Urological diagnostic procedures include urinalysis, ultrasonography, intravenous (IV) pyelogram, and computed tomography (CT) scan of the kidneys. Renal biopsy is used to diagnose the extent of kidney disease. A uroflow is an assessment procedure used to determine the rate of urine flow. The child voids into a receptacle, and a uroflowmeter graphs the volume and pressure. This is useful in diagnosing stricture or scarring. Cytoscopy is useful for investigating congenital abnormalities or acquired lesions in the bladder and lower urinary tract. Radiographic examination of the bladder and urethra before and during **micturition** (voiding) is called *voiding cystourethrography*. The **cystometrogram** and the urethral pressure profile assess bladder capacity and function. Both tests require catheterization and infusion of sterile water. The minimum urine output for infants and toddlers is 2 to 3 mL/kg/hr; for preschoolers and young school-age children, the minimum is 1 to 2 mL/kg/hr; and for school-age children and adolescents, the minimum is 0.5 to 1 mL/kg/hr. Common laboratory tests are reviewed in Table 29-1.

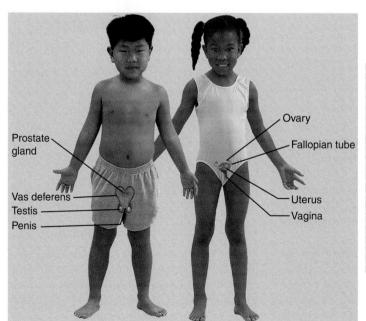

Prostate gland
Vas deferens
Testis
Penis

Ovary
Fallopian tube
Uterus
Vagina

REPRODUCTIVE SYSTEM

- The genitals in preterm females may appear swollen. The labia minora may protrude beyond the labia majora.
- The testicles may appear large at birth in proportion to the size of the infant. They may fail to move into the scrotum, causing a condition termed *undescended testes*.
- The foreskin may be tight at birth, causing phimosis.
- The sex organs do not mature until the onset of puberty.
- Secondary sex characteristics occur with the onset of puberty.

FIGURE 29-3 Summary of some reproductive system differences between the child and the adult male and female. Each reproductive system consists of gonads and associated structures. The reproductive system maintains sexual characteristics and provides for perpetuation of the species. (Art overlay courtesy Observatory Group, Cincinnati, Ohio.)

Table 29-1	Common Laboratory Tests for Urinary Tract Function	
TEST	**NORMAL LEVELS***	**SIGNIFICANCE OF DEVIATION**
Blood		
Blood urea nitrogen (BUN)	Newborn: 3-12 mg/dL Child: 5-18 mg/dL	High BUN level indicates renal disease, dehydration, need for steroid therapy
Uric acid	Child: 2-5 mg/dL	Renal disease
Creatinine	Infant: 0.2-0.4 mg/dL Child: 0.3-0.7 mg/dL Adolescent: 0.5-1.0 mg/dL	Severe renal disease
Urine		
Red blood cells	<2 per HPF	Trauma, infection, stones
Bacteria	Few	Infection
Casts	Occasional	Glomerular disease, pyelonephritis
White blood cells	<5 per HPF	Infection
Ketones	0	Stress; diabetes mellitus
Glucose	0	Diabetes mellitus
Protein	0	Glomerular kidney disease
pH	Newborn: 5-7 Child: 4.8-7.8	Potassium deficiency, electrolyte imbalance
Specific gravity	Newborn: 1.001-1.020 Child: 1.001-1.030	Dehydration Overhydration, renal disease, pituitary malfunction

*Values for different age groups are indicated only when relevant. *HPF*, High-powered field.

Terms commonly used to describe urinary dysfunction include the following:

- **Dysuria**: difficulty in urination
- **Frequency**: abnormal number of voidings in a short period
- **Urgency**: strong urges to void, often despite inability to do so
- **Nocturia**: awakening during the night to void
- **Enuresis**: uncontrolled voiding after bladder control has been established
- **Polyuria**: increased urine output
- **Oliguria**: decreased urine output

ANOMALIES OF THE URINARY TRACT

PHIMOSIS

Pathophysiology. **Phimosis** is a narrowing of the preputial opening of the foreskin, which prevents the foreskin from being retracted over the penis (Figure 29-4). This is normal in newborns and usually disappears by 3 years of age. In some children this narrowing may obstruct the stream of urine, causing dribbling or irritation. Circumcision can correct the condition.

Treatment and Nursing Care. When circumcision is performed on an older boy, careful explanations and reassurance are provided. The nurse is sensitive to the child's embarrassment and fear. Postoperatively the penis is covered with a petroleum gauze. The penis is tender and may burn on urination.

Cleansing of the uncircumcised penis and retraction of the foreskin are discussed in Chapter 12. Forcible retraction of a tight foreskin is avoided because it can

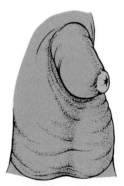

FIGURE 29-4 Phimosis. The foreskin is advanced and fixed; it cannot be retracted over the glans.

lead to **paraphimosis** (Figure 29-5). When this occurs, the foreskin cannot be returned to its normal position. There may be swelling and impaired circulation caused by the constriction. This condition necessitates immediate evaluation by a physician.

HYPOSPADIAS AND EPISPADIAS

Pathophysiology. **Hypospadias** is a congenital defect in which the urinary meatus is located not at the end of the penis but on the lower shaft. In mild cases it lies just below the tip of the penis, but it may be found at the midshaft or near the penile–scrotal junction. With **epispadias**, the opening of the urinary meatus is on the upper surface of the penis. Unlike epispadias, hypospadias is fairly common, occurring in 1 out of 250 to 500 newborn boys (Elder, 2011). Hypospadias may be accompanied by **chordee**, a downward curvature of the penis caused by a fibrotic band of tissue (Figure 29-6).

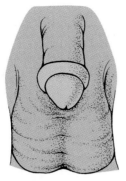

FIGURE 29-5 Paraphimosis. The foreskin is retracted and fixed; it cannot be returned to its original position. Constriction impedes circulation.

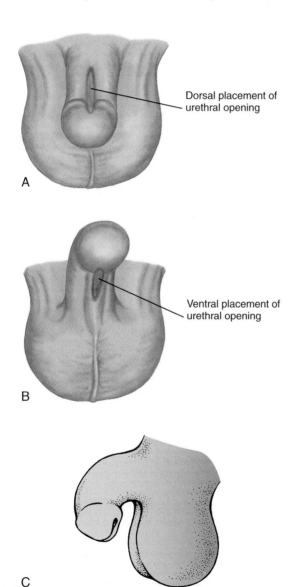

A — Dorsal placement of urethral opening

B — Ventral placement of urethral opening

C

FIGURE 29-6 A, Epispadias. **B,** Hypospadias. **C,** Chordee. (From James SR, Nelson KA, Murray SS, Ashwill JW: *Nursing care of children: principles and practice*, ed 4, St Louis, 2013, Saunders.)

Treatment and Nursing Care. The alert nurse may discover hypospadias or epispadias in the nursery during neonatal assessment. In many mild cases surgery is not necessary for either condition unless the location and extent of the defect are such that the child will not be able to stand to void or the defect would cause psychological problems or difficulties in future sexual relations. Treatment consists of surgical repair and is usually performed before age 18 months. It is sometimes done in stages depending on the associated defects. Most techniques can be performed during same-day surgery. Routine circumcision is avoided in these children, because the foreskin may be useful in the repair. A urinary catheter may be required after surgery. Parents are instructed in the home care of the catheterized child. Medication for bladder spasms may be required.

This condition is corrected at a time in childhood when fears of separation and mutilation are great, and therefore attention is directed to psychological considerations. In the older child, questions about virility and reproduction may surface and need to be addressed.

EXSTROPHY OF THE BLADDER

Pathophysiology. In exstrophy of the bladder the lower portion of the abdominal wall and the anterior wall of the bladder are missing. As a result, the bladder lies open and exposed on the abdomen. Exstrophy is caused by a failure of the midline to close during embryonic development. Other congenital anomalies may also be present. This anomaly occurs in 1 out of 40,000 live births and is more common in boys than in girls.

Manifestations. This disorder is noticeable by fetal sonogram. The defect may range from a small cutaneous fistula in the abdominal wall to complete exstrophy (the turning inside out of an organ). Urine leaks continually from the bladder. The skin around the bladder becomes excoriated. Other anomalies are common.

Treatment and Nursing Care. The bladder is covered with a plastic shield or appropriate dressing to protect its mucosa but still to allow for urinary drainage. This also protects the bladder from irritation by bedclothes or diapers. A suitable ointment is applied to protect the skin. Diapers are generally placed under rather than around the infant. The infant is positioned on his or her back or side so that urine drains freely. Antibiotics are given to prevent infection. Surgical closure is ideally performed during the first 48 hours of life.

OBSTRUCTIVE UROPATHY

Pathophysiology. Many conditions, such as calculi (stones), tumors, strictures, and scarring, may cause an obstruction of the normal flow of urine. These conditions may be congenital or acquired, and blockage may be either partial or complete. One or both kidneys may be affected. The pathological changes depend on the nature and location of the problem. **Hydronephrosis** (*hydro*, "water," and *nephro*, "kidney") is the distention of the renal pelvis as a result of an obstruction. The pelvis of the kidney becomes enlarged, and cysts form. This may eventually damage renal nephrons, resulting

Table 29-2	Surgical Procedures Used in Urinary Diversion
PROCEDURE	**DEFINITION**
Ureterostomy	Ureters are surgically diverted to opening (stoma) on outside abdominal wall. This allows urine to drain into a collection device.
Ileal or colon conduit (artificial channel)	Conduit diverts urine at ureter, bypassing bladder and urethra; ureters are removed from bladder and attached to ileum or colon, which then acts as bladder; there is no voluntary control of voiding. Patient has stoma, which is larger and not as prone to stenosis as a ureterostomy; child wears ileostomy appliance. NOTE: Urine from conduit may appear cloudy from secretions of bowel conduit; this is not a sign of urinary tract infection.
Nephrostomy	Tube passes through flank into pelvis of kidney; this allows urine to be drained from pelvis (bypassing ureter, bladder, and urethra; drains into ostomy bag).
Suprapubic tube placement	A suprapubic tube is placed above symphysis pubis into bladder to provide urinary drainage.
Vesicostomy*	A surgical opening is made into bladder between umbilicus and pubis; bladder wall is brought to surface of abdomen.

*Vesico, "bladder," and stoma, "passage."

in deterioration of the kidneys. *Polycystic kidney* refers to a condition in which large, fluid-filled cysts form in place of healthy kidney tissue in the fetus. This is inherited as an autosomal recessive trait. Kidney damage can result in an inability of the kidney to concentrate urine, resulting in metabolic acidosis. Urine that is not excreted promptly can promote the growth of organisms that cause urinary tract infection.

Treatment and Nursing Care. Urinary diversion is necessary in certain conditions and may be accomplished by several procedures (Table 29-2). This type of surgery is a source of great apprehension for parents. The physical care of the child with a urinary stoma (artificially created opening or passage) presents hygiene problems, skin problems, and difficulties in leaving the infant in the care of others. Frequent trips to the health care provider add to the strain of everyday life.

Stress from the urinary diversion is age related. The toddler may be unable to attain independence in toilet training. The school-age child suffers from being different and may have a distorted body image. The adolescent may have lowered self-esteem and is concerned about sexuality. Parents with affected newborns grieve for the loss of a perfect child and experience concerns about the length and quality of the infant's life. The nurse anticipates the impact of this type of diagnosis and incorporates suitable psychological interventions into daily care. Providing emotional support and teaching parents how to prevent infection are priorities of care.

Assessing for a distended bladder. To assess for a distended bladder, the nurse gently palpates below the umbilicus, moving toward the symphysis pubis. The normal bladder is not palpable because it lies behind the symphysis pubis.

> **Nursing Tip**
>
> The bladder capacity of a child can be approximated by the following formula:
>
> Age in years + 2 = Ounces of bladder volume or capacity

ACUTE URINARY TRACT INFECTION

Pathophysiology. Urinary tract infections (UTIs) are common in children. They are more common in girls than in boys (except during the neonatal period) and occur predominantly in children 7 to 11 years of age. Of all infections, 75% to 90% are caused by *Escherichia coli,* followed by *Klebsiella* and *Proteus* (Kligman et al, 2011). The nurse will note that the following terms are used to describe the location and nature of urinary tract disturbances:

- ***Urethritis***: infection of the urethra
- *Cystitis:* inflammation of the bladder
- *Bacteriuria:* bacteria in the urine
- ***Pyelonephritis***: infection of the kidney and the renal pelvis
- ***Ureteritis***: infection of the ureters
- ***Vesicoureteral reflux***: backward flow of urine into the ureters

Several factors account for the preponderance of UTIs in girls. These include a shorter urethra, the location of the urethra closer to the anus, the wearing of close-fitting nylon underwear, the use of bubble baths, the retention of urine, and vaginitis. Incest or other sexual abuse should be considered in young girls with repeated infections. In boys, the longer male urethra and the antibacterial properties of prostatic secretions inhibit the entry of pathogens.

Certain chemical and physical factors are important. Normal urine is acidic. Alkaline urine favors pathogens.

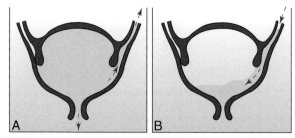

FIGURE 29-7 Vesicoureteral reflux. **A,** Congenital abnormalities of the junction between the bladder and the ureters can force urine to flow backward into the ureters during voiding. **B,** After voiding, residual urine from the ureter remains in the bladder.

Urine that remains in the bladder for a prolonged time serves as an excellent medium for bacterial growth. In certain conditions such as *vesicoureteral reflux*, the urine is forced backward from the bladder and into the ureters during urination (Figure 29-7).

Vesicoureteral reflux. *Vesicoureteral reflux (VUR)* refers to the abnormal retrograde flow of urine from the bladder to the ureters during a void (see Figure 29-7). After the void, urine flows back into the bladder, where urinary stasis occurs that allows growth of bacteria leading to UTI. The bacteria have access to the kidneys during subsequent reflux; pyelonephritis and renal scarring can result.

Manifestations and Diagnosis. The signs and symptoms of UTI are age dependent. The infant may be admitted with high fever, vomiting, and chills. A urine specimen for culture is obtained before antibiotics are administered. Specimens must be processed promptly or refrigerated to prevent contamination. Urine specimens should not be collected from the diaper because the chemicals and gels contained in the diaper fabric may alter the results of some tests. In toilet-trained children, a midstream urine specimen is obtained after cleansing the urethral meatus and rinsing with sterile water. A renal/bladder ultrasound is recommended, and a voiding cystourethrogram (VCUG) may be ordered if the ultrasound is abnormal (Roberts, 2011).

Treatment and Nursing Care. Infants less than 1 year of age are usually hospitalized and observed. Treatment with daily low-dose antimicrobial medications may be required to keep the urine sterile and to prevent kidney infection. Infants usually outgrow the reflux, but they are monitored regularly as outpatients. For severe reflux, an endoscopic procedure injects a bulking agent via a subtrigonal injection (STING) into the mucous membrane of the ureter to prevent retrograde flow of urine. Open surgical intervention is reserved mostly for significant anatomical defects.

Acute cystitis is treated promptly to prevent development of pyelonephritis and kidney damage. Until the specific organism causing the infection is identified, broad-spectrum antibiotics are initially prescribed.

Methods of preventing UTIs are taught to parents and to the patient, if age appropriate. The nurse stresses the need for proper amounts of fluid to maintain sterility and flushing of the bladder. Nursing Care Plan 29-1 presents the nursing considerations appropriate for these patients. The prognosis is excellent with prompt treatment. Monitoring vital signs, including blood pressure, and providing anticipatory guidance help to decrease the stress levels of the children and parents.

🔼 Nursing Tip

Interventions to prevent urinary tract infection (UTI) include:
- Cleanse perineum with each diaper change
- Wipe perineum from front to back
- Avoid bubble baths
- Have child urinate immediately after a bath
- Use white, cotton underwear
- Use loose-fitting pants
- Offer adequate fluid intake (diuresis increases antibacterial properties of the renal medulla)

NEPHROTIC SYNDROME (NEPHROSIS)

Pathophysiology. **Nephrotic syndrome** refers to a number of different types of kidney conditions that are distinguished by the presence of marked amounts of protein in the urine, edema, and hypoalbuminemia. *Minimal change nephrotic syndrome* (MCNS), found in approximately 85% of cases, is discussed in this section.

Nephrosis is more common in boys than in girls and is seen most often in children 2 to 7 years of age. The specific cause is unknown but may be related to a thymus T-cell dysfunction. The prognosis is good in steroid-responsive patients. Most children experience periods of relapse until the disease resolves itself. There is an 80% favorable prognosis over the long term.

Manifestations. The characteristic symptom of nephrosis is edema. This occurs slowly; the child does not appear to be sick. It is first noticed around the eyes and ankles and later becomes generalized. The edema shifts with the position of the child during sleep. The child gains weight because of the accumulation of fluid. The abdomen may become distended (ascites). The child is pale, irritable, listless, and has a poor appetite. Blood pressure is usually normal.

Urine examination shows massive albumin (protein) and a few red blood cells. The **glomeruli**, the working units of the kidneys that filter the blood, become damaged and allow albumin and blood cells to enter the urine. The level of protein in the blood falls; this is termed **hypoalbuminemia** (*hypo*, "below," *albumin*, and *emia*, "blood").

Treatment. The goals of treatment include minimizing edema, preventing infection, reducing the loss of protein in the urine, and preventing toxicity from the medication prescribed.

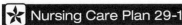

PATIENT DATA A school-age female child is brought to the clinic complaining of burning on urination. Her mother states the child fears going to the bathroom because "it will hurt."

Selected Nursing Diagnosis: Impaired urinary elimination related to dysuria, incontinence

Goals	Nursing Interventions	Rationales
Child will not complain of frequency, urgency, or pain on urination. Child will not strain or fret before voiding. Child will verbalize reasons for frequent bladder emptying.	Administer antibiotics as prescribed.	Antibiotics are chosen according to urine culture and sensitivity; phenazopyridine (Pyridium) may be given to decrease dysuria.
	Encourage complete bladder emptying; explain necessity for this, as age appropriate.	Retained urine in the bladder is very susceptible to the growth of organisms.
	Remind child to void frequently; anticipate incontinence.	Under normal conditions the bladder flushes away organisms by regularly ridding itself of urine; this prevents organisms from accumulating and invading nearby structures. The convalescent bladder is less resistant to invasion than is a healthy bladder.
	Encourage fluids.	Child may be febrile; increasing fluids decreases the concentration of solutes and alleviates urinary stasis.
	Keep accurate intake and output records.	This is essential to determine the progress of treatment, because the kidneys and bladder play an important part in fluid balance.
	Teach child how to collect urine specimens, if age appropriate.	Education ensures that the specimen will be correctly obtained without contamination.
	Provide privacy.	Children must be given the same courtesy as adults because they are sensitive and embarrassed by body exposure and body functions.

Selected Nursing Diagnosis: Deficient knowledge related to hygiene measures useful in prevention of urinary tract infection

Goals	Nursing Interventions	Rationales
Girl will demonstrate on doll how to wipe herself after voiding. Child will verbalize methods to accomplish this.	Instruct girl of importance of wiping self from front to back.	Good perineal hygiene prevents fecal contamination of urethra.
	Emphasize need to avoid bubble baths, water softeners.	The oils in these products are known to irritate the urethra.
	Encourage the use of showers.	These hygienic measures are helpful in preventing infection.
	Explain the need for cotton underwear.	Cotton underwear is more absorbent.
	Suggest juices (e.g., apple, cranberry) to maintain acidity of urine. Diet of meats, cheese, prunes, cranberries, plums, and whole grains is also beneficial (acid ash–producing foods).	Acidifying urine decreases the rate of bacterial multiplication.
	Recommend frequent pad change for menstruating girls and proper genital cleansing during period.	Old, pooled blood fosters the growth of organisms; proper cleansing helps to prevent irritation.

Selected Nursing Diagnosis: Deficient parental knowledge related to follow-up care

Goals	Nursing Interventions	Rationales
Parents will verbalize necessity for continued supervision and medication.	Instruct parents to administer medication as prescribed and to continue for time recommended by the physician.	Typical course of antibiotic treatment is 7-10 days; emphasize the need to complete prescribed dosage.
	Suggest that patient avoid hot tubs or whirlpool baths.	May be potential sources of infection.
	Remind parents of necessity of adequate hydration for child.	Children dehydrate very quickly.
	Instruct parents that recurrence is most likely within 3-12 months after infection and is often asymptomatic.	Emphasize the need for routine office visits to test for asymptomatic infections.
	Explain necessity for periodic follow-up urine cultures.	Recurrence is common; a urine culture obtained approximately 1 week after medicine use is discontinued will determine if medication has eradicated bacteria.

Critical Thinking Question

1. A mother comes to the clinic with her 5-year-old child who has a urinary tract infection for the second time in 3 months. You notice that the child is wearing spandex sports shorts and is carrying a doll. She is holding a bottled water container that is filled with fruit punch. What teaching interventions could the nurse initiate?

Control of edema. The child with nephrosis is given medications designed to reduce proteinuria and, consequently, edema. Steroid therapy is currently used for this purpose. Oral prednisone is initially given. The dosage is reduced for maintenance therapy, which continues for 1 to 2 months. Because steroids mask signs of infection, the patient must be watched closely for more subtle symptoms of illness. Children are prone to infection when absolute granulocyte counts fall below 1000 cells/mm³. This is called **neutropenia**.

The child's skin is examined at sites of punctures, wounds, pierced ears, body piercings, and catheters. The nurse watches for temperature variations and changes in behavior. Suspicions are promptly reported, because septicemia is life threatening. Prompt antimicrobial therapy is begun when an acute infection is recognized. Generally, diuretics have not been effective in reducing nephrotic edema. Immunosuppressive therapy (e.g., cyclophosphamide [Cytoxan] and chlorambucil) is used for some steroid-resistant children.

 Safety Alert!

When steroids are administered, the immune system is depressed. Care should be taken to limit exposure to infections.

Diet. An attractively served, well-balanced diet is desirable because appetite is often poor. Parents are instructed to avoid adding salt to foods served whenever edema is present. Fluids are not usually restricted except when massive edema is present. A normal protein intake is recommended.

Nursing Care. The nursing care of the child with nephrosis is of the greatest significance because the disease necessitates long-term therapy. The child is periodically hospitalized and becomes a familiar personality to hospital personnel.

The nurse provides supportive care to the parents and child throughout the course of this disease. The child is treated at home whenever possible and is brought to the hospital for special therapy only. Parents are instructed to keep a daily record of the child's weight, urinary protein levels, and medications. Signs of infection, abnormal weight gain, and increased protein in the urine must be reported promptly. Good skin care is especially important during periods of marked edema. After the acute stage of the illness subsides, the child is allowed to participate in normal childhood activities.

Positioning. The child is turned frequently to prevent respiratory tract infection. A pillow placed between the knees when the child is lying on the side prevents pressure on the edematous skin surfaces. The child's head is elevated from time to time during the day to reduce edema of the eyelids and to make him or her more comfortable. Swelling impairs the circulation of the lacrimal secretions. It may therefore be necessary to bathe the eyes to prevent the accumulation of exudate.

Monitoring intake and output. The child's intake and output are strictly charted. This is the responsibility of the nurse, regardless of who feeds the patient. Parents are instructed to inform the nurse of how much fluid has been taken. The importance of keeping proper fluid balance sheets (i.e., intake and output records) for patients with diseases of the kidneys cannot be overemphasized.

As stated, the patient's urine output must be carefully measured. Diapers may be weighed on a gram scale before application and after removal (1 g = 1 mL). The dry weights are marked on the diaper. A careful check of the number of voidings is of particular value. The character, odor, and color of the urine are also important. If a 24-hour urine collection is ordered, *every* voided specimen within that time must be saved, or the test will not be valid. The specimens are collected in a large bottle or container that is correctly labeled. Some tests require special care or certain preservatives be added to the container; these instructions are clarified before the procedure begins.

Nursing Tip

Remember to measure and record urine specimens sent to the laboratory.

Weight and protection from infection. The patient is weighed two or three times weekly to determine changes in the degree of edema. The child is weighed on the same scale each time and at about the same time of day. Abdominal girth (circumference) should also be measured daily.

Nurses make every effort to protect the child from exposure to upper respiratory tract infections. Children who are active must not be allowed to wander into areas where they would be in danger of contracting an infection. **No vaccinations or immunizations should be administered** while the disease is active and during immunosuppressive therapy.

The vital signs of a patient with nephrosis are taken regularly. Ordinarily, there is no temperature elevation unless an infection is present. Blood pressure remains normal. All members of the nursing team provide parental guidance and support. The child with nephrosis is kept under close medical supervision throughout an extended period. Home care during remissions is preferred, with parents being taught monitoring skills.

ACUTE GLOMERULONEPHRITIS

Pathophysiology. **Acute glomerulonephritis** (AGN), formerly called Bright's disease, is an allergic reaction (antigen-antibody) to a group A beta-hemolytic streptococcal infection. It may appear after the patient has had scarlet fever or skin infections. The body's immune mechanisms appear to be important in its development. Antibodies produced to fight the invading organisms also react against the glomerular tissue. Glomerulonephritis is the most common form of nephritis in

Table 29-3	Comparison Between Nephrosis and Acute Glomerulonephritis	
	NEPHROSIS	**ACUTE GLOMERULONEPHRITIS**
Cause	Unknown, may be thymus T-cell dysfunction	Response to infection with group A beta-hemolytic streptococci
Edema	Massive edema Anasarca: whole-body edema Ascites: fluid in abdominal cavity	Periorbital edema (puffiness of eyes)
Blood pressure	Usually normal	Usually moderately elevated
Urine tests	Proteinuria Trace of blood	Trace of protein Hematuria (resolves within 1 month, but urinary symptoms may persist for 1 year)
Pallor	Degree of pallor is greater than expected in relation to degree of anemia (appearance resulting from edematous tissue)	Pallor related to anemia

NOTE: The signs and symptoms of nephrosis and acute glomerulonephritis are similar. Careful analysis and comparisons show significant differences. Either condition can lead to renal failure and its consequences.

children, and it occurs most often in boys 3 to 7 years of age. Both kidneys are usually affected.

The nephron is the working unit of the kidneys. Nephrons number in the millions. Within the bulb of each nephron lies a cluster of capillaries called the *glomerulus.* It is these structures that are affected, as the name implies. They become inflamed and sometimes blocked, permitting red blood cells and protein (which are normally retained) to enter the urine. The kidneys become pale and slightly enlarged. Table 29-3 compares nephrosis with AGN.

The prognosis for AGN is excellent. Patients with mild cases of the disease may recover within 10 to 14 days. Patients with protracted cases may show urinary changes for as long as 1 year, but they experience complete recovery. The possibility of complications involving hypertensive changes such as brain ischemia necessitates careful monitoring and care of each patient.

Manifestations. From 1 to 3 weeks after a streptococcal infection has occurred, the parent may notice that the child has periorbital edema when awakening in the morning and that the child's urine is smoky brown or bloody. This is frightening to the parent and child, and most parents immediately seek medical advice. Urine output may be decreased. The urine specific gravity is high, and albumin, red and white blood cells, and casts may be found on examination. The blood urea nitrogen (BUN) level is elevated, as are the serum creatinine level and the sedimentation rate. The serum complement level (C3) is usually reduced. **Hyperkalemia** (excessive potassium in the blood) may produce cardiac toxicity. Hypertension may occur. An antistreptolysin (ASO) titer, if positive, evidences a recent streptococcal infection.

Treatment and Nursing Care. Although children may feel well, activity is limited until gross hematuria subsides. The urine is examined regularly. Every effort is made to prevent children from becoming overly tired, chilled, or exposed to infection. Because renal function is impaired, there is a danger of accumulating nitrogenous wastes and sodium in the body. Dietary sodium and fluid restrictions are based on the hypertension and edema present. Foods high in potassium, such as bananas, are restricted during periods of oliguria.

Nursing care is supportive. Prevention of infection and fatigue, maintenance of accurate intake and output records, and frequent monitoring of vital signs are essential.

Although glomerulonephritis is generally benign, it can be a source of anguish for the parents and child. If the patient is treated at home, the parents must plan quiet activities to keep the child occupied. They must understand the importance of continued medical supervision, because follow-up urine and blood tests are necessary to assess progress toward recovery. All children with hypertension should be monitored for signs of increased intracranial pressure. Most children recover completely with no sequelae.

WILMS' TUMOR

Pathophysiology. **Wilms' tumor**, or *nephroblastoma* (*nephro,* "kidney," *blasto,* "bud," and *oma,* "tumor"), is one of the most common malignancies of early life. It is an embryonal adenosarcoma (*adeno,* "glandular," and *sarcoma,* "cancer of connective tissue") that is now known to be associated with certain congenital anomalies, particularly of the genitourinary tract. It is thought to have a genetic basis.

About two thirds of these growths are discovered before the child is 3 years of age. As with some other malignancies, there are few or no symptoms during the early stages of growth. A mass in the abdomen is generally discovered by a parent or by the physician during a routine checkup. Radiographic examinations of the kidneys (most importantly, IV pyelograms) show a growth and verify that the remaining kidney is normal. The tumor compresses kidney tissue and is usually encapsulated. Renal damage may cause hypertension. Chest x-ray films, ultrasonography, bone surveys, liver scan, and CT may also be indicated. Wilms' tumor seldom affects both kidneys.

Treatment and Nursing Care. Treatment of patients with Wilms' tumor consists of a combination of surgery, radiation therapy, and chemotherapy. The kidney and tumor are removed as soon as possible after the diagnosis has been confirmed. It is important to prepare the parents and the child for the extent of the incision, which is considerable.

General nursing measures for the comfort of the patient are implemented. One important consideration pertaining to this condition is the avoidance of all unnecessary handling of the abdomen, because it can cause the tumor to spread. The physician explains this to the parents, and in the hospital a sign is placed on the crib: "Do not palpate abdomen." Nursing Care Plan 29-2 outlines care for a child undergoing surgery of the renal system. Chemotherapy and radiation therapy after surgery are usually completed at a specialized cancer center. Postoperatively, contact sports should be avoided to prevent damage to the remaining kidney.

> **⚠ Safety Alert!**
>
> Abdominal palpation as part of the daily assessment of a child with Wilms' tumor is omitted.

✷ Nursing Care Plan 29-2 | Child Undergoing Surgery of the Renal System

PATIENT DATA A preadolescent boy is admitted for elective kidney surgery. The child asks his parents to stay and asks the nurse many questions about the planned surgery.

Selected Nursing Diagnosis: Anxiety related to surgical experience

Goals	Nursing Interventions	Rationales
Parents will state ways they are coping with the stress of this surgery.	Provide surgical tour; include wake-up room.	Explanations and familiarity with physical surroundings may decrease apprehension.
	Encourage parents to remain with child, as appropriate.	Child is more secure when parents are nearby.
Child will verbalize an understanding of procedure, as age appropriate.	Explain mask and anesthesia equipment.	It is frightening to have something placed over the face; equipment is intimidating.
	Determine the small child's words for *penis* and *urination*.	This will promote understanding postoperatively.
	Provide support and reassurance.	Urinary surgery may raise anxiety about sexual function, which parents or patients are often unable to express.

Selected Nursing Diagnosis: High risk for ineffective airway clearance related to poor cough effort associated with postanesthesia, postoperative immobility, pain

Goals	Nursing Interventions	Rationales
Child will maintain airway patency as evidenced by clear lung sounds and vital signs within normal range.	Assist child to turn, cough, and deep breathe; reposition infants.	Prolonged postoperative immobility leads to decreased chest expansion, pooling of mucus in bronchi, and hypostatic pneumonia. In nephrectomy patients, the incision is close to the diaphragm, making breathing painful; allow infants to cry for a few seconds to ensure deep breathing; if secretions are present, coughing will generally follow. Ambulate as ordered.
	Monitor vital signs frequently.	Monitoring vital signs permits assessment of cardiovascular function and tissue perfusion.
	Teach splinting of incision preoperatively.	Splinting incision lessens pain.
	Teach incentive spirometry preoperatively.	Spirometry promotes alveolar inflation, restores and maintains lung capacity, and strengthens respiratory muscles; it also provides immediate feedback about the effectiveness of deep breathing.
	Observe and medicate for bladder spasm and incisional pain.	Postoperative pain and discomfort may make patients reluctant to turn, cough, and deep breathe.

Continued

⭐ Nursing Care Plan 29-2　Child Undergoing Surgery of the Renal System—cont'd

Selected Nursing Diagnosis: High risk for deficient fluid volume, related to patient's age, surgery, catheters, or refusal to drink

Goals	Nursing Interventions	Rationales
Vital signs will remain within normal limits. Child's hydration and acid-base balance will remain stable as evidenced by laboratory reports.	Regulate intravenous (IV) fluids.	Child will probably take nothing by mouth for a brief period before and after surgery. IV fluids maintain hydration and replace lost electrolytes.
	Keep accurate intake and output records.	Careful monitoring of fluid intake and output will show early renal complications.
	Weigh infants daily.	Daily weights in infants aid in monitoring underhydration or overhydration. Comparison with preoperative weight permits assessment of infant's nutritional progress.
	Record separate output for each drainage tube.	An unexpected reduction in urine flow necessitates prompt intervention. Each catheter drains into its own collection bag, so the source of reduced flow will be immediately noticed.
	Observe tissue turgor and fontanelles of infants.	Depressed fontanelles, sunken eyeballs, lack of tears, dark circles around eyes, and poor skin turgor denote dehydration, which can occur quickly in infants and children.
	Begin clear oral fluids gradually.	Replacement of fluids and electrolytes by mouth is generally considered to be the safest method; clarify ambiguous orders, such as "force fluids," "restrict fluids," particularly in infants and small children with, for example, urological disorders or cardiac conditions.
Child's temperature will remain at or below 38° C (100.4° F); incision site will not be erythematous or foul-smelling.	Observe for signs of infection.	Fever, incisional tenderness, redness, drainage from incisions, and lethargy indicate infection.
	Observe and record patency, color, amount, and consistency of drainage.	Catheters can become plugged by mucus shreds, blood clots, and chemical sediment; plugging of conduits can lead to infection of urinary tract, urine stasis, and, if obstruction persists, hydronephrosis.
	Obtain urine cultures as indicated.	Pathogens in urine are most specifically determined by culture; goal is to obtain urine that is uncontaminated by organisms outside the urinary tract.
	Maintain aseptic closed drainage system.	Maintaining a closed drainage system aids in preventing infection; careful handwashing before and after handling of catheter or drainage system is also important.

Critical Thinking Question

1. The parents of a postoperative patient who has undergone renal surgery appear anxious and upset. When questioned, they state that: they both work, cannot afford to take the time off from work to stay with their child, and are also worried that he will fail in school and no longer be able to travel with his friends in a carpool. They do not know how they will manage. What is the best response of the nurse?

HYDROCELE

Pathophysiology. A **hydrocele** (*hydro,* "water," and *cele,* "tumor") is an excessive amount of fluid in the sac that surrounds the testicle, and it causes the scrotum to swell (Figure 29-8). When the testes descend into the scrotum in utero, the *processus vaginalis* (a fold of tissue) precedes them. This tissue ordinarily fuses, separating the peritoneal cavity from the scrotum. When this fusion does not take place, however, peritoneal fluid may enter the inguinal canal. Its appearance in the newborn is not uncommon, and in many cases the condition corrects itself by 1 year of age.

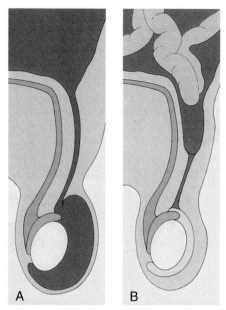

FIGURE 29-8 Hydrocele. **A,** Simple hydrocele. **B,** Hydrocele with herniation of the bowel into the scrotum. (From Zitelli BJ, Davis HW, editors: *Atlas of pediatric physical diagnosis*, ed 4, St Louis, 2002, Mosby.)

Treatment. A chronic hydrocele that persists beyond 1 year is corrected by surgery. Routine postoperative nursing care is provided. This is outlined in Chapter 22. Same-day surgery may be arranged.

CRYPTORCHIDISM

Pathophysiology. The testes are the male sex glands. These two oval bodies begin their development in the embryo within the abdominal cavity, just below the kidneys. Their function is to produce spermatozoa (male sex cells) and male hormones, particularly testosterone. Toward the end of the seventh fetal month, the testes begin to descend along a pathway into the scrotum. If this descent does not take place normally, the testes may remain in the abdomen or the inguinal canal. This condition is common in approximately 30% of low-birth-weight infants (Latendresse, 2010). When one or both testes fail to lower into the scrotum, the condition is termed **cryptorchidism** (*kryptos,* "hidden," and *orchi,* "testis"). The unilateral form is more common.

Because the testes are warmer in the abdomen than in the scrotum, the sperm cells begin to deteriorate. If both testes are affected, sterility results. *Inguinal hernia* often accompanies this condition. Acute scrotal pain may indicate a **testicular torsion** (twisting), which necessitates immediate surgery to preserve testicular function.

Treatment and Nursing Care. Occasionally, a testis or the testes spontaneously descend during the first year of life. An operation called an **orchiopexy** (*orchio,* "testicle," and *pexy,* "fixation") may be performed.

Although an orchiopexy improves the condition, the fertility rate among these patients may be reduced, even when only one testis is undescended. In addition, the incidence of testicular tumors is increased in these patients during adulthood (Latendresse, 2010). Parents are told to teach the growing child the importance of self-examination of the testes. When the child returns from surgery, care is taken to prevent contamination of the suture line, and scrotal support is maintained.

> ### Home Care Considerations
>
> Monitoring of the urine output and prevention of infection should be taught to parents. Self-image support may be needed (Latendresse, 2010).

The psychological approach of the nurse to the patient and his family is important because of the embarrassment they may feel. People may ask the child why he is undergoing surgery when there is no visible evidence of trauma. This problem is often compounded by the fact that the older child may have been told not to discuss his condition; in addition, his understanding of his problem and just what is going to happen in surgery may be vague. Therefore the nurse caring for the child should know what he has been told and how he feels about his operation to give emotional support. Terminology is clarified. The nurse assures the child that his penis will not be involved in the surgery.

The parents, too, may have anxieties that they cannot verbalize. It is difficult for many of them to communicate with their child about such matters. A thoughtful, sensitive nurse who tries to anticipate related feelings and fears promotes the child's adjustment.

IMPACT OF URINARY OR GENITAL SURGERY ON GROWTH AND DEVELOPMENT

Surgery of the urinary or genital tract affects growth and development. Preschoolers may perceive the treatment as punishment. Separation anxiety during hospitalization peaks, and preventive strategies should be explained to the parents. The body image of the child must be assertively maintained whenever surgery is delayed beyond infancy. Between 3 and 6 years of age, the child becomes curious about sexual differences and may masturbate. Surgical interventions during this stage of development necessitate guidance and preparation to minimize the negative impact on growth and development.

During home care, tub baths may be contraindicated, dressings to "private parts" of the body must be inspected daily, and restrictions on play activities that involve straddle toys (e.g., tricycles, rocking horses) are necessary. Adolescents may be concerned about the effects of surgery on their appearance and sexual abilities.

Get Ready for the NCLEX® Examination!

Key Points

- The functional unit of the kidney is the nephron.
- Children with hypospadias are born with the urethral opening on the undersurface of the penis.
- Bladder exstrophy is a serious congenital defect in which the bladder lies exposed on the lower portion of the abdominal wall. Surgical correction of this defect is lifesaving.
- Obstruction of the urinary tract may lead to hydronephrosis, a distention of the kidney pelvis. This is a serious condition because it could eventually lead to kidney failure if left untreated.
- To prevent fecal contamination of the urinary tract, girls are taught to wipe the perineal area from front to back after urination.
- Ascites is an abnormal collection of fluid in the peritoneal cavity. It is seen in advanced cases of nephrosis and in other conditions.
- The accurate charting of intake and output for patients with kidney problems is absolutely essential to their treatment and recovery. This includes ostomy and urinary drainage.
- Accurate blood pressure measurements will detect hypertension, a condition often associated with kidney problems.
- Normally urine flows from the ureters into the bladder, and almost no flow reenters the ureters.
- Repeated urinary tract infections or improper position of the ureters or sphincters in the bladder at birth may result in the reflux of urine into the ureters.
- Good health habits include assessing one's own body, including the genitalia.
- Routine abdominal palpation is omitted for a child diagnosed with Wilms' tumor.
- Early treatment of cryptorchidism is necessary to preserve testicular function.
- A hydrocele is an excessive amount of fluid in the sac that surrounds the testicle. This causes the scrotum to swell.
- Undescended testes (cryptorchidism) refers to a condition in which the testes do not lower into the scrotum during the fetal period but remain in the abdomen or the inguinal canal after birth.
- The minimum urine output for infants and toddlers is 2 to 3 mL/kg/hr; for preschoolers, the minimum is 1 to 2 mL/kg/hr; and for school-age children and adolescents, the minimum is 0.5 to 1 mL/kg/hr.

Additional Learning Resources

SG Go to your Study Guide for additional learning activities to help you master this chapter content.

evolve Go to your Evolve website (http://evolve.elsevier.com/Leifer) for the following learning resources:
- Animations
- Answer Guidelines for Critical Thinking Questions

- Answers and Rationales for Review Questions for the NCLEX® Examination
- Glossary with English and Spanish pronunciations
- Interactive Review Questions for the NCLEX® Examination
- Patient Teaching Plans in English and Spanish
- Skills Performance Checklists
- Video clips and more!

 Online Resources
- Hypospadias: www.urologychannel.com/pediatric/hypospadias.shtml
- Phimosis: www.healthscout.com/ency/68/360/main.html
- Urinary tract infections: www.pediatrics.org/cgi/content/full/103/4/e54
- Vesicoureteral reflux: www.findarticles.com/cf_dls/g2601/0014/2601001452/p1/article.jhtml
- National Kidney Foundation: www.kidney.org

Review Questions for the NCLEX® Examination

1. The nurse understands that genitourinary surgery affects growth and development. When caring for a 4-year-old child postoperatively, a priority nursing responsibility would include:
   1. strategies to preserve the child's body image.
   2. assurances that appearance and sexual function will not be affected.
   3. providing age-appropriate toys such as tricycles.
   4. preventing embarrassment by limiting visitation of family and friends.

2. The administration of prednisone to children with nephrosis creates the problem of:
   1. intolerance to foods.
   2. increased risk of infection.
   3. increased periorbital edema.
   4. weight loss.

3. Daily weights are obtained in children with nephrosis to monitor:
   1. weight loss from a low-protein diet.
   2. accuracy of fluid balance sheets.
   3. changes in the amount of edema.
   4. percentile on the growth grid.

4. A priority nursing responsibility in the care of a child with Wilms' tumor is to:
   1. maintain accurate intake and output records.
   2. omit abdominal palpation during daily assessments.
   3. maintain strict bed rest.
   4. assess neurological function.

5. The nurse is caring for a child diagnosed with nephrosis. Symptoms that are characteristic of nephrosis include (select all that apply):
   1. massive proteinuria.
   2. edema.
   3. a positive antistreptolysin titer.
   4. bacteriuria.

The Child with a Skin Condition

Objectives

1. Define each key term listed.
2. Recall the differences between the skin of the infant and that of the adult.
3. Identify common congenital skin lesions and infections.
4. Describe two topical agents used to treat acne.
5. Summarize the nursing care for a child who has infantile eczema. State the rationale for each nursing measure.
6. Differentiate four types of topical medication.
7. Discuss the nursing care of various microbial infections of the skin.
8. Discuss the prevention and care of pediculosis and scabies.
9. Differentiate among first-, second-, and third-degree burns: the anatomical structures involved, the appearance, the level of sensation, and the first aid required.
10. Identify the principles of topical therapy.
11. Describe how the response of the child with burns differs from that of the adult.
12. Examine the emergency treatment of three types of burns.
13. List five objectives of the nurse who is caring for the burned child.
14. Discuss the prevention and treatment of sunburn and frostbite.

Key Terms

allergens (ĂL-ŭr-jĕnz, p. 689)
alopecia (ăl-ō-PĒ-shă, p. 693)
autograft (ĂW-tō-grăft, p. 698)
chilblain (CHĬL-blān, p. 701)
comedo (KŎM-ĕ-dō, p. 688)
crust (p. 685)
Curling's ulcer (KŬR-lĭngz ŬL-sŭr, p. 698)
debridement (dĕ-BRĒD-mnt, p. 698)
dermabrasion (dŭrm-ă-BRĀ-zhŭn, p. 688)
ecchymosis (ĕk-ĭ-MŌ-sĭs, p. 685)
emollient (ĕ-MŎL-ē-ŭnt, p. 689)
eschar (ĔS-kăhr, p. 697)
exanthem (ĕg-ZĂN-thŭm, p. 684)
frostbite (p. 701)
heterograft (HĔT-ŭr-ō-grăft, p. 698)
hives (p. 684)

homografts (HŌ-mō-grăfts, p. 698)
ileus (ĬL-ē-ŭs, p. 698)
isograft (Ī-sō-grăft, p. 698)
macule (MĂK-yūl, p. 685)
methicillin-resistant *Staphylococcus aureus* (MRSA) (mĕth-ĭ-SĬL-ĭn rē-zĭs-tĕnt stăf-ĭ-lō-KŎK-ŭs ĂW-rē-ŭs, p. 692)
papule (PĂP-yūl, p. 685)
pediculosis (pĕ-dĭk-yū-LŌ-sĭs, p. 694)
pruritus (prū-RĪ-tŭs, p. 686)
pustule (PŬS-tyūl, p. 685)
sebum (p. 688)
stye (p. 684)
total body surface area (TBSA) (p. 694)
vesicle (VĔS-ĭ-kŭl, p. 685)
wheal (WĒL, p. 685)
xenografts (ZĒ-nō-grăfts, p. 698)

SKIN DEVELOPMENT AND FUNCTIONS

The main function of the skin is protection. It acts as the body's first line of defense against disease. It prevents the passage of harmful physical and chemical agents and prevents the loss of water and electrolytes. It also has a great capacity to regenerate and repair itself. The skin and the structures derived from it, such as hair and fingernails, are known as the integumentary system. Figure 30-1 depicts these structures and how they differ in the developing child and in the adult.

Maintaining skin integrity is important to self-esteem and therefore has both a psychological and a physiological component. This is particularly evident in patients with facial disfiguration. Four basic skin sensations—pain, temperature, touch, and pressure—are felt by the skin in conjunction with the nervous system. The skin also secretes sebum, which helps to protect and maintain its texture. The outer surface of the skin is acidic, with a pH of 4.5 to 6.5, to protect the skin from pathological bacteria that thrive in an alkaline environment.

The skin is composed of two layers: the epidermis (derived from the ectoderm) and the dermis (derived from the mesoderm). Vernix caseosa is a cheeselike substance that covers the fetus until birth. This protects the fetal skin from maceration as the fetus floats in its watery home. The fetal skin is at first so transparent that blood vessels are clearly visible. Downy lanugo hair

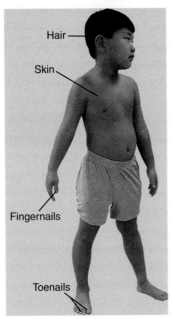

Hair

Skin

Fingernails

Toenails

INTEGUMENTARY SYSTEM

- The thin epidermis in infants blisters easily, absorption is dramatically greater, and infections occur more readily.
- Sebaceous glands do not begin producing sebum until about 8 to 10 years of age. Without lubrication, the skin is more dry and chaps more easily.
- Skin infections are more likely to produce systemic symptoms.
- Preterm and term newborns have less subcutaneous fat; therefore they are more sensitive to heat and cold.
- At birth the skin is alkaline, increasing susceptibility to infection.
- The ability to perspire through the skin matures by 3 years of age, and axillary perspiration begins near puberty. Therefore thermoregulation may be a problem in children.

FIGURE 30-1 Summary of some *integumentary system* differences between the child and the adult. The integumentary system consists of the skin and the structures derived from it. This system protects the body, helps to regulate body temperature, and receives stimuli such as pressure, pain, and temperature. (Art overlay courtesy Observatory Group, Cincinnati, Ohio.)

begins to develop at about 13 to 16 weeks, especially on the head. At 21 to 24 weeks the skin is reddish and wrinkled, with little subcutaneous fat. Adipose tissue forms during later weeks. At birth the subcutaneous glands are well developed, and the skin is pink and smooth and has a polished look. It is thinner than the skin of an adult.

SKIN DISORDERS AND VARIATIONS

Certain skin conditions in children may be associated with age, as in the case of milia in infants and acne in adolescents. A skin condition may be a manifestation of a systemic disease, such as chickenpox. Some lesions, such as strawberry nevi and mongolian spots, are congenital. Other skin lesions, such as those seen in rubella and fifth disease, are self-limited and do not necessitate treatment.

There are great individual differences in skin texture, color, pH, and moisture. Skin color is an important diagnostic criterion in cases of liver disease, heart conditions, child abuse, and for overall assessment. Complete blood counts and serum electrolyte levels are helpful in diagnosing skin conditions. Skin tests are used in diagnosing allergies. The purified protein derivative (PPD) test is useful in screening for tuberculosis. Skin scrapings are used for microscopic examination. The *Wood's light* is an instrument used to diagnose certain skin conditions. It reflects a particular color according to the organism present.

Hair condition is important to observe. Hair is inspected for color, texture, quality, distribution, and elasticity. Hair may become dry and brittle and may lack luster owing to inadequate nutrition. Hair may begin to fall out or even change color during illness or the ingestion of certain medications.

Skin conditions may be acute or chronic. The nurse should describe the lesions with regard to size, color, configuration (e.g., butterfly rash), presence of pain or itching, distribution (e.g., arms, legs, behind ears), and whether the rash is general or local. **Hives**, a general rash that appears abruptly, is often an allergic or medication reaction. The condition of the skin around the lesions is also significant, as is the skin turgor. Managing itching is a key component in preventing secondary infection that can result from scratching. Dressings and ointments are applied as prescribed. Preventing infections is a consideration in the case of open wounds. Mongolian spots and physiological jaundice are covered in Chapter 12. The communicable diseases are discussed in Chapter 32.

Many childhood infectious diseases, such as measles, German measles, and chickenpox, involve the presence of an **exanthem** (a skin rash). Box 30-1 identifies terms used to describe some conditions of the skin that the nurse may witness. Some rashes begin as one lesion and evolve into others. For example, the sequence of chickenpox rash is macule to papule, to vesicle, and then to crust. A **stye** is an infection of the sebaceous gland of the eyelash (Figure 30-2).

CONGENITAL LESIONS

Strawberry Nevus

The strawberry nevus (Figure 30-3) is a common hemangioma (consists of dilated capillaries in the dermal space) that may not become apparent for a few weeks

Box 30-1   Terms Used to Describe Skin Conditions

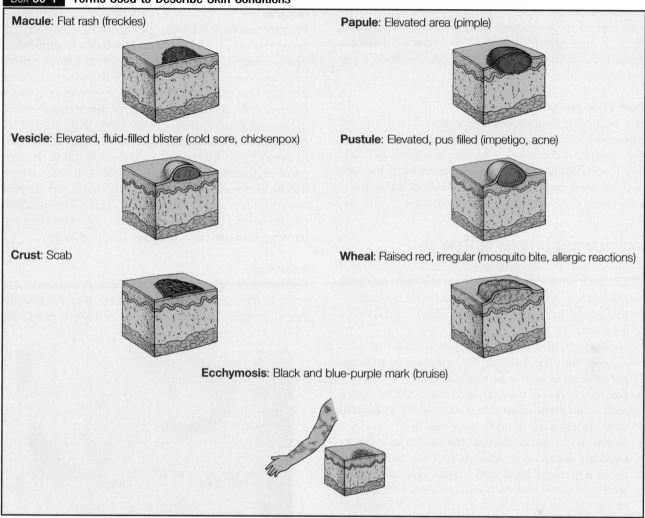

Macule: Flat rash (freckles)

Papule: Elevated area (pimple)

Vesicle: Elevated, fluid-filled blister (cold sore, chickenpox)

Pustule: Elevated, pus filled (impetigo, acne)

Crust: Scab

Wheal: Raised red, irregular (mosquito bite, allergic reactions)

Ecchymosis: Black and blue-purple mark (bruise)

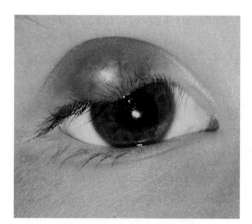

FIGURE 30-2 A *stye,* or *hordeolum,* is an inflammation of the sebaceous gland of the eyelid commonly seen in infants and children. (From Zitelli BJ et al: *Zitelli and Davis' atlas of pediatric physical diagnosis,* ed 6, St Louis, 2012, Saunders.)

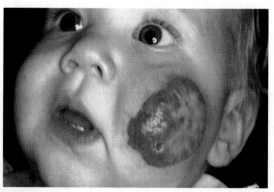

FIGURE 30-3 Strawberry nevus. This minor lesion can result in major psychological problems. (From Swartz MH: *Textbook of physical diagnosis: history and examination,* ed 7, Philadelphia, 2014, Saunders.)

after birth. Although it is harmless and usually disappears without treatment, it is disturbing to parents, especially when it appears on the head or face. At first it is flat, but it gradually becomes raised. The lesion is bright red, elevated, and sharply demarcated. The lesions gradually blanch, with 60% disappearing spontaneously by 5 years of age and 90% disappearing by 9 years of age. Laser treatment or excision may be considered if the area becomes ulcerated. Parents are often quizzed about the growth by insensitive persons, and they may be advised about various unorthodox treatments. The nurse offers support and reassurance to parents and corrects misinformation. After laser surgery, the skin may appear black for 7 to 10 days. Salicylates should be avoided, and sun exposure should be minimized.

Port-Wine Nevus

Port-wine nevi (Figure 30-4) are present at birth and are caused by dilated dermal capillaries. The lesions are flat, sharply demarcated, and purple to pink in color. The lesion darkens as the child grows older. If the area is small, cosmetics may disguise the lesion. If the area is large, laser surgery may be indicated.

SKIN MANIFESTATIONS OF ILLNESS

- *Café au lait macules* occur in 10% to 20% of people and are light brown, oval patches on the skin. Multiple café au lait macules are associated with neurofibromatosis (a chromosomal abnormality) and tuberous sclerosis.
- *Hypopigmented macules* are whitish oval- or leaf-shaped macules. Multiple hypopigmented macules are associated with tuberous sclerosis.
- *Butterfly rash* over the nose and cheeks can be associated with photosensitivity and may be associated with systemic lupus erythematosus (SLE).
- *Scaling skin eruption* around the mouth in a horseshoelike distribution around the chin and cheeks, or as a perianal rash and involving papules and scales, is associated with zinc deficiency in infants. It also is associated with diarrhea and failure to thrive.
- *Vascular birth marks* such as hemangioma resemble a bruise that changes in appearance through the years. Hemangiomas around the chin may be associated with airway problems, and those appearing around the lumbar region may be associated with spinal problems.

INFECTIONS

Miliaria

Pathophysiology. Miliaria (prickly heat) refers to a rash caused by excess body heat and moisture (Figure 30-5). There is retention of sweat in the sweat glands, which have become blocked or inflamed. Rupture or leakage into the skin causes the inflamed response. It appears suddenly as tiny, pinhead-sized, reddened papules with occasional clear vesicles. It may be accompanied by **pruritus** (itching). It is seen in infants during hot weather or in newborns that sleep in overheated rooms. It often occurs in the diaper area or in the folds of the skin where moisture accumulates. Plastic enclosures on diapers hold in body warmth that results in a rash. This harmless condition may be reversed by removing extra clothing, bathing, skin care, and frequent diaper changes.

Intertrigo

Pathophysiology. Intertrigo (*in*, "into," and *terere*, "to rub") is the medical term for chafing. It is a dermatitis that occurs in the folds of the skin (Figure 30-6). The

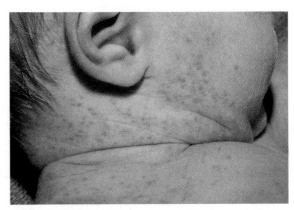

FIGURE 30-5 Miliaria. Note the many tiny pustular lesions in the folds of the neck. (From Zitelli BJ et al: *Zitelli and Davis' atlas of pediatric physical diagnosis*, ed 6, St Louis, 2012, Saunders.)

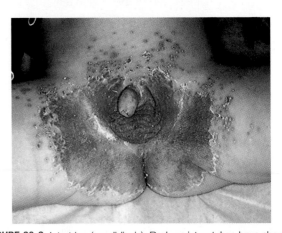

FIGURE 30-6 Intertrigo (candidiasis). Red, moist patches have sharply demarcated borders and some loose scales, usually in the genital area and extending along the inguinal and gluteal folds. Urine, feces, heat, and moisture aggravate this lesion. (From Hurwitz S: *Clinical pediatric dermatology: a textbook of skin disorders of childhood and adolescence*, ed 2, Philadelphia, 1993, Saunders.)

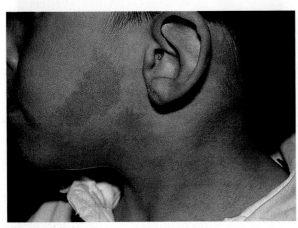

FIGURE 30-4 Port-wine stain. (From Weston WL, Lane AT, Morelli JG: *Color textbook of pediatric dermatology*, ed 4, St Louis, 2007, Mosby.)

patches are red and moist and are usually located along the neck and in the inguinal and gluteal folds. Urine, feces, heat, and moisture aggravate this condition. Obese children are more prone to intertrigo. Prevention consists of keeping the affected areas clean and *dry*. The child is allowed to be out of diapers to expose the area to air and light. Maceration of the skin can lead to secondary infections.

Seborrheic Dermatitis

Pathophysiology. Seborrheic dermatitis (cradle cap) is an inflammation of the skin that involves the sebaceous glands (Figure 30-7). Thick, yellow, oily, adherent, crustlike scales on the scalp and the forehead characterize this condition. The skin beneath the patches may be red (erythematous). Less often it may involve the eyelids, the external ear, and the inguinal area. Secondary bacterial and yeast infections may occur. It is seen in newborns, in infants, and at puberty. In newborns it is commonly known as "cradle cap." It is seen in infants with sensitive skin, even when the head and hair are washed frequently. Seborrhea resembles eczema, but it usually does not itch and there is a negative family history. In adolescence it is more localized and is usually confined to the scalp. A condition resembling seborrheic dermatitis is common in children and adolescents infected with the human immunodeficiency virus (HIV).

Treatment. Treatment consists of shampooing the hair on a regular basis. Applying baby oil to the head the evening before and shampooing in the morning may soften scales that are particularly stubborn in newborns. The scalp is rinsed well. A soft brush is helpful in removing loose particles from the hair. The nurse teaches the parent how to shampoo an infant's head using the football hold (see Skill 12-5). A dandruff-control shampoo containing selenium such as Selsun is used for adolescents. The response to therapy is usually rapid.

Diaper Dermatitis

Pathophysiology. Diaper dermatitis (diaper rash) is a commonly seen condition that results from prolonged contact of the skin to a mixture of urine and feces. The urine increases the pH of the skin, resulting in increased sensitivity to fecal enzymes. If the skin remains moist inside the soiled diaper, the skin may become more likely to develop a *Candida albicans* infection. The rash of simple diaper dermatitis may appear as an erythema (redness); however, a beefy red rash in the diaper area may be indicative of a *Candida* (thrush) infection and necessitates prompt treatment (Figure 30-8). Disposable diapers contain a super-absorbent gel material that helps maintain normal skin pH and therefore reduces the occurrence of diaper dermatitis.

Treatment and Nursing Care. It is easier to prevent diaper rash than to cure it. Prevention is accomplished by frequent diaper changes to limit the skin's exposure to moisture. The diaper is periodically removed to expose the skin to light and air. With each diaper change, the perineal area is gently and thoroughly cleansed (preferably with warm water) and gently dried. After bowel movements, the area is cleansed with mild soap and water. The skin folds are thoroughly washed, rinsed, and dried. A cloth, non–alcohol-containing wipe, or a cosmetic pad may be used to remove feces from the skin. Some common over-the-counter ointments for prevention of diaper dermatitis include ointments with the active ingredients of vitamins A and D and lanolin, and other products containing zinc oxide. A thick layer of zinc oxide (Desitin) should be applied for an erythematous rash; an antifungal cream (Nystatin) may be added if there is evidence of candida; and for denuded (open) skin diaper rash a triple paste (Liex) and Vaseline may be used to protect the skin (Hiemall, 2013). Aggressive scrubbing of the skin should be avoided. Mineral oil can aid in removing sticky ointments. The use of

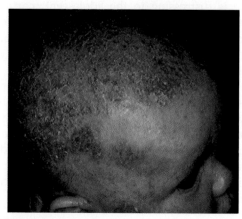

FIGURE 30-7 Seborrheic dermatitis (cradle cap). Thick, yellow, greasy adherent scales appear on the scalp and forehead. There is no itching (pruritus). (From Hurwitz S: *Clinical pediatric dermatology: a textbook of skin disorders of childhood and adolescence,* ed 2, Philadelphia, 1993, Saunders.)

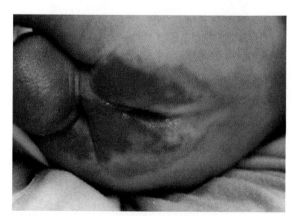

FIGURE 30-8 Diaper rash (diaper dermatitis). A red, moist maculopapular rash with poorly defined borders appears in the diaper area. The infant may have a history of infrequent diaper changes or the use of snug rubber/plastic pants. The inflammation results from ammonia, heat, and moisture. (From Bowden VR, Dickey SB, Greenberg SC: *Children and their families: the continuum of care,* Philadelphia, 1998, Saunders.)

corticosteroid ointments in an occluded diaper area should be avoided because skin absorption can cause systemic complications (Eichenfeld, 2008).

Acne Vulgaris

Pathophysiology. Acne is an inflammation of the sebaceous glands and hair follicles in the skin (Figure 30-9). Because of hormonal influence, the sebaceous glands enlarge at puberty and secrete increased amounts of a fatty substance called **sebum.** Genetic factors and stress are also thought to play a part in acne's etiology. The course of acne may be brief or prolonged (lasting 10 years or longer). Preadolescent and premenstrual acne in girls is not uncommon. The principal lesions include comedones, papules, and nodulocystic growths.

A **comedo** (plural, *comedones*) is a plug of keratin, sebum, or bacteria. Keratin is a protein substance and is the main constituent of epidermis and hair. There are two types of comedones: open and closed. In the open comedo, or *blackhead,* the surface is darkened by melanin. Closed comedones, or *whiteheads,* are responsible for the inflammatory process of acne. With continued buildup, the walls of the follicle rupture, releasing their irritating contents into the surrounding skin. A pustule may appear when this develops near the exterior. This process occurs no matter how carefully the teenager washes, because surface bacteria are not involved in the pathogenesis. Acne is usually seen on the chin, the cheeks, and the forehead. It can also develop on the chest, the upper back, and the shoulders. It usually is more severe in winter.

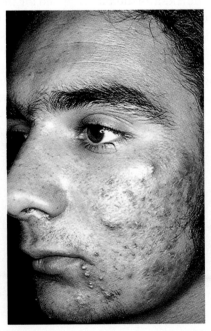

FIGURE 30-9 Acne. Acne is the most common skin problem of adolescence. An increase in sebaceous gland activity creates increased oiliness. Open comedones (blackheads) and closed comedones (whiteheads) are common. Severe acne includes papules and nodules. The lesions can appear on the face, chest, back, and shoulders. (From Hurwitz S: *Clinical pediatric dermatology: a textbook of skin disorders of childhood and adolescence,* ed 2, Philadelphia, 1993, Saunders.)

Treatment. The basic treatment of acne has changed considerably during the past few years. It is no longer thought that certain foods trigger the condition; therefore the restriction of chocolate, peanuts, and cola drinks is unwarranted. A regular, well-balanced diet is encouraged. General hygienic measures of cleanliness, rest, and the avoidance of emotional stress may help to prevent exacerbations.

Routine skin cleansing with a gentle soap-free, pH balanced cleanser is helpful. Excessive cleansing of the skin can irritate and dry the tissues. Squeezing pimples ruptures intact lesions and causes local inflammation. Facial toners can remove make-up or dirt. Oil-free concealer make-up can be used to enhance self-image. The topical preparations that can be obtained over-the-counter include products that contain salicylic acid, sulfur, sodium sulfacetamide, benzoyl peroxide, and resorcinol, and they are somewhat effective. Retinoids reduce peeling of follicular epithelium and help to clear existing lesions. Retinoids are available as gels, creams, and liquids and can be combined with moisturizers to reduce the side-effects of burning, dryness, and scaling. Oral antibiotics may be prescribed for inflammatory acne, and extended-release minocycline is the only FDA-approved antibiotic for acne treatment in children older than 8 years of age (Eichenfeld, 2013). Isotretinoin (Accutane) is given to patients with severe pustulocystic acne who have been unable to benefit from other types of treatment. It has many side effects; thus the patient must be carefully monitored with liver studies and lipid levels. **It is not prescribed during pregnancy or to those at risk for pregnancy because of the possibilities of fetal deformity.** Planing of the skin to minimize scarring (**dermabrasion**) is done selectively, because it is not always successful. Oral contraceptives (OCs) such as Ortho Tri-Cyclen (norgestimate and ethinyl estradiol) may also be given, because sebum production is controlled by androgens, and these OCs reduce androgen levels.

Acne is distressing to the adolescent, particularly when the face is extensively involved. Sometimes even a minimal problem is seen as disastrous when it happens before an important event. The self-conscious young person feels different and embarrassed. The nurse who is attuned to the feelings of individuals can provide understanding support. Although the adolescent is educated to assume responsibility for the regimen, including the parents in the education helps to prevent conflict surrounding the regimen. Drug-induced acne can occur in children taking long-term steroids, phenobarbital, phenytoin, lithium, vitamin B_{12}, or medications containing iodides or bromides.

> **Nursing Tip**
>
> Topical benzoyl peroxide and Retin-A neutralize each other when applied together.

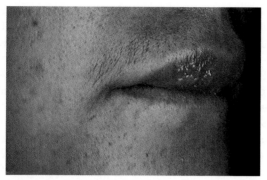

FIGURE 30-10 Herpes simplex (cold sores). These begin with tingling skin and sensitivity, and they erupt with tight vesicles, then pustules, and then a crust. Lesions commonly appear on the upper lip. (From Hurwitz S: *Clinical pediatric dermatology: a textbook of skin disorders of childhood and adolescence,* ed 2, Philadelphia, 1993, Saunders.)

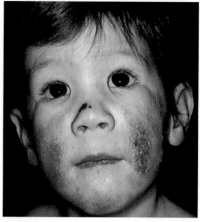

FIGURE 30-11 Infantile eczema (atopic dermatitis) is characterized by erythematous papules and vesicles with weeping, oozing, and crusts on the face and body. Severe itching is common. There is often a family history of allergy. (From Hurwitz S: *Clinical pediatric dermatology: a textbook of skin disorders of childhood and adolescence,* ed 2, Philadelphia, 1993, Saunders.)

Herpes Simplex Type I

Pathophysiology. **Herpes simplex type I**, a viral infection, is commonly known as a cold sore or fever blister. It may begin with a feeling of tingling, itching, or burning on the lip. Vesicles and crusts form (Figure 30-10). Spontaneous healing occurs in about 8 to 10 days. Communicability is highest early in the formation and is spread by direct contact. Recurrence is common, because the virus lies dormant in the body until it is activated by stress, sun exposure, menstruation, fever, and other causes. Patients must become familiar with their own personal triggers. Herpes can be serious in newborns and in the patients who are immunocompromised.

Treatment and Nursing Care. Topical acyclovir may reduce viral shedding and hasten healing. In the hospital, ointments are applied with gloved hands. Contact and protective environment precautions should be followed (see Appendix A). Patients are instructed not to pick at lesions, because this may produce spreading to other sites. They should not share lipstick and should avoid kissing while lesions are active. Sensitivity to the self-conscious adolescent who has a cold sore is important. Genital herpes caused by the herpes virus type II, and spread by sexual contact, are discussed in Chapter 11 and Table 11-1. The distinction between the two types has become less clear because of an increase in the practice of oral–genital sex.

Infantile Eczema (Atopic Dermatitis)

Pathophysiology. Infantile eczema, or atopic dermatitis, is an inflammation of genetically hypersensitive skin (Figure 30-11). The pathophysiology is characterized by local vasodilation in affected areas. This progresses to *spongiosis,* or the breakdown of dermal cells and the formation of intradermal vesicles. Chronic scratching produces weeping and results in lichenification, or coarsening, of the skin folds. The exact cause of this condition is difficult to pinpoint because it is thought to be caused mainly by allergy. Infantile

eczema is rarely seen in breastfed infants until they begin to eat additional food. It seems to follow a definite familial history of allergies; emotional factors are often involved.

Eczema is actually a symptom rather than a disorder. It indicates that the infant is oversensitive to certain substances called **allergens**, which enter the body via the digestive tract (food), by inhalation (dust, pollen), by direct contact (wool, soap, strong sunlight), or by injections (insect bites, vaccines). Some children develop the triad of atopic dermatitis, asthma, and hay fever.

Manifestations. Although infantile eczema can occur at any age, it is more common during the first 2 years of the infant's life. The pruritic lesions form vesicles that weep and develop a dry crust. They are more severe on the face but may occur on the entire body, particularly in the skin folds. Eczema is worse in the winter than in the summer and has periods of temporary remission.

The infant scratches because the itching is constant, and he or she is irritable and unable to sleep. Bacterial or viral agents easily infect the lesions. Infants and children with eczema should not be exposed to adults with cold sores because the children may develop a systemic reaction with high fever and multiple vesicles on the eczematous skin. Eczema may flare up after immunization. Laboratory studies may show an increase in immunoglobulin E (IgE) and eosinophil levels.

Treatment and Nursing Care. Treatment of the child with infantile eczema is aimed at relieving pruritus (itching), hydrating and lubricating the skin, relieving inflammation, and preventing infection. Efforts should be made to identify triggers of recurrent relapses. An **emollient** bath is sometimes ordered for its soothing effect on the skin. Oatmeal and a mixture of cornstarch and baking soda are examples of emollients prescribed. The infant's hair is washed with a soap substitute rather than a shampoo. Some dermatologists think that bathing should be kept to a minimum. The physician may suggest that a bath oil such as Alpha Keri Therapeutic Bath Oil be used as the lesions begin to heal. This prevents the skin from becoming too dry. For correct use, bath oils should be added after the patient has soaked for a while and the skin is hydrated. In this way, moisture is sealed rather than excluded, as it is when oil is added before the patient gets into the tub.

Whenever possible, patients are treated at home because of the danger of infection in the hospital. When soap is used, a mild, nonperfumed soap such as Dove or Neutrogena is used. Glycerin-based lubricants are preferred over lanolin, which may be an irritant to an infant who is allergic to wool (Perry et al, 2010). Aquaphor and Eucerin are creams that can be used to enhance skin hydration. White petroleum (Vaseline) costs less and is effective.

Corticosteroids may be administered systemically or locally. Antibiotics are needed if infection is present. Medication to help relieve itching is ordered for the patient. A child who is uncomfortable and unable to sleep may receive sedation.

The nurse plays a vital role in the treatment of patients with skin problems (Nursing Care Plan 30-1). The nurse should assess the family's ability to cope with the care of this child at home. Techniques of home bathing or application of soaks combined with quiet playtime enhances family coping. Control of itching is essential. Ointments are applied with a gloved hand to minimize contact with the skin. The fingernails of the child are kept short, and cotton gloves or socks can be used to prevent scratching. Appropriate dress is advised, as is using cotton fabric and avoiding wool and stuffed animals because of their allergy potential. Clothes should be laundered using mild soaps, avoiding products that contain fragrances or harsh chemicals. Parents should be taught the principles of general hygiene to prevent secondary infection of the open skin lesions. A hypoallergenic formula and a plan to identify possible food allergens are explained to parents. When a food allergen is the cause of eczema, stopping the food results in a clearing of the skin; however, restarting the food after a time may cause an anaphylactic reaction. The types of topical medications are listed in Table 30-1.

Parent teaching concerning topical therapy. Skin lesions can be pruritic (itchy), scaling, weeping, or crusted. Most skin lesions cause psychological stress, which should be addressed for both the parents and the child with the skin lesion. Prevention of secondary infection is essential, and the nurse should help the parent to understand the signs of inflammation or infection. When topical medication is applied, the lesions may change in form or color as they heal. Parents should be advised of changes to expect and when to seek follow-up advice. The nurse should teach parents the principles and techniques of applying topical medication:

- Absorption is best when an ointment is applied after a warm bath.
- Medication should be applied by stroking in the direction of hair growth. (Circular or rubbing motions can inflame hair follicles.)
- Teach how much ointment to apply (e.g., pea-sized bead).

★ Nursing Care Plan 30-1 | The Child with Eczema

PATIENT DATA An 18-month-old child is brought to the clinic by his parents. The child has many open lesions on the skin and is diagnosed with eczema.

Selected Nursing Diagnosis: Impaired skin integrity related to inflammation

Goals	Nursing Interventions	Rationales
Child's skin will not show signs of irritation or infection.	Describe the types of lesions and their configuration and location.	Eczema has a typical pattern of distribution; vesicles, oozing, and crusting may denote infection.
	Provide supervision rather than restraints whenever possible.	Elbow restraints may aid in preventing self-inflicted skin damage caused by scratching and picking; restriction of movement to infants has been related to learning difficulties and other problems; therefore application of any restraint must be judicious.
	Keep fingernails short.	Trimming fingernails and covering hands with "sock mittens" reduces excoriation from scratching.
	Administer medicated baths such as with Aveeno.	Medicated baths soothe and rehydrate the skin.
	Apply wet dressings.	Wet dressings promote cooling of the skin, which decreases inflammation and itching (pruritus).
	Administer oral antibiotics and sedatives as prescribed.	Systemic antibiotics such as erythromycin may be prescribed if there is an infection; sedatives reduce itching.
	Apply steroid ointments as prescribed.	Steroid ointments reduce inflammation.

Continued

★ Nursing Care Plan 30-1   The Child with Eczema—cont'd

Selected Nursing Diagnosis: Risk for imbalanced nutrition, less than body requirements related to irritability, sensitivity to certain foods

Goals	Nursing Interventions	Rationales
Child will eat portions of each meal and maintain weight.	Serve hypoallergenic diet if prescribed.	This is a basic diet in which only one new food is added at a time to determine whether the infant is allergic to it.
Child will receive adequate nutrition as evidenced by growth charts and other parameters.	Determine specific food sensitivities from parents if child is not on a diet.	Parents have the most knowledge from experience with their child.
	Observe child for food sensitivities.	Any food can produce allergic symptoms, but some are thought to be highly allergenic. Certain antigens (foreign protein) may enter the bloodstream and activate antibody formation of the immune system. One reason this occurs during infancy is that an infant's gastrointestinal tract is immature. The allergy may be outgrown as body systems mature.
	Administer vitamins and mineral supplements as prescribed.	Child may be deficient in nutrients owing to irritability and food restrictions. Adequate intake of vitamins and minerals is essential to the maintenance of healthy skin (particularly vitamins A, B, and C).
	Provide adequate fluids.	Adequate hydration prevents drying of the skin and pruritus, and it makes the skin less prone to breaks, which can become infected.

Selected Nursing Diagnosis: Deficient parental knowledge related to nature of disorder

Goals	Nursing Interventions	Rationales
Parents will verbalize understanding of potential allergens. Parents will state they have an understanding of the disease process.	Advise parents to remove articles that irritate skin (e.g., wool) and to provide loose cotton clothing.	Clothing with rough and tightly woven fibers will prevent natural evaporation from skin; wool may cause an allergic reaction. Sweating increases itching.
	Encourage parents to use mild detergents and to rinse clothes thoroughly.	Avoiding strong detergents and rinsing clothing thoroughly will prevent skin flare-ups.
	Expose child to sunlight, but monitor carefully.	Although sunlight is beneficial, overexposure to ultraviolet rays can seriously damage the skin. Infants and young children require special protection from the sun because their epidermis is thin; exposure time should be brief, even on hazy days.
	Help parents identify products in which wheat, milk, and eggs may not be readily apparent.	Food labels are read carefully to determine content.
	Advise parents to expect exacerbations and remissions.	Eczema is a chronic disease that takes time and energy to control.

Critical Thinking Question

1. Parents bring their child to the clinic. This child has a history of long-term asthma and eczema. The child is dressed in a wool jacket and is eating from a bag of peanuts. The mother states she has been using a lanolin lotion for dry skin that her friend gave to her, but the child's skin lesions have only become worse. What teaching interventions by the nurse would be appropriate?

- The use of elbow restraints can prevent an infant from scratching while allowing freedom of movement.
- Do not use topical steroids when a viral infection is present.

Over-the-counter skin products. Parents should be guided in the use of over-the-counter products that affect skin health. Simple ointments such as petrolatum,

A+D, and zinc oxide are helpful only if they are washed off completely between diaper changes. Frequent diaper changes are essential. High-absorbency disposable diapers decrease wetness on the skin and may help to prevent diaper dermatitis. Home-laundered diapers are not subject to high temperatures, and soaps often contain fragrances that may be irritating. Commercially prepared wipes sometimes contain

Table 30-1	Types of Topical Medications
TYPE	**DEFINITION**
Cream	A water-based emulsion of oil in water that is nongreasy for use on weeping lesions
Ointment	An oil-based emulsion of water in oil that is clear and greasy; used on dry skin; does not rub off easily
Lotion	A suspension of powder in water that should be shaken well before using; may cause drying of skin; often used on scalp lesions
Aerosol spray	Suspension of medication in an alcohol base; alcohol evaporates, leaving medication on the skin; effective for hairy areas
Gel	A clear, semisolid emulsion; liquefies when applied to skin
Bath oils	Bath oils are not used in pediatrics because they lubricate the sides of the tub, causing falls and injuries; the value of the treatment must be weighed against the risks involved; colloidal oatmeal baths may be soothing

perfumes and can leave the skin moist; warm water and a mild soap are less irritating. If paper towels are used, prints should be avoided because the color dyes can be irritating to the skin. Cortisone creams should be avoided because cortisone may temporarily clear the rash but does not resolve the underlying cause that will prevent recurrence.

> **◈ Nursing Tip**
>
> Parents should be taught that the "kiss to make it better" can introduce organisms into a wound that can cause infection.

Staphylococcal Infection

Pathophysiology. The genus of bacteria called *Staphylococcus* comprises common bacteria that are found in dust and on the skin. Under normal conditions, they do not present a problem to the healthy body's defenses. Skin infections may occur if the number of organisms increases in preterm infants and newborns, whose general resistance is low. An abscess may form, and infection may enter the bloodstream. This condition is called *septicemia*. Pneumonia, osteomyelitis, or meningitis may result. Primary infection of the newborn may develop in the umbilicus or circumcision wound. It may occur while the newborn is in the hospital or after discharge. This infection spreads readily from one infant to another. Small pustules on the newborn must be reported immediately.

Treatment and Nursing Care. Antibiotics effective against the appropriate strain of *Staphylococcus* are administered. Ointments may be locally applied.

In past years the staphylococci that invaded the body developed resistance to the drugs in current use. **Methicillin-resistant *Staphylococcus aureus* (MRSA)** infections are resistant to certain antibiotics and are handled under strict contact isolation precautions. The use of disposable individual equipment for patients and aseptic techniques can decrease health care–associated spread of infection.

Scalded skin syndrome is caused by *S. aureus*. The lesions begin with a mild erythema with sandpaper texture; vesicles appear and rupture, and peeling occurs, exposing a bright red surface. The skin looks as though it has been scalded, and child abuse is often suspected. Intravenous (IV) antibiotics, strict isolation, and prevention of secondary infection are priorities. Maintaining warmth and fluid-electrolyte balance are also important in the plan of care. Healing usually takes place without scarring.

Impetigo

Pathophysiology. Impetigo is an infectious disease of the skin caused by staphylococci or by group A beta-hemolytic streptococci. It results when the organism comes in contact with a break in the skin, such as an insect bite. The bullous form seen primarily in infants is usually staphylococcal, whereas nonbullous types, more commonly seen in children and young adults, can harbor either organism. The newborn is susceptible to this infection because resistance to skin bacteria is low. Impetigo tends to spread from one area of skin to another and is contagious.

Manifestations. The first symptoms of a bullous lesion are red papules (Figure 30-12). These eventually become small vesicles or pustules surrounded by a reddened area. When the blister breaks, the surface beneath is raw and weeping. The lesions may occur anywhere but are most often found around the nose and mouth and in moist areas of the body, such as the creases of the neck, the axilla, and the groin. A crust may form in older children, and scratching may cause further infection.

> **Safety Alert!**
>
> If an infant/child has recurrent impetigo, the caregiver may be a nasal carrier of *S. aureus* (Zajac, 2009).

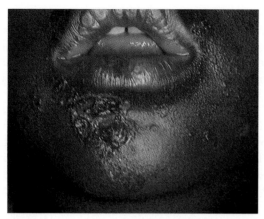

FIGURE 30-12 Impetigo. This consists of moist, thin-roofed vesicles with an erythematous base. The vesicles rupture to form a thick, honey-colored crust. It is a contagious bacterial infection of the skin that is most common in infants and children. (From Hurwitz S: *Clinical pediatric dermatology: a textbook of skin disorders of childhood and adolescence,* ed 2, Philadelphia, 1993, Saunders.)

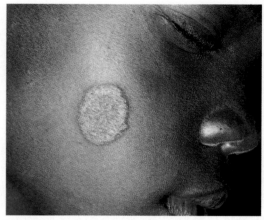

FIGURE 30-13 Tinea corporis (ringworm of the body). Scales, hyperpigmented in Caucasians and depigmented in dark-skinned children, appear on the face, chest, abdomen, or arms, forming multiple circular lesions with clear centers. (From Hurwitz S: *Clinical pediatric dermatology: a textbook of skin disorders of childhood and adolescence,* ed 2, Philadelphia, 1993, Saunders.)

Treatment and Nursing Care. Systemic antibiotics are administered either orally or parenterally. Parents are instructed to wash the lesions 3 or 4 times daily to remove crusts. Ointments such as mupirocin (Bactroban) may be prescribed for topical application. Prevention of the disease by treating small cuts promptly is important. The prognosis with proper treatment is good. Nursing care consists primarily of preventing this disease.

Education of parents includes reminding them of the necessity for prompt attention to minor cuts and bites. In diagnosed cases, compliance with the treatment regimen is needed to prevent the spread of infection to other children and family members. If the diagnosis is made in the newborn nursery, the infant is isolated to prevent other newborns from becoming infected. Nephritis may occur as a complication of group A beta-hemolytic streptococcal infections.

Fungal Infections

Pathophysiology. Fungal infections are caused by several closely related fungi that have a preference for invading the stratum corneum, the hair, and the nails. The word *tinea* comes from the Latin "worm." The common name for this infection is ringworm. Fungi are larger than bacteria. Some fungi may be transmitted from person to person and others from animal to person. The name denotes the part of the body involved.

Tinea capitis. Tinea capitis ("ringworm of the scalp") is seen in school-age children. Patches of **alopecia** (hair loss) characterize this condition. The hair loses pigment and may break off. The papules become pustules, which progress to red scales. There are areas of circular balding.

Diagnosis is made by history and appearance. Some strains of tinea capitis glow green under a Wood's light. This condition is treated with griseofulvin (Fulvicin, Grisactin), which is administered by mouth. It is given with or after meals to avoid gastrointestinal irritation and increase absorption. Suspensions should be well shaken. Parents are instructed to continue therapy as long as ordered and that they should not miss a dose. Exposure to the sun is avoided. Treatment may be necessary for 8 to 12 weeks. Children may go to school but are warned not to exchange hats, combs, or other personal items. Selenium sulfide shampoos are also used, which may eliminate the spores. This infection can be stubborn and may take several weeks to clear.

Tinea corporis. Tinea corporis ("ringworm of the skin") is evident as an oval scaly inflamed ring with a clear center. It is seen on the face, neck, arms, and hands (Figure 30-13). Infected pets can transmit it. Treatment consists of local application of an antifungal preparation such as clotrimazole for 2 to 4 weeks.

Tinea pedis. Tinea pedis refers to *athlete's foot.* Lesions are located between the toes, on the instep, and on the soles. There is accompanying pruritus. It occurs more often in preadolescents and adolescents. Direct microscopic scrapings of the lesions provide the diagnosis. Treatment consists of topical therapy with an antibacterial or antifungal preparation such as econozole or clotrimazole.

Because this condition is aggravated by heat and moisture, the feet must be carefully dried, especially between the toes. Clean socks are worn. Shoes need to be well ventilated. Plastic shoes that retain heat are avoided. Recurrences are common.

Tinea cruris. Tinea cruris ("thigh") affects the groin area and is commonly referred to as "jock itch." It occurs on the inner aspects of the thighs and scrotum. The initial lesion is small, raised, and scaly. It spreads, and tiny vesicles occur at the margins of the rash. Local application of the antifungal clotrimazole may be effective. General hygiene should be stressed.

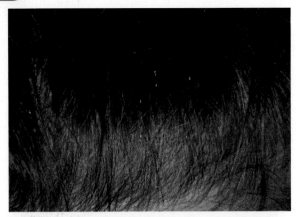

FIGURE 30-14 Pediculosis. White nits or eggs of the head lice are attached to the hair. (Courtesy Dr. Michael Sherlock. In Zitelli BJ et al: *Zitelli and Davis' atlas of pediatric physical diagnosis*, ed 6, St Louis, 2012, Saunders.)

Pediculosis

The infestation of humans by lice is termed **pediculosis**. There are three types: pediculosis capitis (head lice), pediculosis corporis (body lice), and pediculosis pubis (crabs or pubic lice). The various types usually remain in the part of the body designated by their name. They are transmitted from person to person or by contact with contaminated articles. Their survival depends on the blood they extract from the infected person. Severe itching in the affected area is the main symptom. In all cases, treatment is aimed at ridding the patient of the parasite, treating the excoriated skin, and preventing the infestation of others. The most common form seen in children is head lice (Figure 30-14).

Pediculosis Capitis

Pathophysiology. Pediculosis capitis, which is commonly known as head lice, affects the scalp and hair. The louse lays eggs (nits) that attach to the hair and hatch within 3 or 4 days. Head lice are more common in girls than in boys because of hair length and the tendency to share combs and hair ornaments. The parasite may be acquired from hats, combs, or hairbrushes. It is easily transferred from one child to another and is seen most often in the school-age child and in preschool children who attend day care centers.

Manifestations. Children with pediculosis capitis suffer from severe itching of the scalp. They scratch their heads frequently and often cause further irritation. The hair becomes matted. Pustules and excoriations may be seen about the face. Nurses admitting patients to pediatric units should be on the alert for head lice. In particular, the nurse inspects the hairline at the back of the neck and about the ears. Crusts, pediculi, nits, and dirt may cause matting of the hair and a foul odor. When the condition is discovered, it is handled with discretion so as not to embarrass the child or parents.

Treatment and nursing care. Treatment is directed toward killing the lice, getting rid of the nits, and managing any infections of the face and scalp. Family members and playmates of the child should be examined and treated as necessary. Shampoos such as Nix are commonly used. Retreatment may be necessary in 1 week to 10 days. It has been reported that lindane (Kwell) has neurotoxic effects, and it is no longer used (AAP, 2012).

If the eyebrows and eyelashes are involved, a thick coating of petroleum jelly (Vaseline) may be applied, followed by removal of the remaining nits. Nits on the head are removed by combing the hair with a fine-toothed comb dipped in a 1:1 solution of white vinegar and water. The hair is then washed. In some cases, recovery is hastened by cutting the hair. Transmission-based contact isolation precautions should be followed. A commercial machine that uses hot air to kill lice has been developed and will be available for use by trained workers (Frankowski, 2010).

Children should be cautioned against swapping caps, headscarves, and combs. Parents are instructed to inspect the child's head regularly. Parents are encouraged to report infestations to the school nurse, because widespread outbreaks are periodically encountered.

Scabies

Pathophysiology. Scabies is a parasitic infection caused by the itch mite, *Sarcoptes scabiei*. It is seen worldwide. The adult female mite, who burrows under the skin and lays eggs, causes scabies. The mite has a round body and four pairs of legs and is visible by microscopic examination. A characteristic burrow is sometimes seen under the skin, particularly between the fingers. Burrows contain the eggs and feces of the mite. Itching is intense, especially at night. A vesiculopustular lesion can occur in children.

Scabies may occur anywhere on the body but is seldom seen on the face. It thrives in moist body folds, but in young children the lesions may appear on the head, the palms, and the soles of the feet. It is spread by close personal contact, including sexual relations. It is rarely transmitted by fomites because the isolated mite dies within 2 to 3 days.

Treatment and Nursing Care. Treatment consists of the application of permethrin (Elimite). It can be used for children older than 2 months of age. Parents are instructed to follow the directions carefully. All family members, babysitters, and close associates require treatment. Transmission-based contact isolation precautions are followed (see Appendix A). An oral antiparasitic agent *ivermectin* has been approved for use in children weighing more than 15 kg in cases where the response to other methods is deficient (Orrico, 2010).

INJURIES

Burns

Pathophysiology. Burns often occur during childhood. They are the leading cause of accidental death in the home for children between 1 and 4 years of age.

Sometimes burns are a result of child abuse and neglect. The two times of day during which burns are most likely to occur are the early morning hours before parents awaken and after school. There are several types of burns:

- *Thermal:* caused by fire or a scalding vapor or liquid
- *Chemical:* caused by a corrosive powder or liquid
- *Electrical:* caused by electrical current passing through the body
- *Radiation:* caused by x-rays or radioactive substances

Burns can involve the skin or mucous membranes. When a child is burned by fire near the face, the flames may be *inhaled,* causing a burn of the mucous membrane lining the airway. Assessing for resulting edema and respiratory distress is a priority. When a formula or food is heated in the microwave oven, "hot spots" occur that can cause burns to the mucous membranes lining the mouth.

The differences in responses of children to a burn are as follows:

- The child's skin is thinner than that of the adult, leading to a more serious depth of burn with lower temperatures and shorter exposure than with adults.
- The large body surface area of the child results in greater fluid, electrolyte, and heat loss.
- Immature response systems in young children can cause shock and heart failure.
- The increased basal metabolic rate (BMR) of a child results in increased protein and calorie needs.

- Less muscle and fat in the body results in protein and caloric deficiencies when oral intake is limited.
- The skin is more elastic in children, causing pulling on the scarring areas and resulting in formation of a larger scar.
- The immature immune system predisposes the child to developing infections that complicate burn treatment.
- The prolonged immobilization and treatment required for burns adversely affects growth and development.

> **!** **Safety Alert!**
>
> The small child should be taught to stop, drop, and roll if the clothes become ignited.

Classification. The severity of a burn depends on the area, extent, and depth of involvement. The size of the burn is calculated as a percentage of **total body surface area (TBSA)**. Age-related charts are used for children, because their body proportions differ from those of adults, and a standard (rule of nines) cannot be applied (Figure 30-15). The terms *partial thickness* and *full thickness* describe the extent of destruction of the skin. In partial-thickness burns, only some of the skin layers are damaged. Full-thickness burns are deeper and more extensive and may necessitate skin grafting. The classification of and first aid treatment for burns are

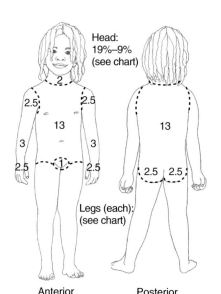

Head: 19%–9% (see chart)

2
2.5   2.5
13   13
3   3
2.5   1   2.5   2.5   2.5

Legs (each): (see chart)

Anterior   Posterior

Child Burn Size Estimation Table
(percent total body surface area)

	Age (yr)					
	<1	1	5	10	15	Adult
Head	19	17	13	11	9	7
Neck	2	2	2	2	2	2
Anterior trunk	13	13	13	13	13	13
Posterior trunk	13	13	13	13	13	13
Buttock	2.5	2.5	2.5	2.5	2.5	2.5
Genitalia	1	1	1	1	1	1
Upper arm	2.5	2.5	2.5	2.5	2.5	2.5
Lower arm	3	3	3	3	3	3
Hand	2.5	2.5	2.5	2.5	2.5	2.5
Thigh	5.5	6.5	8	8.5	9	9.5
Leg	5	5	5.5	6	6.5	7
Foot	3.5	3.5	3.5	3.5	3.5	3.5

FIGURE 30-15 Body surface area (BSA) charts. This chart is used to determine the developmentally related percentage of body surface area burned. The percent of BSA involved is the basis for determining the fluid and nutritional needs of the burned child. In children younger than 3 years of age, the "rule of nines" assigns the infant's head as 18% of total BSA (TBSA) and the lower extremities as 14% TBSA, with 9% assigned to each arm and 1¼% to the hands or palms. This chart is also referred to as the *Lund and Browder chart.* (From Wong DL, Hockenberry MJ, Wilson D, Perry SE, Lowdermilk DL: *Maternal-child nursing care,* ed 3, St Louis, 2006, Mosby.)

Table 30-2 Classification and First Aid Treatment of Burns

DEGREE	ANATOMY AND DEPTH	APPEARANCE AND SENSATION	FIRST AID TREATMENT
Superficial (first)	Epidermis only	Skin red but blanches easily on pressure and refills quickly; painful, indicating tissue viability	Immerse in cold water to halt burning process; apply an antimicrobial ointment.
Partial thickness (second)	Epidermis and much of dermis; partial thickness	Blistered, moist, pink, or red; painful, indicating tissue viability	If area is small, treat as if for first-degree burn and apply antimicrobial ointment; otherwise treat as if for deep dermal burn.
Deep dermal (deep partial thickness)	Extends deep into dermis; partial thickness but can become full thickness with infection, trauma, or poor blood supply	Mottled; red, tan, or dull white; blisters; painful, indicating tissue viability	Immerse in cold water to halt burning process; cover with sterile dressing or clean cloth to prevent contamination and decrease pain from contact with air; avoid breaking blisters; seek medical attention immediately.
Full thickness (third)	Subdermal; involves entire skin and all its structures; full thickness	Tough, leathery, dry; does not blanch or refill; dull brown, tan, black, or pearly white; painless to touch, indicating death of tissue	Halt the burning process by immersing in cold water or rolling in blanket or rug; wrap in clean sheet or other sterile dressing; provide blanket for warmth; have victim lie down; *do not* apply ointment or any other substance to burned area; take patient to nearest emergency treatment center immediately. Skin graft may be needed.
Fourth	All skin and nerve endings destroyed and includes muscle and bone destruction	Blood vessels and bone may be visible. Necrosis occurs.	

summarized in Table 30-2. One can survive a rather extensive superficial burn, whereas a deep burn involving a smaller surface area can threaten the patient's life. Table 30-3 discusses children's response to burn injuries.

Burns can also be complicated by fractures, soft tissue injury, or preexisting conditions such as diabetes, obesity, epilepsy, and heart or renal disease. Moderate burns are considered to be: (1) partial-thickness burns involving 15% to 30% of body surface, or (2) full-thickness burns involving less than 10% of body surface. Major burns are: (1) partial-thickness types involving 30% or more of body surface or (2) full-thickness burns involving 10% or more of body surface. Partial-thickness and full-thickness burns must be regarded as open wounds that include the added danger of infection. The "6 Cs" of burn care include clothing, cooling, cleaning, chemoprophylaxis, covering, and comforting or pain relief (Herndon, 2007). Burn treatment can be administered in an outpatient clinic, in a general hospital, or at a specialized burn center.

Treatment

Care of electrical burns. When electricity is the cause of the injury, the child should be assessed for entry and exit lesions that may appear as a small erythematous area. The locations of the entry and exit wounds indicate the path of electricity through the body

Table 30-3 Response to Burn Injury in Children*

RESPONSE	EFFECT
Capillary permeability increases, and hypovolemia occurs.	There is a loss of plasma, proteins, and fluids; shock occurs.
Blood flow to vital organs increases, and blood flow to periphery of body and nonvital organs decreases.	Peristalsis ceases (ileus). Curling's ulcer can form in stomach.
Body metabolism increases to maintain heat.	Increased basal metabolic rate (BMR) can strain the heart by causing increased cardiac output.
Damage to red blood cells and hemolysis results in anemia.	Anemia causes increased cardiac output to maintain perfusion.
Open wounds of burn can predispose to infection. Dead tissue provides a medium for bacterial growth.	Immature immune system can be overwhelmed, and sepsis can result.
Waste products accumulate in the blood because of anemia and slow perfusion of nonvital organs.	Renal failure, cardiac failure, and pulmonary edema can complicate toxicity from burn injury.

*Thermal injuries produce both local and systemic effects.

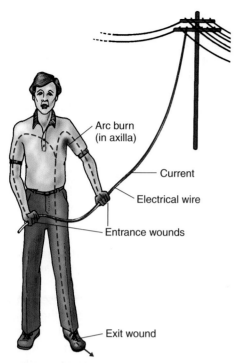

FIGURE 30-16 Mechanism of electrical injury. The electrical current enters the body and travels through the heart before exiting the body. All patients with electrical injuries should have their cardiac enzymes monitored to determine if heart damage has occurred. (From Ignatavicius DD, Workman ML: *Medical-surgical nursing: patient-centered collaborative care*, ed 7, St Louis, 2013, Saunders.)

(Figure 30-16). Muscle damage can occur, and if the electrical current passes through the heart, cardiac muscle damage can result. Deep muscle damage can cause renal impairment from myoglobinuria. The child should be observed closely for responses with electrocardiography (ECG) monitors, the recording of vital signs, and assessment of cardiac enzymes before discharge.

> ### Nursing Tip
>
> Electrical burns of the mouth are common in small children, who put everything into their mouths. Biting into electrical cords is not unusual. Such wounds are usually deep and leave an entrance and an exit burn. They are subject to bleeding for several weeks.

Emergency care. Community education programs emphasize the response to a child with a burn injury. The school nurse plays a major role in the education process, as follows:

- *Stop the burning process.* Stop, drop, and roll is the sequence of care. Rolling the child in a blanket smothers the flames. A caustic powder should be brushed off before water is used to wash the area; this prevents spreading the caustic substance and enlarging the area of contact. Electricity should be turned off before touching a child who has been electrocuted.
- *Evaluate the injury.* Check the "ABCs" (**a**irway, **b**reathing, **c**irculation) of the victim. Cardiopulmonary

resuscitation (CPR) is initiated as appropriate. Minor burns can be treated; a physician should assess major burns.

- *Cover the burn.* The burned area should be covered with a clean cloth to minimize contact with air, reduce pain, minimize hypothermia, and prevent contamination of the wound. Burned clothing and jewelry should be removed, because metal retains heat and continues the burn injury.
- *Transport to a hospital.* Do not give any fluids by mouth, because peristalsis may have diminished in response to the burn injury. If available, IV fluids and oxygen should be administered and the child comforted and reassured.

Care of minor thermal burns. Minor burns are treated at home and followed with clinic visits until healing is complete. The wound is cleansed and an antimicrobial ointment applied with a loose dressing. Blisters are not disturbed unless a chemical burn occurred. Dressings are changed as prescribed, and the parent is advised to report any sign of infection. The status of tetanus immunization is reviewed and updated as needed. Pain relief is administered as needed. The wound of a minor burn is usually completely healed within 20 days. Evaluation of scarring and effect on range of motion (ROM) will determine future follow-up needs.

Care of major burns. The physician, nurse, and respiratory therapist and other specialists in the emergency department or, in some instances, the operating room, handle the immediate treatment of shock in cases of severe burns. Priorities include establishing an airway in patients with facial burns or smoke inhalation, instituting IV lines, and assessing burn wounds and other, perhaps initially unrecognized, injuries. At times, some of these procedures are performed simultaneously.

> ### Nursing Tip
>
> A severe burn can cause a loss of function in two of the most important properties of the skin: the ability to protect against infection and the ability to prevent loss of body fluid.

Establishing an airway. Cyanosis, singed nasal hairs, charred lips, and stridor are indications that flames may have been inhaled. An endotracheal tube is inserted to maintain an adequate airway, although this is not required for all patients. This permits the delivery of humidified air with oxygen, easy removal of secretions from respiratory passages, and use of a pressure ventilator if needed. Sedation is administered with caution to prevent further respiratory inhibition.

If **eschar** (*eschara,* "scab") from burns on the trunk inhibits respirations, an incision called an *escharotomy* is made to prevent the restriction of chest movement. Blood gas levels, including level of carbon monoxide, are ascertained. The child is placed on sterile sheets. Attendants wear a facemask, sterile gown, and gloves.

IV infusions are begun to prevent intravascular dehydration and electrolyte imbalance. Ringer's lactate solution is often used initially. Albumin or plasma may be used when capillary permeability is restored (within 24 to 48 hours).

Laboratory studies include hematocrit and sodium chloride, potassium, carbon dioxide, blood urea nitrogen, creatinine, and serum protein levels. Blood typing and cross matching are performed. Fluid therapy requires close monitoring throughout hospitalization. To determine urine volume and characteristics, a urinary catheter is inserted and an intake and output record is maintained.

The loss of fluid causes renal vasoconstriction, leading to depressed glomerular filtration and oliguria. Acute renal failure can develop without adequate therapy. Urine output is observed hourly. It varies considerably, but on the average 20 to 30 mL/hr for patients older than 2 years of age is considered adequate during the resuscitative stage. The patient's weight is recorded and used as baseline data for determining adequacy of ongoing treatment.

A nasogastric tube is inserted and is attached to low wall suction. This empties the stomach and prevents complications such as gastric dilation, vomiting, and paralytic **ileus** (intestinal muscle paralysis). The patient has nothing by mouth for the first 24 hours. Sporadic bleeding as a result of **Curling's ulcer** (stress ulcer) is not uncommon in patients with severe burns; the administration of IV antacids such as cimetidine has helped to reduce its incidence. Pain control and close monitoring is essential.

Wound care. The goals of wound care include the removal of necrotic tissue to allow healing to take place, the maintenance of moist conditions and adequate circulation, the conservation of body heat and fluids, the prevention of infection, and the minimization of scar formation. A partial thickness burn is treated with antibacterial agents such as silver sulfadiazine (Silvadene), mafenide acetate (Sulfamylon), or bacitracin after initial assessment and cleaning. Cleaning a burn wound can be painful, and measures for pain relief should be taken. The black eschar of necrotic tissue can be debrided via whirlpool. Yellow eschar is not removed. Dressings may be applied. Aquacel AG and Acticoat are silver-based antimicrobial dressings that provides a long-acting and sustained pain-relief and bacteriocidal effect, and the dressing can remain in place for several days.

Immediate care of the wound itself includes cleansing and **debridement** (removal of dried crusts) of necrotic tissue. The loss of skin increases the threat of infection, and fluid loss caused by evaporation can be significant. The immune system is depressed. Strict asepsis is maintained, and the wound site is treated in accordance with the physician's instruction. A tetanus immunization history is obtained, and tetanus prophylaxis is administered as required. Low doses of antibiotics may be prescribed to prevent streptococcal infection.

A semiopen method of burn dressing may be used, although exposure methods may be useful on accessible areas such as the face. The wound is covered by a few layers of sterile gauze that has been saturated with antibacterial ointment or cream. The gauze may be held in place by elastic netting (Figure 30-17). When the wound is being dressed, *no two burn surfaces should touch.* A sterile blanket may be used to prevent chilling. The wound is cleansed by tub baths or, in many cases, whirlpool baths are used to soften necrotic areas and debride the wound. Surgical debridement is done when needed to cleanse the wound and prepare the new granulation tissue for grafting. Ointments such as Sulfamylon or Silvadene may be prescribed for use. A biological dressing or a synthetic dressing may be used to prevent fluid loss and to promote healing. The burn area is closed and resurfaced by grafting.

Skin grafts. Temporary grafts are used during the acute stage of recovery. They protect the wound from infection and reduce fluid loss but are eventually rejected by the body. Temporary grafts include **homografts** (usually tissue from disease-free cadavers) and **heterografts** (tissues obtained from different species). Heterografts are also referred to as **xenografts** (*xeno,* "foreign," and *graft,* "slice of skin").

Many grafts are derived from pigskin, which is available commercially either fresh or frozen; these biological dressings are often used in children and are called *porcine xenografts.* They are particularly useful in partial-thickness or deep dermal burns and have greatly improved burn management. Deep dermal wounds may be preceded by tangential (*merely touching*) excision, which is a surgical technique of removing burned eschar with a dermatome. Thin layers are shaved down to the live tissues, and temporary porcine grafts are applied.

There are two types of permanent grafts: autografts and isografts. An **autograft** (*auto,* "self") is healthy tissue obtained from another part of the patient's body. An **isograft** (*iso,* "equal") is obtained from the patient's identical twin or genotype. Permanent grafts are performed during the rehabilitative stage of the patient's illness to improve appearance and function. The site from which the tissue is removed is called the donor area.

Advances in grafting techniques have improved the overall prognosis in burn patients and have helped to minimize scarring. A split-thickness skin graft can be prepared with the use of a dermatome. For extensive burns, it is sometimes difficult to find enough intact skin for use. Special methods such as the Tanner mesh graft may be used. In this method a strip of split-thickness skin is run through a special cutting machine that makes multiple slits; this expands the skin to provide more coverage, which in some cases is as much as 9 times the original area of the skin. The graft is sutured in place to maintain tension.

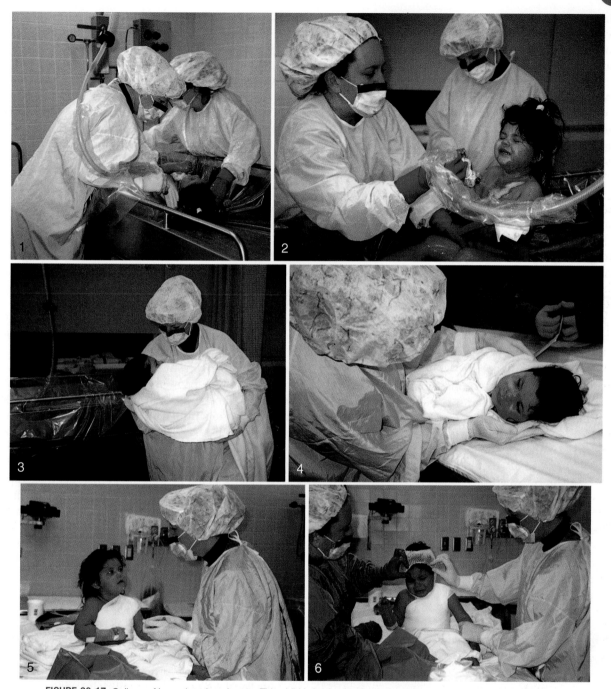

FIGURE 30-17 Collage of burn dressing change. This child is having her burn dressings changed and is undergoing whirlpool bath debridement. She is gently dried with sterile towels, and a pressure dressing is reapplied. (Photos courtesy Pat Spier, RN-C.)

The "postage stamp" graft consists of small pieces of donor skin placed on the granulation tissue. Spaces between grafts allow for drainage and healing. Full-cover grafts are sheets of skin placed intact over the wound. These are cosmetically more effective than patch and mesh grafts but are not always available. The donor site is covered with xenograft or fine mesh gauze; it heals in about 2 weeks. Newly grafted areas are covered with sterile dressings. Every effort is made to prevent bleeding and infection. The areas surrounding the wound are observed for edema and impaired circulation. Hyperbaric therapy can enhance the healing of grafts (see Chapter 34).

Biological dressings. Biological dressings can be applied to a noninfected burn wound within 6 hours of the injury and will peel off as the wound heals. Dressing changes are not necessary. The dressings are made from neonatal foreskin fibroblast cells combined in a nylon mesh that is sterile and frozen for storage. After thawing, they cannot be refrozen. The dressings, Biobrane or TransCyte with bismuth-impregnated petrolatum gauze, contain human or pigskin products, and hypersensitivity should be considered before use.

Vacuum-assisted wound closure is negative pressure applied to a wound after the wound is packed and sealed. Fluid from the wound exits via a suction tube into a canister. The vacuum draws out fluid, increases blood perfusion to the tissues, and decreases bacterial contamination and scarring while enhancing healing. It is used in older children and adolescents but the FDA has not yet approved the device for use with young children (USFDA, 2011).

Posthealing care. After basic healing has occurred, a nonperfumed moisturizer cream such as Eucerin or Nivea, or cocoa butter, may be recommended to maintain skin moisture. Ointments containing lanolin are not advised. Sun block should be used to prevent hyperpigmentation of the newly healed skin. It may take 2 years for complete healing to occur. Systemic antihistamines such as diphenhydramine (Benadryl) or hydroxyzine (Atarax) may be prescribed to control itching. Bicarbonate of soda baths are soothing.

 Nursing Tip

Disorientation, fever, and diminished bowel sounds may be early signs of sepsis.

Nursing Care of the Burned Child. Children who have suffered extensive burns and survive the early dangers face a long period of hospitalization and require specialized care. The various aspects of nursing care differ with the age of the patient, the area of the burn, and the type of treatment used. Box 30-2 lists some topical agents used in treating burn patients.

Protective isolation (expanded precautions) is instituted. All instruments that come in contact with the wound must be sterile. Ointments are applied with a sterile gloved hand or sterile tongue depressor. Care must be taken to prevent injury to granulation tissue.

The nurse immediately reports signs of infection: elevations of temperature, pulse, and respiration;

Box **30-2**   Topical Agents Used to Treat Burn Patients
SILVER SULFADIAZINE CREAM 1% (SILVADENE) Cream is effective against gram-negative and gram-positive bacteria and yeast (*Candida albicans*). Do not use if patient is allergic to sulfa drugs. Cream does not sting; it softens eschar. Do not waste; cream is expensive. Gently remove old cream before reapplying. **MAFENIDE ACETATE 10% (SULFAMYLON)** Agent is effective against gram-positive and gram-negative organisms; penetrates eschar. Agent is painful because it draws water out of the tissues; pain may last 15 to 30 minutes or longer. Remain with child after application for comfort and diversion. Do not apply to face. There is a potential for metabolic acidosis. **BACITRACIN** Agent is painless and is applied twice daily. Agent is a low-cost prophylactic antibiotic.

---

restlessness and confusion; pain; purulent drainage; and an odor emanating from the wound dressing. A careful description of the wound in the nurse's notes facilitates daily comparison and determination of progress. All infection must be cleared before skin grafting can be performed.

The nurse remains alert for signs of fluid overload, in particular, behavioral changes and altered sensorium. Although initially restricted to prevent nausea and vomiting, oral fluids are necessary during the convalescent stages to prevent kidney damage and to maintain body fluid requirements. The nurse must use ingenuity to persuade the child to take sufficient amounts of fluids. An accurate record of intake and output of fluids is kept.

The demands on the metabolism as it copes with this trauma are increased, and more calories are spent as water evaporates from the wound site. Frequent feedings of foods high in calories, protein, and iron are therefore necessary. A high-protein diet—a normal diet with added amounts of meat, milk, eggs, fish, or poultry—is usually prescribed. Iron therapy may be initiated if anemia begins to develop. Eggnogs are nourishing between-meal drinks for burn patients with such needs. Small amounts are offered frequently. Vitamins A, B, and C and zinc sulfate are given to hasten healing and to stimulate the appetite. Gavage feedings may be necessary. Accurate daily records of foods consumed, calorie count, and patient's weight will help to determine the nutritional status.

The nurse bears in mind that other, unaffected parts of the body need exercise and proper positioning to prevent painful contractures. The child's position is changed every 2 to 4 hours unless contraindicated. A footboard is used to prevent foot drop. Support should be provided by means of pillows, sandbags, and rolled towels as necessary.

The physical therapist attends to the child regularly for exercise and to keep the joints limber and healthy. The child begins to ambulate as soon as possible. Self-help activities and mobility are encouraged. Pressure splints or elasticized garments help to reduce scar tissue and are sometimes worn for months after discharge.

Emotional support. A burn injury is taxing to the child and parents. It requires long periods of hospitalization and frequent readmissions. The accident itself is terrifying for the child but is made even worse if caused by disobedience. Nurses encourage children to express their feelings. Analgesics are administered *before* painful procedures. The long-term patient requires diversions of various types. School tutors are requested, and contact is maintained with peers through cards or e-mail.

Nurses give constant support to the parents, who usually feel guilty if the child was injured in an accident. Nurses indicate by their manner that they do not blame the parents for what has happened. Preparation for discharge begins early. The multidisciplinary health care team includes the physician, the nurse, the school nurse, the schoolteacher, the physiotherapist,

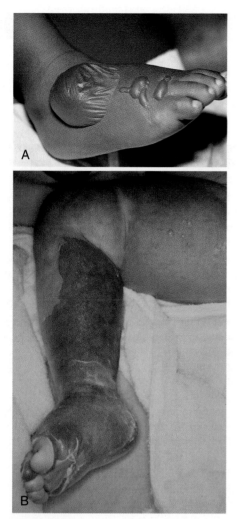

FIGURE 30-18 Scald burns. **A,** An accidental scald burn. Note the droplet pattern indicating a splash. **B,** Nonaccidental scald burn. An inflicted scald reveals severe extensive second-degree burns on the entire leg. (From Zitelli BJ et al: *Zitelli and Davis' atlas of pediatric physical diagnosis,* ed 6, St Louis, 2012, Saunders.)

and the psychologist. Instructions are provided regarding wound care, diet, exercise, and rest. Return appointments are made, and referral agencies are contacted. Methods to improve the physical appearance of the patient are discussed. The importance of burn prevention cannot be overemphasized. Figure 30-18 shows the difference in appearance of a scald burn wound from an accidental spill and a scald wound that was inflicted (child abuse).

> **Nursing Tip**
>
> In cases of car, house, or airplane fires, patients may face additional crises, such as the loss of relatives, pets, and possessions.

Sunburn

Sunburn is a common skin injury caused by overexposure to the sun, especially at midday. Sunburn can be a minor epidermal burn or a more serious partial-thickness burn with blistering. Goals of treatment include stopping sun exposure, treating inflammation, and rehydrating the skin. Immersion in a tepid water bath (36.7° C [98° F]) for 15 to 20 minutes is the initial treatment. A bland oil-in-water moisturizing lotion can be applied. Education is the key to preventing sunburn. Covering the skin with clothing, wearing a hat, and using sunscreen liberally is recommended. Two types of products are available. Topical sunscreen partially absorbs ultraviolet (UV) light, and sunblocks reflect sunlight. Zinc oxide and titanium dioxide are effective sunblocks. Sunscreens have a sun protection factor (SPF) rating to evaluate effectiveness at blocking the sun's rays. If individuals normally burn in sun exposure after 10 minutes, use of an SPF 15 sunscreen will allow 10×15, or 150, minutes of sun exposure before burning occurs. Sunscreens with para-aminobenzoic acid (PABA) are very effective, but some children are sensitive or can have an allergic reaction. Sunscreens are not recommended for infants younger than 6 months of age. Small infants should be physically protected from excessive sun exposure. Melanoma is a common form of cancer that occurs as a result of frequent sun exposure without protection. Avoiding sunburn in children is very important.

Frostbite

Frostbite is the result of the freezing of a body part. **Chilblain** is a cold injury with erythema and the formation of vesicles and ulcerative lesions that occur as a result of vasoconstriction. Education to prevent cold injury is essential for those living in or visiting cold climates. School nurses play a vital role in educating parents and children. Adequate layered clothing, including hats and gloves (wool over cotton), is preferred.

In exposure to extreme cold, warmth is lost in the periphery of the body before the core temperature drops, and the extremities can suffer considerable damage before the onset of potentially fatal hypothermia. Therefore, in extreme cases of exposure to freezing temperatures, the head and the torso should be warmed before the extremities to ensure survival with minimal consequences. Frostbitten extremities appear pale and hard and are without sensation. Sensitive skin should be handled gently. Massage is contraindicated. Dry clothing should be applied and muscle activity encouraged. Blankets or sleeping bags are initially used to start rewarming. Warm, moist oxygen; warming blankets; and warming baths of 37.8° to 42.2° C (100° to 108° F) are used. A deep purple flush appears with the return of sensation, which is accompanied by extreme pain. Pain relief and monitoring of vital signs are essential. Blistering and ulcers can occur and are treated with whirlpool soaks. Skin damage is similar to that incurred with burns. Frostbite can result in *necrosis* (death) of tissue and may necessitate amputation of the extremity.

Get Ready for the NCLEX® Examination!

Key Points

- The skin is the body's first line of defense against disease.
- Certain skin conditions are symptoms of systemic disease.
- Common skin problems in infants are diaper dermatitis, seborrheic dermatitis, and atopic dermatitis (eczema).
- A strawberry nevus is an example of a hemangioma.
- Pediculosis is the term for lice. Lice may occur on the head, body, or pubic area.
- Tinea pedis, or athlete's foot, is prevented by drying the feet well, particularly between the toes, and wearing well-ventilated footwear.
- A severe burn can cause a loss of function in two of the most important properties of the skin: the ability to protect against infection and the ability to prevent the loss of body fluid.
- Electrical burns carry the risk of thrombosis and tissue damage in other parts of the body.
- The severity of a burn depends on the area, extent, and depth of involvement.
- Preventing infection is an important nursing intervention for patients with burns or any skin lesion.
- A sunburn can be a minor epidural burn or a partial-thickness burn with blisters.
- Topical sunscreens partially absorb the sun's UV rays and have ratings to evaluate the effectiveness of blocking these rays. Sun blockers reflect sunlight.
- Frostbite can cause tissue damage similar to burns.
- Absorption of a topical hydrating medication is best when applied after a warm bath.
- Types of burns include thermal, electrical, chemical, and radiation.

Additional Learning Resources

SG Go to your Study Guide for additional learning activities to help you master this chapter content.

evolve Go to your Evolve website (http://evolve.elsevier.com/Leifer) for the following learning resources:
- Animations
- Answer Guidelines for Critical Thinking Questions
- Answers and Rationales for Review Questions for the NCLEX® Examination
- Glossary with English and Spanish pronunciations
- Interactive Review Questions for the NCLEX® Examination
- Patient Teaching Plans in English and Spanish
- Skills Performance Checklists

 Online Resources
- American Academy of Dermatology: www.aad.org/index.html
- Burn awareness and prevention: www.shrinershq.org/Hospitals/BurnAwareness

Review Questions for the NCLEX® Examination

1. Why is pain relief important for the burn patient?
   1. It prevents discomfort.
   2. The child must be kept from crying.
   3. Parents become upset.
   4. Pain contributes to shock.

2. The principles of care in the treatment of infantile eczema include (select all that apply):
   1. hydrate skin, prevent infection, relieve itching.
   2. keep skin dry, clean with mild soap.
   3. use elbow restraints to prevent scratching, increase fluid intake.
   4. dress warmly, bathe often with clear water, administer antibiotics.

3. When caring for a child newly admitted with a major burn injury, the priority nursing responsibilities include which of the following interventions? (Select all that apply.)
   1. Prevent infection.
   2. Maintain accurate intake and output.
   3. Provide daily baths for cleanliness
   4. Provide a high carbohydrate diet.

4. What is contained in an emollient bath often prescribed for children with eczema?
   1. Bath oil
   2. Glycerin soap
   3. Oatmeal
   4. Salt or saline solution

5. When instructing parents who plan to take their 5-month-old infant sunbathing at the beach, it is most important to emphasize which of the following:
   1. Use a sunscreen with a SPF greater than 15 over exposed areas of the infant's skin.
   2. Reapply sunscreen after playing in the water.
   3. Use sunglasses to protect eyes.
   4. Use light clothes and a hat to protect against sun exposure.

The Child with a Metabolic Condition

Objectives

1. Define each key term listed.
2. Relate why growth parameters are of importance to patients with a family history of endocrine disease.
3. List the symptoms of hypothyroidism in infants.
4. Discuss the dietary adjustment required for a child with diabetes insipidus.
5. Differentiate between type 1 and type 2 diabetes mellitus.
6. List three precipitating events that might cause diabetic ketoacidosis.
7. Compare the signs and symptoms of hyperglycemia and hypoglycemia.
8. List a predictable stress that the disease of diabetes mellitus has on children and families during the following periods of life: infancy, toddlerhood, preschool age, elementary school age, puberty, and adolescence.
9. Outline the educational needs of the parents and the child with diabetes mellitus in the following areas: nutrition and meal planning, exercise, blood tests, glucose monitoring, administration of insulin, and skin care.
10. Discuss the preparation and administration of insulin to a child, highlighting any differences between pediatric and adult administration.
11. List three possible causes of insulin shock.
12. Explain the Somogyi phenomenon.

Key Terms

antidiuretic hormone (p. 705)
dawn phenomenon (p. 716)
gestational diabetes mellitus (GDM) (p. 707)
glucagon (p. 716)
glycosuria (glī-kō-SYŪ-rē-ă, p. 708)
glycosylated hemoglobin test (HgbA$_{1c}$) (glī-kō-sī-lā-tĭd HĒ-mō-glō-bĭn tĕst, p. 709)
hormones (p. 703)
hyperglycemia (hī-pŭr-glī-SĒ-mē-ă, p. 708)
hypoglycemia (hī-pō-glī-SĒ-mē-ă, p. 715)

hypotonia (hī-pō-TŌ-nē-ă, p. 705)
ketoacidosis (kē-tō-ă-sǐ-DŌ-sǐs, p. 709)
lipoatrophy (lǐp-ō-ĂT-rō-fē, p. 714)
polydipsia (pŏl-ē-DǏP-sē-ă, p. 708)
polyphagia (pŏl-ē-FĀ-jhă, p. 708)
polyuria (pŏl-ē-YŪ-rē-ă, p. 708)
Somogyi phenomenon (sō-mō-gēē p. 716)
target organ (p. 703)
vasopressin (vāz-ō-PRĔS-ĭn, p. 705)

INTEGRATION OF THE NERVOUS AND ENDOCRINE SYSTEMS

The two major control systems that monitor the functions of the body are the nervous system and the endocrine system. These systems are interdependent. The endocrine, or ductless, glands regulate the body's metabolic processes. They are primarily responsible for growth, maturation, reproduction, and the response of the body to stress. Figure 31-1 depicts the organs of the endocrine system and outlines how this system in children differs from that in adults. **Hormones** are chemical substances produced by the glands. They pour their secretions directly into the blood that flows through them. An organ specifically influenced by a certain hormone is called a **target organ**. Too much or too little of a given hormone may result in a disease state.

Most of the glands and structures of the endocrine system develop during the first trimester of fetal development. Hormonal control is immature until at least 18 months of age, and therefore infants are more prone to problems related to the functioning of the endocrine system. Maternal endocrine dysfunction may affect the fetus; therefore an in-depth maternal history is a valuable tool in data collection.

The absence or deficiency of an enzyme that has a role in metabolism causes a defect in the metabolism process; this can result in illness. Most inborn errors of metabolism can be detected by clinical signs or screening tests that can be performed in utero. Lethargy, poor feeding, failure to thrive, vomiting, and an enlarged liver may be early signs of an inborn error of metabolism in the newborn. When clinical signs are not manifested in the neonatal period, an infection

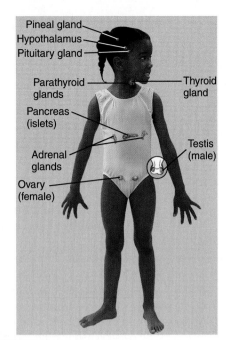

Pineal gland
Hypothalamus
Pituitary gland

Parathyroid glands
Thyroid gland

Pancreas (islets)

Adrenal glands
Testis (male)

Ovary (female)

ENDOCRINE SYSTEM

- The endocrine system of the newborn is supplemented by maternal hormones that cross the placental barrier. In males and females, this may result in swelling of the breasts and genital changes.
- Hormone disturbances during childhood may cause disrupted growth patterns, resulting in short stature or gigantism.
- Congenital hypothyroidism may occur as a result of an absent, nonfunctioning thyroid gland.
- In childhood the pancreas may be deficient in insulin, causing type 1 (insulin-dependent) diabetes.

FIGURE 31-1 Summary of some endocrine system differences between the child and the adult. The endocrine system consists of the ductless glands that release hormones. It works with the nervous system to regulate metabolic activities. (Art overlay courtesy Observatory Group, Cincinnati, Ohio.)

or body stress can precipitate symptoms of a latent defect in the older child. Unexplained mental retardation, developmental delay, convulsions, an odor from the body or from the urine, or episodes of vomiting may be subtle signs of a metabolic dysfunction. Phenylketonuria (PKU), galactosemia, and maple syrup urine disease are discussed in Chapter 14. Cystic fibrosis is discussed in Chapter 25.

Radiographic studies to determine bone age are valuable diagnostic tools. Serum electrolytes and glucose, hormonal, and calcium level tests may be required. PKU testing of newborns is an important screening device for identifying an enzyme deficiency. Chromosomal studies and tissue biopsy are other diagnostic tools. Sexual maturation and skin texture, pigment, and temperature may be indicators of specific disorders. Thyroid function tests may be required. Ultrasonography is helpful in determining the size and character of adrenal glands, ovaries, and other organs. A 24-hour urine specimen may provide important data. Genetic counseling can help prevent some disorders. Most endocrine dysfunctions involve chronic problems and call for long-term nursing management. The nurse must assess the effect on growth and development, advocate for early detection and intervention, and promote comprehensive follow-up care that will minimize complications.

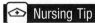 Nursing Tip

Growth hormone is administered at bedtime to simulate the natural timing of hormone release.

DISORDERS AND DYSFUNCTION OF THE ENDOCRINE SYSTEM

INBORN ERRORS OF METABOLISM

Archibald Garrod coined the term *inborn errors of metabolism* at the turn of the twentieth century. There are literally hundreds of these hereditary biochemical disorders that affect body metabolism. The pattern of inheritance is generally autosomal recessive. These conditions range from mild to severe.

Tay-Sachs Disease

Pathophysiology. Tay-Sachs disease involves a deficiency of lysosomal-beta-*hexosaminidase*, an enzyme necessary for the metabolism of fats. Lipid deposits accumulate on nerve cells, causing both physical and mental deterioration. This is a disease found primarily in the Ashkenazi Jewish population. It is an autosomal recessive trait carried by 1 in 30 of the Ashkenazi Jewish population, resulting in an occurrence of 1 in 320,000 live births (Pastores, 2011).

Manifestations. The infant with Tay-Sachs disease is normal until about age 5 to 6 months, when physical development begins to slow. There may be head lag or an inability to sit. The disease progresses, and when deposits occur on the optic nerve, blindness may result. Mental retardation eventually develops because the brain cells become damaged. Most children with Tay-Sachs disease die before 5 years of age from secondary infection or malnutrition.

Treatment and Nursing Care. There is no treatment for this devastating disease. The nursing care is mainly palliative. Most care is administered in the home, with periodic hospitalization for complications such as pneumonia. Chapter 27 discusses the care of the dying child. Carriers can be identified by screening tests in the first trimester of pregnancy. Genetic testing and prenatal counseling have markedly decreased the occurrence of Tay-Sachs disease.

ENDOCRINE DISORDERS

Hypothyroidism

Pathophysiology. Hypothyroidism occurs when there is a deficiency in the secretions of the thyroid gland. It may be congenital or acquired. It is one of the more common disorders of the endocrine system in children. The thyroid gland controls the rate of metabolism in the body by producing thyroxine (T_4) and triiodothyronine (T_3). In congenital hypothyroidism, the gland is absent or not functioning. The symptoms of hypothyroidism may not be apparent for several months.

The older child acquires juvenile hypothyroidism. It may be caused by a number of conditions, the most common being lymphocytic thyroiditis. Often it appears during periods of rapid growth. Infectious disease, irradiation for cancer, certain medications containing iodine, and lack of dietary iodine (uncommon in the United States) may predispose the child. The symptoms, diagnosis, and treatment are similar to those for congenital hypothyroidism. Because brain growth is nearly complete by 2 to 3 years of age, mental retardation and neurological complications are not seen in the older child.

Manifestations. The infant with hypothyroidism is very sluggish and sleeps a lot. The tongue becomes enlarged, causing noisy respiration (Figure 31-2). The skin is dry, there is no perspiration, and the hands and feet are cold. The infant feels floppy when handled. This **hypotonia** also affects the intestinal tract, causing chronic constipation. The hair eventually becomes dry and brittle. If hypothyroidism is left untreated, irreversible mental retardation and physical disabilities result.

Treatment and Nursing Care. Early recognition and diagnosis are essential to prevent the developing sequelae. A screening test for hypothyroidism is mandatory in the United States and is performed at birth. This is generally part of an overall screen for other metabolic defects. Treatment involves the administration of the synthetic hormone called sodium levothyroxine (Synthroid, Levothroid). Hormone levels are monitored regularly. Therapy reverses the symptoms and prevents further mental retardation but does not reverse existing retardation; therefore early detection of congenital hypothyroidism is very important.

The medication is taken at the same time each day, preferably in the morning. Parents are cautioned not

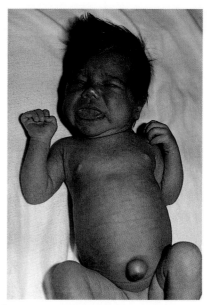

FIGURE 31-2 An infant with hypothyroidism. Note the large head and tongue, puffy face, broad nasal bridge, and relaxed abdominal muscles resulting in an umbilical hernia. The infant is not alert and feeds poorly. (Courtesy Dr. TP Foley, Jr, Pittsburgh, Pa. In Zitelli BJ, et al: *Zitelli and Davis' atlas of pediatric physical diagnosis,* ed 6, St Louis, 2012, Saunders.)

to interchange brands. Children may experience reversible hair loss, insomnia, and aggressiveness, and their schoolwork may decline during the first few months of therapy. This is temporary. It may take 1 to 3 weeks for the medication to reach the full therapeutic effect. Medication is not to be discontinued, because hormone replacement for hypothyroidism is lifelong. Parents should be taught the signs and symptoms of overdose, which include rapid pulse rate, dyspnea, irritability, weight loss, and sweating. Signs of inadequate dosage or noncompliance are fatigue, sleepiness, and constipation. Parents are instructed about these issues and are advised to consult their physician before giving other medications.

COMMON METABOLIC DYSFUNCTIONS

Other common metabolic dysfunctions, their manifestations, and their treatments are discussed in Table 31-1.

Diabetes Insipidus

Pathophysiology. Diabetes insipidus can be hereditary (autosomal dominant) or acquired as the result of a head injury or tumor. It is the consequence of posterior pituitary *hypofunction* that results in a decreased secretion of **vasopressin**, the **antidiuretic hormone**. A lack of antidiuretic hormone results in uncontrolled diuresis. The kidney does not concentrate the urine during dehydration episodes.

Manifestations. *Polydipsia* and *polyuria* are the initial signs. The infant cries and prefers water to milk formula. Loss of weight, growth failure, and dehydration

Table 31-1 Metabolic Dysfunctions

GLAND	PROBLEM	INVOLVED HORMONE	MANIFESTATION	THERAPY
Pituitary— anterior	Decreased: hypopituitarism	Growth hormone	Short stature, dwarfism	Synthetic growth hormone replacement
	Increased: hyperpituitarism	Growth hormone	Before epiphyseal closure, gigantism After epiphyseal closure, acromegaly Sexual precocity (puberty before 8 to 9 years of age)	Cryosurgery, irradiation Radioactive implants Monthly hormone injection to control secretions until puberty
Pituitary— posterior	Decreased: hypopituitarism	Decreased antidiuretic hormone	Diabetes insipidus (see p. 705)	Vasopressin by injection or nasal spray Provide adequate fluids
	Increased: hyperpituitarism (SIADH)	Increased antidiuretic hormone	SIADH Decreased urine output Edema Fluid overload	Fluid restriction and hormone antagonists
Parathyroid	Decreased: hypoparathyroidism	Decreased parathyroid hormone	Decreased blood calcium and increased phosphorus levels, causing tetany and laryngospasm	Calcium gluconate, vitamin D supplements
	Increased: hyperparathyroidism	Increased parathormone	Elevated blood calcium and lowered phosphorus levels, causing spontaneous fractures and CNS problems	Restore calcium balance, excise tumor, vitamin D, low phosphorus diet
Adrenal	Decreased: adrenal cortical insufficiency (Addison's disease)	Decreased steroids, sex steroids, epinephrine	Craving for salt, seizures, neurological and circulatory changes, decreased sexual development	Replace cortisol and aldosterone, genetic sexual assessment
	Increased: hyperadrenalism (Cushing's disease)	Increased cortisol	Cushing's syndrome, hyperglycemia, electrolyte problems, pheochromocytoma	Depends on cause, tumor removal, and hormone replacement

CNS, Central nervous system; *SIADH*, syndrome of inappropriate antidiuretic hormone.

occur rapidly. As the child grows older, enuresis may be a problem. Excessive thirst and the search for water overshadow the desire to play, explore, eat, learn, or sleep. Perspiration is deficient, and the skin is dry.

Treatment and Nursing Care. Treatment involves hormone replacement of vasopressin in the form of desmopressin by subcutaneous injection or DDAVP (desmopressin acetate) nasal spray. Parents should be taught to monitor for signs of overdose, which include symptoms of water intoxication (edema, lethargy, nausea, central nervous system signs). Children with diabetes insipidus who are admitted to the hospital in an unconscious state and are unable to express thirst are at great risk. A medical identification bracelet should be worn. School personnel should be advised of the child's needs. School protocol often limits children's access to bathrooms and water fountains, even during or after physical activity. Such restrictions could be life threatening to a child with diabetes insipidus. The child's nurse should contact the school nurse and physical education instructors and educate parents concerning the child's needs and the lifelong administration of the medication.

Home care instructions should include recognizing the signs of water intoxication and dehydration.

Diabetes Mellitus
Pathophysiology. Diabetes mellitus (DM) is a chronic metabolic syndrome (group of symptoms) in which the body is unable to use carbohydrates (CHO) properly, leading to an impairment of glucose transport (sugar cannot pass into the cells). The body is also unable to store and use fats properly. There is a decrease in protein synthesis. When the blood glucose level becomes dangerously high, glucose spills into the urine, and diuresis occurs. Incomplete fat metabolism produces ketone bodies that accumulate in the blood. This is termed *ketonemia* and is a serious complication. DM affects the physical and psychological growth and development of children because it requires lifestyle alterations (diet, glucose monitoring, and insulin administration). There are also many long-term complications related to hyperglycemia that result in blindness, circulatory problems, kidney disease, and neuropathy that loom in the future for these children. Treatment is designed to optimize growth and development and to minimize complications.

Classification. The major forms of diabetes mellitus have been classified according to those caused by a deficiency of insulin secretion because of pancreatic beta cell damage and those that are a consequence of insulin resistance. Type 1 diabetes is the most common metabolic disorder of children, with an occurrence of 1:300 in the United States (Kliegman, 2011). Diabetes comes with a high degree of risk for long-term complications that may manifest in adulthood. Although there is a genetic susceptibility to type 1 diabetes, a large percentage of affected children have no known family history. Genetic studies have implicated chromosome #6 and #11, but other genetic risk factors have been identified, and environmental factors such as viruses may play a role in triggering diabetes. Diet may also play a role in autoimmunity, such as the timing of introducing new foods in infancy, but no conclusive findings have been found. Research is ongoing.

The accepted criterion for diagnosing diabetes mellitus is a fasting blood glucose level of 126 mg/dL or higher after no caloric intake for 8 hours (Kliegman, 2011).

The classifications of diabetes mellitus (Table 31-2) pertinent to pediatrics include:

- **Type 1,** formerly known as *insulin-dependent diabetes mellitus (IDDM)* and *juvenile-onset diabetes mellitus:* Type 1 DM is an autoimmune condition that occurs when a child with a genetic predisposition is exposed to an environmental factor such as a viral infection that triggers the syndrome by causing destruction of beta cells in the pancreas and resulting in insufficient insulin production. Drugs, chemicals, and ionizing radiation may cause beta cell destruction in some cases (Kliegman, 2011).

Table 31-2	Classification of Diabetes Mellitus
Type 1	Destruction of beta cells in pancreas results in lack of insulin production Formerly known as insulin-dependent diabetes mellitus (IDDM) or juvenile-onset diabetes mellitus
Type 2	Involves insulin resistance or *decreased* insulin production Formerly known as non–insulin-dependent diabetes mellitus (NIDDM) or adult-onset diabetes mellitus Associated with obesity and elevated blood lipids
Gestational diabetes	Transient form of diabetes mellitus that is triggered by pregnancy Resolves after delivery but may reoccur several years later (see Chapter 5)
Other genetic defects	Defects in chromosomes 6, 7, 12, and 20 and other genetic disorders are associated with diabetes mellitus syndrome

Table 31-3	Clinical Features of Type 1 and Type 2 Diabetes	
FEATURE	**TYPE 1**	**TYPE 2**
Onset	Abrupt; patient can often state week of onset	Insidious; often found by screening tests
Body size	Normal or thin	Often obese
Blood glucose level	Fluctuates widely with exercise and infection	Fluctuations are less marked
Ketoacidosis	Common	Infrequent
Sulfonylurea responsiveness	Rare	>50%
Insulin required	Almost all	<25%
Insulin dosage	Increases until glucose control is stable	May remain stable

- **Type 2,** formerly known as *non–insulin-dependent diabetes mellitus (NIDDM)* or adult-onset DM or *maturity-onset DM:* Type 2 DM involves a resistance to insulin. It is often triggered by a sedentary lifestyle and obesity. It also occurs more frequently in certain ethnic groups, such as African American and Pacific Islanders, especially those who have hypertension and elevated blood lipid levels. *Acanthosis nigricans* (a dark pigmentation in the flexor creases of the skin) may be a cutaneous marker for patients with type 2 DM.
- **Gestational diabetes mellitus (GDM)** is the appearance of symptoms for the first time during pregnancy (see Chapter 5).

Table 31-3 lists the clinical features of types 1 and 2 DM. Lifestyle intervention is the cornerstone of preventing or delaying the onset of type 2 diabetes mellitus in susceptible individuals.

Type 1 Diabetes Mellitus

Incidence. Approximately 12 million Americans have diabetes mellitus. In the United States, the annual incidence is about 1 newly diagnosed case of type 1 DM per 500 children (Kliegman et al, 2011). The frequency is increasing. Symptoms of type 1 DM may occur at any time in childhood, but the rate of occurrence of new cases is highest among 5- and 7-year-old children and pubescent children 11 to 13 years of age. In the former group, the stress of school and the increased exposure to infectious diseases may be the precipitating event that triggers the onset.

During puberty, rapid growth, increased emotional stress, and insulin antagonism of sex hormones may be implicated as contributing to development of diabetes. DM occurs in both sexes with equal frequency. The disease is more difficult to manage in childhood because the patients are growing, expend a great deal of energy, have varying nutritional needs, and face a lifetime of diabetic management. Young children with type 1 often do not demonstrate the typical "textbook" picture of the disorder. The initial diagnosis may be determined when the child develops ketoacidosis. Therefore the nurse must be particularly astute in subjective and objective observations.

Manifestations. Children with diabetes mellitus present a classic triad of symptoms: polydipsia, polyuria, and polyphagia. The symptoms appear more rapidly in children. The patient complains of excessive thirst (**polydipsia**), excretes large amounts of urine frequently (**polyuria**), and is constantly hungry (**polyphagia**). An insidious onset with lethargy, weakness, and weight loss is also common. The child who is toilet trained may begin wetting the bed or have frequent "accidents" during play periods, may lose weight, and is irritable. The skin becomes dry. Vaginal yeast infections may be seen in the adolescent girl. There may be a history of recurrent infections. The symptoms may remain unrecognized until an infection becomes apparent or coma results. Laboratory findings indicate glucose in the urine (**glycosuria**). **Hyperglycemia** (*hyper,* "above," *gly,* "sugar," and *emia,* "blood") is also apparent. Hyperglycemia occurs because glucose cannot enter the cells without the help of insulin, and therefore glucose remains in the bloodstream. The cells use protein and fat for energy; therefore protein stores in the body are depleted. The lack of glucose in the cells triggers the body to develop polyphagia and the increase in glucose intake further increases glucose levels in the blood. Hyperglycemia is the cause of the many complications associated with uncontrolled diabetes mellitus.

The honeymoon period. When type 1 is initially diagnosed and the child is stabilized by insulin dosage, the condition may appear to improve. Insulin requirements decrease and the child feels well. This phenomenon supports the parent's phase of "denial" in accepting the long-term diagnosis of DM for their child. The "honeymoon period" lasts a short time (a few months), and parents must be encouraged to closely monitor blood glucose levels to prevent complications.

> **Nursing Tip**
>
> A period of remission, or the "honeymoon" phase of the disease, may occur within a few weeks of beginning insulin administration. There is a decline in insulin need and improved metabolic control. This phase, however, is temporary.

Diagnostic Blood Tests

Blood glucose. A random blood glucose level may be obtained at any time and requires no preparation of the patient. The results should be within the normal limits for both nondiabetic patients and diabetic patients who have good control of their disease.

- *Fasting blood glucose.* A fasting blood glucose level is a standard and reliable test for diabetes. The blood glucose level is measured in the fasting patient, usually immediately on awakening in the morning. The results of the test will not be accurate if the patient is receiving a dextrose intravenous solution. If the child is known to have diabetes, food and insulin are withheld until after the test. If a person's fasting blood glucose level is greater than 126 mg/dL on two separate occasions and the history is positive, the patient is considered to have diabetes mellitus and requires treatment.

- *Glucose tolerance test.* Another test to determine the amount of glucose in the blood is the glucose tolerance test (GTT). The results are plotted on a graph (Figure 31-3). This procedure is time-consuming, and therefore is no longer in routine use because the glycosylated hemoglobin test is fast and accurate

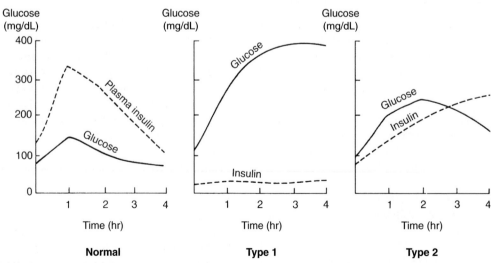

FIGURE 31-3 The glucose tolerance test: *Left,* normal; *center,* type 1 diabetes; *right,* type 2 diabetes. The graphs show the relationship between the ingestion of glucose and the level of plasma insulin during 4 hours in a normal person and in persons with type 1 and type 2 diabetes. (Modified from Waechter EH, Blake FG: *Nursing care of children,* ed 9, Philadelphia, 1976, Lippincott.)

and shows longer-term elevation of glucose levels. A blood glucose concentration greater than 200 mg/dL is considered positive. Normal values may not return for more than 3 hours.

- *Glycosylated hemoglobin test.* The **glycosylated hemoglobin test (HgbA$_{1c}$)** reflects glycemic levels throughout a period of months. Values are found to be elevated in virtually all children with newly diagnosed diabetes. This study also helps to confirm the results of blood and urine tests performed either at home or by the physician. Glucose in the bloodstream constantly enters red blood cells and links with, or glycosylates, molecules of hemoglobin. The more glucose in the blood, the more hemoglobin becomes coated with glucose. The red blood cells carry this glucose until cells with fresh hemoglobin replace them. This process takes about 3 to 4 months. Values vary according to the measurement used. Values of 6% to 9% represent very good metabolic control. Values greater than 12% indicate poor control.
- *The future of testing.* The Human Genome Project has identified the genes responsible for many diseases. Because DM is considered an autoimmune response, it is possible to predict the occurrence risk of DM by use of genetic, immunological, and metabolic markers. Research is ongoing concerning the screening techniques and preventive immunotherapy. C-peptide (connecting chains of insulin peptides) may also be measured to determine how much insulin the body is producing (endogenous). This is of particular value during the honeymoon period of the disease.

Diabetic Ketoacidosis.

Diabetic **ketoacidosis** (DKA) is also referred to as diabetic coma, although a person may have DKA with or without being in a coma. It is manifested by ketonemia and may be precipitated by a secondary infection. It may also occur if the disease proceeds unrecognized; this happens fairly often in children with diabetes. Even minor infections, such as a cold, increase the body's metabolic rate and thereby change the body's demand for insulin and the severity of diabetes. Ketoacidosis is the end result of the effects of insulin deficiency.

Symptoms of ketoacidosis are compared with those of hypoglycemia in Table 31-4; signs and symptoms include a fruity odor to the breath, nausea, decreased level of consciousness, and dehydration. Lab values include ketonuria, decreased serum bicarbonate concentration (decreased CO_2 levels) and low pH, and hypertonic dehydration. Diabetic teaching should include this information. The symptoms range from mild to severe and occur within hours to days.

Treatment and Nursing Care.

The three goals of treatment in type 1 diabetes mellitus are the following:

1. Ensure normal growth and development through metabolic control.

Table 31-4	Hyperglycemia and Hypoglycemia
HYPERGLYCEMIA (KETOACIDOSIS)	**HYPOGLYCEMIA**
Cause	
Inadequate insulin Excess CHO intake	Excess exercise Too little CHO intake Insulin overdose
Signs and Symptoms	
Blood glucose levels >160 mg/dL Polyuria, polydipsia, polyphagia Fruity odor to breath Fatigue Abdominal pain Red lips, flushed face Dehydration Disorientation Drowsiness progressing to coma Deep, rapid (Kussmaul's) respirations	Blood glucose <70 mg/dL Fatigue, hunger Pale, clammy skin Diaphoresis Tremors Lethargy Headache Irritability Tachycardia
Treatment	
Regular insulin	Administer glucagon IM, orange juice, or CHOs orally or IV glucose

CHO, carbohydrate; *IM,* by intramuscular route; *IV,* by intravenous route.

2. Enable the child to cope with a chronic illness, have a happy and active childhood, and be well integrated into the family.
3. Prevent complications.

Maintaining the blood glucose at consistently normal levels can minimize complications. Teaching ideally begins when the diagnosis is confirmed. A planned educational program is necessary to provide a consistent body of information, which can then be individualized. The patient's age and financial, educational, cultural, and religious background must be considered. Many hospitals hold group clinics for diabetic patients and their relatives. These sessions are conducted by the multidisciplinary health care team and include the diabetes nurse educator, dietitian, and pharmacist. Patients who are living with the disease provide encouragement and help by sharing concerns. Health professionals become directly involved with the patient's progress and can offer necessary feedback and support. Continuous follow-up is essential.

Because children with diabetes are growing, additional dimensions of the disorder and its treatment become evident. Growth is not steady but occurs in spurts and plateaus that affect treatment. Infants and toddlers may have hydration problems, especially during illness. Preschool children have irregular activity and eating patterns. School-age children may grieve over the diagnosis and ask, "Why me?" They may use their illness to gain attention or to avoid responsibilities. The onset of puberty may require insulin adjustments as a result of growth and the antagonistic effect of the sex hormones on insulin. Adolescents often resent this condition, which deviates from their concept of the "body ideal." They have more difficulty in resolving their conflict between dependence and independence. This may lead to rebellion against parents and treatment regimens.

The impact of the disease on the rest of the family must also be considered. Parents may feel guilty for having passed the disease on to their child. Siblings may feel jealous of the attention the patient receives. The sharing of responsibility by parents is ideal but not necessarily a reality. Some may have difficulty accepting the diagnosis and the more regimented lifestyle it imposes. Family members must cope with their individual reactions to the stress of the illness.

Children must assume responsibility for their own care gradually and with a minimum of pressure. Overprotection can be as detrimental as neglect. Parents who have received satisfaction from their child's dependence on them may need help "letting go." The diabetic camp experience is helpful in this respect. A medical identification bracelet should be worn.

The nursing management of childhood diabetes requires knowledge of growth and development, pathophysiology, blood glucose self-monitoring, nutritional management, insulin management, insulin shock, exercise, skin and foot care, infections, effects of emotional upsets, and long-term care. Nursing Care Plan 31-1 lists interventions for the child with diabetes.

Teaching Plan for Children with Diabetes Mellitus. The patient and family are instructed about the location of the pancreas and its normal function. The nurse explains the relationship of insulin to the pancreas, differentiating between type 1 and type 2 diabetes. All information is provided gradually and at the level of understanding of the child and family. Audiovisual aids and pamphlets are incorporated into the session. If the patient is newly diagnosed, hospitalization offers opportunities for instruction.

Blood Glucose Self-Monitoring. Patients can test their own blood glucose level in the home. While still being supervised by and consulting with the physician, the patient can make rational changes in insulin dosage (sliding scale dosage) based on home blood glucose tests, nutritional requirements, and daily exercise. This is of great psychological value to the child, adolescent, and parents because it reduces feelings of helplessness and complete dependence on medical personnel. Home glucose monitoring should be taught to all young patients and their caregivers. The patient not only must be skilled in the techniques but also should understand the results and how to incorporate them into daily regimens. This means involving the entire health care team in ongoing supervision, demonstrations, and support.

Although instructions are included with the various products, patients need individual training.

Glucometer systems provide readouts and automatically store data by time and date. Some also keep track of diet and the amount of exercise for the day. They can be connected to a computer or computer printer for review or to an insulin pump. Records can be transmitted electronically to the physician.

Obtaining blood specimens before meals and at bedtime has been simplified by the use of capillary bloodletting devices such as the Glucolet. This device automatically controls the depth of penetration of the lancet into the skin. Other brands include Hamlet, Autoclix, Monoject, Autolet, and Accu-Chek. The sides of the fingertips are recommended testing sites because there are fewer nerve endings and more capillary beds in these areas. The best fingers to use are the middle, ring, or little fingers on either hand. The finger will bleed more easily if the child washes the hands in warm water for about 30 seconds. To perform the test, a drop of blood is put on a chemically treated reagent strip. The test strip with a drop of blood is inserted into the glucometer, and the blood glucose reading appears.

Noninvasive devices to assess blood glucose levels also have been developed. One system is worn on the wrist like a watch and uses infrared technology to provide noninvasive glucose monitoring. The FDA has approved the "At Last" glucose monitor (Amira) that has a lancet built in and takes a sample from the forearm or the thigh. It is less painful than the fingertip devices.

The methods of glucose monitoring provide different information. The fingerstick method of glucose monitoring shows the glucose level at a moment in time. The $HgbA_{1c}$ value shows a history of several weeks' pattern of glucose control. Continuous glucose monitoring measures levels within the interstitial tissues and shows trends in glucose levels but does not completely replace glucometers.

Cost, convenience, and portability are factors to consider when selecting glucometers. Most products can be obtained at the local pharmacy. Newer and more precise instruments are being developed constantly. Frequency of use is determined by the amount of diabetes control required by the particular child.

Continuous Glucose Monitoring. The continuous glucose monitor consists of a sensor placed subcutaneously in the abdomen that transmits interstitial blood glucose levels every 10 to 60 seconds to a monitor worn on the clothing of the patient. This technique helps identify fluctuation and trends that cannot be picked up by the standard $HgbA_{1c}$ test or intermittent finger-stick measurements. The continuous glucose monitoring system is used to devise an individualized treatment plan for the patient. In 2008, the FDA approved a Continuous Glucose Monitoring System that was intended for use by children age 7 years and older. The goal was

⭐ Nursing Care Plan 31-1 | The Child with Diabetes Mellitus

PATIENT DATA A 10-year-old boy is admitted with new-onset diabetes mellitus. An insulin regimen is prescribed. The child states that he wishes to return to a normal life with his peers.

Selected Nursing Diagnosis: Risk for injury related to hypoglycemia or diabetic ketoacidosis (hyperglycemia)

Goals	Nursing Interventions	Rationales
Child will be able to measure blood glucose level with glucometer, as age appropriate.	Teach child home glucose monitoring.	Self-care increases feelings of control.
	Record vital signs regularly.	Vital signs detect infection and illness, which affect diabetes; in ketoacidosis, Kussmaul's respirations may be seen until blood pH and serum bicarbonate levels normalize.
Child will be adequately hydrated as evidenced by good tissue turgor and intake and output records.	Monitor fluid intake and output.	Dehydration may occur as a result of vomiting, polyuria, and hyperglycemia.
	Serve meals and snacks on time.	Serving meals on time prevents hypoglycemia and minimizes hyperglycemia.
	Administer or have patient administer insulin as ordered.	Insulin is individualized to meet the response of patients. It cannot be taken by mouth because stomach juices would destroy it before it could be used.
	Determine level of consciousness.	Both hypoglycemia and hyperglycemia affect sensorium, depending on stage of reaction.
Child will be asymptomatic of hypoglycemia or hyperglycemia.	Carefully observe patient for signs of hypoglycemia or hyperglycemia.	Factors such as diet, increased exercise, or illness can contribute to the body's balance of insulin and glucose; changes in hormone levels that accompany menstruation can cause swings of high or low blood glucose levels.

Selected Nursing Diagnosis: Deficient knowledge related to exercise

Goals	Nursing Interventions	Rationales
Child will describe physical exercise program.	Determine child's activity level as age appropriate.	Exercise increases glucose use.
	Explain that exercise lowers the blood glucose level and in this respect acts like more insulin.	Patient may need to adjust insulin dose for days when involved in high-impact exercise.
Child will be prepared for hypoglycemia should it occur.	Teach symptoms of hypoglycemia, such as irritability, shakiness, hunger, headache, and altered levels of consciousness.	Early recognition and prompt treatment will prevent injury.
	Teach child importance of carrying extra sugar when exercising or playing sports.	Taking sugar reverses symptoms of hypoglycemia.
	Teach child the dangers of swimming alone.	Child could drown if symptoms occur.

Selected Nursing Diagnosis: Deficient knowledge related to identification

Goals	Nursing Interventions	Rationales
Child will state understanding of importance of wearing proper identification bracelet.	Child demonstrates proper identification.	Diabetes symptoms may be mistaken for other conditions, such as flu.
Family will acquire identification bracelet.	Encourage purchase of means of identification.	Child may be unconscious or too young to inform others of condition.

Critical Thinking Question

1. A child comes to the clinic for follow-up after discharge from the hospital with a diagnosis of diabetic ketoacidosis. He states he is excited about returning to school and rejoining his cross-country team with his friends. His father states he wants his son to stay home and do more sedentary activities to prevent any more health problems. What is the best response of the nurse?

to provide a closed loop wireless system that provides glycemic control with minimum intervention by connecting the glucose monitor to the insulin pump that more closely mimics normal physiology (Carchidi, 2013) (see Insulin Management section).

Diet Therapy for Children with Diabetes Mellitus

Nutrition management. The triad of diabetes management consists of a well-balanced diet, precise insulin administration, and regular exercise. The importance of glycemic control in decreasing the incidence of symptoms and complications of the disease has been established. The advent of blood glucose self-monitoring is affecting food intake in that diets can be fine-tuned and more flexible while the cornerstone of *consistency* (in amount of food and time of feeding) is maintained. Contrary to popular belief, there is no scientific evidence indicating that persons with diabetes require special foods. In fact, if it is good for the diabetic patient, it is good for the entire family. The nutritional needs of diabetic children are essentially no different from those of nondiabetic children. The timing of food consumption has to be correlated with the time and action of the type of insulin prescribed so that blood glucose levels will not be abnormally high or abnormally low.

The goals of nutrition management in children are to ensure normal growth and development, to distribute food intake so that it aids metabolic control, and to individualize the diet in accordance with the child's ethnic background, age, gender, weight, activity, family economics, and food preferences. Total estimated caloric intake is based on body size or surface area and can be obtained in standard tables. The recommended intake is 50% carbohydrates (mostly complex carbohydrates), 30% fat, and 20% protein (Kliegman, 2011). Most of the carbohydrate intake should consist of complex carbohydrates that absorb slowly and do not cause sudden and wide elevation of blood glucose level. The various types of insulin allow flexibility in diet intake and improve the quality of life. There are many "sugar free" products on the market, but sorbitol and xylitol should not be used as artificial sweeteners because they may contribute to diabetic complications (Kliegman, 2011). Dietary fat from animal sources should be limited and replaced with polyunsaturated fats found in vegetables. Occasional excesses for birthdays or special occasions can be accommodated to prevent rebellion and to promote compliance. Special supplements may be required to accommodate the exercise patterns and growth needs of children. After a diet prescription is received from the physician, the dietitian assists the family in designing an individualized diet plan. The dietitian also explains the use of exchange lists.

Carbohydrate counting provides flexibility in meal planning, using one carbohydrate choice to equal 15 g of carbohydrate. Generally, one unit of insulin covers 15 g of carbohydrate. A general nutrition plan can be created for a child using foods they like, including snacks. The diet prescription usually includes carb values. Carb counting offers adolescents control and involvement in their need to maintain a positive self-concept and self-esteem that promotes compliance. The My Plate food guide (www.choosemyplate.gov) may be used to guide the child and family concerning portion control and selection of foods.

Education of the patient is ongoing. Too much information given at one time may overwhelm the parents and discourage the child. Well-informed nurses can offer much reinforcement and support. They can clarify terms such as dietetic, sugar free, juice-packed, water-packed, and unsweetened. Meal trays in the hospital provide an excellent opportunity for teaching. Children should bring their lunches to school. Respecting cultural patterns and personal preferences is important. The content of foods that are commonly found in fast-food chain restaurants is available through the American Diabetes Association.

The importance of fiber in diets is well documented. In the diabetic patient, soluble fiber has been shown to reduce blood glucose levels, lower serum cholesterol values, and sometimes reduce insulin requirements. Fiber appears to slow the rate of absorption of sugar by the digestive tract. Raw fruits and vegetables, bran cereals, wheat germ, beans, peas, and lentils are good sources of soluble fiber.

> **! Safety Alert!**
>
> Instruct the patient and family to read food labels carefully. The word *dietetic* does not mean *diabetic*. Dietetic merely means something has been changed or replaced; for example, the food may contain less salt or less sugar.

Glycemic index of foods. The glycemic index for selected foods has an impact on the manipulation of dietary needs (Table 31-5). The *glycemic index* is the impact of a portion of food on the blood glucose as compared to the same portion of pure glucose. The glycemic index may be higher for the liquid form (apple juice) than the same carbohydrate in solid form (whole apple). The fiber content of the food can lower the glycemic index. Some chocolate may have a low glycemic index, but the high saturated fat content limits its nutritional and health value. The *glycemic load* takes into account the amount of glucose in a food combined with the total carbohydrate content of a serving portion. Foods with a low glycemic index (less than 55) takes longer to increase the glucose levels in the blood. Foods that have a high glycemic index (more than 70) increase blood glucose more rapidly. Use of this knowledge enables a person to select optimal foods to eat before, during, and after exercise. The size of portions, the type of processing or cooking, and the combinations of foods have also been shown to have a bearing on glucose responses.

Table 31-5   Glycemic Index of Selected Foods

FOOD	GLYCEMIC INDEX*
All-Bran cereal	60
Apple	36
Baked potato	78
Banana	51
Carrots	39
Corn flakes	81
French baguette bread	95
Cranberry juice cocktail	68
Cola	65+
Sports beverages	75+
Peach	43
Peanuts	17
Skim milk	37
Spaghetti	58
Watermelon	72
White bread	70

*Foods with a low glycemic index take a longer time to increase the glucose levels in the blood.
Data from Atkinson F, Foster-Powell R, Brand-Miller J: International table of glycemic index and glycemic load values, *Diabetic Care* 31(12):2281-2283, 2008; Dudek S: *Nutrition essentials for nursing practice*, ed 7, Philadelphia, 2014; Lippincott; Mahan L, Escott-Stump S: *Krause's food, nutrition, and diet therapy*, ed 13, Philadelphia, 2012, Saunders.

◈ Nursing Tip

Take snacks seriously—they are an important part of the day's food supply.

◈ Nursing Tip

Avoid the use of sorbitol or xylitol as artificial sweeteners in the diets of children with diabetes (Kliegman et al, 2011).

Insulin management. Insulin is used principally as a specific drug for the control of DM. When injected into the diabetic patient, it enables the body to burn and store sugar. Current data emphasize the importance of blood glucose control in the prevention of microvascular disease.

The dose of insulin is measured in units, and special syringes are used in its administration. U-100 (100-unit) insulin is the standard form. All vials of U-100 insulin have color-coded caps, and all labels bear black printing on a white background.

It is important to teach the parents and child about the administration of insulin. Insulin cannot be taken orally because it is a protein and would be broken down by the gastric juices. The usual method of administration is subcutaneous injection (Figure 31-4). When injected at a 90-degree angle, the short needle enters the subcutaneous space. This technique may be easier for the child to learn because it takes less coordination to administer than a 45-degree-angle technique.

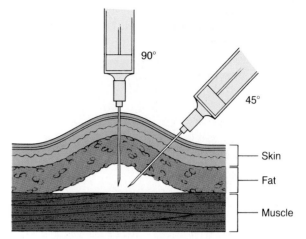

FIGURE 31-4 Subcutaneous injection of insulin.

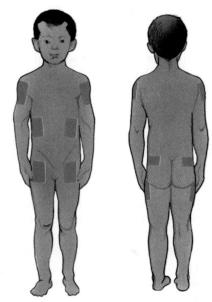

FIGURE 31-5 Sites of injection of insulin. (From McKinney ES, James SR, Murray SS, Ashwill JW: *Maternal-child nursing*, ed 2, Philadelphia, 2005, Saunders.)

⚠ Medication Safety Alert!

Human insulin and pork insulin are *not* interchangeable.

The site of the injection is rotated to prevent poor absorption and injury to tissues (Figure 31-5). Injection model forms made from construction paper and site rotation patterns are useful. One suggested site rotation pattern is to use one area for 1 week. A different site within that area is used for each injection. Injections should be about 1 inch apart. The young child and parents can use a doll or a simulator to practice self-injection.

Insulin should not be injected into an area in which circulation is temporarily increased. In such areas, a more rapid than expected absorption and effect can trigger hypoglycemia. For example, a more rapid circulation to the legs can be expected in a child who is riding

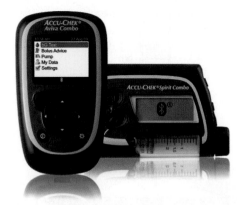

FIGURE 31-6 The ACCU-CHEK Combo System consists of an insulin pump and a glucose monitor that act together via *Bluetooth*® technology. This is a subcutaneous insulin infusion system that eliminates the need for frequent injections. A small, battery-powered pump holds a cartridge of fast-acting insulin. A catheter attaches to a needle that is inserted into the subcutaneous tissue and is secured with transparent tape. This combined unit allows discreet bolus programming with a wireless smart meter that uses *Bluetooth*® wireless technology. The units work together to provide prescribed amounts of insulin around the clock with required changes made by remote control. This smart meter can also provide useful reminders such as the need to check insulin-delivered blood glucose levels and doctor appointments. (Courtesy of Roche Diagnostics Corp.)

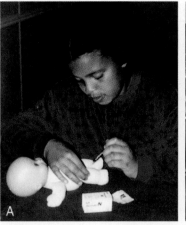
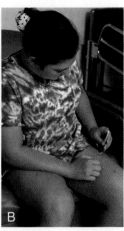

FIGURE 31-7　A, By giving injections to dolls or puppets, children can be prepared for this procedure and may be less frightened by it. **B,** A child 7 years of age or older can take the responsibility for self-injection with proper supervision. (**A** courtesy Pat Spier, RN-C; **B** from McKinney ES et al: *Maternal-child nursing*, ed 4, St. Louis, 2013, Saunders.

a tricycle; therefore the thigh should not be selected as a site for injection after such activity. If a teen returns from playing tennis, the upper arm is avoided as an injection site for the same reason.

The insulin pump. The insulin pump offers continuous subcutaneous insulin infusion without the need for frequent injections. A small, pager-sized, battery-powered, programmable pump holds a cartridge supply of insulin. A catheter attaches to a needle that is inserted into the subcutaneous tissue and is secured with transparent tape. An insulin pump can deliver a 24-hour cycle of fast-acting insulin plus manual delivery of bolus doses as needed. When connected by wireless technology to a glucose monitor, changes in insulin doses can be programmed and automatic reminders for appropriate actions offered (Figure 31-6). The insulin pump may need to be disconnected for more than 2 hours if an MRI is needed, and other sources of insulin must be provided (Carchidi, 2013).

In general, a child can be taught to perform self-injection after 7 years of age (Figure 31-7). The physician prescribes the type and amount of insulin and specifies the time of administration.

Lipoatrophy (*lipo*, "fat," and *atrophy*, "loss of") and lipohypertrophy (*lipo*, "fat," and *hypertrophy*, "increase of") refer to changes that can occur in the subcutaneous tissue at the injection site. Proper rotation of sites and the availability of the newer purified insulins have helped to eliminate this condition. The child is taught to "feel for lumps" every week and to avoid using any sites that are suspicious.

The various types of insulin and their action are listed in Table 31-6. The main differences between

insulins are the amount of time required for the insulin to take effect and the duration of the protection provided. The values listed in the table are only *guidelines*. The response of each diabetic child to any given insulin dose is highly individual and depends on many factors, such as site of injection, local destruction of insulin by tissue enzymes, and insulin antibodies.

Human insulin manufactured by biosynthesis is the treatment of choice. It is available in rapid-acting,

Table 31-6　Types of Insulin*

TYPE	ONSET	APPROXIMATE PEAK	APPROXIMATE DURATION
Short-Acting			
Regular	30-60 min	2-5 hr	5-8 hr
Rapid-Acting			
Insulin Lispro	15-30 min	30-90 min	3-5 hr
Aspart	10-20 min	40-50 min	3-5 hr
Intermediate-Acting			
Neutral protamine Hagedorn (NPH)	1-2 hr	4-12 hr	14+ hr
Isophane suspension (NPH)	1-2 hr	4-12 hr	14+ hr
Long-Acting			
Insulin glargine†	1 hr	Relatively flat	20-24 hr
Detemir†	1 hr	Relatively flat	24 hr

*There are many combined mixtures of insulin available commercially. Synthetic insulin, free of animal impurities, is used for children.
†Do not mix with other insulins.
Data from *Physician's desk reference,* ed 65, Montvale, N.J., 2012, PDR Network; Kapustin J: Uncomplicating insulin therapy, *Adv NPs PAs* 3(5):20-27, 2012; Lewis S, Dirksen S, Heitkemper M, Bucher L, Camera I: *Medical-surgical nursing,* ed 9, St Louis, 2014, Elsevier; Clayton B, Willihnganz W: *Basic pharmacology for nurses,* ed 16, St Louis, 2013, Elsevier.

1. Wash your hands.
2. Gently rotate the intermediate insulin bottle.
3. Wipe the tops of the insulin vials with an alcohol sponge.
4. Draw back an amount of air into the syringe equal to the total dose.
5. Inject air equal to the NPH dose into the NPH vial. Remove the syringe from the vial.

7. Invert the regular insulin bottle and withdraw the regular insulin dose.

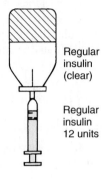

Regular insulin (clear)

Regular insulin 12 units

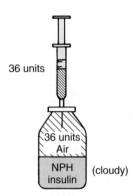

36 units

36 units Air

NPH insulin   (cloudy)

6. Inject air equal to the regular dose into the regular vial.

8. Without adding more air to the NPH vial, carefully withdraw the NPH dose.

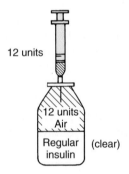

12 units

12 units Air

Regular insulin   (clear)

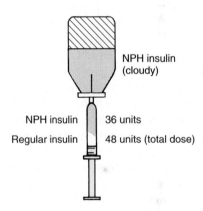

NPH insulin (cloudy)

NPH insulin   36 units

Regular insulin   48 units (total dose)

FIGURE 31-8 Mixing insulin. This step-order process avoids the problem of contaminating the regular insulin with the intermediate-acting insulin. If contamination of the regular insulin does occur, the rapid-acting effect of this drug is diminished, and it is unreliable as a quick-acting insulin in an acute situation such as diabetic ketoacidosis. (From Bowden VR, Dickey SB, Greenberg SC: *Children and their families: the continuum of care*, Philadelphia, 1998, Saunders.)

short-acting, intermediate-acting, and long-acting preparations. Extreme temperatures (below [2.2° C, or 36° F] or above [29.4° C, or 85° F]) can destroy insulin. Insulin potency can be decreased if the bottle has been opened longer than 1 month.

The physician often orders a combination of short-acting and intermediate-acting insulin; for example, "Give 10 units of NPH insulin and 5 units of regular insulin at 7:30 AM." This offers the patient immediate and longer-lasting protection. Neutral protamine Hagedorn (NPH) insulin may be administered in the same syringe as regular or crystalline insulin (Figure 31-8). Long-acting types of insulin are seldom given to children because of the danger of **hypoglycemia** during sleep. Stable, premixed insulins are available. Insulin

"pens" and injectors for insulin are available alternatives for the traditional syringe technique of administering insulin. Insulin analogs such as Glargine and Detemir more closely mimic human insulin but studies of these drugs in the pediatric population are not currently available (Zeitler, 2012).

> **⚠ Medication Safety Alert!**
>
> When mixing insulin, always withdraw the regular insulin first and then add the long-acting insulin into the syringe.

Inhaled or oral insulin. Inhaled insulin has been under study and appears effective. Continued FDA study is needed to determine long-term effects on the lung tissue before it is released for general use. Oral insulin is currently under study but is not yet available for general use in pediatrics (Kliegman, 2011). An insulin patch is under development but is not yet fully approved by the FDA.

Insulin shock. Insulin shock, also known as *hypoglycemia* (*hypo*, "below," *glyco*, "sugar," and *emia*, "blood"), occurs when the blood glucose level becomes abnormally low. Too much insulin causes this condition. Factors that may account for this imbalance include poorly planned exercise, reduced diet, and errors made because of improper knowledge of insulin and the insulin syringe.

Children are more prone to insulin reactions than adults because of the following:

- The condition itself is more unstable in young people.
- Children are growing.
- Children's activities are more irregular.

Poorly planned exercise is often the cause of insulin shock during childhood. Hospitalized patients who are being regulated must be observed frequently during naptime and at night. The nurse becomes suspicious of problems if there is difficulty in arousing the patient or if the child is perspiring heavily.

The symptoms of an insulin reaction, which range from mild to severe, are generally noticed and treated in the early stages. They appear suddenly in the otherwise well person. Examination of the blood would show a lowered blood glucose level. The child becomes irritable, may behave poorly, is pale, and may complain of feeling hungry and weak. Sweating occurs. Symptoms related to disorders of the nervous system arise because glucose is vital to the proper functioning of nerves. The child may become mentally confused and giddy, and muscular coordination is affected. If insulin shock is left untreated, coma and convulsions can occur.

The immediate treatment consists of administering sugar in some form, such as ½ cup of orange juice, hard candy, a small box of raisins, or a commercial (glucose tablet) product. The patient begins to feel better within a few minutes and at that time may eat a small amount of protein or starch (sandwich, milk, cheese) to prevent another reaction. **Glucagon** is recommended for the treatment of severe hypoglycemia. It quickly restores the child to consciousness in an emergency; the child can then consume some form of sugar or a planned meal.

The **Somogyi phenomenon** (rebound hyperglycemia) occurs when blood glucose levels are lowered to a point at which the body's counterregulatory hormones (epinephrine, cortisol, glucagon) are released. Glucose is released from muscle and liver cells, which precipitates a rapid rise in blood glucose levels. It is generally the result of chronic insulin use, especially in patients who require fairly large doses of insulin to regulate their blood glucose levels. Hypoglycemia during the night and high glucose levels in the morning are suggestive of the phenomenon. The child may awaken at night or have frequent nightmares and experience early morning sweating and headaches. The child actually needs less insulin, not more, to rectify the problem.

The *Somogyi* phenomenon differs from the **dawn phenomenon**, in which early morning elevations of blood glucose occur *in the absence of* preceding hypoglycemia and may be a response to growth hormone secretion that occurs in the early morning hours. Together the *Somogyi* and *dawn* phenomena are the most common causes of instability in diabetic children. Testing blood glucose levels around 3 AM helps to differentiate the two conditions and aids in regulating insulin dosage. Whenever the insulin regime is changed, close monitoring of blood glucose levels is essential to detect the *dawn* and *Somogyi* effects that are common with children.

Home Management of Children with Diabetes Mellitus

Exercise. Exercise is important for the patient with diabetes because it causes the body to use sugar and promotes good circulation. It lowers the blood glucose level, and in this respect it acts like more insulin. The diabetic patient who has planned vigorous exercise should carry extra sugar to avoid insulin reactions. The patient should also carry money for candy or a drink and, if possible, should also carry a cell phone. The blood glucose level is high immediately after meals, and the child can participate in active sports at such times. Games enjoyed directly before meals should be less active. The diabetic child is able to participate in almost all active sports. Poorly planned exercise, however, can lead to difficulties.

Skin care. The patient is instructed to bathe daily and dry well, especially between the toes. Cleansing of the inguinal area, axillae, perineum, and inframammary areas is especially important because yeast and fungal infections tend to occur at these sites. The skin is inspected for cuts, rashes, abrasions, bruises, cysts, or boils. These lesions are managed promptly. If skin is very dry, an oil such as Alpha Keri may be used in the bath water. Adolescents are taught to use electric razors. Exposing the skin to extremes in temperatures is avoided. Injection sites are inspected for lumps.

Foot care. Although circulatory problems of the feet are less common in children, proper habits of foot hygiene must be established. Patients are instructed to wash and dry their feet well each day. The feet are inspected for interdigital cracking, and the condition of the toenails is checked. Nails are trimmed straight across. Socks are changed daily, and tight socks or large ones that bunch up are avoided. Shoes are replaced often as the child grows. The child should not go barefoot.

Infections. Immunizations against communicable diseases are essential (see Chapter 32). Meticulous skin care and care of needles and insulin equipment can prevent infections.

Emotional upsets. Emotional upsets can be as disturbing to the patient as an infection and may necessitate food adjustments, insulin adjustments, or both. Table 31-7 lists nursing interventions for stress on the child and family related to type 1 diabetes.

Urine checks. Routine urine checks for sugar are being replaced by the more accurate glucose blood monitoring. However, this procedure does not test for acetone level, which the patient may need to determine, particularly during illness and when the blood glucose level is high. When urine checks are advocated for patients, saying urine "check" rather than "test" is less confusing to young children.

Glucose-insulin imbalances. The patient is taught to recognize the signs of insulin shock and ketoacidosis (see Table 31-4). Early attention to changes and daily record keeping are stressed. Many excellent teaching films and brochures are available. The child should wear a bracelet identifying him or her as having diabetes. Wallet cards are also available. Teachers, athletic coaches, and guidance personnel are informed about the disease and should have the telephone numbers of the patient's parents and health care provider.

Travel. With planning, children can enjoy travel with their families, and older adolescents can travel alone. Before leaving on a trip, the child should be seen by

Table 31-7	Nursing Interventions for Predictable Types of Stress on a Child with Type 1 Diabetes and on the Family	
AGE	**ISSUE**	**NURSING INTERVENTION**
Infant	Trust versus mistrust Onset and diagnosis particularly difficult during infancy; anxiety can be transmitted to infant	Stress consistency in fulfilling needs. Involve both parents in education. Avoid information overload. Instill hope and confidence. Focus on child rather than disease. Review normal growth and development of infancy. Assist in problem solving (e.g., babysitters, difficulty in obtaining specimens, baby food exchange lists).
Toddler	Autonomy versus shame and doubt Is this a temper tantrum or high or low blood glucose?	Prepare child for procedures or separations. Encourage exploration of environment. Stress limit setting as a form of love. Admit it is difficult to distinguish temper tantrums from symptoms. If behavior worsens or is prolonged or if physical symptoms appear, check blood glucose level. Provide 24-hr telephone number for advice from nurse.
Preschool	Initiative versus guilt May view injections as punishment May view denial of sweets as lack of love "Picky eater"	Foster sense of competence. Educate parents to provide consistent warmth, reassurance, and love. Discuss feelings about child's life and diabetes. Avoid use of words with a negative connotation, such as "bad blood test" or "cheating." Help parents sort out child's fantasies. Plan favorite party dishes on occasion. Invite a playmate for lunch. Suggest alternative nutritious snacks.
Elementary school	Industry versus inferiority Patients may feel they will be cured by hospitalization Grief over lack of cure Rebellion about treatment regimen Rebellion regarding food plan Anxiety about disclosure of condition to friends Embarrassed about reactions in school, missed days Unpredictable effects of exercise	Assist child in how to respond to teasing from peers ("Yecch, needles"). Explain "honeymoon" stage of disease. Accept child's disappointment. Gradually promote self-management of insulin and specimen tests; this increases feelings of mastery and control. Provide lists of fast-food exchanges. Provide group-related education with diabetic peers. Promote open dialogue among health personnel and teachers, school nurse, and fellow students. Continually reinforce treatment principles with specific regard to hypoglycemia or hyperglycemia and emergencies.
Puberty	"Bouncing" blood glucose levels may make adolescent feel out of control Anger at the disease: "Why must I be different?" More frequent hospitalizations	Explain that growth and sex hormones affect blood glucose levels. Girls, in particular, experience difficulties during the time of menstruation. Adjustments in insulin and food are common for most diabetic patients at this stage. Assist patient in acceptable ways of expressing anger; discuss anger with parents, because parents are often its target. Provide encouragement and support; be alert to marital stress and sibling deprivation.

the physician for a checkup and prescriptions for supplies. A written statement and a card identifying the child as having diabetes should be carried. Time changes may affect meals. Additional supplies of insulin, sugar, glucagon, and food are kept with the child. These are never checked with luggage, especially on an airplane, because they may be lost. If foreign travel is planned, parents must become familiar with the food in the visited area so that dietary requirements can be met. Local chapters of the American Diabetes Association or the Juvenile Diabetes Foundation can help vacationing families in an emergency.

Follow-up care. The child must see the physician regularly. The child should also be taught to visit the dentist regularly for cleaning of teeth and gums. Brushing and flossing daily are essential. Eyes should be examined regularly; blurry vision must not be ignored. There are many brochures, books, and journals that offer excellent suggestions and guidance at an age-appropriate level.

Illness or surgery. When illness occurs, close glucose monitoring and control is essential. Hyperglycemia causes diuresis and dehydration, and ketosis can involve vomiting. Counteracting regulatory hormones that are secreted during periods of stress interfere with the effectiveness of insulin, resulting in increased glucose levels. Modification of insulin doses may be necessary. The patient with diabetes usually tolerates surgery well. Insulin may be given before, during, or after the operation. If the patient is restricted to nothing by mouth, calories may be supplied by intravenous glucose. Details vary according to the procedure and the patient's treatment for diabetes. Careful review of the patient's history helps in formulating nursing care plans and provides a basis for teaching.

Prospects for the Future. Diabetic research is being conducted on many fronts. Geneticists have determined how diabetes is inherited, and soon they will be able to alter genes or prevent the condition for those at risk. Pancreas transplantation has been performed, and in vitro and in vivo regeneration therapy is under study. The laser beam has aided the treatment for complicated eye conditions. Such advances hold promise for resolving or eradicating the dilemma of diabetes.

Type 2 Diabetes Mellitus. Type 2 diabetes is thought to be caused by insulin resistance and decreased insulin secretion. It is precipitated by obesity, low physical activity, and a lipid-rich diet resulting in insulin resistance. Type 2 diabetes mellitus is becoming more prevalent in children and young adults. Risk factors include the following:
- Family history of type 2 diabetes mellitus
- Signs of insulin resistance
- *Acanthosis nigricans* (a dark pigmentation of the flexure creases of the skin and back of neck)
- Hypertension

Nutrition Considerations
Diet Therapy in Pediatric Metabolic Disorders

DISORDER	MAJOR SIGNS AND SYMPTOMS	DIETARY REGIMEN
Phenylketonuria (PKU)	Mental retardation	Low phenylalanine diet, Lofenalac formula for infants
Celiac disease	Chronic diarrhea, irritability, distention, failure to thrive	Eliminate gluten; use corn flour and vitamin B supplements
Cystic fibrosis	Thick mucus causes obstruction of pancreatic enzymes and poor absorption of nutrients, flatulence, and foul-smelling stools	Pancreatic enzyme replacement with normal meals
Lactose intolerance	Abdominal distention, cramps, diarrhea, failure to thrive	Lactose-free diet; use ProSobee, soy formulas; avoid milk and milk products
Galactose intolerance	Jaundice, vomiting, convulsions, lethargy, blindness	No galactose or lactose in diet; use milk substitutes
Fructose intolerance	Vomiting, diarrhea, failure to thrive	Fructose-free diet; avoid honey, fruit, sorbitol, and sucrose; offer vitamin C and vegetables
Maple syrup urine disease	Acidosis, convulsions	Low-leucine and low-valine diet
Urea cycle defect	Lethargy	Low-protein diet
Acidemia	Seizures, elevated ammonia levels	May need to restrict meat proteins
Diabetes insipidus	Inability to concentrate urine, diuresis	Unrestricted water intake
Diabetes mellitus	Inability to produce insulin to metabolize sugar, protein, and fat	Controlled sugar intake regulated with insulin administration; high-fiber, balanced diet

- Increased lipids (hyperlipidemia)
- Repeated vaginal monilial (Candida) infections resulting from chronic glycosuria
- Obesity (body mass index [BMI] 35 to 39 kg/m^2 or weight and height or greater than the 120th percentile for the ideal weight for height)

The oral glucose tolerance test has little value in diagnosing type 2 diabetes. In 2010, the American Diabetes Association added a hemoglobin A_{1c} of 6.5% or higher in obese adolescents as a diagnostic criterion. However, conditions such as iron-deficiency anemia, sickle cell disease, or thalassemia can alter the HgbA$_{1c}$. A fasting serum insulin is also not diagnostic of type 2 diabetes or prediabetes (Zeitler, 2012). Asymptomatic adolescents are often not diagnosed until diabetic ketoacidosis occurs.

Treatment guidelines for type 2 diabetes mellitus include lifestyle changes to reduce obesity and antidiabetic medication such as Metformin, which is the only oral antidiabetic agent approved for children and adolescents (Zeitler, 2012). Newer antidiabetic drugs have been developed for adult use but the risks and benefits must be closely evaluated before use in the pediatric setting (Sisson, 2012). A combination therapy of Metformin and insulin may be required for adequate glucose control.

When metformin is prescribed, the creatinine level and kidney function should be monitored and metformin should be temporarily discontinued during radiologic tests that include IV iodized contrast dyes.

Blood glucose monitoring and family education and support are essential to follow-up care.

Nutrition counseling should be focused around patient and family food preferences and should include fruits and vegetables, a decrease in fats, and a reduction in sugary drinks. The diet should include about 1200 calories a day for adolescents. Moderate to vigorous physical activity for 1 hour per day and fewer than 2 hours of nonacademic screen time per day are recommended (Copeland, 2013).

Get Ready for the NCLEX® Examination!

Key Points

- The two major systems that control and monitor the functions of the body are the nervous system and the endocrine system.
- The term *inborn error of metabolism* refers to a group of inherited biochemical disorders that affect body metabolism.
- Screening programs for early detection of inborn errors are important because some conditions can cause irreversible neurological damage.
- Diabetes mellitus type 1 is the most common endocrine disorder of children. The body is unable to use carbohydrates properly because of a deficiency of insulin, which is an internal secretion of the pancreas.
- The symptoms of diabetes mellitus appear more rapidly in children. Three symptoms are polydipsia, polyuria, and polyphagia.
- Insulin resistance causes type 2 diabetes mellitus. It is precipitated by obesity, a lipid-rich diet, and inactivity, and it is becoming more prevalent in children.
- The mainstays of the management of diabetes mellitus are insulin replacement, diet, and exercise.
- Diabetic ketoacidosis is a serious complication that may become life threatening.
- The Somogyi phenomenon and the dawn phenomenon are common causes of glucose instability in children.
- Self-management to maintain glucose control and to prevent complications is a major goal of education of the child with diabetes mellitus.
- A continuous glucose monitoring system can be programmed to meet individual needs.
- An insulin pump provides subcutaneous doses of insulin controlled by a computerized monitor.
- The glycosylated hemoglobin test (HgbA$_{1c}$) reflects glucose control through time.
- Sugar substitutes such as sorbitol and xylitol should not be provided to children.
- A child with diabetes insipidus requires unlimited access to water.
- Growth hormone is administered at bedtime to simulate the natural time of hormone release.
- A deficiency in the secretions of the thyroid gland is termed *hypothyroidism*. It may be congenital or acquired and necessitates lifelong treatment by the oral administration of a synthetic thyroid hormone.

Additional Learning Resources

SG Go to your Study Guide for additional learning activities to help you master this chapter content.

evolve Go to your Evolve website (http://evolve.elsevier.com/Leifer) for the following learning resources:
- Animations
- Answer Guidelines for Critical Thinking Questions
- Answers and Rationales for Review Questions for the NCLEX® Examination
- Glossary with English and Spanish pronunciations
- Interactive Review Questions for the NCLEX® Examination
- Patient Teaching Plans in English and Spanish
- Skills Performance Checklists

 Online Resources
- *Acanthosis nigricans:* www.cdc.gov/diabetes/news/docs/an.htm
- American Diabetes Association: www.diabetes.org
- Diabetes Public Health Resource: www.cdc.gov/diabetes/index.htm
- International Society of Pediatric and Adolescent Diabetes: www.ispad.org/index_html

Review Questions for the NCLEX® Examination

1. What is an important aspect of a teaching plan for the parent of a child with hypopituitarism?
   1. The child should be enrolled in a special education program at school.
   2. The routine administration of growth hormone should be performed at bedtime.
   3. All family members should have an endocrine workup.
   4. The routine medication should be administered before the school day starts.

2. A child who has diabetes mellitus asks why he cannot take insulin orally instead of by subcutaneous injection. The best response of the nurse would be that:

 1. pills are only for adults.
 2. digestive enzymes destroy insulin.
 3. insulin can cause a stomach ulcer.
 4. insulin interacts with food in the stomach.

3. What may indicate a need for insulin in a diabetic child?

 1. Diaphoresis and tremors
 2. Red lips and fruity odor to the breath
 3. Confusion and lethargy
 4. Headache and pallor

4. The nurse teaches the diabetic child to rotate sites of insulin injection so as to:

 1. prevent subcutaneous deposit of the drug.
 2. prevent lipoatrophy of subcutaneous fat.
 3. decrease the pain of injection.
 4. increase absorption of insulin.

5. Kussmaul's respirations are seen in diabetic children with:

 1. neuropathy.
 2. ketoacidosis.
 3. hypoglycemia.
 4. retinopathy.

Objectives

1. Define each key term listed.
2. Discuss the characteristics of common childhood communicable diseases.
3. Interpret the detection and prevention of common childhood communicable diseases.
4. Discuss three principles involved in standard and transmission-based precautions used to prevent the transmission of communicable diseases in children.
5. Discuss national and international immunization programs.
6. Describe the nurse's role in the immunization of children.
7. Understand the vulnerability of pregnant women, young infants, and children to exposure to bioterrorism agents.
8. Understand the role of the nurse in the hospital and in the community in preventing and responding to disaster events.
9. Demonstrate a teaching plan for preventing sexually transmitted infections (STIs) in an adolescent.
10. Formulate a nursing care plan for a child with acquired immunodeficiency syndrome (AIDS).

Key Terms

acquired immunity (p. 726)
active immunity (p. 726)
body substance (p. 725)
communicable disease (kŏ-MYŪ-nĭ-kă-būl dĭ-ZĒZ, p. 725)
endemic (ĕn-DĔM-ĭk, p. 725)
epidemic (ĕp-ĭ-DĔM-ĭk, p. 725)
erythema (ĕr-ĭ-THĒ-mă, p. 727)
fomite (FŌ-mīt, p. 725)
health care–associated infection (p. 726)
incubation period (p. 725)
macule (MĂK-yūl, p. 727)
natural immunity (p. 726)
opportunistic infections (ŏp-pŏr-tū-NĬS-tĭk ĭn-FĔK-shŭnz, p. 725)
pandemic (păn-DĔM-ĭk, p. 725)

papule (PĂP-yūl, p. 727)
passive immunity (p. 726)
pathogens (PĂTH-ō-jĕnz, p. 725)
pathognomonic (păth-ŏg-nō-MŎN-ĭk, p. 727)
portal of entry (p. 725)
portal of exit (p. 725)
prodromal period (prō-DRŌ-mŭl PĒ-rē-ŏd, p. 725)
pustule (PŬS-tyūl, p. 727)
reservoir for infection (p. 725)
scab (p. 727)
standard precautions (p. 726)
transmission-based precautions (p. 726)
vector (VĔK-tŭr, p. 725)
vesicle (VĔS-ĭ-kŭl, p. 727)

There have been only a few brief periods in history when infectious disease did not dominate the attention of health care professionals. Despite immunization, sanitation, antimicrobial drugs, and other controls, the world continues to face infectious agents such as human immunodeficiency virus (HIV), hepatitis, tuberculosis, and sexually transmitted infections (STIs). Despite our knowledge of immunizations, some children still suffer from common communicable diseases. Antimicrobial drug-resistant organisms are increasing in number and virulence, and immunocompromised patients are threatened by nonpathogenic organisms. Prevention and control are key factors in managing infectious disease.

COMMON CHILDHOOD COMMUNICABLE DISEASES

The incidence of common childhood communicable diseases has dramatically decreased as immunological agents have been developed. Diseases such as smallpox have declined to a point worldwide that routine immunizations are no longer recommended. (A brief review of smallpox is presented in this chapter because the nurse must be able to identify a smallpox lesion, and promptly isolate the patient and arrange for *immediate* follow-up care to prevent an outbreak of this deadly illness.) Providing all children with the appropriate immunizations is the health care challenge of today. Air travel is commonplace, and rapid transmission of

Communicable Diseases of Childhood

DISEASE	CAUSATIVE ORGANISM	SIGNS AND SYMPTOMS	INCUBATION PERIOD	PREVENTION AND/OR TREATMENT	HOW LONG CONTAGIOUS	NURSING INTERVENTIONS
Chickenpox (varicella) (Figure 32-1)	Varicella-zoster virus	Prodromal signs include mild fever followed by macules, papules, vesicles, pustules, and scabs. All stages of lesion are present on the body at the same time.	2-3 weeks (13-17 days average)	Vaccine available—2 doses are given at the same time as MMR (12-18 months, and preschool age); acyclovir (Zovirax) or immune globulin (VZIG) is given to immunosuppressed children who are exposed.	6 days after appearance of rash	Trim fingernails to prevent scratching. (Removal of scabs may cause scars.) Calamine lotion may reduce itching. Airborne isolation precautions. Monitor Acyclovir side-effects.
Smallpox (variola)	Virus	Child's condition appears toxic. Macules, papules, vesicles, pustules, and scabs appear. Only one stage of the lesion at a time is present on the body.	6-18 days (12 days average)	Routine smallpox vaccination is no longer recommended unless a bioterrorism event involving smallpox occurs. Vaccination may be effective if administered within 2 days of exposure.	Highly contagious; notification to local public health department is required	This is a toxic illness with a high mortality rate. Strict isolation is required, preferably in a negative pressure room and with restricted number of caregivers.
German measles (rubella) (Figure 32-2)	Rubella virus	Mild fever and cold symptoms precede a rose-colored, maculopapular rash. Glands at ears and back of neck are enlarged.	2-3 weeks (18 days average)	All infants should receive vaccine at 12-18 months of age, with boosters at preschool age.	Until rash fades (5 days) Contact precautions for congenital rubella for 1 year or 3 months of negative cultures (AAP, 2012)	Provide symptomatic treatment and comfort measures. Avoid exposing any woman who might be in the early months of pregnancy, because rubella can cause fetal anomalies. Droplet precautions.
Measles (rubeola) (Figure 32-3)	Virus	Fever, cough, and conjunctivitis are followed by small white (Koplik) spots on inner cheeks (enanthem); maculopapular rash (exanthem) then erupts.	1-2 weeks (10 days average)	All infants should receive vaccine at 15 months and boosters at preschool age. Gamma globulin may be given after exposure. Vitamin A is recommended to reduce morbidity in severe cases in some children with certain health problems, such as a low retinol level.	From 4 days before to 5 days after rash appears	Provide symptomatic care. Airborne isolation precautions and provide quiet activities. Use measures to reduce eyestrain caused by photophobia. Give detailed oral care. Avoid use of soap.
Fifth disease (erythema infectiosum)	Human parvovirus B19	Child has "slapped cheek" appearance. Generalized rash appears, subsides, and reappears if skin is irritated by sun or heat.	4-14 days	None.	During incubation period	This is a benign condition unless child is immunocompromised. Isolation is not required other than standard precautions. Condition may last 1-3 weeks. Use oatmeal baths for itching.
Roseola (sixth disease) (exanthem subitum)	Herpesvirus 6 (HSV-6) or 7 (HHV-6 or 7)	Persistent high fever (39.4° to 40.5° C [103° to 105° F]) is present, then drops rapidly as the rash appears. The maculopapular rash is nonpruritic and blanches easily.	2 weeks	None; high fever may precipitate convulsions.	Until rash fades	Rest and quiet should be provided. Teach parents temperature-reducing techniques and prevention of seizures. Use standard precautions. Rarely hospitalized.

🏃 Health Promotion

Communicable Diseases of Childhood—cont'd

DISEASE	CAUSATIVE ORGANISM	SIGNS AND SYMPTOMS	INCUBATION PERIOD	PREVENTION AND/OR TREATMENT	HOW LONG CONTAGIOUS	NURSING INTERVENTIONS
Mumps (parotitis)	Paramyxovirus	Fever, headache, glands near ear and toward jawline ache and develop painful swelling. Parotid gland is enlarged. Condition may be bilateral.	14-21 days (18 days average)	Vaccine (MMR) is given after 15 months of age.	Until swelling subsides Keep out of school.	Encourage fluids, apply ice compresses to neck for comfort. Use droplet precautions if hospitalized. Avoid citrus and spices that stimulate salivary flow.
Whooping cough (pertussis)	*Bordetella pertussis*	Fever, cold, and cough are present. Spells of coughing are accompanied by a noisy gasp for air that creates a "whoop."	5-21 days (10 days average)	Vaccinate all infants with series (DTaP). May administer erythromycin to exposed, unvaccinated child. Cool mist tent and antibiotics are used for treatment.	Several weeks	Droplet precautions until 5 days after antibiotics. Encourage bed rest, provide abdominal support during coughing spell. Re-feed child if he or she vomits. Observe for airway obstruction and O₂ saturations.
Polio (infantile paralysis; poliomyelitis)	Enterovirus	Fever, headache, stiff neck and stiff back, paralysis.	1-2 weeks	Start complete series of polio vaccines in infancy. May necessitate respirator care.	1 week for throat secretions; 4 weeks for feces	Standard precautions. Encourage bed rest, observe for respiratory distress. Provide positioning, physiotherapy, and range-of-motion exercises.
Infectious mononucleosis (glandular fever)	Epstein-Barr virus (EBV) Type 4	Low-grade fever, malaise, jaundice, enlarged spleen.	2-6 weeks	Limit contact with saliva. Do not share eating utensils.	Spread by direct contact only Return to school when fever and swallowing are normal.	Provide rest and supportive treatment. Standard precautions. Provide school tutoring to maintain grade level. Contact sports avoided until spleen and liver lab tests normal.
Hepatitis A	Enterovirus 72	Fever, anorexia, headache, abdominal pain, malaise, jaundice, dark urine, and chalklike stools.	15-45 days	Hepatitis A vaccine is recommended for children traveling to endemic areas. Gamma globulin is provided if child is exposed.	Virus may be shed for up to 6 months in neonates.	Educate family and community concerning the ingestion of contaminated water or shellfish from contaminated water or swimming in contaminated water. Proper hand hygiene is essential. Standard and contact precautions are essential.
Hepatitis B	HBV virus	Symptoms are the same as type A. Can manifest liver pathology.	30-180 days	Hepatitis B vaccine (HepB) series is provided during newborn period or for health care workers or travelers. Interferon or reverse transcriptase inhibitors may be an effective treatment. Liver transplant may be necessary. Immune globulin may be indicated for exposed, susceptible children.	May persist in carrier state	Prevent contact with blood or blood products. Identify high-risk mothers and newborns. Educate concerning need for vaccination.

Continued

🏃 Health Promotion

Communicable Diseases of Childhood—cont'd

DISEASE	CAUSATIVE ORGANISM	SIGNS AND SYMPTOMS	INCUBATION PERIOD	PREVENTION AND/OR TREATMENT	HOW LONG CONTAGIOUS	NURSING INTERVENTIONS
Lyme disease	*Borrelia burgdorferi*	Skin lesions at site of tick bite. Macule with raised border and clear center (target or bulls-eye appearance that is 2 inches or 5 cm in diameter). May "burn." Fever, arthralgia. May lead to heart and neurological involvement.	3-32 days	Wear protective clothing in wooded area. Inspect for ticks after play when camping. Light-colored clothing makes tick more noticeable. Remove tick with tweezers. Inspect pets. Treat with amoxicillin or doxycycline.	Spread by infected tick	Educate concerning the prevention of exposure. Use standard precautions. Avoid sun if patient is treated with doxycycline. Insect repellant containing 20% DEET and Permethrin on skin and clothes and camping gear is advised (Marchese, 2013).
Tuberculosis	*Mycobacterium tuberculosis*	Low-grade fever, malaise, anorexia, weight loss, cough, night sweats. Children are often asymptomatic. Adenopathy, pneumonia, and positive tuberculin skin test.	2-10 weeks (airborne droplet infection)	Early detection is through routine PPD skin test. Examine contacts. Exposed children may receive isoniazid (INH), rifampin, and pyrazinamide (PZA), administered for several months.	After treatment when cough subsides	Isolate newborn from infected mother. Identify contacts. Isolate, using special mask (see Appendix A).
Diphtheria	*Corynebacterium diphtheriae*	Common cold with purulent nasal discharge. Malaise, sore throat. White or gray membrane forms in throat, causing respiratory distress.	2-5 days	DTaP vaccine is given to all infants. Intravenous antibiotics, antitoxin, tracheotomy required. Provide oxygen and suction as needed.	Until 4 days after antibiotic therapy	Observe for respiratory, cardiac, and central nervous system involvement. Have emergency airway equipment available. Droplet precautions. Identify contacts for treatment.
Scarlet fever	Group A beta-hemolytic *Streptococcus*	Tachycardia, strawberry tongue, pinpoint rash, circumoral pallor, desquamation	2-5 days	Penicillin therapy is provided for 10 days. Culture for and treat streptococcal infections.	During incubation and clinical illness; may become a carrier	Provide bed rest and quiet activity. Teach regarding prevention of streptococcal infections and culture of sore throats.

DTaP, Diphtheria-tetanus–acellular pertussis vaccine; *MMR,* measles-mumps-rubella vaccine; *PPD,* purified protein derivative; *VZIG,* varicella-zoster immune globulin.
NOTE: DTaP is administered to infants and children up to age 10; Tdap (tetanus-diphtheria–acellular pertussis vaccine) is provided to children age 11 and older.

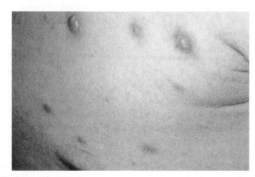

FIGURE 32-1 Chickenpox. (From Feigin RD, Cherry JD: *Textbook of pediatric infectious diseases,* ed 2, Philadelphia, 1987, Saunders.)

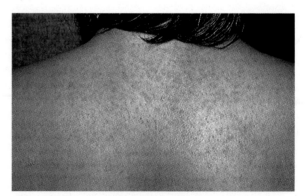

FIGURE 32-2 German measles. (From Hurwitz S: *Clinical pediatric dermatology: a textbook of skin disorders of childhood and adolescence,* ed 2, Philadelphia, 1993, Saunders.)

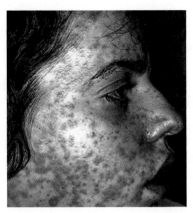

FIGURE 32-3 Measles. (From Hurwitz S: *Clinical pediatric dermatology: a textbook of skin disorders of childhood and adolescence,* ed 2, Philadelphia, 1993, Saunders.)

contagious diseases from around the world makes alert assessment by the nurse and all health care workers essential.

REVIEW OF TERMS

A **communicable disease** is one that can be transmitted, directly or indirectly, from one person to another. Organisms that cause disease are called **pathogens**.

The **incubation period** is the time between the invasion by the pathogen and the onset of clinical symptoms. The **prodromal period** refers to the initial stage of a disease: the interval between the earliest symptoms and the appearance of a typical rash or fever. Children are often contagious during this time, but because the symptoms are not specific they may attend preschool or another group program and spread the disease. A **fomite** is any inanimate material that absorbs and transmits infection. A **vector** is an insect or animal that carries and spreads a disease. A **pandemic** is a worldwide high incidence of a communicable disease. An **epidemic** is a sudden increase of a communicable disease in a localized area. **Endemic** refers to a continuous incidence of a communicable disease expected in a localized area.

Body substance refers to moist secretions or parts of the body that can contain microorganisms. Emesis, saliva, sputum, semen, urine, feces, and blood are examples of body substances. Body substance precautions indicate the need to wear disposable protective gloves and/or garments when coming in contact with these body substances. A **portal of entry** is a route by which the organisms enter the body (e.g., a cut in the skin). A **portal of exit** is the route by which the organisms exit the body (e.g., feces or urine). A **reservoir for infection** is a place that supports the growth of organisms (e.g., standing, stagnant water). The *chain of infection* refers to the way in which organisms spread and infect the individual (Figure 32-4). Standard precautions are found in Appendix A. Careful hand hygiene is basic and essential to prevent the spread of infection.

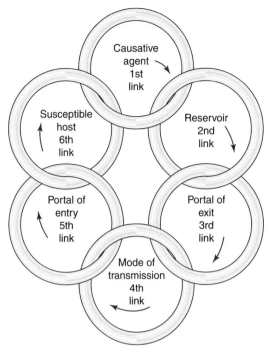

FIGURE 32-4 The chain of infection. The process by which pathogens are transmitted from the environment to a host, invade the host, and cause infection. (From Leahy J, Kizilay P: *Foundations of nursing practice: a nursing process approach,* Philadelphia, 1998, Saunders.)

HOST RESISTANCE

Many factors contribute to the virulence of an infectious disease. The age, sex, and genetic makeup of the child have a bearing on the degree of resistance. The nutritional status of the person, as well as physical and emotional health, is also important. The efficiency of the blood-forming organs and of the immune systems affects resistance. Important factors in host resistance to disease include the following:

- *Intact skin and mucous membranes:* A break in the skin can be a portal of entry for an organism that can cause illness.
- *Phagocytes* in the blood attack and destroy organisms.
- The functioning *immune system* in the body responds to fight infection. Some factors in this immune response include interferon, T cells, B cells, and antibodies. Vaccinations assist the body to manufacture antibodies that can help the child to resist infections.

The child who has an underlying condition such as diabetes, cystic fibrosis, burns, or sickle cell disease may be more susceptible to certain organisms. Children with HIV or acquired immunodeficiency syndrome (AIDS) or cancer and children receiving steroid or immunosuppressive drugs often have depressed immune systems. This makes them very susceptible to **opportunistic infections** (an *opportunistic infection* is caused by organisms **normally** found in the environment that the immune-suppressed individual cannot resist or fight). An infection acquired in a health care facility during hospitalization is termed a **health care–associated infection**.

TYPES OF IMMUNITY

Immunity is the *natural* or *acquired* resistance to infection. In **natural immunity**, resistance is inborn. Some races apparently have a greater natural immunity to certain diseases than other races. Immunity also varies from person to person. If two persons are exposed to the same disease, one may become very ill and the other may show no evidence of the disease.

Acquired immunity is not the result of inherited factors but is gained as a result of having the disease or is artificially acquired by receiving vaccines or immune serums. Vaccines contain live attenuated (weakened) or dead organisms that are not strong enough to cause the disease but stimulate the body to develop an immune reaction and antibodies. When the person produces his or her own immunity, it is called **active immunity**.

If a person is exposed and needs immediate protection from a specific infectious disease, antibodies can be obtained in immune serums; most are from animals, but some are from humans. For example, tetanus serum (used to prevent lockjaw) is procured from the horse, but gamma globulin, which is rich in antibodies, is obtained from human blood. This type of immunity, known as **passive immunity**, acts immediately but does not last as long as immunity actively produced by the body. Passive immunity provides the antibody. It does not stimulate the system to produce its own antibodies.

A *carrier* is a person who is capable of spreading a disease but does not show evidence of it. Typhoid fever is an example of a disease spread by a carrier.

TRANSMISSION OF INFECTION

Infection can be transmitted from one person to another by *direct* or *indirect* means. *Direct transmission* involves contact with the person who is infected (the body fluids of that person, such as nasal discharge or an open lesion). *Indirect transmission* involves contact with objects that have been contaminated by the infected person. These objects are called *fomites*. Bedrails, intravenous (IV) pumps, overbed tables, door handles, used tissues, countertops, and toys are examples of fomites. For example, the respiratory syncytial virus (RSV) lives on dry soap for several hours. Therefore picking up soap used by a person infected with RSV transmits the organism. This is one of the reasons why the use of liquid soap is advocated. The chain of infection transmission is shown in Figure 32-4. Preventing the spread of infection depends on breaking the chain.

Various tests are available to determine whether an individual has been exposed to a particular disease, such as the *Mantoux* intradermal purified protein derivative (PPD) skin test or a blood serum test called the QuantiFERON-TB Gold test, for tuberculosis. The *Schick test* for diphtheria and the *Dick test* for scarlet fever have been replaced by serum DNA-PCR (DNA polymerase chain reaction) testing.

MEDICAL ASEPSIS, STANDARD PRECAUTIONS, AND TRANSMISSION-BASED PRECAUTIONS

The purpose of medical aseptic techniques used with *all* patients is to prevent the spread of infection from one person to another. A person or object is considered *contaminated* if he, she, or it has touched the infected patient or any equipment or fomite that has come in contact with the patient or his or her bodily fluids.

Articles that have come in direct contact with the patient must be disinfected before others can use them. When something is disinfected, the microorganisms in or on it are killed by physical or chemical means. The autoclave, which uses steam under pressure, is considered effective in killing most microbes when the article is adequately exposed and sterilized for the proper length of time.

All children suspected of having a communicable disease who are admitted to the hospital are placed on both standard and transmission-based precautions until a definite diagnosis is established. A private room or negative-pressure room (prevents air from flowing out of the room when the door is opened) may be assigned. (See Appendix A for specific transmission-based precautions and the practices required.)

Disposable items are used when a child is placed on transmission-based precautions; these include tissues, suction catheters, thermometers, suture sets, nursing bottles, and blood pressure cuffs. They are disposed of according to hospital protocol.

The nurse must understand the importance of protecting himself or herself and others from a contagious patient. This is accomplished by specific precautions, called **standard precautions**. The Centers for Disease Control and Prevention (CDC) recommend that *standard* precautions be used for *all* patients; these involve, at minimum, hand hygiene and the use of disposable gloves. In addition to these precautions, **transmission-based precautions** are designed according to the method of spread of infection, such as airborne infection isolation (AII), contact, and *droplet* (see Appendix A).

Airborne infection isolation precautions are used for patients with conditions such as tuberculosis, varicella (chickenpox), and rubeola (measles). Small airborne particles floating in the air can be inhaled any place in the room. The use of negative-pressure rooms and respirator masks (e.g., N95 particulate masks) are required when entering the room. The respirator masks are removed when exiting the room.

Contact precautions are used when the condition causes organisms to be transmitted via skin-to-skin contact or through indirect touch of a contaminated fomite. Gloves and a cover gown are worn for close contact with patients with RSV, patients with hepatitis A who are incontinent, patients with contagious skin diseases such as impetigo, and patients with wound infections. It is important to note that some diseases may have more than one mode of spread and therefore necessitate more than one precaution technique.

Droplet precautions are used with diseases such as pertussis and influenza. When the patient coughs or sneezes, the droplets can contaminate an area 3 feet around the patient. Beyond the 3-foot radius, a mask and gown are not usually necessary.

Standard precautions are discussed in Appendix A along with the protocols for the use of masks, gowns, gloves, and other protective equipment. Personal protective equipment (PPE) should be worn when *anticipating* the risk of exposure to blood, body fluids, or other potentially infectious materials.

 Safety Alert!

Disposable gloves should be worn whenever touching something that is moist and not yours.

PROTECTIVE ENVIRONMENT ISOLATION

Protective environment isolation precautions (previously called reverse isolation) are used for patients who are *not* communicable but have a lowered resistance, perhaps because of neutropenia, and are highly susceptible to infection. This simple procedure reduces the incidence of health care–associated infections. The patient is placed in a private room with the door closed. It is recommended that all persons wear a gown, a mask, and gloves when attending the child. Both the child and family need adequate explanations concerning the protective environment precautions.

HAND HYGIENE

The nurse must perform hand hygiene on his or her hands between patients and after removing gloves. Hospital-approved antibacterial soaps and lotions are used. The use of hot water, instead of warm water, can irritate skin and may promote the development of resistant strains of microorganisms. Self-contained liquid soap dispensers are preferable to bar soap that can harbor organisms. Alcohol-based hand sanitizers can be used as long as the hands are not visibly soiled. Artificial fingernails, including tips, wraps, and nail jewelry, are not permitted in patient care areas. Refer to hospital infection prevention and control protocol. Caregivers with skin lesions on exposed areas of their bodies should not provide direct patient care until the lesions are completely cleared.

 Safety Alert!

Alcohol-based hand sanitizers should not be used when caring for a patient diagnosed with *Clostridium difficile* diarrhea because this organism is spore forming and resistant to alcohols. Soap and water must be used after every contact.

 Nursing Tip

Teaching children and their families to wash their hands before meals and after using the toilet, blowing their noses, sneezing, or handling soiled objects is important to minimize the spread of infection and to promote healthy living. Making hand hygiene fun for children can motivate them to wash appropriately for a minimum of 15 seconds.

FAMILY EDUCATION

Education of family members must be ongoing. Factors to be emphasized include the necessity for immunization of children, proper storage of food (particularly perishables), use of pasteurized milk, proper cooking of meats, cleanliness in food preparation, and proper hand hygiene. The nurse must review the ways in which infectious diseases are spread. Children must be taught to avoid using community hand towels. Other modes of transmission, such as crowded living conditions, insects, rodents, and sandboxes, may also be discussed.

RASHES

Many infectious diseases begin with a rash. Rashes tend to be itchy (pruritic) and uncomfortable. Symptomatic care is provided by prescribing acetaminophen (Tylenol) and diphenhydramine (Benadryl), or topical lotions. Rashes can be described as follows (see Box 30-1):
- **Erythema:** Diffused reddened area on the skin
- **Macule:** Circular reddened area on the skin
- **Papule:** Circular reddened area on the skin that is elevated
- **Vesicle:** Circular reddened area on the skin that is elevated and contains fluid
- **Pustule:** Circular reddened area on the skin that is elevated and contains pus
- **Scab:** Dried pustule that is covered with a crust
- **Pathognomonic:** Term used to describe a lesion or symptom that is *characteristic* of a specific illness (e.g., Koplik spots are pathognomonic for measles)

 Safety Alert!

Apply lotions to open lesions sparingly to prevent absorption that could lead to drug toxicity.

Worldwide travel makes it a priority for the nurse to be able to communicate with patients in different languages concerning signs and symptoms that may indicate the presence of a communicable disease. Appendix F is an example of a multilingual list of common symptoms related to communicable diseases that can be used by health care personnel.

WORLDWIDE IMMUNIZATION PROGRAMS

HEALTHY PEOPLE 2020

Federally funded programs to provide vaccines and to educate are already in place. The effort of the World Health Organization (WHO) and the United Nations Children's Fund (UNICEF) has resulted in dramatic declines in vaccine-preventable illnesses worldwide, especially in developing countries. New vaccines are developed and assessed for routine use in endemic areas.

At a meeting in Switzerland of the Strategic Advisory Group of Experts (SAGE) in 2012, concerning immunization practices around the world, new recommendations and guidelines were endorsed by the WHO and the American Academy of Pediatrics (AAP). Recommendations included the development of a global vaccine action plan; identification of regional challenges; and an establishment of a storage stockpile for cholera vaccines as well as research priorities (AAP, 2013).

Table 32-1 presents types of immunization agents. The influenza vaccine, the pneumococcal vaccine, the varicella vaccine, and RSV immune globulin (Respi-Gam) are available for children. Vaccines for cholera and yellow fever are available for families traveling to endemic areas. The CDC provides advice concerning vaccinations needed for persons traveling to various parts of the world.

THE NURSE'S ROLE

Worldwide immunization practices have eliminated smallpox as a threat. However, nurses must remain alert to signs and symptoms of communicable diseases, including smallpox. The threat of bioterrorism increases the risk of these and other diseases reemerging.

Table 32-1	Types of Immunization Agents
AGENT	**DESCRIPTION**
Vaccine	A suspension of weakened or inactivated (killed) organisms that stimulate immune bodies to form A form of **active** immunity
Toxoid	A modified toxin that stimulates the production of antitoxin A form of **active** immunity
Immune globulin	A solution containing antibodies extracted from human or animal blood Provides **passive** immunity
Specific immune globulins or antitoxins	Special preparations obtained from blood donors selected for their high antibody level against a specific disease Provides **passive** immunity to the specific disease

Measles is rarely seen in developed countries. Current vaccinations against varicella, hepatitis, influenza (for children 6 months of age and older or high-risk children), and pneumonia (for children greater than 2 years of age) are available, and the challenge is to make them accessible. The nurse is a vital link in educating parents about the need for immunizations. The U.S. Public Health Service has forms listing the benefits and risks of immunizations that are available to aid in parent education. Parental consent is required before a child is vaccinated, and appropriate vaccine information statements (VISs) should be provided and reviewed with the parents before administration of the vaccine.

VACCINES

In newborn infants, the presence of passively acquired immunity from the mother may inhibit the infant's natural immune response to vaccines. Therefore, routine immunizations are not started until 2 months of age, unless a high risk of infection exists. Because hepatitis B is a continuing problem in the United States, the immunization series for hepatitis B is often started before the newborn is discharged to the home.

Most antibodies cannot reach intracellular sites of infection but can prevent spread from the site of entry into the body to a target organ. For that reason, vaccinations prevent the disease, but most cannot be used to treat the disease after cellular penetration of the organism has occurred. For some diseases, postexposure immunization is recommended; immune globulins are most often the choice.

Multiple doses of a vaccine at predetermined intervals may be needed to achieve an immunity status. The nurse can educate parents and school personnel about immunization schedules and should assess the immunization status of each child at every clinic visit (Figure 32-5).

Routes of Administration

The correct *route of administration* is important to achieve immunization. The oral, subcutaneous, and intramuscular routes are used for various vaccines. The route of administration of a vaccine influences the response of the infant. The recommended route must be used to obtain optimum response. For example, the administration of hepatitis B vaccine into the buttock will not result in the same optimal level of immunity as administration of the vaccine into the deltoid muscle (Mandell, 2005). Refer to Chapter 22 for principles and techniques if administering intramuscular injections to pediatric patients.

Nursing Tip

The earliest age a vaccine should be administered is the youngest age at which the infant can respond by developing antibodies to that illness.

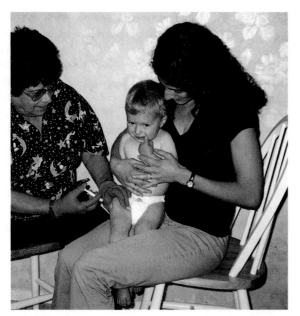

FIGURE 32-5 The "hug" restraining position for administration of vaccinations. Note that the mother restrains the arms, and the child's legs are restrained between the mother's knees. The mother comforts the child during the procedure and may breastfeed after the procedure. The site for intramuscular injections in infants is the thigh, and the nurse wears a protective glove. The use of aerosol sprays, EMLA cream or distraction techniques may reduce the pain of multiple injections in infants and children.

Storage and Handling

Correct *storage* of vaccines is essential to ensure their potency. The nurse should check the label to determine what type of refrigeration is needed. Proper storage and handling of vaccines ensures that potency is maintained. Improper temperatures can reduce the potency of the vaccine, and there are often no visible signs of these changes. Vaccines should not be stored in the doors of refrigerators or freezers, near the cold air vents in the refrigerator, or in storage bins; and they must be placed in the center of shelves to allow the free flow of air around the vaccines. Most vaccines are stored inside the refrigerator at 1.6° to 7.7° C (35° to 46° F). Varicella vaccine (Varivax) and live attenuated influenza virus (LAIV) are very fragile. The varicella and LAIV must be stored in the freezer at −15° C (5° F) or lower and used within 30 minutes of reconstitution. *The vaccines cannot be refrozen after they have been thawed.* Inactivated vaccines can be harmed if frozen, and live vaccines are harmed by heat and light. This information is especially important to know when participating in outdoor mass immunization programs. In clinic or office settings, the refrigerator temperatures must be documented at the beginning and the end of each workday, and the records must be kept on file for at least 3 years. Refrigerator-freezers with automatic defrost cycles are not appropriate for vaccine storage because temperatures may not be held stable as required (Kroger, 2011).

Emergency Preparedness

Most parts of the United States are threatened at times by sudden and unexpected power outages caused by storms, earthquakes, and other events. To minimize the potential for vaccine loss, preventive steps should be taken in preparation for such an emergency. These steps include keeping several bottles of water and cold packs in the freezer to help maintain the temperature of the vaccines if power is disrupted.

Allergies and Adverse Responses

Allergies. Children who have a history of allergy to neomycin should notify the health care provider before receiving the inactivated poliovirus vaccine (IPV), the measles-mumps-rubella vaccine (MMR), the varicella vaccine, and some influenza vaccines (Fluvirin). An allergy to eggs should also be reported before receiving MMR, varicella, or influenza vaccines. Epinephrine should be available in the unit where vaccines are administered, and the child should be observed for a minimum of 20 minutes before he or she leaves the area.

A serious allergy to baker's yeast should be reported to the health care provider before recombinant hepatitis B immunization is administered. The influenza vaccine should be administered with caution to persons who are allergic to eggs. Varicella vaccine, if not given on the same day as MMR, must be given *no less* than 28 days later. A tuberculin test should not be administered within 6 weeks of receiving an MMR or varicella immunization, because the results will not be accurate.

Mercury Toxicity. Thimerosal is a mercury-containing preservative used in some multidose vials of vaccines, and there is some concern about the rise of mercury contamination in the environment and exposure to children. The American Academy of Pediatrics (AAP) recommends that Comvax, a thimerosal-free hepatitis B vaccine, be used within 12 hours after birth for all high-risk newborn infants born in the United States. The pneumococcal vaccine (Prevnar 13) does not contain thimerosal and is effective in preventing common childhood pneumonia and otitis media. Thimerosal-free vaccines are used for pregnant women. The U.S. Food and Drug Administration (FDA) urges the elimination of mercury in medical equipment, such as thermometers and blood-pressure machines. Parents should be counseled about reducing exposures to other sources of mercury. In 2013, the AAP endorsed the WHO Strategic Advisory Group (SAGE) recommendations on immunizing children and concluded that the use of thimerosal in multidose vials for children is safe at this time. Research concerning alternative preservatives and their effect on the efficacy of the immunization products are ongoing (AAP, 2013). More information concerning mercury, animal proteins, and chemical contents in vaccines can be accessed at www.know-vaccines.org/?page_id=309.

On some occasions vaccines may elicit a hypersensitivity response or may block the body's immune defenses. Rotavirus is a live, attenuated oral vaccine recommended by the AAP to be given in a three-dose schedule (RV-5) or a two-dose schedule (RV-1) depending on the type of vaccine used. The vaccine is not recommended for immune-compromised children or children with latex allergy because the RV-1 applicator contains latex. The vaccine is given between 6 weeks and 32 weeks of age with at least a 1-month interval between doses. There is little value of rotovirus vaccines in children older than 15 months (AAP, 2014).

The hepatitis A vaccine is not licensed for use before 2 years of age. The AAP endorses the WHO recommendation that the one-dose inactivated hepatitis A vaccine be used for people who travel in high risk endemic areas and others who are at high risk (AAP, 2014). Serious adverse events occurring within a designated time after vaccination should be reported to the national Vaccine Adverse Events Reporting System (VAERS) (www.vaers.hhs.gov) or by calling 1-800-822-7967. The National Childhood Vaccine Injury Act of 1986 contains a provision for compensation in some cases of specific vaccine injuries. All patients should be directly observed for 15 to 20 minutes after receiving an immunization, and appropriate equipment for the treatment of anaphylaxis should be immediately available.

Refusal of Vaccination

When a parent refuses immunizations for a child, the nurse should listen carefully for the reason and offer appropriate education. Some vaccines contain heavy metals, antibiotics, and animal products (Grabenstein, 2009). Animal products contained in a vaccine may present a problem for parents with specific cultural beliefs. The nurse should be culturally sensitive and offer education concerning the values of the vaccine as well as options. Detailed information concerning contents of vaccines can be obtained online (see Online Resources at the end of the chapter).

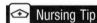 **Nursing Tip**

Some vaccines contain heavy metals, antibiotics, or animal products, which may be a problem for parents with specific cultural beliefs.

Nursing Responsibilities in Vaccine Administration

The nurse must be aware of when the vaccines are due to be scheduled for administration, the immunization history of the child, the vaccines that can be given together, contraindications, the route of administration, and the proper equipment needed. Epinephrine should be on hand for emergencies, and the child should remain in the clinic under observation for at least 20 minutes.

Reducing pain at the site of injection, especially when multiple injections are required, should be considered. The use of vapocoolant sprays or EMLA cream

(see Figure 21-3) is effective. Using the proper technique of injection of vaccines is important. The *Haemophilus influenzae* type B (Hib) vaccine must be dispensed in a separate syringe from other vaccines administered at the same clinic visit. The varicella vaccine is given subcutaneously, whereas the diphtheria-tetanus–acellular pertussis (DTaP) vaccine causes significant tissue irritation if given subcutaneously, and careful intramuscular (IM) technique is essential. Combination vaccines have been developed that reduce the number of injections required at each clinic visit.

The CDC and the AAP approve the recommended immunization program in the United States (Box 32-1). Advances in the field of immunology may change recommendations for existing policies and cause new policies to be developed (see the sites listed in Online Resources for updates). Alternative methods of vaccine delivery are being developed, including use of the intranasal route and transdermal techniques (Sharts-Hopko, 2009).

Before a vaccine is administered to a child, the nurse should provide a vaccine information statement (VIS) to the parent, discuss the vaccine, and obtain consent. VISs are printed in several different languages and can easily be obtained online (see Online Resources).

Box 32-1 **Highlights of the 2014 Vaccine Guidelines (AAP, 2014)**

- Pregnant adolescents should receive Tdap vaccination for each pregnancy at 27-36 week gestation regardless of previous Td or Tdap history to protect the newborn against pertussis until immunization can be given.
- New guidelines for influenza vaccination dosages for infants 6 months to 9 years of age are presented in the footnotes.
- Two new meningococcal conjugate vaccines are available for infants 2 months of age with a 3 dose plus booster regime designated for high risk infants and children including those with Sickle Cell disease.
- HPV vaccine intervals are clarified. The third dose should be administered 12 weeks after the second dose and at least 24 weeks after the first dose. The HPV quadrivalent vaccine is recommended for boys and either the quadrivalent or the bivalent vaccine can be used for girls.
- The footnotes to Figure 32-6 clarify use of pneumococcal vaccine (PCV13) and the 23 valent polysaccharide vaccine (PPSV23) use in children at increased risk.
- Doses of any vaccine administered more than 5 days earlier than the minimal interval between doses, or minimal age are not counted as valid doses.
- Rotavirus vaccine can be administered as early as 6 weeks of age but should not be started after 15 weeks of age.
- A single dose of Tdap is recommended for children at 11-12 years of age who have completed the childhood series.

Data from the AAP: Committee on Infectious Disease 2014: ACIP Releases 2014 Pediatric Vaccine Schedule, *Pediatrics* 133(2): 357-363, 2014 and www.cdc.gov/vaccines/acip.

Nursing Tip

There should be a 3- to 11-month interval between the administration of an immune globulin and administration of a live-virus vaccine (AAP, 2012).

Immunization Schedule for Children. Informed consent concerning the potential risks and the documentation of immunization are essential. Parents should have copies of their child's immunization records. The immunization program for children in the United States is described in Figure 32-6.

Contraindications to live virus vaccine administration may include the following:

- Immunocompromised state (necessitates individual evaluation by the health care provider)
- Pregnancy
- Bacteremia or meningitis
- Immunocompromised caregiver in the home (necessitates individual evaluation by the health care provider)
- Corticosteroid therapy (necessitates individual evaluation)
- History of high fever (40.5° C [105° F]) after previous vaccinations

A subcutaneous injection should be administered with a 3⅝-inch, 23- to 25-gauge needle; an IM injection should be administered with a 1- to 1½-inch, 22- to 25-gauge needle; and an intradermal injection should be administered with a ⅜- to ¾-inch, 25- to 27-gauge needle with the bevel up and parallel to the volar surface of the forearm.

Children from 4 months to 18 years of age who start the immunization process late or are more than 1 month behind should adhere to the catch-up schedule (Figure 32-6).

 Nursing Tip

An interrupted vaccination series can usually continue without restarting the entire series.

‼ **Safety Alert!**

If the MMR and the Varivax vaccine are not administered on the same day, they must be spaced at least 28 days apart. A tuberculin (TB) test may be given the same day as MMR or must be spaced at least 4 to 6 weeks later.

THE FUTURE OF IMMUNOTHERAPY

Research concerning the development of new vaccines and the refinement of established vaccines continues at an amazing pace. The use of transgenic plants for oral administration of bacterial and viral antigens would enable low-cost, effective distribution. Research in the field of transcutaneous immunization involves the application of an antigen with an adjuvant to the intact skin. Recombinant DNA technology and the use of adjuvants are being developed for rheumatic fever and malaria. Alum is an adjuvant currently used in the vaccine against hepatitis B to increase its effectiveness. RNA and DNA viruses are being developed for use as carriers (vectors) of other antigens. Forms of bacterial DNA are also being developed as carriers of antigens. A "gene gun" that blasts the vaccine through intact skin is also in the development stage. The techniques in research may hold promise for developing effective vaccines against influenza A virus, HIV type 1 (HIV-1), malaria organisms, and the Ebola virus. A catalogue of genes that code for viruses and potential immunogens is being studied.

The most exciting development in immunology is the use of immunotherapy for noncommunicable diseases. An example would be the mucosal administration of myelin in multiple sclerosis and a type 2 collagen for rheumatic arthritis. The possibility of preventing specific types of cancer has been recognized, and the challenge of developing tumor antigens that lyse tumor cells is also a clear possibility. In Alzheimer's disease the formation of neurotoxic plaques in the brain causes the loss of mental function. Early immunization with amyloid B may prevent or lyse the plaque formation and prevent the devastating problems of this disease.

The use of immunotherapy for autoimmune diseases is promising. The greatest achievement of the twentieth century was the eradication of smallpox and the development of many safe vaccines for children. Perhaps the achievement of the twenty-first century will be the development of immunotherapy for noncommunicable diseases such as Alzheimer's disease and cancer.

BIOTERRORISM AND THE MATERNAL–CHILD PATIENT

THE NURSE'S ROLE IN THE HOSPITAL SETTING

All nurses play a key role in assuring a coordinated and efficient response to natural and man-made disasters. Whether it is a summer tornado, a winter ice storm, an earthquake, or a man-made terrorist attack, all nurses must have basic knowledge of what to do.

‼ **Safety Alert!**

Although the United States has a response plan for identified incidences of bioterrorism, the nurse should maintain a high level of suspicion when many children with the same signs and symptoms present in school, or seek care in a health care facility, and he or she should call attention to that observation.

A basic knowledge of symptoms of exposure/infection, the medical supplies that may be needed, the drugs that may be used, and self-protection that may be essential is important for all nurses at all levels of

Text continued on p. 737

These recommendations must be read with the footnotes that follow. For those who fall behind or start late, provide catch-up vaccination at the earliest opportunity as indicated by the green bars in Figure 32-6, A. To determine minimum intervals between doses, see the catch-up schedule (Figure 32-6, B). School entry and adolescent vaccine age groups are in bold.

Vaccine	Birth	1 mo	2 mos	4 mos	6 mos	9 mos	12 mos	15 mos	18 mos	19–23 mos	2-3 yrs	4-6 yrs	7-10 yrs	11-12 yrs	13-15 yrs	16-18 yrs
Hepatitis B[1] (HepB)	1st dose	←2nd dose→			←————— 3rd dose —————→											
Rotavirus[2] (RV) RV1 (2-dose series); RV5 (3-dose series)			1st dose	2nd dose	See footnote 2											
Diphtheria, tetanus, & acellular pertussis[3] (DTaP: <7 yrs)			1st dose	2nd dose	3rd dose		←——— 4th dose ———→					5th dose				
Tetanus, diphtheria, & acellular pertussis[4] (Tdap: ≥7 yrs)														(Tdap)		
Haemophilus influenzae type b[5] (Hib)			1st dose	2nd dose	See footnote 5		←— 3rd or 4th dose, See footnote 5 →									
Pneumococcal conjugate[6] (PCV13)			1st dose	2nd dose	3rd dose		←— 4th dose —→									
Pneumococcal polysaccharide[6] (PPSV23)																
Inactivated poliovirus[7] (IPV) (<18 yrs)			1st dose	2nd dose	←————— 3rd dose —————→							4th dose				
Influenza[8] (IIV; LAIV) 2 doses for some: See footnote 8					Annual vaccination (IIV only)						Annual vaccination (IIV or LAIV)					
Measles, mumps, rubella[9] (MMR)							←— 1st dose —→					2nd dose				
Varicella[10] (VAR)							←— 1st dose —→					2nd dose				
Hepatitis A[11] (HepA)							←— 2-dose series, See footnote 11 —→									
Human papillomavirus[12] (HPV2: females only; HPV4: males and females)														(3-dose series)		
Meningococcal[13] (Hib-MenCY ≥ 6 weeks; MenACWY-D ≥9 mos; MenACWY-CRM ≥ 2 mos)					See footnote 13									1st dose		Booster

Legend:
- Range of recommended ages for all children
- Range of recommended ages for catch-up immunization
- Range of recommended ages for certain high-risk groups
- Range of recommended ages during which catch-up is encouraged and for certain high-risk groups
- Not routinely recommended

This schedule includes recommendations in effect as of January 1, 2014. Any dose not administered at the recommended age should be administered at a subsequent visit, when indicated and feasible. The use of a combination vaccine generally is preferred over separate injections of its equivalent component vaccines. Vaccination providers should consult the relevant Advisory Committee on Immunization Practices (ACIP) statement for detailed recommendations, available online at http://www.cdc.gov/vaccines/hcp/acip-recs/index.html. Clinically significant adverse events that follow vaccination should be reported to the Vaccine Adverse Event Reporting System (VAERS) online (http://www.vaers.hhs.gov) or by telephone (800-822-7967). Suspected cases of vaccine-preventable diseases should be reported to the state or local health department. Additional information, including precautions and contraindications for vaccination, is available from CDC online (http://www.cdc.gov/vaccines/recs/vac-admin/contraindications.htm) or by telephone (800-CDC-INFO [800-232-4636]).

This schedule is approved by the Advisory Committee on Immunization Practices (http://www.cdc.gov/vaccines/acip), the American Academy of Pediatrics (http://www.aap.org), the American Academy of Family Physicians (http://www.aafp.org), and the American College of Obstetricians and Gynecologists (http://www.acog.org).

A

The figure below provides catch-up schedules and minimum intervals between doses for children whose vaccinations have been delayed. A vaccine series does not need to be restarted, regardless of the time that has elapsed between doses. Use the section appropriate for the child's age. Always use this table in conjunction with Figure 32-6, A and the footnotes that follow.

Vaccine	Minimum Age for Dose 1	Minimum Interval Between Doses			
		Dose 1 to dose 2	Dose 2 to dose 3	Dose 3 to dose 4	Dose 4 to dose 5
Persons aged 4 months through 6 years					
Hepatitis B[1]	Birth	4 weeks	8 weeks and at least 16 weeks after first dose; minimum age for the final dose is 24 weeks		
Rotavirus[2]	6 weeks	4 weeks	4 weeks[2]		
Diphtheria, tetanus, & acellular pertussis [3]	6 weeks	4 weeks	4 weeks	6 months	6 months[3]
Haemophilus influenzae type b[5]	6 weeks	4 weeks If first dose administered at younger than age 12 months / 8 weeks (as final dose) if first dose administered at age 12 through 14 months / No further doses needed If first dose administered at age 15 months or older	4 weeks[5] if current age is younger than 12 months and first dose administered at <7 months old / 8 weeks (as final dose)[5] if current age is younger than 12 months and first dose administered between 7 through 11 months (regardless of Hib vaccine (PRP-T or PRP-OMP) used for first dose); OR if current age is 12 through 59 months and first dose administered at younger than age 12 months; OR first 2 doses were PRP-OMP and administered at younger than 12 months. No further doses needed if previous dose administered at age 15 months or older	8 weeks (as final dose) This dose only necessary for children aged 12 through 59 months who received 3 (PRP-T) doses before age 12 months and started the primary series before age 7 months	
Pneumococcal[6]	6 weeks	4 weeks If first dose administered at younger than age 12 months / 8 weeks (as final dose for healthy children) if first dose administered at age 12 months or older / No further doses needed for healthy children if first dose administered at age 24 months or older	4 weeks if current age is younger than 12 months / 8 weeks (as final dose for healthy children) if current age is 12 months or older / No further doses needed for healthy children if previous dose administered at age 24 months or older	8 weeks (as final dose) This dose only necessary for children aged 12 through 59 months who received 3 doses before age 12 months or for children at high risk who received 3 doses at any age	
Inactivated poliovirus[7]	6 weeks	4 weeks[7]	4 weeks[7]	6 months[7] minimum age 4 years for final dose	
Meningococcal[13]	6 weeks	8 weeks[13]	See footnote 13	See footnote 13	
Measles, mumps, rubella[9]	12 months	4 weeks			
Varicella[10]	12 months	3 months			
Hepatitis A[11]	12 months	6 months			
Persons aged 7 through 18 years					
Tetanus, diphtheria; tetanus, diphtheria, & acellular pertussis[4]	7 years[4]	4 weeks	4 weeks If first dose of DTaP/DT administered at younger than age 12 months / 6 months if first dose of DTaP/DT administered at age 12 months or older and then no further doses needed for catch-up	6 months If first dose of DTaP/DT administered at younger than age 12 months	
Human papillomavirus[12]	9 years	Routine dosing intervals are recommended[12]			
Hepatitis A[11]	12 months	6 months			
Hepatitis B[1]	Birth	4 weeks	8 weeks (and at least 16 weeks after first dose)		
Inactivated poliovirus[7]	6 weeks	4 weeks	4 weeks[7]	6 months[7]	
Meningococcal[13]	6 weeks	8 weeks[13]	See footnote 13		
Measles, mumps, rubella[9]	12 months	4 weeks			
Varicella[10]	12 months	3 months If person is younger than age 13 years / 4 weeks if person is aged 13 years or older			

NOTE: The above recommendations must be read along with the footnotes of this schedule.

B

FIGURE 32-6, A, Recommended immunization schedule for persons aged 0 through 18 years—United States, 2014. Hib is given intramuscularly. MMR and IPV are given subcutaneously. **B**, Catch-up immunization schedule for children 4 months to 18 years who start late or who are more than 1 month behind schedule, United States, 2014. *DTaP/Tdap*, Diphtheria toxoids, pertussis, and tetanus and tetanus–diphtheria–acellular pertussis vaccine; *HepB*, hepatitis B vaccine; *Hep*, hepatitis; *Hib*, *Haemophilus influenzae* type b vaccine; *IPV*, inactivated poliovirus vaccine; *MMR*, measles-mumps-rubella vaccine.

Continued

For further guidance on the use of the vaccines mentioned below, see: http://www.cdc.gov/vaccines/hcp/acip-recs/index.html.
For vaccine recommendations for persons 19 years of age and older, see the adult immunization schedule.

Additional Information

- For contraindications and precautions to use of a vaccine and for additional information regarding that vaccine, vaccination providers should consult the relevant ACIP statement available online at http://www.cdc.gov/vaccines/hcp/acip-recs/index.html.
- For purposes of calculating intervals between doses, 4 weeks = 28 days. Intervals of 4 months or greater are determined by calendar months.
- Vaccine doses administered 4 days or less before the minimum interval or minimum age should not be counted as valid doses and should be repeated as age-appropriate. The repeat dose should be spaced after the invalid dose by the recommended minimum interval. For further details, see MMWR, General Recommendations on Immunization and Reports / Vol. 60 / No. 2; Table 1. Recommended and minimum ages and intervals between vaccine doses available online at http://www.cdc.gov/mmwr/pdf/rr/rr6002.pdf.
- Information on travel vaccine requirements and recommendations is available at http://wwwnc.cdc.gov/travel/destinations/list.
- For vaccination of persons with primary and secondary immunodeficiencies, see Table 13, "Vaccination of persons with primary and secondary immunodeficiencies," in General Recommendations on Immunization (ACIP), available at http://www.cdc.gov/mmwr/pdf/rr/rr6002.pdf.; and American Academy of Pediatrics. Immunization in Special Clinical Circumstances, in Pickering LK, Baker CJ, Kimberlin DW, Long SS eds. Red Book: 2012 report of the Committee on Infectious Diseases. 29th ed. Elk Grove Village, IL: American Academy of Pediatrics.

1. Hepatitis B (HepB) vaccine. (Minimum age: birth)
   Routine vaccination:
   At birth:
   - Administer monovalent HepB vaccine to all newborns before hospital discharge.
   - For infants born to hepatitis B surface antigen (HBsAg)-positive mothers, administer HepB vaccine and 0.5 mL of hepatitis B immune globulin (HBIG) within 12 hours of birth. These infants should be tested for HBsAg and antibody to HBsAg (anti-HBs) 1 to 2 months after completion of the HepB series, at age 9 through 18 months (preferably at the next well-child visit).
   - If mother's HBsAg status is unknown, within 12 hours of birth administer HepB vaccine regardless of birth weight. For infants weighing less than 2,000 grams, administer HBIG in addition to HepB vaccine within 12 hours of birth. Determine mother's HBsAg status as soon as possible and, if mother is HBsAg-positive, also administer HBIG for infants weighing 2,000 grams or more as soon as possible, but no later than age 7 days.

   Doses following the birth dose:
   - The second dose should be administered at age 1 or 2 months. Monovalent HepB vaccine should be used for doses administered before age 6 weeks.
   - Infants who did not receive a birth dose should receive 3 doses of a HepB-containing vaccine on a schedule of 0, 1 to 2 months, and 6 months starting as soon as feasible. See Figure 2.
   - Administer the second dose 1 to 2 months after the first dose (minimum interval of 4 weeks), administer the third dose at least 8 weeks after the second dose AND at least 16 weeks after the first dose. The final (third or fourth) dose in the HepB vaccine series should be administered no earlier than age 24 weeks.
   - Administration of a total of 4 doses of HepB vaccine is permitted when a combination vaccine containing HepB is administered after the birth dose.

   Catch-up vaccination:
   - Unvaccinated persons should complete a 3-dose series.
   - A 2-dose series (doses separated by at least 4 months) of adult formulation Recombivax HB is licensed for use in children aged 11 through 15 years.
   - For other catch-up guidance, see Figure 2.

2. Rotavirus (RV) vaccines. (Minimum age: 6 weeks for both RV1 [Rotarix] and RV5 [RotaTeq])
   Routine vaccination:
   Administer a series of RV vaccine to all infants as follows:
   1. If Rotarix is used, administer a 2-dose series at 2 and 4 months of age.
   2. If RotaTeq is used, administer a 3-dose series at ages 2, 4, and 6 months.
   3. If any dose in the series was RotaTeq or vaccine product is unknown for any dose in the series, a total of 3 doses of RV vaccine should be administered.

   Catch-up vaccination:
   - The maximum age for the first dose in the series is 14 weeks, 6 days; vaccination should not be initiated for infants aged 15 weeks, 0 days or older.
   - The maximum age for the final dose in the series is 8 months, 0 days.
   - For other catch-up guidance, see Figure 2.

**3. Diphtheria and tetanus toxoids and acellular pertussis (DTaP) vaccine. (Minimum age: 6 weeks.
   Exception: DTaP-IPV [Kinrix]: 4 years)**
   Routine vaccination:
   - Administer a 5-dose series of DTaP vaccine at ages 2, 4, 6, 15 through 18 months, and 4 through 6 years. The fourth dose may be administered as early as age 12 months, provided at least 6 months have elapsed since the third dose.

   Catch-up vaccination:
   - The fifth dose of DTaP vaccine is not necessary if the fourth dose was administered at age 4 years or older.
   - For other catch-up guidance, see Figure 2.

4. Tetanus and diphtheria toxoids and acellular pertussis (Tdap) vaccine. (Minimum age: 10 years for Boostrix, 11 years for Adacel)
   Routine vaccination:
   - Administer 1 dose of Tdap vaccine to all adolescents aged 11 through 12 years.
   - Tdap may be administered regardless of the interval since the last tetanus and diphtheria toxoid-containing vaccine.
   - Administer 1 dose of Tdap vaccine to pregnant adolescents during each pregnancy (preferred during 27 through 36 weeks gestation) regardless of time since prior Td or Tdap vaccination.

   Catch-up vaccination:
   - Persons aged 7 years and older who are not fully immunized with DTaP vaccine should receive Tdap vaccine as 1 (preferably the first) dose in the catch-up series; if additional doses are needed, use Td vaccine. For children 7 through 10 years who receive a dose of Tdap as part of the catch-up series, an adolescent Tdap vaccine dose at age 11 through 12 years should NOT be administered. Td should be administered instead 10 years after the Tdap dose.
   - Persons aged 11 through 18 years who have not received Tdap vaccine should receive a dose followed by tetanus and diphtheria toxoids (Td) booster doses every 10 years thereafter.
   - Inadvertent doses of DTaP vaccine:
     - If administered inadvertently to a child aged 7 through 10 years may count as part of the catch-up series. This dose may count as the adolescent Tdap dose, or the child can later receive a Tdap booster dose at age 11 through 12 years.
     - If administered inadvertently to an adolescent aged 11 through 18 years, the dose should be counted as the adolescent Tdap dose.
   - For other catch-up guidance, see Figure 2.

5. Haemophilus influenzae type b (Hib) conjugate vaccine. (Minimum age: 6 weeks for PRP-T [ACTHIB, DTaP-IPV/Hib (Pentacel) and Hib-MenCY (MenHibrix)], PRP-OMP [PedvaxHIB or COMVAX], 12 months for PRP-T [Hiberix])
   Routine vaccination:
   - Administer a 2- or 3-dose Hib vaccine primary series and a booster dose (dose 3 or 4 depending on vaccine used in primary series) at age 12 through 15 months to complete a full Hib vaccine series.
   - The primary series with ActHIB, MenHibrix, or Pentacel consists of 3 doses and should be administered at 2, 4, and 6 months of age. The primary series with PedvaxHib or COMVAX consists of 2 doses and should be administered at 2 and 4 months of age; a dose at age 6 months is not indicated.
   - One booster dose (dose 3 or 4 depending on vaccine used in primary series) of any Hib vaccine should be administered at age 12 through 15 months. An exception is Hiberix vaccine. Hiberix should only be used for the booster (final) dose in children aged 12 months through 4 years who have received at least 1 prior dose of Hib-containing vaccine.

FIGURE 32-6, cont'd Footnotes—Recommended immunization schedule—2014.

For further guidance on the use of the vaccines mentioned below, see: http://www.cdc.gov/vaccines/hcp/acip-recs/index.html.

5. **Haemophilus influenzae type b (Hib) conjugate vaccine (cont'd)**
- For recommendations on the use of MenHibrix in patients at increased risk for meningococcal disease, please refer to the meningococcal vaccine footnotes and also to MMWR March 22, 2013; 62(RR02);1-22, available at http://www.cdc.gov/mmwr/pdf/rr/rr6202.pdf.

Catch-up vaccination:
- If dose 1 was administered at ages 12 through 14 months, administer a second (final) dose at least 8 weeks after dose 1, regardless of Hib vaccine used in the primary series.
- If the first 2 doses were PRP-OMP (PedvaxHIB or COMVAX), and were administered at age 11 months or younger, the third (and final) dose should be administered at age 12 through 15 months and at least 8 weeks after the second dose.
- If the first dose was administered at age 7 through 11 months, administer the second dose at least 4 weeks later and a third (and final) dose at age 12 through 15 months or 8 weeks after second dose, whichever is later, regardless of Hib vaccine used for first dose.
- If first dose is administered at younger than 12 months of age and second dose is given between 12 through 14 months of age, a third (and final) dose should be given 8 weeks later.
- For unvaccinated children aged 15 months or older, administer only 1 dose.
- For other catch-up guidance, see Figure 2. For catch-up guidance related to MenHibrix, please see the meningococcal vaccine footnotes and also MMWR March 22, 2013; 62(RR02);1-22, available at http://www.cdc.gov/mmwr/pdf/rr/rr6202.pdf.

Vaccination of persons with high-risk conditions:
- Children aged 12 through 59 months who are at increased risk for Hib disease, including chemotherapy recipients and those with anatomic or functional asplenia (including sickle cell disease), human immunodeficiency virus (HIV) infection, immunoglobulin deficiency, or early component complement deficiency, who have received either no doses or only 1 dose of Hib vaccine before 12 months of age, should receive 2 additional doses of Hib vaccine 8 weeks apart; children who received 2 or more doses of Hib vaccine before 12 months of age should receive 1 additional dose.
- For patients younger than 5 years of age undergoing chemotherapy or radiation treatment who received a Hib vaccine dose(s) within 14 days of starting therapy or during therapy, repeat the dose(s) at least 3 months following therapy completion.
- Recipients of hematopoietic stem cell transplant (HSCT) should be revaccinated with a 3-dose regimen of Hib vaccine starting 6 to 12 months after successful transplant, regardless of vaccination history; 3 doses should be administered at least 4 weeks apart.
- A single dose of any Hib-containing vaccine should be administered to unimmunized* children and adolescents 15 months of age and older undergoing an elective splenectomy; if possible, vaccine should be administered at least 14 days before procedure.
- Hib vaccine is not routinely recommended for patients 5 years or older. However, 1 dose of Hib vaccine should be administered to unimmunized* persons aged 5 years or older who have anatomic or functional asplenia (including sickle cell disease) and unvaccinated persons 5 through 18 years of age with human immunodeficiency virus (HIV) infection.
*Patients who have not received a primary series and booster dose or at least 1 dose of Hib vaccine after 14 months of age are considered unimmunized.

6. **Pneumococcal vaccines. (Minimum age: 6 weeks for PCV13, 2 years for PPSV23)**

Routine vaccination with PCV13:
- Administer a 4-dose series of PCV13 vaccine at ages 2, 4, and 6 months and at age 12 through 15 months.
- For children aged 14 through 59 months who have received an age-appropriate series of 7-valent PCV (PCV7), administer a single supplemental dose of 13-valent PCV (PCV13).

Catch-up vaccination with PCV13:
- Administer 1 dose of PCV13 to all healthy children aged 24 through 59 months who are not completely vaccinated for their age.
- For other catch-up guidance, see Figure 2.

Vaccination of persons with high-risk conditions with PCV13 and PPSV23:
- All recommended PCV13 doses should be administered prior to PPSV23 vaccination if possible.
- For children 2 through 5 years of age with any of the following conditions: chronic heart disease (particularly cyanotic congenital heart disease and cardiac failure); chronic lung disease (including asthma if treated with high-dose oral corticosteroid therapy); diabetes mellitus; cerebrospinal fluid leak; cochlear implant; sickle cell disease and other hemoglobinopathies; anatomic or functional asplenia; HIV infection; chronic renal failure; nephrotic syndrome; diseases associated with treatment with immunosuppressive drugs or radiation therapy, including malignant neoplasms, leukemias, lymphomas, and Hodgkin disease; solid organ transplantation; or congenital immunodeficiency:
  1. Administer 1 dose of PCV13 if 3 doses of PCV (PCV7 and/or PCV13) were received previously.
  2. Administer 2 doses of PCV13 at least 8 weeks apart if fewer than 3 doses of PCV (PCV7 and/or PCV13) were received previously.

6. **Pneumococcal vaccines (cont'd)**
  3. Administer 1 supplemental dose of PCV13 if 4 doses of PCV7 or other age-appropriate complete PCV7 series was received previously.
4. The minimum interval between doses of PCV (PCV7 or PCV13) is 8 weeks.
5. For children with no history of PPSV23 vaccination, administer PPSV23 at least 8 weeks after the most recent dose of PCV13.
- For children aged 6 through 18 years who have cerebrospinal fluid leak; cochlear implant; sickle cell disease and other hemoglobinopathies; anatomic or functional asplenia; congenital or acquired immunodeficiencies; HIV infection; chronic renal failure; nephrotic syndrome; diseases associated with treatment with immunosuppressive drugs or radiation therapy, including malignant neoplasms, leukemias, lymphomas, and Hodgkin disease; generalized malignancy; solid organ transplantation; or multiple myeloma:
  1. If neither PCV13 nor PPSV23 has been received previously, administer 1 dose of PCV13 now and 1 dose of PPSV23 at least 8 weeks later.
  2. If PCV13 has been received previously but PPSV23 has not, administer 1 dose of PPSV23 at least 8 weeks after the most recent dose of PCV13.
  3. If PPSV23 has been received but PCV13 has not, administer 1 dose of PCV13 at least 8 weeks after the most recent dose of PPSV23.
- For children aged 6 through 18 years with chronic heart disease (particularly cyanotic congenital heart disease and cardiac failure), diabetes mellitus, alcoholism, or chronic liver disease, who have not received PPSV23, administer 1 dose of PPSV23. If PCV13 has been received previously, then PPSV23 should be administered at least 8 weeks after any prior PCV13 dose.
- A single revaccination with PPSV23 should be administered 5 years after the first dose to children with sickle cell disease or other hemoglobinopathies; anatomic or functional asplenia; congenital or acquired immunodeficiencies; HIV infection; chronic renal failure; nephrotic syndrome; diseases associated with treatment with immunosuppressive drugs or radiation therapy, including malignant neoplasms, leukemias, lymphomas, and Hodgkin disease; generalized malignancy; solid organ transplantation; or multiple myeloma.

7. **Inactivated poliovirus vaccine (IPV). (Minimum age: 6 weeks)**

Routine vaccination:
- Administer a 4-dose series of IPV at ages 2, 4, 6 through 18 months, and 4 through 6 years. The final dose in the series should be administered on or after the fourth birthday and at least 6 months after the previous dose.

Catch-up vaccination:
- In the first 6 months of life, minimum age and minimum intervals are only recommended if the person is at risk for imminent exposure to circulating poliovirus (i.e., travel to a polio-endemic region or during an outbreak).
- If 4 or more doses are administered before age 4 years, an additional dose should be administered at age 4 through 6 years and at least 6 months after the previous dose.
- A fourth dose is not necessary if the third dose was administered at age 4 years or older and at least 6 months after the previous dose.
- If both OPV and IPV were administered as part of a series, a total of 4 doses should be administered, regardless of the child's current age. IPV is not routinely recommended for U.S. residents aged 18 years or older.
- For other catch-up guidance, see Figure 2.

8. **Influenza vaccines. (Minimum age: 6 months for inactivated influenza vaccine [IIV], 2 years for live, attenuated influenza vaccine [LAIV])**

Routine vaccination:
- Administer influenza vaccine annually to all children beginning at age 6 months. For most healthy, nonpregnant persons aged 2 through 49 years, either LAIV or IIV may be used. However, LAIV should NOT be administered to some persons, including 1) those with asthma, 2) children 2 through 4 years who had wheezing in the past 12 months, or 3) those who have any other underlying medical conditions that predispose them to influenza complications. For all other contraindications to use of LAIV, see MMWR 2013; 62 (No. RR-7):1-43, available at http://www.cdc.gov/mmwr/pdf/rr/rr6207.pdf.

For children aged 6 months through 8 years:
- For the 2013–14 season, administer 2 doses (separated by at least 4 weeks) to children who are receiving influenza vaccine for the first time. Some children in this age group who have been vaccinated previously will also need 2 doses. For additional guidance, follow dosing guidelines in the 2013-14 ACIP influenza vaccine recommendations, MMWR 2013; 62 (No. RR-7):1-43, available at http://www.cdc.gov/mmwr/pdf/rr/rr6207.pdf.
- For the 2014–15 season, follow dosing guidelines in the 2014 ACIP influenza vaccine recommendations.

For persons aged 9 years and older:
- Administer 1 dose.

Continued

FIGURE 32-6, cont'd Footnotes—Recommended immunization schedule—2014.

For further guidance on the use of the vaccines mentioned below, see: http://www.cdc.gov/vaccines/hcp/acip-recs/index.html.

9. **Measles, mumps, and rubella (MMR) vaccine. (Minimum age: 12 months for routine vaccination)**

Routine vaccination:
- Administer a 2-dose series of MMR vaccine at ages 12 through 15 months and 4 through 6 years. The second dose may be administered before age 4 years, provided at least 4 weeks have elapsed since the first dose.
- Administer 1 dose of MMR vaccine to infants aged 6 through 11 months before departure from the United States for international travel. These children should be revaccinated with 2 doses of MMR vaccine, the first at age 12 through 15 months (12 months if the child remains in an area where disease risk is high), and the second dose at least 4 weeks later.
- Administer 2 doses of MMR vaccine to children aged 12 months and older before departure from the United States for international travel. The first dose should be administered on or after age 12 months and the second dose at least 4 weeks later.

Catch-up vaccination:
- Ensure that all school-aged children and adolescents have had 2 doses of MMR vaccine; the minimum interval between the 2 doses is 4 weeks.

10. **Varicella (VAR) vaccine. (Minimum age: 12 months)**

Routine vaccination:
- Administer a 2-dose series of VAR vaccine at ages 12 through 15 months and 4 through 6 years. The second dose may be administered before age 4 years, provided at least 3 months have elapsed since the first dose. If the second dose was administered at least 4 weeks after the first dose, it can be accepted as valid.

Catch-up vaccination:
- Ensure that all persons aged 7 through 18 years without evidence of immunity (see *MMWR* 2007; 56 [No. RR-4], available at http://www.cdc.gov/mmwr/pdf/rr/rr5604.pdf) have 2 doses of varicella vaccine. For children aged 7 through 12 years, the recommended minimum interval between doses is 3 months (if the second dose was administered at least 4 weeks after the first dose, it can be accepted as valid); for persons aged 13 years and older, the minimum interval between doses is 4 weeks.

11. **Hepatitis A (HepA) vaccine. (Minimum age: 12 months)**

Routine vaccination:
- Initiate the 2-dose HepA vaccine series at 12 through 23 months; separate the 2 doses by 6 to 18 months.
- Children who have received 1 dose of HepA vaccine before age 24 months should receive a second dose 6 to 18 months after the first dose.
- For any person aged 2 years and older who has not already received the HepA vaccine series, 2 doses of HepA vaccine separated by 6 to 18 months may be administered if immunity against hepatitis A virus infection is desired.

Catch-up vaccination:
- The minimum interval between the two doses is 6 months.

Special populations:
- Administer 2 doses of HepA vaccine at least 6 months apart to previously unvaccinated persons who live in areas where vaccination programs target older children, or who are at increased risk for infection. This includes persons travelling to or working in countries that have high or intermediate endemicity of infection; men having sex with men; users of injection and non-injection illicit drugs; persons who work with HAV-infected primates or with HAV in a research laboratory; persons with clotting-factor disorders; persons with chronic liver disease; and persons who anticipate close, personal contact (e.g., household or regular babysitting) with an international adoptee during the first 60 days after arrival in the United States from a country with high or intermediate endemicity. The first dose should be administered as soon as the adoption is planned, ideally 2 or more weeks before the arrival of the adoptee.

12. **Human papillomavirus (HPV) vaccines. (Minimum age: 9 years for HPV2 [Cervarix] and HPV4 [Gardasil])**

Routine vaccination:
- Administer a 3-dose series of HPV vaccine on a schedule of 0, 1-2, and 6 months to all adolescents aged 11 through 12 years. Either HPV4 or HPV2 may be used for females, and only HPV4 may be used for males.
- The vaccine series may be started at age 9 years.
- Administer the second dose 1 to 2 months after the first dose (minimum interval of 4 weeks), and administer the third dose 24 weeks after the first dose and 16 weeks after the second dose (minimum interval of 12 weeks).

Catch-up vaccination:
- Administer the vaccine series to females (either HPV2 or HPV4) and males (HPV4) at age 13 through 18 years if not previously vaccinated.
- Use recommended routine dosing intervals (see above) for vaccine series catch-up.

13. **Meningococcal conjugate vaccines. (Minimum age: 6 weeks for Hib-MenCY [MenHibrix], 9 months for MenACWY-D [Menactra], 2 months for MenACWY-CRM [Menveo])**

Routine vaccination:
- Administer a single dose of Menactra or Menveo vaccine at age 11 through 12 years, with a booster dose at age 16 years.
- Adolescents aged 11 through 18 years with human immunodeficiency virus (HIV) infection should receive a 2-dose primary series of Menactra or Menveo with at least 8 weeks between doses. See below.
- For children aged 2 months through 18 years with high-risk conditions, see below.

Catch-up vaccination:
- Administer Menactra or Menveo vaccine at age 13 through 18 years if not previously vaccinated.
- If the first dose is administered at age 13 through 15 years, a booster dose should be administered at age 16 through 18 years with a minimum interval of at least 8 weeks between doses.
- If the first dose is administered at age 16 years or older, a booster dose is not needed.
- For other catch-up guidance, see Figure 2.

Vaccination of persons with high-risk conditions and other persons at increased risk of disease:

- Children with anatomic or functional asplenia (including sickle cell disease):
  1. For children younger than 19 months of age, administer a 4-dose infant series of MenHibrix or Menveo at 2, 4, 6, and 12 through 15 months of age.
  2. For children aged 19 through 23 months who have not completed a series of MenHibrix or Menveo, administer 2 primary doses of Menveo at least 3 months apart.
  3. For children aged 24 months and older who have not received a complete series of MenHibrix or Menveo or Menactra, administer 2 primary doses of either Menactra or Menveo at least 2 months apart. If Menactra is administered to a child with asplenia (including sickle cell disease), do not administer Menactra until 2 years of age and at least 4 weeks after the completion of all PCV13 doses.

- Children with persistent complement component deficiency:
  1. For children younger than 19 months of age, administer a 4-dose infant series of either MenHibrix or Menveo at 2, 4, 6, and 12 through 15 months of age.
  2. For children 7 through 23 months who have not initiated vaccination, two options exist depending on age and vaccine brand:
     a. For children who initiate vaccination with Menveo at 7 months through 23 months of age, a 2-dose series should be administered with the second dose after 12 months of age and at least 3 months after the first dose.
     b. For children who initiate vaccination with Menactra at 9 months through 23 months of age, a 2-dose series of Menactra should be administered at least 3 months apart.
  c. For children aged 24 months and older who have not received a complete series of MenHibrix, Menveo, or Menactra, administer 2 primary doses of either Menactra or Menveo at least 2 months apart.

- For children who travel to or reside in countries in which meningococcal disease is hyperendemic or epidemic, including countries in the African meningitis belt or the Hajj, administer an age-appropriate formulation and series of Menactra or Menveo for protection against serogroups A and W meningococcal disease. Prior receipt of MenHibrix is not sufficient for children traveling to the meningitis belt or the Hajj because it does not contain serogroups A or W.
- For children at risk during a community outbreak attributable to a vaccine serogroup, administer or complete an age- and formulation-appropriate series of MenHibrix, Menactra, or Menveo.
- For booster doses among persons with high-risk conditions, refer to *MMWR* 2013; 62(RR02);1-22, available at http://www.cdc.gov/mmwr/preview/mmwrhtml/rr6202a1.htm.

Catch-up recommendations for persons with high-risk conditions:
1. If MenHibrix is administered to achieve protection against meningococcal disease, a complete age-appropriate series of MenHibrix should be administered.
2. If the first dose of MenHibrix is given at or after 12 months of age, a total of 2 doses should be given at least 8 weeks apart to ensure protection against serogroups C and Y meningococcal disease.
3. For children who initiate vaccination with Menveo at 7 months through 9 months of age, a 2-dose series should be administered with the second dose after 12 months of age and at least 3 months after the first dose.
4. For other catch-up recommendations for these persons, refer to *MMWR* 2013; 62(RR02);1-22, available at http://www.cdc.gov/mmwr/preview/mmwrhtml/rr6202a1.htm.

For complete information on use of meningococcal vaccines, including guidance related to vaccination of persons at increased risk of infection, see *MMWR* **March 22, 2013; 62(RR02);1-22, available at** http://www.cdc.gov/mmwr/pdf/rr/rr6202.pdf.

FIGURE 32-6, cont'd Footnotes—Recommended immunization schedule—2014.

Box 32-2	The Nurse's Role During Disaster in the Maternal–Child Units

1. Have a disaster plan in place and know where to find it; know who the leader on the unit is; have protective gear available to wear.
2. The Federal Emergency Management Agency (FEMA) and the Occupational Safety and Health Administration (OSHA) have publications available to help design a plan. The National Incident Management System (NIMS) also has training for disaster events. All nurses should participate in training sessions on a regular basis.
3. Maintain communication with hospital and community. Everyone should wear a picture ID.
4. Know where emergency outlets are located; they should be clearly marked for use with generator for priority equipment.
5. Have bag-valve self-inflating masks available and oxygen cylinders and regulators available on the unit.
6. Provide for gravity-assisted IV and enteral feedings.
7. Use available daylight and have flashlights with batteries available on crash cart.
8. Document on paper forms until computers are working.
9. Have extra blankets on hand—use kangaroo care for infants as needed.
10. Use manual override for electronic medical dispensing systems.
11. Have minimum supply of formulas on hand for infants.
12. Have a supply of waterless hand cleaners, diapers, bottles, and nipples.
13. Be sure each infant has proper ID bands or secure identifying information on Tegaderm and paste to infant's back during evacuations.
14. Keep patients away from windows.
15. Keep parents and infants together whenever possible.
16. Identify safe areas within unit for babies, parents, and staff.

care to know so as to work effectively within a health care team in a time of emergency or disasters. See Box 32-2 concerning details of the nurse's role in maternal–child units during a disaster.

Physiological Effects of Biological Agents on Infants and Children

Children are generally more vulnerable to biological warfare, because their immune systems are not fully developed. They are also closer to the ground, so heavy particles from an aerosol-propelled agent may reach them in higher doses than a taller adult. All new drugs are tested on adults as they are being developed, and it sometimes takes many years to determine safety for the pediatric patient. Therefore a new drug that is developed to treat a bioterror or chemical agent may in reality be more harmful than beneficial to the pediatric patient. The large head and body surface area in relation to weight and the low body-fat content makes the child more vulnerable to develop hypothermia, which can be life threatening in the pediatric age group. Therefore the routine "hazmat" decontamination procedure of stripping and total body washing may not be suitable for the pediatric patient.

The thin skin of the pediatric patient may make dermal chemicals, such as mustard gas, more dangerous to children than adults. A relatively small blood volume makes children more susceptible to fluid losses caused by cholera or other gastrointestinal toxins. Smallpox vaccine cannot be given to pregnant women, and other vaccines, such as anthrax, may not be useful for children. Gas masks are often not available in pediatric sizes, and the national disaster medical system protocol may not make provisions for pediatric beds.

Table 32-2 lists common diseases (and their symptoms) that are spread through bioterrorism. Chemical agents that may be used in a terrorist attack may include *pulmonary* agents such as chlorine, *cyanide* agents such as sulfur mustard, *nerve* agents such as

sarin, or *incapacitating* agents such as the military glycolate anticholinergic compound coded BZ by the North Atlantic Treaty Organization (NATO). The local health department's bioterrorism branch should be contacted concerning the management of victims.

The Mental Health Needs of Parents and Children

Terrorist acts in the form of chemical warfare or physical assaults such as bombings can be brought into the home via television from remote locations in the United States, thus violating a child's personal feeling of safety. Children listen to television and to their trusted adults who are expressing fears, they perhaps lose loved ones or friends, and they may play out their own fears with toys, in art, or through altered behavior.

The mental health needs of parents and children after a disaster can be anticipated and include physical and mental acute distress, increased risk-taking behaviors such as the use of alcohol or substance abuse, or the manifestation of a specific mental health disorder. Pregnant women are at increased risk of mental health problems and altered pregnancy outcomes. The basic role of the nurse is to establish safety. Move patients to safe areas, and help families care for themselves in a calm manner, maximizing positive thoughts. Help the families maintain a routine for sleep and meals and keep them informed about the situation and what they can and should do to obtain food and supplies and to vent their emotions. Available counseling options should be provided. Children may not understand what is happening and they may be separated from familiar places and faces, but they can respond positively to helpful adults around them. Families should be kept together whenever possible and children should have ID tags affixed and secured. Nurses can help parents meet the developmental needs of their children during and after disaster strikes. Online resources to prepare for disaster can be accessed at www.bt.cdc.gov/bioterrorism.

Table 32-2   Common Diseases/Response to Agents That Can Be Spread Through Bioterrorism

BIOTERRORISM AGENTS	SYMPTOMS AND MANAGEMENT	INCUBATION PERIOD
Anthrax	Flulike symptoms that improve, after which respiratory and circulatory collapse occurs; chest x-ray film shows widened mediastinum caused by thoracic edema; skin lesions involve vesicles with a black eschar center and enlarged adjacent lymph nodes. Management includes ciprofloxacin or doxycycline (ciprofloxacin should be avoided in pregnant women). Vaccine approved for age older than 18 years.	1-14 days
Botulism	Difficulty speaking and swallowing, blurred or double vision, respiratory distress; descending muscular paralysis. NOTE: Inhaled form has **no** gastrointestinal symptoms. Management includes IV equine antitoxins and diphenhydramine for serum sickness.	1-5 days
Ebola virus *(Filovirus)*	Abrupt onset of fever, headache, muscle pain, gastrointestinal upset, maculopapular rash on the trunk, petechiae, and progressive bleeding. Management includes supportive care. Ribovirin used outside United States.	4-10 days
Lassa fever *(Arenavirus)*	Fever, retrosternal pain, tremor of tongue and hands, hearing loss.	7-16 days
Plague	Fever, mucopurulent sputum, chest pain, hemoptysis, purpura. Management includes gentamycin, streptomycin; ciprofloxacin.	2-3 days
Smallpox	"Chickenpox–like" lesions starting on the face and extremities, with each stage of the lesions progressing from one state to the next **together**. Management: Vaccine can be effective if administered 2-3 days after exposure. Vaccine not safe during pregnancy.	12 days (average)
Tularemia	Fever, pneumonitis, nonproductive cough, periorbital edema. Management: Streptomycin, gentamycin, ciprofloxin, and supportive care. Does not require isolation.	3-5 days
Nerve agents: Sarin	Copious secretions; altered mental status; paralysis Respiratory arrest. Nurses need to wear self-contained breathing apparatus, and full protective gear.	Decontaminate with soap and water. Atropine preparation administered.
Respiratory agents: Phosgene	Hives on skin; tearing; blindness; respiratory distress. Smells like newly mowed hay. Agent is heavier than air, therefore ambulatory children may receive higher exposure. Nurses must wear full protective gear.	Decontaminate. Supportive care.
Vesicants Mustard gas	Photophobia; sunburn-like rash. Agent is heavier than air, therefore ambulatory children may be exposed to larger dose. Nurses must wear full protective gear.	Decontaminate with soap and water. Flush eyes. Treat similar to burns. Provide respiratory support.

Data adapted from Schultz R, Paulestsos C, Combs A: Considerations for emergencies and disasters in the NICU, *MCN* 33(4):204-210, 2008; Marirose B, Matthews P: Evacuation of maternal-newborn area during hurricane Katrina, *MCN* 33(4):213-220, 2008; Teran-MacKiver M, Larson M: Implications of chemical bioterrorism events for children and pregnant women, *MCN* 33(4):224-230, 2008; Carrarino J: Disaster related mental health needs of women and children, *MCN* 33(4):242-246, 2008: Collister L: Among the most vulnerable: women and children in global disasters, *MCN* 33(4):263, 2008; Cieslak T, Henretig F: Biological and chemical terrorism. In Kliegman R, Stanton B, St Geme III J, Schor N, Behrman R: *Nelson textbook of pediatrics,* ed 19, Philadelphia, 2011, Saunders; National Center for Bioterrorism, www.ncbi.nim.nih.gov, accessed December 2013.

The Nurse's Role in the Community

Emergency Preparedness. The nurse can assist families to prepare for natural disasters, such as hurricanes or floods, or manmade disasters, such as bioterrorist attacks or bombings. The American Medical Association (AMA) office guidelines for preparing a family and community disaster plan state that the family should keep several days' supply of food, water, pet food, warm clothing, blankets, copies of vital documents, and toiletries on hand. A battery-powered radio and extra medications, eyeglasses, and basic first aid supplies are also essential. Disaster drills held on a regular schedule should include emergency plans, exit strategies, and out-of-state family contact phone numbers or email addresses. Children should be taught the importance of keeping personal identification with them at all times (perhaps an ID bracelet for infants or small children) and how to call for help when needed (see Online Resources).

Initial Observation. Although the ABCs of emergency triage for adults apply to children, a pediatric quick examination includes the following:

- *Airway:* Assess for blockage or obstruction that may be present
- *Breathing (respiratory effort):* Tachypnea may indicate shock, whereas retractions may indicate a lung problem
- *Circulation:* Circulatory problems causing cyanosis, pallor, mottling, capillary refill time (CFT) more than 2 seconds
- *Mental status:* Alert, aware of surroundings, interacting

The initial examination of a patient after suspected exposure to a biological agent may be delayed between exposure and the development of symptoms (incubation period). Tentative triage categories for victims of bioterrorist attacks may include *immediate* (requiring prompt intervention), *delayed* (care can wait for a short time), *minimal* (only outpatient care is required), and *expectant* (moribund victims unlikely to survive lifesaving measures) (Armstrong, 2002).

A heightened awareness by health care professionals plays a critical role in facilitating early recognition of the release of a biological agent as a weapon. The health care professional must immediately notify the infection prevention and control department of the hospital, which will work with hospital administration and the local health department. The CDC in Atlanta will be notified of the suspected or confirmed event by the state health department. It is very important that the reporting chain of command be followed. A 24-hour local health department contact number is available to the health care professional.

The Pediatric Patient in a Disaster Setting

The pediatric patient has a proportionately larger body surface area and thinner skin than an adult. Children may also suffer increased pulmonary problems from the same exposure as adults. Children are closer to the ground and may be more readily exposed to vaporized agents of terror. The immature blood–brain barrier and increased central nervous system (CNS) receptor sensitivity may increase susceptibility of children to the effects of nerve agents. Vascular access may be difficult in the pediatric patient, and dosage calculations for varied kilogram weights increase the challenge for safe medical therapy for this population. Pediatric autoinjectors of low-dose atropine and pralidoxime are available for treatment of children with severe clinical

symptoms after nerve agent exposure. Drs. Jim Broselow and Bob Luten have developed a color-coding system (the Broselow tape) to reduce medication errors in children. Their systems include a water-resistant "Pediatric Antidotes for Chemical Warfare tape," which measures the child's length to determine weight and color zones that correlate to safe dosages of specific emergency drugs commonly used in bioterrorism attacks. This tape is used as a guide in emergency care in the field or hospital emergency rooms.

SEXUALLY TRANSMITTED INFECTIONS

OVERVIEW

Sexually transmitted infection (STI) is the general name given to infections spread through direct sexual activity. This term replaces the terms *sexually transmitted disease* and *venereal disease*. STIs can be transmitted by a pregnant woman to her unborn child and can cause serious problems in the fetus such as blindness, birth defects, or death (Table 32-3). The occurrence of an STI in a prepubertal patient should always prompt investigation into the possibility of sexual abuse. Sexually transmitted infections in adults are discussed in Chapter 11.

> **Nursing Tip**
>
> The use of condoms to prevent STIs, although recommended, is not considered 100% effective because condoms are apt to slip or break during intercourse and can be damaged by oil-based lubricants.

NURSING CARE AND RESPONSIBILITIES

Regardless of the medical professional's feelings about the changes in society and sexual permissiveness, the consequences of these changes must be recognized and managed. Nurses who wish to help adolescents with STIs must create an environment in which the adolescent feels safe and at ease. Adolescents need emotional support, which the nurse can provide through listening and maintaining a nonjudgmental attitude. The nurse is also responsible to stay up to date on CDC changes in recommended vaccine protocols.

The nurse sensitively approaches the patient, recognizing that the adolescent is embarrassed and in need of privacy, especially during examinations. Girls are often afraid and always nervous about a pelvic examination. This is true even when their outward manner may seem otherwise. Careful explanations are needed. The patient is draped appropriately, and the nurse remains during the examination to provide reassurance. The findings are discussed with the patient, and questions are encouraged. Most adolescents need to be drawn out and do not readily ask questions, even when they do not understand.

The requirement to report sexual contacts is an emotionally charged topic that often prevents patients

Table 32-3	Nursing Care to Prevent and Treat Sexually Transmitted Infections

Nursing Goals

- To provide anticipatory guidance concerning sexuality at a level that the child or young person can comprehend throughout developmental cycle
- To prevent infection
- To identify early symptoms and provide prompt treatment if infection occurs
- To prevent sequelae

CONCERN	NURSING INTERVENTIONS
Children less than 12 years of age	Provide age-appropriate instruction concerning sexuality; also explore expected patterns that might occur before next visit.
Puberty and adolescence	Review structure and function of reproductive systems; review personal hygiene; discuss values and decision making, possible sexual behavior and consequences, and prevention of pregnancy and sexually transmitted infections (STIs).
Self-concept: anticipate evidence of fear, embarrassment, anger, and decreased self-esteem on suspicion of infection	Create nonjudgmental atmosphere; listen, assess level of knowledge, observe nonverbal behavior, establish confidentiality; provide privacy when assisting with pelvic or genital examination; provide appropriate draping of patient; realize anger is often a mask for depression, grief—do not take personally.
Skin and hair	It is not uncommon to see skin rashes, "crabs" (pubic lice), or scabies (mites).
Sexual partners	Determine sexual preference; investigate and direct to treatment; persons at particular risk are those who have multiple sexual partners, are homosexuals, are with new partners, or have a history of previous STI.
Sexual intercourse	Encourage patient to abstain during treatment; use condom to prevent reinfection.
Medication	Encourage patient to take all of prescribed medication; if taking tetracycline, advise to take 1 hour before or 2 hours after meals (on empty stomach); avoid dairy products, antacids, iron, and sunlight.
Compliance with treatment	Stress importance of follow-up and routine annual Papanicolaou (Pap) smears.
Sequelae	Discuss the possible complications of specific disorders such as birth defects and infertility.

from seeking help. The person who is assured of confidentiality and who has been treated in a dignified manner is more apt to cooperate. Girls who are sexually active must be taught to take responsibility for their own health. Young people must be made aware of the fact that sex with only one partner does not eliminate the risk, because this partner may have had contact with others; the partner needs to have had only one sexual experience with one infected person to transmit disease.

The nurse assesses the person's level of knowledge and provides information at an understandable level. Many young people have little knowledge of their body and their developing sexuality. Others have mild to deep-seated emotional problems that must be addressed. They may be using sex to escape from reality, to express hostility or rebellion, or to call attention to themselves. They may be involved in relationships they no longer desire and therefore need help in formulating positive attitudes toward themselves. They also need help understanding their behavior and that of others. In particular, adolescents must learn that they are responsible for their own actions if they choose to be sexually active.

Prevention of STIs is discussed in Chapter 11.

 Nursing Tip

Sex education is not limited to the mechanics of intercourse but rather includes the feelings involved in a sexual experience: expectations, fantasies, fulfillments, and disappointments.

Human Papillomavirus

The most common STI in adolescents in the United States is human papillomavirus (HPV) (CDC, 2011). This condition has become endemic in the United States. It is contracted via direct sexual contact, and the risk is increased when multiple sexual partners are involved. Many types of HPV are associated with the development of cancer in both males and females, but HPV may be a significant cause of cervical cancer in women (CDC, 2011).

Manifestations. Manifestations include the development of clusters of flesh-colored cauliflower-shaped warts in the perineal area. Contact with the warts results in spreading the condition.

Prevention. There are 2 licensed vaccines in the United States that can prevent the development of certain strains of HPV if taken before exposure (Friedman, 2011): the quadrivalent Guardasil HPV 6/11/16/18, and the bivalent Cervatrix HPV 16/18. The CDC recommends both males and females receive the 3-dose regime between 9 and 26 years of age.

Treatment. The warts can be removed with cryotherapy (freezing the lesion) or electrocautery. Topical treatment with podofilox gel or sinecatechins ointment may also be prescribed. These treatments are not cures, and reoccurrence is possible. All sexual contact partners also need to be treated.

HIV/AIDS IN CHILDREN

Pediatric HIV/AIDS is a worldwide public health problem with a devastating outcome. Children usually acquire the HIV infection through the following:

- Contact with an infected mother at birth (approximately 90% of cases in infants)
- Sexual contact with an infected person
- Use of contaminated needles or contact with infected blood

A challenge for public health authorities includes educating the public about the role of unprotected sex and intravenous drug abuse in increasing the risk of HIV infection. The recommended HIV counseling and testing for pregnant women and the highly active antiretroviral therapy (HAART) has played an important role in preventing perinatal transmission (Hahn, 2009).

AIDS is caused by a retrovirus known as HIV-1 that attacks lymphocytes (the white blood cells that protect against disease). It appears to cause an imbalance between the helper T cells (CD4) that support the immune system and the suppressor T cells that shut it down. In a person not infected with HIV, the number of CD4 cells remains constant throughout time. In an HIV-infected person, the number of CD4 cells drops as the months and years pass. The CD4 cell count is a measure of the damage to the immune system caused by HIV and of the body's ability to fight infection. A physician uses the CD4 cell count to help determine the best medical treatments for the individual.

A series of terms for this disorder have been developed, but the disease is now classified along a continuum of categories by the CDC:

- *Asymptomatic infection (Category N).* This refers to a latent period. Individuals in this category may have positive antibody tests, indicating exposure to the virus, but they are not ill.
- *Symptomatic HIV infection (May be categories A or B).* Many individuals have this earlier and milder condition (compared with AIDS). This was formerly referred to as AIDS-related complex (ARC).
- *AIDS.* This refers to the most advanced involvement, which includes the finding of HIV antibodies in the patient's blood, the presence of complicating opportunistic infections, and other criteria.

Children do not contract AIDS from casual relationships at schools and medical facilities or through family living. The virus is infectious but not highly contagious, and the circumstances for acquiring it are specific, as previously indicated. Improved attention to hygiene practices in response to this disease can only be applauded.

Because passive transmission of antibodies from the mother occurs, infants are born with antibodies that crossed the placenta. Some infants' systems become clear of antibodies in about 15 months, whereas other infants eventually experience the infection. Because of the transference of antibodies, the standard enzyme-linked immunosorbent assay (ELISA) and Western blot tests that are used to diagnose HIV infection in older children and adults are less reliable until the child is at least 15 months of age.

Manifestations. The CDC has outlined criteria for the disease in children. Initial symptoms in infancy are vague and include failure to thrive, lymphadenopathy (enlarged lymph glands), chronic sinusitis, and nonresponse to the treatment of infections. The patient becomes subject to overwhelming infection. Opportunistic infections such as oral thrush, *Pneumocystis jiroveci* (formerly called *Pneumocystis carinii*) pneumonia, herpes viruses, and cytomegalovirus take advantage of the body's depressed immune system. Kaposi's sarcoma, a rare type of skin cancer, appears to be less common in children than in adults. Serious bacterial infections such as meningitis, impetigo, and urinary tract problems are reported in children. In general, the symptoms of HIV infection develop more rapidly in infants, and this may be attributed to the infant's immature immune system. The CDC considers that a child less than 13 years of age is HIV-infected if four symptoms meet the CDC criteria (AAP, 2009b).

Treatment and Nursing Care. The goals of care are to slow the growth of the virus, prevent opportunistic infections, and provide adequate nutrition and supportive therapy. Assessment and care of the child with HIV/AIDS are critically important. Education concerning long-term compliance with prescribed antiviral drugs and supportive care to promote growth and development are essential. The CD4 and lymphocyte counts are normally high in infancy and decline to adult levels when a child is approximately 6 years old. Common tests include a CDC 4 cell count; Western Blot Test; Rapid HIV Test; enzyme immunoassay (EIA); and enzyme-linked immunoassay (ELISA) (Hahn, 2009). Nursing Care Plan 32-1 provides selected nursing diagnoses and interventions for a newborn or infant with HIV/AIDS.

Psychological support for these children is paramount. Sensory stimulation and touching are especially important for infants. The effects of isolation can be physically and emotionally devastating to the developing child. Many infants are abandoned, outlive their mothers, or must live in foster care. Unique programs

⭐ Nursing Care Plan 32-1 | The Infant with HIV

PATIENT DATA An infant boy, who is positive for human immunodeficiency virus (HIV), has been admitted with an upper respiratory infection; his mother is rooming in.

Selected Nursing Diagnosis: Risk for infection related to HIV attack on T cells and the suppression of antibody function

Goals	Nursing Interventions	Rationales
Patient will be free from infection as evidenced by intact skin, absence of respiratory distress, and normal laboratory findings.	Anticipate opportunistic infections because patient's immune system is depressed.	Opportunistic infections are those that occur because of the opportunity afforded by poor health of patient. Newborns and preterm infants have immature immune systems and are particularly susceptible; once infected, they have few reserves to fight illness.
	Monitor respiratory status closely; watch for restlessness, apprehension.	Lungs are a target for infection; patients are subject to pneumonia, particularly *Pneumocystis jiroveci (carinii)*.
	Examine patient regularly for infection (puncture sites, mouth, rectum, pierced ears).	Thrush and herpes simplex are common in children; the perianal region is in danger of secondary infection from feces.
	Reposition frequently.	Frequent repositioning reduces pooling of secretions in lungs.
	Administer antipyretics and antimicrobials as prescribed.	These will increase patient comfort and may help to ward off infection. Pneumonia necessitates aggressive efforts to identify pathogen; fever is common.

Selected Nursing Diagnosis: Imbalanced nutrition, less than body requirements, related to anorexia, anemia, thrush

Goals	Nursing Interventions	Rationales
Nutrition will be maintained as evidenced by normal healing, muscle tone, and body weight.	Offer small portions of high-calorie, bland foods often.	Infant may have a poor appetite and mouth sores.
	Provide oral formula to infants as prescribed.	Infant must have sufficient nutrients to meet growth and development needs and to maintain body expenditures. Breastfeeding is contraindicated.
	Administer nasogastric tube feedings if ordered.	Preterm and weakened infants may require nasogastric feedings.
	Provide total parenteral nutrition (TPN) therapy if ordered.	Nutritional supplements may be necessary as disease progresses; prognosis may be poor despite aggressive management.
	Provide for mobility to ensure muscle strength.	Immobility contributes to wasted muscles; infants and toddlers need to be up and around as condition permits.
	Chart intake and output, daily weights.	These patients become easily dehydrated. Daily weights will demonstrate nutritional progress.

Selected Nursing Diagnosis: Risk for injury related to changes in central nervous system and related to decreased blood components

Goals	Nursing Interventions	Rationales
Parents will become aware of potential sources of injury; parents will recognize signs of bleeding. Child will not show signs of injury as evidenced by absence of petechiae.	Provide developmentally safe environment.	Children are accident-prone; normal cuts and abrasions become easily infected; impetigo can be very dangerous for this child.
	Observe skin for petechiae and bruising; explain to parents.	Thrombocytopenia is common. Kaposi's sarcoma, a form of skin cancer, is rare in children but may be seen in adolescents; looks like a bruise in early stages.
	Monitor laboratory reports (e.g., prothrombin times, hematocrit).	Cultures of blood, urine, throat, and stool may be ordered; child may be unable to generate a white cell response great enough to be detected in laboratories, and there may also be an abnormal response of cells.

Selected Nursing Diagnosis: Risk for impaired skin integrity related to immunosuppression

Goals	Nursing Interventions	Rationales
Skin will remain intact; patient is able to eat without discomfort.	Inspect mouth often for lesions (*Candida albicans*).	Mouth sores may prevent child from eating.
	Observe frequently for diaper rash; apply prescribed ointment; maintain skin intactness by thorough, gentle cleansing.	Skin is subject to breakdown and infection.
	Apply nystatin suspension if ordered.	Nystatin may soothe skin and promote healing.

⭐ **Nursing Care Plan 32-1**	**The Infant with HIV—cont'd**

Selected Nursing Diagnosis: Deficient family knowledge related to care of the infant after hospitalization

Goals	Nursing Interventions	Rationales
Family will verbalize understanding of the disease process, transmission, and necessary precautions.	Clarify misconceptions about the disease. Help to prepare parents for possible need for long-term follow-up care. Prepare parents adequately for discharge from hospital. Encourage parents to stay abreast of current, unfolding information. Provide ongoing support services.	Misconceptions create anxiety; there are many misconceptions about HIV/AIDS. Prognosis involves remissions and exacerbations; anti-HIV medication "cocktails" have helped to delay the onset of full-blown AIDS. Children should remain with their families and, if possible, should be managed out of the hospital with medical and social support. Newer developments may change the outcome of disease; this instills some hope in family. Because of the stigma, possible duration, and prognosis of this disease, families require much support.

Selected Nursing Diagnosis: Fear (parents and patient) related to loss of normal life or possible death

Goals	Nursing Interventions	Rationales
Parents will verbalize fears; families will develop coping skills that assist them in managing stress related to life-threatening disease.	Encourage family to support one another and keep lines of communication open. Alert parents to self-help groups. Acquire accurate knowledge about disease. Dispel inordinate fears that are common to the general public.	Fear is reduced if it can be shared. HIV/AIDS support groups or hospice can be helpful. Discuss the value of life-support measures; families may be faced with this and similarly difficult decisions. There is much inaccurate information about how HIV/AIDS is acquired and transmitted. It is important that pediatric nurses be well informed about the disease.

Critical Thinking Question

1. A new mother has been diagnosed with AIDS and is rooming-in with her infant in the pediatric unit. The mother states she wants to breastfeed her infant because she feels well enough. Her CD4+ levels are high. She states she wants herself and the infant to adhere to normal routine practices like other healthy newborns. What nursing response is appropriate?

such as Children's AIDS Program (CAP) provide a homelike respite care environment and day care. The goal of the program is to help families living with HIV/AIDS infection to stay together.

The nurse anticipates interventions related to the care of the child with a life-threatening disease. Efforts to support families in crisis are particularly pertinent. Often the extended family must take over. Many families have few financial resources and are exhausted from the child's frequent hospitalizations and physical care. They need to be introduced to such agencies as social service, financial aid, HIV/AIDS and grief support groups, home health, nutritional programs such as Women, Infants, and Children (WIC), and hospice.

Several medications are used to manage HIV/AIDS in children. A fungal infection caused by *P. jiroveci* may be the first opportunistic infection to affect the pediatric patient. Prophylactic medications are available. The nurse should be alert for central nervous system involvement such as motor deficits or a failure to achieve developmental milestones. RSV, pneumonia, renal failure, and gastrointestinal malfunction often plague the child with HIV/AIDS.

Children with HIV/AIDS should be assessed for the need to update routine immunizations. Tuberculosis testing is done routinely and as needed. Several antiviral drugs are being tested in children. Early diagnosis and treatment can improve the quality and length of life for many children.

🔖 **Nursing Tip**

Rapid HIV tests are offered to high-risk patients and include a blood sample or oral swab with results available within ½ hour. Traditional tests are used to confirm positive results. Counseling should be available to all patients.

Prevention. Prevention is the core of education related to HIV/AIDS. Education of adolescents should include methods of transmission, hazards of IV and illicit drug use, and safe sex practices. The strict use of standard precautions when caring for all patients is essential, especially when handling blood and other body fluids. The health education curriculum in elementary school for students and staff should include information concerning HIV/AIDS prevention. Nurses should encourage high-risk adolescents to undergo counseling and testing with the hope of modifying risky behaviors. Infants born to mothers with HIV may be treated with antivirals early and are monitored long-term.

Get Ready for the NCLEX® Examination!

Key Points

- *Standard precautions* are techniques recommended by the CDC to prevent the transmission of communicable diseases.
- *Body substance* refers to moist secretions of the body that can contain microorganisms.
- An *opportunistic infection* is caused by organisms normally found in the environment that the immunosuppressed child cannot fight.
- Immunization programs in the United States provide *active* immunity for children.
- Proper hand hygiene is the basic essential factor in preventing the transmission of infection.
- Proper storage of vaccines and appropriate routes of administration are essential to ensure the potency of the vaccine.
- Education of parents about the need for immunizations against common childhood communicable diseases is a primary nursing responsibility.
- It is the responsibility of the nurse to know when the immunizations are due, the immunization history of the child, contraindications, routes of administration, and which vaccines can be given together. The child should be observed for untoward reactions for at least 20 minutes following immunization.
- Koplik spots are white spots on the mucous membrane of the oral cavity that occur before a skin rash and are indicative of measles (rubeola) infection.
- In chickenpox (varicella), all stages of the skin lesions are present on the skin at the same time.
- A woman in the early months of pregnancy should not care for a child with German measles (rubella), because the virus can cause fetal anomalies.
- In children with roseola, a persistently high fever *suddenly* drops as the rash erupts.
- Gamma globulin offers *passive* immunity for exposed children who are immunosuppressed.
- The AMA and CDC offer guidelines to help families to prepare for community disasters.
- All nurses must understand their role in the hospital unit when disaster strikes.
- Maternity and pediatric nurses must understand the special vulnerability of pregnant women and small infants to agents of terrorism.
- Listening skills and a nonjudgmental attitude are essential when caring for adolescents with sexually transmitted infections (STIs).
- Children acquire the HIV/AIDS infection by contact with an infected mother at birth, sexual contact with an infected person, or use of contaminated needles during drug use.
- The long-term nursing goals in the care of a child with AIDS are to promote compliance for long-term drug therapy and to provide support to maintain optimum growth and development.

Additional Learning Resources

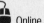
Review Questions for the NCLEX® Examination

1. The nurse is caring for a newborn with HIV/AIDS. What is the priority goal?
   1. Encourage breastfeeding.
   2. Prevent infections.
   3. Provide initial immunizations.
   4. Notify social services.

2. An adolescent diagnosed with AIDS asks about the mode of transmission for the illness. An accurate response is that it was most likely through:
   1. casual contact with a friend who is HIV-positive.
   2. a latent response to an inherited predisposition.
   3. use of a contaminated toilet seat.
   4. contact with contaminated body substance through sex or intravenous needle use.

3. When providing play therapy for a child with a communicable disease who is in an isolation room, what would be one priority principle or rationale for toy selection?

   1. The toy should be selected from the hospital playroom.
   2. Most children love books.
   3. It is best to bring the child's favorite toy from home.
   4. The toy should be washable.

4. A parent brings a 4-month-old infant to the clinic for the second in the routine immunization series. The nurse should prepare for administration of which immunizations?

   1. DTaP, Hib, polio
   2. DTaP, polio, MMR
   3. DTaP, polio, varicella
   4. Td, hepatitis, MMR

5. The DTaP immunization is administered:

   1. orally.
   2. subcutaneously.
   3. intramuscularly.
   4. intravenously.

Objectives

1. Define each key term listed.
2. Differentiate among the following terms: psychiatrist, psychoanalyst, clinical psychologist, and counselor.
3. Discuss the impact of early childhood experience on a person's adult life.
4. Discuss the effect of childhood Autism Spectrum Disorders on growth and development.
5. Discuss behavioral therapy and how it is applied to obsessive-compulsive disorders and depression in children.
6. List the symptoms of potential suicide in children and adolescents.
7. Discuss immediate and long-range plans for the suicidal patient.
8. List four behaviors that may indicate substance abuse.
9. Name two programs for members of families of alcoholics.
10. Discuss the problems facing children of alcoholics.
11. List four symptoms of attention-deficit hyperactivity disorder.
12. Describe techniques of helping children with attention-deficit hyperactivity disorder to adjust to the school setting.
13. Compare and contrast the characteristics of bulimia nervosa and anorexia nervosa.

Key Terms

art therapy (p. 747)
behavior modification (p. 747)
bibliotherapy (p. 747)
Diagnostic and Statistical Manual of Mental Disorders (5th ed., text revision) *(DSM-5)* (p. 746)
dysfunctional (p. 747)
family therapy (p. 747)

intellectual disability (p. 746)
intervention (p. 747)
milieu therapy (mēl-yoo THĔR-ă-pē, p. 747)
play therapy (p. 747)
psychosomatic (sī-kō-sō-MĂ-tĭk, p. 748)
recreation therapy (p. 747)
sibling rivalry (p. 758)

THE NURSE'S ROLE

The nurse is often the person who has the greatest amount of contact with the family. Assessing child–parent relations is an important and ongoing aspect of care. To work effectively with children with emotional or behavioral conditions, nurses first must understand the types of behavior considered within normal range. The *Diagnostic and Statistical Manual of Mental Disorders* (5th ed., text revision) *(DSM-5)* published by the American Psychiatric Association (APA) in 2013 is a resource that defines mental disorders and is used by health professionals to aid in diagnoses of specific mental health conditions. The *DSM-5* standardizes criteria alongside the World Health Organization (WHO) international classification of diseases. The *DSM-5* also identifies symptom severity for individual disorders and is compatible with disabilities resulting from the disorders as described in the International Classification of Functioning Disabilities and Health (ICF). The term **"intellectual disability"** or "intellectual

developmental disorder" replaces the term "mental retardation" and involves impairment of general mental ability that impairs functioning related to everyday tasks; this includes language, reading, math, reasoning, memory, social skills and judgment, communication skills, and self-management impairment with onset before 18 years of age. It may include an IQ below 70 and performance at least 2 standard deviations below age-appropriate norms of development. A history and physical exam, chromosomal assays of the genome, or karyotyping may be used to assist in diagnosis and early intervention.

Nurses are valuable members of the multidisciplinary health care team in that they work closely with hospitalized acutely ill children, long-term chronically ill children, and children in school. Nurses should keep a careful record of behavior and note relationships with members of the family. Such notations are meaningful to the physician and other staff members, who are as concerned with prevention of problems as they are with treating them.

Every day, everywhere, children are trying to cope with stress. Many succeed and grow stronger; some do not. Early childhood intervention programs are helpful in preventing major problems that affect growth and development. Parenting classes teach what to expect at various ages and stages. They also stress the importance of age-appropriate discipline and guidance. Parent groups provide education, socialization, and support. Other agencies provide a variety of services. Some services include the National Alliance for the Mentally Ill (NAMI), Family Service Association of America, Tough Love parenting, and National Center for Prevention of Youth Suicide. Nurses must be aware of such resources to guide parents appropriately.

When parents request guidance, the nurse encourages them to seek help from their family physician or pediatrician or from a community mental health center. In the hospital, a psychiatric clinical nurse specialist (CNS) is an excellent resource. If the child is in school, the services of the school psychologist or guidance counselor may prove valuable. Some religious centers employ counselors who are available free of charge to parishioners. Families who lack adequate financial resources can be directed to the appropriate agencies. Some agencies not only provide emergency funds but also can establish a budgeting system for those receiving minimum wages. This is particularly helpful when the parents are young adolescents.

No matter how dysfunctional the parent–child relationship, most children consciously and unconsciously identify with parental values. If the health care provider discredits the parents' values it threatens the child's security and creates anxiety. The nurse reassures parents and helps them regain or maintain confidence in their parenting role. In addition, because children do not seek treatment on their own, the nurse should assist parents in becoming invested in the treatment modality. Finally, as a professional, the nurse supports organizations concerned with mental health, votes on issues that are pertinent to the welfare of children in the community, and offers services when needed.

> ### 🏠 Nursing Tip
>
> Parents provide important assessment data about the child that the young child cannot provide. They are also important because they bring the child to therapy. Discrediting parents threatens the child and is not therapeutic.

TYPES AND SETTINGS OF TREATMENT

The basic staff of the modern child guidance clinic is composed of a psychiatrist, a psychologist, a social worker, a pediatrician, and the nurse. Usually the child guidance clinic provides diagnostic and treatment services. It may be part of a hospital, school, court, or public health or welfare service, or it may be an independent agency.

The *psychiatrist* is a medical doctor who specializes in mental disorders. The psychoanalyst is usually a psychiatrist but may be a psychologist; all psychoanalysts have advanced training in psychoanalytic theory and practice. The *clinical psychologist* has an advanced degree in clinical psychology from a recognized university. Many of these specialists work in the school system with children, teachers, and families to prevent or resolve problems. A *counselor* is a professional with a master's degree from an accredited institution. Many counselors specialize in a specific area, such as substance abuse or counseling of children. In most states, counselors must be licensed.

Children who do not respond well to individual outpatient therapy may require the type of care provided in residential treatment centers. Their home situations may be so disruptive that they might benefit from a change of environment. This alternative also provides a cooling-down period for the family. **Family therapy** is begun and includes all family members. The length of stay for the child varies from 1 to 3 weeks. Partial hospitalization programs in which the child attends therapy during the day and returns home at night are popular.

An **intervention** is a planned event by others to get someone into professional counseling for addiction or a life crisis. It may be direct (confrontational) or indirect (referral) and may involve individual, family, or group therapy; behavior modification; or milieu therapy. It may also involve a combination of these therapies. **Behavior modification** focuses on modifying specific behaviors by means of stimulus and response conditioning. **Milieu therapy** refers to the physical and social environment provided for the child. **Art therapy**, *music therapy,* and **play therapy** are particularly helpful for interacting with younger children who have difficulty expressing themselves. **Recreation therapy** is also valuable. **Bibliotherapy**, the reading of stories about children in a situation similar to the child's situation, is also therapeutic. Creating an *emotionally safe environment* is basic to all forms of therapy.

ORIGINS OF EMOTIONAL AND BEHAVIORAL CONDITIONS

Early childhood experiences are critical to personality formation. Situations that disrupt family patterns can have a lasting impact on the child. Children who come from these **dysfunctional** families may experience any of the following: failure to develop a sense of trust (in their caregivers and environment), excessive fears, misdirected anger manifested as behavioral problems, depression, low self-esteem, lack of confidence, and feelings of lack of control over themselves and their environment. These and other manifestations may make children feel negative about themselves and the world. They experience guilt and may blame themselves when confronted with disappointment and failure.

Growing up can be painful even under the best circumstances. It is difficult for the child in the early school years to live up to so many rapidly developing standards. Guilt and anxiety develop. Finger sucking, nail biting, excessive fears, stuttering, and conduct problems are reflections of nervous tension.

The current trend toward prevention by identifying risk factors and advocating early intervention is a major goal of children's mental health services. The term **psychosomatic** has come to refer to the dysfunctions of the body that seem to have an emotional or a mental root. Each person has a different potential for coping with life. Truancy, lying, stealing, failure in school, and a crisis such as death or divorce of parents are but a few of the difficulties that may necessitate intervention.

ORGANIC BEHAVIORAL DISORDERS

Mental health and cognition differ in children and adults because the various stages of growth and development impact the perceptions and responses of the child. The brain matures, experiences expand, and interactions with others all build mental health. Early bonding and attachment are essential parts of developing positive mental health. Children must rely on adults for their experiences, and the environment, as well as genetics, plays a role in mental health. The nurse assesses the level of development, social skills, affect, eye contact, face and body expressions, appearance, and behavior. The main goal of therapy is to assist the family to promote an optimal level of functioning. A thorough understanding of growth and development, developmental needs, expectations, and abilities is essential.

AUTISM SPECTRUM DISORDERS (ASD)

The CDC has shown that 1 in 88 or 1% of children has ASD, which represents a 23% increase from 2009 and a 78% increase from 2007 (Peterson, 2013). ASD is a group of neurodevelopmental disorders characterized by difficulties in social interaction and communication, repetitive behaviors, and stereotyped interests and activities (Peterson, 2013). Three types have been identified:

1. Classic autism
2. Asperger syndrome
3. Pervasive developmental disorders

The cause is unknown, although some studies suggest an association with neonatal jaundice or older fathers (Lindstrom, 2010). However, a genetic link has been identified (Devlin, 2012). The Childhood Autism Risk from Genetics and Environment (CHARGE) studied preschool children with autism and has shown the role of prenatal vitamins in early pregnancy. There is the possibility that ASD might be prevented with the intake of folic acid supplements for 3 months before pregnancy begins (Lockwood, 2013). There are several genetic syndromes that exhibit symptoms similar to autism, such as Rett syndrome, fragile X syndrome, and Prader-Willi syndrome, but the relationship is unclear. Parents need to be educated concerning normal growth and development so they can recognize deviations and seek early interventions. Red flags to report include:

- No babbling or pointing by 12 months
- No 2-word spontaneous phrases by 24 months
- Loss of social skills or language previously attained

Routine screening before 2 years of age during scheduled clinic visits is advised. The Modified Checklist for Autism in Toddlers (M-CHAT) and the Ages and Stages questionnaire are two popular screening tools. Federal law funds early intervention programs for identified at-risk children. The website www.healthychildren.org is a referral source for parents. Peer-related social behavior normally develops early in the preschool period, with symbolic play normally emerging by 2 years of age. ASD children do not show interest in other children and have difficulty engaging in pretend play. Solitary play is the preference of the child with ASD.

Treatment of ASD involves providing well-structured home and school environments, behavior modification, and in some cases the use of specific drugs to manage specific behavioral problems. The goal of therapy is to maximize the ability to live independently.

Drug therapy of ASD is not curative. A multidisciplinary approach to care is essential. The nurse's role is to identify abnormal behavior as early as possible, refer for follow-up care, and monitor the side effects of prescribed medications.

The nurse's approach to the patient should be slow paced, with few distractions. The child should be allowed to become familiar with the office, room, or equipment. Permission should be asked of the child before touching him or her, and sudden movements or loud noise should be avoided. Safety and family support are priorities. The development of meaningful language by 5 years of age is a favorable prognosis.

OBSESSIVE-COMPULSIVE DISORDERS IN CHILDREN

With obsessive-compulsive disorder (OCD), a recurrent, persistent, repetitive thought invades the conscious mind (obsession), or a ritual movement or activity (not related to adapting to the environment) assumes inordinate importance (compulsion). The rituals or movements may involve touching an object, saying a certain word, or washing the hands repetitively. OCD in children differs from OCD in adults in that the children's symptoms are not usually part of an obsessive personality. The behavior may start as early as 4 years of age but may not be noticed as interfering with daily functioning until 10 years of age or older.

OCD does not involve an impairment of cognitive function or interpersonal relationships. Poor school performance is related to compulsive repetitive behavior rather than a deficit in intelligence. Family conflicts arise to compound the problem.

Behavior therapy combined with medication provides the best results. The treatment involves exposure to the stressor or obsession and prevention of the compulsory response. For behavior therapy to be successful, however, the child must be motivated and capable of following directions. Parent and sibling involvement and support are essential. The nurse's role is to assess normal growth and development and to understand that ritualistic behavior that is normal at 3 years of age is normally replaced by hobbies of collecting and special interests by 8 years of age. Prolonged ritualistic behavior should be referred for follow-up care. Assessing the response to and side effects of medications used to treat OCD is an important nursing role. In *DSM-5*, several other disorders have been listed under OCD. They include: body dysmorphic disorder, trichotillomania (hair-pulling disorder), hoarding disorder, and excoriation disorder (skin picking).

ATTENTION-DEFICIT HYPERACTIVITY DISORDER (ADHD)

***Pathophysiology. Attention-deficit hyperactivity disorder** (ADHD)* refers to a developmentally inappropriate degree of gross motor activity, impulsivity, and inattention in the school or home setting that begins before age 7 years, lasts more than 6 months, and is not related to the existence of any other central nervous system illness. It occurs more often in some families, which suggests a genetic connection. ADHD that occurs together with ASD may have more serious cognitive disabilities. The *DSM-5* (2013) has defined the condition and has established specific criteria for diagnosis. ADHD can persist through adulthood.

Manifestations. The childhood criteria for diagnosis of ADHD include at least 6 symptoms, and adulthood criteria require 5 symptoms for diagnosis.

Learning disability is an educational term; however, learning disabilities often occur in children with ADHD. Although these children may have average or above-average intellectual ability, they experience difficulties in areas such as the following:

- *Receptive language:* listening and understanding
- *Expressive language:* an inability to express ideas
- *Information processing:* differentiating words that look or sound alike
- *Memory:* remembering personal information or spelling
- *Motor coordination:* copying forms, printing, writing
- *Orientation:* confusing left and right
- *Behavioral problem:* difficulty in concentrating, impatience

Dyslexia (reading difficulties) and *dysgraphia* (writing difficulties) may be apparent. These children may transpose letters; for example, they may read "pot" for "top." They may also have difficulty in expressing themselves. Some symptoms include:

- *Inattention* (at least three of the following): is easily distracted, needs a calm atmosphere in which to work, fails to complete work, does not appear to listen, has difficulty concentrating unless instruction is one-to-one, needs information repeated
- *Impulsivity* (at least three of the following): is disruptive with other children, talks out in class, is extremely excitable, cannot wait turn, is overly talkative, requires a lot of supervision
- *Hyperactivity* (at least two of the following): climbs on furniture, fidgets, is always "on the go," cannot stay seated, does things in a loud and noisy way

In 2013, the FDA approved a noninvasive brainwave test to assist in the diagnosis of ADHD. The Neuropsychiatric EEG Assessment Aid (NEBA) detects elevated theta brain waves that occur with ADHD (Lockwood, 2013b).

 Nursing Tip

ADHD is characterized by inattention, hyperactivity, impulsivity, and distractibility.

The history of the ADHD patient involves a description of the child's behavior and responses, an observation of parenting style, and an understanding of the existing family stresses. The coping strategies of the child should be observed, and input from schoolteachers is sought. Psychologists may interpret behavior-rating scales administered to the child.

Management. The management of ADHD is multidisciplinary. Family education to manage their knowledge deficit about the condition, counseling to help the family and child cope with the problems encountered, and medication to help control some symptoms are the core of therapy.

Health Promotion

Emphasizing the strengths of the child rather than the problems is essential to any plan of care.

Various support groups can aid parents in their coping skills. The school nurse can help teachers develop strategies for managing children with ADHD in the classroom (see Health Promotion box). Increasing positive interactions, providing tutoring, giving computer assistance, and using behavioral management strategies under the supervision of a professional psychologist are helpful approaches to care. ADHD is a chronic condition that can persist through adulthood. Some children who are "labeled" in school develop low self-esteem and antisocial behavior.

ANOREXIA NERVOSA

Pathophysiology. **Anorexia nervosa** (*anorexia,* "want of appetite," and *nervosa,* "nervous") is a form of self-starvation seen mostly in adolescent girls. Only 10% of patients with eating disorders are male. The criteria for this disorder are well outlined in the *DSM-5* (APA, 2013). It is classified under *"Binge eating disorder,"* and it is characterized by the following:

- Failure to maintain the minimum normal weight for age and height (less than 85% of expected weight)
- An intense fear of gaining weight
- Excess influence of body weight on self-evaluation
- Amenorrhea

The adolescents characteristically have average to superior intelligence and are overachievers who expect to be perfect in all areas. For young people with the disorder, their own emerging sexuality is very threatening. They experience anxiety and guilt over an imagined or a real fear of intimacy. They have low self-esteem, are obedient, and are nonassertive and shy.

Families of these young people are often dysfunctional. They may exhibit such abnormal behaviors as overprotectiveness, rigidity, lack of privacy, and inability to resolve conflicts. There is often a power struggle between child and parent. Children may feel that the only thing they can control in their environment is what they put into their mouth. Affluent families may be at high risk when the concept of being thinner rules and the focus is on diet and exercise.

Manifestations. The primary symptom of anorexia nervosa is severe weight loss. Adolescents who wish to be fashion models or actresses or who participate in sports, dance, or gymnastics activities may be at risk for developing an eating disorder. On physical examination, some of the following conditions may be evident: dry skin, amenorrhea, lanugo hair over the back and extremities, cold intolerance, low blood pressure, abdominal pain, and constipation.

Adolescents with anorexia experience feelings of helplessness, lack of control, low self-esteem, and depression. Socialization with peers diminishes. Mealtime becomes a family battleground. The body image becomes increasingly disturbed (Figure 33-1), and there is a lack of self-identity. The young person remains egocentric and unable to complete normal adolescent tasks. Although eating less, the anorexic

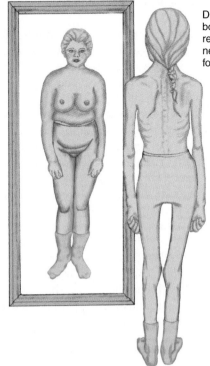

Distorted body image results in extreme need to control food intake.

Amenorrhea
Lanugo
Fatigue
Constipation
Dry, flaky skin
Severe caries
Dull, brittle hair
Muscle wasting

FIGURE 33-1 Adolescents with eating disorders often have a disturbed self-image. (From McKinney ES, James SR, Murray SS, et al: *Maternal-child nursing,* ed 4, St. Louis, Saunders.)

individual is preoccupied with food and its preparation. Hunger is denied. The patient complains of bloating and abdominal pain after ingesting small amounts of food.

Treatment and Nursing Care. The treatment of anorexia nervosa is complex and involves several modalities. Some hospitals have eating disorder units. A brief period of hospitalization may be necessary to correct electrolyte imbalance, establish a minimum restoration of nutrients, and stabilize the patient's weight. It also provides a time-out from a dysfunctional home environment.

Therapies include individual and family psychotherapy, behavior therapy, and pharmacological therapy (Lock, 2011). Antidepressant medications may be helpful (Flament, 2012). The nurse plays an important role in ensuring that the atmosphere is relaxed and nonpunitive. Follow-up after discharge from the unit is essential. Individual and family therapy is continued.

Nurses working with adolescents in any capacity must be alert to the symptoms of this condition; a lack of recognition is one of the biggest obstacles to treatment. In the early stages, dissatisfaction with body image, amenorrhea, and social isolation are suspect. Young people must be educated about the seriousness of the disorder. Educational materials, referral sources, and counseling are available from the National Association of Anorexia Nervosa and Associated Disorders.

Encouragement and support from self-help groups are also valuable.

Prognosis. Most patients gain weight in the hospital regardless of the type of therapy. However, this may not predict future success. Complications include gastritis, cardiac dysrhythmias, inflammation of the intestine, and kidney problems. Fatalities do occur, particularly in untreated persons. Approximately 50% of patients are cured, approximately 30% improve but continue to have dysfunctional eating problems and a distorted body image (although they function well in school and at work), and approximately 15% remain chronically ill through adulthood.

BULIMIA

Bulimia, or compulsive eating, is recognized by the *DSM-5* as a *"Binge eating disorder."* It has been estimated that as many as 5% of college women and 1% of college men have this condition. It is characterized by recurrent episodes of uncontrolled eating of more food in a short time than is considered normal and is followed by self-induced vomiting and the misuse of laxatives and/or diuretics on a weekly basis for more than 3 months duration.

Family dysfunctions are usually present in children with bulimia; unlike with anorexia, however, the mother–daughter relationship is usually distant or strained. Depression and alcoholism may be a family problem. The binge–purge cycle is thought to be a coping mechanism for handling guilt, depression, and low self-esteem. Impulsive behaviors are characteristic of adolescents with bulimia.

Persistent vomiting can cause erosion of tooth enamel and eventual tooth loss. The use of laxatives and self-induced vomiting can cause electrolyte imbalance. Muscle weakness will result if emetics are routinely used to induce vomiting. The HEADSSS (**H**ome, **E**mployment or **E**ducation, **A**ctivities, **D**rugs, **S**exual activity, **S**uicidal ideas, **S**afety) format of interviewing adolescents is helpful in obtaining a detailed assessment.

The nursing role in coping with adolescents with eating disorders is to educate, prevent, identify, and refer. It is very difficult to identify an adolescent with a weight obsession in a society in which weight and thinness define beauty. This concept is reinforced in movies and magazines. The nurse should maintain a supportive and respectful, but firm, manner. Establishing trust with the adolescent is the first step in education, referral, and treatment. Adolescents with eating disorders must maintain a sense of control in their therapy for success to be achieved. Compromise and contracts must replace authoritative restrictions on diet and activity. A referral to support groups and child and family counseling groups is helpful. A multidisciplinary approach with nurse, pediatrician, nutritionist, psychiatrist, and social worker helps to achieve a positive outcome.

Other identified conditions listed in the *DSM-5* 2013 that may be found in the pediatric population include, but are not limited to the following disorders, which have been defined but are awaiting evidence-based management strategies.

DISRUPTIVE MOOD REGULATION DISORDER

This disorder is characterized by a daily persistently irritable or angry mood between the ages of 6 and 18 years that lasts more than one year and is evident in both home and nonhome settings.

OPPOSITIONAL DEFIANT DISORDER (ODD)

ODD is described as an ongoing pattern of anger-guided disobedience or a hostile or defiant response to authority. **Bipolar disorder** may include behaviors described previously but they occur *episodically* rather than daily and may not be as serious as ODD or disruptive mood regulation disorders.

CONDUCT DISORDER

This disorder is characterized by behavior that violates the rights of others or rules of society. It evidences an unemotional interpersonal style with limited empathy or concern for others.

INTERNET GAMING DISORDER

This is not yet included in *DSM-5* as a formal disorder but is identified as needing further research and study. The condition involves compulsive Internet game playing that excludes other interests, endangers academics or employment, and results in withdrawal symptoms if stopped.

ENVIRONMENTAL OR BIOCHEMICAL BEHAVIORAL DISORDERS

Social anxiety disorders affect 1 in 10 adolescents but only 1 in 5 are ever diagnosed or treated for social anxiety (Burstein, 2012). Many adolescents are shy, but social anxiety disorders are marked by fear or anxiety in social situations that involve observation and possible criticism by others (Burstein, 2012). The adolescent fears embarrassment or rejection to the extent they may avoid social situations. Basic shyness can be a totally normal characteristic and should not be confused with a social anxiety disorder, which most often involves distress that impairs functioning.

DEPRESSION

Depression in a child is not as easy to identify as depression in an adult. Many children have difficulty expressing their feelings and often "act out" their concerns. Depression is an emotion common to childhood. Sadness caused by receiving poor grades, moving to a new community, or losing a pet may trigger a depressive mood that results in either a dependent type or a disruptive type of behavior. These manifestations are resolved in a short time and are considered perfectly normal.

Manifestations. A major depressive or mood disorder is usually characterized by a prolonged behavioral change from baseline that interferes with schooling, family life, and/or age-specific activities. Symptoms can include loss of appetite, sleep problems, lethargy, social withdrawal, and sudden drop in grades. In young children, head banging, truancy, lying, and stealing can occur. If left untreated, depressive behavior can lead to substance abuse and/or suicide. Inheritance factors, organic factors, and environmental factors all contribute to major depressive disorders in children. Treatment of depressive disorders is often on an outpatient basis and may include prescribed drugs.

Management. Nursing responsibilities include recognizing the signs of depression and initiating appropriate and prompt referral (Nursing Care Plan 33-1). Educating parents and school personnel concerning the identification of children at risk is an important nursing function in the community and in the hospital setting. A depression toolkit for professionals is available free at www.depression-primarycare.org/clinicians/toolkits/full/. The toolkit contains evidence-based practice information concerning the approach and treatment of depression and sample patient questionnaires that can be used.

Tricyclic antidepressant medication is often prescribed for children and adolescents diagnosed with depression.

⭐ Nursing Care Plan 33-1 | The Depressed Adolescent

PATIENT DATA An adolescent is admitted with a diagnosis of depression after a failed suicide attempt

Selected Nursing Diagnosis: Risk for self-directed violence related to depression and stress

Goals	Nursing Interventions	Rationales
Adolescent will state whether suicide is contemplated. Adolescent does not harm self. Adolescent will verbalize acceptance of protective measures. Family will verbalize seriousness of suicidal threats.	Ask adolescent if suicidal thoughts are present.	This information is important to know because it will determine intervention; most depressed adolescents are filled with contradictory feelings; talking honestly about feelings helps to clarify them.
	Inquire about precipitating event (e.g., broken romance, poor grades).	Suicidal reactions are associated with feelings of hopelessness, often related to the loss of a significant or valued relationship or to a disappointment.
	Determine if the adolescent has specific suicidal plan.	How person plans to take his or her life is one of the most significant criteria for assessing suicidal potential; more specific plans are a more dangerous threat.
	Determine if the adolescent has a history of suicidal attempts.	The situation is considered more critical if the adolescent has made serious attempts in the past.
	Determine if the adolescent has a history of emotional instability.	A history of emotional instability is more dangerous.
	Determine if the adolescent has the means available to injure himself or herself.	If the means to commit suicide are available (e.g., drugs, gun), the threat is imminent and more serious.
	Provide supervision as outlined by the physician or institution.	Surveillance and support by staff and family are important.
	Determine if a "safe contract" has been signed and discussed with the adolescent.	This is a written agreement that the adolescent will contact a nurse, counselor, or crisis line or go to an emergency department before harming self.
	The family will attend team conferences as appropriate.	It is wise to have available as many persons as possible to support one another and to share the stress of the situation.
	Administer antidepressants if ordered.	Antidepressants elevate the mood of the patient; unfortunately, most antidepressants must be taken for 3 to 4 weeks before a therapeutic response is evident; some require monitoring of blood values.
	Monitor room for potentially dangerous articles.	Belts, glasses, rope, and other materials may be used to self-destruct.
	Explain precautions to the adolescent and family members.	Explanations will lessen fear and increase compliance.
	Reinforce to parents the seriousness of the adolescent's suicidal threat.	All suicidal threats need to be taken seriously.

⭐ **Nursing Care Plan 33-1**   **The Depressed Adolescent—cont'd**

Selected Nursing Diagnosis: Ineffective coping related to poor self-esteem, isolation, and inability to handle painful feelings

Goals	Nursing Interventions	Rationales
Adolescent will make a positive statement about self. Adolescent will accept positive statements from others. Adolescent will accept the presence of the nurse, peers, or significant others.	Have the adolescent list two positive things about self and reinforce daily. Instruct the adolescent to draw "how I see myself" and "how others see me."	Determines adolescent's strengths so the nurse can build on them. Provides valuable information about the adolescent's self-esteem. Self-destructive behavior reflects underlying depression related to low self-esteem and anger directed inward. Drawing offers a release from feelings, helps to clarify emotions, and is a vehicle for discussion between the patient and the nurse.
	Build extra time into visits so that the adolescent does not feel rushed; give your undivided attention.	This indicates that you are truly interested; a ringing telephone and personal interruptions devalue the visit.
Adolescent will gradually cope with painful feelings by sharing and expressing them either verbally or nonverbally.	Instruct the adolescent to draw a box and put things that bring happy feelings in the box; then instruct to draw another box and place things that cause sadness in that box. Encourage the adolescent to verbalize feelings about drawings; respect the adolescent's wish not to talk should this occur.	Drawings help adolescents to distance themselves from the problem and see it more clearly.
Adolescent will speak in future terms. Adolescent states two healthy coping measures.	Review methods of coping.	Discovering how the adolescent coped in the past when he or she was less distressed is of importance so that these methods can be reinforced.
	Suggest healthy methods of coping such as exercise, relaxation tapes, and talking things out with parents or peers.	Many adolescents are not aware of healthy coping methods.

The nurse should be alert for side effects such as cardiac changes and increase in blood pressure and should report deviations promptly. An SSRI medication blocks reuptake of serotonin so that serotonin levels increase to improve mood and behavior. A serious side effect of SSRI medication is "serotonin syndrome," which is manifested by muscle twitching, GI upset, and dizziness that is caused by overstimulation of serotonin receptors. At highest risk for this complication are adolescents who use alcohol, diet pills, over-the-counter medications, or recreational drugs. Close monitoring is essential.

SUICIDE

Suicide is the third leading cause of death in adolescents after accidents and homicide. Completed suicides are more common in boys than in girls, but girls make more attempts using less lethal means. Many adolescent suicides are not intended to end in death but instead are a cry for help that may end tragically. The risk of a successful suicide increases when there is a plan of action, a means to carry out the plan, and an absence of obvious resources to turn to for help. The breakdown of family ties, pressure to succeed, or foiled relationships may trigger a low self-esteem or frustration that results in the turning of feelings of hostility or hopelessness inward.

Suicidal behaviors can be identified as *suicidal ideation,* which involves thoughts about suicide; *suicidal gestures,* which are an attempt at a suicidal action that does not result in injury; and a *suicidal attempt,* an action that is seriously intended to cause death (although it may be unsuccessful). Some adolescents may exhibit rage behavior or an emotional outburst that results in an *impulsive act* that can result in accidental death. Some adolescents display a chronic type of high-risk behavior that can lead to serious injury or death. The nurse's role lies in education, prevention, and identification of those children at risk and prompt referral for follow-up care.

 Safety Alert!

Every threat of suicide must be taken seriously.

Some manifestations of suicidal behavior include a flat affect or a "fixed" facial expression, a deterioration in school performance, isolation from friends and family, changes in physical appearance, giving away of cherished possessions, and talk of death. The nurse is a vital link in working with school personnel to develop peer support groups and educate families concerning the available community resources. Mental health associations, hotlines, drop-in centers, safe houses, and free clinics are community resources that can be helpful to use. The USDHHS offers free publications that can be used as a suicide prevention toolkit, containing valuable patient management tools. A pocket guide for medical professionals is available from Western Interstate Committee for Higher Education. The 5 steps of the SAFE-T program include:

1. Identifying risk (warning signs)
2. Identifying protective factors (coping strategies; support persons)
3. Suicide inquiry (identify plans)
4. Determine risk level (interventions)
5. Document and follow-up

Further details about the toolkits can be accessed at www.SPRC.org/for-providers.

The suicide hotline should be well publicized for all teens at 1-800-273-TALK.

Nursing Tip

When an adolescent feels hopeless and talks about feeling useless or worthless, do not contradict what he or she is saying. Instead listen, indicate your understanding, and encourage the expression of feelings.

SUBSTANCE ABUSE

Substance abuse is the illegal use of drugs, alcohol, or tobacco for the purpose of producing an altered state of consciousness. Substances may be ingested, injected, or inhaled to produce the desired effect. Four levels of substance abuse have been established: *experimentation, controlled use, abuse,* and *dependence.* Although there is often a fine line between controlled use and abuse, frequency may be a major signal. This is especially true when accompanied by inappropriateness, such as "getting stoned" at the weekend party versus on the way to school.

There are two types of dependence: *psychological* and *physical.* Psychological dependence includes a craving for and a compulsive need to use a substance. Physical dependence occurs with drugs such as heroin and alcohol. People become "hooked on the drug" and experience physical withdrawal symptoms in addition to psychological dependence. *Tolerance* develops when a user's body becomes accustomed to certain drugs. The person must then increase the dose each time to maintain its effect. Life-threatening reactions to synthetic cannabinoids resulted in almost 3000 calls to

the poison control center in 2010 and almost 7000 calls in 2011 (Saha, 2011), and these cannabinoids are advertised on the Internet and easily available in head shops and tobacco stores. Bath salts are packaged in colorful packets resembling tea and are more potent than plant-based products. They can be snorted, eaten, taken rectally, or injected. Bath salts cause euphoria, nausea, tachycardia, headache, panic, agitation, hallucinations, self-injury, and seizures (Saha, 2012). Drugs of abuse often have "nicknames." Bath salts are also known as "Bliss," "Blue silk," "Purple wave," and "Vanilla Sky" (McGraw, 2012).

Almost every drug of abuse harms some tissue or organ in addition to the brain, but the developing brain of the child and adolescent may suffer more injury than the mature brain and organs of the adult. Table 33-1 summarizes the characteristics of some of the more commonly abused drugs and the adolescent's reactions to them. Table 33-2 lists street names for some of these drugs.

Alcohol

Experimentation with alcohol has traditionally been accepted as a normal part of growing up. Most states have legal drinking age laws that are well defined and enforced. However, studies have shown that many eighth-grade children have experimented with beverages containing alcohol. Nurses must educate the public that alcoholism is a disease with established criteria that are both treatable and preventable. The devastating physical consequences of alcohol abuse as well as the increased risk of accidents and injury should be discussed with children as early as elementary-school age. School nurses and parent–teacher associations can work together to prevent alcohol abuse and identify alcohol abusers who can be referred for follow-up care. Al-Anon, Alateen, and Alcoholics Anonymous (AA) are programs listed on the Internet and in most local telephone directories in the United States, and they welcome the young adolescent seeking help with an alcohol problem. Alcoholism is often a family disease. Adults often serve alcohol freely at social events in the home and therefore offer mixed messages about alcohol use to their children.

Cocaine

The easy availability of cocaine and the affordability of "crack" cocaine are the causes of increased experimentation by children. The drug can be snorted, smoked, or used intravenously. The drug can cause life-threatening systemic responses as well as aggressive, antisocial behavior. Acute overdose can result in death. Treatment usually necessitates inpatient residential care.

Gateway Substances

Gateway substances are common household products and alcohol that can be abused to achieve an altered state of consciousness, or a "high" (Figure 33-2).

Table 33-1 **Characteristics of Abused Drugs and Their Acute Reactions in Adolescents***

CLASS	EXAMPLE	ROUTE	BEHAVIORAL SIGNS	PHYSICAL SIGNS	MEDICAL COMPLICATIONS
Opiates	Heroin, methadone, morphine	Subcutaneous, intranasal, intravenous	Euphoria, lethargy to coma	Constricted pupils, respiratory depression, cyanosis, rales, needle marks	Injection site infection, hepatitis, bacterial endocarditis, amenorrhea, peptic ulcer, pulmonary edema, tetanus
Hypnotics, sedatives	Barbiturates, glutethimide	Oral, intravenous	Slurred speech, ataxia, short attention span, drowsiness, combativeness, violence	Constricted pupils (barbiturates), dilated pupils (glutethimide), needle marks	Injection site infection, hepatitis, endocarditis
	Alcohol	Oral	As above		Gastritis, CNS infection, depression
Stimulants	Amphetamines	Oral, subcutaneous, intravenous	Hyperactivity, insomnia, anorexia, paranoia, personality change, irritability	Hypertension, weight loss, dilated pupils	Injection site infection, hepatitis, endocarditis, psychosis, depression
	Cocaine	Intravenous, intranasal	Restlessness, hyperactivity, occasional depression or paranoia	Hypertension, tachycardia	Nausea, vomiting, inflammation or perforation of nasal septum
Hallucinogens	LSD, THC, PCP, STP (DOM), mescaline, DMT	Oral, inhaled	Euphoria, dysphoria, hallucinations, confusion, paranoia	Dilated pupils, occasional hypertension, hyperthermia, piloerection	Primarily psychiatric with high risk to individuals with unrecognized or previous psychiatric disorder
Hydrocarbons, fluorocarbons	Glue (toluene)	Inhalant	Euphoria, confusion, general intoxication	Nonspecific	Secondary trauma, asphyxiation from plastic bag used to inhale fumes
	Cleaning fluid (trichloroethylene)	Inhalant	Euphoria, confusion, general intoxication, vomiting, abdominal pain	Oliguria, jaundice	Hepatitis, renal injury
	Aerosol sprays, Freon	Inhalant	Euphoria, dysphoria, slurred speech, hallucinations	Nonspecific	Psychiatric
Cannabis	Marijuana, hashish, THC	Smoke, oral	Mild intoxication and simple euphoria to hallucination (dose-related)	Occasional tachycardia, delayed response time, poor coordination	Occasionally psychiatric, with depressive or anxiety reactions

CNS, Central nervous system; *DMT*, dimethyltryptamine; *LSD*, lysergic acid diethylamide; *PCP*, phencyclidine hydrochloride; *STP* (DOM), 2,5-dimethoxy-4-methylamphetamine; *THC*, tetrahydrocannabinol.

*Data modified from Kliegman R et al: *Nelson essentials of pediatrics,* ed 6, Philadelphia, 2005, Saunders; Kliegman R et al: *Nelson textbook of pediatrics,* ed 19, Philadelphia, 2011, Saunders; Endo Pharmaceuticals National Supporter: *Drug Guide for Parents;* www.Timetotalk.org, accessed December 2013; www.drugfree.org/drug_chart_10.25, accessed January 2014.

Table 33-2	Street Names for Commonly Abused Drugs*
STREET NAME	**DRUG**
Ice; chalk; crystal; speed	Methamphetamine
Apache; goodfella; TNT	Fentanyl
Angel dust; cliffhanger	Phencyclidine hydrochloride (PCP)
Bin laden*; brown sugar; smack	Heroin (after September 11, 2001)*
Acid; boomers; cubes; crack	Lysergic acid diethylamide (LSD)
Charlie, coke; candy; snow	Cocaine
Downers	Barbiturates or tranquilizers
E hug-drug; Adam; bean	Ecstasy (methylenedioxymethamphetamine)
Gamma; cherry meth; soap oh scoop	Gamma hydroxybutyrate (GHB)
Goof ball	Cocaine mixed with heroin; depressants
K2; spice; JWH	Synthetic cannabinoids (packed to resemble tea or incense)
Bath salts; goob; cat; gaggers	Cathinones (from khat plant)
Joint; grass; pot; ditch	Marijuana cigarette
Kicker	Oxycontin
Pikachu	Pills containing PCP and ecstasy
Roofies; circles; woolfies	Rohypnol
Vitamin K; ket; purple	Ketamine
Yellow jackets	Pentobarbital

*These names often change and vary within subcultures.
Data from http://casapalmera.com/top-20-drugs-and-their-street-names/ accessed 12/13; Endo Pharmaceuticals, National Supporter: *Drug guide for parents*; National Institute of Drug Abuse. 2010; Saha S, Willson J, Adger H: K2 spice and bath salts: new drugs of abuse, *Pediatrics* 29(10):22-31, 2012; Kliegman R et al: *Nelson textbook of pediatrics*, ed 19, Philadelphia, 2011, Saunders.

A feeling of euphoria can be followed by central nervous system depression, seizures, and cardiac arrest. "Huffing" substances include cleaning fluid, glue, lighter fluid, paints, shoe polish, various aerosols, and gasolines that are inhaled in various ways. They are called gateway substances because their use often leads to the abuse of stronger drugs (such as cocaine) and drug addiction.

⚠ Safety Alert!

It has been estimated that more than 2 million people in the United States use cocaine on a regular basis. "Crack" is a popular form of cocaine and can be extremely addictive.

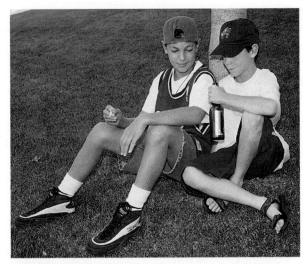

FIGURE 33-2 Beer and cigarettes used by young adolescents are considered "gateway" substances that can lead to other illegal substances. (From Bowden VR, Dickey SB, Greenberg SC: *Children and their families: the continuum of care*, Philadelphia, 1998, Saunders.)

Marijuana

Marijuana is a hemp plant *(Cannabis sativa)*. Hashish, the portion of the plant that is most potent, is smoked or ingested and rapidly absorbed by the body and metabolized by the liver. Asthmatic children can have serious reactions because of the bronchoconstriction that occurs when smoking this substance. A loss of inhibitions, euphoria, and a loss of coordination and of goal-direction are associated with the use of this substance. Users should be referred for professional counseling.

Opiates

Heroin is the most common opiate abused by adolescents. Because opiate users often drop out of school, statistics concerning use by children in school are lacking. The main consequence of heroin abuse is related to the sharing of unsterile needles, which places the adolescent at risk for human immunodeficiency virus (HIV) infection. Hepatitis and other infections are also common among heroin users. Long-term treatment programs are the therapy of choice for adolescents.

Prevention and Nursing Goals

The prevention of substance abuse begins by helping expectant parents to develop good parenting skills. It is imperative that children learn to feel good about themselves very early in life. They need a safe environment and adults whom they can trust and who serve as good role models. As orderly development proceeds, the growing child learns to interact with others and develops a sense of identity. A positive self-image and feelings of self-worth help adolescents fine-tune their adaptive coping skills. In time, they rely on their own problem-solving abilities and ideally do not need chemicals to manage the complexities of life. Nurses in their various settings can contribute to this process.

They can also educate their patients about the seriousness of substance abuse.

Although it is generally true that problem drinkers cannot be helped unless they want to be helped, more *intervention* is now being performed. Most adolescents involved in substance abuse do not choose to enter treatment but are coerced by family members or the juvenile justice system. Although the issue is controversial, clinical experience in substance abuse treatment settings has shown that many adolescents become interested in treatment and make behavioral changes after they have been required to enter a treatment program.

Children of Alcoholics

Pathophysiology. Until recently, little attention has been shown to children of alcoholics. This trend is changing, and support groups such as Adult Children of Alcoholics are more numerous. This discussion is directed to young children of alcoholics, although unresolved issues are similar in adults. Pediatric nurses are in an excellent position to recognize and intervene in cases in which physical or emotional neglect exists because of parental alcoholism. These problems stem from the parents' preoccupation with the disease. It is not unusual for both parents to be users.

Children of alcoholics are often confused by the unpredictability of family life. They do not understand why their needs are not being met. In some families there is a role reversal, with the child being forced to act maturely and make decisions ordinarily assumed by a parent. Often these children believe they are responsible for the disruptive environment. They are at high risk for emotional or physical abuse, including sexual abuse. Children of alcoholics are also strong candidates for becoming alcoholics as adults. Role models are distorted or lacking. A parent may try to cover up for the alcohol-abusing partner by lying to employers and relatives but may punish the child for the same behavior. The child may become isolated from peers while trying to avoid embarrassment at home.

Four predominant coping patterns of children of alcoholics are flight, fight, the perfect child, and the super coper or family savior (Figure 33-3). The child who flees may do so literally or emotionally. The goal is to get away; as the child grows older, more and more time is spent away from home. Feelings are buried and left unexpressed. The child fighter is aggressive and displays acting-out behavior. The perfect child tries to gain love by never causing any trouble; he or she is obedient and is generally a good student. The savior

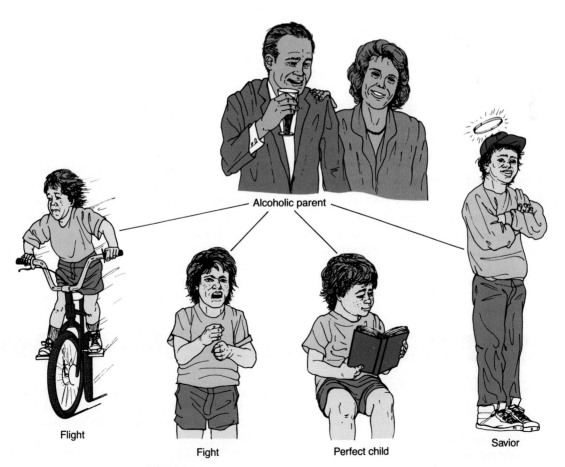

Alcoholic parent

Flight   Fight   Perfect child   Savior

FIGURE 33-3 Some defense patterns of children of alcoholics.

or super coper feels overly responsible, often has a job to help out, and tries to do everything perfectly.

Manifestations, Nursing Care, and Treatment. Early recognition of and intervention for children of alcoholics are paramount. The astute nurse with a heightened awareness of alcoholism can expand admission observations and nursing history. Some clues that may or may not be related to this problem include a refusal to talk about family life, poor school grades or overachievement, an unusual need to please, fatigue, passive or acting-out behavior, or maturity beyond the child's years. Treatment is multifold. One immediate priority is to teach the child how to get help in an emergency and to put him or her in touch with someone from the extended family, the school, or another suitable agency. Cultural diversities must be incorporated into treatment plans.

MINIMIZING THE IMPACT OF BEHAVIORAL DISORDERS IN CHILDREN

The primary care physician gathers data concerning behavioral problems based on the *Developmental Troubleshooters Eclectic Checklist for Kids and Teenagers (D-TECKT)*, a comprehensive guide offering approaches to care developed by the American Academy of Pediatrics (Tellerman, 2005). The guide includes a database of parental concerns and an assessment of developmental issues (such as development of trust, handling separation, toddler autonomy, magical thinking of preschoolers, peer issues with school-age children, independence issues in adolescence, and sexual identity). Data concerning environmental issues, discipline techniques, family dynamics, and communication issues are also collected. After the source of the problem is identified, a combination of mental health interventions can be implemented or the child can be referred as needed.

EFFECT OF THE ILLNESS ON GROWTH AND DEVELOPMENT

Children respond to traumatic events in their life and to stressors within the family, in the school, and within the peer or social group. The duration and intensity of the stressful event and the child's coping skills determine the impact on the growth and development process.

Knowledge of normal growth and development throughout childhood combined with good observation and listening skills can enable the nurse to play a major role in minimizing the negative impact of behavioral problems on growth and development. Because outpatient services play a significant role in health care today, nurses must be aware of agencies and support groups available to children with behavioral disorders and their parents. Prompt early referral and treatment can improve the prognosis of emotional and behavioral disorders, enabling children to reach their potential in growth and development.

Children's behavioral problems necessitate a total family approach to care. Education of the community (school personnel), family (parents and siblings), and child is an essential nursing responsibility. Patient advocacy with a focus on prevention and long-term management are goals of care. A knowledgeable, caring, understanding, and supportive nature is valuable for any nurse caring for children with behavioral disorders.

EFFECT OF THE ILLNESS ON SIBLINGS

Most siblings of children with emotional disorders either suffer emotional scars or develop protective coping mechanisms to handle their experiences. Siblings of children with long-term illness are at risk for developing poor self-esteem and problems with their own peer relationships. Some siblings, however, are resilient and develop strength and positive coping mechanisms. **Sibling rivalry**, a competition between siblings for the attention or love of parents, is a normal part of growth and development, but guilt on the part of the other sibling enters the picture when one sibling becomes ill. Sibling rivalry teaches interactive social skills that will be used with friends and at work later in life. A child who is left at home with a babysitter while the parents tend to an ill sibling in the hospital may feel abandoned and often is burdened with extra household responsibilities that may add to the stress. Some children may react negatively to the stress of making dinner for the rest of the family, whereas other children react positively and develop positive self-esteem, knowing they are trusted with such a task.

The nurse can provide support for the family system, identify available resources, and collaborate with the health care team to meet total family needs.

Get Ready for the NCLEX® Examination!

Key Points

- Early childhood experiences are critical to personality formation.
- The child's environment must be safe, and the child must be able to trust caretakers.

- Nurses play an important role in the mental and emotional assessment of children because they often have the most contact with the hospitalized child and family.
- Talk of suicide must always be taken seriously.

- The risk of suicide increases when there is a definite plan of action, the means are available, and the person has few resources for help and support.
- Substance abuse is the number one problem of American adolescents.
- Al-Anon and Alateen are two excellent resources for family members of alcoholics.
- The *Diagnostic and Statistical Manual of Mental Disorders (DSM-5)* (APA, 2013) lists specific criteria for diagnosing various mental conditions seen in children and adults.
- Attention-deficit hyperactivity disorder is characterized by a developmentally inappropriate degree of gross motor activity, impulsivity, distractibility, and inattention in school or at home.
- Behavioral problems can be caused by the stresses accompanying the transition from childhood to adulthood or by genetic or biochemical factors.
- Children with ASD do not show interest in other children, do not make eye contact, and do not engage in "pretend" play.
- Sudden movements and loud noises should be avoided when caring for children with ASD.
- Obsessive-compulsive disorders in children do not involve impaired cognitive functioning.
- Ritualistic behavior may interfere with daily activities.
- A major depressive disorder is characterized by a prolonged behavioral change from baseline that interferes with school or age-specific activities.
- Substances abused by children and adolescents may be inhaled, injected, or ingested. The practice of sharing unsterile needles may lead to HIV infection.
- Emphasizing the strengths of the child rather than the weaknesses is essential when caring for a child with a behavioral disorder.
- Anorexia nervosa can lead to starvation and death.
- Bulimia is an eating disorder that involves bingeing and purging and can result in deterioration of teeth and electrolyte imbalance.
- Education, prevention, identification, and referral are essential nursing functions in the care of the child with a behavioral disorder.

Additional Learning Resources

SG Go to your Study Guide for additional learning activities to help you master this chapter content.

evolve Go to your Evolve website (http://evolve.elsevier.com/Leifer) for the following learning resources:
- Animations
- Answer Guidelines for Critical Thinking Questions
- Answers and Rationales for Review Questions for the NCLEX® Examination

- Glossary with English and Spanish pronunciations
- Interactive Review Questions for the NCLEX® Examination
- Patient Teaching Plans in English and Spanish
- Skills Performance Checklists
- Video clips and more!

 Online Resources
- Agency for Healthcare Research and Quality: http://ahrq.gov/clinic
- Autism Research Center: www.autismresearchcenter.com
- Autism Society: www.autism-society.org
- International Dyslexia Association: www.interdys.org
- National Center for Learning Disabilities: www.ncld.org
- Educational poster re suicide: www.sprc.org/sites/sprc.org/files/library/er_SuicideRiskPosterVert2.PDF.

Review Questions for the NCLEX® Examination

1. The adolescent with anorexia nervosa has a body self-image characteristically expressed by:
   1. wearing tight clothing to emphasize thinness.
   2. increasing elation as weight is lost.
   3. feeling "fat" even when appearing thin.
   4. efforts to achieve specific figure measurements.

2. A priority goal in the approach to a child with anorexia nervosa is to:
   1. encourage weight gain.
   2. prevent depression.
   3. limit exercise.
   4. correct malnutrition.

3. A child with suspected bulimia should be assessed for:
   1. abnormal weight gain.
   2. abnormal weight loss.
   3. erosion of tooth enamel.
   4. amenorrhea.

4. An important approach to the care of a 7-year-old child diagnosed with attention-deficit hyperactivity disorder (ADHD) is to encourage:
   1. a diet high in processed foods.
   2. regular use of sedatives.
   3. strict discipline.
   4. a structured, one-on-one environment.

5. When assessing an 8-year-old child with obsessive-compulsive disorder (OCD), the nurse would expect to find:
   1. an intelligence deficit.
   2. ritualistic behavior.
   3. antisocial behavior.
   4. combative behavior.

Complementary and Alternative Therapies in Maternity and Pediatric Nursing

Objectives

1. Define each key term listed.
2. Define complementary and alternative medicine (CAM) therapy.
3. Identify the role of the nurse in CAM therapy.
4. Discuss the integration of CAM therapy into nursing practice.
5. Discuss the impact on nursing care of patients who use CAM therapy.
6. State three herbs that should be discontinued 2 weeks before surgery.
7. Describe the involvement of the federal government in CAM therapy.
8. State the use of meridians, dermatomes, and reflexology lines in CAM therapy.
9. State five types of CAM therapy in common use.
10. State three herbal products contraindicated in pregnancy.
11. State three herbal products commonly used in pediatrics.
12. State popular herbs used during menopause.
13. Discuss the use of hyperbaric oxygen therapy in the care of carbon monoxide poisoning and necrotic ulcers.

Key Terms

alternative therapy (p. 760)
aromatherapy (p. 765)
coin-rubbing (p. 763)
complementary therapy (p. 760)
dermatomes (DŬR-mă-tōmz, p. 764)
herbal medicine (p. 765)

hyperbaric oxygen therapy (HBOT) (p. 769)
meridians (mě-RĬD-ē-ănz, p. 764)
reflexology (p. 763)
Rolfing (RŎL-fĭng, p. 763)
shiatsu (shē-ĂHT-sū, p. 765)

COMPLEMENTARY AND ALTERNATIVE THERAPIES

Complementary therapy refers to nontraditional (non-Western medical) therapy that is used *with* traditional or conventional (Western medical) therapy. An example would be the treatment of hypertension with medication *plus* relaxation or biofeedback techniques. **Alternative therapy** refers to unconventional or nontraditional therapy that *replaces* conventional or traditional therapy. Complementary and alternative medicine (CAM) therapies are also known as *integrative therapy, integrative healing,* and *holistic healing.* Although CAM therapy is used throughout the lifespan, this chapter focuses only on the common gynecological, obstetric, and pediatric practices.

PEDIATRIC USE

Infants and children are not small adults and their immature development can result in responses that are different than expected in the adult patient. Some side-effects can be dangerous for children. There is limited research available concerning CAM therapy for infants and children and many parents are influenced by testimonials which often do not provide evidence-based information.

The Task Force on Complementary and Alternative Medicine has reviewed the status of CAM research (Kemper, 2008). The American Academy of Pediatrics (AAP) recognizes the increasing use of complementary and alternative therapies for pediatric patients and has developed resources to educate professionals and consumers, as well as review legal and ethical considerations (Vohra, 2012). CAM therapies are used effectively and often integrated with traditional Western medicine in the United States. For example, the ketogenic diet has proven effective in some seizure disorders, and chiropractic care for children is common practice, although evidence-based research and randomized controlled trials on both are ongoing. Meditation, guided imagery, and biofeedback have been useful in managing and controlling pain, anxiety, sleep disorders, asthma, and many other conditions. Acupuncture has been successful in the treatment of some headaches in children, and many pediatricians and gastroenterologists now recommend probiotics for gastrointestinal problems (Johnston, 2012).

Herbal therapy is used for children with ADHD (Sarris, 2011) and the use of complementary and alternative medicine in pregnancy is well documented (Bishop, 2011). Continued research and documentation of CAM therapies that are currently in use is needed to build an evidence base for continued care (Edwards, 2013).

The National Center for Complementary and Alternative Medicine awarded a grant to the University of Arizona to study pediatric CAM practices, and in 2004, an Integrative Pediatric Council was formed to compile evidence-based practices in pediatrics. In 2007, Duke University Medical School designed a "living laboratory" to study effective use of CAM therapies. More comprehensive integration of evidence-based CAM practices in obstetrics and pediatrics is on the horizon.

THE NURSE'S ROLE

Many CAM therapies are based on accepted theories such as the gate control theory of pain relief (see Chapter 7). Nurses have used complementary therapies such as imagery, journaling, therapeutic touch, humor, and support groups and therefore have an integral role in the development and assessment of CAM therapy. A large proportion of people worldwide use some sort of CAM therapy for adults and children, with complementary therapy readily accepted in Europe (Corrigan and Alfers, 2007). Knowledge concerning CAM therapy expands knowledge about health care practices used in many cultures. *Cultural competence* is sensitivity to and respect for practices and philosophies different from one's own; the awareness and understanding of CAM therapy can enhance the cultural competence of nurses.

 Cultural Considerations

Popular Cultural Folk Healers

Mexican: *Curanderos*
African American: Root doctor
Asian and Chinese: Herbalist
Puerto Rican: *Espiritistas* or *santiguadoras*
Navajo: Singers

The focus of health care has changed, moving from the patient in the hospital to the patient in the home. The hospital setting is a somewhat controlled environment, but nursing care in the home brings new challenges. As nurses enter this health care environment within the community, familiar equipment, practices, and support personnel will no longer surround them. Instead they will encounter some *alternative health care* practices involving patients who want increasing

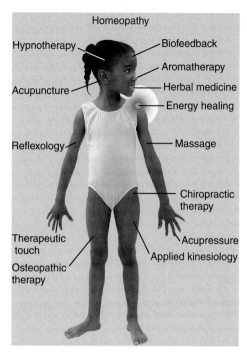

FIGURE 34-1 Alternative health care. (Art overlay courtesy Observatory Group, Cincinnati, Ohio.)

control over their health problems, need to be a part of the decision-making process, and want to incorporate cultural beliefs and traditions into their care. In addition to accepting treatment prescribed by a traditional health care provider, the patient may also be consulting other healing authorities such as holistic practitioners, naturopaths, and nutritional consultants (Figure 34-1). Food therapy, vitamin and mineral supplements, herbal therapy, and acupressure are common forms of alternative therapies practiced in many homes.

The greater acceptance of CAM therapies by the layperson and the inclusion of CAM therapies in medical curricula and practice have resulted in the need for nurses to understand CAM therapy, how it can be used, and how it may interact with or enhance traditional medical or nursing care (Table 34-1). It is important to note that not all alternative therapists are licensed, not all alternative medicines are regulated, and much of the practice may not be evidence-based.

Many pharmacies sell herbal medications, but few pharmacists have continuing education concerning herbal products and supplements. This may mean they have knowledge of the use of herbal medications but at the same time need increased understanding of possible adverse interactions and side effects for the individual patient. Many health food stores sell herbal products and supplements with unlicensed employees offering advice.

Box 34-1 lists some cautions concerning the use of CAM therapy. CAM therapy is not currently viewed as part of routine health care, but its popularity and some limited research has resulted in some insurance companies offering coverage for selected practices,

Table 34-1 Herbs That Should Be Discontinued Two Weeks Before Surgery

HERB	SIDE EFFECTS	PROBLEM DURING SURGERY
Echinacea	Unpleasant taste sensation, potential liver toxicity	May potentiate barbiturate toxicity
Garlic	Increased bleeding time, hypotension	Increased risk of intraoperative hemodynamic instability
Ginger	Increased bleeding time	Increased risk of intraoperative hemodynamic instability
Ginkgo biloba	Platelet dysfunction	Increased intraoperative and postoperative bleeding tendencies; may decrease effectiveness of intravenous barbiturates
St. John's wort	Dry mouth, dizziness, constipation, nausea	Increases risk of bleeding and increases metabolism of select medications, including altering effects of anesthetic agents
Ginseng	Hypertension, insomnia, headache, vomiting, epistaxis, prolonged bleeding time, hypoglycemia	Increased risk of intraoperative hemodynamic instability
Kava kava	Characteristic scaling of the skin	Increases level of sedation; can lead to coma; interacts with other drugs and can cause liver failure
Feverfew	Mouth ulcers, gastrointestinal irritability, headache	Increased risk of intraoperative hemodynamic instability
Ephedra (ma huang)	Hypertension, tachycardia, stroke, dysrhythmias	May interact with volatile anesthetic agents (e.g., halothane) to cause fatal cardiac dysrhythmias; profound intraoperative hypotension

NOTE: The nurse must also be alert to the effects of CAM therapy on traditional medical or nursing care.

Box 34-1 Cautions in Complementary and Alternative Medicine Therapy

- Herbs can interact with cardiac drugs.
- Herbs can affect glucose control in patients with diabetes.
- Herbs can lower the concentration of some synthetic drugs.
- Herbs can lower the blood level of some medications used for human immunodeficiency virus (HIV) and/or acquired immunodeficiency syndrome (AIDS).
- Polypharmacy (the use of many medicines) should be avoided; the use of some drugs in tandem with herbal remedies can be dangerous.

and some CAM practices have filtered into accepted nursing practice (e.g., massage, imagery, acupressure and aromatherapy). It is likely that nurses today and in the future will encounter CAM therapy as part of the health care delivery system. Therefore it is essential that nurses understand basic underlying philosophies and beliefs concerning CAM interventions. The nurse's role is not to promote the acceptance of CAM therapy but to recognize and respect its use by patients and to use critical thinking skills to determine interactions with traditional therapy. Healing is best achieved with the patient as a partner and by giving consideration to the cultural and environmental influences that affect the overall health and wellness of the patient and family. When documenting a patient's health history, questions should be asked concerning the family's use of CAM therapies.

FEDERAL REGULATIONS

There are more than 1800 identified CAM therapies practiced in the United States. The practices are not standardized, and often there is a lack of research-based evidence concerning their mechanism of action, effectiveness, or safety. In 1938 the Federal Food, Drug, and Cosmetic Act required all drugs, including herbs, to be safe before sale. In 1962 the Kefauver-Harris Drug Amendment required proof to the U.S. Food and Drug Administration (FDA) of drug effectiveness before placing agents on the market for sale. Manufacturers of herbal products declared their products to be "dietary supplements" and therefore not subject to this law. In 1976 the Proxmire amendment prevented the FDA from regulating supplement potency. In 1994 the Dietary Supplement Health and Education Act defined the term *dietary supplement* and prohibited claims of medicinal value. There have been requests by many health groups for closer regulation of dosages, warnings, and contraindications for dietary supplements, but the FDA has not yet regulated the herbal industry. For this reason, many dietary supplements and herbal remedies vary in their strengths and ingredients.

In 1992 the National Institutes of Health (NIH) created the Office of Alternative Medicine to evaluate the various CAM therapies. It has since been renamed the National Center for Complementary and Alternative Medicine (NCCAM). This Center serves as a public clearinghouse and resource for research concerning CAM therapies. There are 14 university-affiliated or medical center–affiliated research facilities for alternative medicine in the United States today. The more popular herbs and oils have been the first to be researched in centers such as the University of California, Los Angeles (UCLA), and the University of Chicago.

In 1994 the Dietary Supplement Health and Education Act (DSHEA) required regulations in the marketing of dietary supplements that include plant extracts, vitamins, minerals, and herbs that are available to consumers without a prescription. Claims on labels must show that they are *not* FDA approved.

In 1999 the NIH directed the NCCAM to work together with the Office of Dietary Supplements in research programs concerning the safety and efficacy of alternate medications. A journal, *The Scientific Review of Alternative Medicine*, is an example of a publication dedicated to evaluating CAM therapies based on review of medical studies.

COMMON ALTERNATIVE HEALTH CARE PRACTICES

Massage

An underlying premise of some alternative healing techniques is that the symptoms are the result of a problem in the body that may not be related to the specific symptom manifested. The body is thought to have a self-healing ability that can be aided by spinal or energy manipulation. Soft-tissue massage is thought to bolster the immune response. Fascia pressure, stretching, and manipulation, known as **Rolfing**, are thought to improve muscle and bone function. "Cao-gio," or **coin-rubbing**, is a form of skin manipulation thought to help bring the body into healthy alignment (Figure 34-2). Neuromuscular massage helps to relieve muscle tension and the trigger points of pain and generally improves circulation. Perineal massage during

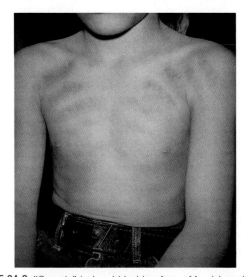

FIGURE 34-2 "Cao-gio" (coin-rubbing) is a form of fascial manipulation believed to bring the body in alignment with gravity. It is a form of CAM therapy that can easily be mistaken for child abuse because of the lingering marks on the skin after treatment. (From Shah BR, Laude TA: *Atlas of pediatric clinical diagnosis*, Philadelphia, 2000, Saunders.)

pregnancy and before delivery may prevent the need for an episiotomy during delivery, thereby reducing perineal trauma. *Effleurage* is a form of massage used during labor (see Figure 7-3). Foot message, often given with pedicures, can stimulate preterm labor in susceptible women.

Massage therapy is often used for children with asthma, arthritis, and eating disorders. Gentle touch massage therapy has had positive effects on premature infants. Massage and manipulative therapy is contraindicated in patients with cancer, osteoporosis, localized infection, and cardiac and circulatory disorders because of the increase it causes in blood flow to affected areas. Children with Down syndrome are particularly prone to cervical spine anomalies and may be injured by manual manipulative therapy. Children who have a history of sexual abuse do not usually respond favorably to touch therapy.

Osteopathy

Osteopaths combine manipulative therapy with traditional (allopathic) medicine. Pressure point therapy is based on the theory that certain areas of the body are connected to specific identified pressure points such as the feet, the hands, and the ears. It is believed that channels conduct vital energy through the body. The osteopath can guide a woman with previous back problems to select a birthing position that will not aggravate the problem. Many osteopaths currently practice in the mainstream of Western medicine.

Energy Healing

Energy healing involves the belief that an electromagnetic flow emerges from the therapist's hands and can funnel energy into the patient. Some believe that repatterning a patient's own energy field can aid in healing. The body, mind, spirit, and emotions are usually involved in this type of therapy.

A wristband that uses transcutaneous electrical nerve stimulation (TENS) placed on identified trigger points can prevent nausea and vomiting during chemotherapy and pregnancy-induced nausea and vomiting (Figure 34-3). TENS, shen, reiki, and the use of magnets are other forms of energy therapy. Magnets should not be used over the abdominal area during pregnancy.

Light therapy or sunlight is an ancient form of healing therapy. Light therapy is used in the treatment of jaundiced newborn infants (hyperbilirubinemia; see Chapter 13) and is also used in treating persons with seasonal affective disorder.

Reflexology

Reflexology deals with reflex points in the hands and feet that are thought to correspond to every organ or part of the body. The foot or hand represents a map of the entire body linked by energy pathways (Figure 34-4). Massaging these reflex points can relieve specific problems.

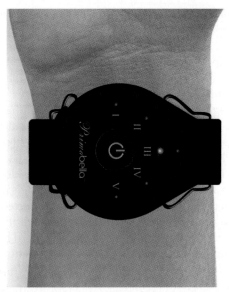

FIGURE 34-3 PrimaBella is a noninvasive transdermal device cleared by the FDA for treatment of pregnancy-induced nausea and vomiting (morning sickness). The device is applied to the ventral side of the wrist, where the median nerve is closest to the surface of the skin. It emits a programmed pulse that stimulates the nerve to create electrical signals that travel to the central nervous system to restore normal gastric rhythm. (Photo courtesy Neurowave Medical Technologies.)

Acupuncture and Acupressure

Acupuncture is an ancient Chinese practice that works on the principle that the body has complex **meridians**, which are imaginary lines that are thought to be pathways carrying energy to specific organs or parts of the body. These meridians surface at specific locations called *acupuncture points*. It is at these 150 points on the 12 meridian sites that positive or negative energy can be realigned through stimulation. "Chi" energy is thought to regulate proper body function, and acupuncture or acupressure is applied to restore a balance of chi energy. In acupuncture, hair-thin needles are applied to specific meridians and may stimulate nerve cells to release endorphins.

A **dermatome** is a specific area of the skin that is supplied by a sensory neuron that originates from a specific single spinal nerve root. The general dermatome pattern is similar for all people although the specific area of innervation within that pattern might be unique to the individual. Obstructing the dermatome line can anesthetize that area of the skin. These areas can be manipulated by chiropractors.

Acupressure uses finger pressure and massage on the meridian sites (see Figure 34-4) rather than needles. Acupuncture and acupressure have achieved

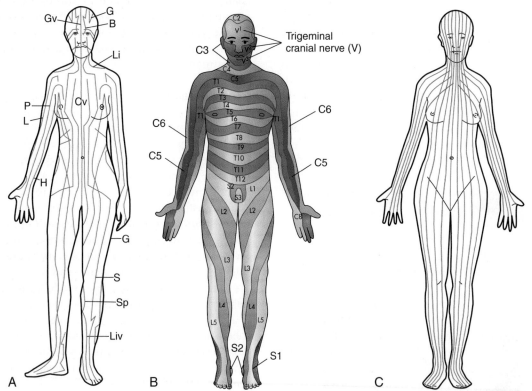

FIGURE 34-4 A, Meridians. Acupuncture is based on the belief that the correct flow of energy through meridians (invisible tracks running through the body) controls the health of all vital organs. Stimulating any of the 12 meridians with heat, electricity, needles, or pressure can affect corresponding parts of the body. **B,** Dermatomes. The areas of the skin innervated by the dorsal roots of the spinal cord are called dermatomes. Obstructing one dermatome line can anesthetize that segment of the skin and adjacent structures (although some dermatome lines from adjacent dorsal roots of the spine can overlap). **C,** Reflexology lines. *Reflexology lines* divide the body into 10 zones of longitudinal lines. Blockage of the lines is thought to obstruct vital energy pathways. Stimulating the area around the anklebone can affect the uterus and pelvic organs and relieve pain during labor. (**A** and **C** from Moore S, editor: *Understanding pain and its relief in labour,* London, 1997, Churchill Livingstone. **B** from Patton KT, Thibodeau GA: *Anatomy & physiology,* ed 8, St Louis, 2013, Mosby.)

popularity in the Western world and can be used during pregnancy to control nausea, backache, and pain. Acupressure wristbands are available for use to prevent nausea and vomiting during travel or pregnancy. These techniques have also been useful for minor postpartum problems such as constipation. Acupoints to avoid during pregnancy include the bottom of the foot, the inner lower leg, the base of the thumb, and most areas over the abdomen, because pressure here may result in negative outcomes such as premature labor. **Shiatsu** is a finger pressure used with an emphasis on preventing disease rather than treating symptoms. Pressure is applied to achieve a level of sensation between pain and pleasure in the individual.

Homeopathy

Homeopathy accounts for approximately 25% of pediatric visits to alternative health practitioners. Homeopathy uses plants, herbs, and earth minerals that are thought to stimulate the body's immune system to manage specific health problems. The homeopathic philosophy involves the belief that disease is an energy imbalance and that prescribed remedies assist the body to reestablish correct balance. Homeopathic remedies are taken sublingually and should not be combined with caffeine, alcohol, or traditional Western medications. Some homeopathic medicines are alcohol based, and some contain mercury or arsenic bases that can cause toxicity or allergic responses in children. Only one remedy is administered at a time, and minimum dosage is the principle of most practitioners.

Ayurveda

Ayurveda is an ancient Hindu healing regimen that deals with the biological rhythms of nature and can include music, herbs, massage, aromatherapy, and a diet tailored to the specific body type.

Aromatherapy

Aromatherapy is an ancient practice that involves concentrated fluid or the essence of specific herbs that are combined with steams or baths to inhale or bathe the skin. Essential oils are concentrated and, if undiluted, are usually used in 2- to 5-drop doses. Often a few drops of the herbal oil are added to soaps or regular lotions immediately before use. Concentrated oils are volatile and must be freshly prepared and stored properly. Some essential oils are contraindicated for use during pregnancy because of the effect on the mother or fetus; these include anise, juniper, thyme, wintergreen, nutmeg, pennyroyal, and mugwort. Aromatherapy under the supervision of a trained aromatherapist with oils such as jasmine, citrus, clary sage, lavender, and peppermint has been useful during labor and delivery to relieve anxiety, reduce nausea, and improve the general feeling of well-being.

Nursing Tip

Lavender, chamomile, and sandalwood essential oils are useful in aromatherapy for children with chronic pain.

Hypnotherapy

In *hypnotherapy*, the patient enters a hypnotic state of induced sleep. Under the guidance of the practitioner, specific and potentially long-lasting suggestions are given to the patient. Smoking cessation and pain control have been successfully achieved using this method. Some patients resist the trance state and are not candidates for hypnotherapy.

Hydrotherapy

Hydrotherapy is the therapeutic use of water to promote relaxation. It is often used during labor in the form of showers (see Box 7-1). In some independent birthing centers, delivery is accomplished under water under the direction of certified nurse midwives (CNMs).

Guided Imagery

Guided imagery is based on the ancient Greek belief that the mind can influence the body. Asking the patient to focus on a specific image can result in the reduction of stress and increased performance. This technique is most often combined with breathing and relaxation techniques to manage the discomforts of labor (see Box 7-1).

Biofeedback

Biofeedback is a type of relaxation therapy that enables the patient to recognize tension in the muscles via responses on an electronic machine and visual electromyography responses. Traditional health care providers also use the process for conditions such as drug addiction and chronic pain control.

Chiropractic Care

Chiropractic care concerns the relationship between the spinal column and the nervous system and involves nerve energy thought responsible for restoring and maintaining health. During pregnancy, circulating hormones such as relaxin increase the mobility of joint capsules and pelvic joint structures that affect the musculoskeletal system. Vigorous manipulation should be avoided between the twelfth and sixteenth weeks of pregnancy to avoid stimulating a miscarriage or premature labor.

Most chiropractors also use massage, diet, nutritional, and enzyme therapy for a more comprehensive approach. Chiropractors offer well-child care by preventive manipulation.

Herbal Remedies

The World Health Organization (WHO) reports that herbal remedies are often used worldwide and are the first-line treatment for most children in developing countries. **Herbal medicine** has been used for thousands of years in many countries. Herbs are powerful nutritional agents, and most are safe to ingest. Occasionally an allergic type of reaction is encountered, possibly because of differences in processing or storing of the products. Herbal products are sold in stores, but the processes of growth, processing, storage, and prescription are not regulated the way they are for traditional drugs. However, there are general guidelines for their use, including dosages and the recommendation that herbal mixtures are preferred to single-herb products to avoid overdosing on single ingredients.

Many current medications are related to herbal remedies. Digitalis originates from foxglove, opiates originate from poppy flowers, and quinine originates from the cinchona tree. However, some herbs, such as ephedra, can be fatal to children. Herbal remedies consumed during pregnancy can cross the placenta and reach the fetus. Breastfeeding mothers who use herbal remedies can pass the substance to their nursing infants. Home-grown herbs, such as chamomile used for tea, can be contaminated with botulism. Taking time to elicit an accurate history from parents may reveal their practice of using herbal remedies for the family.

Herbal capsules are about 4 times stronger than herbal teas, and *herbal extracts* are about 4 to 8 times stronger than capsules. Most extracts should not be taken for longer than 6 consecutive days. *Herbal tinctures* contain a high amount of alcohol and are not often recommended. *Herbal baths* are relaxing and soothing, and herbal salves, oils, compresses, and poultices use the skin as the body's organ of ingestion. Most practitioners emphasize that herbal dosage is determined by body weight and that megadoses can be harmful.

Herbs and Obstetrics. CAM therapy for obstetrics helps some women feel a sense of control over their well-being. Because many women view CAM therapy and herbal remedies as "natural remedies," they may not be aware of the possible dangers to themselves or their growing fetus. The patient may have been using herbal products before becoming pregnant, and the question of whether or not to continue during pregnancy, labor, and delivery must be discussed with the health care provider. Table 34-2 lists commonly used herbs that are contraindicated for use during pregnancy.

Table 34-2 Common Herbs Contraindicated in Pregnancy and Lactation

HERB	USE	CONTRAINDICATION
Aloe vera	Treats constipation Aids wound healing	Causes engorgement of pelvic vessels that can result in increased bleeding and spontaneous abortion; avoid during pregnancy.
Garlic, ginkgo biloba	Decreases cholesterol Prevents motion sickness Lessens depression	Avoid in pregnancy; do not use with other antiplatelet medications.
St. John's wort	Lessens depression	Avoid exposure to sun. Increases tone of uterus. Use with caution in pregnancy. Interacts with alcohol, cold and flu medications, chocolate, aged cheese, and beer.
Angelica (dong quai)	Used for gynecological disorders, menstrual discomfort, and postmenopausal symptoms	Avoid in pregnancy and breastfeeding because of uterine stimulation. Prolongs prothrombin time and causes poor glycemic control in diabetics.
Chamomile	Prevents urinary tract infections, gastrointestinal spasms; used for sedation	Avoid in pregnancy. May cause abortion and teratogenic effects on fetus.
Feverfew	Used for migraine headache and menstrual problems	Avoid use during pregnancy and lactation. Can cause withdrawal symptoms.
Flax (flaxseed)	Used for bowel problems	Contraindicated in pregnancy; potential for toxicity. Must be refrigerated.
Ginseng	Aids resistance to stress Used to increase stamina	Avoid in pregnancy and lactation. May be toxic. Central nervous system effects increase when used with coffee or tea. Interacts with St. John's wort and monoamine oxidase inhibitors (MAOIs).
Kava kava	Reduces anxiety and stress	Avoid in pregnancy and lactation. May cause nutritional deficiencies or blood dyscrasias.
Ma huang (ephedra)	Used as central nervous system stimulant	Avoid use during pregnancy. Can cause cardiac dysrhythmia, urinary retention, and uterine contractions.
Nettle	Used as diuretic	Diuresis can cause electrolyte imbalance.

Data from Loo M: *Integrative medicine*, Philadelphia, 2008, Saunders; *PDR for herbal medicines*, Montvale, N.J., 2010, Medical Economics; Rakel D: *Philosophy of integrative medicine*, ed 2, Philadelphia, 2012, Saunders; Skidmore-Roth L: *Handbook of medicinal herbs*, Philadelphia, 2009, Saunders.

Box **34-2**	Some Herbs That Promote Menstruation and May Cause Miscarriage

- Cascara
- Cohosh
- Goldenseal
- Juniper
- Marjoram
- Motherwort
- Mugwort
- Pennyroyal
- Sage
- Senna
- Wormwood

In general, herbs that promote menstruation are contraindicated for use in pregnancy (Box 34-2). It should be remembered that tannic acid and bran decrease the absorption of iron from foods, and therefore tea with meals should be avoided during pregnancy when blood volume increases and hemoglobin levels may fall into the anemic zone. The use of herbal products for neonates is contraindicated unless carefully monitored by a licensed herbalist and neonatologist. The ingestion of high levels of vitamin C by a breastfeeding mother can result in colic in the newborn infant.

Herbs and Pediatrics. The use of CAM therapy has increased for children with various chronic disorders. Chiropractic, biofeedback, homeopathy, and herbal-food supplements are popular treatments for children. Parents sometimes prefer "natural remedies" such as herbs to prescription medicines for their children diagnosed with attention-deficit hyperactivity disorder (ADHD). Herbal treatments focus on improving cognition, producing sedation, or alleviating anxiety. These herbs are obtained without a prescription, and their use is often not supported by scientific studies concerning effectiveness or safety. Some herbs are contained in flavored tea sold in supermarkets. Parents often do not discuss CAM therapy that they used for their children unless directly asked by the nurse or health care provider. Table 34-3 reviews herbs commonly used for children, and the Online Resources section at the end of this chapter lists several websites to help parents and healthcare providers find reliable information.

Herbs and Menopause. Menopause is a stage of health within the health–illness continuum in a woman's life. It is not approached as a disease or illness but rather as a unique stage of life and as a normal, healthy process. The physiological alterations that occur as a woman reaches and enters menopause result in minor discomforts such as hot flashes, night sweats, and insomnia. Traditionally, hormone replacement therapy (HRT) has been the most popular approach to managing menopausal symptoms. Recently, more "natural" paths of management have developed:

- Exercise, such as weight-bearing or water aerobic exercise programs
- Relaxation techniques, including breathing, biofeedback, and hypnosis
- A low-fat, high-fiber, soy diet
- Herbs (Table 34-4)

Table **34-3**	Herbs Commonly Used in Pediatrics	
HERB	**USE**	**TOXICITY OR CAUTIONS**
Blue-green algae (*Cyanobacteria spirulina*)	Stimulates tumor necrosis Antiinflammatory Antiviral Antifungal Used in children with ADHD	There are no clinical studies supporting cognitive improvement in children. Contaminated source of collection can cause toxicity, liver failure, and cholera. Should not be used in children with phenylketonuria. Nutritional value is limited in humans.
Chamomile (*Matricaria recutita*)	Used to calm infants with colic Used as an antispasmodic, reduces anxiety	Use with caution if allergic to ragweed.
Ephedra (ma huang)	Used for asthma; decongestant; central nervous system stimulant	Often used by adolescents as an illegal stimulant. Can cause hypertension, anxiety, and toxic psychosis. Overdose can be deadly.
Echinacea	Thought to be an immune enhancer	Increases barbiturate toxicity. Do not use with immunosuppressant therapy.
Evening primrose oil (*Oenothera biennis*)	Relieves eczema, asthma, and diabetic retinopathy	Nausea, diarrhea, and headache can occur.
Fennel seed oil	Reduces stomach spasms and increases colon motility	Do not use if allergic to carrots or celery.

Continued

Table 34-3   **Herbs Commonly Used in Pediatrics—cont'd**

HERB	USE	TOXICITY OR CAUTIONS
Feverfew (*Tanacetum parthenium*)	Migraine relief	Contraindicated during pregnancy and lactation, and in children less than 2 years of age. Can cause mouth ulcers; may interact with antithrombotic drugs.
Fish oil	Improves visual processing and coordination Reduces asthma risk	Flatus, bad breath can occur. Do not use with anticoagulants or in bleeding disorders.
Ginger (*Zingiber officinale*)	Used for nausea and motion sickness	In large doses can cause heartburn and diarrhea.
Ginkgo biloba	Thought to improve alertness and memory Possibly decreases hypoxia damage to brain	Headache, dizziness can occur. Decreases the effectiveness of barbiturates. Do not use with aspirin or in persons with bleeding disorders.
Siberian ginseng (*Eleutherococcus senticosus*)	Stimulant Aids resistance to stress Used in ADHD	Potentiates the effect of caffeine and other stimulants. Not to be taken with steroids or hormones.
Kava kava (*Piper methysticum*)	Thought to reduce anxiety	Scaly skin rash can occur. Enhances barbiturate levels. Can cause oculomotor problems. Do not use with sedatives or anticoagulants. Increases high-density lipoproteins (HDLs).
Lemon balm (*Melissa officinalis*)	Used for nervous stomach complaints, nausea, and sleep disorders	May inhibit thyroid hormones.
Licorice (*Glycyrrhiza glabra*)	Treatment of asthma and stomach problems	Contraindicated for use in persons with hypertension or kidney and heart disease.
Melatonin (*N*-acetyl-5-methoxytryptamine)	Antioxidant Sleep-cycle disorders	Reduced alertness, headache, irritability, possible suppression of puberty can occur. Use with caution in children with seizures.
Peppermint (*Mentha piperita*)	Used for newborn colic, flatulence, nausea, indigestion Slows colon motility	Should not be used in persons with gastroesophageal reflux disease (GERD).
Probiotics (*Lactobacillus* species, *Saccharomyces boulardii*, *Bifidobacterium* species) (Found in yogurt, buttermilk, kefir, miso, sauerkraut)	Found in some yogurt Used for antibiotic-induced diarrhea or traveler's diarrhea, irritable bowel syndrome, and viral gastroenteritis	
Psyllium (*Plantago ovata*)	Used for constipation	Inadequate fluid intake can lead to intestinal obstruction or fecal impaction.
Pycnogenol (oligomeric proanthocyanidin; OPC)	Antioxidant Improves behavior in ADHD	Avoid use in bleeding disorders. Do not use with anticoagulants.
Siete Jarabes (commercial syrup)	Used as expectorant and laxative Relieves asthma and congestion	Is a combination of sweet almond, castor oil, licorice, honey, and other products. May cause diarrhea or hypertension.
St. John's wort (*Hypericum perforatum*)	Antidepressant	Can cause photosensitivity. Do not use with nasal decongestants, asthma medications, MAOIs, or drugs with phenylalanine content. Can cause high blood pressure.
Valerian (*Valeriana officinalis*)	Sleep disorders Used for complaints of anxiety	Gastrointestinal upset, headache can occur. Do not use with other sedatives.

ADHD, Attention-deficit hyperactivity disorder; *MAOIs,* monoamine oxidase inhibitors.
Data from *PDR for herbal medicines:* Montvale, N.J., 2010, Medical Economics; Gardiner P, Kemper K: For GI complaints: which herbs and supplements spell relief? *Contemp Pediatr* 22(8):50-55, 2005; Reddy P, Devi S: Herbal therapy for children with ADHD and depression, *Internet J Alt Med* 4(1), 2007; Rakel D: *Integrative medicine,* ed 3, Philadelphia, 2012, Saunders.

Table 34-4   **Popular Herbs Used in Menopause**

HERB	USES AND CONTRAINDICATIONS
Black cohosh (*Cimicifuga racemosa*)	Diminishes hot flashes by reducing luteinizing hormone (LH); reduces joint pain, hot flashes, and other menopausal discomforts
Sage (*Salvia officinalis*)	Contains phytosterols and bioflavonoids; effective for night sweats and hot flashes and has been used to decrease breast milk production
Dong quai (*Angelica sinensis*)	Contains phytoestrogens; contraindicated for use in presence of midcycle spotting and fibroids
Chasteberry (*Vitex agnus-castus*)	Reduces hot flashes and dizziness caused by high levels of follicle-stimulating hormone (FSH); balances hormonal fluctuations when combined with other herbs
Motherwort (*Leonurus cardiaca*)	Relieves hot flashes and moodiness; reduces anxiety and insomnia

Data from *PDR for herbal medicines*, Montvale, N.J, 2010, Medical Economics; Rakel D: *Integrative medicine,* ed 3, Philadelphia, 2012, Saunders.

Hyperbaric Oxygen Therapy

Hyperbaric oxygen therapy (HBOT) uses an airtight enclosure to provide compressed air or oxygen under increased pressure. HBOT is used to revive children with carbon monoxide poisoning, to aid wound healing, and to treat the diving syndrome known as decompression illness. Many hospitals currently use hyperbaric oxygen therapy as a standard treatment for diabetic wound healing and other specific problems. HBOT is also used as CAM therapy in private centers. HBOT is contraindicated during pregnancy, because the increased oxygen saturation can cause the ductus arteriosus to close, resulting in fetal death.

Research concerning the use and the effects of HBOT is ongoing.

Sauna/Heat Therapy

Overheating the body has long been used to speed up metabolism and inhibit the replication of viruses and bacteria. The sweating that results from the sauna is thought to help eliminate body waste. Patients should monitor their pulse during treatment. Some medical conditions can inhibit the ability to perspire, and heat can adversely affect the cardiac status of some patients. Therefore medical guidance should be sought before using this type of therapy. Sauna/heat therapy is contraindicated during pregnancy.

Get Ready for the NCLEX® Examination!

Key Points

- To promote positive outcomes, nurses must be well informed about the use and validity of complementary and alternative medicine (CAM) practices and understand the potential interactions with prescribed medications and treatments.
- Complementary therapies are treatments used **in conjunction with** traditional medicine.
- Alternative therapies are treatments that **replace** traditional medical therapy.
- The National Center for Complementary and Alternative Medicine, part of the National Institutes of Health, was created to conduct and review research concerning the efficacy and dangers of CAM therapy.
- Many herbal preparations do not have research-based data to guide determination of safe dosage and use.
- Many CAM therapies are used effectively and integrated with traditional Western medicine.
- Nurses have successfully used some CAM therapies, such as guided imagery, massage, and therapeutic touch, for many years.
- It is likely that nurses today and in the future will encounter some form of CAM therapy as part of the health care delivery system.
- Transcutaneous electrical nerve stimulation (TENS) is a form of energy therapy used to prevent nausea in labor, after surgery, and during chemotherapy.
- Nurses must use critical thinking skills to determine the interactions between CAM therapy and traditional prescribed treatments.
- Coin-rubbing is a type of CAM therapy that can be mistaken for child abuse because of lingering skin marks after treatment.
- Meridians are invisible (imaginary) lines running through the body that are thought to control the health of vital organs. Stimulation of any of the 150 pressure points on the 12 meridian sites is the basis of acupressure and acupuncture.
- Dermatomes are areas of the skin that are innervated by the dorsal roots of the spinal cord and affect specific segments of the skin and adjacent structures. These areas are manipulated by chiropractors.

- Reflexology lines divide the body into 10 zones of longitudinal lines. Blockage is thought to obstruct energy pathways; this is the basic concept of reflexology.
- As part of routine history data collection, nurses should ask all patients if they use a form of CAM therapy; this information should be recorded on the chart.

Additional Learning Resources

SG Go to your Study Guide for additional learning activities to help you master this chapter content.

evolve Go to your Evolve website (http://evolve.elsevier.com/Leifer) for the following learning resources:
- Animations
- Answer Guidelines for Critical Thinking Questions
- Answers and Rationales for Review Questions for the NCLEX® Examination
- Glossary with English and Spanish pronunciations
- Interactive Review Questions for the NCLEX® Examination
- Patient Teaching Plans in English and Spanish
- Skills Performance Checklists
- Video clips and more!

 Online Resources
- Attention deficit hyperactivity disorder: www.adhd.org
- Herbs and supplements: www.nlm.nih.gov/medlineplus/druginfo/herb_All.html
- National Center for Complementary and Alternative Medicine: www.nccam.nih.gov
- What Is CAM?: http://nccam.nih.gov/health/whatiscam/
- http://nccam.nih.gov/health/providers/digest
- http://nccam.nih.gov/health/pediatrics
- www.aap.org/en-us/professional-resources/research/pages/PS49

Review Questions for the NCLEX® Examination

1. The nurse should communicate to parents that herbal medicines sold over the counter:
   1. are harmless to children.
   2. are effective substitutes for traditional medication.
   3. can interact with prescribed medications and produce adverse effects.
   4. should never be given to children.

2. What instruction would a nurse give a patient who is using an herbal product?
   1. Take high doses of single herb to maximize effectiveness.
   2. Depend on the label for claims of benefits of use.
   3. Buy the least expensive brand of the product.
   4. Inform the health care provider of all herbal products used.

3. A patient in the prenatal clinic asks the nurse about the use of alternative or complementary therapies during her pregnancy. What would be the most appropriate response of the nurse?
   1. Discussing CAM therapy is not within the scope of practice of the licensed practical or vocational nurse (LPN/LVN).
   2. All CAM therapies should be stopped during pregnancy, labor, and delivery.
   3. Many complementary therapy techniques are taught in prenatal classes; some forms of alternative therapies may be contraindicated during pregnancy, labor, and delivery.
   4. Only those herbs approved by the FDA should be used during pregnancy, labor, or delivery.

4. What is the branch of the federal government that conducts research concerning the safety and efficacy of specific CAM therapies?
   1. Department of Health and Human Services
   2. National Center for Complementary and Alternative Medicine (NCCAM)
   3. Food and Drug Administration (FDA)
   4. Drug Enforcement Agency (DEA)

5. The role of the nurse in CAM therapy is to:
   1. encourage the use of CAM therapy in maternity and pediatric patients.
   2. discourage the use of CAM therapy in maternity and pediatric patients.
   3. discuss the impact or interaction of the CAM therapy with prescribed therapy.
   4. provide a resource of certified CAM therapists for maternity and pediatric patients.

Critical Thinking Questions

1. Explain the way in which complementary and alternative therapies can be used during labor.

2. Identify complementary and alternative techniques taught to women during most prenatal classes.

All health care providers must apply standard precautions to all patients regardless of diagnosis, disease, or infection status. The health care provider should perform appropriate barrier precautions to prevent exposure to skin or mucous membranes, especially when contact with blood, body fluids, secretions, and/or excretions is anticipated:

- Perform hand hygiene before and immediately after performing a task or procedure.
- Clean gloves should be worn whenever touching blood, body fluids, secretions, and/or excretions is anticipated. They should also be worn when handling items or surfaces soiled with blood or body fluids and when performing venipuncture and/or vascular access. Gloves must be changed and hand hygiene performed after contact with each and every patient.
- Personal protective equipment (PPE) such as face masks, protective eyewear (goggles) and/or face shields, and fluid-repelling gowns should be worn for procedures that are likely to generate droplets of blood or exposure to body fluids, secretions, and/or excretions. If mouth-to-mouth resuscitation is needed, always use a resuscitation mask or bag-valve mask to prevent direct contact with the patient's mucous membranes.
- All health care providers should take precautions to prevent injuries that can be caused from inappropriate handling of needles, scalpels, and other sharp instruments. After sharp items are used, they must be placed in PUNCTURE-RESISTANT containers nearby.

Transmission-based precautions (TBPs) are for patients with a suspected and/or diagnosed infection by an organism with a high risk of transmission. In such cases, both standard precautions and transmission-based precautions must be used. There are three types of transmission-based precautions:

1. Airborne infection isolation (AII) precautions (5 micrometers [μm] or smaller) must be used whenever working with a patient who has pulmonary tuberculosis (TB), chicken pox (varicella), measles (rubeola), smallpox (variola), and specific respiratory infections. The health care provider or others in the room can inhale these infecting microorganisms. Therefore N-95 respirator face masks must be worn, and special ventilation and air-handling protocols must be used to prevent transmission of the microorganism. Patients are placed in a private room, and specific air-circulation requirements and/or filtration of air particles must be done. All health care providers coming in contact with the TB-positive patient MUST be fitted for and wear an N-95 face mask or positive airway pressure respirator.

2. Droplet precautions (5 μm or larger) are used when the microorganism is spread through talking, coughing, or sneezing. Haemophilus influenzae type B, pertussis (whooping cough), scarlet fever, pneumonia, and rubella fall into this category. Transmission of these large droplets requires contact within 3 feet, because the large size does not stay suspended in the air for an extended period. Droplet precautions necessitate a separate room but do not necessitate special ventilation or air handling. When working within 3 feet of a patient with a droplet infection, using standard precautions and wearing a disposable face mask are recommended.

3. Contact precautions are used to reduce the spread of infectious organisms by direct or indirect contact. They are used when skin-to-skin contact may occur, such as when turning or bathing a patient. When possible, these patients are placed in a private room or in a room with another patient who has the same infection. On entering the room, the health care provider should wear clean gloves and a fluid-resistant cover gown. While performing care on this patient, gloves should be changed after having any contact with blood, body fluids, secretions, or excretions that may have a high concentration of the infecting organism. Health care providers must be sure to remove their gloves and their cover gown BEFORE leaving the patient's room and they must be sure to perform hand hygiene. They must be careful not to touch anything in the patient's room as they leave.

All patients on TBPs should be transported from the room only for essential purposes. Patients under airborne precautions should wear a regular, surgical face mask during transport.

The Centers for Disease Control and Prevention (CDC) in Atlanta, Georgia, provides guidelines for infection prevention and control, and the Occupational Health and Safety Commission (OSHA) establishes legal requirements for infection prevention and control. Employers are mandated to provide personal protective equipment at no cost to the employee.

Sequence for Donning and Removing Personal Protective Equipment (PPE)

http://evolve.elsevier.com/Leifer

SEQUENCE FOR DONNING PERSONAL PROTECTIVE EQUIPMENT (PPE)

The type of PPE used will vary based on the level of precautions required; e.g., Standard and Contact, Droplet or Airborne Infection Isolation.

1. GOWN
- Fully cover torso from neck to knees, arms to end of wrists, and wrap around the back
- Fasten in back of neck and waist

2. MASK OR RESPIRATOR
- Secure ties or elastic bands at middle of head and neck
- Fit flexible band to nose bridge
- Fit snug to face and below chin
- Fit-check respirator

3. GOGGLES OR FACE SHIELD
- Place over face and eyes and adjust to fit

4. GLOVES
- Extend to cover wrist of isolation gown

USE SAFE WORK PRACTICES TO PROTECT YOURSELF AND LIMIT THE SPREAD OF CONTAMINATION
- Keep hands away from face
- Limit surfaces touched
- Change gloves when torn or heavily contaminated
- Perform hand hygiene

SECUENCIA PARA PONERSE EL EQUIPO DE PROTECCIÓN PERSONAL (PPE)

El tipo de PPE que se debe utilizar depende del nivel de precaución que sea necesario; por ejemplo, equipo Estándar y de Contacto o de Aislamiento de infecciones transportadas por gotas o por aire.

1. BATA
- Cubra con la bata todo el torso desde el cuello hasta las rodillas, los brazos hasta la muñeca y dóblela alrededor de la espalda
- Átesela por detrás a la altura del cuello y la cintura

2. MÁSCARA O RESPIRADOR
- Asegúrese los cordones o la banda elástica en la mitad de la cabeza y en el cuello
- Ajústese la banda flexible en el puente de la nariz
- Acomódesela en la cara y por debajo del mentón
- Verifique el ajuste del respirador

3. GAFAS PROTECTORAS O CARETAS
- Colóquesela sobre la cara y los ojos y ajústela

4. GUANTES
- Extienda los guantes para que cubran la parte del puño en la bata de aislamiento

UTILICE PRÁCTICAS DE TRABAJO SEGURAS PARA PROTEGERSE USTED MISMO Y LIMITAR LA PROPAGACIÓN DE LA CONTAMINACIÓN
- Mantenga las manos alejadas de la cara
- Limite el contacto con superficies
- Cambie los guantes si se rompen o están demasiado contaminados
- Realice la higiene de las manos

SEQUENCE FOR REMOVING PERSONAL PROTECTIVE EQUIPMENT (PPE)

Except for respirator, remove PPE at doorway or in anteroom. Remove respirator after leaving patient room and closing door.

1. GLOVES
- Outside of gloves is contaminated!
- Grasp outside of glove with opposite gloved hand; peel off
- Hold removed glove in gloved hand
- Slide fingers of ungloved hand under remaining glove at wrist
- Peel glove off over first glovet
- Discard gloves in waste container

2. GOGGLES OR FACE SHIELD
- Outside of goggles or face shield is contaminated!
- To remove, handle by head band or ear pieces
- Place in designated receptacle for reprocessing or in waste container

3. GOWN
- Gown front and sleeves are contaminated!
- Unfasten ties
- Pull away from neck and shoulders, touching inside of gown only
- Turn gown inside out
- Fold or roll into a bundle and discard

4. MASK OR RESPIRATOR
- Front of mask/respirator is contaminated — DO NOT TOUCH!
- Grasp bottom, then top ties or elastics and remove
- Discard in waste container

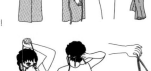

PERFORM HAND HYGIENE IMMEDIATELY AFTER REMOVING ALL PPE

SECUENCIA PARA QUITARSE EL EQUIPO DE PROTECCIÓN PERSONAL (PPE)

Con la excepción del respirador, quítese el PPE en la entrada de la puerta o en la antesala. Quítese el respirador después de salir de la habitación del paciente y de cerrar la puerta.

1. GUANTES
- ¡El exterior de los guantes está contaminado!
- Agarre la parte exterior del guante con la mano opuesta en la que todavía tiene puesto el guante y quíteselo
- Sostenga el guante que se quitó con la mano enguantada
- Deslice los dedos de la mano sin guante por debajo del otro guante que no se ha quitado todavía a la altura de la muñeca
- Quítese el guante de manera que acabe cubriendo el primer guante
- Arroje los guantes en el recipiente de deshechos

2. GAFAS PROTECTORAS O CARETA
- ¡El exterior de las gafas protectoras o de la careta está contaminado!
- Para quitárselas, tómelas por la parte de la banda de la cabeza o de las piezas de las orejas
- Colóquelas en el recipiente designado para reprocesar materiales o de materiales de deshecho

3. BATA
- ¡La parte delantera de la bata y las mangas están contaminadas!
- Desate los cordones
- Tocando solamente el interior de la bata, pásela por encima del cuello y de los hombros
- Voltee la bata al revés
- Dóblela o enróllela y deséchela

4. MÁSCARA O RESPIRADOR
- La parte delantera de la máscara o respirador está contaminada — ¡NO LA TOQUE!
- Primero agarre la parte de abajo, luego los cordones o banda elástica de arriba y por último quítese la máscara o respirador
- Arrójela en el recipiente de deshechos

EFECTÚE LA HIGIENE DE LAS MANOS INMEDIATAMENTE DESPUÉS DE QUITARSE CUALQUIER EQUIPO DE PROTECCIÓN PERSONAL

The Joint Commission's List of Dangerous Abbreviations, Acronyms, and Symbols

The Joint Commission (TJC) has approved a "minimum list" of dangerous abbreviations, acronyms, and symbols. The items in Table 1 must be included on each accredited organization's "Do Not Use" list.

The Institute for Safe Medication Practices (ISMP) has published a list of dangerous abbreviations (available at www.ismp.org) relating to medication use that it recommends should be explicitly prohibited. Two nurses must double-check the following before administration: heparin, insulin, parenteral chemotherapeutic agents, patient-controlled analgesia, and epidural pumps.

The Health Insurance Portability and Accountability Act (HIPAA) privacy requirements state that patient information concerning name, age, diagnosis, and other personal information should not be posted. Charts and medication records must be kept in a confidential area.

TABLE 1 The Joint Commission Minimum "Do Not Use" List of Abbreviations

DO NOT USE	POTENTIAL PROBLEM	USE INSTEAD
U (unit)	Mistaken for "0" (zero), "4" (four), or cc	Write "unit"
IU (international unit)	Mistaken for IV (intravenous) or the number 10 (ten)	Write "international unit"
Q.D., QD, q.d., qd (daily)	Mistaken for each other	Write "daily"
Q.O.D., QOD, q.o.d., qod (every other day)	Period after the Q mistaken for "I" and the "O" mistaken for "I"	Write "every other day"
Trailing zero (X.0 mg) [NOTE: Prohibited only for medication-related notations] Lack of leading zero (.X mg)	Decimal point is missed	Never write a zero by itself after a decimal point (X mg), and always use a zero before a decimal point (0.X mg)
MS	Can mean "morphine sulfate" or "magnesium sulfate"	Write "morphine sulfate" or "magnesium sulfate"
MSO_4 and $MgSO_4$	Confused for one another	

The Joint Commission, 2012. Reprinted with permission.

AB	abortion	G	gravida (number of pregnancies)
AC	abdominal circumference	GDM	gestational diabetes mellitus
AGA	appropriate for gestational age	GER	gastroesophageal reflux
AGE	acute gastroenteritis	GH	gestational hypertension
AROM	artificial rupture of membranes	GI	gastrointestinal
BCP	birth control pill	GIFT	gamete intrafallopian transfer
BMR	basal metabolic rate	GnRH	gonadotropin-releasing hormone
BOM	bilateral otitis media	GTPAL	gravida, term, premature, abortion, living children
BOW	bag of waters		
Bpd	biparietal diameter	GTT	glucose tolerance test
BPD	bronchopulmonary dysplasia (infants)	H&H	hemoglobin and hematocrit
bpm	beats per minute (beats/min)	H&P	history and physical
BRP	bathroom privileges	HBO	hyperbaric oxygen
BS	bowel sounds	HC	head circumference
BSA	body surface area	hCG	human chorionic gonadotropin
BSE	breast self-examination	HELLP	*hemolysis, elevated liver enzymes, low platelet count*
BTB	breakthrough bleeding		
BW	birth weight	Hib	*Haemophilus influenzae* type B conjugate vaccine
C/S	cesarean section		
CAN	child abuse and neglect	HPL	human placental lactogen
cp	cerebral palsy	HR	heart rate
CNS	central nervous system	HRT	hormone replacement therapy
CNS	clinical nurse specialist	I&D	incision and drainage
CPD	cephalopelvic disproportion	IM	intramuscular
CRL	crown–rump length	I/O	intake and output
CST	contraction stress test	IUD	intrauterine device
CX	cervix	IUGR	intrauterine growth restriction
D&C	dilation and curettage	IVF	in vitro fertilization
D&E	dilation and evacuation	KUB	kidneys, ureters, bladder
DFA	diet for age	KVO	keep vein open
DOB	date of birth	L&D	labor and delivery
EBL	estimated blood loss	LBW	low birth weight
EDC	estimated date of confinement	LDR	labor-delivery room
EDD	estimated date of delivery	LGA	large for gestational age
EFM	external fetal monitor	LH	luteinizing hormone
EFW	estimated fetal weight	lmp	last menstrual period
EGA	estimated gestational age	LMP	left mentoposterior
ENT	ear, nose, and throat	LNMP	last normal menstrual period
FAS	fetal alcohol syndrome	LOM	left otitis media
FB	foreign body	MAS	meconium aspiration syndrome
FHR	fetal heart rate	MDI	metered dose inhaler
FHS	fetal heart sound	med neb	nebulized medication
FHT	fetal heart tone	mL	milliliter(s)
FSH	follicle-stimulating hormone	MRCP	mental retardation with cerebral palsy
FTT	failure to thrive	N/V/D/C	nausea, vomiting, diarrhea, constipation
FUO	fever of unknown origin	NCP	nursing care plan
Fx	fracture	NKDA	no known drug allergies

NPO	nothing by mouth	SAT	saturation
NST	non–stress test	SGA	small for gestational age
NSVD	normal spontaneous vaginal delivery	SIDS	sudden infant death syndrome
NTT	nasotracheal tube	SL	sublingual (under the tongue)
NV	neurovascular	SOAP	subjective/objective/assessment and planning
OB	obstetric		
OC	oral contraceptive	SOB	shortness of breath
OE	otitis externa	SPROM	spontaneous premature rupture of membranes
ORIF	open reduction internal fixation		
OTC	over-the-counter (nonprescription drug)	S/S	signs and symptoms
PAR	postanesthesia recovery	SubQ	subcutaneous
Para	woman who has given birth to a viable infant (number increases by 1 for each such birth)	STAT	at once
		STD	sexually transmitted disease
		TKO	to keep open
PDA	patent ductus arteriosus	TO	telephone order
PEG	percutaneous endoscopic gastrostomy	TPN	total parenteral nutrition
PERRLA	*p*upils *e*qual, *r*ound, *r*eactive to *l*ight, and *a*ccommodation	TRA	to run at
		TSS	toxic shock syndrome
PICC	peripherally inserted central venous catheter	UC	uterine contractions
		VBAC	vaginal birth after cesarean
PID	pelvic inflammatory disease	VDRL	Venereal Disease Research Laboratories
PKU	phenylketonuria	VLBW	very low birth weight
PMDD	premenstrual dysphoric disorder	VO	verbal order
PMS	premenstrual syndrome	W-D	well developed
PP	postpartum	WIC	Women, Infants, Children
PPD	tuberculin test	wn	well nourished
PROM	premature rupture of membranes	WNL	within normal limits
PT	prothrombin time	y/o	year old
PTT	partial thromboplastin time	YOB	year of birth
RAD	reactive airway disease	ZIFT	zygote intrafallopian transfer
RDA	recommended daily allowance	↑	increase
RDI	recommended daily intake	↓	decrease
RDS	respiratory distress syndrome	+	positive, plus
REM	rapid eye movement	<	less than
R/O	rule out	>	greater than
ROM	range of motion	~	approximate
ROM	rupture of membranes	Δ	change

Is there someone with you who speaks English?
¿Hay alguien con usted que hable inglés?
Ah-ee ahl-gee-ehn kohn oos-tehd keh ah-bleh een-glehs?

I am the nurse.
Soy la enfermera.
Soy lah ehn-fehr-meh-rah.

Sit down, please.
Siéntese, por favor.
See-ehn-teh-seh, pohr fah-bohr.

Lie down.
Asuéstese.
Ah-kwehs-teh-seh.

Turn on your right (left) side.
Voltéese del lado derecho (izquierdo).
Bohl-teh-eh-seh dehl lah-doh deh-reh-choh (ees-kee-her-doh).

Lie on your back.
Acuéstese boca arriba.
Ah-kwehs-teh-seh boh-kah ah-ree-bah.

Lie on your stomach.
Acuéstese boca abajo.
Ah-kwehs-teh-seh boh-kah ah-bah-hoh.

You need to take medicine (medication).
Usted necesita tomar medicina.
Oos-tehd neh-seh-see-tah toh-mahr meh-dee-see-nah.

Show me with one finger where you have the pain.
Enséñeme con un solo dedo dónde tiene el dolor.
Ehn-seh-nyeh-meh kohn oon soh-loh deh-doh dohn-deh tee-eh-neh ehl doh-lohr.

Do you have nausea?
¿Tiene náusea?
Tee-eh-neh nah-oo-seh-ah?

Do you have vomiting?
¿Tiene vómito?
Tee-eh-neh boh-mee-toh?

When was the last time that you ate?
¿Cuándo fue la última vez que comió?
Kwahn-do fweh lah ool-tee-mah behs keh koh-mee-oh?

Do you have diarrhea?
¿Tiene diarrea?
Tee-eh-neh dee-ah-reh-ah?

Are you constipated?
¿Está estreñido (-a)?
Ehs-tah ehs-treh-nyee-doh (-dah)?

Are you passing gas?
¿Está pasando gas?
Ehs-tah pah-sahn-doh gahs?

Does it burn when you urinate?
¿Le arde cuando orina?
Leh ahr-deh kwahn-doh oh-ree-nah?

Bend your knees.
Doble las rodillas.
Doh-bleh lahs roh-dee-yahs.

Do you have pain here?
¿Tiene dolor aquí?
Tee-eh-neh doh-lohr ak-kee?

Breathe deeply.
Respire profundo.
Rehs-pee-reh proh-foon-doh.

Drink clear liquids.
Tome líquidos claros.
Toh-meh lee-kwee-dohs klah-rohs.

Can you give us a stool sample?
¿Puede darnos una muestra de excremento?
Pweh-deh dahr-nohs oo-nah mwehs-trah deh eks-kreh-mehn-toh?

When was the last time you had a bowel movement?
¿Cuándo fue la última vez que obró (que usó el baño)?
Kwahn-doh fweh lah ool-tee-mah behs keh oh-broh (keh oo-soh ehl bah-nyoh)?

Drink eight glasses of water a day.
Tome ocho vasos de agua al día.
Toh-meh oh-choh bah-sohs deh ah-gwah ahl dee-ah.

Do you have sexual relations with men (women, prostitutes)?
¿Tiene usted relaciones sexuales con hombres (mujeres, prostitutas)?
Tee-eh-neh oos-tehd rel-lah-see-oh-nehs sek-soo-ah-lehs kohn ohm-brehs (moo-heh-rehs, prohs-tee-too-tahs)?

Are you allergic to any medicine or food?
¿Es alérgica a alguna medicina o alimento?
Ehs ah-lehr-hee-kah ah al-goo-nah meh-dee-see-nah oh ah-lee-mehn-toh?

Do you take medicine?
¿Toma usted medicina?
Toh-mah oos-tehd meh-dee-see-nah?

Do you have the medicine with you?
¿Trae la medicina con usted?
Trah-eh lah meh-dee-see-na kohn oos-tehd?

Take your medication.
Tome su medicina.
Toh-meh soo meh-dee-see-nah.

I am going to give you pain medicine.
Le voy a dar medicina para el dolor.
Leh boy ah dahr med-dee-see-nah pah-rah ehl doh-lohr.

Do you have shortness of breath?
¿Tiene falta del aire?
Tee-ehn-eh fahl-tah deh ay-reh?

We need a urine sample.
Necesitamos una muestra de orina.
Neh-seh-see-tah-mohs oo-nah mwehs-trah deh oh-ree-nah.

You need a catheter in your bladder.
Usted necesita una sonda en la vejiga.
Oos-tehd neh-seh-see-tah oo-nah sohn-dah ehn lah beh-hee-gah.

Have you lost weight?
¿Ha perdido peso?
Ah pehr-dee-doh peh-soh?

How long have you had the discharge?
¿Cuánto tiempo tiene con el deshecho (flujo)?
Kwahn-toh tee-ehm-poh tee-eh-neh kohn ehl dehs-eh-choh (floo-hoh)?

What do you use to prevent pregnancy?
¿Qué clase de anticonceptivo usa para prevenir el embarazo?
Keh klah-seh deh ahn-tee-kohn-sept-tee-boh oo-sah pah-rah preh-beh-neer ehl ehm-bah-rah-soh?

When was your last period?
¿Cuándo fue su última regla (menstruación)?
Kwahn-do fweh soo ool-tee-mah reh-glah (mehns-troo-ah-see-ohn)?

Are your periods regular?
¿Sus reglas (menstruaciones) son regulares?
Soos rehs-glahs (mehns-troo-ah-see-oh-nehs) sohn reh-goo-lah-rehs?

Are you pregnant?
¿Esta embarazada?
Ehs-tah ehm-bah-rah-sah-dah?

How many times have you been pregnant?
¿Cuántas veces ha esado embarazada?
Kwahn-tahs beh-sehs ah ehs-tah-doh ehm-bah-rah-sah-dah?

How many children do you have?
¿Cuántos hijos tiene?
Kwahn-tohs ee-hohs tee-eh-neh?

Have you received prenatal care?
¿Ha recibido cuidado prenatal?
Ah reh-see-bee-doh kwih-dah-doh preh-nah-tahl?

When was the last time you visited your doctor?
¿Cuándo fue la última vez que visitó a su médico?
Kwahn-doh fweh lah ool-tee-mah behs keh bee-see-toh ah soo meh-dee-koh?

How long have you had vaginal bleeding?
¿Por cuánto tiempo ha tenido sangrado vaginal?
Pohr kwahn-toh te-ehm-poh ah teh-nee-doh sahn-grah-doh bah-hee-nahl?

How many sanitary pads did you use today?
¿Cuántas toallas femininas usó hoy?
Kwhan-tahs toh-ah-yahs feh-meh-nee-nahs oo-soh oh-ee?

Are you having contractions?
¿Tiene contracciones?
Tee-eh-neh kohn-trahk-see-ohn-ehs?

How many minutes do the contractions last?
¿Cuántos minutos le duran las contracciones?
Kwahn-tohs mee-noo-tohs leh doo-rahn lahs kohn-trakh-see-ohn-ehs?

Did your bag of water break?
¿Se le rompió la fuente del agua?
Seh leh rohm-pee-oh lah fwehn-teh dehl ah-gwah?

When did your bag of water break?
¿Cuándo se le reventó la fuente del agua?
Kwahn-doh seh leh reh-behn-toh lah fwehn-teh dehl ah-gwah?

(Don't) push.
(No) Empuje.
(Noh) Ehm-poo-heh.

I am going to listen to the baby's heartbeat.
Voy a escuchar los latidos del corazón del bebé.
Boh-ee ah ehs-koo-chahr lohs lah-tee-dohs dehl koh-rah-sohn dehl beh-beh.

Do you want me to call a friend or relative for you?
¿Quiere que yo le llame a una amistad o pariente?
Kee-eh-reh keh yoh leh yah-meh ah oo-nah ah-mees-tahd oh pah-ree-ehn-teh?

I need to comb your hair.
Necesito peinarle el pelo.
Neh-seh-see-toh peh-ee-nahr-leh ehl peh-loh.

Do you know if you have diabetes?
¿Usted sabe si tiene diabetes?
Oos-tehd sah-beh see tee-eh-neh dee-ah-beh-tehs?

Do you take insulin (diabetic pills)?
¿Toma insulina (píldoras para la diabetes)?
Toh-mah een-soo-lee-nah (peel-doh-rahs pah-rah lah dee-ah-beh-tehs)?

What type of insulin do you take? Regular? NPH? Humulin 70/30?
¿Qué tipo de insulina toma? ¿Regular? ¿NPH? ¿Humulina 70/30?
Keh tee-poh deh een-soo-lee-nah toh-mah? Reh-goo-lahr? Eh-neh Peh Ah-cheh? Oo-moo-lee-nah seh-tehn-tah treh-een-tah?

How many units of insulin do you take in the morning (evening)?
¿Cuántas unidades de insulina toma en la mañana (tarde)?
*Kwahn-tahs oo-nee-**dah**-dehs deh een-soo-**lee**-nah **toh**-mah ehn lah mah-**nyah**-nah (**tahr**-deh)?*

Do you check your blood sugar level at home?
¿Usted revisa en casa el nivel de azúcar de la sangre?
*Oos-**tehd** reh-**bee**-sah ehn **kah**-sah ehl nee-**behl** deh ah-soo-kahr deh lah **sahn**-greh?*

What was the blood sugar when you checked it?
¿Cuánto fue el azúcar cuándo lo revisó?
*Kwahn-toh fweh ehl ah-soo-kahr **kwan**-doh loh reh-bee-**soh**?*

When was the last time you took your medicine?
¿Cuándo fue la última vez que tomó su medicina?
*Kwahn-doh fweh lah **ool**-tee-mah behs keh toh-**moh** soo meh-dee-**see**-nah?*

(X) hours (days, weeks) ago.
(X) hora (días, semanas).
*(X) oh-rahs (**dee**-ahs, seh-**mah**-nahs).*

Have you eaten breakfast?
¿Ha desayunado?
*Ah dehs-ah-yoo-**nah**-doh?*

Have you eaten lunch?
¿Ha almorzado (merendado, tomado el lonche)?
*Ah ahl-mohr-**sah**-doh (meh-rehn-**dah**-doh, toh-**mah**-doh ehl **lohn**-cheh)?*

Have you eaten dinner (supper)?
¿He cenado (tomado la comida)?
*Ah seh-**nah**-doh (toh-**mah**-doh lah koh-**mee**-dah)?*

When did the accident occur?
¿Cuándo ocurrió el accidente?
*Kwahn-doh **oh**-koo-ree-oh ehl ak-see-**dehn**-teh?*

Did you lose consciousness?
¿Perdió el conocimiento?
*Pehr-dee-**oh** ehl koh-noh-see-mee-**ehn**-toh?*

When was the last time you received a tetanus vaccine?
¿Cuándo fue la última vez que recibió una vacuna del tétano?
*Kwahn-doh fweh lah **ool**-tee-mah behs keh reh-see-bee-**oh** oo-nah bah-**koo**-nah dehl **teh**-tah-noh?*

Does the baby sleep more than usual?
¿El (La) bebé duerme más de lo normal?
*Ehl (Lah) beh-**beh** dwehr-meh mahs deh loh nohr-**mahl**?*

Does the baby cry more than usual?
¿El (La) bebé llora más de lo normal?
*Ehl (Lah) be-**beh** yoh-rah mahs deh loh nohr-**mahl**?*

Do you have difficulty waking up the child?
¿Tiene dificultad para despertar al niño (a la niña)?
*Tee-**eh**-neh dee-fee-kool-**tahd** pah-rah dehs-pehr-**tahr** ahl nee-nyoh (ah lah **nee**-nyah)?*

When was the last time you gave him (her) medicine for the fever?
¿Cuándo fue la última vez que le dio medicina para la fiebre?
*Kwahn-doh fweh lah **ool**-tee-mah behs keh leh dee-**oh** meh-dee-**see**-nah **pah**-rah lah fee-**eh**-breh?*

Be sure he (she) drinks plenty of fluids.
Asegure que tome muchos líquidos.
*Ah-seh-**goo**-reh keh **toh**-meh **moo**-chohs **lee**-kee-dohs.*

Give him (her) Tylenol every four hours.
Dele Tylenol cada cuatro horas.
*Deh-leh **tay**-leh-nohl **kah**-dah koo-**ah**-troh oh-rahs.*

Is he (she) acting normally?
¿Está actuando normalmente?
*Ehs-**tah** ahk-too-**ahn**-doh nohr-mahl-**mehn**-teh?*

When he (she) vomits, does the emesis shoot out in projectile form?
Cuándo vomita, ¿sale disparado el vómito en forma proyectil?
*Kwahn-doh boh-**mee**-tah, sah-leh dees-pah-**rah**-doh ehl **boh**-mee-toh en **fohr**-mah proh-yek-**teel**?*

When was the last time he (she) vomited?
¿Cuándo fue la última vez que vomitó?
*Kwahn-doh fweh lah **ool**-tee-mak behs keh-boh-mee-**toh**?*

Has the baby lost weight?
¿Ha perdido peso el (la) bebé?
*Ah pehr-**dee**-doh **peh**-soh ehl (lah) beh-beh?*

Have you recently traveled outside the country?
¿Recientemente ha viajado fuera del país?
*Reh-see-ehn-teh-**mehn**-teh ah bee-ah-**hah**-doh fweh-rah dehl pah-**ees**?*

Have you changed his (her) formula?
¿Le ha cambiado la fórmula?
*Leh ah kahm-bee-**ah**-doh lah **fohr**-moo-lah?*

What brand of formula does he (she) take?
¿Qué marca de fórmula toma?
*Keh **mahr**-kah deh **fohr**-moo-lah toh-mah?*

Do you give him (her) cow's milk?
¿Le da leche de vaca?
*Leh dah **leh**-chech deh bah-kah?*

Does the baby vomit only when you give him (her) milk?
¿El (La) bebé vomita solamente cuándo le da leche?
*Ehl (Lah) beh-**beh** boh-**mee**-tah soh-lah-**mehn**-teh **kwahn**-doh leh dah **leh**-cheh?*

Is there another person in the house with the same symptoms?
¿Hay otra persona en casa con los mismos síntomas?
*Ah-ee oh-trah pehr-**soh**-nah ehn **kah**-sah kohn lohs **mees**-mohs **seen**-toh-mahs?*

Does he (she) have a history of asthma?
¿Tiene una historia de asma?
*Tee-**eh**-neh oo-nah ees-**toh**-ree-ah deh **ahs**-mah?*

We need to do an x-ray of his (her) chest.	**Necesitamos hacerle una radiografia del pecho.** *Neh-seh-see-**tah**-mohs ah-**sehr**-leh **oo**-nah rah-dee-oh-grah-**fee**-ah dehl **peh**-choh.*
When did the convulsion occur?	**¿Cuándo le ocurrió la convulsión?** *Kwahn-doh leh oh-koo-ree-**oh** lah kohn-bool-see-**ohn**?*
How long did the convulsion last?	**¿Cuánto tiempo duró la convulsión?** *Kwahn-toh tee-**ehm**-poh doo-**roh** lah kohn-bool-see-**ohn**?*
Did the child lose consciousness?	**¿Perdió el ninó (la niná) el conocimiento?** *Pehr-dee-**oh** ehl **nee**-nyoh (lah **nee**-nyah) ehl koh-noh-see-mee-**ehn**-toh?*
When did the rash appear?	**¿Cuándo empezó la erupción?** *Kwahn-doh ehm-peh-**soh** lah eh-roop-see-**ohn**?*
Do you have a new dog or cat at home?	**¿Tienen un nuevo perro o gato en casa?** *Tee-**eh**-nehn oon **nweh**-boh **peh**-roh oh **gah**-toh ehn **kah**-sah?*
Have you used a new soap, shampoo, detergent, or lotion?	**¿Ha usado un nuevo jabón, champú, detergente, o loción?** *Ah oo-**sah**-doh oon **nweh**-boh hah-**bohn,** chahm-poo, deh-tehr-**hehn**-teh, oh loh-see-**ohn**?*
Are your child's shots up to date?	**¿Está al corriente con sus vacunas su hijo (-a)?** *Ehs-**tah** ahl koh-ree-**ehn**-teh kohn soos bah-**koo**-nahs soo **ee**-hoh (-hah)?*
Is he (she) teething?	**¿Le están saliendo los dientes?** *Leh ehs-**tahn** sah-lee-**ehn**-doh lohs dee-**ehn**-tehs?*
Does he (she) have problems swallowing?	**¿Tiene problemas al tragar?** *Tee-**eh**-neh proh-**bleh**-mahs ahl trah-**gahr**?*
How long has he (she) had trouble walking?	**¿Cuánto tiempo lleva con dificultad al caminar?** *Kwahn-toh tee-**ehm**-poh **yeh**-bah kohn dee-fee-kool-**tad** ahl kah-mee-**nahr**?*
Did he (she) fall?	**¿Se cayó?** *Seh kah-**yoh**?*

Modified from Nasr I, Cordero M: *Medical Spanish: an instant translator,* Philadelphia, 1996, Saunders.

glossary of Symptoms

Symptom	Definition		Spanish	Chinese	Korean	Japanese	Tagalog
Abnormal Bleeding	Unusual loss of blood from stools, urine, bleeding gums, internal organs.		Sangrado anormal	異常出血	비정상 출혈	異常出血	Di-normal na Pagdugo
Chills	A feeling of being cold and shivering, usually with pale skin and a high temperature.		Escalofrio	寒顫	오한	悪寒	Ginaw
Cough	Rapid expulsion of air from the lungs in order to clear fluid, mucus, or phlegm.		Tos	咳嗽	기침	咳	Ubo
Diarrhea	Having loose and watery stools (bowel movements) often.		Diarrea, excrementos liquidos	腹瀉	설사	下痢	Pagtatae
Disorientation	To lose a sense of time, place, and one's personal identity.		Desorientación, confusión mental	定向障礙	방향 감각 상실	方向感覚の喪失	Pagkalito
Dizziness	A feeling of unsteadiness.		Sentirese desmayado	頭暈	현기증	めまい	Pagkahilo
Dyspnea	Shortness of breath or difficulty breathing.		Dificultad de respirar	呼吸困難	호흡 곤란	呼吸困難	Pangangapos ng Hininga
Fever	A rise in the temperature of the body above normal, usually when the body has an infection. (A temperature taken by mouth greater than 100.4° Fahrenheit means you have a fever.)		Fiebre	發燒	열	発熱	Lagnat
Headache	A pain located in the head, as over the eyes, at the temples, or at the bottom of the skull.		Dolor de cabeza intenso	頭痛	두통	頭痛	Sakit ng Ulo
Hemoptysis	Coughing up blood (or bloody mucus).		Tos con sangre	咯血	객혈	血を吐く	Pag-ubo ng Dugo
Jaundice	Yellowing of eyes, skin.		Piel y ojos de color amarillo (ictericia)	黃疸	황달	黄疸	Paninilaw ng Mata at Balat
Loss of Appetite	No desire to eat.		Pérdida del apetito	食欲不振	식욕 부진	食欲不振	Pagkawala ng Ganang Kumain
Loss of Consciousness (Unconscious)	Not responsive, not aware, not feeling, not thinking (sometimes as a result of fainting).		Desmayarse	失去知覺	무의식	意識不明	Pagkawala ng Malay
Malaise	Feeling generally weak and tired, and bodily discomfort.		Indisposición o malestar	不舒服	권태감	倦怠感	Panlulupaypay
Nausea	An unpleasant feeling in the stomach, with an urge to vomit (throw up).		Ganas de vomitar o náuseas	噁心	메스꺼움	吐き気	Nasusuka
Pain	An unpleasant feeling in the body that can range from being mild to extremely painful. The pain can be physical or emotional. Body pain is physical pain, usually due to tissue damage.		Dolor	疼痛	통증	痛み	Masakit
Rash	Red bumps (or flaky patches) on the body that are sometimes itchy.		Erupción o sarpullido	皮疹	발진	発疹	Singaw sa Balat
Sore Throat	Pain or discomfort in swallowing.		Dolor de garganta	喉嚨痛	목앓이	喉の痛み	Masakit na Lalamunan
Tremor	An uncontrollable trembling, shaking, or quivering from physical weakness, emotional stress, or disease.		Temblor continuo	震顫	떨림	震え	Pangangatal
Vomiting	To throw up what is inside the stomach through the mouth.		Vómito	嘔吐	구토	嘔吐	Pagsusuka

Division of Communicable Disease Control

IMM-835 (3/05)

glossary of *Symptoms* (Cont.)

Symptom	Cambodian	Hmong	Laotian	Vietnamese	Arabic	Farsi	Armenian	Russian	Punjabi
Abnormal Bleeding	ឈាមហូរខុសធម្មតា	Los ntshav			Chảy Máu Bất Thường	نزيف شديد غير طبيعي	خونریزی غیرعادی (ب ترمال بلیدینگ)	Արատավոր Արյունահոսություն	Кровотечение в брюшную полость	ਬਹੁਤ ਖੂਨ ਪੈਣਾ
Chills	ត្រជាក់	No		Ớn Lạnh	قشعريرة	لرز (چیلز)	Սարսուռներ	Озноб	ਪਾਲਾ
Cough	ក្អក	Hnoos		Ho	سعال / كحة	سرفه (کاف)	Հազ	Кашель	ਖੰਘ
Diarrhea	រាគ	Thoj plab		Tiêu Chảy	إسهال	اسهال (دایریا)	Լուծ	Понос	ਟੱਟੀਆਂ ਲੱਗਣਾ
Disorientation	ងឿងឆ្ងល់	Feeb tsis meej		Bối Rối / Mất Định Hướng	توهان	اختلال در جهت یابی (دیس أیینتیشن)	Ապակողմնորոշում	Дезориентация	ਭੌਂਦਲਣਾ
Dizziness	វិលមុខ	Kiv taubhau		Chóng mặt	دوخة/دوار	سرگتخه	Գլխապտույտ	Головокружение	ਚੱਕਰ ਆਉਣੇ
Dyspnea	ពិបាកដកដង្ហើម	Txog Siav		Hụt Hơi / Khó Thở	ضيقة نفس / صعوبة في التنفس	تنگی نفس (دیسپینا)	Դժվարաշունչ Շնչառություն	Одышка	ਸਾਹ ਲੈਣ ਵਿਚ ਮੁਸ਼ਕਲ
Fever	គ្រុន	Kub cev		Sốt	سخونة شديدة	تب (فیور)	Ջերմություն	Жар	ਬੁਖਾਰ
Headache	ឈឺក្បាល	Mob taubhau		Nhức Đầu	صداع	سردرد (هد إک)	Գլխացավ	Головная боль	ਸਿਰਦਰਦ
Hemoptysis	ក្អកផ្ដាច់ឈាម	Hnoos tau ntshav		Ho / Khạc Ra Máu	سعال مع بصق الدم / كحة مع بصق الدم	خلط خونی (همپتا یسیس)	Արյունախառն Հազ	Кровохарканье	ਖੰਘ ਨਾਲ ਖੂਨ ਆਉਣਾ
Jaundice	ជម្ងឺខាន់លឿង	Daj ntseg		Vàng Da	الصفراء	یرقان . زردی (جاندیس)	Դեղնախտ	Желтуха	ਪੀਲੀਆ
Loss of Appetite	ឥតឃ្លានអាហារ	Tsis qab los		Biếng ăn	فقدان الشهية/عدم الرغبة في الطعام	بی اشتهایی	Ախորժակի Կորուստ	Потеря аппетита	ਭੁੱਖ ਨਾ ਲੱਗਣਾ
Loss of Consciousness (Unconscious)	សន្លប់	Looj lawm		Bất Tỉnh	فقدان الوعي (فاقد الوعي)	ناموشیاری (آنکانسیس نس)	Ուշագնացություն (Ուշաթափում Չկա)	Потеря сознания	ਬੇਹੋਸ਼ੀ
Malaise	ឈឺថ្ងាល់	Nkees		Mệt Mỏi / Uể Oải	تعب في الجسم كله	احساس بیحالی و ناخوشی عمومگی (میلز)	Թուլություն	Недомогание	ਕਮਜ਼ੋਰੀ
Nausea	ចង់ក្អួត	Xeev siab		Buồn Nôn	ميل للتقيؤ/ غثيان	حال بهم خوردگی، تهوع (نازیا)	Սրտախառնություն	Тошнота	ਜੀਅ ਕੱਚਾ ਹੋਣਾ
Pain	ឈឺ	Mob		Đau Nhức	ألم	درد (پین)	Ցավ	Боль	ਦਰਦ
Rash	កន្ទួលឡើងស្បែក	Ua xua		Da nổi mụn đỏ	طفح	جوش و دانه های قرمز روی پوست (رَش)	Ցան	Сыпь	ਧੱਫੜ
Sore Throat	ឈឺបំពង់ក	Mob cajpas		Đau Cổ Họng	ألم في الزور	گلو درد (سُرترُت)	Կոկորդի Բորբոքում	Больное горло	ਗਲਾ ਦੁਖਣਾ
Tremor	ញ័រក្បាល	Tshee		Run Rẩy	رعشة	لرزش و تکان غیر ارادی (ترمُر)	Դող	Дрожь	ਕੰਬਣਾ
Vomiting	ក្អួត	Ntuav		Ói Mửa	تقيؤ	استفراغ (وامیتینگ)	Փսխումներ	Рвота	ਉਲਟੀਆਂ

Division of Communicable Disease Control   IMM-835 (3/05)

	OUNCES															
POUNDS	0	1	2	3	4	5	6	7	8	9	10	11	12	13	14	15
0	—	28	57	85	113	142	170	198	227	255	283	312	336	369	397	425
1	454	482	510	539	567	595	624	652	680	709	737	765	794	822	850	879
2	907	936	964	992	1021	1049	1077	1106	1134	1162	1191	1219	1247	1276	1304	1332
3	1361	1389	1417	1446	1474	1503	1531	1559	1588	1616	1644	1673	1701	1729	1758	1786
4	1814	1843	1871	1899	1928	1956	1984	2013	2041	2070	2098	2126	2155	2183	2211	2240
5	2268	2296	2325	2353	2381	2410	2438	2466	2495	2523	2551	2580	2608	2637	2665	2693
6	2722	2750	2778	2807	2835	2863	2892	2920	2948	2977	3005	3033	3062	3090	3118	3147
7	3175	3203	3232	3260	3289	3317	3345	3374	3402	3430	3459	3487	3515	3544	3572	3600
8	3629	3657	3685	3714	3742	3770	3799	3827	3856	3884	3912	3941	3969	3997	4026	4054
9	4082	4111	4139	4167	4196	4224	4252	4281	4309	4337	4366	4394	4423	4451	4479	4508
10	4536	4564	4593	4621	4649	4678	4706	4734	4763	4791	4819	4848	4876	4904	4933	4961
11	4990	5018	5046	5075	5103	5131	5160	5188	5216	5245	5273	5301	5330	5358	5386	5415
12	5443	5471	5500	5528	5557	5585	5613	5642	5670	5698	5727	5755	5783	5812	5840	5868
13	5897	5925	5953	5982	6010	6038	6067	6095	6123	6152	6180	6209	6237	6265	6294	6322
14	6350	6379	6407	6435	6464	6492	6520	6549	6577	6605	6634	6662	6690	6719	6747	6776
15	6804	6832	6860	6889	6917	6945	6973	7002	7030	7059	7087	7115	7144	7172	7201	7228
	0	1	2	3	4	5	6	7	8	9	10	11	12	13	14	15
	OUNCES															

*To convert the weight known in grams to pounds (lb) and ounces (oz), for example, for a baby weighing 3717 g, glance down columns to find the figure closest to 3717, which is 3714. Refer to the number at the far left or right of the column for pounds and the number at the top or bottom for ounces to obtain 8 lb, 3 oz.

Conversion formulas:
Pounds × 453.6 = grams
Ounces × 28.35 = grams
Grams ÷ 453.6 = pounds
Grams ÷ 28.35 = ounces

Normal Vital Signs and Temperature Equivalents of Infants and Children

Normal Pediatric Vital Signs

AGE	HEART RATE (beats/min)	RESPIRATORY RATE (breaths/min)	BLOOD PRESSURE (mm Hg)*
Newborn	110-160	40-60	65-85/45-55
1-3 months	100-150	35-55	65-85/45-55
3-6 months	90-120	30-45	70-90/50-65
6-12 months	80-120	25-40	80-100/55-65
1-3 years	70-110	20-30	90-105/55-70
3-6 years	65-110	20-25	95-110/60-75
6-12 years	60-95	14-22	100-120/60-75
>12 years	55-85	12-18	110-135/65-85

*A blood pressure cuff should cover approximately two thirds of the extremity for accuracy.
From Kliegman R, Stanton B, St. Geme III J, Schor N, Behrman R: *Nelson textbook of pediatrics,* ed 19, Philadelphia, 2011, Saunders.

Temperature Equivalents

CELSIUS	FAHRENHEIT	CELSIUS	FAHRENHEIT	CELSIUS	FAHRENHEIT
34.0	93.2	37.2	98.9	40.2	104.3
34.2	93.6	37.4	99.3	40.4	104.7
34.4	93.9	37.6	99.6	40.6	105.1
34.6	94.3	37.8	100.0	40.8	105.4
34.8	94.6	38.0	100.4	41.0	105.8
35.0	95.0	38.2	100.7	41.2	106.1
35.2	95.4	38.4	101.1	41.4	106.5
35.4	95.7	38.6	101.4	41.6	106.8
35.6	96.1	38.8	101.8	41.8	107.2
35.8	96.4	39.0	102.2	42.0	107.6
36.0	96.8	39.2	102.5	42.2	108.0
36.2	97.1	39.4	102.9	42.4	108.3
36.4	97.5	39.6	103.2	42.6	108.7
36.6	97.8	39.8	103.6	42.8	109.0
36.8	98.2	40.0	104.0	43.0	109.4
37.0	98.6				

Conversion formulas:
Fahrenheit to Celsius: $(°F - 32) \times \frac{5}{9} = °C$
Celsius to Fahrenheit: $(°C \times \frac{9}{5}) + 32 = °F$

Pediatric Laboratory Values Reference

TEST	AGES	NORMAL RANGE
WBCs $(\times 10^3/mm^3)^6$	Birth	18.9 (9.4-34000/mm^3)
	6 months	11.9 (6-17,.500/mm^3)
	2-6 years	8.5 (5-15,.500 mm^3)
	6-12 years	8.1 (4.5-10000 mm^3)
RBCs $(\times 10^6/\mu L)$	1 month	4.0-6.0
	3-6 months	3.5-5.5
	6 months-2 years	3.5-5.2
	2-6 years	4.0-5.5
	>6 years	4.0-5.5
Hgb	Newborn	13.5-22 g/dL
	2 months	11.2 g/dL
	6 months-2 years	10.5-13 g/dL
	2-6 years	12.5 g/dL
	6-13 years	13.5 g/dL
Hct	2 months	28%-42%
	6 months-2 years	33%-36%
	2-6 years	34%-37%
	6-12 years	35%-43%
MCV	6 months-2 years	70-78 fL
	6-12 years	77 fL
	12-18 years	78-88 fL
MCHC	Birth	30-36 g/dL
	2 months	28.3-37.8 g/dL
	6 months-2 years	30-37 g/dL
	2-6 years	31-34 g/dL
	6-12 years	31-34 g/dL
	12-18 years	31-37 g/dL
Reticulocyte	Newborn	0.4%-6.0%
	1-4 weeks	1.8%-4.6%
	6 months	0.7%-3.1%
	2-12 years	0.5%-1.0%
	>12 years	0.8%-2.5%
Platelet $(\times 10^9/L)$	Newborn	150-350
	6 months-2 years	150-450
Neutrophils $(\times 10^3/mm^3)^6$	Birth	11 (6-26)
	2 weeks	4.5 (1-9.5)
	6 months	3.8 (1-8.5)
	4 years	3.8 (1.5-8.5)
	8 years	4.4 (1-5.7)
Lymphocytes (%)	Birth	5.5 (2-11) mm^3
	6 months	7.3 (4-13) mm^3
	4 years	4.5 (2-8) mm^3
	6 years	3.5 (1-5.7) mm^3
Monocytes $(\times 10 (9)/L)$	Birth	1.1
	1 month	0.7-1.1
	6 years	0.0-0.8
	>6 years	0.4-0.9

Continued

TEST	AGES	NORMAL RANGE
Eosinophils	Birth 6 months >6 years	0.4 mean 0.3 mean 0.2 mean or <3%
Glucose	Cord 1 day Newborn >1 day Child Thereafter	45-96 mg/dL 40-60 mg/dL 50-90 mg/dL 60-100 mg/dL 70-110 mg/dL
HgbA$_{1c}$		5.0%-7.0% of total Hgb
Antistreptolysin O titer Titer	Infant 2-4 years 5-12 years	<50 todd units <160 todd units 170-330 todd units
Acid phosphatase	Newborn 2-13 years Adult	7.4-19.4 u/mL 6.4-15.2 u/mL 0.2-11 u/L
Ammonia	Newborn Child Adolescent	70-150 mcg/dL 40-50 mcg/dL 0-60 mcg/dL
LDH	Newborn Infant Child	160-450 u/L 100-250 u/L 60-170 u/L
Amylase	<2 years 1-3 years Adult	0-20 u/L 8-75 u/L 30-102 u/L
Phosphorus	Newborn Child	4.3-9.3 mg/dL 3.2-5.5 mg/dL
Alkaline phosphatase	1-2 years 2-8 years 9-15 years	80-283 u/L 65-210 u/L 100-311 u/L (44-147 international units)
Total bilirubin	**Full Term** Cord 0-1 day 1-2 days 2-5 days >5 days	 <2.0 mg/dL <6.0 mg/dL <8.0 mg/dL <11.7 mg/dL <1.0 mg/dL
Cholesterol	Newborn Infant	53-135 mg/dL 70-170 mg/dL
Uric acid	Newborn Child Adult	2.0-6.2 mg/dL 2.5-5.5 mg/dL 2.4-6.4 mg/dL
Basophils		0-0.75%
Sodium	Newborn Infant Child Thereafter	134-140 mEq/L 139-146 mEq/L 138-145 mEq/L 135-145 mEq/L
Chloride	Cord Newborn Thereafter	96-106 mEq/L 97-110 mEq/L 98-106 mEq/L
Potassium	Newborn Child	3.0-6.0 mEq/L 3.4-4.7 mEq/L
CO_2	Cord Preemie Newborn Infant/Child	14-22 mEq/L 14-27 mEq/L 13-22 mEq/L 20-28 mEq/L
Calcium (Total)	Cord Newborn	9.0-11.5 mg/dL 7.6-10.4 mg/dL

Continued

TEST	AGES	NORMAL RANGE
	4-7 days	9.0-10.9 mg/dL
	Child	8.8-10.8 mg/dL
	Thereafter	8.4-10.0 mg/dL
INR	1-5 years	0.96-1.04
	11-16 years	0.93-1.2
PT	Newborn	10.1-13.9 seconds
	1-10 years	11-12.1 seconds
PTT	Newborn	31.3-45.3 seconds
	1-10 years	24-36 seconds
BUN	Newborn	3-12 mg/dL
	Infant/child	5-18 mg/dL
	Adult	7-18 mg/dL
Creatinine	Newborn	0.3-0.9 mg/dL
	Infant/child	0.3-0.7 mg/dL
	Adolescent	0.5-1.3 mg/dL
Thyroxin (TBG)	Cord	19-39 mg/dL
	1-11 months	16-36 mg/dL
	1-9 years	12-28 mg/dL
Bicarbonate	Infant	17-24 mEq/L
	>2 years	22-26 mEq/L
Fibrinogen	Newborn	1.76-3.09 g/L
	1-10 years	1.7-4.0 g/L
Erythrocyte sedimentation rate (ESR)	Child	4-20 mm/hr
	1-10 years	1-13 mm/hr
Phenylalanine	Newborn	1.2-3.4 mg/dL
	Adult	0.8-1.8 mg/dL
Lead		<10 mg/dL
Total protein	Newborn	4.6-7.4 g/dL
	1-7 years	4.9-8.10 g/dL
	8-12 years	6.4-8.1 g/dL
	13-19 years	6.6-8.0 g/dL
Albumin	Newborn	3.2-4.8 g/dL
	Infant	3.9-5 g/dL
	Child	4-4.9 g/dL
Blood gas arterial	Newborn	7.26-7.29 pH
		60 PAO_2
		55 $PaCO_2$
		19 HCO_2
	Infant	7.4 pH
		90 PAO_2
		34 $PaCO_2$
		20 HCO_2
	Child	7.35 pH
		96 PAO_2
		37 $PaCO_2$
		22 HCO_2
	Adult	7.35-7.45 pH
		90-110 PAO_2
		35-45 $PaCO_2$
		22-26 HCO_2

NOTE: Results of laboratory tests are method dependent or instrument dependent. Measurements are approximate.
Data from Kee J: *2010 laboratory and diagnostic tests,* ed 8, Upper Saddle River, N.J., 2010, Pearson; Kliegman R, Stanton B, St. Geme III J, Schor N, Behrman R: *Nelson textbook of pediatrics,* ed 19, Philadelphia, 2011, Saunders; Soldin SJ, Wong EC, Brugnara C, Soldin OP (editors): *Pediatric reference ranges,* ed 7, Washington D.C., 2011, AACC Press; Schudy M, Arcara K: *The Harriet Lane handbook,* ed 19, St Louis, 2011, Mosby.

Blood Pressure Classifications in Children

Girls SBP by Age and Height
(Normal SBP is less than the prehypertensive result.)

Age	BP Classification	Systolic BP (mmHg)						
3	Height (cm)	91	92	95	98	100	103	105
	Prehypertension	100	100	102	103	104	106	106
	Stage 1 HTN	104	104	105	107	108	109	110
	Stage 2 HTN	116	116	118	119	120	121	122
4	Height (cm)	97	99	101	104	108	110	112
	Prehypertension	101	102	103	104	106	107	108
	Stage 1 HTN	105	106	107	108	110	111	112
	Stage 2 HTN	117	118	119	120	122	123	124
5	Height (cm)	104	105	108	111	115	118	120
	Prehypertension	103	103	105	106	107	109	109
	Stage 1 HTN	107	107	108	110	111	112	113
	Stage 2 HTN	119	119	121	122	123	125	125
6	Height (cm)	110	112	115	118	122	126	128
	Prehypertension	104	105	106	108	109	110	111
	Stage 1 HTN	108	109	110	111	113	114	115
	Stage 2 HTN	120	121	122	124	125	126	127
7	Height (cm)	116	118	121	125	129	132	135
	Prehypertension	106	107	108	109	111	112	113
	Stage 1 HTN	110	111	112	113	115	116	116
	Stage 2 HTN	122	123	124	125	127	128	129
8	Height (cm)	121	123	127	131	135	139	141
	Prehypertension	108	109	110	111	113	114	114
	Stage 1 HTN	112	112	114	115	116	118	118
	Stage 2 HTN	124	125	126	127	128	130	130
9	Height (cm)	125	128	131	136	140	144	147
	Prehypertension	110	110	112	113	114	116	116
	Stage 1 HTN	114	114	115	117	118	119	120
	Stage 2 HTN	126	126	128	129	130	132	132
10	Height (cm)	130	132	136	141	146	150	153
	Prehypertension	112	112	114	115	116	118	118
	Stage 1 HTN	116	116	117	119	120	121	122
	Stage 2 HTN	128	128	130	131	132	134	134
11	Height (cm)	136	138	143	148	153	157	160
	Prehypertension	114	114	116	117	118	119	120
	Stage 1 HTN	118	118	119	121	122	123	124
	Stage 2 HTN	130	130	131	133	134	135	136
12	Height (cm)	143	146	150	155	160	164	166
	Prehypertension	116	116	117	119	120	120	120
	Stage 1 HTN	119	120	121	123	124	125	126
	Stage 2 HTN	132	132	133	135	136	137	138
13	Height (cm)	148	151	155	159	164	168	170
	Prehypertension	117	118	119	120	120	120	120
	Stage 1 HTN	121	122	123	124	126	127	128
	Stage 2 HTN	133	134	135	137	138	139	140
14	Height (cm)	151	153	157	161	166	170	172
	Prehypertension	119	120	120	120	120	120	120
	Stage 1 HTN	123	123	125	126	127	129	129
	Stage 2 HTN--	135	136	137	138	140	141	141
15	Height (cm)	152	154	158	162	167	171	173
	Prehypertension	120	120	120	120	120	120	120
	Stage 1 HTN	124	125	126	127	129	130	131
	Stage 2 HTN	136	137	138	139	141	142	143
16	Height (cm)	152	154	158	163	167	171	173
	Prehypertension	120	120	120	120	120	120	120
	Stage 1 HTN	125	126	127	128	130	131	132
	Stage 2 HTN	137	138	139	140	142	143	144
17	Height (cm)	152	155	159	163	167	171	174
	Prehypertension	120	120	120	120	120	120	120
	Stage 1 HTN	125	126	127	129	130	131	132
	Stage 2 HTN	138	138	139	141	142	143	144

Boys SBP by Age and Height
(Normal SBP is less than the prehypertensive result.)

Age	BP Classification	Systolic BP (mmHg)						
3	Height (cm)	92	94	96	99	102	104	106
	Prehypertension	100	101	103	105	107	108	109
	Stage 1 HTN	104	105	107	109	110	112	113
	Stage 2 HTN	116	117	119	121	123	124	125
4	Height (cm)	99	100	103	106	109	112	113
	Prehypertension	102	103	105	107	109	110	111
	Stage 1 HTN	106	107	109	111	112	114	115
	Stage 2 HTN	118	119	121	123	125	126	127
5	Height (cm)	104	106	109	112	116	119	120
	Prehypertension	104	105	106	108	110	111	112
	Stage 1 HTN	108	109	110	112	114	115	116
	Stage 2 HTN	120	121	123	125	126	128	128
6	Height (cm)	110	112	115	119	122	126	127
	Prehypertension	105	106	108	110	111	113	113
	Stage 1 HTN	109	110	112	114	115	117	117
	Stage 2 HTN	121	122	124	126	128	129	130
7	Height (cm)	116	118	121	125	129	132	134
	Prehypertension	106	107	109	111	113	114	115
	Stage 1 HTN	110	111	113	115	117	118	119
	Stage 2 HTN	122	123	125	127	129	130	131
8	Height (cm)	121	123	127	131	135	139	141
	Prehypertension	107	109	110	112	114	115	116
	Stage 1 HTN	111	112	114	116	118	119	120
	Stage 2 HTN	124	125	127	128	130	132	132
9	Height (cm)	126	128	132	136	141	145	147
	Prehypertension	109	110	112	114	115	117	118
	Stage 1 HTN	113	114	116	118	119	121	121
	Stage 2 HTN	125	126	128	130	132	133	134
10	Height (cm)	130	133	137	141	146	150	153
	Prehypertension	111	112	114	115	117	119	119
	Stage 1 HTN	115	116	117	119	121	122	123
	Stage 2 HTN	127	128	130	132	133	135	135
11	Height (cm)	135	137	142	146	151	156	159
	Prehypertension	113	114	115	117	119	120	120
	Stage 1 HTN	117	118	119	121	123	124	125
	Stage 2 HTN	129	130	132	134	135	137	137
12	Height (cm)	140	143	148	153	158	163	166
	Prehypertension	115	116	118	120	120	120	120
	Stage 1 HTN	119	120	122	123	125	127	127
	Stage 2 HTN	131	132	134	136	138	139	140
13	Height (cm)	147	150	155	160	166	171	173
	Prehypertension	117	118	120	120	120	120	120
	Stage 1 HTN	121	122	124	126	128	129	130
	Stage 2 HTN	133	135	136	138	140	141	142
14	Height (cm)	154	157	162	167	173	177	180
	Prehypertension	120	120	120	120	120	120	120
	Stage 1 HTN	124	125	127	128	130	132	132
	Stage 2 HTN	136	137	139	141	143	144	145
15	Height (cm)	159	162	167	172	177	182	184
	Prehypertension	120	120	120	120	120	120	120
	Stage 1 HTN	126	127	129	131	133	134	135
	Stage 2 HTN	139	140	141	143	145	147	147
16	Height (cm)	162	165	170	175	180	184	186
	Prehypertension	120	120	120	120	120	120	120
	Stage 1 HTN	129	130	132	134	135	137	137
	Stage 2 HTN	141	142	144	146	148	149	150
17	Height (cm)	164	166	171	176	181	185	187
	Prehypertension	120	120	120	120	120	120	120
	Stage 1 HTN	131	132	134	136	138	139	140
	Stage 2 HTN	144	145	146	148	150	151	152

Complete Bibliography and Reader References

Chapter 1: The Past, Present, and Future

Alfaro-LeFevre, R. (2011). *Critical thinking and clinical judgment: A practical approach* (4th ed.). Philadelphia: Saunders.

American Academy of Pediatrics. (2011). *Car seat safety: Information for families 2011*. Retrieved February 2013, from www.healthychildren.org.

Bulechek, G., Butcher, H., & Dochterman, J. (2012). *Nursing interventions classification (NIC)*. St. Louis: Elsevier.

Forum on Child and Family Statistics. (2011). *American child: Key national indicators of well being 2011*. Retrieved February 2013, from www.childstats.gov.

Hamric, A., Sprouse, J., & Hansen, C. (2008). *Advanced practice nursing: An integrative approach* (4th ed.). Philadelphia: Saunders.

Healthy People 2020. (2010). Retrieved February 2013, from www.HealthyPeople.gov/HP2020.

Institute of Medicine (IOM). (2011). *IOM clinical practice guidelines*. Retrieved February 2013, from www.iom.edu.

Johnson, M., Moorehead, S., Bulechek, G., Butcher, H., Maas, M., & Swanson, E. (2011). *Nursing diagnosis outcomes and interventions: NANDA, NOC & NIC* (3rd ed.). St. Louis: Mosby.

Kliegman, R., Stanton, B., St. Geme, J., III, Schor, N., & Behrman, R. (2011). *Nelson textbook of pediatrics* (19th ed.). Philadelphia: Saunders.

London, M., Ladewig, P., Ball, J., Bindler, R., & Cowen, K. (2011). *Maternal-child nursing* (3rd ed.). Englewood Cliffs, NJ: Prentice-Hall.

Moorehead, S., Johnson, M., Maas, M., & Swanson, E. (2012). *Nursing outcomes classification (NOC)* (4th ed.). St. Louis: Mosby.

National Center for Health Statistics, Health US. (2007). Government Printing Office. Retrieved June 13, 2010, from www.cdc.gov/nchs/data/hus/hus07.pdf.

National Institute of Health, (NIH). (2012). *Deaths under one years of age due to cardiovascular and lung diseases, 2007–2011*. Retrieved June 2013, from NIH.org.

National Vital Statistics Reports. (2012). *Preliminary data for 2011*. Retrieved February 2013, from www.cdc.gov/NCHS/data/NVSR/NVSR61/NVSR61_05_tables.pdf.

North American Nursing Diagnosis Association International. (2009–2011). *NANDA I Nursing diagnoses: Definitions and classification 2009–2011*. Hoboken, NJ: Wiley-Blackwell.

Pregnancy Activity Surveillance in United States. Retrieved February 2013, from www.cdc.gov/mmwr/pdf/ss/ss.

Raikkonen, K., Personen, A., & Heinonen, K. (2009). Maternal licorice consumption and detrimental cognitive and psychiatric outcomes in children. *American Journal of Epidemiology, 130*, 1137.

Rayburn, W. F., Klagholz, J. C., Murray-Krezan, C., Dowell, L. E., & Strunk, A. L. (2012). Summary of access to care statistics. *American Journal of Obstetrics and Gynecology, 119*(5), 1017–1022.

U.S. Department of Health and Human Services. (2010). *Healthy People 2020: National health promotion and disease prevention objectives*. Washington, DC: U.S. Government Printing Office.

U.S. National Commission on the International Year of the Child. (March 1980). *Report to the President*. Washington, DC: U.S. Government Printing Office. (Classic reference)

Chapter 2: Human Reproductive Anatomy and Physiology

Creasy, R., Resnick, R., Iams, J., Lockford, C., & Moore, T. (2009). *Maternal-fetal medicine* (6th ed.). Philadelphia: Saunders.

Blackburn, S. (2013). *Maternal, fetal and neonatal physiology: A clinical perspective*. Philadelphia: Saunders.

Gabbe, S., Niebyl, J., Simpson, J., Landon, M., Galan, H., Jauniaux, E., et al. (2012). *Obstetrics: Normal and problem pregnancies*. St. Louis: Elsevier.

Hacker, N., Gambone, L., & Hobel, C. (2010). *Essentials of obstetrics and gynecology* (5th ed.). Philadelphia: Saunders.

Hall, J. (2011). *Guyton and Hall textbook of medical physiology* (12th ed.). Philadelphia: Saunders.

Kliegman, R., Stanton, B., St. Geme, J., III, Shor, V., & Behrman, R. (2011). *Nelson's textbook of pediatrics* (19th ed.). Philadelphia: Saunders.

Leifer, G. (2011). *Maternity nursing* (11th ed.). Philadelphia: Saunders.

Mattson, S., & Smith, J. (2011). *AWHONN core curriculum for maternal newborn nursing* (4th ed.). Philadelphia: Saunders.

Moore, K., & Persaud, T. (2011). *Before we are born: Essentials of embryology and birth defects* (8th ed.). Philadelphia: Saunders.

Patton, K., & Thibodeau, G. (2010). *Anatomy and physiology* (7th ed.). St. Louis: Mosby.

Thibodeau, G., & Patton, K. (2010). *The human body in health and disease* (5th ed.). St. Louis: Mosby.

Chapter 3: Fetal Development

Creasy, R., Resnick, R., Iams, J., Lockford, C., & Moore, T. (2009). *Maternal-fetal medicine* (6th ed.). Philadelphia: Saunders, St. Louis: Elsevier.

Gabbe, S., Niebyl, J., Simpson, J., Landon, M., Galan, H., Jauniaux, E., et al. (2012). *Obstetrics: Normal and problem pregnancies*. Philadelphia: Saunders.

Hall, J. (2011). *Guyton and Hall textbook of medical physiology* (12th ed.). Philadelphia: Saunders.

Kliegman, R., Stanton, B., St. Geme, J., III, Shor, W., & Behrman, R. (2011). *Nelson's textbook of pediatrics* (19th ed.). Philadelphia: Saunders.

Leifer, G. (2011). *Maternity nursing* (11th ed.). Philadelphia: Saunders.

Moore, K., & Persaud, T. (2011). *Before we are born: Essentials of embryology and birth defects* (8th ed.). Philadelphia: Saunders.

Moore, K., & Persaud, T. (2009). *The developing human: Clinically oriented embryology* (9th ed.). Philadelphia: Saunders.

Thibodeau, G., & Patton, K. (2010). *The human body in health and disease* (5th ed.). St. Louis: Mosby.

Walsh, D., & Adzick, S. (2000). Fetal surgical intervention. *American Journal of Perinatology, 17*(6), 277–283.

Chapter 4: Prenatal Care and Adaptations to Pregnancy

ACOG. (2009). Practice bulletin #106: Intrapartum fetal monitoring. *American Journal of Obstetrics and Gynecology, 114*(1), 192–202.

ACOG. (2009). Travel during pregnancy: ACOG committee opinion #443: *Journal of the American College of Obstetricians and Gynecologists, 114*, 954–955.

ACOG. (2010). Practice bulletin #116: Management of intrapartum fetal heart tracings. *American Journal of Obstetrics and Gynecology, 116*(5), 1232–1240.

ACOG. (2010). Committee opinion #468: Influenza vaccination during pregnancy. *American Journal of Obstetrics and Gynecology, 116*(4), 1006–1007.

ACOG. (2012). *Guidelines for perinatal care* (7th ed.). Washington, DC: ACOG Author.

American Academy of Pediatrics & American College of Obstetricians and Gynecologists. (2007). Maternal and newborn nutrition. In *Guidelines for perinatal care* (6th ed.). Elk Grove Village, IL: American Academy of Pediatrics.

American Diabetes Association. (2010). *Living with diabetes: Prenatal care*. Retrieved April 10, 2010, from www.diabetes.org.

Ashmead, G. (2011). Fetal heart monitoring update: The good, the bad, and the atypical. *The Female Patient, 36*, 14–18.

Blackburn, S. (2013). *Maternal, fetal and neonatal physiology: A clinical perspective* (4th ed.). Philadelphia: Saunders.

Brown, H., Ahmadzia, H., & Heine, R. (2013). GBS screening: An update on guidelines. *Contemporary Ob/Gyn*, July 1.

Centers for Disease Control and Prevention. (2009). *Spina bifida*. Retrieved April 10, 2010, from www.cdc.gov/ncbddd/birthdefects/spinabifida.htm.

Centers for Disease Control and Prevention. (2010). *Folic acid: Questions and answers*. Retrieved January 12, 2013, from http://www.cdc.gov/ncbddd/folicacid/faqs.html.

Centers for Disease Control and Prevention. (2010). Planning for a healthy pregnancy while traveling. In CDC (Ed.). *Yellow book: CDC health information for international travel*. Washington, DC: U.S. Government Printing Office.

Centers for Disease Control and Prevention (CDC). (2011). Updated recommendations for use of tetanus toxoid, reduced diptheria toxoid and acellular pertussis TDaP vaccine in pregnant women and persons with close contact with infants under 12 months of age. Advisory Committee on Immunization Practices. *MMWR. Morbidity and Mortality Weekly Report, 60*(41), 1424–1426.

Creasy, R., Resnick, R., Iams, J., Lockford, C., & Moore, T. (2009). *Maternal-fetal medicine* (6th ed.). Philadelphia: Saunders.

Deane, R. (2010). Cultural competence: Nursing in a multicultural society. *Nursing and Women's Health, 14*(1), 50–59.

Dog, T. (2009). The use of botanicals during pregnancy and lactation. *Alternative Therapies in Health and Medicine, 15*(1), 54–56.

Gabbe, S., Niebyl, J., Simpson, J., Landon, M., Galan, H., Jauniaux, E., et al. (2012). *Obstetrics: Normal and problem pregnancies* (6th ed.). Philadelphia: Saunders.

Grodner, M., Roth, S., & Walkingshaw, B. (2012). *Foundations and clinical applications of nutrition: A nursing approach* (5th ed.). Philadelphia: Mosby.

Guyton, A. C., & Hall, J. E. (2011). *Textbook of medical physiology* (12th ed.). Philadelphia: Saunders.

Hacker, N., Gambone, L., & Hobel, C. (2010). *Essentials of obstetrics and gynecology* (5th ed.). Philadelphia: Saunders.

Hodgson, B., & Kizior, R. (2013). *Nursing drug handbook*. Philadelphia: Saunders.

Immunization Action Coalition. (2010). *Vaccine information for health professionals*. Retrieved January 1, 2010, from www.vaccineinformation.org.

Institute of Medicine (IOM). (2009). *Weight gain during pregnancy: Reexamining the guidelines*. Washington, DC: National Academy Press. Retrieved June 13, 2010, from www.aap.edu.

Institute of Medicine. (2010). *Food and nutrition board: DRI for calcium and vitamin D*. Washington, DC: National Academies Press.

Josefson, J. (2011). The impact of pregnancy nutrition on offspring obesity. *Journal of the American Dietetic Association, 111*(1), 50–52.

Kinser, P., & Williams, C. (2008). Prenatal yoga: Benefits and recommendations. *Advance for Nurse Practitioners, 16*(5), 59–61.

Kliegman, R., Stanton, B., St. Geme, J., III, Shor, W., & Behrman, R. (2011). *Nelson's textbook of pediatrics* (19th ed.). Philadelphia: Saunders.

Kramer, J., Bowen, A., Stewart, N., & Muhajarine, N. (2013). Nausea and vomiting of pregnancy: Prevalence, severity and relation to psychosocial health. *MCN. The American Journal of Maternal Child Nursing, 38*(1), 21–27.

Lathian, J. (2006). Birth plans: The good, the bad and the future. *Journal of Obstetric, Gynecologic, and Neonatal Nursing, 35*(2), 265–270.

Leifer, G. (2011). *Maternity nursing* (11th ed.). Philadelphia: Saunders.

Lewis, B., Avery, M., Jennings, E., Sherwood, N., Martinson, N., & Crain, L. (2008). The effect of exercise during pregnancy on maternal outcomes: Practical implications for practice. *American Journal of Lifestyle Medicine, 2*(5), 441–455.

Lockwood, C. J. (2013). Autism and the obstetrician. *Contemporary Ob/Gyn, 58*(5), 12–14.

London, M., Ladewig, P., Ball, J., & Bindler, R. (2011). *Maternal-child nursing* (3rd ed.). Englewood Cliffs, NJ: Prentice-Hall.

Lucock, M., & Yates, Z. (2009). Folic acid fortification: A double edged sword. *Current Opinion in Clinical Nutrition and Metabolic Care, 12*(6), 555–564.

Mahan, L., & Escott-Stump, S. (2012). *Krause's food, nutrition, and diet therapy* (13th ed.). Philadelphia: Saunders.

Mathews, T., Manino, A., & Osterman, K. (2011). Annual summary of vital statistics. *Pediatrics, 127*(1), 146–157.

Mattola, M. (2009). Exercise prescription for overweight and obese women: Pregnancy and postpartum. *Obstetrics and Gynecology Clinics of North America, 36*(2), 301–316.

Mattson, S., & Smith, J. (2011). *AWHONN core curriculum for maternal-newborn nursing* (4th ed.). Philadelphia: Saunders.

McKinney, E., James, S., Murray, S., & Ashwill, J. (2013). *Maternal-child nursing* (4th ed.). Philadelphia: Saunders.

Moore, M., Moos, M., & Callister, L. (2010). *Cultural competence: An essential journey for perinatal nurses*. White Plains, NY: March of Dimes.

Moore, K., & Persaud, T. (2011). *Before we are born: Essentials of embryology and birth defects* (8th ed.). Philadelphia: Saunders.

Pagana, K., & Pagana, T. (2012). *Mosby diagnostic and laboratory test reference* (10th ed.). St. Louis: Mosby.

Phelan, S. (2012). Pregnancy: A teachable moment for weight control and obesity management. *American Journal of Obstetrics and Gynecology, 135e*, 20j0.

Rubin, R. (1984). *Maternal identity and the maternal experience*. New York: Springer. (Classic reference)

Simmons, S. (2013). Folic acid: Friend or foe? *Nursing, 43*(3), 55–60.

Skidmore-Roth, L. (2010). *Mosby drug reference* (24th ed.). Philadelphia: Mosby.

Skidmore-Roth, L. (2010). *Mosby handbook of herbs and natural supplements* (4th ed.). Philadelphia: Mosby.

U.S. Department of Agriculture. (2010). *USDA national nutrient database for standard reference*. Retrieved January 2013, from www.ARS.usda.gov/service/docs.htm?docid=20958.

U.S. Department of Agriculture. (2012). *MyPlate*. Washington, DC: Author. Retrieved December 1, 2012, from www.myplate.gov.

U.S. Department of Health and Human Services. (2010). *Healthy people 2020*. Washington, DC: Author.

U.S. Preventive Services Task Force. (2008). Screening for bacterial vaginosis in pregnancy to prevent preterm delivery: U.S. Preventive Services Task Force recommendation statement. *Annals of Internal Medicine, 148*(3), 214–219.

Verani, J., McGee, L., & Schrag, S. (2010). Prevention of perinatal GBS disease: Revised guidelines from CDC. *MMWR. Recommendations and Reports: Morbidity and Mortality Weekly Report, 59*(RR-10), 1–36.

Chapter 5: Nursing Care of Women with Complications During Pregnancy

American College of Obstetricians and Gynecologists. (2011). Committee opinion #504: Screening and diagnosis of gestational diabetes mellitus. *American Journal of Obstetrics and Gynecology, 118*, 751–753.

American College of Obstetricians and Gynecologists. (2010). ACOG practice bulletin #33: *Diagnosis and management of preeclampsia and eclampsia.* Washington, DC: Author.

American College of Obstetricians and Gynecologists. (2010). ACOG practice bulletin #30: *Gestational diabetes.* Washington, DC: Author.

American College of Obstetricians and Gynecologists. (2010). ACOG practice bulletin #29: *Chronic hypertension in pregnancy.* Washington, DC: Author.

American College of Obstetricians and Gynecologists. (2011). ACOG practice bulletin #52: *Nausea and vomiting of pregnancy.* Washington, DC: Author.

American College of Obstetricians and Gynecologists. (2012). *Guidelines for perinatal care* (7th ed.). Washington, DC: ACOG Author.

American College of Obstetricians and Gynecologists. (2009). Practice bulletin #101: Ultrasonography in pregnancy. *J Obstet Gynecol, 113,* 451.

American Diabetes Association. (2009). Standards of diabetes care. *Diabetes Care, 32*(Suppl.), s13–s61.

American Diabetes Association. (2011). Diagnosis and classification of diabetes mellitus. *Diabetes Care, 34*(Suppl. 1), s62–s69.

Amiel, A., Liberman, M., Pomerantz, M., et al. (2005). "Genetic pap" at 5-12 gestational weeks: A new screening method for Down syndrome. *Journal of the Society for Gynecologic Investigation, 12S,* 290 (abstr 644).

Andrews, J. (2011). Hepatitis viral infections. In D. James, C. Steer, & C. Weiner (Eds.), *High risk pregnancy: Management options.* Philadelphia: Saunders.

Arslaneum-Engoren, C. (2011). Women's risk factors and screening for coronary heart disease. *Journal of Obstetric, Gynecologic, and Neonatal Nursing, 40*(3), 337–347.

Ashoor, G., Syngelabe, A., Wagner, M., Birder, C., & Necolaides, K. (2012). Chromosome selective sequencing of maternal plasma cell free DNA for first trimester detection of trisomy 21 and 18. *American Journal of Obstetrics and Gynecology, 286*(4), 322–325.

Blackburn, S. (2013). *Maternal, fetal and neonatal physiology: A clinical perspective.* St. Louis: Mosby.

Bobrowski, R. (2011). Trauma in pregnancy. In D. James, P. Steer, & C. Weiner (Eds.), *High risk pregnancy: Management options* (4th ed.). Philadelphia: Saunders.

Brown, H., Ahmadzia, H., & Heine, R. (2013). GBS screening: An update on guidelines. *Contemporary Ob/Gyn, 1*(1318).

Callaghan, W. (2010). Delivery is not the end of the story: Follow-up of women with GDM. *Contemporary Ob/Gyn, 55* (4), 40–46.

Centers for Disease Control and Prevention. (2009). National Center for Health Statistics: Deaths, final data for 2006. *National Vital Statistics Report, 57*(14), April 17, 2009.

Centers for Disease Control and Prevention. (2010). *ACIP: Guidelines for vaccinating pregnant and breastfeeding women.* Atlanta: CDC. Retrieved January 2013, from www.cdc.gov.

Centers for Disease Control and Prevention. (2012). Prevention of perinatal group B streptococcal disease: Revised guidelines. *MMWR, 59*(RR-10). Retrieved January 2013, from www.cdc.gov/mmwr.

Clausens, T., Mathiesen, E., & Hansen, T. (2009). Overweight and metabolic syndrome in adult offspring of women with diet treated GDM or type 1 diabetes. *The Journal of Clinical Endocrinology and Metabolism, 94,* 2464.

Cousins, L., Smok, D., Lovett, S., & Poeltler, D. (2005). AmniSure placental alpha microglobulin-1 rapid immunoassay versus standard diagnostic methods for detection of ruptured membranes. *American Journal of Perinatology, 22,* 317–320.

Creasy, R., Resnick, R., Iams, J., Lockford, C., & Moore, T. (2009). *Maternal-fetal medicine* (6th ed.). Philadelphia: Saunders.

Dotti, J. (2005). Terrorism and the pregnant woman. *Journal of Perinatal and Neonatal Nursing, 19*(3), 226–237.

Gabbe, S., Niebyl, J., Simpson, J., Landon, M., Galan, H., Jaunioux, E., et al. (2012). *Obstetrics: Normal and problem pregnancies.* Philadelphia: Saunders/Elsevier.

Hacker, N., Gambone, L., & Hobel, C. (2010). *Essentials of obstetrics and gynecology* (5th ed.). Philadelphia: Saunders.

Hoyert, D., & Xu, J. (2012). Deaths: Preliminary data for 2011. *National Vital Statistics Report, 61*(6), Hyattsville, MD.

Kitzman, J., Snyder, M., & Ventura, M. (2012). Noninvasive whole genome sequencing of human fetus. *Science Translational Medicine, 4*(137), 137–176.

Kliegman, R., Stanton, B., St. Geme, J., III, Shor, W., & Behrman, R. (2011). *Nelson's textbook of pediatrics* (19th ed.). Philadelphia: Saunders.

Langen, J., & James, D. (2005). *Preparing nurses for disaster management.* Upper Saddle River, NJ: Prentice-Hall Health.

Mahan, L., & Escott-Stump, S. (2012). *Krause's food, nutrition, and diet therapy* (13th ed.). Philadelphia: Saunders.

Mattson, S., & Smith, J. (2011). *AWHONN core curriculum for maternal-newborn nursing* (4th ed.). Washington, DC: Association of Women's Health, Obstetric, and Neonatal Nurses.

Moore, T. (2010). Fetal exposure to GDM contributes to subsequent adult metabolic syndrome. *American Journal of Obstetrics and Gynecology, 202*(6), 643–649.

Moore, L., Clokey, D., Rappaport, V., & Curet, L. (2010). Metformin compared to glyburide in GDM: A randomized trial. *J Obstet Gynecol, 115,* 55.

Simpson, J. (2013). Non-invasive fetal diagnosis: Promise versus practicality. *Contemporary Pediatrics, 1*(13), 13.

Spong, C., Signore, C., & Freeman, R. (2009). Antenatal testing: A re-evaluation. *J Obstet Gynecol, 113,* 687.

Verani, J., McGee, L., & Schrag, S. (2010). Prevention of perinatal GBS disease: Revised guidelines from CDC. *MMWR. Recommendations and Reports: Morbidity and Mortality Weekly Report, 59*(RR-10), 1–36.

Wittendorf, D., & Muenke, M. (2005). Fetal alcohol spectrum disorders. *American Family Physician, 72*(2), 279–285.

Chapter 6: Nursing Care of Mother and Infant During Labor and Birth

ACOG. (2009). *Standards for professional nurse practice in care of women and newborns* (7th ed.). Washington, DC: Author.

Adams, E., & Bianchi, A. (2008). A practical approach to labor support. *Journal of Obstetric, Gynecologic, and Neonatal Nursing, 37*(1), 106–122.

American College of Obstetricians and Gynecologists. (2010). Practice Bulletin: Vaginal birth after previous cesarean section delivery. *J Obstet Gynecol, 116*(2), 450–462.

American College of Obstetricians and Gynecologists. (2012). *Guidelines for perinatal care* (7th ed.). Washington, DC: ACOG Author.

American College of Obstetricians and Gynecologists. (2010). Practice bulletin #116: *Management of intrapartum fetal monitoring.* Washington, DC: ACOG Author.

American College of Obstetric and Gynecologic Nursing. (2009). Intrapartum fetal heart rate monitoring: Nomenclature, interpretation, and general management principles. Practice bulletin #106: *Obstetrics and Gynecology, 114*(1), 136–138.

AWHONN. (2009). *Fetal heart monitoring: Principles and practice* (4th ed.). Dubuque, IA: Kendall/Hunt.

Blackburn, S. (2012). *Maternal and neonatal physiology* (4th ed.). St. Louis: Saunders.

Chalmers, B. (2012). Childbirth across cultures: Research and practice. *Women's Health Nursing, 39*(4), 276–280.

Clark, S., Simpson, K., Knox, G., & Garite, G. (2009). Oxytoxin: New perspectives on an old drug. *American Journal of Obstetrics and Gynecology, 200,* 35.

Crawford, C., & Johnson, J. (2012). To aspirate or not: An integrative review of the evidence. *Nursing, 4*(3), 20–25.

Creasy, R., Resnick, R., Iams, J., Lockford, C., & Moore, T. (2009). *Maternal-fetal medicine* (6th ed.). Philadelphia: Saunders.

D'Avanzo, C. (2007). *Mosby's pocket guide to cultural health assessment* (4th ed.). St. Louis: Mosby.

Einstein, F., & Merkatz, I. (2008). An obstetricians guide to cord blood banking. *Contemporary Pediatrics,* October(Suppl.), 1–16.

Field, T. (2008). Alternative therapy in pregnancy and labor. *Alternative Therapies in Health and Medicine, 14*(5), 12–16.

Gabbe, S., Simpson, J., Niebyl, J., Galan, H., Goetzl, L., Jauniaux, E., et al. (2012). *Obstetrics: Normal and problem pregnancies* (6th ed.). Philadelphia: Elsevier.

Giger, J., & Davidhizar, R. (2008). *Transcultural nursing: Assessment and intervention* (5th ed.). St. Louis: Mosby.

Hall, J. (2011). *Guyton and Hall textbook of medical physiology* (12th ed.). Philadelphia: Saunders.

Halper, S., & Abdullah, F. (2010). Effect of labor analgesia on labor outcome. *Current Opinion in Anaesthesiology, 23,* 317.

Hensel, D., Morson, G., & Preusse, E. (2013). Best practices in newborn injection. *MCN. The American Journal of Maternal Child Nursing, 38*(3), 163–167.

Ho, M., Cheng, S., & Tsai-Chung, L. (2010). Titrated oral misoprostol solution compared with oxytoxin for labor augmentation. *Journal of Obstetrics and Gynecology, 116*(3), 612–618.

Immunization Action Coalition. (2009). *Administering vaccines: Dose, route, site and needle size.* Retrieved May 2013, from www.immunize.org/CATG.D/p3085.PDF.

Imo, A., Ugiou, A., & Okoye, I. (2009). Sonographic evaluation of cervical length during normal pregnancy. *Internet Journal of Medical Update, 4*(1).

Keil, S., Anjema, K., Francjan, J., Vanspronsen, F. J., Lambruschini, N., Burlina, A., et al. (2013). Long term follow-up and outcome of PKU patients on sapropterin. *Pediatrics, 131,* 1881–1888.

Kelly, H., Johnson, E., & Lee, V. (2010). Delayed VS immediate pushing in second stage of labor. *MCN. The American Journal of Maternal Child Nursing, 35*(2), 81–88.

Kliegman, R., Stanton, B., St. Geme, J., III, Shor, W., & Behrman, R. (2011). *Nelson's textbook of pediatrics* (19th ed.). Philadelphia: Saunders.

Lawrence, A., Lewis, L., & Hofmeyer, G. (2009). Maternal position and mobility during first stage of labor. *The Cochrane Database of Systematic Reviews.*

Leifer, G. (2011). *Maternity nursing* (11th ed.). Philadelphia: Saunders.

Mattson, S., & Smith, J. (2011). *AWHONN core curriculum for maternal newborn nursing* (4th ed.). Philadelphia: Saunders.

Moore, M., Moos, M., & Callister, L. (2010). *Cultural competency: An essential journey for perinatal nurses.* New York: March of Dimes.

Moore, K., & Peters, L. (2012). Implementing baby friendly practices: Strategies for success. *MCN. The American Journal of Maternal Child Nursing, 37*(4), 228–230.

Murasaki, S. (1996). *Diary of lady murasaki.* New York: Penguin Press (Classic reference).

Perlman, J., Wiley, J., & Hankel, J. (2010). International consensus on cardiopulmonary resuscitation and emergency cardiovascular care science with treatment recommendations. *Pediatrics, 126*(5), 1319–1344.

Perry, S., Hockenberry, M., Lowdermilk, D., & Wilson, D. (2010). *Maternal child nursing care* (4th ed.). St. Louis: Mosby.

Selby, C., Valencia, S., Garcia, L., Keep, D., Overcash, J., & Jackson, J. (2011). Activity level during one hour labor check evaluation: Walking vs bedrest. *MCN. The American Journal of Maternal Child Nursing, 37*(2), 101–107.

Shrivastava, V., Garite, T., & Jenkins, S. (2009). A randomized double blinded controlled trial comparing parenteral normal saline with and without dextrose on course of labor in nulliparas. *American Journal of Obstetrics and Gynecology, 20,* 379.

Simpson, K. (2008). Fetal assessment during labor. In K. Simpson, & B. Creehan (Eds.), *AWHONN perinatal nursing* (pp. 399–442). (3rd ed.). Philadelphia: Lippincott Williams & Wilkins.

Simpson, K. (2009). Fresh perspectives on intrapartum nursing care. *MCN. The American Journal of Maternal Child Nursing, 34*(1), 5–6.

Spector, R. (2009). *Cultural diversity in health and illness* (7th ed.). Upper Saddleback River, NJ: Prentice-Hall.

VandeVusse, L. (1999). The essential forces of labor revisited. *MCN. The American Journal of Maternal Child Nursing, 24*(4), 176–184. (Classic reference)

Chapter 7: Nursing Management of Pain During Labor and Birth

American College of Obstetricians and Gynecologists. (2010). Obstetric analgesia and anesthesia. In ACOG Practice bulletin #36. Washington, DC: Author.

American College of Obstetricians and Gynecologists. (2012). *Guidelines for perinatal care* (7th ed.). Washington, DC: ACOG Author.

AWHONN. (2011). *Evidence based clinical practice guideline: Nursing care of women receiving regional analgesia/anesthesia in labor* (2nd ed.). Washington, DC: Author.

Blackburn, S. (2013). *Maternal, fetal and neonatal physiology: A clinical perspective* (4th ed.). Philadelphia: Saunders.

Creasy, R., Resnick, R., Iams, J., Lockford, C., & Moore, T. (2009). *Maternal-fetal medicine* (6th ed.). Philadelphia: Saunders.

Gabbe, S., Simpson, J., Niebyl, J., Galan, H., Goetzl, L., Jauniaux, E., et al. (2012). *Obstetrics: Normal and problem pregnancies* (6th ed.). Philadelphia: Saunders.

Hawkins, J. (2010). Epidural anesthesia for labor and delivery. *The New England Journal of Medicine, 362,* 1503.

Kliegman, R., Stanton, B., St. Geme, J., III, Shor, W., & Behrman, R. (2011). *Nelson's textbook of pediatrics* (19th ed.). Philadelphia: Saunders.

McKinney, E., James, S., Murray, S., & Ashwill, J. (2013). *Maternal-child nursing* (4th ed.). Philadelphia: Saunders.

Micozzi, M. (2011). *Fundamentals of complementary and integrative medicine* (4th ed.). St. Louis: Mosby.

Sawhney, M. (2012). Epidural analgesia: What every nurse should know. *Nursing, 42*(8), 36–41.

Simpson, K., & Creehan, P. (2008). *AWHONN perinatal nursing* (3rd ed.). Philadelphia: Lippincott Williams & Wilkins.

The Joint Commission. (2011). *Facts about pain management.* Retrieved January 2013, from www.jointcommission.org.

Chapter 8: Nursing Care of Women with Complications During Labor and Birth

Abdel-Aleem, H. (2011). Misoprostol for cervical ripening and induction of labor: RHL commentary 5/1/2011. In *WHO Reproductive Health Library.* Geneva: WHO.

ACOG. (2010). ACOG practice bulletin #31: *Assessment of risk factors for preterm birth.* Washington, DC: Author.

ACOG. (2010). ACOG practice bulletin #22: *Fetal macrosomia.* Washington, DC: Author.

ACOG. (2010). ACOG practice bulletin #40: *Shoulder dystocia.* Washington, DC: Author.

ACOG. (2010). ACOG practice bulletin #115: *Vaginal birth after cesarean section. American Journal of Obstetrics and Gynecology, 116,* 540.

ACOG. (2011). ACOG practice bulletin #49: *Dystocia: The augmentation of labor.* Washington, DC: Author.

ACOG. (2011). ACOG practice bulletin #43: *Management of preterm labor.* Washington, DC: Author.

ACOG. (2011). ACOG committee opinion #291: *Use of progesterone to reduce preterm births.* Washington, DC: Author.

American College of Obstetricians and Gynecologists. (2012). *Guidelines for perinatal care ACOG*. Washington, DC: Author.

Berman, M. (2009). Finding the right words after pregnancy loss. *Contemporary Ob/Gyn, 54*(3), 46–50.

Clark, S., Meyers, J., & Frye, D. (2011). Patient safety series: Patient safety in obstetrics. Hospital Corporation of America. *American Journal of Obstetrics and Gynecology, 204*(4), 283–287.

Clavreul, G. (2011). Beyond baby blues: How nurses can recognize post partum depression. *Working Nurse Magazine, 4/11 P,* 12–14.

Creasy, R., Resnick, R., Iams, J., Lockford, C., & Moore, T. (2009). *Maternal-fetal medicine* (6th ed.). Philadelphia: Saunders.

Evans-Lynn, C. (2012). Does restrictive movements result in higher cesarean section rates? *Advance for NP's and PA's, 3*(10), 29–37.

Gabbe, S., Simpson, J., Niebyl, J., Galan, H., Goetzl, L., & Jauniaux, E., et al. (2012). *Obstetrics: normal and problem pregnancies* (6th ed.). Philadelphia: Saunders.

Gee, H. (2011). Dysfunctional labor. In D. James, P. Steer, & C. Weiner (Eds.), *High risk pregnancy management options* (4th ed). Philadelphia: Saunders.

Gilbert, E. (2011). *Manual of high risk pregnancies and deliveries* (5th ed.). St. Louis: Mosby.

Hacker, N., Gambone, J., & Hobel, C. (2010). *Essentials of obstetrics and gynecology* (5th ed.). Philadelphia: Saunders.

Hamilton, B., Martin, J., & Ventura, S. (2010). Births: Preliminary data for 2009. *Vital statistics reports:* Hyattsville, MD: National Center for Health Statistics, *59*(3), 1.

Hamilton, E., & Mark, P. (2012). Computerized interpretation of intrapartum fetal heart rate monitoring and predictor of neonatal outcomes. *American Journal of Obstetrics and Gynecology, 208*(11), S316–S317.

Healthy People 2020. (2010). Retrieved February 2013, from www.HealthyPeople.gov/HP2020.

Institute of Medicine (IOM). (2011). *IOM clinical practice guidelines.* Retrieved February 2013, from www.IOM.edu.

Kliegman, R., Stanton, B., St. Geme, J., III, Shor, W., & Behrman, R. (2011). *Nelson's textbook of pediatrics* (19th ed.). Philadelphia: Saunders.

Leifer, G. (2012). *Maternity nursing* (11th ed.). Philadelphia: Saunders.

Mattson, S., & Smith, J. (2011). *AWHONN core curriculum for maternal-child nursing* (4th ed.). St. Louis: Mosby.

National Center for Health Statistics. (2008). Retrieved June 13, 2010, from www.cdc.gov/nchs.

Oyelese, Y., & Anath, C. (2010). Post partum hemorrhage: Epidemiology, risk factors and causes. *Clinical Obstetrics and Gynecology, 53*(1), 147–156.

Simpson, K., & Knox, G. (2009). Oxytocin as a high alert medication: Implications for perinatal patient safety. *MCN. The American Journal of Maternal Child Nursing, 34*(1), 8–15.

U.S. Food and Drug Administration. (2011). *Drug safety communication: New warnings against use of terbutaline to treat preterm labor.* Retrieved January 2013, from www.fda.gov.

U.S. Food and Drug Administration. (2013). *Magnesium sulfate drug safety communication recommends against prolonged use in preterm labor: Drug safety communication.* Retrieved May 30, 2013, from www.FDA.gov.

Watkins, S., Meltzer-Brady, S., & Zolnoun, D. (2012). Early breastfeeding experience and post-partum depression. *J Obstet Gynecol, 118*(2), 214–221.

World Health Organization. *Recommendations for induction of labor.* Geneva WHO. Retrieved from http://whqlibdoc.WHO.INT/publications/2011/9789241150156_Eng.pdf.

Wilhite, L., & Melander, S. (2008). Amniotic fluid embolism: A case study. *The American Journal of Nursing, 108*(7), 83–85.

Chapter 9: The Family After Birth

Academy of Breastfeeding Medicine. (2011). ABM clinical protocol #10: Breastfeeding the late preterm infant. *Breastfeeding Medicine, 6*(3), 151–156.

Academy of Breastfeeding Medicine. (2010). Clinical protocol #22: Guidelines for management of jaundice in breastfeeding infants. *Breastfeeding Medicine, 5*(2), 175–182.

ACOG. (2011). ACOG practice bulletin #123: *Thromboembolism in pregnancy.* Washington, DC: Author.

American Academy of Pediatrics. (2012). Policy statement: Breastfeeding and use of human milk. *Pediatrics, 129*(3), 827–830.

American Academy of Pediatrics. (2011). *Car seat safety: Information for parents 2011.* Retrieved January 29, 2013, from www.HealthyChildren.org.

American College of Obstetricians and Gynecologists. (2012). *Guidelines for perinatal care* (7th ed.). Washington, DC: ACOG Author.

Association of Women's Health, Obstetric, and Neonatal Nurses. (2007). *Evidence-based clinical practice guideline: Neonatal skin care* (2nd ed.). Washington, DC: Author.

Blackburn, S. (2013). *Maternal, fetal and neonatal physiology* (4th ed.). St. Louis: Mosby.

Centers for Disease Control and Prevention. (2009). *Guide to vaccines, contraindications and precautions 2009.* Atlanta: Author.

Centers for Disease Control and Prevention (CDC). (2011a). *Breastfeeding report card: U.S. 2011.* Retrieved January 29, 2013, from www.cdc.gov/breastfeeding/data/reportcard.htm.

Centers for Disease Control and Prevention (CDC). (2011b). Vital signs: Hospital practice to support breastfeeding in U.S. 2008–2009. *MMWR Weekly Report, 60*(30), 1020–1025.

Espey, E., Ogburn, T., & Leeman, L. (2012). Effect of progestin compared with combined oral contraceptives on lactation: A randomized controlled trial. *J Obstet Gynecol, 119,* 5.

Hancock, M., & Brown, J. (2010). Formula feeding safety: What nurses need to teach parents who choose to formula feed. *Nursing for Women's Health, 14*(4), 302–309.

Healthy People 2020. (2010). Retrieved February 2013, from www.HealthyPeople.gov/HP2020.

Institute of Medicine (IOM). (2011). *IOM clinical practice guidelines.* Retrieved February 2013, from www.IOM.edu.

Huber, C., & Blanco, E. (2009). Expressed breast milk: Safety in the hospital. *The American Journal of Nursing, 109*(2), 54–55.

Johnson, T., & Strube, K. (2011). Breast care during pregnancy. *Journal of Obstetric, Gynecologic, and Neonatal Nursing, 40*(2), 144–148.

Kliegman, R., Stanton, B., St. Geme, J., III, Shor, W., & Behrman, R. (2011). *Nelson's textbook of pediatrics* (19th ed.). Philadelphia: Saunders.

Lawrence, R. A., & Lawrence, R. M. (2011). *Breastfeeding: A guide for medical professionals* (7th ed.). St. Louis: Mosby.

Leifer, G. (2011). *Maternity nursing* (11th ed.). Philadelphia: Saunders.

Lockwood, S., & Anderson, K. (2013). Postpartum safety: A patient centered approach to fall prevention. *MCN. The American Journal of Maternal Child Nursing, 38*(1), 15–19.

London, M., Ladewig, P., Ball, J., & Bindler, R. (2011). *Maternal-child nursing* (3rd ed.). Englewood Cliffs, NJ: Prentice-Hall.

Mann, J., Mannan, J., & Quinones, L. (2010). Religious, spiritual, social support and perceived stress in pre- and postpartum women. *Journal of Obstetric, Gynecologic, and Neonatal Nursing, 39*(6), 645–657.

Martin, J., Hamilton, B., & Ventura, S. (2011). *Births: Final data for 2009 neonatal vital statistics reports 60(1).* Hyattsville, MD: National Center for Health Statistics.

Mattson, S., & Smith, J. (2011). *AWHONN core curriculum for maternal-newborn nursing* (4th ed.). St. Louis: Saunders.

McKinney, E., James, S., Murray, S., & Ashwill, J. (2013). *Maternal-child nursing* (4th ed.). Philadelphia: Saunders.

Menacker, F., & Hamilton, B. (2010). NCHS data brief #35: *Recent trends in cesarean section delivery in the United States.* Hyattsville, MD: National Center for Health Statistics.

Moon, R. (2011). AAP task force on SIDS and other related infant deaths: Expansion of recommendations for a safe infant sleeping environment. *Pediatrics*, 128(5), 1030–1039.

Moore, K., & Peters, L. (2012). Implementing baby friendly practices: Strategies for success. *MCN. The American Journal of Maternal Child Nursing*, 37(4), 228–230.

Moore, M., Moos, M., & Callister, L. (2010). *Cultural competence: An essential journey for perinatal nurses*. White Plains, NY: March of Dimes.

Morin, K. (2009). Breastfeeding immediately after birth. *MCN. The American Journal of Maternal Child Nursing*, 34(1), 63.

Norman, E., Sherburn, M., & Osborne, R. (2010). An exercise and education program improves the well-being of new mothers: A randomized controlled trial. *Physical Therapy*, 90, 348.

Phelan, S. (2010). Pregnancy: A "teachable moment" for weight control and obesity prevention. *American Journal of Obstetrics and Gynecology*, 135(1), 1.

Rubin, R. (1967). Attainment of the maternal role, part 1: Process. *Nursing Research*, 16, 237–245 (Classic reference).

Schuman, A. (2012). Best new technology products. *Contemporary Pediatrics*, 29(12), 50.

Simpson, K. (2010). Quality measures for perinatal care. *MCN. The American Journal of Maternal Child Nursing*, 35(1), 64.

Skidmore-Roth, L. (2010). *Mosby's handbook of herbs and natural supplements* (4th ed.). St. Louis: Mosby.

Spatz, D. (2010). The critical role of nurses in lactation support. *Journal of Obstetric, Gynecologic, and Neonatal Nursing*, 39(5), 499–500.

Thung, S., & Norwitz, E. (2010). Postpartum care: We can and should do better. *J Obstet Gynecol*, 202, 1.

Trask, B., Sell, S., Carter, S., & Kindred, C. (2009). Circumcision care. *RN*, 72(2), 22–24.

U.S. Department of Health and Human Services. (2011). *Surgeon General's call to action to support breastfeeding*. Washington, DC: USDHHS Office of Surgeon General.

U.S. Department of Health and Human Services. (2011). *Your guide to breastfeeding*. Washington, DC: USDHHS Office of Women's Health.

Wambock, K. (2010). *Breastfeeding and human lactation* (4th ed.). Sadbury MA: Jones & Bartlett.

Chapter 10: Nursing Care of Women with Complications After Birth

American College of Obstetricians and Gynecologists. (2011). Practice bulletin #123: Thromboembolism in pregnancy. *American Journal of Obstetrics and Gynecology*, 118(3), 718–729.

American College of Obstetricians and Gynecologists. (2012). *Guidelines for perinatal care* (7th ed.). Washington, DC: ACOG Author.

American Psychiatric Association. (2012). *DSM V major depressive episode*. APA.

Association of Women's Health, Obstetric, and Neonatal Nurses. (2007). *Evidence-based clinical practice guideline: Neonatal skin care* (2nd ed.). Washington, DC: Author.

Blackburn, S. (2013). *Maternal, fetal and neonatal physiology* (4th ed.). St. Louis: Mosby.

Blomberg, M. (2011). Maternal obesity and risk of postpartum hemorrhage. *American Journal of Obstetrics and Gynecology*, 118(3), 56–58.

Hacker, N., Gambone, J., & Hobel, C. (2010). *Essentials of obstetrics and gynecology* (5th ed.). Philadelphia: Saunders.

Kliegman, R., Stanton, B., St. Geme, J., III, Shor, W., & Behrman, R. (2011). *Nelson's textbook of pediatrics* (19th ed.). Philadelphia: Saunders.

Laird, R., & Carabine, U. (2008). Recombinant factor VIIa for major obstetrical hemorrhage in a Jehovah's Witness. *International Journal of Obstetric Anesthesia*, 17(2), 193–194.

McKinney, E., James, S., Murray, S., & Ashwill, J. (2013). *Maternal-child nursing* (4th ed.). Philadelphia: Saunders.

Perry, S., Hockenberry, M., Lowdermilk, D., & Wilson, D. (2010). *Maternal child nursing care* (4th ed.). St. Louis: Mosby.

Skopp, R., & Nelson, A. (2009). Transdermal contraceptive patches: Current status and future potential. *Expert Review of Clinical Pharmacology*, 2(6), 601–607.

Chapter 11: The Nurse's Role in Women's Health Care

American Cancer Society. (2007). Guidelines still advise yearly mammography for women aged 40 to 49 years. *CA: A Cancer Journal for Clinicians*, 57, 187–188. Retrieved April 20, 2010, from http://caonline.amcancersoc.org/cgi/content/full/57/4/187.

American Cancer Society. (2012). Bulletin #131: Screening for cervical cancer. *Contemporary Ob/Gyn*, 58(6), 47–52.

American Cancer Society. (2010). *Cervical cancer: Prevention and early detection*. Retrieved May 2013, from www.cancer.org.

American College of Obstetricians and Gynecologists. (2010). Practice bulletin #28: *Use of botanicals for management of menopausal symptoms*. Washington, DC: ACOG Author.

American College of Obstetricians and Gynecologists. (2012). Practice bulletin #131: *Screening for cervical cancer*. Washington, DC: ACOG Author.

American College of Obstetricians and Gynecologists. (2013). Committee on gynecologic practice: Postmenopausal estrogen therapy: Route, administration, and risk of thromboembolism. *J Obstet Gynecol*, 121, 887.

Bond, S. (2013). Transexamic acid is safe and effective for treatment of heave menstrual bleeding. *Journal of Midwifery & Women's Health*, 58(2), 227–228.

Centers for Disease Control and Prevention. (2008). *Gonorrhea, syphilis, and chlamydia*. Retrieved June 13, 2010, from www.cdc.gov/std/stats07/trends.htm.

Centers for Disease Control and Prevention. (2010). *Division of Reproductive Health, National Center for Chronic Disease Prevention and Health Promotion: Assisted reproductive technologies*. Retrieved June 2013, from www.cdc.gov/art/index.htm.

Centers for Disease Control and Prevention. (2011). *What is assisted reproductive technology?* Retrieved May 2013, from www.cdc.org.

Chichester, M., & Ciranni, P. (2011). Approaching menopause (but not there yet). *Nursing for Women's Health*, 15(4), 320–324.

Cleland, K. (2012). The efficacy of intrauterine devices for emergency contraception. *Human Reproduction*, 27, 1994.

Cohen, J., & Farias-Eisner, R. (2013). Cancer screening: Better patient care with fewer Pap smears. *Contemporary Ob/Gyn*, 58(6), 47–52.

Cruz, M., & Bair-Merritt, M. (2013). Screening and intervention for intimate partner violence. *Contemporary Pediatrics*, 30(5), 12–15.

DiGuilio, M., Wiedasech, S., & Monchek, R. (2012). Understanding hydatidform mole. *MCN. The American Journal of Maternal Child Nursing*, 37(1), 30–34.

Federal Drug Administration (FDA). (2013). *FDA approves plan B one-step emergency contraception for women 15 years and older*. Retrieved June 2013, from http://Viajnat.ch/130wg6q.

Fehring, R. J., Schneider, M., & Barron, M. L. (2008). Efficacy of the Marquette method of natural family planning. *MCN. The American Journal of Maternal Child Nursing*, 33(6), 348–354.

Fischer, M. (2008). Implanon: A new contraceptive implant. *Journal of Obstetric, Gynecologic, and Neonatal Nursing*, 37(3), 361–367.

Flowers, J. (2009). An overview of uterine fibroids. *The Nurse Practitioner*, 16(10), 36–41.

Fontenot, H., & Harris, A. (2008). The latest advances in hormonal contraception. *Journal of Obstetric, Gynecologic, and Neonatal Nursing*, 37(3), 369–373.

Fraser, I., Critchley, H., Brader, M., & Munro, M. (2011). Recommendations on terminologies and definitions for normal and abnormal menstrual bleeding. *Seminars in Reproductive Medicine, 29*(5), 383–390.

Freeman, S. (2008). Continuous use oral contraceptives. *NP, 16*(8), 36–39.

Geraghty, P. (2009). Beyond birth control. *Advance for Nurse Practitioners, 17*(2), 47–49.

Girard, S. (2012). Contraception counseling. *Advance for NP's and PA's, 3*(5), 28–38.

Hacker, N., Gambone, J., & Hobel, C. (2010). *Essentials of obstetrics and gynecology* (5th ed.). Philadelphia: Saunders.

Hatcher, R. A., Trussell, J., Nelson, A. L., Cates, W., Kowal, D., & Policar, M. (2011). *Contraceptive technology* (20th ed.). New York: Ardent Media.

Holland-Hall, G. (2012). Heavy menstrual bleeding in adolescents: Normal variant or bleeding disorder? *Contemporary Pediatrics, 29*(11), 24–40.

Isely, M., & Edelman, A. (2008). Extended continuous oral contraceptives dosing regimes. *Contemporary Ob/Gyn, 53*(7), 50–53.

Ishitani, K. (2008). Caffeine consumption and the risk of breast cancer in a large prospective cohort of women. *Archives of Internal Medicine, 168*(10), 20–22.

Judge, D. (2013). Emergency contraception: What it is, how it works, and how to get it. *Journal Watch: The New England Journal of Medicine, 18*(5), 35–36.

Kaplan, C. (2008a). Condoms for women. *Advance for Nurse Practitioners, 16*(12), 44–46.

Kaplan, C. (2008b). Diagnosing STD. *NP, 16*(6), 30.

McFarland, C. (2012). Treating polycystic ovarian syndrome and infertility. *MCN. The American Journal of Maternal Child Nursing, 37*(2), 116–121.

Micozzi, M. (2006). *Fundamentals of complementary and integrative medicine*. Philadelphia: Saunders.

Naoulou, B., & Tsai, M. (2012). Efficacy of tranexamic acid in treatment of idiopathic and non-functional heavy menstrual bleeding: A systematic review. *Acta Obstetricia et Gynecologica Scandinavica, 91*(5), 529–537.

National Center for Health Statistics. (2010). *Health in United States 2010*. Hyattsville MD: NCHS.

Ortho-McNeil-Janssen Pharmaceuticals, Inc. (2009). *The patch*. Retrieved June 15, 2010, from www.orthoevra.com/index.html.

Pallone, S., & Bergus, G. (2009). Fertility awareness-based method: Another option for family planning. *Journal of the American Board of Family Medicine, 22*(2), 147–157.

Priestley, C., Jones, B., Dhar, J., & Goodwin, L. (1997). What is normal vaginal flora? *Genitourinary Medicine, 13*, 23–28.

Speroff, L., & Darney, P. (2011). *Clinical guide for contraception* (5th ed.). Philadelphia: Lippincott Williams and Wilkins.

Stermer, C. (2008). Helping your patient after breast reconstruction. *Nursing, 38*(8), 28–32.

Stewart, C. (2012). Assessment of self-taken swab cultures versus clinician taken swab cultures for diagnosis of gonorrhea in women: Single centre diagnostic study. *BMJ, 345*, 8107.

Theroux, R. (2008). The hysteroscopic approach to sterilization. *Journal of Obstetric, Gynecologic, and Neonatal Nursing, 37*(3), 356–360.

U.S. Department of Health and Human Services. (2010). *Healthy People 2020: National health promotion and disease prevention objectives*. Washington, DC: U.S. Government Printing Office.

Zinaman, M. (2009). Using cervical mucus and other easily observed biomarkers to identify ovulation in prospective pregnancy trials. *Paediatric & Perinatal Epidemiology, 20*(S1), 26–29.

Chapter 12: The Term Newborn

American Academy of Pediatrics. (2007). Position statement: Principles and guidelines for early hearing detection and intervention programs. *Pediatrics, 120*(4), 898–921.

American Academy of Pediatrics. (2013). Weighing pediatric patients in kilograms. *Pediatrics, 3*(1), 2012–3057.

American Academy of Pediatrics, Committee on Fetus and Newborn, and American College of Obstetricians and Gynecologists. (2012). *Guidelines for perinatal care* (7th ed.). Evanston, IL: Author.

Anand, K., & Stevens, B. (2007). *Pain in neonates* (3rd ed.). St. Louis: Elsevier.

Association of Women's Health and Neonatal Nursing. (2007). *Evidence-based clinical practice guidelines: Neonatal skin care*. Washington, DC: Author.

Brazelton, T. B. (1973). *The neonatal behavioral assessment scale*. Philadelphia: Lippincott (Classic reference).

Gottesman, M. (2008). Choosing the right infant formula. *Advance for Nurse Practitioners, 16*(5), 47–50.

Gray, L., & Watt-Blas, E. (2008). Skin to skin contact is analgesic in healthy newborns. *Pediatrics, 105*(1), 110–111.

Harrison, D., Stevens, B., Bueno, M., Yamada, J., Adams-Webber, T., Bayene, J., et al. (2010). Efficacy of sweet solutions for analgesia in infants between 1 and 12 months of age: A systematic review. *Archives of Disease in Childhood, 95*(5), 36–40.

Hensel, D., Morson, G., & Preusse, E. (2013). Best practices in newborn injection. *MCN. The American Journal of Maternal Child Nursing, 38*(3), 163–167.

Hummel, P., Puchalski, M., Creech, S., & Weiss, M. (2008). Clinical reliability and validity of N-PASS: Neonatal pain, agitation and sedatrion scale with prolonged pain. *Journal of Perinatology: Official Journal of the California Perinatal Association, 28*, 55–60.

Kliegman, R., Stanton, B., St. Geme, J., III, Shor, W., & Behrman, R. (2011). *Nelson's textbook of pediatrics* (19th ed.). Philadelphia: Saunders.

Maisels, M. J., Ostrea, E. M., Jr., Touch, S., Clune, S. E., Cepeda, E., Kring, E., et al. (2004). Evaluation of new transcutaneous bilirubinometer. *Pediatrics, 1131*, 1638–1645.

Moore, K., & Peters, L. (2012). Implementing baby friendly practices: Strategies for success. *MCN. The American Journal of Maternal Child Nursing, 37*(4), 228–230.

Morin, K. (2007). Infant nutrition: What about bottled water for babies? *MCN. The American Journal of Maternal Child Nursing, 32*(1), 57.

Morin, K. (2013). Embracing the U.S. Surgeon General's call to increase breastfeeding. *MCN. The American Journal of Maternal Child Nursing, 37*(1), 64–65.

National Center for Health Statistics. (2008). Retrieved June 15, 2010, from www.cdc.gov/nchs.

Neu, M., Robinson, J., & Schmiege, S. (2013). Infant holding practice in preterm infant development. *MCN. The American Journal of Maternal Child Nursing, 38*(3), 136–143.

Rohan, A., & Golombek, S. (2009). Hypoxia in the term newborn: Part one—Cardiopulmonary physiology and assessment. *MCN. The American Journal of Maternal Child Nursing, 34*(2), 106–112.

Thomas, D. (2010). Implementing the IOM recommendations for improving pediatric emergency care in your ED: Start from where you are. *Journal of Emergency Nursing, 36*(4), 375–378.

U.S. Department of Health and Human Services. (2010). *Healthy People 2020: National health promotion and disease prevention objectives*. Washington, DC: U.S. Government Printing Office.

Chapter 13: Preterm and Postterm Newborns

American Academy of Pediatrics. (2013). Screening premature infants for ROP. *Pediatrics, 131*(1), 189–195.

American College of Obstetricians and Gynecologists. (2011). Practice bulletin #475: Corticosteroid use for fetal maturation. *J Obstet Gynecol, 117*(2), 422–424.

Association of Women's Health and Neonatal Nursing. (2007). *Evidence-based clinical practice guidelines: Neonatal skin care*. Washington, DC: Author.

Blackburn, S. (2013). *Maternal, fetal, and neonatal physiology* (4th ed.). Philadelphia: Saunders.

Creasy, R., Resnick, R., Iams, J., Lockford, C., & Moore, T. (2009). *Maternal-fetal medicine* (6th ed.). Philadelphia: Saunders.

Dodd, V. (2005). Implications of kangaroo care for growth and development of preterm infants. *Journal of Obstetric, Gynecologic, and Neonatal Nursing, 34*(2), 218–229.

Gabbe, S., Niebyl, J., Simpson, J., Landon, M., Galan, H., Jauniaux, E., et al. (2012). *Obstetrics: Normal and problem pregnancies* (6th ed.). Philadelphia: Saunders.

Hubbard, E., Stellwagen, L., & Wolf, A. (2009). The late preterm infant: A little baby with big needs. *Contemporary Pediatrics, 240*(11), 51–59.

Kliegman, R., Stanton, B., St. Geme, J., III, Shor, W., & Behrman, R. (2011). *Nelson's textbook of pediatrics* (19th ed.). Philadelphia: Saunders.

McMullen, S. (2013). Transitioning premature infants supine: State of the science. *MCN. The American Journal of Maternal Child Nursing, 38*(1), 8–13.

Mintz-Hittner, M., Kennedy, H., & Chuang, A. (2011). Efficacy of intravitreal bevacizumab for stage 3 and ROP. *The New England Journal of Medicine, 364*(7), 603–615.

Morin, K. (2007). Infant nutrition: What about bottled water for babies? *MCN. The American Journal of Maternal Child Nursing, 32*(1), 57.

Neu, M., Robinson, J., & Schmiege, S. (2013). Influence of holding practice on preterm infant development. *MCN. The American Journal of Maternal Child Nursing, 38*(3), 136–138.

Rohan, A., & Golombek, S. (2009). Hypoxia in the term newborn: Part one—Cardiopulmonary physiology and assessment. *MCN. The American Journal of Maternal Child Nursing, 34*(2), 106–112.

Schuman, A. (2012). Best new technology products. *Contemporary Pediatrics, 29*(12), 50.

Tomasheck, M., & Wallman, I. (2007). Cobedding twins and higher-order multiples in a hospital setting. *Pediatrics, 120*(6), 1359–1366.

Chapter 14: The Newborn with a Perinatal Injury or Congenital Malformation

Carey, W., Feldman, H., Coleman, W., Crocker, A., & Elias, E. (2009). *Developmental-behavioral pediatrics* (5th ed.). Philadelphia: Saunders.

Cassell, C., Daniels, J., & Meyer, R. (2009). Timelines of cleft lip surgery and cleft palate craniofacial surgery. *Cleft Palate Craniofacial Journal, 46*(6), 588–597.

Correa, A. (2008). Diabetes mellitus and birth defects. *American Journal of Obstetrics and Gynecology, 199*, 237.

Gabbe, S., Niebyl, J., Simpson, J., Landon, M., Galan, H., Jauniaux, E., et al. (2012). *Obstetrics: Normal and problem pregnancies.* St. Louis: Elsevier.

Husser, D. (2008). New drugs: Sapropterin dihydrochloride first on the market to treat an inherited disorder. *Nursing, 38*(7), 46–47.

Hyunkyung, C., & VanRiper, M. (2013). Siblings of children with Down syndrome: An integrative review. *MCN. The American Journal of Maternal Child Nursing, 38*(2), 72–78.

Jackson, P., Vessey, J., & Schapiro, N. (2009). *Primary care of the child with a chronic condition* (5th ed.). St. Louis: Mosby.

Johns Hopkins Hospital. (2011). *Harriet Lane handbook* (18th ed.). St. Louis: Mosby.

Keil, S., Anjema, K., Francjan, J., van Spronsen, F. J., Lambruschini, N., Burlina, A., et al. (2013). Long term follow-up and outcome of PKU patients on sapropterin. *Pediatrics, 131*(6), 1881–1888.

Kliegman, R., Stanton, B., St. Geme, J., III, Shor, W., & Behrman, R. (2011). *Nelson's textbook of pediatrics* (19th ed.). Philadelphia: Saunders.

Lockwood, J. (2013). Scientists take notable step toward potential Down syndrome treatment. *Contemporary Pediatrics, 30*(7).

Moise, K. (2005a). Fetal RhD typing with free-DNA in maternal plasma. *American Journal of Obstetrics and Gynecology, 192*, 663–665.

Moise, K. (2005b). Fetal RhD genotyping via maternal serum analysis: A two-year experience. *American Journal of Obstetrics and Gynecology, 192*, 666–669.

National Down Syndrome Society. (2013). *Down syndrome fact sheet.* Retrieved April 2013, from www.NDSS.org.

Skotko, B., & Levene, S. (2006). What the other children are thinking: Brothers and sisters of Down syndrome. *American Journal of Medical Genetics, Part C.* http://dx.doi.org/10.1002 AJMG C 30101.

Wong, R., Bhutani, V., Vreman, H., & Stevenson, D. (2007). TIN mesopoporhyrin for the prevention of severe neonatal hyperbilirubinemia. *NeoReviews, 8*(2), e77.

World Health Organization. (2012). *Genes and chromosomal disease: Down syndrome.* U.S. World Health Organization. Retrieved April 2013, from www.WHO.INT/genomics/public/geneticdiseases/en/index.html.

Chapter 15: An Overview of Growth, Development, and Nutrition

Akers, S., & Groh-Wargo, S. (2005). Normal nutrition during infancy. In P. Q. Samour, K. Helm, & E. Lang (Eds.), *Handbook of pediatric nutrition* (pp. 65–97) (3rd ed.). Sudbury, MA: Jones & Bartlett.

Booth, S., Sallas, J., Rittenbaugh, C., Hill, J., Birch, L., & Frank, L. (2001). Environmental and societal factors affecting food choices and physical activity: Rationale, influence and leverage points. *Nutrition Reviews, 59*(2), s21–s39.

Carey, W., Feldman, H., Coleman, W., Crocker, A., & Elias, E. (2009). *Developmental-behavioral pediatrics* (5th ed.). Philadelphia: Saunders.

Hesselman, B., Sjoberg, F., Saalman, R., Aberg, N., Adlerberth, I., & Wold, A. E. (2013). Pacifier cleaning practices and allergy development. *Pediatrics, 131*(6), 1829–1837.

Hofman, R. (2008). Letting go of sippy cups. *Contemporary Pediatrics, 25*(12), 12.

Kliegman, R., Stanton, B., St. Geme, J., III, Shor, W., & Behrman, R. (2011). *Nelson's textbook of pediatrics* (19th ed.). Philadelphia: Saunders.

Leifer, G., & Fleck, E. (2012). *Growth and development across the lifespan: A health promotion focus.* Philadelphia: Saunders.

Lipson, J., & Dibble, S. (2005). *Culture and nursing care.* San Francisco: UCSF Press.

Mahan, L., & Escott-Stump, S. (2012). *Krause's food, nutrition, and diet therapy* (13th ed.). Philadelphia: Saunders.

Makinen, K., & Bennett, C. (2008). Xylitol chewing gum and caries rates, a 40-month cohort study. *Journal of Dental Research, 1995* (74), 1904.

Meltzer, D. (2006). Complications of body piercing. *American Family Physician, 72*(10), 2029–2035.

Ogden, C., Carroll, M., Kit, B., & Flegal, K. (2012). Prevalence of obesity and trends in BMI among U.S. children and adolescents 1999–2010. *JAMA, 307*(5), 483–490.

Smilkstein, G., Ashworth, C., & Montano, D. (1984). The validity and reliability of the family APGAR as a test of family function. *The Journal of Family Practice, 15*, 303. (Classic reference)

U.S. Department of Health and Human Services. (2012). *Oral health in America: A report of the Surgeon General.* Rockville, MD: National Institute of Dental and Craniofacial Research. Retrieved June 13, 2013, from www.mypyramid.gov.

Wagner, R., & Oskouians, R. (2008). Are you missing the diagnosis of the most chronic disease in childhood?: Tooth caries. *Contemporary Pediatrics, 25*(9), 60–82.

Wang, X., & Perry, A. (2004). Metabolic and physiologic responses to video-game play in 7-10 year old boys. *Archives of Pediatrics & Adolescent Medicine, 160,* 411–415.

Yang, Q. (2012). Sodium intake and blood pressure among U.S. children and adolescents. *Pediatrics, 130,* 611.

Chapter 16: The Infant

Abbott Laboratories Product Comparison. Retrieved July 1, 2011, from http://Abbottnutrition.com/products.

American Academy of Pediatrics. (2009). *Pediatric nutrition handbook* (6th ed.). Elk Grove Village, IL: American Academy of Pediatrics Committee on Nutrition.

American Academy of Pediatrics. (2011). *Amount and schedule of formula feedings.* Retrieved May 2013, from www.healthychildren.org/english/ages-stages/baby/feeding-nutrition/pages/default.aspx.

Anderson, J. (2008). Discipline techniques for the 12 month old. *Contemporary Pediatrics, 25*(9), 84–86.

Bartram, J., & Montoya, C. (2013). Infant formulas: Partnering with parents for rational decision making. *Advance for NP's and PA's, 4*(7), 31–36.

Bolte, R. (2007). The crying child: What are they trying to tell you? *Contemporary Pediatrics, 24*(5), 74–81.

Bright Beginnings formula product information. Retrieved July 1, 2011, from www.BrightBeginnings.com.

Carey, W., Feldman, H., Coleman, W., Crocker, A., & Elias, E. (2009). *Developmental-behavioral pediatrics* (5th ed.). Philadelphia: Saunders.

Craig, G., & Dunn, W. (2010). *Understanding growth and development* (2nd ed.). Upper Saddle River, NJ: Pearson, Prentice-Hall.

Fowles, E. (1999). The Brazelton Neonatal Behavior Scale and maternal identity. *MCN. The American Journal of Maternal Child Nursing, 24*(6), 287–293, (Classic reference).

Fleischer, D. (2013). Primary prevention of allergic disease through nutritional interventions. *The Journal of Allergy and Clinical Immunology. In practice, 1,* 29.

Hockenberry, M., & Wilson, D. (2010). *Wong's essentials of pediatric nursing* (9th ed.). St. Louis: Mosby.

Junsdottir, O. (2012). Timing and introduction of complimentary foods in infants: A randomized control trial. *Pediatrics, 130,* 1038.

Kliegman, R., Stanton, B., St. Geme, J., III, Schor, N., & Berman, R. (2011). *Nelson's textbook of pediatrics* (19th ed.). Philadelphia: Saunders.

Leise, A., Weis, K., Schulz, M., & Tooze, J. (2009). Food intake patterns associated with incident type 2 diabetes. *Diabetes Care, 32*(2), 263–268.

Lester, B., & Sparrow, J. (2010). *Nurturing children and families: Building on the legend of T. Berry Brazelton.* Hoboken, NJ: Wiley Blackwell.

Mahan, L., & Escott-Stump, S. (2012). *Krause's food, nutrition, and diet therapy* (13th ed.). Philadelphia: Saunders.

Mead-Johnson Company Product Information. (2013). Retrieved January 4, 2014, from www.meadjohnson.com.

Moon, R. (2011). AAP task force on SIDS and other sleep related infant deaths: Expansion of recommendations for a safe infant sleeping environment. *Pediatrics, 128*(5), 1030–1039.

Morin, K. (2008). What is bisphenol-A and why are parents worried? *MCN. The American Journal of Maternal Child Nursing, 33*(3), 189.

Morin, K. (2009). Organic baby food: What do you tell parents? *MCN. The American Journal of Maternal Child Nursing, 34*(2), 129.

Mugambi, M., Musikiwa, A., Lombard, M., Young, M., & Young, T. (2012). Synbiotics, probiotics, in infant formula for full term infants: A systematic review. *Nutrition Journal, 11,* 81.

Mundy, P., & Jarrold, W. (2010). Infant joint attention, neural networks, and social cognition. *Neurology Networks, 23*(8–9), 985–987.

Nestle infant formula products. (2013). Retrieved January 4, 2014, from www.nestle-infantnutrition.com.

Rojas, M., Lozano, J., Rojas, M., Rodriguez, V., Rondon, M., Bastidasm, J., et al. (2012). Prophylactic probiotics to prevent death and nosocomial infection in preterm infants. *Pediatrics, 730*(5), 1113–1120.

United States Department of Agriculture. (2011). *Guidelines and standards for organic produce and meat.* Retrieved 2013, from www.USDA.gov.

Zeigler, A. G., Schmid, S., Huber, D., Hummel, M., & Bonifacio, E. (2003). Early infant feeding and risk of developing type 1 diabetes-associated autoantibodies. *JAMA, 290,* 1721–1728.

Chapter 17: The Toddler

American Academy of Pediatrics. (2011). *Committee on injury, violence and poison prevention: Car passenger safety—A guide for families.* Retrieved June 27, 2013, from http://Pediatrics.AAPpublications.org/content/early/2011/03/21/peds2011-0213.full.pdf+html.

American Speech and Lung Association. (2011). *How does your child hear and talk?* Retrieved May 2013, from www.ASHA.org/public/speech/development/chart.htm.

Anderson, J. (2009). Behavior of the 2 year old. *Contemporary Pediatrics, 26*(6), 50–55.

Biagioli, F. (2005). Child safety seat counseling: 3 keys to safety. *American Family Physician, 72*(3), 473–478.

Carey, W., Feldman, H., Coleman, W., Crocker, A., & Elias, E. (2010). *Developmental-behavioral pediatrics* (6th ed.). Philadelphia: Saunders.

Craig, G., & Dunn, W. (2010). *Understanding growth and development* (2nd ed.). Upper Saddle River, NJ: Pearson, Prentice-Hall.

Hockenberry, M., & Wilson, D. (2010). *Wong's essentials of pediatric nursing* (9th ed.). St. Louis: Mosby.

Kliegman, R., Stanton, B., St. Geme, J., III, Schor, N., & Behrman, R. (2011). *Nelson's textbook of pediatrics* (19th ed). Philadelphia: Saunders.

Kreipe, R., & Palomaki, A. (2012). Beyond picky eating. *Current Psychiatry Reports, 14*(4), 421–431.

Lester, B., & Sparrow, J. (2010). *Nurturing children and families: Building on the legend of T. Berry Brazelton.* Hoboken, NJ: Wiley Blackwell.

Mahan, L., & Escott-Stump, S. (2012). *Krause's food, nutrition, and diet therapy* (13th ed.). Philadelphia: Saunders.

Montgomery, T. (1994). When not talking is the chief complaint. *Contemporary Pediatrics, 11*(9), 49 (Classic reference).

Neumann, B. (2009). Management of dog and cat bites. *Advance for Nurse Practitioners, 17*(3), 53–54.

Santrock, J. (2011). *Child development* (13th ed.). New York: McGraw-Hill.

Chapter 18: The Preschool Child

Allsman, L. (2009). Breath holding spells in children. *NP, 16*(6), 53–55.

Brazelton, T. (1993). *Touchpoints: Your child's emotional and behavioral development.* Reading, MA: Addison-Wesley (Classic reference).

Carey, W., Feldman, H., Coleman, W., Crocker, A., & Elias, E. (2009). *Developmental-behavioral pediatrics* (5th ed.). Philadelphia: Saunders.

Craig, G., & Dunn, W. (2010). *Understanding growth and development* (2nd ed.). Upper Saddle River, NJ: Pearson, Prentice-Hall.

Ferguson, C. (2011). Influence of television and videogames on attention and school problems: A multivariate analysis with other risk factors controlled. *Journal of Psychiatric Research, 45*, 808–813.

Hockenberry, M., & Wilson, D. (2010). *Wong's essentials of pediatric nursing* (9th ed.). St. Louis: Mosby.

Kerwin, M., & Eicher, P. (2011). Behavioral intervention and prevention of feeding difficulties in infants and toddlers. *Journal of Early and Intensive Behavioral Interventions, 1*(2), 129–140.

Kliegman, R., Stanton, B., St. Geme, J., III, Shor, W., & Behrman, R. (2012). *Nelson's textbook of pediatrics* (19th ed.). Philadelphia: Saunders.

Kriepe, R., & Palomari, A. (2012). Beyond picky eating: Avoidant/restrictive food intake disorder. *Current Psychiatry Reports, 14*, 421–431.

Lester, B., & Sparrow, J. (2010). *Nurturing children and families: Building on the Legend of T. Berry Brazelton.* Hoboken, NJ: Wiley Blackwell.

McCormick, V., & Markowitz, G. (2013). Picky eater or feeding disorder. *Advance for NP's and PA's, 4*(3), 18–22.

Montgomery, T. (1994). When children do not talk. *Contemporary Pediatrics, 11*(9), 49. (Classic reference)

Pickering, L. (2008). Exposure to non-traditional pets at home and animals in public settings: Risks to children. *Pediatrics, 122*, 876.

Santrock, J. (2011). *Child development* (13th ed.). New York: McGraw-Hill.

Tienstra, J., & Crawford, C. (2011). A translational research intervention to reduce screen behavior and promote physical activity among children: Switch-2-activity. *Health Promotion International, 263*, 11–21.

Toomey, K. (2012). *Sequential oral sensory approach to feeding.* Nutrition. Retrieved April 2013, from www.nutrition411.com/TKcenter/article.php?ID=K-0621.

USDHHS. (2012). *National Center for Health Statistics. Health United States 2011.* Hyattsville MD: USDHHS.

Chapter 19: The School-Age Child

American Medical Association. (2009). *Expert committee recommendations on childhood obesity (revised 2008).* Retrieved July 1, 2009, from www.ama-association.org.

Craig, G., & Dunn, W. (2010). *Understanding growth and development* (2nd ed.). Upper Saddle River, NJ: Pearson, Prentice-Hall.

Ernst, L. (2012). Animal assisted therapy. *Nursing 2012, 42*(10), 54–61.

Ferguson, C. (2011). Influence of television and videogames on attention and school problems: A multivariate analysis with other risk factors controlled. *Journal of Psychiatric Research, 45*, 808–813.

Hockenberry, M., & Wilson, D. (2009). *Wong's essentials of pediatric nursing* (8th ed.). St. Louis: Mosby.

Kliegman, R., Behrman, R., Jenson, H., & Stanton, B. (2007). *Nelson's textbook of pediatrics* (18th ed.). Philadelphia: Saunders.

Leifer, G. (2011). *Maternity nursing* (11th ed.). Philadelphia: Saunders.

Lester, B., & Sparrow, J. (2010). *Nurturing children and families: Building on the legend of T. Berry Brazelton.* Hoboken, NJ: Wiley Blackwell.

Mahan, L., & Escott-Stump, S. (2012). *Krause's food, nutrition, and diet therapy* (13th ed.). Philadelphia: Saunders.

Ogden, C., Carroll, M., Kat, B., & Flegal, B. (2012). Prevention of obesity and trends in body mass index among U.S. children and adolescents 1999–2010. *JAMA, 307*(5), 483–489.

Parish-Plass, N. (2008). Animal assisted therapy with children suffering from insecure attachment due to abuse and neglect: A method to lower risk of intergenerational transmission of abuse. *Clinical Child Psychology and Psychiatry, 13*(1), 7–30.

Pickering, L. (2008). Exposure to non-traditional pets at home and to animals in public settings: Risks to children. *Pediatrics, 122*, 876–878.

Santrock, J. (2011). *Child development* (13th ed.). New York: McGraw-Hill.

Tienstra, J., & Crawford, C. (2011). A translational research intervention to reduce screen behavior and promote physical activity among children: Switch-2-activity. *Health Promotion International, 263*, 11–21.

U.S. Department of Health and Human Services. (2012). *Healthy People 2020: National health promotion and disease prevention objectives.* Washington, DC: U.S. Government Printing Office.

USDHHS. (2012). *National Center for Health Statistics. Health United States 2011.* Hyattsville MD: USDHHS, 2012.

Chapter 20: The Adolescent

American Cancer Society. (2010). Retrieved May 28, 2010, from www.cancer.org/docroot/PED/content/PED_2_3X_Do_I_Have_Testicular_Cancer.asp.

American Psychiatric Association. (2012). *Diagnostic and statistical manual of mental disorders DSM V.* Washington, DC: Author.

Burstein, M. (2012). When to get anxious about social anxiety disorders. *Contemporary Pediatrics, 29*(12), 32–42.

Burstein, M., Ameli-Grillon, L., & Merikangas, K. (2011). Shyness versus social phobia in U.S. youth. *Pediatrics, 128*(5), 917–925.

Centers for Disease Control and Prevention. (2013). *10 Leading causes of death in the U.S. in the 12–21 age group—2010 data.* Atlanta: Author.

Carey, W., Crocker, A., Elias, E., Feldman, H., & Coleman, W. (2009). *Developmental behavioral pediatrics* (5th ed.). Philadelphia: Saunders.

Dartmouth-Hitchcock Medical Center. (2010). *High-fiber diet for children.* Retrieved May 28, 2010, from www.dhmc.org/webpage.cfm?site_id=2&org_id=372&morg_id=0&sec_id=0&gsec_id=39122&item_id=39147.

Donaldson, A., & Gordon, C. (2013). Bone health in adolescents. *Contemporary Pediatrics, 30*(4), 14–16.

Hockenberry, M., & Wilson, D. (2010). *Wong's essentials of pediatric nursing* (9th ed.). St. Louis: Mosby.

Kliegman, R., Stanton, B., St. Geme, J., III, Schor, N., & Behrman, R. (2011). *Nelson's textbook of pediatrics* (19th ed.). Philadelphia: Saunders.

Leifer, G., & Fleck, E. (2013). *Growth and development across the lifespan: A health promotion focus.* Philadelphia: Saunders.

Loman, D. (2009). Promoting physical activity in teenage girls. *MCN. The American Journal of Maternal Child Nursing, 33*(5), 294–296.

Mahan, L., & Escott-Stump, S. (2012). *Krause's food, nutrition, and diet therapy* (13th ed.). Philadelphia: Saunders.

McCartney, P. (2012). Social networking safety for children and adolescents. *MCN. The American Journal of Maternal Child Nursing, 37*(1), 65.

Ogden, C., Carroll, M., Kat, B., & Flegal, B. (2012). Prevention of obesity and trends in body mass index among U.S. children and adolescents 1999–2010. *JAMA, 307*(5), 483–489.

Saglimbeni, A. (2010). *Sports physicals.* Retrieved May 28, 2010, from http://emedicine.medscape.com/article/88972(overview).

Schwartz, R. (1997). Are you ready to deal with a pot-smoking patient? *Contemporary Pediatrics, 11*(4), 85. (Classic reference)

Silk, H., & Romao-Clarke, G. (2009). The 7 tenets to teen oral health. *Contemporary Pediatrics, 26*(6), 50–55.

Tanner, J. M. (1962). *Growth of adolescence* (2nd ed.). Oxford: Blackwell Scientific. (Classic reference)

U.S. Department of Health and Human Services. (2010). *Healthy People 2020: National health promotion and disease prevention objectives.* Washington, DC: U.S. Government Printing Office.

Wisnieski, D., & Matzo, M. (2013). Evidence for excellence: Promoting healthy sexual behavior in adolescents. *The American Journal of Nursing, 113*(6), 67–69.

Chapter 21: The Child's Experience of Hospitalization

American Academy of Pediatrics (AAP). (2005). *Pediatric pain management for primary care.* Elk Grove Village, IL: Author.

American Academy of Pediatrics. (2012). Relief of pain and anxiety in pediatric patients in EMS. *Pediatrics, 122*(2), 450.

Hockenberry, M., & Wilson, D. (2010). *Wong's essentials of pediatric nursing* (9th ed.). St. Louis: Mosby.

Jackson, P., Vessey, J., & Schapiro, N. (2009). *Primary care of the child with a chronic condition* (5th ed.). St. Louis: Mosby.

Kliegman, R., Stanton, B., St. Geme, J., III, Schor, N., & Behrman, R. (2011). *Nelson's textbook of pediatrics* (19th ed.). Philadelphia: Saunders.

Chapter 22: Health Care Adaptations for the Child and Family

AAP. (2013). Weighing patients in kilograms. *Pediatrics, 3*(1), 2012–3057.

Armstrong, M. (2009). The whole picture: Risks, decision making, purpose, regulations and the future of body piercing. *Clinics in Dermatology, 25*(4), 398–406.

Braverman, P. (2006). Body art: Piercing, tattooing, and scarification. *Adolescent Medicine, 17,* 505–519.

Broselow, J., Luten, A., & Schuman, A. (2008). Preventing death by a decimal point. *Contemporary Pediatrics, 25*(7), 38.

Crawford, C., & Johnson, J. (2012). To aspirate or not: An integrative review of the evidence. *Nursing 2012, 42*(3), 20–25.

Crocetti, M., & Serwirt, J. (2005). Fever: Separating fact from fiction. *Contemporary Pediatrics, 22*(1), 34–42.

DeBoer, S., Seaver, M., Angel, E., & Armstrong, M. (2008). Puncturing myths about body piercing and tattooing. *Nursing Made Incredibly Easy, 7*(3), 34–39.

DeBoer, S., McNeil, M., & Amundson, T. (2008). Body piercing and airway management: A photo guide to tongue jewelry removal techniques. *AANA Journal, 76*(1), 19–23.

Hensel, D., Morson, G., & Preuss, E. (2013). Best practice in newborn injections. *MCN. The American Journal of Maternal Child Nursing, 38*(3), 163–167.

Hockenberry, M., & Wilson, D. (2010). *Wong's essentials of pediatric nursing* (9th ed.). St. Louis: Mosby.

Immunization Action Coalition. (2009). *Administering vaccines: Dose, route, site and needle size.* Retrieved May 2013, from www.immunize.org/CATG.D/P3085.pdf.

Kliegman, R., Stanton, B., St. Geme, J., III, Schor, N., & Behrman, R. (2011). *Nelson's textbook of pediatrics* (19th ed.). Philadelphia: Saunders.

Rushing, J. (2009). Using a mummy restraint. *Nursing, 39*(1), 18.

Thomas, J. (2010). Implementing the IOM recommendations for improved pediatric emergency care in your ED: Start from where you are. *Journal of Emergency Nursing, 36*(4), 375–378.

Chapter 23: The Child with a Sensory or Neurological Condition

American Academy of Otolaryngology, Head and Neck Surgery. (2012). *Tonsillectomy pain management.* Retrieved April 2013, from www.entnet.org/aboutUs/q-a-taPainManagement.cfm.

American Association of Endodontists. (2010). *Emergency steps for saving a knocked out tooth.* Retrieved April 2013, from www.AAE.org/patients/patientinfo/references/avulsed.htm.

American Association on Intellectual and Developmental Disabilities. Retrieved May 28, 2010, from www.aamar.org.

American Psychiatric Association. (2012). *Diagnostic and statistical manual of mental disorders DSM V* (5th ed.). Washington, DC: Author.

Blumberg, S. (2013). Changes in prevalence of parent reported autism spectrum disorder in school aged U.S. school children 2007–2012. *National Health Statistics Report, 265,* 1–2.

Carey, W., Crocker, A., Elias, E., Feldman, H., & Coleman, W. (2009). *Developmental behavioral pediatrics* (5th ed.). Philadelphia: Saunders.

Chou, R., Dana, T., & Bougastos, C. (2011). *Screening for visual impairment in children aged 1-5 years: Systemic review.* Agency for Health Care Research and Quality, Report #11-05151-EF-1.

Clare, E. (2010). Seizure precautions for bedside nurses. *Pediatric Nursing, 36*(4), 191–194.

Cohen, S. (2011). Orbital cellulitis as a complication of sinusitis. *The Journal for Nurse Practitioners, 7,* 38–44.

Epilepsy Foundation. (2010). *Ketogenic diet.* Retrieved from www.epilepsyfoundation.org/aboutepilepsy/treatment/ketogenicdiet.

Freeman, J., Kossoff, E., & Hartman, A. (2007). The ketogenic diet: One decade later. *Pediatrics, 119*(3), 535–543.

Haberman, A., Paradise, I., Rockette, H., Shaikh, N., Wald, E., Kearnen, D., et al. (2011). The treatment of acute otitis media in children under two years of age. *The New England Journal of Medicine, 364,* 105–115.

Hockenberry, M., & Wilson, D. (2010). *Wong's essentials of pediatric nursing* (9th ed.). St. Louis: Mosby.

Horeccko, T., & Kupperman, N. (2012). Minor head trauma in your office, clinic or ED: Do I scan? *Contemporary Pediatrics, 29*(8), 40–47.

Kliegman, R., Stanton, B., St. Geme, J., III, Schor, N., & Behrman, R. (2011). *Nelson's textbook of pediatrics* (19th ed.). Philadelphia: Saunders.

Kuhn, F. (2009). Eye and vision assessment. *NP, 17*(10), 43–45.

Leifer, G. (2001). Hyperbaric oxygen therapy: What every nurse should know. *The American Journal of Nursing, 101*(8), 36.

Levy, R., & Cooper, P. (2008). Ketogenic diet for epilepsy. *Cochrane Database of Systematic Reviews,* (Issue 3), http://dx.doi.org/101002/14651858CD001903, CD: 001903.

Mahan, L., & Escott-Stump, S. (2012). *Krause's food, nutrition, and diet therapy* (13th ed.). Philadelphia: Saunders.

McGuire, C., & McCambridge, T. (2011). Concussion in the young athlete: Diagnosis, management and prevention. *Contemporary Pediatrics, 28*(5), 30–40.

Norton, C., Feltz, S., Brocker, A., & Granitto, M. (2013). Tackling long term consequences of concussion. *Nursing, 43*(1), 5053.

Rosenbaum, P., Paneth, N., Leviton, A., Goldstein, M., Bax, M., & Damiano, D. (2007). A report: The definition and classification of cerebral palsy. *Developmental Medicine and Child Neurology, 49*(s109), 1–44.

Rosenfeld, R., Schwartz, S., & Pynnonen, M. (2013). Clinical practice guideline: Tympanostomy tubes in children. *Otolaryngology—Head and Neck Surgery, 149,* s1–s35.

Wilson, B., Shannon, M., & Shield, K. (2011). *Nurses drug guide.* Upper Saddle River, NJ: Pearson, Prentice-Hall.

Wolff, R., Hommerich, J., Riemsma, R., Antes, G., Lange, S., & Kleijnen, J. (2010). Hearing screening in newborns: Systematic review of accuracy, effectiveness, and effects of interventions after screening. *Archives of Disease in Childhood, 95,* 130–135.

Chapter 24: The Child with a Musculoskeletal Condition

American Academy of Pediatrics. (2006). School health assessments. *Pediatrics, 118*(3), 1266–1267.

Chen, C., & Chan, G. (2009). Musculoskeletal effects of obesity. *Current Opinion in Pediatrics, 21,* 65–70.

Davis, R. (2000). International scene: Cultural health care or child abuse: The practice of cao gio. *Journal of the American Academy of Nurse Practitioners, 12*(3), 89–95.

DiMarco, M., & Melnyk, B. (2009). The mental health needs of children and adolescents. *Archives of Psychiatric Nursing, 23*(3), 210–219.

Hockenberry, M., & Wilson, D. (2010). *Wong's essentials of pediatric nursing* (9th ed.). St. Louis: Mosby.

Jackson, P., Vessey, J., & Schapiro, N. (2009). *Primary care of the child with a chronic condition* (5th ed.). St. Louis: Mosby.

Kemp, C. (1962). Battered child syndrome. *JAMA, 181,* 17–24. (Classic reference)

Kliegman, R., Stanton, B., St. Geme, J., III, Schor, N., & Behrman, R. (2011). *Nelson's textbook of pediatrics* (19th ed.). Philadelphia: Saunders.

Moxley, R. T., Ashwal, S., Pandya, S., Connolly, A., Florence, J., Mathews, K., et al. (2005). Practice parameter: Corticosteroid treatment of Duchenne dystrophy. *Neurology, 64*(1), 13–20.

Nistala, K., Woo, P., & Wedderburn, I. (2009). Juvenile idiopathic arthritis. In R. Firestein, E. Budd, J. Harris, & S. McInnes (Eds.), *Kelly's textbook of rheumatology* (p. 1637) (8th ed) St. Louis: Elsevier.

Nooner, K. B., Litrownik, A. J., Thompson, R., Margolis, B., English, D. J., Knight, E. D., et al. (2010). Youth self-report of physical and sexual abuse: A latent class analysis. *Child Abuse & Neglect, 34*(3), 146–154.

Perry, D., & Hall, A. (2011). The epidemiology and etiology of Perthes disease. *The Orthopedic Clinics of North America, 42,* 279–283, Elsevier.

Santrock, J. (2011). *Child development* (13th ed.). New York: McGraw-Hill.

Sarnat, H. (2007). Neuromuscular disorders. In R. Kliegman, R. Behrman, H. Jenson, & B. Stanton (Eds.), *Nelson's textbook of pediatrics* (18th ed.). Philadelphia: Saunders.

Stanley, I., & Ward-Smith, P. (2011). The diagnosis and management of juvenile idiopathic arthritis. *Journal of Pediatric Health Care, 25,* 191–194.

Storch, E., & Elder, J. (2009). Introduction to a special series on child and adolescent mental health. *Journal of Pediatric Nursing, 24,* 1–2.

U.S. Preventive Services Task Force. (2005). Screening for idiopathic scoliosis in adolescents: Recommendations. *American Family Physician, 71*(10), 1975–1976.

Chapter 25: The Child with a Respiratory Disorder

American Academy of Pediatrics. (2012). *Redbook 2012: Report of committee on infectious disease* (29th ed.). Elk Grove Village, IL: Author.

Banasiak, N., & Bolster, A. (2008). Pediatric asthma. *RN, 71*(7), 26–31.

Banfield, J., & Murphy, K. (2013). COPD management and the 2011 GOLD guidelines. *Advance for NP's and PA's, 4*(3), 15–17.

Caliskan, M. (2013). Rhinovirus wheezing illness and genetic risk of childhood onset asthma. *The New England Journal of Medicine, 10,* 1056.

Centers for Disease Control and Prevention (CDC). (2009). *SIDS and sudden unexpected infant death.* Retrieved June 20, 2010, from www.cdc.gov/sids/index/htm.

Cystic Fibrosis Foundation. (2011). *Screening for cystic fibrosis.* Retrieved May 2013, from www.cff.org/aboutcf/testing/newbornscreening/screeningforcf.

D'Augustino, J. (2010). Pediatric airway nightmares. *Emergency Medicine Clinics of North America, 28,* 119–126.

Darge, K., & Chen, A. (2013). Ultrasonography of the lung and pleurae for diagnosis of pneumonia in children: Prime time for routine use. *JAMA, 167,* 187.

Gott, K., & Froh, D. (2010). Alterations in pulmonary function in children. In K. McCance, & S. Huether (Eds.), *Pathophysiology: The biological basis for disease in adults and children* (6th ed.). St. Louis: Mosby.

Kliegman, R., Behrman, R., Jenson, H., & Stanton, B. (2007). *Nelson's textbook of pediatrics* (18th ed.). Philadelphia: Saunders.

Leiberthal, A. (2013). Clinical practice guidelines: The diagnosis and management of acute otitis media. *Pediatrics, 131,* e964.

Lenney, W., Boner, A. L., Bont, L., Bush, A., Carlsen, K. H., Eber, E., et al. (2009). Medicines used in respiratory diseases only seen in children. *The European Respiratory Journal, 34*(3), 531–551.

Meissner, H., & Bocehini, J. (2009). AAP modifies recommendation for use of palivizumab in high risk infants and young children. *AAP News, 30*(7), 1.

McCance, K., & Huether, S. (2010). *Pathophysiology: The biological basis for disease in adults and children* (6th ed.). Philadelphia: Mosby.

Moon, R. (2011). AAP task force on SIDS and other sleep related infant deaths: Expansion of recommendations for a safe infant sleeping environment. *Pediatrics, 128*(5), 1030–1039.

National Center of Health Statistics. (2006). *Health Statistics 2006* (DHHS Publication 2006 1232). Washington, DC: U.S. Government Printing Office.

Plaut, T. (1999). *The peak flow diary for adults, teens, and children over 5.* Amherst, MA: Pediapress. (Classic reference)

Sexton, S., & Natale, R. (2009). The risks and benefits of pacifiers. *American Family Physician, 79*(8), 681–685.

Shah, V. (2013). Prospective evaluation of point-of-care ultrasonography for diagnosis of pneumonia in children and young adults. *JAMA, 167,* 119.

Sobol, S., & Zapata, S. (2008). Epiglottitis and croup. *Otolaryngology Clinics of North America, 41,* 551–556.

Sorce, L. (2009). RSV: From primary care to critical care. *The Journal of Pediatric Health Care, 23*(2), 101–108.

Todd, F., Roberg, K., & Welliver, R. (2010). Preventing RSV infection in at-risk infants: Current and emerging strategies. *Journal of Pediatric Nursing, Supplement, 25*(5), 1–16.

USDA. (2010). *FDA drug safety communication: New safety requirements for long acting inhaled asthma medications called LABA's.* Retrieved May 2013, from www.fda.gov/Drugs/Drugsafety/PostmarketDrugsafetyinformationforPatientandProviders/UCM200776.htm.

Vanhoose, K., & Wood, A. (2009). Current insight into childhood asthma: Implications for practice. *The American Journal for Nurse Practitioners, 13*(9), 10–18.

Ventre, K., & Randolph, A. (2007). Ribavirin for RSV infection in lower respiratory tract in infants and young children. *Cochrane Database of Systematic Reviews, 24*(1), CD000181.

Zagaria, M. (2010). Inhalent agents for asthma, bronchospasm, and COPD: Focus on delivery devices and inhalation technique. *The American Journal for Nurse Practitioners, 14*(3), 21–25.

Chapter 26: The Child with a Cardiovascular Disorder

American Heart Association. (2006). *Step I, step II and the TLC Diet.* Retrieved June 4, 2010, from www.americanheart.org/presenter.jhtml?identifier=4764.

Conway, J., & Dipchand, A. (2010). Heart transplants in children. *Pediatric Clinics of North America, 57,* 353–373.

Gahart, B., & Nazareno, A. (2012). *IV medications* (28th ed.). St. Louis: Elsevier.

Gidding, S. (2012a). An emerging dyslipidemia: Assessing future cardiovascular risk in children. *Contemporary Pediatrics, 29*(6), 14–20.

Gidding, S. (2012b). An emerging dyslipidemia: New NHLBI and NLA treatment guidelines. *Contemporary Pediatrics, 29*(7), 24–31.

Gill, V., & Edelson, M. (2012). Pediatric hypertension: A cause for concern. *Nursing 2012, 42*(3), 54–57.

Gnouchi, Y. (2012). Genetics of Kawasaki disease: What we know and don't know. *Circulation Journal, 76*(7), 1581–1586.

Holcomb, S. (2009). Common herb-drug interactions: What you should know. *Nursing Practice, 34*(5), 25–29.

Kliegman, R., Stanton, B., St. Geme, J., III, Shor, W., & Behrman, R. (2011). *Nelson's textbook of pediatrics* (19th ed.). Philadelphia: Saunders.

Lee, Y., Kuo, H., & Chang, J. (2012). Two new susceptibility loci for Kawasaki disease identified through genome-wide association. *Nature Genetics, 44*(5), 522–525.

National Institutes of Health. (2009). *What are congenital heart defects?* Bethesda, MD: Author. Retrieved June 1, 2010, from www.nhlbi.nih.gov/health/dci/Diseases/chd/chd_what.html.

Rowley, A. (2012). Kawasaki disease: Genetics, pathology and a need for earlier diagnosis. *Contemporary Pediatrics, 29*(12), 18–31.

Son, M., & Newburger, J. W. (2012). Management of Kawasaki disease: Corticosteroids revisited. *Lancet, 379*(9826), 1571–1572.

Zideman, D., & Hazinski, M. (2008). Background and epidemiology of pediatric cardiac arrest. *Pediatric Clinics of North America, 55*, 847–859, St. Louis: Elsevier.

Chapter 27: The Child with a Condition of the Blood, Blood-Forming Organs, or Lymphatic System

Alvarez, O., Rodriguez-Cortez, H., Robinson, N., Lewis, N., Sang, C., Lopez-Mitnik, G., et al. (2009). Adherence to deferasirox in children and adolescents with sickle cell disease during the first year of therapy. *Journal of Pediatric Hematology/Oncology, 31*(10), 739–744.

American Sickle Cell Anemia Association. (2010). *How common is sickle cell anemia.* Retrieved May 2013, from www.ASCAA.org/How-common_is_sickle_cell_anemia.asp.

Diesen, L. (2006). Helping children live with death and loss. *Journal of Pediatric Nursing, 20*(5), 372–374.

Ellison, A. (2012). Sickle cell disease. *Contemporary Pediatrics, 29* (9), 18–21.

Gill, V., & Edelman, M. (2012). Pediatric hypertension: A cause for concern. *Nursing 2012, 42*(9), 48–51.

Greenbaum, L. (2011). Vitamin K deficiency. In B. Kliegman, J. Stanton, J. St. Geme, III, N. Schor, & R. Behrman (Eds.), *Nelson's textbook of pediatrics* (19th ed.). Philadelphia: Saunders.

Jackson, P., Vessey, J., & Schapiro, N. (2009). *Primary care of the child with a chronic condition* (5th ed.). St. Louis: Mosby.

Jacobs, H. (2005). Ethics in pediatrics end of life care. *Journal of Pediatric Nursing, 20*(5), 360–365.

Johnson, M., & Robin, N. (2000). Pediatrics and the human genome project. *Contemporary Pediatrics, 17*(5), 100, (Classic reference).

Kliegman, R., Marcdante, K., Jenson, H., & Behrman, R. (2005). *Essentials of pediatrics* (5th ed.). Philadelphia: Saunders.

Kliegman, R., Stanton, J., St. Geme, J., III, Schor, N., & Behrman, R. (2011). *Nelson's textbook of pediatrics* (19th ed.). Philadelphia: Saunders.

Kubler-Ross, E. (1969). *On death and dying.* New York: Macmillan. (Classic reference)

Kubler-Ross, E. (1975). *Death: The final stage of growth.* Englewood Cliffs, NJ: Prentice-Hall. (Classic reference)

Kubler-Ross, E. (1982). *On children and death.* New York: Macmillan. (Classic reference)

Leifer, R. (1997). *The happiness project: Transforming the three poisons that cause suffering we inflict on ourselves and others.* Ithaca, NY: Snow Lion. (Classic reference)

London, M., Ladewig, P., Ball, J., Bindler, R., & Kowen, K. (2011). *Maternal-child nursing care* (3rd ed.). Upper Saddle River, NJ: Prentice-Hall.

Mahan, C., & Escott-Stump, S. (2012). *Krause's food, nutrition, and diet therapy* (13th ed.). Philadelphia: Saunders.

Matrai, J., Chuah, M., Vander, D., & Reissch, T. (2010). Preclinical and clinical progress in hemophilia gene therapy. *Current Opinion in Hematology, 17*, 387–392.

Muncie, H., & Campbell, J. (2009). Alpha and beta thalassemia. *American Family Physicians, 80*(4), 339–344.

Nordquist, J. (2013). *FDA approves hemophilic B drug rixubis.* Retrieved from www.medicalnewstoday.com/articles/252610.php.

Rabin, K., & Poplack, D. (2011). Management strategies in ALL. *Oncology, 25*, 328–335.

Rees, D., Williams, T., & Gladwin, M. (2010). Sickle cell disease. *Lancet, 376*, 2018–2031.

Scott, J., & Montgomery, R. (2011). Factor VIII or factor IX deficiency (hemophilia A or B). In R. Kliegman, J. Stanton, J. St. Geme, III, N. Schor, & R. Behrman (Eds.), *Nelson's textbook of pediatrics* (19th ed.). Philadelphia: Saunders.

Thompson, C. (2008). Additional antihemophilic factor to be available. *American Journal of Health-System Pharmacy, 65*, 592.

Tubergen, D., Bleyer, A., & Ritchey, A. (2011). The leukemias. In R. Kliegman, J. Stanton, J. St. Geme, III, N. Schor, & R. Behrman (Eds.), *Nelson's textbook of pediatrics* (19th ed.). Philadelphia: Saunders.

Waxman, J., Hochberg, J., & Cairo, M. (2011). Lymphoma. In R. Kliegman, J. Stanton, J. St. Geme, III, N. Schor, & R. Behrman (Eds.), *Nelson's textbook of pediatrics* (19th ed.). Philadelphia: Saunders.

Chapter 28: The Child with a Gastrointestinal Condition

American Academy of Pediatrics. (2013). Policy statement: *Clostridium difficile* in infants and children. *Pediatrics, 131*(1), 196–200.

American Academy of Pediatrics. (2011). *Amount and schedule of formula feedings.* Retrieved May 2013, from www.healthychildren.org/English/ages-stages/baby/feeding-nutrition/pages/default.aspx.

Aschenbrenner, D. (2012). Drug watch: Prevention of infection from over-the-counter nasal spray and eye-drops. *The American Journal of Nursing, 113*(3), 23.

Barclay, L., & Nghiem, H. (2009). Management of common childhood poisoning. *American Family Physician, 79*, 397–403.

Bender, B., Skal, C., & Ozuah, P. (2005). Oral rehydration therapy: The clear solution to fluid loss. *Contemporary Pediatrics, 22*(4), 72–76.

Borowitz, S., Cox, D., Kovatcher, B., Ritterbrand, L., Sheen, J., & Sutphen, J. (2005). Treatment of childhood constipation by primary care physicians: Efficacy and predictors of outcome. *Pediatrics, 115*, 873–877.

Brown, H. (2005). Actions stat: Venomous snake bite. *Nursing, 35* (5), 88.

Centers for Disease Control and Prevention (CDC). (2013). Lead blood levels in children aged 1–5 years in the United States 1999–2019. *MMWR, 62*, 245–248.

Chao, H., & Vandenplas, Y. (2007). Cereal thickened formula and upright position for regurgitation, gastric emptying and weight gain in infants with regurgitation. *Nutrition, 23*(1), 23–31.

Cleveland, L., Minter, M., Cobb, K., Scott, A., & German, V. (2008). Lead hazards for pregnant women and children. *The American Journal of Nursing, 108*(11), 40–47.

Cohen, S., Ephrath, H., Lewis, J., Klevins, A., Bergwerk, A., & Lui, S. (2012). Pediatric capsule endoscopy: A review of small bowel and patency capsules. *Journal of Pediatric Gastroenterology and Nutrition, 54*(3), 409–413.

Collopy, K., & Friese, G. (2010). Pediatric drug administration. *Journal of Emergency Medical Services, 39*(6), 52–57.

DeLoach, R., & Farber, J. (2013). Intussusception. In N. Browne, C. Flannigan, & M. Comisky (Eds.), *Nursing care of pediatric surgical patients* (pp. 399–406) (3rd ed.). Sudbury, MA: Jones and Bartlett.

Frischknecht, J. (2013). Setting the standard of treatment of acetaminophen toxicity. *Advance for NP's and PA's, 4*(3), 34–38.

Hawke, M. (2005). A call for help. *Pediatrics: Specialty guide—January 2005*, 14–16.

Hellekson, K. (2005). AHRQ releases practice guidelines for celiac disease screening. *American Family Physicians, 71*(9), 1814–1816.

Hill, I. (2011). Searching for celiac disease: Who to test, how to test. *Contemporary Pediatrics, 28*(5), 20–29.

Hill, K., & Hill, I. (2005). Celiac disease: Fundamentals for pediatrics. *Contemporary Pediatrics, 22*(10), 65–67.

Hockenberry, M., & Wilson, D. (2009). *Wong's essentials of pediatric nursing* (8th ed.). St. Louis: Mosby.

Isbister, G., & Kumar, K. (2011). Indications for single dose activated charcoal administration in acute overdose. *Current Opinion in Critical Care, 17*(4), 351–357.

Jangi, S., & LaMont, J. (2010). Asymptomatic colonization by *C. difficile* in infants: Implications for disease in later life. *Journal of Pediatric Gastroenterology and Nutrition, 51*(1), 2–7.

Johnston, B. (2012). Probiotics for the prevention of *C. difficile* diarrhea: A systematic review and meta-analysis. *Annals of Internal Medicine*, Retrieved April 2013, from http://annals.org/article.aspx?articleID=1390418.

Jonsdottir, O. (2012). Timing of introduction of complimentary foods in infancy: A randomized controlled trial. *Pediatrics, 130*, 1038.

Karri, S., Saper, R., & Kates, S. (2008). Lead encephalopathy due to traditional medicine. *Current Drug Safety, 3*, 54–59.

Khan, S., & Orenstein, S. (2011). Esophageal atresia and tracheoesophageal fistula. In R. Kliegman, B. Stanton, J. St. Geme, III, N. Schor, & R. Behrman (Eds.), *Nelson's textbook of pediatrics*. (19th ed.). Philadelphia: Saunders.

Kliegman, R., Stanton, J., St. Geme, J., III, Shor, W., & Behrman, R. (2011). *Nelson's textbook of pediatrics* (19th ed.). Philadelphia: Saunders.

Krogh, C. (2012). Bottle feeding and the risk of pyloric stenosis. *Pediatrics, 130*(4), 943–949.

Krogh, C., Biggar, R., Fischer, T., Lindholm, M., & Wohlfhart, M. (2012). Bottle feeding and risk of pyloric stenosis. *Pediatrics, 130*(4), 943–949.

Lightsdale, J. (2013). Clinical report: Gastroesophageal reflux—Management guidance for the pediatrician. *Pediatrics, 131* (May), e1684.

Mahan, L., & Escott-Stump, S. (2012). *Krause's food, nutrition, and diet therapy* (13th ed.). Philadelphia: Saunders.

Mayo Clinic. (2011). *Gluten-free diet: What is allowed and what is not.* Retrieved April 2013, from www.mayoclinic.com/health/gluten-free-diet/MYO1140.

Mays, D. (1995). Turn ABGs into child's play. *RN, 58*(1), 36–39 (Classic reference).

McCabe, M., Toughill, E., Parkhill, A., Bassett, M., Jevic, M., & Nye, M. (2012). Celiac disease: A medical puzzle. *The American Journal of Nursing, 112*(10), 34–43.

McCartney, P. (2013). Pediatric capsule endoscopy: The pill camera. *MCN. The American Journal of Maternal Child Nursing, 38* (4), 252.

McGuire, J. (2013). The relationship between cow's milk and stores of vitamin D and iron in early childhood. *Pediatrics, 131*, 144.

Minkes, R., Bechtel, K., Bellmire, D., Freitas, M., Glick, P., Hennelley, K., et al. (2011). *Pediatric appendicitis.* Retrieved May 2013, from www.emedicine.medscape.com/article/926795-overview.

Misurac, J. (2012). Risk of kidney injury in use of NSAIDs in children who are dehydrated. *J Ped, 11*, 69.

Nylund, C., Gaudie, A., Garza, A., Fairbrother, C., & Cohen, M. (2011). *C. difficile* in hospitalized children in United States. *Archives of Pediatrics & Adolescent Medicine, 16*(4), 604–609.

Osterhardt, K. (2000). The toxic toddler: Drugs that can kill in small doses. *Contemporary Pediatrics, 17*(3), 73.

Payne, D. (2013). Norovirus and medically attended gastroenteritis in U.S. children. *The New England Journal of Medicine, 368*, 1121.

Perry, S., Hockenberry, M., Lowdermilk, D., & Wilson, D. (2010). *Maternal child nursing care* (4th ed.). St. Louis: Mosby.

Pietzak, M. (2012). Celiac disease: Wheat allergy and gluten sensitivity: When gluten free is not a fad. *Journal of Parenteral and Enteral Nutrition, 36*(1 Suppl.), 685–755.

Reignier, J. (2013). Effect of not monitoring residual gastric volume in risk of ventilator associated pneumonia in adults receiving mechanical ventilation and early enteral feeding: A randomized controlled trial. *JAMA, 309*, 249.

Rowley, A. (2012). Kawasaki disease. *Contemporary Pediatrics, 29* (12), 18–24.

Sapone, A. (2012). Spectrum of gluten-related disorders: A new nomenclature and classification. *BMC Medicine, 10*(13), 685–700.

Uyemura, M. (2005). Foreign body ingestion in children. *American Family Physician, 72*(2), 287–293.

Weill, V. (2008). Gastroesophageal reflux in infants. *Advance for Nurse Practitioners, 5*(1), 45–49.

Zhao, Z. Y., Liang, L., Fan, X., Yu, Z., Hotchkiss, A. T., Wilk, B. J., et al. (2008). The role of modified citrus pectin as an effective chelator of lead in children. *Alternative Therapies in Health and Medicine, 14*(4), 34–38.

Chapter 29: The Child with a Genitourinary Condition

Chung, E., & Brock, G. (2011). Cryptorchism and its impact on male fertility: A state of the art review of current literature. *Canadian Urological Association Journal, 5*(3), 210–213.

Elder, J. (2011). Urologic disorders in infants and children. In R. Kliegman, B. Stanton, J. St. Geme, III, N. Schor, & R. Behrman (Eds.), *Nelson's textbook of pediatrics* (19th ed.). Philadelphia: Saunders.

Friedman, A. (2008). Acute UTI: What you want to know. *Contemporary Pediatrics, 25*(10), 68–76.

Helming, M. (2009). GU problems in children. *Advance for Nurse Practitioners, 17*(3), 24–26.

Herreros, F. (2013). A new technique for fast and safe collection of urine in newborns. *Archives of Disease in Childhood, 98*, 27.

Jackson, P., Vessey, J., & Schapiro, N. (2009). *Primary care of the child with a chronic condition* (5th ed.). St. Louis: Mosby.

Kliegman, R., Stanton, B., St. Geme, J., III, Shor, W., & Behrman, R. (2011). *Nelson's textbook of pediatrics* (19th ed.). Philadelphia: Saunders.

Latendresse, G., McCance, A., & Morgan, K. (2010). Alterations in the reproductive system. In K. McCance & S. Huether (Eds.), *Pathophysiology: The biological basis for disease in adults and children* (pp. 816–992) (6th ed.). St. Louis: Mosby.

Mahan, L., & Escott-Stump, S. (2012). *Krause's food, nutrition, and diet therapy* (13th ed.). Philadelphia: Saunders.

Pais, P., & Avener, E. (2011). Nephrotic syndrome. In R. Kliegman, B. Stanton, J. St. Geme, III, N. Schor, & R. Berhman (Eds.), *Nelson's textbook of pediatrics* (19th ed.). Philadelphia: Saunders.

Penson, D., Krishnaswami, S., & Jules, A. (2013). Effectiveness of hormonal and surgical treatment for cryptorchidism. *Pediatrics, 131*(6), 1897–1907.

Perry, S., Hockenberry, M., Lowdermilk, D., & Wilson, D. (2010). *Maternal child nursing care* (4th ed.). St. Louis: Mosby.

Roberts, K. (2011). Urinary tract infections in infants: Clinical practice guidelines for diagnosis and management of initial UTI in febrile infants and children 2 to 24 months. *Pediatrics, 128*(3), 595–610.

Wan, J., Skoog, S., & Hulburt, W. (2012). Executive committee secretary on urology AAP section on urology response to new guidelines for diagnosis and management of urinary tract infections. *Pediatrics, 129*(4), 1051–1053.

Chapter 30: The Child with a Skin Condition

Adam, R. (2008). Skin care of the diaper area. *Pediatric Dermatology, 25*(4), 427–433.

American Academy of Pediatrics Committee on Infectious Diseases. (2012). *Redbook 2012: Report of committee on infectious diseases* (29th ed.). Elk Grove Village, IL: Author.

Eichenfeld, L., Frieden, V., & Esterly, N. (2008). *Neonatal dermatology* (2nd ed.). Philadelphia: Saunders.

Eichenfield, L. (2013). Evidence based recommendations for the diagnosis and treatment of pediatric acne. *Pediatrics, 131*, S163.

Frankowski, B., Bocchini, J., & Council on School Health and Common Infectious Diseases. (2010). Clinical report. *Pediatrics, 126*(2), 392–403.

Friedlander, S. F., Eichenfield, L. F., Leyden, J., Shu, J., & Spellman, M. C. (2009). Diaper dermatitis: Appropriate evaluation and management. *Contemporary Pediatrics*, 1–15, April (Spec Sec).

Heimall, L., Storey, B., Stellar, J., & Davis, K. (2013). Beginning at the bottom: Evidence based care of diaper dermatitis. *MCN. The American Journal of Maternal Child Nursing, 37*(1), 10–15.

Herndon, D., & Jones, J. (Eds.), (2007). *Total burn care* (3rd ed.). St. Louis: Saunders.

Jackson, P., Vessey, J., & Schapiro, N. (2009). *Primary care of the child with a chronic condition* (5th ed.). St. Louis: Mosby.

Kliegman, R., Behrman, R., Jenson, H., & Stanton, B. (2007). *Nelson's textbook of pediatrics* (18th ed.). Philadelphia: Saunders.

Marchese, N., & Primer, S. (2013). Targeting lyme disease. *Nursing 2013, 43*(5), 28–30.

Morel, K., Hogeling, M., & Eichenfield, L. (2005). More than skin deep: Cutaneous signs of systemic disease. *Contemporary Pediatrics, 22*(2), 48–56.

Orrico, J., & Kraus-Parello, C. (2010). Facts, fiction and figures of the sarcoptes scabies infection. *The Journal of School Nursing: The Official Publication of the National Association of School Nurses, 26*(4), 260–266.

Perry, S., Hockenberry, M., Lowdermilk, D., & Wilson, D. (2010). *Maternal child nursing care* (4th ed.). St. Louis: Mosby.

U.S. Department of Health and Human Services. (2007). *Guidelines for isolation precautions in hospitals: Hospital Infection Control Practices Advisory Committee*. Atlanta: Author.

USFDA. (2011). *FDA safety communication: Update on serious complications associated with negative pressure wound therapy systems*. Retrieved May 2013, from www.FDA.gov/MedicalDevices/safety/alertsandnotices/UCM244211.htm.

Zajac, L. (2009). Impetigo: Taking on a common skin infection. *Clinical Advisor, 12*(7), 30–34.

Chapter 31: The Child with a Metabolic Condition

American Academy of Pediatrics. (2009). *Pediatric nutrition handbook* (6th ed.). Elk Grove Village, IL: Author, pp. 873–699.

American Diabetes Association. (2011). Diagnosis and classification of diabetes mellitus. *Diabetic Care, 34*(Suppl.), S62–S69.

Carchidi, C., Holland, C., Minnock, P., & Boyle, D. (2012). New technologies in pediatric diabetic care. *MCN. The American Journal of Maternal Child Nursing, 36*(1), 32–40.

Clayton, B., Stock, Y., & Cooper, S. (2010). *Basic pharmacology for nurses* (15th ed.). St. Louis: Elsevier.

Copeland, K. (2013). Management of newly diagnosed type 2 diabetes mellitus (T2DM) in children and adolescents. *Pediatrics, 131*, 364.

Crawford, A., & Harris, H. (2012). SIADH: Fluid out of balance. *Nursing, 42*(9), 50.

Dea, T. (2012). Pediatric obesity and type 2 diabetes. *MCN. The American Journal of Maternal Child Nursing, 36*(1), 42–45.

DeFronzo, R. (2005). Efficacy of inhaled insulin in patients with type 2 diabetes not controlled with diet and exercise: A 12-week randomized comparative trial. *Diabetic Care, 28*, 1922–1928, Aug.

Ehehalt, S., Gauger, N., Blumenstock, G., & Diary-Group Baden Wuerhenburg. (2011). Hemoglobin ALC as reliable criterion for diagnosing diabetes in childhood and adolescence. *Pediatric Diabetes, 11*(7), 446–449.

Hatfield, L., Schwoebel, A., & Lynyak, C. (2012). Caring for the infant of a diabetic mother. *MCN. The American Journal of Maternal Child Nursing, 36*(1), 10–13.

Howe, C., Ratcliffe, S., Tuhle, A., Dougherty, S., & Lipman, T. (2012). Needle anxiety in children with type 1 diabetes and their mothers. *MCN. The American Journal of Maternal Child Nursing, 36*(1), 25–30.

Hughes, L. (2012). Assessing a patient with an insulin pump. *Nursing 2012, 42*(9), 63–65.

Hussar, D. (2008). Sapropterin dihydrochloride: First on the market to treat an inherited disorder. *Nursing, 38*(7), 46–47w.

Jackson, P., Vessey, J., & Schapiro, N. (2009). *Primary care of the child with a chronic condition* (5th ed.). St. Louis: Mosby.

Kliegman, R., Stanton, J., St. Geme, J., III, Shor, W., & Behrman, R. (2011). *Nelson's textbook of pediatrics* (19th ed.). Philadelphia: Saunders.

Lalau, J. (2010). Lactic acid acidosis induced by metformin: Incidence, management and prevention. *Drug Safety, 33*(9), 727–740.

Lewis, S., Heitkemper, M., Dirksen, S., O'Brien, G., & Bucher, L. (2011). *Medical-surgical nursing* (8th ed.). St. Louis: Elsevier.

Mahan, L., & Escott-Stump, S. (2012). *Krause's food, nutrition, and diet therapy* (13th ed.). Philadelphia: Saunders.

McHugo, J., & Harden, A. (2011). Diabetes insipidus: Navigating troubled waters. *Advance for NP's and PA's, 2*(4), 20–24.

Montvale, N. J., & Kapustin, J. (2012). Uncomplicating insulin therapy. *Advance for NP's and PA's, 3*(5), 20–27.

Nowicka, P., Santoro, N., & Liu, H. (2011). Utility of hemoglobin ALC for diagnosing prediabetes and diabetes in obese children and adolescents. *Diabetes Care, 34*(12), 2597–2602.

Pastores, G., & Hughes, D. (2011). *Gaucher's disease in gene reviews and gene tests: Medical genetics information resource*. Retrieved May 2013, from www.ncbi.nlm.nih.gov/books/NBK1269.

Perry, S., Hockenberry, M., Lowdermilk, D., & Wilson, D. (2010). *Maternal child nursing care* (4th ed.). St. Louis: Mosby.

Rearson, M., McNight-Menci, H., & Steinkrauss, L. (2012). Neonatal diabetes: Current trends in diabetes management. *MCN. The American Journal of Maternal Child Nursing, 36*(1), 17–20.

Sisson, E., Mills, J., & Chin, L. (2012). Recent safety updates on diabetes medications. *The American Journal of Nursing, 112*(12), 49–51.

U.S. Department of Agriculture and USDHHS. (2011). Retrieved May 2013, from www.choosemyplate.gov.

Zeitler, P. (2012). Type 2 diabetes mellitus: Challenges in diagnosis and treatment. *Contemporary Pediatrics, 29*(7), 16–23.

Chapter 32: Childhood Communicable Diseases, Bioterrorism, Natural Disasters, and the Maternal–Child Patient

American Academy of Pediatrics. (2009a). American Academy of Pediatrics update: Guidelines for use of rotavirus vaccines. *Pediatrics, 123*, 1412–1420.

American Academy of Pediatrics. (2009b). *Report of the Committee on Infectious Diseases*. Elk Grove Village, IL: Author.

American Academy of Pediatrics. (2012). *Common infectious diseases 2012: Redbook* (29th ed.). Elk Grove Village, IL: Author.

American Academy of Pediatrics. (2013). Statement of endorsement of recommendations of WHO Strategic Advisory Group (SAGE) on immunization practices. *Pediatrics, 131*(1), 2012–2262.

Armstrong, J. (2002). Chemical warfare. *RN, 65*(4), 32–39.

Bell, E. (2010). DTaP or TDAP: Vaccine and drug name confusion. *Infectious Disease of Children, 23*(10), 12.

Bruhn, K., & Tillett, J. (2009). Administration of vaccinations in pregnancy and postpartum. *MCN. The American Journal of Maternal Child Nursing, 34*(2), 98–105.

Callister, L. (2008). Among the most vulnerable: Women and children in global disasters. *MCN. The American Journal of Maternal Child Nursing, 33*(4), 263.

Carrarino, J. (2008). Disaster related prenatal health needs of women and children. *MCN. The American Journal of Maternal Child Nursing, 33*(4), 242–246.

Centers for Disease Control and Prevention. (2008). Updated recommendations for isolation for persons with mumps. *MMWR, 57*(40), 1103–1105.

Centers for Disease Control and Prevention. (2010). *Vaccines and preventable diseases: Statement regarding rotarix and rotateq rotovirus vaccine and intussusception*. Retrieved February 2013, from www.gov/vaccines/VPD-VAC/rotavirus/intussusception-studies-acip.htm.

Centers for Disease Control and Prevention. (2011). *HPV vaccine: Questions and answers*. Retrieved May 2013, from www.cdc.org.

Centers for Disease Control and Prevention. (2011). *One test—Two lives: HIV screening for prenatal care*. Retrieved May 2013, from www.cdc.gov/features/test2lives.

Davidhizar, R., & Shearer, R. (2002). Helping children cope with public disasters: Support given immediately after a traumatic event can counteract or even negate long-term adverse effects. *The American Journal of Nursing, 102*(3), 26–33.

Department of Health Services, State of California. (2001, June 16). Vaccine storage and rolling blackouts. *Health Bulletin*, #1.

Friedman, L., Bell, D. L., Kahn, J. A., Marcell, A. V., Middleman, A. B., Rosenthal, S. L., et al. (2011). HPV vaccine: An updated position statement for adolescent health and medicine. *Journal of Adolescent Health, 48*, 215–216.

Grabenstein, J. (2009). *Immunization facts: Vaccines and immunological drugs*. St. Louis: Walters-Kluwer.

Hahn, E. (2009). Incorporating the CDC recommendations for adolescent HIV screening into practice. *Journal of Nursing Practice, 5*(4), 265–273.

Hensley, E., & Briars, C. (2010). Closer look at autism and the measles-mumps-rubella vaccine. *Journal of the American Pharmaceutical Association, 50*(6), 736–741.

Jackson, P., Vessey, J., & Schapiro, N. (2009). *Primary care of the child with a chronic condition* (5th ed.). St. Louis: Mosby.

Kliegman, R., Stanton, B., St. Geme, J., III, Shor, W., & Behrman, R. (2011). *Nelson's textbook of pediatrics* (19th ed.). Philadelphia: Saunders.

Kman, N., & Nelson, R. (2008). Infectious agents of bioterrorism: A review for emergency physicians. *Emergency Medical Clinics of North America, 26*, 517–547.

Kroger, A., Sumaya, C., Pickering, L., & Atkinson, W. (2011). General recommendations on immunization. *MMWR, 60*(2), 1–62.

London, M., Ladewig, P., Ball, J., Bindler, R., & Cowen, K. (2011). *Maternal-child nursing care* (3rd ed.). Upper Saddle River, NJ: Prentice-Hall.

Mandell, G. L., Bennett, J. E., & Dolin, R. (2005). *Principles and practice of infectious diseases* (6th ed.). Philadelphia: Churchill Livingstone.

Marchese, N., & Primer, R. (2013). Targeting lyme disease. *Nursing 2013, 43*(5), 28–33.

Marirose, B., & Mathews, P. (2008). Evacuation of the maternal-newborn area during hurricane Katrina. *MCN. The American Journal of Maternal Child Nursing, 33*(4), 213–220.

McCance, K., & Huether, S. (2010). *Pathophysiology: The biological basis for disease in adults and children* (6th ed.). St. Louis: Mosby.

McCartney, P. (2008). Online resources to prepare families for disaster risks. *MCN. The American Journal of Maternal Child Nursing, 33*(4), 259.

Moran, G., Talan, D., & Abrahamian, F. (2008). Biologic terrorism. *Infectious Disease Clinics of North America, 22*, 145–187.

Morin, M., Meissner, H., & Seward, J. (2008). Varicella prevention in the U.S.: A review of successes and challenges. *Pediatrics, 122e*, 744.

Perry, S., Hockenberry, M., Lowdermilk, D., & Wilson, D. (2010). *Maternal child nursing care* (4th ed.). St. Louis: Mosby.

Saveleyt, V. (2010). Lyme disease: A diagnostic dilemma. *Nurse Practitioner, 35*(7), 44–50.

Sharts-Hopko, N. (2009). Issues in pediatric immunizations. *MCN. The American Journal of Maternal Child Nursing, 34*(2), 80–88, Mar-Apr.

Schultz, R., Paulestsos, C., & Combs, A. (2008). Considerations for emergencies and disasters in the NICU. *MCN. The American Journal of Maternal Child Nursing, 33*(4), 204–210.

Snow, M. (2011). Human rabies: Treatment and prevention. *Nursing 2011, 41*(4), 65–66.

Spicer, K., & Powell, D. (2010). Immunization for internationally adopted children. *Pediatric Annals, 39*(8), 517–524.

Spratling, R., & Carmon, M. (2010). Pertussis—An overview of the disease: Immunization and trends for nurses. *Pediatric Nursing, 36*(5), 239–243.

Teran-MacIver, M., & Larson, K. (2008). Implications of terrorist-biological terrorism events for children and pregnant women. *MCN. The American Journal of Maternal Child Nursing, 33*(4), 224–230.

Veenema, T., Benitz, J., & Benwatre, S. (2007). *Disaster nursing and emergency preparedness*. New York: Springer.

Chapter 33: The Child with an Emotional or Behavioral Condition

Allen, S., & Dalton, W. (2011). Treatment of eating disorders in primary care: A systematic review. *Journal of Health Psychology*, http://dx.doi.org/10:1177/(135910531)1402244.

American Association of Intellectual and Developmental Disabilities. (2012). *FAQ in AAIDD definition of intellectual disability*. Retrieved May 2013, from www.AAIDD.org/intellectualdisabilitybook/content_7473cfm?navID=366.

American Psychiatric Association. (2013). *Diagnostic and statistical manual of mental disorders (DSM-V)* (5th ed.). Washington, DC: Author.

Arora, B., & Kanninnikeswaran, N. (2010). Serotonin syndrome: The need for physician awareness. *International Journal of Emergency Medicine, 3*, 373–377.

ASQ-3. (2013). *Ages and stages questionnaires* (3rd ed.). Retrieved May 2013, from www.agesandstages.com.

Belschner, R. (2007). Stop, assess, and motivate: The SAM approach to autism spectrum disorder. *The American Journal for Nurse Practitioners, 11*(4), 43–50.

Blaylock, R. (2009). A possible central mechanism in autism spectrum disorders: Immunotoxicity. *Alternative Therapies in Health and Medicine, 15*(1), 60–63.

Blumberg, S. (2013). Changes in prevalence of parent-reported autism spectrum disorder in school-aged United States children 2007–2011. *National Health Statistics Report, 265*, 1–2.

Brulotte, J., Bukutu, L., & Vohra, S. (2009). Complimentary, holistic and integrative medicine. *Pediatrics in Review, 30*(4), e29–e33.

Burstein, M. (2012). When to get anxious about social anxiety disorders. *Contemporary Pediatrics, 29*(12), 32–42.

Burstein, M., Ameli-Grillon, L., & Merikangas, K. (2011). Shyness versus social phobia in U.S. youth. *Pediatrics, 128*(5), 917–925.

Centers for Disease Control and Prevention (CDC). (2010). *ASD research*. Retrieved 2013, from www.cdc.gov/ncbddd/autism.

Centers for Disease Control and Prevention (CDC). (2013). *New data on autism spectrum disorder*. Retrieved May 2013, from www.cdc.gov/features/countingAutism/.

Christiansen, J. (2013). Prenatal valproic acid exposure and risk of autism spectrum disorders and childhood autism. *JAMA, 309*, 1696–1703.

Devlin, B., & Scherer, S. (2012). The genetic architecture in ASD. *Current Opinion in Genetics & Development, 22*(3), 229–237.

Flament, M., Bissada, H., & Spettigue, W. (2012). Evidence based pharmacotherapy of eating disorders. *The International Journal of Neuropsychopharmacology, 15*(12), 189–207.

Golnik, A., & MacAbee-Ryboy, N. (2010). Autism: Clinical pearls for primary care. *Contemporary Pediatrics, 42*, 60.

Habela, C., & Hamosh, A. (2013). Genetic testing for intellectual disability. *Contemporary Pediatrics, 30*(6), 21–27.

Inglese, M. (2009). Caring for children with autism spectrum disorder: Screening, diagnosis and management. *Journal of Pediatric Nursing, 24,* 49–59.

Jackson, P., Vessey, J., & Schapiro, N. (2009). *Primary care of the child with a chronic condition* (5th ed.). St. Louis: Mosby.

Kliegman, R., Stanton, B., St. Geme, J., III, Shor, W., & Behrman, R. (2011). *Nelson's textbook of pediatrics* (19th ed.). Philadelphia: Saunders.

Kliegman, R., Marcdante, K., Jenson, H., & Behrman, R. (2005). *Nelson's essentials of pediatrics* (5th ed.). Philadelphia: Saunders.

Leifer, R. (1997). *The happiness project: Transforming the three poisons that cause suffering we inflict on ourselves and others.* Ithaca, NY: Snow Lion (Classic reference).

Lock, J. (2011). Evaluation of family treatment models for eating disorders. *Current Opinion in Psychiatry, 24,* 274–279.

Lockwood, J. (2013a). Autism and the obstetrician. *Contemporary Ob/Gyn, 58*(6), 8–11.

Lockwood, J. (2013b). FDA permits marketing of first brain wave test to help assess children with ADHD. *Contemporary Pediatrics, 30*(7).

Lundstrom, S., Howorth, C., & Carlstrom, E. (2010). Trajectories leading to autism spectrum disorders are affected by paternal age. *Journal of Child Psychology and Psychiatry, and Allied Disciplines, 51*(7), 850–856.

Maimburg, R., Beck, B., Vaeth, M., Moller-Madsen, B., & Olsen, J. (2010). Neonatal jaundice, autism, and other disorders of psychological development. *Pediatrics, 12*(5), 872–878.

May, D., & Kratochvic, C. (2010). ADHD: Recent advances in pediatric pharmacology. *Drugs, 70,* 15–40.

M-CHAT. (2013). *General information.* Retrieved 2013, from https://M-CHAT.org.

McGraw, M. (2012). Is your patient high on bath salts? *Nursing 2012, 42*(1), 26–32.

Perry, S., Hockenberry, M., Lowdermilk, D., & Wilson, D. (2010). *Maternal child nursing care* (4th ed.). St. Louis: Mosby.

Peterson, K., & Barbel, P. (2013). On alert for autism spectrum disorders. *Nursing 2013, 43*(4), 28–34.

Saha, S., Wilson, D., & Adger, H. (2012). K2 spice and bath salts: New drugs of abuse. *Contemporary Pediatrics, 29*(10), 22–37.

Smoller, J. (2013). Identification of risk located with shared effects on 5 major psychiatric disorders: A genome-wide analysis. *Lancet,* http://dx.doi.org/10.1016/SO140-6736(12)62129-1.

Starr, H. (2007). The impact of culture on ADHD. *Contemporary Pediatrics, 24*(12), 38–42.

Suren, P., Roth, C., & Bresnahan, M. (2013). The association between use of folic acid supplements and risk of autism spectrum disorders in children. *JAMA, 309*(6), 570–577.

Chapter 34: Complementary and Alternative Therapies in Maternity and Pediatric Nursing

Arnold, E., Hurt, E., & Lofthouse, N. (2013). ADHD dietary and nutritional treatment. *Child and Adolescent Psychiatric Clinics of North America, 22*(3), 381–402.

Bennett, D. (2009). Alternate therapies/integrated medicine. *RN, 72*(3), 38–41.

Bishop, J., Northstone, K., Green, J., & Thompson, E. (2011). The use of complementary and alternative medicine in pregnancy. *Child and Adolescent Psychiatry, 19*(6), 303–310.

Bland, J. (2008). The future of nutritional pharmacology. *Alternative Therapies in Health and Medicine, 14*(5), 12–16.

Cohen, M., Natbony, S., & Abbot, R. (2013). Complementary and alternative medicine in child and adolescent psychiatry. *Psychiatric Clinics of North America, 22*(3), 493–507.

Corrigan, J., & Alfers, L. (2007). Effect of vitamin E on prothrombin levels in warfarin induced vitamin K deficiency. *Journal of Alternative and Complementary Medicine, 13,* 997–1006.

Dog, T. (2009). The use of botanicals during pregnancy and lactation. *Alternative Therapies in Health and Medicine, 15*(1), 54–56.

Edwards, E., Mischoalon, D., Rapaport, M., Stussman, B., & Weber, W. (2013). Building an evidence base in complementary and alternative health care for child and adolescent psychiatry. *The Psychiatric Clinics of North America, 22*(3), 509–529.

Evans, S., & Tsao, J. (2008). CAM for acute procedural pain in children. *Alternative Therapies in Health and Medicine, 14*(5), 52.

Field, T. (2008). Alternative therapy in pregnancy and labor. *Alternative Therapies in Health and Medicine, 14*(5), 28–30.

Gardiner, P., & Kemper, K. (2005). For GI complaints: Which herbs and supplements spell relief? *Contemporary Pediatrics, 22*(8), 51–55.

Hyman, M. (2009). The map: Integrating integrative medicine. *Alternative Therapies in Health and Medicine, 15*(1), 20–22.

Kemper, K., Vohra, S., & Walls, R. (2008). The use of CAM medicine in pediatrics. *The Journal of Pediatrics, 122*(6), 1374–1386.

Kemper, K., & Breuner, C. (2010). Complimentary, holistic and integrative medicine. *Pediatrics in Review, 32*(2), e17–e23.

Johnston, B. (2012). Probiotics for prevention of *C. difficile* diarrhea: A systematic review. *Annals of Internal Medicine,* Retrieved June 2013, from http://annals.org/article.ASPX?articleID=1390418.

Leifer, G. (2001). Hyperbaric oxygen therapy: What every nurse should know. *The American Journal of Nursing, 101*(8), 36.

Leung, A., & Robson, W. (2005). Factitious dermatitis: Spoon scratching, cupping. *Consultant, 45*(2), 183–185.

Loo, M. (2008). *Integrative medicine for children.* Philadelphia: Saunders.

Micozzi, H. (2011). *Fundamentals of complementary and integrative medicine* (4th ed.). Philadelphia: Saunders.

Morelli, V., & Zoorob, R. (2010). *Complementary and alternative modalities: An issue of primary care clinics in office practice.* Philadelphia: Saunders.

Physician's desk reference for herbal medicines. Montvale, NJ: Medical Economics.

Popper, C. (2013). Mood disorders in youth: Complementary treatment approaches. *Psychiatric Clinics of North America, 22*(3), 403–441.

Rainone, F. (2005). Milk thistle. *American Family Physician, 72*(7), 1285–1287.

Rakel, D. (2012). *Integrative medicine.* Philadelphia: Saunders.

Reilly, A. (2005). Role of massage therapy in patient care. *Advance for Nurse Practitioners, 13*(5), 37–42.

Richardson, M. (2008). Black cohosh: A cautionary tale. *Menopause, 8*(15), 583.

Rindfleisch, A. (2010). *Integrative medicine.* Philadelphia: Saunders.

Roemheld-Hamm, B. (2005). Chasteberry. *American Family Physician, 72*(5), 821.

Sarris, J., Kean, J., Schweitzer, I., & Lake, J. (2011). Complimentary medicine (herbal and nutritional) in treatment of ADHD: A systematic review. *Complimentary Therapies in Medicine, 19*(4), 216–227.

Simkin, D., & Popper, C. (Eds.). (2013). Overview of integrative medicine in child and adolescent psychiatry. In *The Psychiatric Clinics of North America, 22*(3), 375–578.

Skidmore-Roth, L. (2010). *Mosby's handbook of herbs and natural supplements* (4th ed.). St. Louis: Mosby.

Trivedi, H. (Ed.). (2013). Alternative and complementary treatment for children with psychiatric disorders. *Child and Adolescent Clinics of North America, 19*(4), 216–227.

Vohra, S., Surette, S., Mittra, D., Rosen, L., Gardner, P., & Kemper, K. (2012). Is pediatric integrative medicine the newest subspecialty? *BMC Pediatrics, 12,* 123.

Zhao, Z., Liang, L., Fan, X., Yu, Z., Hotchkiss, A. T., Wilk, B. J., et al. (2008). The role of modified citrus pectin as an effective chelator of lead in children. *Alternative Therapies in Health and Medicine, 14*(4), 34–39.

Glossary

A

abdominal delivery A cesarean birth.

abduction A movement away from the midline of the body.

abortion The end of a pregnancy before the fetus is viable, whether spontaneous or elective.

abruptio placentae A premature separation of a normally implanted placenta.

abstinence Voluntarily refraining from participation in sexual intercourse.

abuse To attack or cause injury—physical, sexual, emotional, or spiritual. This term includes nonaccidental injury and neglect.

acceleration A temporary increase of the fetal heart rate over the baseline rate of at least 15 beats/min for at least 15 seconds.

acidosis A condition in which there is either a marked increase in the level of acids in the blood or body tissues or a marked decrease in the alkaline reserve (bicarbonate). The pH in the blood is low.

acini cells Cells that secrete a substance that helps with digestion in the alimentary tract and with breathing in the respiratory tract.

acme The peak, or period of greatest strength, of a uterine contraction.

acrocyanosis A peripheral blueness of the hands and feet due to reduced peripheral circulation (normal in newborns).

active acquired immunity Immunity acquired through vaccination or development of antibodies resulting from exposure to an infectious disease.

acupressure A nursing intervention involving the application of firm, sustained pressure to specific points on the body. Used to relieve pain and promote relaxation.

acupuncture Insertion of thin wire needles into the skin at specific sites along a series of lines called meridians to treat illness and pain. A type of complementary and alternative medical (CAM) therapy.

adduction A movement toward the midline of the body.

adolescence Period of human development beginning with puberty and ending with young adulthood.

advanced practice nurses A term used often to describe the pediatric nurse practitioner (PNP) and the clinical nurse specialist (CNS).

advocacy Speaking or acting in support of a person's rights and needs.

afterbirth The placenta and membranes delivered during the third stage of labor.

afterpains Painful contractions of the uterus that occur for several days after delivery; they occur most often in multiparas and are more painful during breastfeeding.

age of viability The time in a pregnancy when the fetus has reached a point in development where it can potentially survive outside of the uterus after birth. Although 20 weeks gestation is thought to be a baseline age of viability, modern biomedical and technological advances now have an influence on survival and therefore no world-wide specific age of viability can be presently defined.

AIDS Acquired immunodeficiency syndrome; caused by human immunodeficiency virus (HIV); characterized by a depressed immune system and involving a deficiency in the CD4 and T lymphocytes.

airway management A positioning of the head and neck to ensure patency of the airway; may include interventions to ensure adequate oxygenation.

albuminuria The presence of a type of protein in the urine.

allergy An abnormal immune response to a substance that causes an inflammatory response resulting in hypersensitivity.

allopathic care The management of disease or injury with interventions such as medical and surgical treatment.

alpha-fetoprotein (AFP) test A maternal blood test used to diagnose neural tube defects in the developing fetus.

alternative treatment Methods to maintain health in the treatment of disease that differ from the traditionally accepted Western practice of medicine.

alveoli The area in the lungs where the exchange of carbon dioxide and oxygen occurs.

amenorrhea The absence or suppression of menstruation; normal before puberty, during pregnancy and lactation, and after menopause.

amniocentesis Transabdominal puncture of the amniotic sac (fetal membranes) to obtain a sample of amniotic fluid for study.

amnioinfusion The infusion of warmed saline into the uterus to relieve cord compression or to wash meconium out of the cavity to prevent aspiration of it at birth.

amnion The inner of the two fetal membranes; thin and transparent; holds the fetus suspended in amniotic fluid.

amnionitis An inflammation or infection of the membrane closest to the developing fetus.

amniotic fluid A transparent, almost colorless fluid contained in the fetal membranes and amnion; it protects the fetus from injury, maintains an even temperature, and allows fetal movement.

amniotic sac The sac formed by the amnion and the chorion and containing fluid and the fetus; it is commonly known as the "bag of waters."

amniotomy A surgical procedure in which the amniotic sac is ruptured to facilitate delivery of the fetus.

analgesic A drug that relieves pain but does not produce unconsciousness.

anaphylactoid syndrome An unpredictable, catastrophic condition that occurs during labor or delivery in which an amniotic fluid embolism is released into the mother's circulation and causes cardiogenic shock or respiratory failure. It is a leading cause of maternal mortality.

androgen A substance that stimulates masculinization, such as the male hormone testosterone or androsterone.

android pelvis A female pelvis that resembles one of masculine size and shape.

anemia A decrease in the amount of hemoglobin or red blood cells circulating within the body.

anesthesia A partial or complete loss of sensation, especially of pain, with or without the loss of consciousness.

angioma A tumor, usually benign, that is made up chiefly of blood and lymph vessels.

animism A type of thinking characteristic of a period of cognitive development in which the child attributes life to inanimate objects.

anomaly Not normal in form, structure, or position; a congenital anomaly is an abnormality present at birth.

anorexia nervosa A syndrome most often seen in adolescent girls and characterized by an extreme form of self-starvation. Although its onset may be acute, the underlying emotional problem develops over a relatively long time.

anoxia A complete absence of oxygen in the blood.

antenatal Before birth.

antepartum Before the onset of labor.

anterior Pertaining to the front or top of the body.

anterior fontanelle A diamond-shaped area between the two frontal and two parietal bones of the newborn's head; also called the *soft spot.*

anthropoid pelvis A female pelvis with a transverse diameter that is equal to or smaller than the anteroposterior diameter.

antibody A specific protein substance that is formed in the body in response to antigens and restricts or destroys antigens.

antigen A substance that precipitates an immune response, resulting in the formation of antibodies. Antigen-antibody reactions form the basis for immunity.

anuria The lack of urine formation by the kidneys.

Apgar score An evaluation tool with a maximum score of 10; used to assess a newborn at 1 minute and 5 minutes after delivery. Five factors (scored 0, 1, or 2) are heart rate, color, muscle tone, reflex irritability, and respiratory effort.

apnea A cessation of respirations.

areola The pigmented circle of tissue around the nipple of the breast.

AROM Artificial rupture of the (amniotic) membranes with a sterile instrument, such as an Amnihook or Allis clamp.

aromatherapy The absorption of essential oils or their aromas by the lungs or skin for systemic effects.

artificial insemination The mechanical injection of viable semen into the vagina for the purpose of impregnation.

ascariasis Roundworm infestation.

asphyxia An inadequate amount of oxygen or an increased amount of carbon dioxide in the blood and tissues of the body.

asynchrony The lack of concurrence in time. A growing child may look gangling because of asynchrony of growth (i.e., different body parts mature at different rates).

atelectasis An incomplete expansion of the lungs or a collapse of the alveoli after expansion.

atony A lack of muscle tone or strength.

attachment A strong psychological bond of affection between an infant and a significant other.

attitude In obstetrics, the position of the fetus in the uterus (normally one of flexion of the head and extremities).

augmentation of labor The enhancement of labor after it has begun.

autoimmunity A condition in which the body produces antibodies against its own tissues.

autolysis The breakdown or endogenous destruction of cells by enzymes in the body.

autonomy Independent functioning; self-control.

autosomal inheritance Transmission of characteristics on a chromosome other than a sex chromosome.

autosome Any chromosome within the body except the sex chromosomes (X and Y).

B

bacteriuria The presence of bacteria in the urine.

bag of waters The membrane containing the amniotic fluid and the fetus.

ballottement In the uterus: the fetus floats away when palpated and then returns to touch the examiner's fingers.

barrier technique A method of medical asepsis in which various types of isolation precautions or standard precautions are used as recommended by the Centers for Disease Control and Prevention. In contraception, it is a method in which sperm is prevented from entering the cervix.

Bartholin glands Two small mucous glands situated on each side of the vaginal orifice that secrete small amounts of mucus during coitus (intercourse).

basal body temperature chart A written graphic chart of daily body temperature, usually taken on awakening. The temperature usually drops at the beginning of ovulation.

bilirubin An orange or yellowish pigment in bile; a breakdown product of hemoglobin carried by the blood to the liver, where it is chemically changed and excreted in bile or is conjugated and excreted in the stool.

bilirubinemia The presence of bilirubin in the blood.

Billings method A method used to check cervical mucus for elasticity, stickiness, wetness, and lubrication.

biofeedback A method of training designed to help an individual control his or her autonomic (involuntary) nervous system.

biophysical profile (BPP) A system of estimating the status of a fetus by evaluating heart rate, respiratory movement, muscle movement and tone, and amniotic fluid volume. Low scores indicate the need for prompt delivery.

birthing centers Freestanding buildings outside of the hospital that provide comprehensive care, including antepartum, labor and delivery, and postpartum care and mothers' classes, lactation classes, and follow-up family planning.

Bishop score A scoring system that uses cervical dilation, effacement, fetal station, cervical consistency, and position to determine if labor can be safely induced.

blastocyst A stage in embryonic development that follows the morula. Implantation in the uterus generally occurs at this stage.

blastula A phase of the fertilized ovum in which all its cells are arranged into a hollow ball or cavity.

bleb An irregularly shaped elevation of the epidermis; a blister or bulla.

blood patch The injection of the patient's blood into the epidural space in order to seal a dural puncture and prevent leakage of cerebral spinal fluid.

bloody show Appearance of a mixture of blood and mucus from the cervix that often precedes labor.

bonding Attachment; the process whereby a unique relationship is established between two people; used in conjunction with parent-newborn attachment.

bone marrow transplant Transplantation of bone marrow from one person to another; currently used to treat aplastic anemia and leukemia.

booster injection The administration of a substance to renew or increase the effectiveness of a prior immunization injection (e.g., a tetanus booster).

bradycardia A heart rate slower than the expected rate for age. In a newborn, a heart rate less than 110 beats/min; in a child, a heart rate less than 70 beats/min; in an adult, a heart rate less than 60 beats/min.

Braxton Hicks contractions Intermittent contractions of the uterus; they occur more frequently toward the end of pregnancy and are sometimes mistaken for true labor contractions.

breech presentation A birth in which the buttocks or feet (or both) present instead of the head; occurs in approximately 3% of all deliveries.

bronchopulmonary dysplasia A complication of artificial oxygen ventilation characterized by scarring of the lung tissue, which inhibits lung ventilation and perfusion.

Broviac catheter A central venous line used in small children who require total parenteral or continuous intravenous infusion.

brown fat Also called *brown adipose tissue*—forms in the fetus around the kidneys, the adrenals, and the neck; between the scapulae; and behind the sternum. Its dark brown hue is a result of its density, enriched blood supply, and abundant nerve supply. Its main purpose is heat production in the neonate.

Bryant's traction A type of skin traction apparatus commonly used for toddlers with a fractured femur. Vertical suspension is used.

C

café au lait spots Permanent light brown patchy spots on the skin. Large size and numbers may be characteristic of neurofibromatosis.

calendar method A natural method of birth control in which the calendar is used to determine which phase of the menstrual cycle the woman is in.

CAM therapy The use of complementary or alternative treatments. Complementary medicine is therapy used *with* traditional or conventional therapy. Alternative therapy is treatments that are used to *replace* conventional or traditional therapy.

caput The head; the occiput of the fetal head, which appears at the vaginal introitus before delivery of the head.

caput succedaneum Swelling or edema of the newborn scalp that crosses the suture lines; usually simply called *caput*. It is self-limiting and necessitates no treatment.

cardiac decompensation Heart failure.

cardinal movement See mechanisms of labor.

carpal tunnel syndrome Occurs when pressure is placed on the median nerve as it goes through the carpal tunnel into the hand. When compressed, it can cause pain and numbness of the affected extremity. It can occur in pregnancy and/or with repetitive motion (e.g., typing, frequent twisting of the wrist).

cephalic presentation A birth in which the fetal head presents against the cervix.

cephalocaudal development The orderly development of muscular control, which proceeds from head to foot.

cephalohematoma Subperiosteal swelling containing blood, found on the head of some newborns. The swelling does not cross suture lines and therefore often appears unilateral; usually disappears within a few weeks to 2 months without treatment.

cephalopelvic disproportion (CPD) A condition in which the fetus cannot pass through the maternal pelvis; also called *fetopelvic disproportion*.

cerclage Closing of the cervix with a suture to prevent early dilation and spontaneous abortion.

certified nurse-midwife (CNM) A registered nurse who has completed special training approved by the American College of Nurses-Midwives and passed a certification test. The CNM provides care to women who have a normal, uncomplicated pregnancy and delivery.

cerumen Ear wax.

cervical cap A contraceptive device that fits over the cervix.

cervical os The small opening of the cervix that dilates during the first stage of labor.

cervix The lower part of the uterus.

cesarean birth Delivery of the fetus by means of an incision into the abdominal wall and the uterus; abdominal delivery.

Chadwick's sign A violet-blue color of the vaginal mucous membrane caused by increased vascularity; it is a probable sign of pregnancy that is visible about the fourth week of pregnancy.

chignon Newborn scalp edema created by a vacuum extractor.

chloasma gravidarum A yellow-brown pigmentation over the bridge of the nose and cheeks during pregnancy and in some women who are taking oral contraceptives; also known as the *mask of pregnancy*.

chordee A congenital anomaly in which a fibrous strand of tissue extends from the scrotum to the penis, preventing urination with the penis in the normal elevated position; commonly associated with hypospadias.

chorion The fetal membrane closest to the interior uterine wall; it gives rise to the placenta and continues as the outer membrane surrounding the amnion.

chorionic villi Threadlike projections on the chorionic surface of the placenta; they help to form the placenta and secrete human chorionic gonadotropin.

chromosome A structure composed of tightly packed DNA; it is found in the nuclei of plant and animal cells and is responsible for the transmission of hereditary characteristics.

circumcision The surgical removal of the foreskin of the penis.

cleansing breath A slow, deep breath that is taken at the beginning and end of each contraction of labor.

clinical nurse specialist (CNS) The CNS provides care in the hospital or community to patients in specific specialty areas, such as cardiac, neurological, or oncological care.

clinical pathways Also known as *critical pathways, care maps,* or *multidisciplinary action plans,* clinical pathways are collaborative guidelines that define multidisciplinary care in terms of outcomes within a timeline.

clitoris The female organ that is homologous to the male penis; a small oval body of erectile tissue situated at the anterior junction of the vulva.

coitus Sexual intercourse.

coitus interruptus Removal of the erect penis from the vagina before ejaculation.

colostrum A secretion from the breast before the onset of true lactation; it has a high protein content, provides some immune properties, and cleanses the newborn's intestinal tract of mucus and meconium.

colposcopy A special type of scope used to examine the vagina and cervix for unusual changes or neoplasms.

comedo A skin lesion caused by a plug of keratin, sebum, and bacteria; there are two types: blackheads and whiteheads.

complementary therapy Nontraditional treatment method or methods used to maintain health or treat disease; used in conjunction with traditional medical therapy or treatment.

conception The union of the male sperm and female ovum; fertilization.

conceptus The products of conception.

condom A sheath or covering that is usually made from rubber or latex; placed over an erect penis to prevent the ejaculate from entering the vagina. The female condom is inserted into the vagina before penetration and is fitted over the cervix with an inner ring to help hold it in place.

congenital Present at birth.

congenital malformation An anomaly present at birth.

contraception The prevention of conception or impregnation.

contraction Tightening and shortening of uterine muscles during labor, causing effacement and dilation of the cervix; contributes to downward and outward movement of fetus.

contraction stress test (CST) Manual manipulation of the nipple of the breast to stimulate the production of oxytocin and test the fetal response to uterine contractions; used for high-risk pregnancies. See also *oxytocin challenge test (OCT)*.

convection The loss of heat from a warm surface to air currents that are much cooler.

Coombs' test A blood test to determine if Rh antibodies are present in the blood of the mother or neonate.

coping Dealing effectively with stress and problems.

corpus luteum A small endocrine structure that develops inside a ruptured ovarian follicle and secretes both estrogen and progesterone.

cost containment The efficient and effective use of resources.

couvade A syndrome in which the father experiences the symptoms of the pregnant partner.

craniosynostosis Premature closure of the cranial sutures that limits the growth of the brain.

critical thinking Applying creativity and ingenuity to solve the problem: combining basic standard principles with data specific to the patient.

crowning The appearance of the presenting fetal part (head) at the vaginal orifice during labor.

culdocentesis Fluid aspiration from the cul-de-sac of the posterior vagina, either for diagnostic or therapeutic reasons.

cultural awareness A conscious awareness of the cultural values, beliefs, and perceptions of one's self and others.

cultural competence A quality, attained by cultural awareness and sensitivity, that enables health care providers to adapt practices to meet the needs of patients from various cultures.

cultural sensitivity An understanding of and sensitivity to cultural practices and values that differ from one's own.

culture The body of symbols, ideas, values, traditions, and practices shared by a group of people; can also mean the growth of organisms in a special medium.

cyanosis A condition in which the skin takes on a blue, gray, or slate cast or color due to a lack of oxygen in the blood.

D

deceleration A periodic decrease in baseline fetal heart rate; can be early, late, or variable.

decidua basalis The part of the decidua that unites with the chorion to form the placenta. It is shed in lochial discharge after delivery.

deciduous teeth Baby teeth.

decrement A decrease or stage of decline, as in a contraction.

delivery The expulsion of an infant (with the placenta and membranes) from the woman at birth.

Denver Developmental Screening Test (DDST) Assesses the developmental status of a child during the first 6 years of life in five areas: personal, social, fine motor adaptive, language, and gross motor activities.

developmental task A skill whose acquisition falls into a particular time frame or a specific age range and which, when accomplished, provides the basis for future tasks.

diagnosis-related groups (DRGs) These refer to a Medicare system that determines payment for a hospital stay based on the patient's diagnosis.

diagonal conjugate The distance between the sacral promontory and the lowest border of the symphysis pubis; the pelvic diameter.

diaphoresis Profuse sweating.

diaphragm A contraceptive device that is used with a spermicide to prevent sperm from entering the uterus.

dilation of the cervix An expansion of the cervical os that allows passage of the fetus and products of conception.

diploid Cell or organism containing a set of maternal and a set of paternal chromosomes. In humans, the diploid number of chromosomes is 46.

disproportion A term used when the pelvis of the mother is too small or the fetal head is too large for safe vaginal delivery.

dizygotic twins Fetuses that develop from two fertilized ova; fraternal twins.

documentation The written or electronic recording of any action taken by the nurse or other health care provider, including when a medication is given, a treatment performed, etc. This information must be accurately entered on the patient's chart.

doula A labor coach.

duration In obstetrics, the elapsed time from the beginning of a contraction until the end of the same contraction.

dyscrasia A synonym for "disease."

dysfunctional Inadequate, abnormal.

dysmenorrhea Menstruation that is painful.

dyspareunia Painful sexual intercourse.

dystocia Difficult labor due to mechanical factors produced by the fetus or the maternal pelvis or due to inadequate uterine or other muscular activity.

E

early decelerations A decrease in fetal heart rate during a contraction as a result of head compression.

early term infant An infant born between 37 weeks gestation and 38 weeks, 6 days gestation.

eclampsia Pregnancy-induced hypertension complicated by one or more seizures.

ectoderm The outer layer of cells in the developing embryo that gives rise to the skin, nails, and hair.

ectopic pregnancy Implantation of a fertilized ovum outside the uterine cavity; the most common ectopic site is the fallopian tube.

effacement Thinning and shortening of the cervix that occur late in pregnancy and during labor.

effleurage Using the tips of the fingers to lightly stroke the abdomen in a patterned movement; a relaxation technique used to help cope with the pain of active labor.

egocentrism A type of thinking in which a child has difficulty seeing anyone else's point of view; this self-centering is normal in young children.

ejaculation The expulsion of semen and sperm from the penis.

embryo A term used for the developing structure in the early stage of development; in humans, the organism during the period from about 3 to 8 weeks of gestation.

empowerment Providing tools and knowledge to the family to enable informed participation in decision making about health care.

encephalitis Inflammation of the brain.

encopresis The passage of stool in a child's underwear or in other inappropriate places after 4 years of age. Some children display concurrent behavioral problems.

endoderm The inner layer of cells in a developing embryo that gives rise to internal organs such as the intestines.

endometriosis A medical condition in which endometrial tissue is found in areas of the body other than the uterus.

endometritis An inflammation or infection of the uterine lining, usually from bacterial invasion.

endometrium The mucous membrane that lines the inner surface of the uterus.

endorphins A natural body substance secreted by the pituitary gland that is similar in action to morphine. Levels of endorphins increase during pregnancy and peak during the labor process.

en face A position in which the parent and infant have eye-to-eye contact at no more than a 9- to 10-inch distance.

engagement The entrance of the fetal presenting part into the pelvis (e.g., the leading edge of the fetal head is at the level of the maternal ischial spines in a vertex presentation).

engorgement Vascular congestion or distention. In obstetrics, the swelling of breast tissue brought about by an increase in the blood and lymph supply to the breast preceding true lactation.

enuresis The abnormal inability to control urine excretion after the age at which control should be established; may be due to organic, allergic, or psychological problems.

epididymis A structure on the posterior border of the testis, where coiled storage ducts provide for maturation and transport of the spermatozoa.

epidural block A regional anesthetic block achieved by injecting a local anesthetic agent into the space overlying the dura of the spinal cord.

episiotomy An incision of the perineum to facilitate delivery and to prevent laceration of the perineum.

epispadias A congenital anomaly in which the urethral meatus is located on the dorsal surface of the penis.

Epstein's pearls The accumulation of yellow-white epithelial cells on the hard palate of a newborn. They usually disappear within a few weeks of delivery.

estrogen A substance produced by the ovaries; during puberty its production increases, helping to produce the secondary sex characteristics.

ethics A system of moral principles or standards that guide behavior.

ethnicity Term describing classification of groups of people within a culture according to religious, racial, national, or physical characteristics.

evidence-based practice Taking the best evidence obtained from current, valid, published research and combining that information with the nurse's critical thinking process, experiences, and patient needs to plan safe, effective nursing care for the patient.

external os The lower cervical opening.

F

facies Pertaining to the appearance or expression of the face; certain congenital syndromes are typically manifested by a specific facial appearance.

fallopian tubes The tubes that extend from the uterus to the ovaries. They serve as a passageway for ova from the ovary to the uterus and for spermatozoa from the uterus toward the ovary; oviducts; uterine tubes.

false labor Contractions of the uterus (regular or irregular) that may be strong enough to be interpreted as true labor but do not dilate the cervix. See also *true labor.*

family Apgar A screening test that is used as a guide to assess family functioning.

family care plan An expansion of the nursing care plan that includes family members.

fern test, also known as *ferning* A palm-leaf pattern seen on a glass slide that contains dried cervical mucus; can be used to determine what phase of the menstrual cycle the woman is in. See also *Billings method.*

fertilization The union of an ovum and sperm.

fetal alcohol syndrome A group of fetal symptoms that evidences prenatal and postnatal growth retardation; intellectual impairment; and facial abnormalities, including a flat, thin upper lip border and down-slanting eyes that often occurs when a mother drinks alcohol during pregnancy.

fetal attitude A position of the fetus in the uterus; normally one of flexion, with the head flexed forward and the arms and legs flexed.

fetal blood sampling A sample of blood taken from the fetus while in the uterine cavity.

fetal heart rate (FHR) The number of times the fetal heart beats per minute; the normal range at term is 110 to 160 beats/min.

fetal heart tones (FHTs) The fetal heartbeat as heard through the mother's abdominal wall.

fetal lie Describes how the spine of the fetus is oriented in relation to the mother's spine.

fetal position Refers to the orientation of a reference point on the fetal presenting part within the mother's pelvis.

fetoscope A stethoscope specially adapted to facilitate listening to the fetal heart.

fetus A term used for the developing structure from the eighth week after fertilization until birth.

fibrinogen A component found in the blood that aids in blood clotting.

fibrocystic breast A benign disorder of the breast in which cysts arise from glandular tissue.

first stage of labor The stage that begins with the first contractions of true labor and is completed when the cervix is fully dilated to 10 cm.

flexion In obstetrics, a situation that occurs when resistance to the descent of the infant down the birth canal causes its head to flex or bend, with the chin approaching the chest, thus reducing the diameter of the presenting part.

fontanelles Openings at the point of union of skull bones, often referred to as *soft spots.*

footling A breech presentation in which one foot or both feet present.

foramen ovale The opening between the left and right atria in the fetal heart.

forceps Obstetric instruments occasionally used to aid in birth by assisting fetal rotation and/or descent.

foreskin The fold of loose skin covering the end of the penis; prepuce.

fourth trimester The first 12 weeks following birth when family adaptation occurs.

frequency In labor, the period of time from the beginning of one contraction to the beginning of the next.

Friedman curve A tool for describing and recording the progress of labor.

full inclusion The process of fully integrating a physically or mentally challenged child into society.

full term infant An infant born between 39 weeks gestation and 40 weeks, 6 days gestation.

fulminating Occurring rapidly; usually said of a disease.

fundus The upper portion of the uterus between the fallopian tubes.

G

gamete A mature germ cell; an ovum or sperm.

gate control theory Rationale for stimulating larger sensory nerves to obstruct the path of pain stimuli and prevent them from reaching the central nervous system; a method used to cope with pain.

gavage Feeding the patient by means of a stomach tube or a tube passed through the nose, pharynx, and esophagus into the stomach.

gene The smallest unit of inheritance; genes are located on the chromosomes.

genetic code A component in the deoxyribonucleic acid (DNA) structure that determines the amino acid sequence within each DNA strand.

genetics The study of heredity.

genomics The study of the functions of all of the genes in the human body, with a focus on their interactions with each other and the environment.

genotype The genetic makeup of a living being.

gestation The period of intrauterine development from conception through birth; pregnancy.

gestational age The actual time, from conception to birth, that the fetus remains in the uterus.

gestational diabetes mellitus An endocrine disorder that manifests during pregnancy.

gestational trophoblastic disease Hydatidiform mole; occurs when the chorionic villi degenerate into a cystic mass of small sacs resembling tiny grapes. Chromosomal abnormalities are found in many cases.

glucometer A meter used to measure blood glucose.

glucosuria Glucose in the urine (glycosuria).

gonad A sex gland; ovaries in the female and testes in the male.

Goodell's sign A probable sign of pregnancy occurring during the second month of pregnancy that involves a softening of the cervix.

graafian follicle The ovarian cyst containing the ripe ovum; it secretes estrogens.

grasp reflex The neonate's tendency to grasp anything that lightly stimulates the palm; used in determining neurological or muscular maturity of the newborn infant.

gravid Pregnant.

gravida The number of times a woman has been pregnant; a pregnant woman.

guided imagery An alternative therapy in which pleasant mental images of events, feelings, or sensations are employed; used as a distraction method of coping with the pain of labor.

gynecologist A health care provider who specializes in the care and treatment of female reproductive issues including, but not limited to, menstruation, pregnancy, menopause, and various forms of cancer.

H

habilitation A term used to describe the treatment of a patient who is handicapped from birth and therefore is *learning*, not relearning, a task.

habituation In an infant, the ability to become accustomed to certain noises, voices, etc., within the environment.

Health Information Portability and Accountability Act (HIPAA) Enacted in 2003, HIPAA set standards to protect patients' health information and allow patients access to their medical records and control over how their personal information is disclosed.

Health maintenance organization (HMO) A medical care delivery system that offers health services for a fixed premium; serves people who are financially stable.

Healthy People 2020 A statement of national health promotion and disease prevention objectives or goals that should be attained by the year 2020; it is facilitated by the federal government.

heart failure A cardiac output inadequate to meet the metabolic needs of the body.

heel stick (heel puncture) A method of obtaining neonate blood from the heel for testing.

Hegar's sign A probable sign of pregnancy that involves softening of the lower uterine segment found upon palpation in the second or third month of pregnancy.

hemangioma A benign tumor of the skin that consists of blood vessels.

herbal medicine An alternative and/or complementary method for treating various ailments by using herbs and plants.

holism An approach to caring for a person that recognizes and adapts to his or her physical, intellectual, emotional, and spiritual nature; a way of relating to the patient as a whole individual or biopsychosocial being rather than just a person with an ailment.

Homans sign On dorsiflexion of the foot, the patient experiences pain in the calf of the leg; used as an indication of thrombophlebitis.

hormone A substance produced in an organ or gland and conveyed by the bloodstream to another part of the body to exert an effect.

hot flash Facial flushing related to vasomotor response to hormonal changes in the perimenopausal woman.

hotline A telephone number staffed around the clock that provides anonymous communication and professional advice in a crisis.

human chorionic gonadotropin (hCG) The hormone produced by chorionic villi and found in the urine of pregnant women.

human immunodeficiency virus (HIV) The organism that causes AIDS. See also *AIDS*.

hydramnios Polyhydramnios; an excess of amniotic fluid, leading to overdistention of the uterus. Often seen in diabetic pregnant women even if there is no coexisting fetal anomaly.

hydrops fetalis A condition of the fetus in which there is cardiac decompensation, hepatosplenomegaly, and respiratory distress or failure; usually due to erythroblastosis fetalis, infection, or multisystem organ failure of the fetus in utero.

hymen A membranous fold that normally partially covers the entrance to the vagina in a female who has not had vaginal penetration.

hyperbilirubinemia An excessive amount of bilirubin in the blood; more commonly seen in association with hemolytic disorders of the newborn, infection, and extreme cold stress.

hypercapnia An increased amount of carbon dioxide in the blood.

hyperemesis gravidarum Excessive vomiting during pregnancy, leading to dehydration and starvation.

hyperglycemia An excessive amount of glucose in the blood; seen most often in diabetic patients.

hypernatremia An excessive amount of sodium in the blood.

hypokalemia A potassium deficit in the blood.

hypospadias A developmental anomaly in which the urethra opens on the lower surface of the penis.

hypotension Low blood pressure; can cause symptoms ranging from dizziness to actual episodes of syncope.

hypoxia Inadequate oxygenation of the tissues.

hysterectomy The surgical removal of the uterus only.

I

icterus neonatorum Jaundice in the newborn.

immune response The body's response to a substance perceived as foreign.

immunoglobulin A protein within the body that can act as an antibody.

implantation The embedding of a fertilized ovum in the uterine mucosa 6 or 7 days after fertilization.

impotence The inability to achieve and/or maintain an erection in the male.

impregnate To make pregnant or to fertilize.

inborn error of metabolism A deficiency of specific enzymes that are needed for normal metabolism and growth. It develops in utero; may be inherited.

incarcerated Confined, constricted.

incest Sexual activities among family members; often seen in father-daughter relationships and less often in mother-son or sibling relationships.

incompetent cervix A mechanical defect in the cervix, making it unable to remain closed throughout pregnancy and resulting in spontaneous abortion.

increment An increase or addition; to build up, as in a contraction.

induction Artificial initiation of labor.

infant mortality rate The number of deaths that occur in the first 12 months of life per 1000 live births.

infertility The inability to produce offspring.

inlet of the pelvis The upper opening into the pelvic cavity.

innominate bone The ilium, the ischium, and the pubis.

integrative therapy Combines complementary and alternative therapy with traditional medicine to facilitate healing; a biopsychosocial approach to care.

intellectual impairment This term replaces the term "mental retardation." It is defined in the current *DSM-V 2013* as an intellectual developmental disorder that involves impairment of general mental ability that impacts adaptive functioning and may include impairment of concepts and skill in language, reading, writing, math, reasoning and memory; social abilities relating to empathy, and interpersonal communication; and self-management; self-care; organization or school functioning. Symptoms usually begin before developmental maturity and are chronic.

internal os The opening found between the cervix and the uterus.

intrapartum The time of onset of true labor, followed by the delivery of the neonate and finally the placenta.

in vitro fertilization Test tube fertilization in which the ripe ovum is collected and fertilized in vitro (in a glass) by sperm. The embryo is then transferred to a woman's uterus.

involution Rolling or turning inward; reduction in the size of the uterus after delivery.

K

kangaroo care The use of skin-to-skin contact between the neonate or infant and the caregiver; used to promote bonding between the parent and the infant.

karyotype The chromosomal makeup of a body cell, arranged from largest to smallest. The normal number of chromosomes in humans is 46.

Kegel exercise The tightening and relaxing of the pubococcygeal muscles; helps to strengthen the pelvic floor muscles.

kernicterus A grave form of jaundice in the newborn caused by hyperbilirubinemia and resulting in brain damage.

kilogram A unit of measure. One kilogram (kg) is equal to 2.2 pounds (lb), or 1000 mg.

L

labia In obstetrics, the external folds of skin on either side of the vulva.

labia majora The larger, outer folds of skin on either side of the vulva.

labia minora The smaller, inner folds of skin on either side of the vulva.

labor The process by which the fetus is expelled from the uterus; childbirth; confinement; parturition.

labor, delivery, and recovery (LDR) rooms Rooms in which the pregnant patient receives care during labor and delivery and then remains to recover and care for her new infant.

labor dysfunction A pattern of labor that interferes with the normal progression of labor and delivery.

laboring down A process by which a health care team allows a laboring woman whose cervix is 10 cm dilated, to hold back from pushing until she has a natural urge or readiness to deliver is urgent.

laceration In obstetrics, a tear in the perineum, vagina, or cervix.

lactase The enzyme that breaks down lactose.

lactation The process of producing and supplying breast milk.

lactiferous ducts Tiny tubes within the breast that conduct milk from the acini cells to the nipple.

lactose intolerant Having an inability to adequately digest milk products.

Laminaria Type of kelp or seaweed that can be used to help dilate the cervical canal to aid in delivery of the products of conception (neonate).

lanugo Fine, downy hair seen on all parts of the fetus, except the palms of the hands and soles of the feet, by the end of 20 weeks of gestation.

late decelerations A decrease in fetal heart rate during a uterine contraction that continues after the contraction ends.

leiomyoma A tumor in the myometrium of the uterus; also known as a *fibroid*.

Leopold's maneuver A method of abdominal palpation used to determine fetal position or placement within the uterus.

let-down reflex A pattern of stimulation, hormone release, and muscle contraction that forces milk into the lactiferous ducts, making it available to the infant; milk ejection reflex.

letting go A phase in the development of the parental role.

libido The sexual drive, be it unconscious or conscious.

lie The position of the fetus described by the relationship of the long axis of the fetus to the long axis of the mother.

lightening Movement of the fetus and uterus downward into the pelvic cavity.

linea nigra A line of darker pigmentation extending from the pubis to the umbilicus; noted in some women during the later months of pregnancy.

lochia The maternal discharge of blood, mucus, and tissue from the uterus; may last for several weeks after birth.

lochia alba White vaginal discharge that follows lochia serosa and lasts from about the tenth to the twenty-first day after delivery.

lochia rubra Red, blood-tinged vaginal discharge that occurs after delivery and lasts 2 to 4 days.

lochia serosa Pink, serous, and blood-tinged vaginal discharge that follows lochia rubra and lasts until the seventh to tenth day after delivery.

L/S ratio The ratio of the amounts of the phospholipids lecithin and sphingomyelin produced by the fetal lungs; useful in assessing fetal lung maturity.

lunar month A 28-day cycle corresponding to the phases of the moon. A normal pregnancy lasts 10 lunar months.

luteinizing hormone (LH) The anterior pituitary hormone responsible for stimulating ovulation and developing the corpus luteum.

M

macrocephaly An abnormally large skull; can be found in infants with hydrocephalus.

macrosomia An abnormally large infant, or neonatal birth weight above the 90th percentile.

mainstream A term used to describe the process of integrating a physically or mentally challenged child into society.

mammary glands Compound glandular elements of the breast that in the female secrete milk to nourish the infant.

mastectomy Surgical removal of a breast.

maternal mortality rate The number of maternal deaths that occur within 42 days after termination of a pregnancy or delivery of a live fetus within 1 year, per 100,000 live births.

McDonald's sign A probable sign of pregnancy in which the examiner can easily flex the cervix against the body of the uterus.

mechanisms (cardinal movements) of labor The positional changes of the fetus as it moves through the birth canal during labor and delivery.

meconium The first stool of the newborn; a mixture of amniotic fluid and secretions of the intestinal glands.

meconium aspiration syndrome Characteristic symptoms that result from aspiration of meconium in utero. The presence of meconium in the trachea or its appearance on a chest x-ray film helps to confirm this diagnosis.

meconium ileus A condition in which the meconium of the fetus becomes excessively sticky and adheres to the intestinal wall, causing obstruction. It is occasionally seen in babies born with cystic fibrosis.

meconium-stained fluid Amniotic fluid that contains meconium.

megacolon Hirschsprung's disease; congenital absence of ganglionic cells in a segment of the large bowel, which results in massive dilation of the bowel.

meiosis Cell division to halve the number of chromosomes in ova and sperm (gametes) to 23.

menarche The beginning of menstrual and reproductive functions in girls.

meningomyelocele A sac-like cyst containing the meninges, spinal cord, and fluid that has herniated through the spinal column, usually via some form of anatomical defect of the bony spinal canal.

menopause The permanent cessation of menses.

menstrual cycle The cyclic buildup of uterine lining, ovulation, and sloughing of the lining occurring approximately every 28 days in nonpregnant females.

menstruation (menses) The shedding of uterine lining at the end of the menstrual cycle, resulting in a bloody discharge from the vagina.

meridian An imaginary line that encircles the body; used in some forms of alternative or complementary therapies (see Chapter 34).

mesoderm The intermediate layer of germ cells in the embryo that gives rise to connective tissue, bone marrow, muscles, blood, lymphoid tissue, and epithelial tissue.

metered-dose inhaler (MDI) A device that delivers measured puffs of medication for inhalation.

microcephaly A congenital anomaly in which the head of the newborn is abnormally small.

midwives The certified nurse-midwife (CNM) is a registered nurse who has graduated from an accredited midwife program and is nationally certified by the American College of Nurse-Midwives. The CNM provides comprehensive prenatal and postnatal care and attends uncomplicated deliveries.

milia Very small, white, keratin-filled cysts or papules normally found on a neonate's face. They generally disappear if left alone.

miliaria Prickly heat; inflammation of the skin caused by sweating.

miscarriage Lay term for spontaneous abortion.

mitosis Cell division in all body cells other than the gametes (ova and sperm).

molding The shaping of the fetal head to facilitate movement through the birth canal during labor.

mongolian spot A benign, blue-hued pigmentation caused by melanin deposits usually found around the lower back or the buttock. It is seen most often in dark-skinned infants and may fade during childhood.

monozygotic twins Two fetuses that develop from a single divided, fertilized ovum; identical twins.

mons veneris The fleshy tissue over the female symphysis pubis from which hair develops at puberty.

Montgomery's glands (tubercles) Small nodules located around the nipples that enlarge during pregnancy and lactation; secrete a moisturizing substance.

morbidity Term pertaining to incidence of illness and disease.

morning sickness Nausea and vomiting occurring during the first trimester of pregnancy; may occur at any time during the day.

Moro reflex The newborn's symmetrical response, when jarred, to extend and abduct the extremities in an embracing motion, including a spreading apart of the fingers with the thumb and forefinger forming a C shape. Evidences health of the newborn's central nervous system.

mortality Term pertaining to incidence of death.

morula A solid mass of cells that develop from the fertilized ovum.

mucous plug A collection of thick mucus that blocks the cervical canal during pregnancy.

multifetal pregnancy A pregnancy in which the woman is carrying two or more fetuses; also called *multiple gestation* and involve twins, triplets, etc.

multigravida A woman who has previously been pregnant.

multipara A woman who has had more than one pregnancy in which the fetus(es) was (were) viable (20 weeks of gestation).

murmur A sound heard while listening to the heart; caused by blood leaking through openings that have not closed as they should before birth.

mutation A change in genetic material.

N

Nägele's rule A method of determining the estimated date of delivery (EDD); after obtaining the first day of the last menstrual period, subtract 3 months and add 7 days.

narcotic agonist A drug that is used to reverse narcotic effects.

neonate A newborn infant from birth to 28 days of age.

nesting The provision of an enclosed space bounded by a small blanket roll encircling the preterm infant. It helps to provide a calm, supportive environment for the infant. Also used to refer to the sudden burst of energy some women experience shortly before the onset of labor.

neutral thermal environment An environment that is neither too hot nor too cold; thus, the body does not need to overwork itself to deliver oxygen or increase its metabolic rate to maintain a normal body temperature.

nevus (pl, *nevi*) A congenital discoloration of an area of the skin, such as a strawberry mark or mole.

nitrazine paper A specially treated type of paper that turns a specific color in the presence of amniotic fluid.

nonnutritive sucking Any sucking activity that is not related to the intake of nutrients.

nonreassuring fetal heart rate An alteration in the normal fetal heart rate that suggests the placenta is not delivering enough oxygen to the fetus, such as a *late deceleration*.

nonshivering thermogenesis The oxidation of brown fat in the neonate to produce heat to keep warm.

non–stress test (NST) A prenatal assessment method by which the reaction (or response) of the fetal heart rate to fetal movement is evaluated.

nuchal Pertaining to the neck.

nuchal cord A term to describe a situation in which the umbilical cord is wrapped around the fetus's neck.

nuclear family A family unit that consists of one or more parents and one or more of their children.

nulligravida A female who has never been pregnant.

nullipara A female who has not delivered a live fetus.

nursing care plan Developed as a result of the nursing process, the nursing care plan is a written instrument of communication among staff members that focuses on individualized patient care.

nursing process Developed in 1963, this term refers to a series of steps describing the systematic problem-solving approach nurses use to identify, prevent, or treat actual or potential health problems. The steps in the nursing process include assessment, diagnosis, outcome identification, planning, implementation, and evaluation.

O

obstetrician A physician specializing in the care of women during pregnancy, labor, birth, and the postpartum period.

obstetrics The branch of medicine concerned with the care of women during pregnancy, childbirth, and the postpartum period.

occiput The posterior part of the skull.

oligohydramnios A decreased amount of amniotic fluid.

oliguria A decrease in urine secretion by the kidney.

omphalocele A herniation of abdominal contents at the umbilicus.

ophthalmia neonatorum Acute conjunctivitis of the newborn, often caused by gonococci or *Chlamydia*.

opportunistic infection An infection caused by bacteria normally found in the environment that become pathogenic to the body due to a defective immune system; usually seen in immunosuppressed individuals whose CD4 counts have dropped to a critical level, such as patients with cancer or AIDS.

oral contraceptive A medication, taken by mouth, that is used to prevent pregnancy.

orgasm Occurs at the peak or climax of sexual and emotional excitement. In the male, ejaculation generally occurs during orgasm.

orthopnea A condition in which the patient must sit up to breathe.

orthostatic hypotension A decrease in either systolic or diastolic blood pressure while moving from a supine or sitting position to a fully upright position.

Ortolani's maneuver A maneuver performed while examining a newborn to determine the presence or absence of congenital hip dysplasia.

osteoporosis A decrease in the overall mass of bones due to an increase in the trabeculae of the bone. It can be caused by age, sedentary lifestyle, smoking, diet, and many other factors.

ovarian cycle The changes that the ovarian follicles undergo throughout the menstrual cycle. Days 1 to 14 comprise the follicular phase, and days 15 to 28 comprise the luteal phase.

ovulation The normal process of discharging a mature ovum from an ovary approximately 14 days before the onset of menses.

Ovum (pl, *ova*) The female reproductive cell; egg.

oxytocics Drugs that intensify uterine contractions to hasten birth or control postpartum hemorrhage.

oxytocin challenge test (OCT) A method of assessing the fetal response to labor by administering an oxytocic drug to stimulate a few labor contractions; used in high-risk pregnancies. See also *contraction stress test (CST)*.

P

paced breathing A breathing technique used during labor to help the woman relax and to increase her pain tolerance.

para A woman who has borne offspring who reached the age of viability (20 to 24 weeks of gestation).

paraphimosis Impaired circulation of the uncircumcised penis due to improper retraction of the foreskin.

parenteral A medication route other than the gastrointestinal tract; can be intravenous, intramuscular, etc.

parity The condition of having borne offspring who attained the age of viability; the number of pregnancies ending after the age of viability.

parturient Pertaining to the act of childbirth; a woman giving birth.

parturition The process of giving birth.

passive acquired immunity Antibodies to a communicable disease are given to the patient.

pediatric capsule endoscopy The swallowing of a capsule embedded with a camera to provide direct visualization of the gastrointestinal mucosa for the purpose of diagnosis without the need for radiation or procedural sedation.

pediatric nurse practitioner (PNP) The PNP provides ambulatory and primary care for patients.

pediatrics The branch of medicine that deals with the child's development and care and the diseases of childhood and their treatment.

pelvic rocking (tilt) An exercise to help strengthen abdominal muscles and reduce the strain on the lower back.

pelvis The lower portion of the trunk of the body bounded by the hip bones, the coccyx, and the sacrum.

penis The male organ of copulation, reproduction, and urination.

perinatal mortality rate The number of fetal and neonatal deaths in a given period of time per 1000 live births.

perineum The area of tissue between the anus and the scrotum in males or between the anus and the vagina in females.

Pfannenstiel's incision A low, transverse incision into the abdomen that is nearly invisible when healed; often used for cesarean section (surgical) deliveries.

phenotype The entire physical, biochemical, and physiologic makeup of an individual as determined both genetically and environmentally.

phenylketonuria (PKU) A genetic disorder caused by the faulty metabolism of phenylalanine, an amino acid essential to life and found in all protein foods. If left untreated, intellectual impairment can occur.

phimosis Tightening of the prepuce of the uncircumcised penis.

phototherapy The treatment of disease by exposure to light; often used to treat hyperbilirubinemia in the newborn.

pica The eating of substances not ordinarily considered to be edible or to have nutritive value.

pincer grasp The use of the index finger and thumb to grasp an object.

placenta A specialized disk-shaped organ that connects the fetus to the uterine wall for gas, nutrient, and waste exchanges; also called *afterbirth*.

placenta previa The abnormal placental implantation in the lower uterine segment.

placental soufflé Soft blowing sounds produced by blood coursing through the dilated arteries of the uterus; occur at the same rate as the maternal pulse.

polycystic ovary syndrome A common endocrine disorder in women that results in fertility problems due to anovulation; excess androgenic hormones and insulin resistance.

polydactyly A developmental anomaly characterized by the presence of extra fingers or toes.

polyhydramnios An excessive amount of amniotic fluid within the placenta.

postpartum After childbirth.

postpartum hemorrhage Blood loss greater than 500 mL after vaginal birth or 1000 mL after cesarean birth.

precipitate birth A birth that is completed in less than 3 hours, thus often occurring with no trained attendant present.

precipitate labor A labor that begins abruptly and intensifies quickly resulting in rapid passage of the fetus through the birth canal.

preferred provider organization (PPO) A medical care delivery system that contracts with providers for services on a discounted fee-for-service basis for members; serves people who are financially stable.

pregnancy The condition of having a developing embryo or fetus in the body after fertilization of the female egg by the male sperm.

prehension The use of the hands to pick up small objects; grasping.

prenatal Before birth.

presentation The fetal body part that enters the maternal pelvis first.

presenting part The fetal part that first enters the maternal pelvis or that first emerges from the cervix.

presumptive signs of pregnancy Symptoms that suggest pregnancy but do not confirm it, such as cessation of menses, quickening, and morning sickness.

preterm infant Premature infant; an infant born before 37 weeks of gestation.

preterm labor The regular contractions of a pregnant uterus resulting in changes in the cervix (dilation and effacement) that start before 37 weeks gestation.

primigravida A woman who is pregnant for the first time.

primipara A woman who has given birth to her first child (past the point of viability), whether or not that child is living or was alive at birth.

prodromal period The initial symptoms indicating an approaching onset of disease.

progesterone A hormone produced by the adrenal cortex, the corpus luteum, and the placenta. Its function is to stimulate the development of the mammary glands and growth of the endometrium and to maintain a pregnancy.

projectile vomiting Vomiting that occurs with force (vomitus landing 2 to 4 feet away).

prolactin A hormone produced by the anterior pituitary gland that stimulates lactation or milk production.

prolapsed cord An umbilical cord that becomes trapped between the fetal presenting part and the maternal pelvis.

prostaglandin (PG) A type of unsaturated fatty acid that exerts an effect locally on a tissue and then is enzymatically destroyed. In obstetrics, PGE_2 gel is used on the cervix to help induce labor.

proteinuria The presence of protein in the urine.

pseudocyesis A condition in which the woman has symptoms of pregnancy but in which hormonal pregnancy test results are negative; false pregnancy.

psychoprophylaxis Psychophysical training aimed at preparing the expectant parents to cope with the processes of labor and to prevent their concentrating on the discomforts associated with childbirth.

puberty The period during which the secondary sexual characteristics develop and the ability to procreate is attained.

pudendal block The injection of an anesthetizing agent at the pudendal nerve to produce numbness of the external genitals and the lower third of the vagina.

puerperal morbidity Postpartum fever; a temperature of 38 ° C (100.4 ° F) or higher after the first 24 hours and continuing for at least 2 days during the first 10 days after delivery.

puerperium The period after delivery until involution of the uterus is complete, usually 6 weeks.

pulmonary vascular resistance (PVR) In the fetus, PVR is the resistance to the flow of blood in the fetal lung tissue.

pulse oximeter Equipment that uses a sensor placed on the skin to determine the level of blood oxygen saturation.

Q-R

quickening The first fetal movements felt by the pregnant woman, usually occurring between 16 and 18 weeks of gestation.

radiant warmer An infant bed providing infrared heat to warm the infant while permitting access to the infant for care or treatment.

radiation Heat loss from the body to a cooler object within the environment. The object does not necessarily have to be touching the body. It can also refer to a mode of therapy used for cancer.

rapport Harmonious relationship.

reflexology Integrative therapy that uses varying degrees of pressure, usually to the hands or the feet, to promote relaxation.

reflux A backward flow of fluid (e.g., vesicoureteral reflux [urine is forced from the bladder into the ureters], gastric reflux [stomach contents flow into the esophagus; it may or may not enter the oral cavity]).

regression Behavior that is more appropriate to an earlier stage of development; often occurs in children as a response to stress.

relaxin A water-soluble protein secreted by the corpus luteum that causes relaxation of the symphysis pubis and facilitates cervical dilation during birth.

retinopathy of prematurity (ROP) Condition in which there is damage to immature retinal blood vessels, which can lead to blindness; thought to be caused by high oxygen levels of arterial blood. Formerly called *retrolental fibroplasia*.

retractions Abnormal "sucking in" of the chest wall during inspiration; indicates respiratory distress. They can be substernal or intercostal.

Rh factor An antigen present on the surface of blood cells that makes them incompatible with those that do not have the antigen.

rhabdomyosarcoma An extremely malignant neoplasm originating in skeletal muscle.

RhoGAM An immune globulin given to the mother (not the infant) after the delivery of an Rh-positive infant to an Rh-negative mother.

rhythm method A natural form of birth control that requires the woman to chart her menstrual cycles for several months on a calendar. This method is based on the woman ovulating about 14 days *before* the next menstrual cycle begins and involves proper use of contraception or abstinence during the fertile period.

rickets A disease of the bones caused by a lack of calcium or vitamin D.

ritualism A need to maintain strict structure and routine.

rooting reflex The infant's tendency to turn the head and open the lips to suck when that side of the mouth or cheek is touched or stroked.

S

sacrum Five fused vertebrae that form a triangle of bone just beneath the lumbar vertebrae and between the hip bones.

salpingitis Inflammation or infection of a fallopian tube.

SBAR A formal method of providing end-of-shift reports, which includes *s*ituation, *b*ackground, *a*ssessment, and *r*ecommendation.

scoliosis Lateral curvature of the spine.

second stage of labor The stage lasting from complete dilation of the cervix to expulsion of the fetus.

semen Thick, whitish fluid ejaculated by the male during orgasm; contains the spermatozoa and their nutrients.

separation anxiety Distress behavior that occurs when the infant is separated from the parents.

sex chromosomes The X and Y chromosomes that are responsible for sex determination; women have two X chromosomes, and men have one X and one Y chromosome.

sexually transmitted infections (STIs) Refers to infections ordinarily transmitted by direct sexual contact with an infected individual.

shunt A bypass.

Skene's ducts (paraurethral ducts) The ducts located on either side of the urethra; provide lubrication of the urethra.

smegma A cheeselike substance secreted by the sebaceous glands near the clitoris in the female and under the prepuce of an uncircumcised male.

Snellen alphabet chart A device used to measure near and far vision; a variation of the Snellen E chart.

spermatogenesis The process by which mature spermatozoa are formed and during which the number of chromosomes is reduced by half.

spermatozoa Mature sperm cells produced by the testes.

spina bifida A congenital embryonic neural tube defect in which there is an imperfect closure of the spinal vertebrae. There are two types: occulta (hidden) and cystica (sac or cyst).

spinnbarkeit Elasticity seen in cervical mucus at the time of ovulation.

spontaneous abortion The (unintended) loss of the products of conception before 20 weeks of gestation; miscarriage.

standard precautions Infection control guidelines established by the Centers for Disease Control and Prevention to prevent the spread of infection (see Appendix A).

station The relationship of the presenting fetal part to an imaginary line drawn between the pelvic ischial spines.

statistics The science of gathering and analyzing numerical data.

sterility The inability of the male to impregnate a female; the inability of a female to conceive. It can also refer to the absence of live organisms on an object.

stillbirth The delivery of a dead fetus.

strabismus (cross-eye or squint) A condition in which the child is not able to direct both eyes toward an object at the same time due to a lack of muscle coordination.

striae gravidarum Stretch marks; shiny reddish lines that appear on abdomen, breasts, thighs, and buttocks of pregnant women as a result of the skin's stretching.

stridor Emission of a shrill sound during respiration; caused by air passing through a narrowed portion of the respiratory tract.

subinvolution A slower-than-expected return of the uterus to its nonpregnant condition. Infection and a retained placenta are the usual causes.

supine hypotension syndrome The lowering of blood pressure while in a supine position; occurs as a result of pressure or the weight of the pregnant uterus on the inferior vena cava.

surfactant A mixture of lipoproteins secreted in the alveoli and air passages that reduces the surface tension within the alveoli and contributes to the expansion of the lungs.

surrogate mother A fertile woman who is impregnated for the purpose of producing a child for another (infertile) couple.

sutures In obstetrics, separation between fetal skull bones that permits molding during the birth process.

T

taking hold The second phase of maternal adaptation in which the mother assumes control of herself and the infant.

taking in The initial maternal adaptation after birth in which passive acceptance of care occurs.

talipes equinovarus Clubfoot.

teratogen A nongenetic factor that can produce malformations of the fetus.

term infant A live-born infant of 38 to 42 weeks of gestation.

testes The male gonads, in which sperm and testosterone are produced.

testosterone The male hormone; responsible for the development of secondary male characteristics.

therapeutic play Guided play that helps children deal with concerns or disabilities and helps nurses gain insight into needs (e.g., blowing bubbles is postoperative therapeutic play designed to help expand lungs).

third stage of labor The period from delivery of the fetus to the time when the placenta has been completely expelled.

thrombophlebitis Inflammation or the formation of a blood clot in or along a vein.

thrombus A blood clot that moves within the circulation.

tissue perfusion Nutrition and oxygenation of tissue resulting from adequate blood flow.

tocodynamometer External device that can be used to identify the pressure of uterine contractions during labor.

tocolytic A drug that inhibits uterine contractions.

tocotransducer An electronic monitoring device used to measure uterine contractions.

TOLAC See Trial of Labor After Cesarean.

TORCH Acronym used to describe a group of infections that represent potentially severe fetal problems if infection occurs during pregnancy. *T*, toxoplasmosis; *O*, other agents; *R*, rubella; *C*, cytomegalovirus; and *H*, herpesvirus.

toxic shock syndrome (TSS) An infection usually caused by *Staphylococcus aureus* and found most often in women of reproductive age who use tampons.

transition The period of labor in which the cervix is dilated to approximately 8 cm, the contractions are very strong, and the laboring woman feels the urge to push.

transplacental Through the placenta (i.e., the exchange of nutrients, waste products, drugs, and hormones).

triage A process used to prioritize care that determines the urgency of illness.

Trial of Labor After Cesarean A labor experience in which the woman attempts to have a natural labor and birth after a previous cesarean section birth. The birth is known as a VBAC (Vaginal Birth After Cesarean).

trimester One third of the gestational time for pregnancy.

trophoblast Comprises the nutritive relationship with the endometrium of the uterus.

true labor Labor involving contractions that gradually develop a regular pattern, becoming more frequent and stronger and causing effacement and dilation of the cervix. Changes in the cervix provide the key distinction between true and false labor.

turgor Normal elasticity of the skin.

tympanometry The measurement of mobility of the tympanic membrane of the ear and the estimation of middle ear pressure.

U

ultrasound High-frequency sound waves that may be directed (through the use of a transducer) into the maternal abdomen. The ultrasonic sound waves reflected by the underlying structures of varying densities allow maternal and fetal tissues, bones, and fluids to be identified.

umbilical cord The structure connecting the placenta to the umbilicus of the fetus through which nutrients from the woman are exchanged for waste from the fetus.

umbilicus The navel, or "belly button," on the abdomen, which forms the attachment of the umbilical cord during fetal life.

uterine tachysystole An excessively frequent uterine contraction during pregnancy. It can include more than 6 contractions within a 10 minute period; a single contraction lasting more than 2 minutes; or uterine hyperstimulation that results in a non-reassuring fetal heart pattern.

uterus A hollow, muscular organ in which the fertilized ovum is implanted and the developing fetus is nourished until birth.

V

vacuum extractor A device to aid the birth of the fetal head by means of suction.

vagina The musculomembranous tube or passageway located between the external female genitals and the uterus.

Valsalva's maneuver Holding one's breath or bearing down as though passing stool, thereby increasing intraabdominal and intrathoracic pressure.

variability Describes the fluctuations, or constant changes, in the baseline heart rate; results in a fine sawtooth-shaped tracing on a heart monitor.

varicella Chickenpox.

varicose veins Permanently distended veins.

variola Smallpox.

vas deferens A duct that aids in the transport of sperm and semen into the male urethra.

vasectomy A form of male sterilization in which the vas deferens is cut and ligated.

vector A carrier that transmits an infective agent from one host to another.

ventriculography An x-ray examination of the ventricles of the brain after the injection of air into the ventricles.

vernix caseosa A protective cheeselike, whitish substance made up of sebum and desquamated epithelial cells that is present on fetal skin and the skin of the newborn.

version Turning of the position of the fetus in the uterus before birth; can be spontaneous or manually induced.

vertex The top or crown of the head.

viable Capable of living.

volvulus Twisting of the loops of the small intestine, causing obstruction.

vulva The external structure of the female genitals lying between the mons veneris and the anus.

W

warm line A telephone number staffed around the clock that provides communication and professional advice in a noncrisis situation.

Wharton's jelly Yellow-white gelatinous material that surrounds and protects the vessels of the umbilical cord.

wheal A large, slightly raised, red or blistered area of skin; may itch.

Women, Infants, and Children (WIC) program A subsidized supplemental food program for mothers and children.

womb A lay term referring to the uterus.

X-Z

X chromosome The female sex chromosome.

Y chromosome The male sex chromosome.

zygote A fertilized ovum.

Index

Note: Page numbers followed by *b* indicate boxes, *f* indicate figures, and *t* indicate tables.

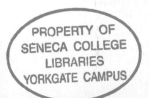